Textbook of Obstetric Anesthesia

Textbook of Obstetric Anesthesia

David J. Birnbach, MD
Director, Obstetric Anesthesiology
St. Luke's–Roosevelt Hospital
Associate Professor, Departments of Anesthesiology and
Obstetrics and Gynecology
Columbia University College of Physicians & Surgeons
New York, New York

Stephen P. Gatt, MD
Head of Division of Anaesthesia and
Intensive Care; Programme Director,
Acute Services Programme,
Prince of Wales, Sydney Children's and
Prince Henry Hospitals, Randwick, Sydney, Australia
Senior Lecturer in Anesthesia
University of New South Wales
Kensington, Sydney, Australia

Sanjay Datta, MD
Professor of Anaesthesia
Harvard Medical School
Director of Obstetric Anesthesia
Brigham and Women's Hospital
Boston, Massachusetts

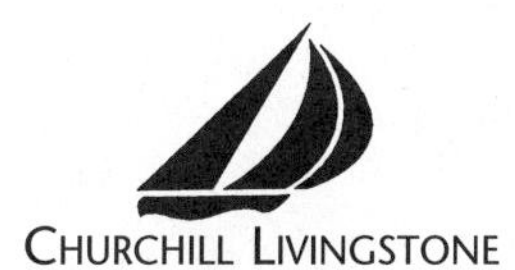

CHURCHILL LIVINGSTONE

A Harcourt Health Sciences Company
New York ■ Edinburgh ■ London ■ Philadelphia

CHURCHILL LIVINGSTONE
A Harcourt Health Sciences Company

The Curtis Center
Independence Square West
Philadelphia, Pennsylvania 19106

Library of Congress Cataloging-in-Publication Data

Textbook of Obstetric Anesthesia/[edited by] David J. Birnbach, Stephen P. Gatt, Sanjay Datta.

p. cm.

ISBN 0–443–06560–8

1. Anesthesia in obstetrics. I. Birnbach, David J. II. Gatt, Stephen P. III. Datta, Sanjay.
[DNLM: 1. Anesthesia, Obstetrical—methods. 2. Analgesia, Obstetrical—methods. 3. Pregnancy Complications. WO 450 T355 2000]

RG732.T49 2000 617.9′682—dc21

DNLM/DLC 99–462024

Acquisitions Editor: Allan Ross
Developmental Editor: Melissa Dudlick
Production Manager: Norman Stellander
Project Manager: Gina Scala
Illustration Coordinator: Walt Verbitski

TEXTBOOK OF OBSTETRIC ANESTHESIA ISBN 0–443–06560–8

Printed in the United States of America.

Last digit is the print number: 9 8 7 6 5 4 3 2 1

To the memory of the two teachers whose wisdom, guidance, and love inspired me and helped to shape me into the person I am today. To my father, Dr. Seymour Birnbach, who taught me to love to learn and to my mentor, Dr. Gerard W. Ostheimer, who taught me to love to teach. They are not forgotten.

DJB

To my wife, companion, best mate and live-in lover
Alice
who had to bear with me while I accrued a sleep debt by working long into the night and over the weekends while I wrote manuscript and revised and copyedited chapters . . .
It is her never-ending, unconditional support which makes all things possible;
And to my children—
Ian McAlister, Andrea Geraldine, Kristina Anne, and Emma Kathleen, for having been graceful and supportive in their fatherlessness for some considerable periods of time.

SPG

To my wife, Gouri, and daughter, Nandini, whose constant support I rely on and count on so heavily.

SD

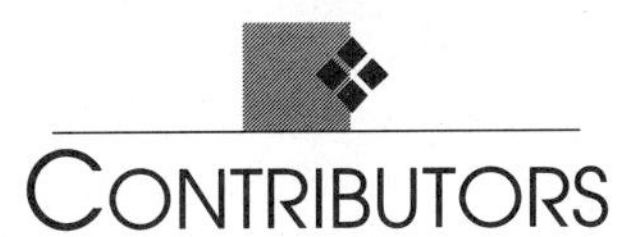

Contributors

Hugo Van Aken, MD, PhD, FRCA, FANZCA
Professor and Senior Lecturer, Westfalische Wilhelms Universität; Staff, Klinik und Poliklinik für Anasthesiologie und Intensivmedizin, Muenster, Germany
The Effects of Drugs Used in Pregnancy

Seppo Alahuhta, MD, PhD
Professor in Anaesthesiology, University of Oulu; Head, Department of Anaesthesiology, Oulu University Hospital, Oulu, Finland
Uteroplacental Blood Flow

John Anthony, MBChB, FCOG
Associate Professor of Obstetrics and Gynaecology, University of Cape Town; Principal Specialist and Head of the Maternity Centre, Groote Schuur Hospital Observatory, Cape Town, South Africa
Critical Care Management of the Pregnant Patient

Valerie A. Arkoosh, MD
Associate Professor, Departments of Anesthesiology and Obstetrics and Gynecology, Interim Chair, Department of Anesthesiology, MCP Hahnemann University, Philadelphia, Pennsylvania
Neonatal Resuscitation

Chakib M. Ayoub, MD
Assistant Professor, Department of Anesthesiology, American University of Beirut, Lebanon
Postcesarean Analgesia: Patient-Controlled Analgesia and Neuraxial Techniques

Dan Benhamou, MD
Professor of Anesthesia and Intensive Care, Universite Paris-Sud, Lekremlin Bicêtre; Chairman, Departement D'Anesthesie-Reanimation, Hôpital Antoine Beclere, Clamart, France
Pulmonary Disease in the Pregnant Patient

Marewenteiti Ali Biribo, DSM (Fiji), DA (UP&FSM), FPBA
Specialist and Consultant, Anaesthesia and Critical Care, Colonial War Memorial Hospital, Suva, Fiji Islands
General Anesthesia for Cesarean Section

David J. Birnbach, MD
Associate Professor, Departments of Anesthesiology and Obstetrics and Gynecology, College of Physicians and Surgeons of Columbia University; Director of Obstetric Anesthesiology, St. Luke's–Roosevelt Hospital Center, New York, New York
Drug Abuse in Pregnancy

Remi Bourlier, MD
Staff Anesthesiologist, Hôpital Robert Debre, Paris, France
Anesthesia for Postpartum Surgery

Christoph A. Brezinka, MD, PhD
Associate Professor of Obstetrics and Gynecology, Leopold Franzens University, Innsbruck University Hospital, Innsbruck, Austria
Multiple Gestation and Fetal Malpresentation

Anton G. L. Burm, MSc, PhD
Department of Anesthesiology, Leiden University Medical Center, Leiden, The Netherlands
Perinatal Pharmacology of Local Anesthetics and Opioids

David C. Campbell, MD, MSc, FRCPC
Associate Professor, Department of Anesthesiology, University of Saskatchewan College of Medicine; Director of Obstetric Anesthesiology, Royal University Hospital, Saskatoon, Saskatchewan, Canada
Musculoskeletal Disorders

Giorgio Capogna, MD
Professor of Obstetric Anesthesia, Midwifery University School, University of Tor Vergata; Director, Obstetric Anesthesia, Ospedale Fatebenefratelli, Isola Tiberina, Rome, Italy
Anesthesia for Vaginal Birth After Cesarean Delivery

José Carvalho, MD, PhD, FANZCA
Professor, Department of Anesthesiology, University of São Paulo; Director, Department of Anesthesiology, Hospital and Maternidade Santa Joana; Medical Superintendent, Maternidade Pro Matre Paulista, São Paulo, Brazil
Cardiovascular Disease in the Pregnant Patient

Alfredo N. Cattaneo, MD
Anesthesiologist, Hospital Español de Mendoza, Mendoza, Argentina
Air and Amniotic Fluid Embolism

Danilo Celleno, MD
Professor of Obstetric Anesthesia, Università Cattolica S Cuore di Roma; Chairman, Department of Anesthesia and Intensive Care, Ospedale Fatebenefratelli, Isola Tiberina, Rome, Italy
Anesthesia for Vaginal Birth After Cesarean Delivery

Y. K. Chan, MBBS(Mal), FFARCSI
Associate Professor, University of Malaya Faculty of Medicine; Consultant Anesthesiologist, University Hospital, Kuala Lumpur, Malaysia
Pulmonary Aspiration

Clive Bourn Collier, MBBS, MD, MRCP, FRCA, FANZCA
Visiting Anaesthetist, Royal Hospital for Women, Sydney, Australia
Complications of Regional Anesthesia

Michael J. Cousins, MBBS, MD (Syd), FANZCA, FRCA, FFPMANZCA
Professor and Head, Department of Anaesthesia and Pain Management, Royal North Shore Hospital, University of Sydney, St. Leonards, New South Wales, Australia
Pain Mechanisms in Labor

David K. Crooke, MBBS, MBiomedE, FANZCA
Lecturer in Anaesthesia/Critical Care, University of New South Wales, Sydney; Director of Obstetric Anaesthesia, Division of Critical Care, Liverpool Hospital, Liverpool, Australia
Ethical Issues and Consent in Obstetric Anesthesia

John A. Crowhurst, BPharm, MB BS, D(Obst) RCOG, FANZCA
Reader in Obstetric Anaesthesia, Imperial College School of Medicine, University of London; Director of Anaesthesia, Queen Charlotte's Hospital, London, United Kingdom
The Combined Spinal-Epidural Technique

Sanjay Datta, MD, FFARCS(Eng)
Professor of Anaesthesia, Harvard Medical School; Director of Obstetric Anesthesia, Brigham & Women's Hospital, Boston, Massachusetts
Anesthetic Management of Diabetic Parturients

Paola Dorato, MD
Research Fellow in Obstetric Anesthesia, Ospedale Fatebenefratelli, Isola Tiberina, Rome, Italy
Anesthesia for Vaginal Birth After Cesarean Delivery

Catherine S. Downs, MBBS (Hons 1), FANZCA
Anaesthesiologist, Royal Hospital for Women; Staff Anaesthesiologist, Department of Cardiothoracic Anaesthesia, Prince of Wales Hospital, Sydney, Australia
Anesthesia for the Parturient with Neurologic Disease

Leon Drobnik, MD, PhD
Professor of Anesthesiology and Co-Chair of Anesthesiology Department, Karol Marcinkowski University Hospital, Poznan, Poland
Nerve Blocks in the Pregnant Patient

Marie-Louise Felten, MD
Department of Anesthesiology, Hôpital Antoine Beclere, Clamart, France
Pulmonary Disease in the Pregnant Patient

Michael Frölich, MD, DEAA
Assistant Professor, Department of Anesthesiology, University of Florida College of Medicine; Attending Physician, Shands Hospital, Gainesville, Florida
Anesthesia for Presumed Fetal Jeopardy

Stephen P. Gatt, MD, OAM, KM, LRCP, MRCS, MRACMA, FFICANZCA, FANZCA, FFA
Senior Lecturer, Anaesthesia, Critical Care and Emergency Medicine, University of New South Wales; Head Division of Anaesthesia and Intensive Care, and Programme Director, Acute Services Programme, Prince of Wales, Sydney Children's and Prince Henry Hospitals, Senior Staff Anaesthetist, Royal Hospital for Women, Randwick, Sydney, Australia
Hypertensive Disorders and Renal Disease in Pregnancy and Labor

Peter Gerner, MD
Instructor in Anaesthesia, Harvard Medical School; Anesthesiologist, Brigham & Women's Hospital, Boston, Massachusetts
Preterm Labor

Tony Gin, MD, MBChB, Dip HSM, FRCA, FANZCA
Professor and Chairman, Department of Anaesthesia and Intensive Care, The Chinese University of Hong Kong; Chief of Service, Department of Anaesthesia and Intensive Care, Prince of Wales Hospital, Shatin, Hong Kong
Nausea and Vomiting

Wiebke Gogarten, MD
Fellow, Westfalische Wilhelms Universität; Staff, Klinik und Poliklinik für Anasthesiologie und Operative Intensivmedizin, Muenster, Germany
The Effects of Drugs Used in Pregnancy

Hans-Fritz Gramke, MD
Fellow, Westfalische Wilhelms Universität; Staff, Klinik und Poliklinik für Anasthesiologie und Operative Intensivmedizin, Muenster, Germany
The Effects of Drugs Used in Pregnancy

Admir Hadžić, MD, PhD
Assistant Professor of Clinical Anesthesiology, College of Physicians and Surgeons, Columbia University; Deputy Associate Director of Anesthesia, Co-Director, Regional Anesthesia, St. Luke's–Roosevelt Hospital Center, New York, New York
Nerve Blocks in the Pregnant Patient

Martin C. Haeusler, MD
Professor of Obstetrics and Gynecology, University Hospital, Graz, Austria
Preterm Labor

Fumi Handa, MD
Department of Anesthesia, Mito Saiseikai General Hospital, Mito, Ibaraki, Japan
Difficult and Failed Intubation

Björn Holmström, MD, PhD
Chairman, Department of Anesthesiology and Intensive Care, Örebro Medical Centre Hospital, Örebro, Sweden
The Combined Spinal-Epidural Technique

Ronald J. Hurley, MD
Assistant Professor, Harvard Medical School; Associate Director of Obstetric Anesthesia, Brigham and Women's Hospital, Boston, Massachusetts
Continuous Spinal Anesthesia Techniques for Labor and Delivery

Peter R. Isert, MBBS (Hons), FANZCA, FFARACS
Senior Lecturer, Faculty of Medicine, University of New South Wales; Senior Staff Anaesthetist, Director of Operating Theatres (Anaesthesia), Prince of Wales and Sydney Children's Hospitals, Sydney, Australia
Intracranial Disease During Pregnancy: Anesthetic Management

M. F. M. James, MBChB, FRCA, PhD
Professor and Head, Department of Anaesthesia, University of Cape Town, Cape Town, South Africa
Critical Care Management of the Pregnant Patient

Mark Johnson, MD
Clinical Associate Professor, Department of Anesthesiology, Tufts University School of Medicine, Boston; Chairman of Anesthesiology, Melrose-Wakefield Hospital, Melrose, Massachusetts
Anesthesia for Fetal Surgery

Kenneth Kardash, MD, FRCPC
Associate Professor, McGill University Faculty of Medicine; Staff Anesthetist and Co-Director, Chronic Pain Management Center, Jewish General Hospital, Montreal, Quebec, Canada
Functional Anatomy of Central Blockade in Obstetrics

Hector J. Lacassie, MD
Instructor, School of Medicine, Pontificia Universidad Católica de Chile, Santiago, Chile
Nonpharmacologic Alternatives for Obstetric Analgesia

Frank Lah, MBBS, FANZCA
Clinical Lecturer, University of Sydney; Consultant Anesthetist, The Canberra Hospital, Canberra, Australia
Intrapartum Fetal Assessment

Say Wan Lim, MBBS, FFARCSI, FRCA, FANZCA, FRCPS(G), FACP (Hon)
Consultant Anaesthesiologist, Pantai Medical Centre, Kuala Lumpur, Malaysia
Regional Anesthesia in the Third World: Is It an Option?

Chong Jin Long, MD
Head of Anaesthesiology Department, Kandang Kerbau Women's and Children's Hospital, Singapore, Singapore
Hepatic Disease

Michael Lottan, MD
The "Sackler" School of Medicine, Tel Aviv University; Director of Anesthesia, "Lis" Hospital, Tel Aviv Sourasky Medical Center; Member of the Central Committee of the Israel Medical Association (HARI), Member of the Central Committee of the Israeli Society of Anesthesiologists, Tel Aviv, Israel
Hematologic Disease

Gordon Lyons, MD, FRCA
Consultant Obstetric Anaesthetist, Department of Anaesthesia, St. James' University Hospital, Leeds, United Kingdom
Pharmacology of Local Anesthetics

Marco A. E. Marcus, MD, PhD
Associate Professor, Westfalische Wilhems Universität; Staff, Klinik und Poliklinik für Anasthesiologie und Intensivmedizin, Muenster, Germany
The Effects of Drugs Used in Pregnancy

Ramon Martin, MD, PhD
Assistant Professor, Harvard Medical School; Staff Anesthesiologist, Brigham and Women's Hospital, Boston, Massachusetts
Fetal Physiology

Roy Mashiach, MD
Department of Obstetrics and Gynecology, The "Lis" Maternity Hospital, Sackler School of Medicine, Tel Aviv University, Tel Aviv, Israel
Hematologic Disease

Fréderic J. Mercier, MD
Staff Anesthesiologist, Hôpital Antoine Beclere, Clamart, France
Pulmonary Disease in the Pregnant Patient

Manfred G. Moertl, MD
Consultant for Anesthesiology, Leopold Franzens University, Innsbruck; Staff Obstetrician and Gynecologist, Department of Obstetrics and Gynecology, Medical Center Klagenfurt, Klagenfurt, Austria
Multiple Gestation and Fetal Malpresentation

Pamela J. Morgan, MD, CCFP, FRCPC
Associate Professor, University of Toronto Faculty of Medicine; Staff Anesthesiologist, Sunnybrook & Women's College Health Sciences Centre, Toronto, Ontario, Canada
Allergic Reactions

Beverly A. Morningstar, MD, FRCP(C)
Assistant Professor, Department of Anesthesia, University of Toronto Faculty of Medicine; Staff Anesthesiologist, Sunnybrook and Women's Health Sciences Centre, Toronto, Ontario, Canada
The Febrile Parturient

Michael Namestnikov, MD
Department of Anesthesia, Tel Aviv Sourasky Medical Center, Sackler School of Medicine, Tel Aviv University, Tel Aviv, Israel
Hematologic Disease

Florian R. Nuevo, MD
Clinical Faculty, Department of Anesthesiology, University of Santo Tomas; Consultant Anesthesiologist, Santo Tomas University Hospital, Manila, Philippines
Anesthesia for Nonobstetric Surgery in the Pregnant Patient

David A. O'Gorman, MD, FFARCSI
Clinical Lecturer, National University of Ireland; Consultant Anaesthetist, University College Hospital, Galway, Ireland
Drug Abuse in Pregnancy

Michael Paech, MBBS, DRCOG, FRCA, FANZCA, FFPWANZCA
Specialist Anaesthetist, Department of Anaesthesia, King Edward Memorial Hospital for Women, Perth, Australia
Patient-Controlled Epidural Analgesia

John Paull, FANZCA, Dip Ed
Consultant Anaesthetist, Launceston General Hospital, Launceston, Tasmania, Australia
Epidural Analgesia for Labor

Michael Peek, MBBS, PhD, FRACOG
Senior Lecturer, University of Sydney; Consultant Obstetrician, The Canberra Hospital, Canberra, Australia
Intrapartum Fetal Assessment

Narinder Rawal, MD, PhD
Professor, Department of Anesthesiology, Örebro Medical Centre Hospital, Örebro, Sweden
The Combined Spinal-Epidural Technique

Jorge Riquelme, MD
Head, Anesthesiology Recovery and Pain Service, Clinica Alemana de Santiago, Santiago, Chile
Nonpharmacologic Alternatives for Obstetric Analgesia

D. Anthony Rocke, MD, FRCP, FCA(SA)
Professor and Head, Department of Anaesthesia, University of Natal Medical School, Durban, South Africa
AIDS and Obstetric Anesthesia

Stephen H. Rolbin, MD, FRCP(C)
Assistant Professor, University of Toronto Faculty of Medicine; Staff Anesthesiologist, Sunnybrook and Women's College Medical Sciences Centre, Toronto, Ontario, Canada
The Febrile Parturient

Andrew Ross, MBBS, FFA, RACS, FANZCA, Grad Dipl Health Med Law, Dipl Psych
Head of Anaesthesia, Mercy Hospital for Women, East Melbourne, Australia
Physiologic Changes of Pregnancy

Christopher C. Rout, MBBS, FRCA
Research Professor, Department of Anaesthetics, Faculty of Medicine, University of Natal; Chief Specialist, King Edward VIII Hospital, Durban, South Africa
Regional Anesthesia for Cesarean Section

Peter Salmon, MSc, DPhil
Professor of Clinical Psychology, University of Liverpool, Liverpool, United Kingdom
Patient Satisfaction: Capturing Patients' Perspective in the Evaluation of Obstetric Care

Michael Schmid, MD
Department of Anesthesiology, University of Basel/Kantonsspital, Basel, Switzerland
Post–Dural Puncture Headache

Markus C. Schneider, MD
Associate Professor, Department of Anesthesiology, University of Basel School of Medicine; Head of Obstetric Anesthesia, University Women's Hospital, Basel, Switzerland
Post–Dural Puncture Headache

Ferne B. Sevarino, MD
Associate Professor, Department of Anesthesiology, Yale University School of Medicine; Director, Section of Obstetrical Anesthesiology, Yale–New Haven Hospital, New Haven, Connecticut
Postcesarean Analgesia: Patient-Controlled Analgesia and Neuraxial Techniques

Graham Sharpe, MBChB, FANZCA
Consultant Anaesthetist, Wellington Hospital, Capital Coast Health, Ltd., Wellington South, New Zealand
Autoimmune Disease

Raymond S. Sinatra, MD, PhD
Professor of Anesthesiology, Yale University School of Medicine; Attending Anesthesiologist and Director of Acute Pain Service, Yale–New Haven Hospital, New Haven, Connecticut
Postcesarean Analgesia: Patient-Controlled Analgesia and Neuraxial Techniques

Usha Singh, MBChB, FCA(SA)
Specialist Anesthesiologist, Department of Anesthetics, University of Natal; Consultant, Obstetric Anesthesia, King Edward VIII Hospital, Durban, South Africa
AIDS and Obstetric Anesthesia

Jonathan H. Skerman, BDSc, MScD, DSc
Professor of Anesthesiology and of Obstetrics and Gynecology, Louisiana State University School of Medicine, Shreveport, Louisiana; Professor and Chairman, Department of Anaesthesia and Intensive Care, Arabian Gulf University, College of Medicine and Medical Sciences, Manama, Bahrain
Anesthesia for Fetal Surgery

Rudolf Stienstra, MD, PhD
Vice Chairman, Department of Anesthesiology, Leiden University Medical Center, Leiden, The Netherlands
Perinatal Pharmacology of Local Anesthetics and Opioids

Peter Stone, MD, MBChB, DDU, FRCOG
Professor, Department of Obstetrics and Gynaecology, University of Auckland, Faculty of Medicine and Health Science; Professor, Maternal Fetal Medicine, National Women's Hospital, Auckland, New Zealand
Autoimmune Disease

Sun Sunatrio, MD
Head Lector, Medical Facility, University of Indonesia; Head, Department of Anesthesiology, Graha Medika Hospital, Metropolitan Medical Center Hospital, Jakarta Islamic Hospital, Djakarta, Indonesia
Inhalation Agents for Labor

Makoto Tanaka, MD
Associate Professor, Department of Anesthesia, Akita University School of Medicine, Akita, Japan
The Obese Parturient

Katsuo Terui, MD
Assistant Professor, Saitama Medical School; Director of Obstetric Anesthesia, Center for Maternal-Fetal-Neonatal Medicine, Saitama Medical Center, Kawagoe, Saitama, Japan
Antepartum Hemorrhage

Trevor A. Thomas, MBChB, FRCA
Honorary Clinical Lecturer, University of Bristol; Senior Consultant Anaesthetist, United Healthcare Trust, St. Michael's Hospital, Bristol, United Kingdom
Maternal Mortality

Lawrence C. Tsen, MD
Assistant Professor in Anesthesia, Harvard Medical School; Attending Anesthesiologist, Department of Anesthesia, Perioperative and Pain Medicine, Brigham & Women's Hospital, Boston, Massachusetts
Anesthesia for Assisted Reproductive Technologies

André Van Zundert, MD, PhD
Vice-Chairman, Department of Anesthesiology, Intensive Care and Pain Therapy, Catharina Hospital, Eindhoven, The Netherlands
The Combined Spinal-Epidural Technique

Shusee Visalyaputra, MD
Associate Professor, Department of Anesthesia, Mahidol University Medical School; Director, Obstetric Anesthesia, Siriraj Hospital, Bangkok, Thailand
Systemic Analgesia for Labor

Jerry D. Vloka, MD, PhD
Assistant Professor of Clinical Anesthesiology, College of Physicians and Surgeons, Columbia University; Director of Regional Anesthesia; St. Luke's–Roosevelt Hospital Center, New York, New York
Nerve Blocks in the Pregnant Patient

M. Elizabeth Ward, MD, FRCPC
Senior Lecturer and Specialist Anaesthetist, Department of Anaesthesia and Pain Management, Royal North Shore Hospital, University of Sydney, St. Leonards, New South Wales, Australia
Pain Mechanisms in Labor

Andrew D. L. Warmington, MBChB, FANZCA
Specialist Anaesthetist, Department of Anaesthesia, National Women's Hospital, Auckland, New Zealand
Postpartum Hemorrhage

Seiji Watanabe, MD, PhD
Anesthetist-in-Chief, Mito Saiseikai General Hospital, Mito, Ibaraki, Japan
Difficult and Failed Intubation; The Obese Parturient

Frank G. Zavisca, MD, PhD
Associate Professor, Department of Anesthesiology, Louisiana State University School of Medicine; Attending Anesthesiologist and Director of Obstetric Anesthesia, Louisiana State University Health Sciences Center Hospital, Shreveport, Louisiana
Anesthesia for Fetal Surgery

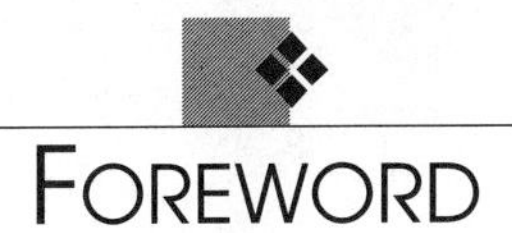

FOREWORD

Obstetric analgesia-anesthesia is unique in that it involves two human beings simultaneously, the mother and her unborn child. Severe and long-lasting complications can affect either or both when attempts to provide anesthesia care are not supported by a foundation of sound knowledge of the special considerations that accompany pregnancy. During the course of gestation, the pregnant woman undergoes anatomic and physiologic changes that can influence the course of anesthesia but may also be affected by it. Anesthetic drugs and techniques can affect the uterus and placenta, the interface between mother and fetus. The resultant changes in blood flow or muscle tone (i.e., uterine contractility) can retard placental exchange of essential nutrients.

These and other considerations unique to the pregnant state are covered extensively in this superb volume. The editors have assembled a truly remarkable group of experts in obstetric anesthesia to present the most up-to-date views on matters pertinent to sound anesthesia practice. Drawn from six continents, the contributors have presented a truly international overview of the problems facing the anesthesiologist in the obstetric suite and the solutions to those problems.

As we embark upon the twenty-first century, the editors and contributors have performed a valuable service not only for the professionals who provide anesthesia care to the parturient, but also for women and their children worldwide who deserve to be the beneficiaries of the knowledge contained within the covers of this book.

Gertie F. Marx, MD
Emeritus Professor of Anesthesiology
Albert Einstein College of Medicine
Bronx, New York

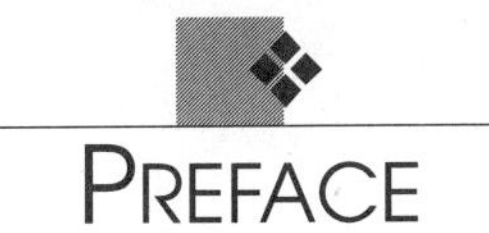

PREFACE

We are living in a world different from that of the previous generation. The "information superhighway" is a reality and has become a tool for instant sharing of vast amounts of information. However, a review of the world's obstetric anesthesia literature clearly illustrates that clinical practice continues to have a huge geographic and cultural component. Dictated by numerous factors, anesthesiologists from different countries often provide dramatically different kinds of anesthesia for the same types of patients. Is there a single "right" way of administering obstetric anesthesia in all countries? Clearly not. However, I would argue that there are many well established and superior techniques that should have already crossed all geographic boundaries, but have failed to do so. Although computer and Internet access has not yet reached all physicians, given the availability of excellent textbooks it is surprising that advancements in this field are not affecting practice throughout the world. To help bridge this gap, this new textbook endeavors to establish a uniformity of clinical approach to obstetric anesthesia that will be appreciated for its distinctly international approach. Many of the world's most respected clinicians and researchers have joined forces and present in this textbook, what I hope the reader will appreciate to be, a unified approach and philosophy. The authors have provided the reader with a balanced view of the many excellent choices available for providing analgesia and anesthesia during pregnancy, regardless of geographic location.

The role of the anesthesiologist in obstetric practice is being redefined, as advances in reproductive medicine have improved obstetric outcome in women despite significant systemic diseases and advancing age. Today, anesthesiologists take a much more active role in labor and delivery suites. Not only do they provide anesthesia and analgesia for the pregnant woman, but also they are an integral part of the team of physicians who care for the high-risk parturient. In keeping with this important new role of the anesthesiologist, in this textbook a significant emphasis is placed on management of the high-risk parturient.

A new philosophy with respect to labor analgesia has evolved. Women in labor and their obstetricians are no longer seeking or expecting labor "anesthesia," but rather "analgesia," and an increasing number of women are requesting that they be allowed to ambulate while in labor. The past decade has brought about a social acknowledgment that labor results in severe pain for most women and that there are now safe and effective means available from which a woman may choose to reduce that pain. The ideal technique should effectively reduce the pain of labor while allowing the parturient to actively participate in the birthing experience. Today's new techniques come close to achieving this laudable goal. Of all the possible methods of pain relief that are now being utilized in labor, neuraxial blockade provides the most effective and least depressant analgesia. The past decade has seen major changes in the practice of Obstretric Anesthesiology, as evidenced by an improved understanding on the part of anesthesiologists of the many disease entities seen in obstetric patients as well as by the enhancements in new neuraxial techniques and drugs. A sizable portion of this textbook is also dedicated to an extensive discussion of these new techniques.

The purposes of this text are multiple: to teach the science of obstetric anesthesia, to provide practical information for the clinical anesthesiologist or obstetrician, to serve as an encyclopedic reference that can be used by residents and fellows, and, perhaps most important, to help bridge the disparate worlds of obstetric anesthesia practice. To achieve these goals, each chapter was prepared by an authority in his or her assigned subject. Each chapter ends with a summary, key reference, and a clinical case stem that will help the reader to recognize how the chapter's information can be applied to a clinical scenario. These stems should also help the resident and fellow who are preparing for oral examination.

The editors hope that the information in this reference textbook will provide a foundation for anesthesiologists as well as obstetricians and that it will find its way into clinical practice throughout the world and improve patient care within our specialty.

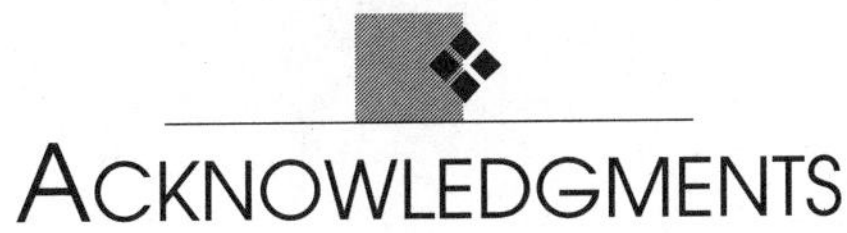

ACKNOWLEDGMENTS

This book was possible only because of the herculean efforts of the many contributors who took valuable time from their busy schedules to participate in this exciting endeavor. My heartfelt thanks to them all and to my colleagues Stephen Gatt and Sanjay Datta for their commitment to this project and for putting up with my persistency as the many deadlines approached. In addition, the help of Melissa Dudlick and Allan Ross from Harcourt was essential to the success of this project. Having survived this one, I'm sure that everyone will agree that Melissa definitely has a future in politics. With contributors from 29 different countries, this obstetric anesthesia mini United Nations would have never been possible without the excellent secretarial skills of Zona Rose. Finally, my deepest thanks to my friend, mentor, and chairman Daniel M. Thys, MD, for his support and encouragement during the three years that saw the concept of this textbook change from dream to reality.

David J. Birnbach

The compilation of this textbook presented an immense logistical and technical task. Now that it is completed, I begin to realize that it would have been impossible without the invaluable help and assistance of so many. My thanks go especially to Kay King, whose dedicated enthusiasm made the mammoth task of rushing page proofs and documents to contributing authors, organizing illustrations, compiling bibliography, and monitoring compliance with deadlines seem like a breeze; to my close friends and fellow-editors David Birnbach and Sanjay Datta for their drive, enthusiasm, and tenacity in seeing this project through to fruition; to Melissa Dudlick and Allan Ross for bearing with us through many a deadline and for keeping us on the straight and narrow; and to the many colleagues and friends who offered helpful criticism and advice.

Stephen P. Gatt

To my mentor, Phillip Bromage, and to my associates who have been a great help to me.

Sanjay Datta

NOTICE

Medicine is an ever-changing field. Standard safety precautions must be followed, but as new research and clinical experience broaden our knowledge, changes in treatment and drug therapy become necessary or appropriate. Readers are advised to check the product information currently provided by the manufacturer of each drug to be administered to verify the recommended dose, the method and duration of administration, and the contraindications. It is the responsibility of the treating physician, relying on experience and knowledge of the patient, to determine dosages and the best treatment for the patient. Neither the publisher nor the editor assumes any responsibility for any injury and/or damage to persons or property.

THE PUBLISHER

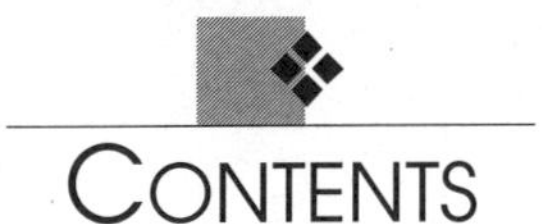

CONTENTS

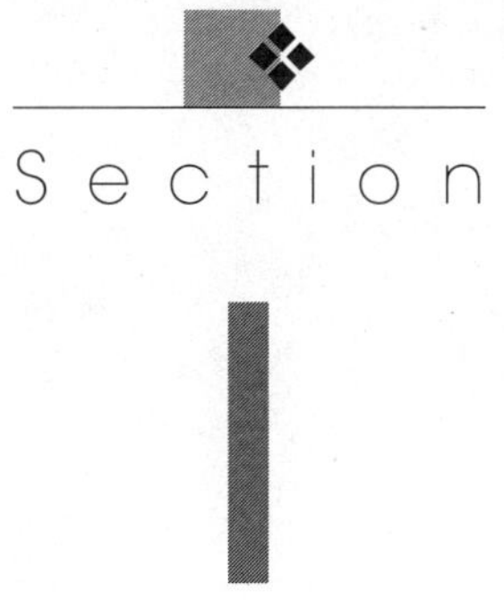

Physiology, Pharmacology, and Anatomy

1

Pain Mechanisms in Labor

M. ELIZABETH WARD, MD, FRCPC

MICHAEL J. COUSINS, MBBS, MD (SYD), FANZCA, FRCA, FFPMANZCA

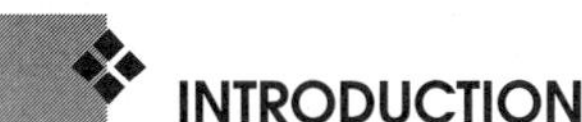

INTRODUCTION

The provision of optimal obstetric anesthetic care of the parturient requires an appreciation of the multidimensional nature of the pain of childbirth. It is essential for the anesthetist to understand the mechanisms of pain transmission during labor and delivery and the many factors that influence pain intensity, duration, distribution, and quality. Pain in childbirth is frequently severe, being rated by many women as the most painful experience of their lives. Variables, such as pain origin and transmission, and the parturient's perception of, and response to, pain, contribute to pain during childbirth. Moreover, the perception and expression of pain is a complex interaction that involves sensory, emotional, behavioral, and environmental factors.[1] Rational pain management requires an awareness of the underlying mechanisms involved and an understanding of how pharmacologic and nonpharmacologic interventions can act to disrupt these mechanisms. Herein lies the challenge for the obstetric anesthetist.

The alleviation of pain and suffering is one of the fundamental principles guiding medical practice, yet the amelioration of pain during childbirth has historically attracted much controversy. In fact, the concept of pain relief during childbirth is a relatively recent one. Development of methods for pain relief has been delayed by folklore, superstition, and religious beliefs, as well as by opposition from members of the medical profession.[2]

Morton's demonstration of the anesthetic properties of ether for the first time in 1846 was hailed by most physicians and by the general population as a great blessing for humanity. Three months later, on January 19, 1847, James Young Simpson, the professor of midwifery at Edinburgh, became the first person to document the use of anesthesia in obstetric practice. He used ether to aid the delivery of a dead fetus after failed internal podalic version in a woman with obstructed labor.[2] However, unlike the enthusiasm that greeted Morton's discovery, the use of ether to relieve the pain of labor evoked strong criticism from the medical and religious communities and from the general public. Many considered anesthesia in childbirth to be unnatural and morally wrong. Whereas Simpson maintained that all pain—labor pain included—was without physiologic value and that it degraded and destroyed those who experienced it,[3] most obstetricians of the day asserted that the pain of childbirth was a "most desirable, salutary, and conservative manifestation of life force" and that "to be in natural labor is the culminating point of the female somatic forces."[4] Many obstetricians predicted that any drug that abolished pain would alter uterine contractions, prolonging delivery, and would have deleterious effects on the mother and the fetus. Some believed that the mother's reaction to labor pain was a valuable guide and argued that it would be dangerous to abolish it[2]; for example, the application of forceps would be made very difficult if there was no pain to guide their placement.[4]

Much more acrimonious debate about the use of anesthesia in childbirth came from those who objected on religious and moral grounds. The clergy, the general public, and many doctors felt that to provide pain relief during labor contravened the word of God. Some translations of the Scriptures implied that labor should be a painful process: "I will greatly multiply thy sorrow and thy conception; in sorrow thou shalt bring forth children" (Genesis 3:16). Various clergy of the day were beset upon to give their interpretation of the scriptures to settle this question.[4]

As medical and religious debate subsided, the use of analgesia for labor gradually became more commonplace, largely as a result of popular demand. By 1860, anesthesia for childbirth had become part of medical practice by public acclaim, just as Simpson had predicted.[3]

Nevertheless, even today, misconceptions and confusion still exist among the public and some physicians, nurses, and midwives about the nature of the pain of childbirth and its treatment. Advocates of "natural childbirth" contend that normal labor need not be painful and that when it is, it is due to the influence of modern cultural and environmental factors.[5] Some believe that because labor is a normal, physiologic process, labor pain is also normal, serving an important biologic function and, as such, should not be interfered with. The public is often inadequately and incorrectly informed about recent advances in knowledge and current therapeutic practice, and this leads to further misunderstanding. There is continued debate among some obstetricians over the issue of whether the use of analgesia and anesthesia for labor and delivery, in particular epidural neural blockade, prolongs the second stage of labor, increasing the rate of instrumental vaginal delivery and cesarean section.[6, 7] Although a recent meta-analysis suggests that epidural analgesia does not increase the risk of cesarean delivery,[8] some still insist that it may contribute to maternal and neonatal morbidity and mortality,[9] although the preponderance of evidence suggests otherwise. In addition, economic constraints at both the governmental level and the individual level may preclude the provision of labor analgesia in certain circumstances.

Despite all of the controversy, there is no doubt that for most women, childbirth is associated with very severe pain, often exceeding all expectations.[10] Indeed, labor pain is one of the most intense pains experienced by women; when compared with several pain syndromes such as back pain, cancer pain, phantom limb pain, or postherpetic neuralgia, and with other sources of acute pain, for example, a fracture or a deep laceration, labor pain has been found to be the most severe (Fig. 1–1).[11, 12] Pain is reported as severe or intolerable in up to two thirds of parturients.[11, 13, 14] A study of women in the first stage of labor used the McGill Pain Questionnaire[15] to evaluate pain; 60% of primiparae described the pain of uterine contractions as being "unbearable, intolerable, extremely severe, or excruciating," and a further 30% described it as being "moderately severe."[11, 16] Among multiparae, 45% had severe or extremely severe pain, 30% had moderate pain, and 25% had mild pain.[16]

Pain is not a necessary accompaniment of childbirth. Although pain serves the important biologic function of indicating the commencement of labor to the parturient, it should be effectively relieved once it has fulfilled this task. Persistent, severe pain has harm-

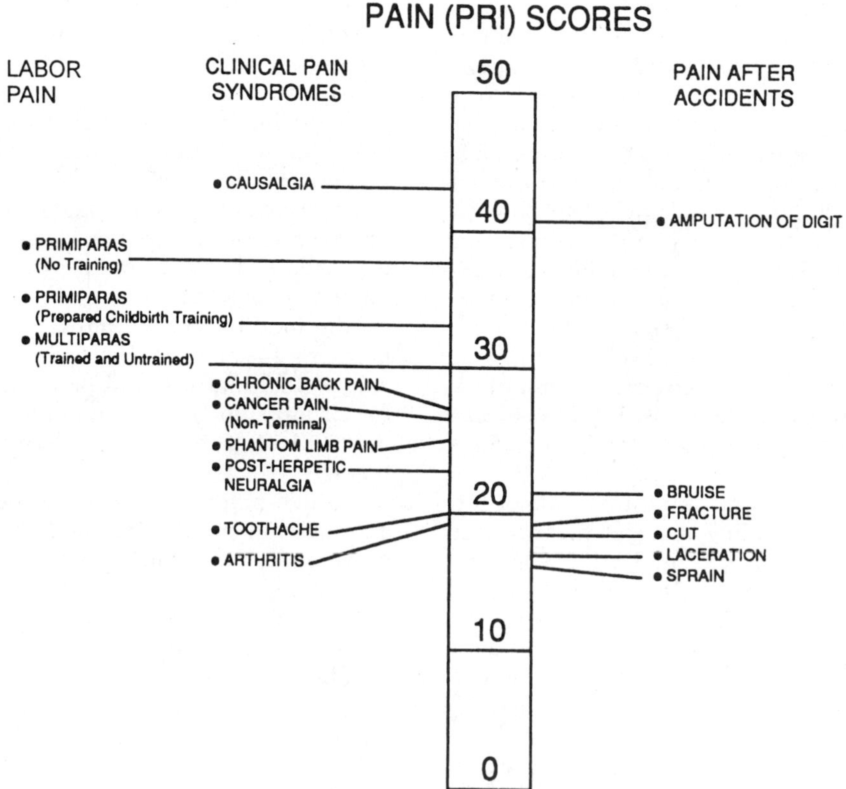

Figure 1–1 Comparison of pain scores, using the McGill Pain Questionnaire, obtained from women during labor and from patients in a general hospital pain clinic and an emergency department. The Pain Rating Index (PRI) represents the sum of the rank values of all the words chosen from 20 sets of pain descriptors. (From Melzack R: The myth of painless childbirth. The John J Bonica Lecture. Pain 1984; 19:321–337, with permission from Elsevier Science; as modified by Bonica JJ: The nature of pain in parturition. *In* Van Zundert A, Ostheimer GW (eds): Pain Relief and Anesthesia in Obstetrics. New York: Churchill Livingstone; 1996:32.)

ful effects on the mother and might also have harmful effects on the fetus and neonate in some instances (see Chapter 4).[17] Moreover, pain during childbirth may be unpleasant and distressing, and the experience of labor may be disappointing for the parturient if she feels she has been unable to cope. There is now overwhelming evidence that properly administered analgesia and anesthesia do *not* contribute to maternal and perinatal morbidity and mortality but may, in fact, help to reduce their occurrence, especially in high-risk pregnancies (see Chapter 10). Maternal-fetal factors and obstetric management appear to be the dominant factors in determining cesarean delivery rates, not epidural analgesia.[18, 19] In addition, women now have better access to information about options for effective pain management, and many women expect—even demand—adequate pain relief during childbirth.

This chapter presents a comprehensive discussion of the various aspects of the pain mechanisms involved in the process of childbirth. The material is organized into two major sections: acute and chronic pain mechanisms, and obstetric pain mechanisms. The pain of childbirth is unique; although it is an acute, normal physiologic process, it includes suffering and pain behavior in many parturients, and these aspects are usually recognized as being associated with chronic pain states.

Initially, a brief account of some historical aspects of pain is presented, followed by a general overview of current concepts of acute and chronic pain mechanisms, including peripheral and dorsal horn mechanisms, ascending tracts, and descending modulatory pathways. Some of the factors implicated in the development of chronic pain are discussed also. This is followed by a detailed description of labor pain mechanisms, neural pathways, and clinical characteristics. Other elements that influence pain perception in the parturient, including physical, psychologic, and cultural factors, are summarized. In addition, recent research pertaining to some of the neurohumoral factors implicated in childbirth pain mechanisms are reviewed.

Discussion of the physiologic and pathophysiologic consequences of the pain of labor and delivery on the mother, the fetus, and the newborn, and their modification by analgesia and anesthesia, is not within the scope of this chapter; this material is presented in detail in Chapter 2.

A BRIEF HISTORY OF PAIN

For centuries, the notion of pain has puzzled, fascinated, and confounded physicians, scientists, and philosophers alike. Many varied and diverse hypotheses have been put forward in an attempt to elucidate the basic nature of pain.[20] From the earliest days, ancient societies thought pain to be an invasion of the body by spirits or objects. In ancient Egypt and Persia, it was believed that pain was the result of magic influences of the dead or of evil spirits. In Hebraic society, pain signified divine retribution inflicted as punishment for sins committed. In early Greek civilization, Plato regarded the heart as the center of all sensations, and both pain and pleasure as "affections" common to the whole body.[20] Aristotle described pain as an affective quality, a "passion of the soul" felt in the heart, a state of feeling opposite to pleasure and the epitome of unpleasantness.[20] Galen postulated that a specific set of nerves, each one dedicated to one of the senses, including pain, transmitted sensory stimulation to the brain via "psychic pneuma."[21]

When physiology emerged as an experimental science in the early part of the 19th century, the study of pain in the modern sense was initiated.[17] The availability of methods for recording nerve impulses made it possible to establish that pain sensation was carried to the brain by specific afferent nerves. Two opposing theories of pain emerged.[20] The *specificity (sensory) theory* stated that pain was a pure sensation with specific receptor organs and conducting pathways, independent of touch and other senses, that transmitted nociceptive information to the brain with little modification. The *intensive (summation) theory* hypothesized that pain resulted from intense stimulation of any nerve and central summation of impulses provoked by the stimuli.

By the mid-20th century, the specificity theory predominated, although it was gradually modified, and pain research became progressively focused on peripheral mechanisms. Up until the 1950s, no theory took into account the reality of human pain as a psychologic experience that depends as much on the subject's disposition and character as on the injury sustained. Wolff and others [17, 20] attempted to explain the importance of environmental and psychologic factors in pain perception, suggesting that the total pain experience incorporates not only the perception of pain, but also the associated emotions and sensations. Beecher[22] postulated that the individual's attitude, judgment, mood, and emotional state at the time of pain perception determine his or her reaction to that pain. This was presumed to explain the variability in pain perception and response to an identical stimulus observed between individuals and even in the same individual at different times.[23] In 1965, the "gate control" theory of Melzack and Wall[24] suggested a possible explanation of how the pain experience might be modulated by other processes. This theory proposed that pain results from activity in several interacting specialized neural systems, and that it is not simply the result of neural activity from an exclusive pain pathway, as implied by the simplistic peripheral-to-central, hard-wired, neural system of the specificity theory.

Still today, the concept of pain, both human and animal, continues to evolve.[21] The use of several experimental approaches, including behavioral studies, in vivo and in vitro electrophysiology, molecular biology, and anatomic studies, has resulted in an improved understanding of nociceptive processing. The classic model of pain transmission and perception has, until recently, been a hard-wired, line-labeled, modality-specific, single pathway leading from stimulus to sensation,[25] but this model is now seen as an oversimplification. Our understanding of pain mechanisms has progressed significantly; in the last three decades, there has been a shift of interest toward including central pain processes and the neurophysiologic basis for pain control. It is now recognized that a single pain mechanism does not exist; rather, noxious stimuli produce a series of dynamic, interlocking, biologic, reactive responses.[25] Thus, the acute pain experience is a multidimensional one, the net effect of many contributing and interacting biologic, psychologic, and environmental mechanisms.

ACUTE AND CHRONIC PAIN MECHANISMS

Pain is a highly complex perception of an adverse sensation originating from a specific region of the body.[26] The International Association for the Study of Pain (IASP) defines pain as "an unpleasant sensory and emotional experience associated with actual or potential tissue damage, or described in terms of such damage."[27]

The term *pain* is used to describe all sensations that hurt or are unpleasant, but it is now recognized that a prolonged insult to the body produces changes in the nervous system that alter the "normal," "physiologic" response to a noxious stimulus. As a result of the recognition of these changes, Woolf[28, 29] has proposed that pain be divided into two entities: (1) physiologic, or brief nociceptive, pain and (2) pathophysiologic, or clinical, pain. The processes that underlie our physiologic experience of a brief noxious stimulus are quite different from the pathophysiologic processes that occur in the clinical situation.

Physiologic (nociceptive) pain describes the situation in which a transient noxious stimulus activates peripheral nociceptors, which then transmit that information through several relays until it reaches the brain, where it is recognized as a potentially harmful stimulus. Whereas a low-intensity, non-noxious stimulus activates low-threshold receptors and is relayed via A-beta fibers to the dorsal horn of the spinal cord,[29] a high-intensity stimulus is transmitted to the dorsal horn by high-threshold, thinly myelinated A-delta and unmyelinated C sensory fibers (Fig. 1–2). The latter type of stimulus is differentiated as transient, well-localized pain. Physiologic pain is a key component of the body's normal defense mechanisms, providing a warning system to protect the body from a potentially harmful external environment by initiating behavioral and reflex avoidance strategies.

More commonly, the insult to the body that produces pain also results in inflammation and tissue and nerve injury. The factors responsible for the development of clinical or pathophysiologic pain result in a stimulus-response system that has characteristics quite different from those of physiologic pain. Inflammation and nerve injury, either peripheral or central, give rise to changes in sensory processing at a peripheral and a central level with a resultant sensitization. Clinical pain is characterized by the presence of ongoing discomfort and abnormal sensitivity.[30] It usually has three general attributes: spontaneous pain (dull, burning, or stabbing); exaggerated pain in response to noxious, suprathreshold stimuli (hyperalgesia); and pain produced by low-intensity, or formerly subthreshold, stimuli (allodynia).[30] Abnormal excitability of both the peripheral

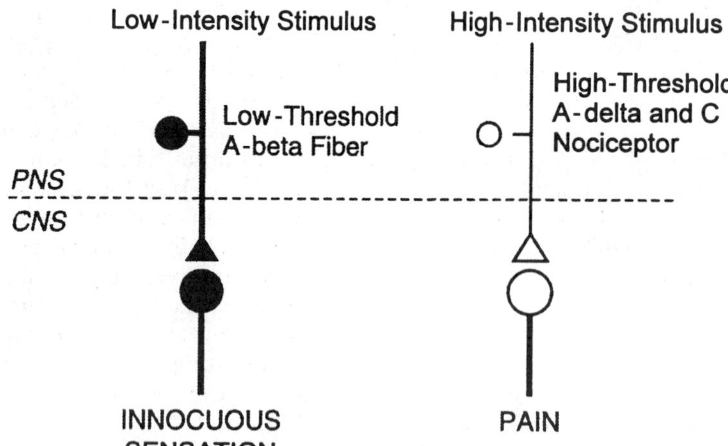

Figure 1–2 Under "physiologic" conditions, low-intensity, non-noxious stimuli activate low-threshold receptors to generate innocuous sensations, and high-intensity, noxious stimuli activate high-threshold nociceptors that may lead to the sensation of pain. PNS, peripheral nervous system; CNS, central nervous system. (From Woolf CJ, Chong MS: Preemptive analgesia—treating postoperative pain by preventing the establishment of central sensitization. Anesth Analg 1993; 77:362–379, as modified by Siddall PJ, Cousins MJ: Introduction to pain mechanisms: implications for neural blockade. *In* Cousins MJ, Bridenbaugh PO (eds): Neural Blockade in Clinical Anesthesia and Management of Pain, 3rd ed. Philadelphia: Lippincott-Raven; 1998:676.)

and the central nervous system is present.[29] A low-intensity stimulus elicits pain via A-delta and C, as well as A-beta fibers; this pathophysiologic pain spreads to nondamaged areas and often outlasts the stimulus (Fig. 1–3). Clinical pain can be acute or chronic.

Pain perception is a dynamic process that involves both peripheral and central mechanisms, and continuous interaction among complex ascending nociceptive and descending antinociceptive systems.[1] Many of the recent findings concerning peripheral and central mechanisms and pathways for pain and its modulation are reviewed below. The organization of some ascending nociceptive pathways is discussed. Structures involved in the descending analgesia systems are described, and the pathways and neurotransmitters used are mentioned. The following discussion of mechanisms involved in pain physiology and pathophysiology is intended to provide the reader with information that will contribute to a more complete understanding and appreciation of factors involved in obstetric pain mechanisms. Where applicable, the clinical implications of recent findings on pain and pain modulation systems for the obstetric patient are discussed.

Peripheral Mechanisms

The primary afferent nociceptor (free nerve endings of A-delta and C fibers) is the initial structure involved in nociceptive processes. It is activated by thermal, mechanical, and chemical stimuli[31]; impulses are propagated along the afferent fiber (A-delta or C fiber) toward the first relay in the dorsal horn of the spinal cord (Fig. 1–4). Peripheral nociceptors are distinguished from other sensory nerve fibers on the basis of morphology, conduction velocity, and responsiveness to mechanical stimuli.[32] Nociceptors have poorly differentiated terminals, slow conduction velocities (unmyelinated C fibers, <2.5 m/sec; myelinated A-delta fibers, 2.5–20.0 m/sec), and are normally activated by potentially damaging or damaging stimuli, that is, stimuli of strong to noxious intensity.[32] Peripheral afferent nociceptors terminate mainly in the superficial (A-delta and C fibers), but also in the deep (A-delta fibers) dorsal horn of the spinal cord, where they release several neurotransmitters (see next paragraph). Most thermal and mechanical pain signaling arises from activation of polymodal nociceptors at peripheral levels; these are innervated by C fibers.[33, 34]

High-threshold sensory nociceptors normally respond to a range of physical (e.g., pressure, extremes of temperature) and chemical stimuli, but their activity and metabolism may be profoundly altered by a variety of mediators generated by tissue injury and inflammation through a process called *peripheral sensitization.* Not only does inflammation stimulate peripheral nerve fibers to induce pain, but also it generates changes in local blood flow and vascular permeability, alters the release of growth and trophic factors from surrounding tissues, and causes activation and migration of immune cells.[35] Thus, the release of intracellular contents from damaged cells and the activation of lymphocytes, mast cells, and macrophages occurs, with the liberation of chemical mediators from inflammatory cells. This leads to alteration of the excitability of sensory and sympathetic nerve fibers. Moreover, primary afferent nociceptors release several neuro-

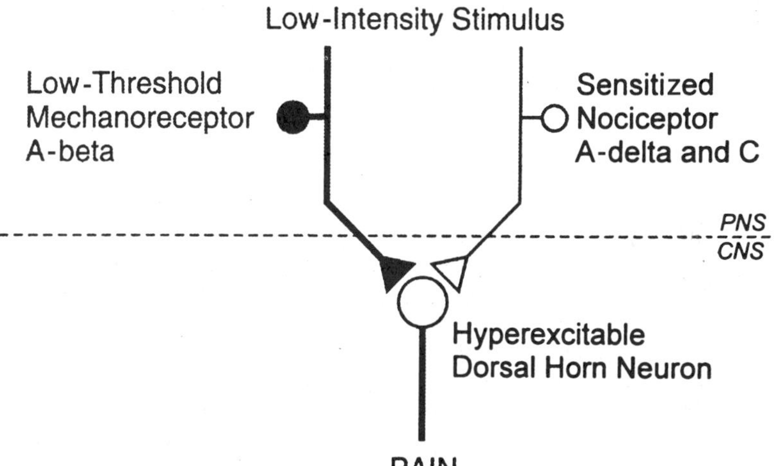

Figure 1–3 In the "pathophysiologic," or clinical situation, central and peripheral changes lead to abnormal excitability in the nervous system. This means that low-intensity stimuli can produce pain. PNS, peripheral nervous system; CNS, central nervous system. (From Woolf CJ, Chong MS: Preemptive analgesia—treating postoperative pain by preventing the establishment of central sensitization. Anesth Analg 1993; 77:362–379, as modified by Siddall PJ, Cousins MJ: Introduction to pain mechanisms: implications for neural blockade. *In* Cousins MJ, Bridenbaugh PO (eds): Neural Blockade in Clinical Anesthesia and Management of Pain, 3rd ed. Philadelphia: Lippincott-Raven; 1998:676.)

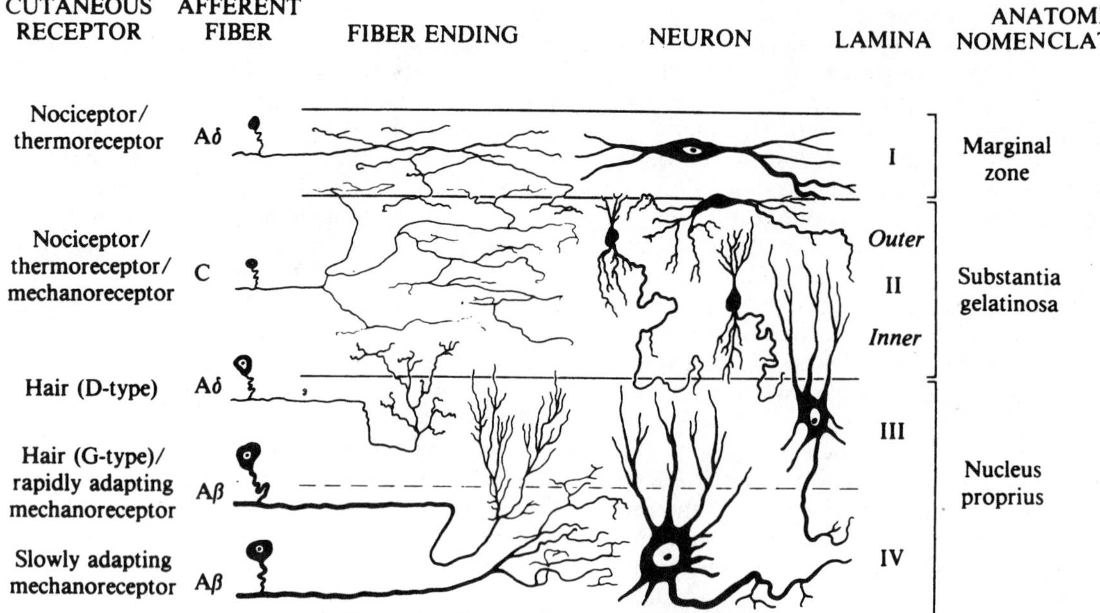

❖ **Figure 1–4** Schematic diagram of the neuronal organization of, and afferent input to, the superficial dorsal horn. The diagram represents an imaginary transverse section of the dorsal horn and illustrates the afferent fiber endings and neuronal elements present in the first four laminae of the dorsal horn. To the left of the diagram the types of afferent fiber and relevant receptor groups associated with them are listed. Fiber endings in the dorsal horn are schematized diagrams taken from published morphologic studies. Neurons in the diagram represent standard types of neuron in the superficial dorsal horn. The following types have been illustrated *(from top to bottom)*: a marginal cell, a substantia gelatinosa (SG)–limiting cell, two SG central cells, and two neurons of the nucleus proprius, the most superficial of which has dendrites penetrating lamina II. Indicated at the right of the diagram are the laminar division of the superficial dorsal horn and corresponding anatomic nomenclature. (From Cervero F, Iggo A: The substantia gelatinosa of the spinal cord: a critical review. Brain 1980; 103:717, with permission of Oxford University Press; as modified by Yaksh TL: Physiologic and pharmacologic substrates of nociception and nerve injury. *In* Cousins MJ, Bridenbaugh PO (eds): Neural Blockade in Clinical Anesthesia and Management of Pain, 3rd ed. Philadelphia: Lippincott-Raven; 1998:740.)

transmitters, including glutamate, an excitatory amino acid (EAA), and the neuropeptides substance P, neurokinin A, and calcitonin gene-related peptide (CGRP).[32, 36] The net effect of these interactions is the generation of a "soup" of inflammatory mediators, including potassium and hydrogen ions, serotonin, bradykinin, substance P, histamine, cytokines, purines, nitric oxide, and products from the cyclooxygenase and lipoxygenase pathways of arachidonic acid metabolism; these substances sensitize high-threshold nociceptors (Fig. 1–5).[37–40] The resulting clinical scenario is one of increased responsiveness to thermal stimuli, with a reduced threshold for pain (primary hyperalgesia) and painful perception of normally non-noxious, low-intensity, mechanical stimuli (allodynia) at the site of injury.

It is important to make mention of the effect of peripheral sensitization on another recently identified class of unmyelinated primary afferent fibers, the "silent nociceptors,"[41] so-named because under normal circumstances, they are quiescent to excessive thermal or mechanical stimuli. However, as a result of chemical sensitization from tissue and nerve injury and inflammation, these nociceptors respond to stimuli by discharging vigorously and continuously, even during ordinary movements; they also display changes in receptive fields.[42] Their properties have yet to be defined, but they have been identified in a number of different tissues and species.

Other Changes Induced by Tissue Damage and Inflammation

Opioid Receptors. Opioids have well-established central analgesic effects. It has also been shown that tissue damage increases peripheral opioid receptor expression on primary afferent nociceptors.[43] Tissue injury and inflammation result in the synthesis of opioid receptors in the cell body of the dorsal root ganglion, and subsequent receptor transport to the central terminal in the dorsal horn, and to the peripheral terminal.[44–46] These receptors are activated by endogenous opioid peptides synthesized and released by immunocompetent cells (monocytes, T cells, B cells, and macrophages) during inflammation.[45] The antinociceptive effect of opioids is due, at least in part, to their action on primary afferent nerve terminals[47] and sympathetic fibers.[48] Opioid receptors have been demonstrated on peripheral sensory axons in opioid-naive animals,[49] in-

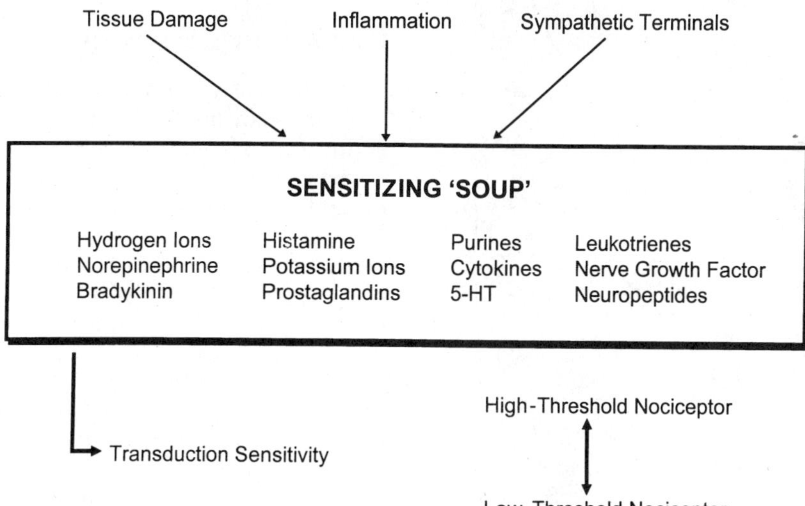

❖ **Figure 1–5** The sensitivity of high-threshold nociceptors can be modified in the periphery by a combination of chemicals that act as a "sensitizing soup." These chemicals are produced by damaged tissue as part of the inflammatory reaction and by sympathetic terminals. 5-HT, 5-hydroxytryptamine. (From Woolf CJ, Chong MS: Preemptive analgesia—treating postoperative pain by preventing the establishment of central sensitization. Anesth Analg 1993; 77:362–379, as modified by Siddall PJ, Cousins MJ: Introduction to pain mechanisms: implications for neural blockade. *In* Cousins MJ, Bridenbaugh PO (eds): Neural Blockade in Clinical Anesthesia and Management of Pain, 3rd ed. Philadelphia: Lippincott-Raven; 1998:677.)

dicating a wider function for opioid receptors than was previously envisioned.

Primary Afferent Fibers. As outlined earlier, peripheral sensitization may induce complex changes in afferent fibers; these include overt activation, sensitization to other stimuli, and alterations in their phenotype and structure (Fig. 1–6).[36, 50–53] These effects are, in part, the result of changes in membrane ion channels that are regulated through receptor-coupled second messenger cascades,[35] which, in turn, may alter gene transcription and ultimately bring about long-term modifications in the biochemistry of sensory neurons.[35]

In addition, biochemical, physiologic, and morphologic changes in injured nerve fibers can act as foci of pain in themselves.[54, 55] One such example is the expression by damaged nerves of nerve growth factor (NGF), a neurotrophin. NGF is essential for the survival and development of sensory neurons and for maintaining their phenotype,[56] acting via a tyrosine kinase receptor (trkA) to regulate specific gene transcription processes. Under usual circumstances, NGF is synthesized by the peripheral target tissues of afferent fibers and by supporting cells, including fibroblasts, Schwann cells, and keratinocytes. However, NGF production, when stimulated by inflammatory substances, such as the cytokines (interleukin-1β [IL-1β] and tumor necrosis factor-α [TNF-α]), leads to the synthesis of several neuropeptides, including neurokinins and CGRP,[57] and abnormal regulation of a number of other proteins, such as the capsaicin receptor, membrane sodium channels, and proton-activated ion channels.[52, 58] In the presence of nerve injury, such changes may be accompanied by increased sensitivity to exogenous stimuli, producing hyperalgesia. Nerve injury can also act as a focus of pain through altered neural response to various stimuli, including spontaneous firing or increased sensitivity to mechanical stimulation.[54] The dorsal root ganglion itself may undergo similar changes.[59] Moreover, ectopic nerve impulses may arise if demyelination occurs as a result of reduced blood supply.

Sympathetic Nervous System. The sympathetic nervous system not only serves to regulate involuntary functions but also appears to play an important part in modulating sensory processing.[60] Nerve damage, including even minor trauma, can bring about a disturbance in sympathetic activity that may give rise to a sustained condition known as "sympathetically maintained pain."[61] An example is the development of a chronic pain state known as "complex regional pain syndrome."[61–63] Various mechanisms have been proposed. Sympathetic fibers are known to release prostanoids during inflammation; these may contribute to sensitization of primary nociceptive afferent fibers.[36] Also, following nerve injury, it appears that stimulation of sympathetic nerves can excite primary nociceptive afferent fibers via α-adrenergic receptors. Moreover, the dorsal root ganglion (DRG) becomes innervated by sympathetic efferent terminals[64] at newly

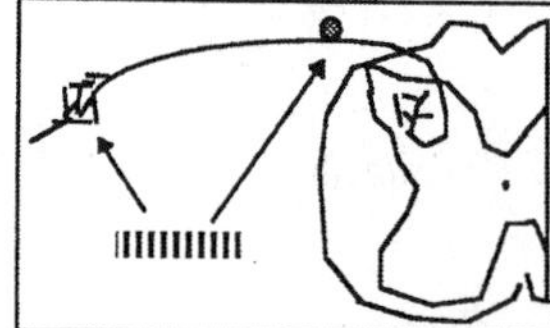

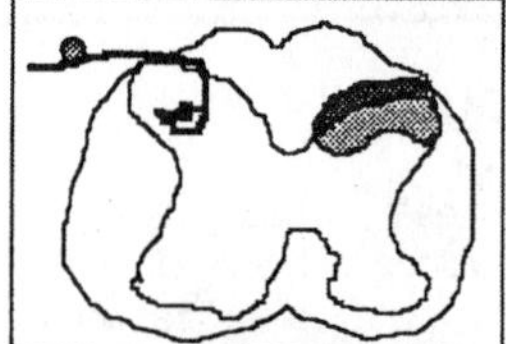

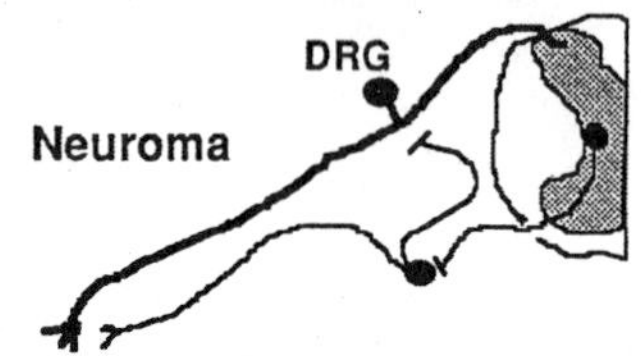

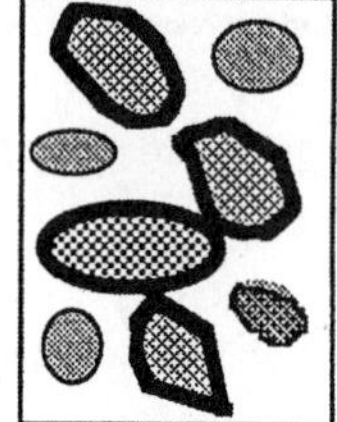

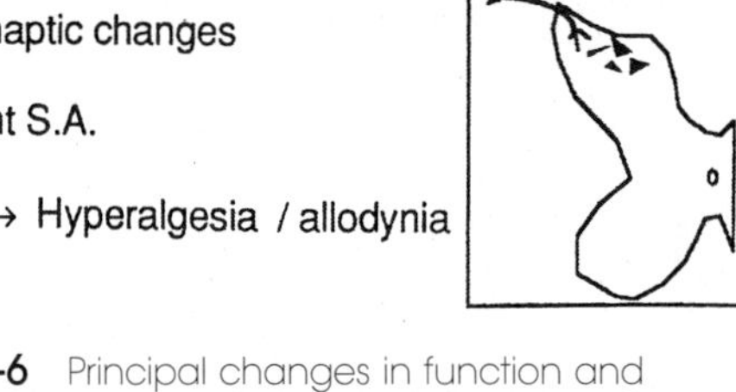

❖ **Figure 1–6** Principal changes in function and connectivity potentially contributing to pain states after peripheral nerve injury. *A*, After nerve injury, spontaneous activity develops in the injured terminal (neuroma), in the dorsal root ganglion (DRG) cell of the injured axon, and in the spinal cord dorsal horn. Sprouted endings may develop sensitivity to a number of humoral factors and display increases in the densities of sodium channels. *B*, Laminae I and II (lam II) receive smaller, unmyelinated axons that are typically high-threshold in character, while larger low-threshold afferents terminate in lamina III (lam III) or deeper. After injury, large afferent terminals sprout into lamina II. *C*, After peripheral nerve injury, there is a significant increase in sympathetic innervation at the neuroma of the resprouting axon. DRG cells display basket-like projections around DRG cells from proliferating postganglionic sympathetic terminals. These projections have been shown to drive activity in DRG cells. *D*, There is an increased incidence of "dark-staining" neurons, suggesting a loss of interneurons (some of which are believed to contain γ-aminobutyric acid and glycine). In addition, after injury, there is an increased release of spinal glutamate, perhaps secondary to loss of inhibitory interneurons and to increased spontaneous afferent drive. Loss of spinal glycine inhibition and/or increased glutamate receptor (Glu-r) activation leads to hyperalgesia and allodynia. (From Yaksh TL: Physiologic and pharmacologic substrates of nociception and nerve injury. *In* Cousins MJ, Bridenbaugh PO (eds): Neural Blockade in Clinical Anesthesia and Management of Pain, 3rd ed. Philadelphia: Lippincott-Raven; 1998:761.)

formed α-adrenergic receptors on the DRG. It is likely that, collectively, these alterations in sympathetic efferent activity result in abnormal responsiveness of the primary afferent fiber (Fig. 1–6). However, more central disturbances usually play a major role (see under Dorsal Horn Mechanisms).

Dorsal Horn Mechanisms

Much of recent pain research has focused on dorsal horn mechanisms.[65] The dorsal horn of the spinal cord is the primary receiving area for somatosensory input. Primary afferent fibers transmitting nociceptive information from the periphery terminate in laminae I and V (A-delta fibers), and in lamina II (C fibers) (Fig. 1–7),[66] synapsing with second-order neurons that either transmit or modulate the information received. Complex interactions among afferent fibers, local intrinsic spinal neurons, and the terminal fibers of descending tracts from higher levels[65] have the potential to alter the relation between the stimulus and the response to pain in the individual. Incoming messages may be attenuated or enhanced. Some of the primary afferents ascend or descend several segments in Lissauer's tract before terminating on neurons that project to higher centers, either directly, or via brain stem relay nuclei, to the thalamus and then on to the cortex, where the sensation of pain is perceived.[67]

Second-order dorsal horn neurons are classified into three main groups, based on location and response properties. The first group are the nociceptive-specific or high-threshold neurons; they are found in superficial laminae and demonstrate a selective response to noxious stimuli.[68] The second group, located in deeper laminae, and termed wide dynamic range (WDR) neurons, responds to a range of noxious and non-noxious stimuli.[67] For example, a tactile stimulus at a non-noxious level would not normally activate a WDR neuron. However, when sensitized, these neurons are hyperresponsive to touch; the stimulus is perceived as painful (allodynia) when the activity of the WDR neuron exceeds threshold.[69] A third class of neurons consists of excitatory and inhibitory interneurons within the spinal cord; they enhance or diminish responsiveness to sensory input from the periphery.[70]

Pharmacologic studies have been important in identifying the many neurotransmitters and neuromodulators that are involved in pain mechanisms in the dorsal horn.[71, 72] These substances, derived from stimulation of myelinated and unmyelinated primary afferent fibers, intrinsic interneurons, and descending fibers, include peptides, such as substance P, neurokinin A and CGRP, and the EAAs, glutamate and aspartate. Both the peptide and amino acid groups fulfil functions in nociceptive transmission in the dorsal horn,[73] acting selectively at a variety of receptor types located presynaptically and postsynaptically at the termination of primary nociceptive afferents.[71] Glutamate elicits fast synaptic responses in second-order neurons that are mediated by at least two EAA receptor subtypes, the AMPA and the NMDA receptors[32] (see next paragraph).

The dorsal horn has been found to contain high concentrations of a large variety of receptors. These receptors tend to congregate in lamina II, which is a

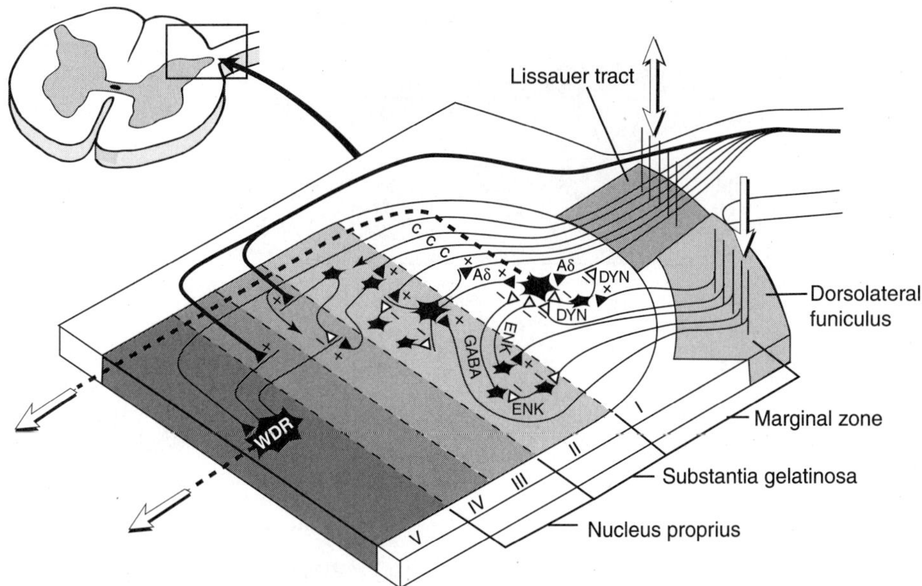

Figure 1–7. Diagrammatic representation of primary afferent nociceptor inputs and connections within the dorsal horn of the spinal cord. Large- and small-diameter primary afferent neurons have their cell bodies in the dorsal root ganglia. On entry to the dorsal horn, large-diameter afferent fibers *(thick solid line)* travel medially and small-diameter afferent fibers *(thin solid lines marked Aδ and C)* travel in the lateral portion of the entry zone. The spinal terminals of the small fibers enter the cord and have collateral branches, which may ascend and descend the spinal cord for several segments, in Lissauer's tract, before synapsing in the dorsal horn. Aδ fiber afferents terminate in lamina I (marginal zone) and C fiber afferents terminate in lamina II (substantia gelatinosa). Local interneurons may produce synaptic inhibition of small-diameter afferents and postsynaptic inhibition of projection neurons. Interneurons may have an excitatory action. Modulation also occurs as a result of descending influences arising from fibers in the dorsolateral funiculus. These descending fibers make contact with either projection neurons or interneurons. Neurotransmitters released from interneurons include γ-aminobutyric acid (GABA), enkephalin (ENK), and dynorphin (DYN). WDR, wide dynamic range neuron. (From Siddall PJ, Cousins MJ: Introduction to pain mechanisms: implications for neural blockade. *In* Cousins MJ, Bridenbaugh PO (eds): Neural Blockade in Clinical Anesthesia and Management of Pain, 3rd ed. Philadelphia: Lippincott-Raven; 1998:686.)

major receiving center for fine, presumably nociceptive, somatosensory input.[72] Dorsal horn receptor organization is remarkably plastic, and many of these receptors undergo rapid reorganization in response to various stimuli or pathologic situations. The receptor types found in the dorsal horn include (1) the excitatory amino acid (EAA) receptors (the ionotropic glutamate receptors: *N*-methyl-D-aspartate [NMDA], (±)-α-amino-3-hydroxy-5-methylisoxazole-4-propionic acid [AMPA], and kainate [the latter two being referred to as non-NMDA receptors], and the metabotropic glutamate receptors); (2) the inhibitory amino acid receptors (γ-aminobutyric acid [GABA] and glycine); (3) the peptide receptors (opioid [μ, δ, and κ], neurokinin, CGRP); (4) the biogenic amine receptors (α-adrenergic, dopaminergic, serotonergic [5-HT]); and (5) the cholinergic receptors (nicotinic, muscarinic) (Fig. 1–8).[70, 72] Although the actions of the EAAs, glutamate and aspartate, are mediated via the NMDA and non-NMDA receptors, substance P and neurokinin A act at neurokinin receptors.[71, 74] A detailed discussion of dorsal horn receptor types and transmitters is not within the scope of this chapter, and the reader is referred to several comprehensive reviews.[34, 71, 72]

Several of these receptor types have been targets for investigation of new pain treatment options. The NMDA receptor has received particular attention. It appears that physiologic processing of sensory information is mediated by non-NMDA receptors, but their prolonged activation caused by the sustained release of EAAs may also result in sensitization of the NMDA receptor. NMDA receptor activation leads to a cascade of secondary events and intracellular changes resulting in increased nociceptive responsiveness.[75] Indeed, NMDA receptors appear to be involved in the development of mechanisms that contribute to the pathophysiologic changes present in chronic pain states; for example, "wind-up,"[76] facilitation, central sensitization,[77] changes in peripheral receptive fields, induction of oncogenes, and long-term potentiation.[78]

Nitric oxide (NO) has also been implicated in chronic pain mechanisms. The production of NO oc-

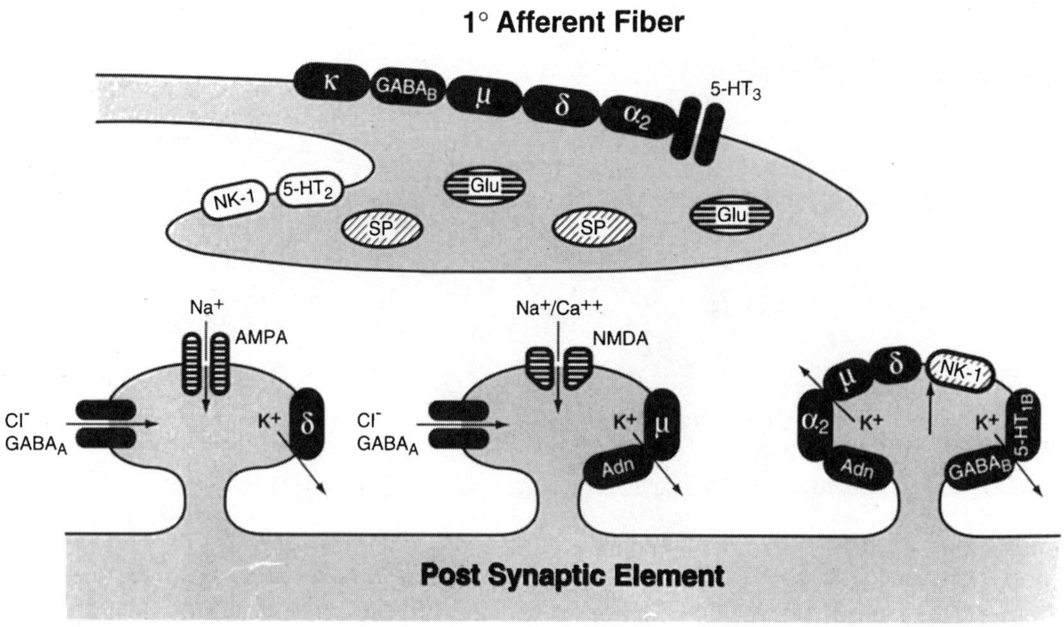

Figure 1–8 Possible arrangement of receptors on pre- and postsynaptic structures in the dorsal horn of the spinal cord. α_2, α_2-adrenergic receptor; Adn, adenosine; AMPA, (±)-α-amino-3-hydroxy-5-methylisoxazole-4-propionic acid; GABA, γ-aminobutyric acid; Glu, glutamate; 5-HT, 5-hydroxytryptamine (serotonin); κ, δ, μ, kappa, delta, mu opioid receptors respectively; NK-1, neurokinin-1; NMDA, *N*-methyl-D-aspartate; SP, substance P. (From Wilcox GL: Excitatory neurotransmitters and pain. *In* Bond MR, Charlton JE, Woolf CJ (eds): Proceedings of the VIth World Congress on Pain. Amsterdam: Elsevier; 1991: 99, as modified by Siddall PJ, Cousins MJ: Introduction to pain mechanisms: implications for neural blockade. *In* Cousins MJ, Bridenbaugh PO (eds): Neural Blockade in Clinical Anesthesia and Management of Pain, 3rd ed. Philadelphia: Lippincott-Raven; 1998:682.)

curs secondary to NMDA receptor activation and calcium ion (Ca^{2+}) influx (Fig. 1–9). In addition to its role in normal cell function, NO has been observed to play a role in nociceptive processing and may act to induce and maintain chronic pain states.[79]

Peripheral injury is associated with an increase in the excitability of neurons in the dorsal horn,[80] a phenomenon known as *central sensitization*.[30, 81–83] This produces allodynia and a zone of secondary hyperalgesia in uninjured tissue surrounding the site of injury. Central sensitization is generated by sustained primary C afferent fiber barrage[84, 85]; the morphologic and biochemical changes produced are expressed as alterations in the spatial extent, responsiveness, and threshold of the receptive fields of dorsal horn neurons.[86] The following changes in dorsal horn neurons occur: (1) expansion in receptive field size, such that a spinal neuron will respond to nociceptive stimuli that would normally be outside its responsive region; (2) increase in the magnitude and duration of the response to stimuli above threshold; and (3) reduction in threshold, such that non-noxious stimuli activate neurons that normally transmit nociceptive information.

Thus, it can be seen that in the presence of pain, the central nervous system is not hard-wired; rather, it is plastic. A simple stimulus-response relationship between nociceptive input and clinical pain does not exist; instead, wind-up of spinal cord neuron activity occurs, resulting in a progressive increase in dorsal horn neuron activity[87] and increased sensitivity to other input. These changes may be important both in acute pain states and in the development of chronic pain[71] and are thought to be mediated by the NMDA receptor.[77, 88] Attempts to modify pain must take these changes into account.

Nerve injury itself results in morphologic changes in the dorsal horn. For example, redistribution of the terminals of myelinated afferents occurs, with sprouting of these terminals from lamina III to lamina II (see Fig. 1–6).[89, 90] Aberrant communication between nerve terminals that usually transmit non-noxious information and neurons that usually receive nociceptive input may explain the symptom of allodynia.

Modulation at the Dorsal Horn Level

Modulation of afferent impulses arriving in the dorsal horn occurs via endogenous and exogenous agents acting on presynaptic and postsynaptic opioid, α-adrenergic, GABA, and glycine receptors (Fig. 1–10). Inhibition, limiting the effect of subsequent impulses, occurs via local inhibitory interneurons and descending pathways from the brain.

It is recognized that an analgesic effect can be produced by activation of spinal cord α-adrenergic

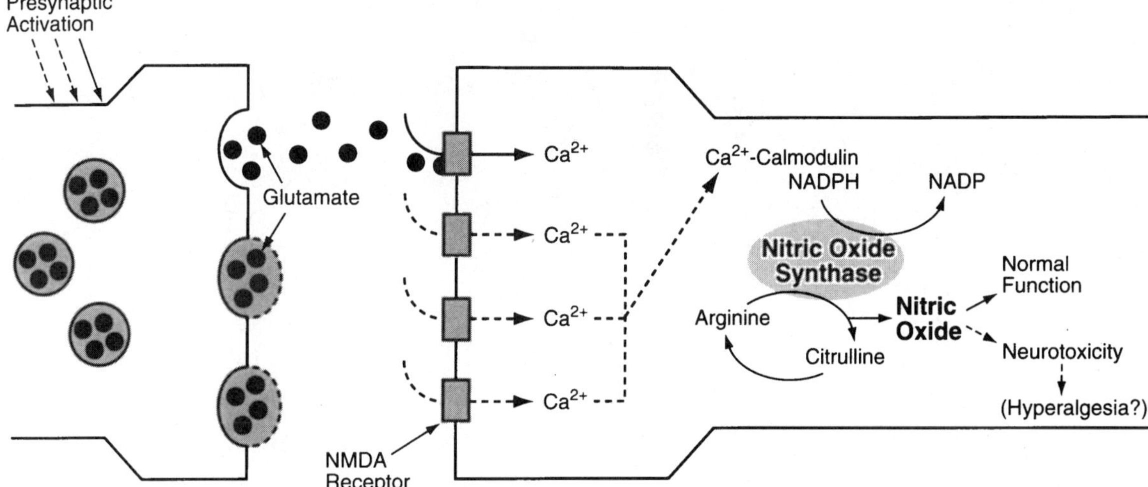

❖ **Figure 1–9** Diagram illustrating postsynaptic events following release of glutamate from central terminals of primary afferents in the spinal cord. Following priming of the *N*-methyl-D-aspartate (NMDA) receptor complex, subsequent glutamate release results in NMDA receptor activation with subsequent calcium influx. Intracellular calcium then acts on a calmodulin-sensitive site to activate the enzyme nitric oxide synthase (NOS). In the presence of the cofactor nicotinamide adenine dinucleotide phosphate, reduced form (NADPH), NOS uses arginine as a substrate to produce nitric oxide and citrulline. Nitric oxide has a role in normal cellular function but increased production may be involved in hyperalgesia and may lead to neurotoxicity. NADP, nicotinamide adenine dinucleotide phosphate. (From Siddall PJ, Cousins MJ: Introduction to pain mechanisms: implications for neural blockade. *In* Cousins MJ, Bridenbaugh PO (eds): Neural Blockade in Clinical Anesthesia and Management of Pain, 3rd ed. Philadelphia: Lippincott-Raven; 1998:683.)

receptors, either by endogenous release of norepinephrine (NE) by brain stem descending pathways, or by exogenous spinal administration of agents such as clonidine.[91] Painful stimulation has been shown to increase spinal cord NE in animals, and spinally released NE induces acetylcholine (ACh) release to cause analgesia.[92, 93] Intrathecal administration of the cholinergic agent neostigmine, a cholinesterase inhibitor, causes analgesia in humans.[94, 95] α-Adrenergic agonists exhibit a synergistic effect with opioids.[96]

Tonic inhibition of nociceptive input involves GABA and glycine. $GABA_A$ and $GABA_B$ receptor–mediated inhibition occurs through presynaptic and postsynaptic sites. $GABA_A$-active drugs have a powerful antinociceptive and antineuropathic effect when given spinally (e.g., midazolam). $GABA_B$ agonists (e.g., baclofen) produce analgesia in some animal studies, but evidence for analgesia in humans is thus far lacking.[97, 98]

Ascending Tracts

Nociceptive projection neurons in the spinal cord transmit information to a number of regions of the brain stem and diencephalon, including the thalamus, periaqueductal gray, parabrachial region, and bulbar reticular formation, as well as to limbic structures in the hypothalamus, amygdaloid nucleus, septal nucleus, and other sites[99] via several pathways, including the spinothalamic, spinoreticular, and spinomesencephalic tracts (Figs. 1–10 and 1–11). These ascend the spinal cord in the contralateral anterolateral quadrant. The spinocervicothalamic and postsynaptic dorsal column pathways are dorsal quadrant pathways.

In the thalamus, there are two main groups of relays. The region concerned with the sensory-discriminative component of pain is located in the ventrocaudal and ventroposterior nuclei, while that involved with the affective-motivational aspect of pain is found in the medial nuclei.[99] Neurons within the ventral posterolateral nucleus respond preferentially to noxious stimuli.[100] Positron emission tomography (PET) has been used to identify subcortical structures that may be involved in nociceptive transmission and pain perception, including the thalamus, putamen, caudate nucleus, hypothalamus, amygdala, periaqueductal gray, hippocampus, and cerebellum.

The role of the cortex in pain perception remains unclear. Recent evidence favors the participation of both the cerebral cortex and the thalamus, not only in the sensory-discriminative aspects of pain but also in the affective-motivational aspects.[101] Using the techniques of PET and functional magnetic resonance imaging, it has been determined that painful stimuli result in activation of sensory, motor, premotor, parietal, frontal, occipital, insular, and anterior cingulate regions of the cortex.[102–104] Sensory inputs may be analyzed, classified, and identified by premotor systems in terms of motor actions that are relevant to the input.[105] It has been postulated that evaluation of the temporal and spatial features of pain may occur in the parietal regions of the cortex, while the emotional response to pain occurs in the frontal cortex, including the anterior cingulate.[104] Evidence from experimental and clin-

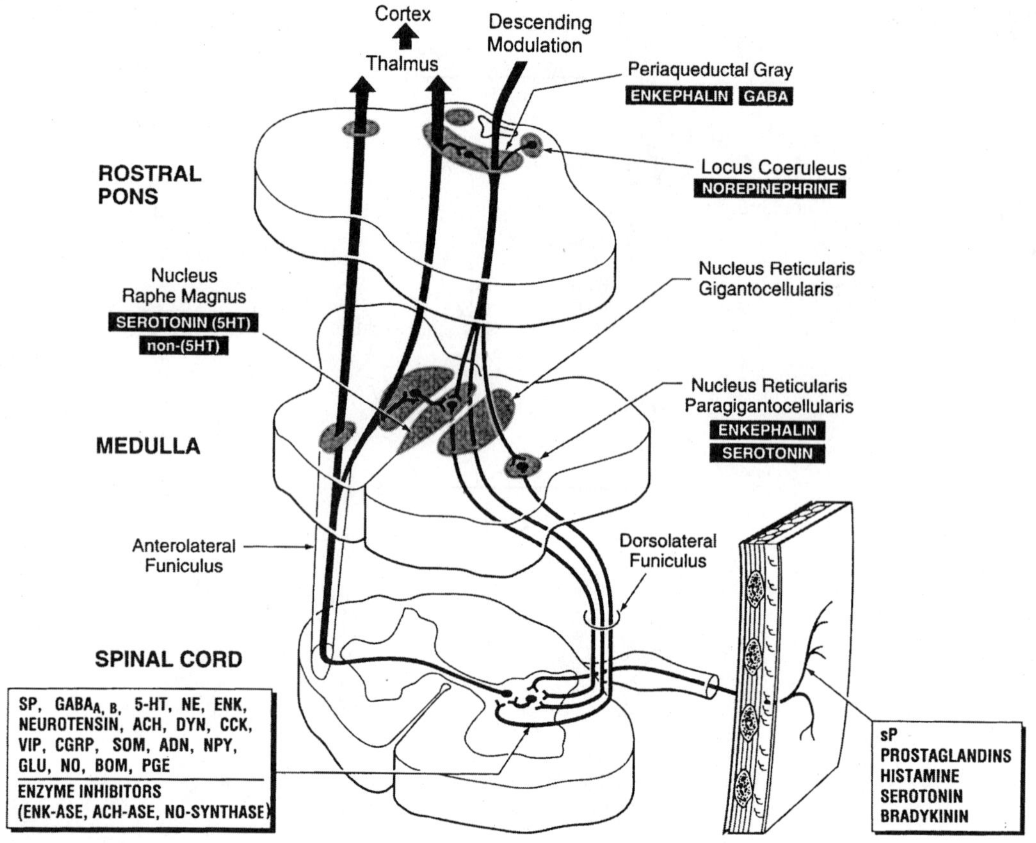

❖ **Figure 1–10** Simplified schema of afferent sensory pathways *(left)* and descending modulatory pathways *(right)*. Stimulation of nociceptors in the skin surface leads to impulse generation in the primary afferent. Concomitant with this impulse generation, increased levels of various endogenous algesic agents (substance P, prostaglandins, histamine, serotonin, bradykinin) are detected near the area of stimulation in the periphery. Primary afferent nociceptors relay to projection neurons in the dorsal horn, which ascend in the anterolateral funiculus to terminate in the thalamus. En route, collaterals of the projection neurons activate multiple higher centers, including the nucleus reticularis gigantocellularis (NRG). Neurons from the NRG project to the thalamus and also activate the nucleus raphe magnus (NRM) and periaqueductal gray (PAG) of the midbrain. Descending fibers from the PAG project to the NRM and reticular formation adjacent to the NRM. These neurons activate descending inhibitory neurons which are located in these regions and travel via the dorsolateral funiculus to terminate in the dorsal horn of the spinal cord. Descending projections also arise from a number of brain stem sites including the locus coeruleus (LC). A number of neurotransmitters are released by afferent fibers, descending terminations, or local interneurons in the dorsal horn and modulate peripheral nociceptive input. These include substance P (SP), γ-aminobutyric acid (GABA), serotonin (5-HT), norepinephrine (NE), enkephalin (ENK), neurotensin, acetylcholine (ACh), dynorphin (DYN), cholecystokinin (CCK), vasoactive intestinal peptide (VIP), calcitonin gene-related peptide (CGRP), somatostatin (SOM), adenosine (Adn), neuropeptide Y (NPY), glutamate (Glu), nitric oxide (NO), bombesin (BOM), and prostaglandins (PGE). Inhibitors of enzymes such as enkephalinase (ENK-ASE), acetylcholinesterase (ACh-ASE) and nitric oxide synthase (NO-SYNTHASE) may act to modify the action of these neurotransmitters. (From Siddall PJ, Cousins MJ: Introduction to pain mechanisms: implications for neural blockade. *In* Cousins MJ, Bridenbaugh PO (eds): Neural Blockade in Clinical Anesthesia and Management of Pain, 3rd ed. Philadelphia: Lippincott-Raven; 1998:687.)

ical studies clearly shows that the basal ganglia (i.e., the striatum, globus pallidus, and substantia nigra) are also involved in nociceptive sensorimotor integration.[106]

Descending Modulatory Pathways

The notion of a descending control system has appeared relatively recently. Not until the late 1960s was it realized that pain sensation is subject not only to modulation during its ascending transmission from the periphery to the cortex, but also to segmental modulation and descending control from higher centers.[107] Our knowledge of the descending endogenous analgesia system is still very incomplete; however, it is recognized that powerful inhibitory descending influences act on nociceptive transmission at many levels of the neuraxis. These inhibitory influences are manifested

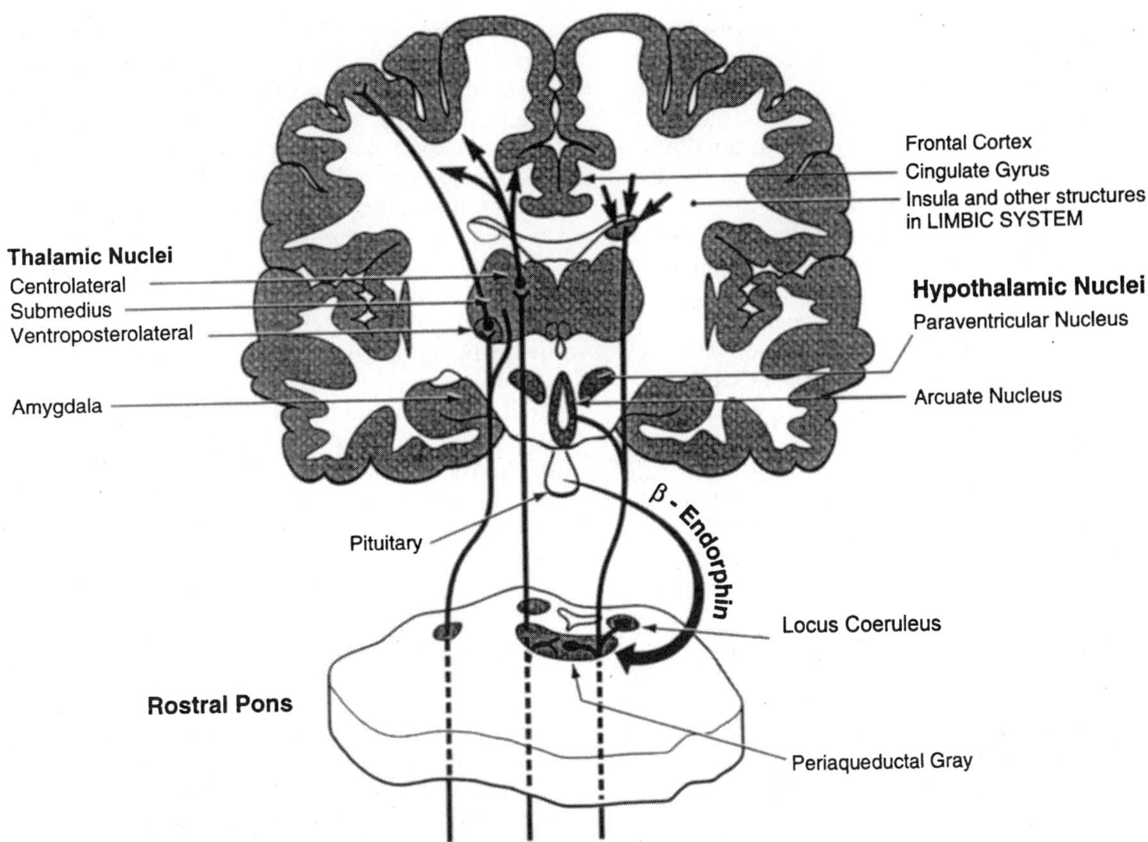

❖ **Figure 1–11** Rostral projections of nociceptive processing. Ascending projections *(left)* traveling in the anterolateral funiculus, as well as projections from the medulla, pons, and midbrain, terminate in the thalamic nuclear complex. The ventroposterolateral (VPL), centrolateral, and submedian nuclei receive nociceptive information. The VPL nucleus projects to the somatosensory cortex. The centromedian nucleus projects more diffusely, including projections to regions of the limbic system. The descending fibers *(right)* inhibit the transmission of nociceptive information between primary afferents and projection neurons in the dorsal horn. The periaqueductal gray (PAG) receives projections from a number of brain regions including the amygdala, frontal and insular cortex, and the hypothalamus. In addition to direct neural connections, endorphins synthesized in the pituitary are released into the cerebrospinal fluid and blood, where they can exert an inhibitory effect at multiple centers including the PAG. (From Siddall PJ, Cousins MJ: Introduction to pain mechanisms: implications for neural blockade. *In* Cousins MJ, Bridenbaugh PO (eds): Neural Blockade in Clinical Anesthesia and Management of Pain, 3rd ed. Philadelphia: Lippincott-Raven; 1998:689.)

via pathways that originate from several of the supraspinal structures, including the cerebral cortex, thalamus, and brain stem (the periaqueductal gray [PAG], raphe nuclei, and locus coeruleus–subcoeruleus complex [LC/SC]) (see Figs. 1–10 and 1–11).[107] These descending pathways have been shown to use several different neurotransmitters, the main ones being NE, serotonin (5-HT), GABA, and the endogenous opioid peptides.

Although 5-HT was initially thought to be the major transmitter mediating inhibitory control at spinal levels, it is clear from more recent work that NE also plays an important part. It is now recognized that both NE and adenosine are endogenous mediators of the antinociceptive action of 5-HT within the dorsal horn of the spinal cord.[108] Opioids and GABA are also involved in descending control at both brain stem and spinal levels, although the relative roles of the different types of opioid and amino acid receptors are unknown. The precise connections and cord synaptology are the basis of ongoing research.[107]

Periaqueductal Gray. The PAG was the first region in the brain where electrical stimulation could be shown to evoke a degree of hypoalgesia adequate for surgical intervention.[109] Since then, much progress has been made in elaborating and understanding topography and pathways of endogenous antinociceptive systems.[110] In the past, most investigations were carried out by means of traumatic lesions and/or reversible local anesthetic blocks of selected brain stem nuclei or fiber tracts; however, current techniques use proto-oncogene *c-Fos* protein expression as a marker of activated neurons.[111]

The PAG is believed to be involved in complex behavioral responses to stressful or life-threatening situations and to promote recuperative behavior after a defense reaction.[101] These behaviors are mediated by activation of complex ascending and descending projections of the PAG.[112, 113] The analgesia that is observed following stimulation of the midbrain PAG is thought to be due to the inhibitory action of the PAG on nociceptive dorsal horn neurons.[101]

One of the key structures in the descending analgesia pathway from the PAG is the nucleus raphe magnus (NRM). It is believed that the antinociceptive effects of stimulation in the PAG are mediated by the NRM. Neurotransmitters involved in the PAG-NRM pathway include endogenous opioids, 5-HT, and NE.[101]

Visceral Pain

Acute and chronic pain may arise from cutaneous, deep somatic, or visceral structures. It is recognized that cutaneous/somatic and visceral pain mechanisms are different; thus, it is not surprising that the nature of pain arising from these two types of tissues exhibits marked differences (Table 1–1).[114] There are several possible reasons for this. Visceral structures have a much less dense innervation, less than 1% of that found in skin.[114] This is likely to account for a certain amount of imprecision of perceived sensations. Moreover, these two tissues possess very different physical properties, affecting the encoding properties of sensory fibers,[115] are exposed to very different types of stimuli, and participate in different behavioral repertoires.

Despite the clinical significance of visceral pain, very little is known about visceral pain mechanisms. Visceral pain is poorly understood, in comparison with various forms of somatic pain.[116, 117]

Visceral nociceptive fibers travel to the spinal cord via the sympathetic chain; however, these are not "sympathetic" fibers, since they do not synapse in sympathetic ganglia and their cell bodies are in the dorsal root ganglion. Convergence of visceral and somatic nociceptive afferents on the same dorsal horn neuron occurs; this may partially explain the concept of "referred pain" (Fig. 1–12). Visceral noxious stimuli are then conveyed, along with somatic noxious stimuli, to the brain along spinothalamic pathways. Although the view has long been held that the dorsal columns of the spinal cord subserve graphesthesia, two-point discrimination, and position sense, recently, the existence of a visceral nociceptive pathway in the dorsal columns involving the postsynaptic dorsal column pathway has been demonstrated.[101, 118–120] Pelvic visceral pain in rats has been shown to be transmitted along a pathway involving neurons of the postsynaptic dorsal column pathway at the L6 to S1 segmental level, axons of these neurons in the fasciculus gracilis, and neurons of the nucleus gracilis and the ventral posterolateral nucleus of the thalamus.[120]

Visceral pain is dull, vague, and very poorly localized because peripheral visceral afferents branch considerably, causing much overlap at the dorsal roots; visceral afferents converge on the dorsal horn over a wide number of segments, and are few in number compared with somatic nociceptor fibers.

Visceral nociceptors are known to respond to injury; peripheral sensitization may occur with visceral pain. Visceral nociceptors can also become sensitized to non-noxious stimuli during the inflammatory process that follows intense noxious stimulation, increasing the excitability of central nociceptive systems and leading to central sensitization.[117]

MECHANISMS OF THE PAIN OF PARTURITION

An understanding of the mechanisms of pain transmission during parturition and the many factors that influence pain intensity, duration, distribution, and quality is essential if optimal labor analgesia is to be provided. Most of these factors vary as labor progresses; thus, the stages of labor are considered separately.

Table 1–1 VISCERAL PAIN COMPARED WITH SOMATIC PAIN

	SOMATIC	VISCERAL
Site	Well-localized	Poorly localized
Radiation	May follow distribution of somatic nerve	Diffuse
Character	Sharp and definite	Dull and vague (may be colicky, cramping, squeezing)
Relation to stimulus	Hurts where the stimulus is; associated with external factors	May be "referred" to another area; associated with internal factors
Temporal quality	Often constant (sometimes periodic)	Often periodic and builds to peaks (sometimes constant)
Associated symptoms	Nausea usually only with deep somatic pain owing to bone involvement	Often nausea, vomiting, sickening feeling

From Siddall PJ, Cousins MJ: Introduction to pain mechanisms: implications for neural blockade. *In* Cousins MJ, Bridenbaugh PO (eds): Neural Blockade in Clinical Anesthesia and Management of Pain, 3rd ed. Philadelphia: Lippincott-Raven; 1998:690.

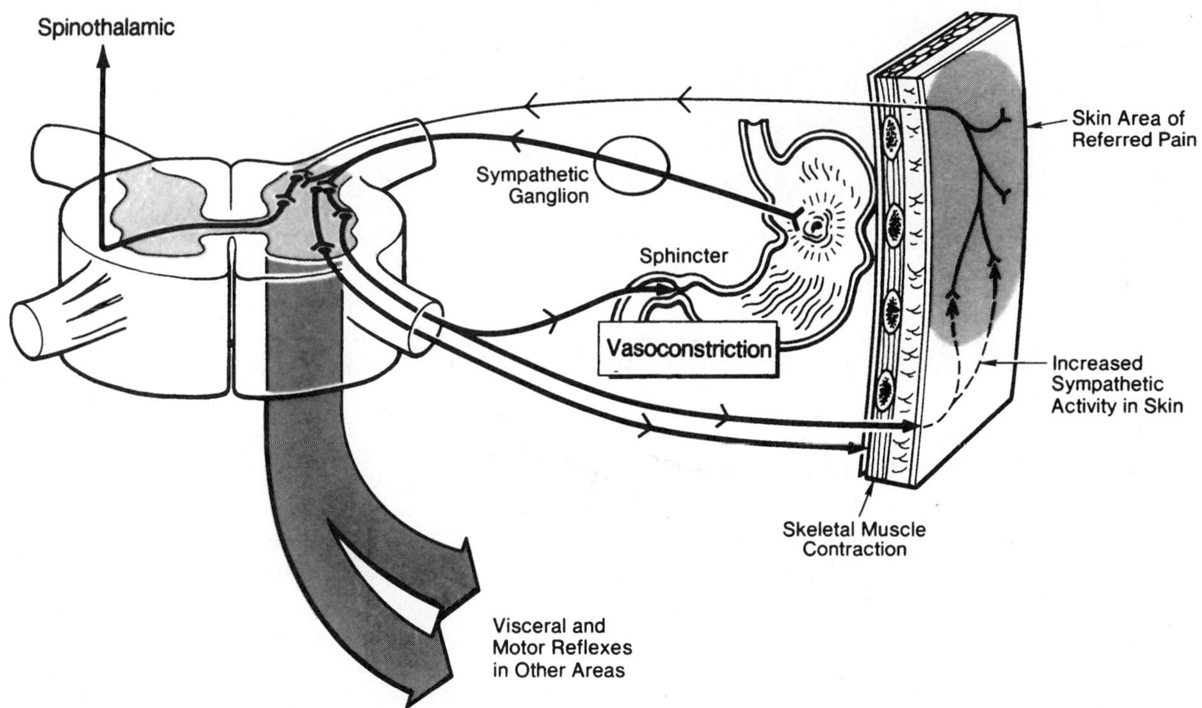

❖ **Figure 1–12** Visceral pain: The convergence of visceral and somatic nociceptive afferents. Visceral nociceptive afferents converge on the same dorsal horn neuron as somatic nociceptive afferents. Visceral noxious stimuli are then conveyed, together with somatic noxious stimuli, by means of the spinothalamic pathways to the brain. Note the following: (1) Referred pain is felt in the cutaneous area corresponding to the dorsal horn neurons on which visceral afferents converge. This is accompanied by allodynia and hyperalgesia in this skin area. (2) Reflex somatic motor activity results in muscle spasm, which may stimulate parietal peritoneum and initiate somatic noxious input to the dorsal horn. (3) Reflex sympathetic efferent activity may result in spasm of sphincters of viscera over a wide area, causing pain remote from the original stimulus. (4) Reflex sympathetic efferent activity may result in visceral ischemia and further noxious stimulation. Also, visceral nociceptors may be sensitized by norepinephrine release and microcirculatory changes. (5) Increased sympathetic activity may influence cutaneous nociceptors, which may be at least partly responsible for referred pain. (6) Peripheral visceral afferents branch considerably, causing much overlap in the territory of individual dorsal roots. Only a small number of visceral afferent fibers converge on dorsal horn neurons compared with somatic nociceptive fibers. Also, visceral afferents converge on the dorsal horn over a wide number of segments. Thus, dull, vague, visceral pain is very poorly localized. This is often called deep visceral pain. (From Siddall PJ, Cousins MJ: Introduction to pain mechanisms: implications for neural blockade. *In* Cousins MJ, Bridenbaugh PO (eds): Neural Blockade in Clinical Anesthesia and Management of Pain, 3rd ed. Philadelphia: Lippincott-Raven; 1998:691.)

First Stage of Labor

Pain during the first stage of labor arises from the uterus and adnexae during contractions, and is visceral in nature. A number of possible mechanisms to explain the origin of uterine nociception have been proposed, but the current view is that pain is largely the result of dilatation of the cervix and lower uterine segment, and their subsequent mechanical distention, stretching, and tearing during contractions.[121, 122] Pain intensity is related to the strength of the contraction and the pressure thus generated.[123] Isometric contractions of the uterus against the obstruction presented by the cervix and perineum probably also contribute to pain.[17] It has also been suggested that several chemical nociceptive mediators contribute to pain, including bradykinin, leukotrienes, prostaglandins, serotonin, lactic acid, and substance P.[123]

Evidence in support of the current hypothesis of uterine nociception origin is based on the following observations; these have been reviewed in detail by Bonica[17]:

1. Visceral pain can be stimulated by stretching the smooth muscle of a hollow viscus.[124, 125]
2. Rapidity of dilatation of the cervix and lower uterine segment is correlated with pain intensity.[122]
3. Time of onset of uterine contractions is related to time of onset of pain (Fig. 1–13).[17] The observed lag time between the two reflects the time needed for a contraction to generate an increase in amniotic fluid pressure to 15 mm Hg above baseline; this is the minimum pressure required to initiate dilatation of the cervix and lower uterine

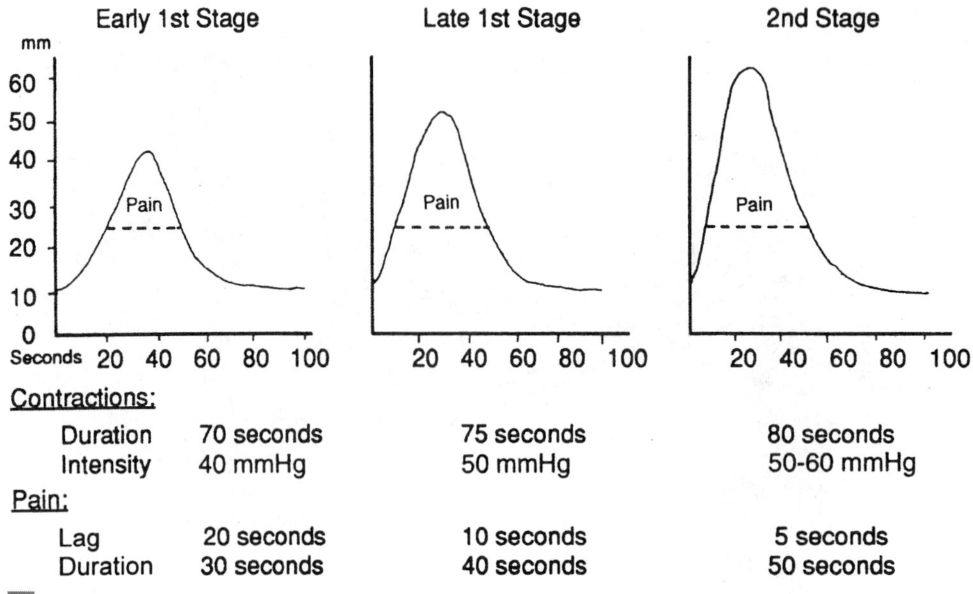

Figure 1-13 Relation between duration of uterine contraction and duration of pain associated with the contraction. Because intensity of contraction must reach 25 mm Hg before pain is evoked, there is a lag of 20 sec during the early phase of the first stage of labor when the buildup of the contraction is slower. As labor progresses, the contraction reaches its peak more rapidly and the lag is shortened. (From Bonica JJ: Principles and Practice of Obstetric Analgesia and Anesthesia. Philadelphia: FA Davis; 1967:104, as modified by Bonica JJ: The nature of pain in parturition. *In* Van Zundert A, Ostheimer GW (eds): Pain Relief and Anesthesia in Obstetrics. New York: Churchill Livingstone; 1996:34.)

segment.[126] Typically, intrauterine pressure must exceed 25 mm Hg before pain is experienced. During early labor, less than 45% of the contraction time is associated with pain, whereas during late first stage, 60% of the contraction time is associated with pain.

4. The unanesthetized uterus can be incised and gently palpated without discomfort to the patient undergoing cesarean delivery under abdominal field block,[121, 127] whereas forceful palpation and stretching of the cervix and lower uterine segment under the same conditions produce pain similar in quality and location to that occurring during labor.[126]
5. Sudden dilatation of the cervix during a gynecologic procedure causes pain similar to that of uterine contractions.[121, 127, 128]

Contractions of the body of the uterus also contribute to labor pain. However, it is interesting to note that Braxton-Hicks contractions are often painless, even though they can attain the intensity of contractions during labor. Similarly, postpartum uterine contractions are of a magnitude two to three times those of active labor, but are associated with much less intense pain. During labor, when the cervix dilates very slowly, or when an abnormal fetal position creates mechanical distortion, strong contractions are associated with very severe labor pain. This is presumably because the uterus is contracting isometrically, against obstruction; these strong uterine contractions present a potent source of pain.[17]

Earlier theories to explain the origins of labor pain have been largely discounted. These are as follows:

1. Pressure on afferent nerve endings located between uterine muscle fibers.[129]
2. Ischemia of the myometrium and cervix caused by blood expulsion with contractions,[121] or by sympathetic hyperactivity causing vasoconstriction[5]; however, it has been shown that myometrial (as opposed to intervillous) blood flow actually increases during uterine contractions.[130]
3. Inflammation of uterine muscle fibers[129]; however, there is no evidence of this.
4. Hyperactivity of the sympathetic nervous system induced by fear, with subsequent contraction of the cervix and lower uterine segment.[5] Evidence in disagreement with this theory is that the cervix is made up of connective tissue, with little muscle[131] and very weak contractile force.[126]

Second Stage of Labor

During the second stage of labor, when the cervix is fully dilated, nociceptive stimulation continues from uterine body contractions and distention of the lower uterine segment. The pain caused by cervical dilatation decreases; however, the progressively increasing pressure of the fetal presenting part on pelvic structures gives rise to somatic pain, with stretching and tearing of fascia and subcutaneous tissues of the lower birth canal, distention of the perineum, and pressure on perineal skeletal muscle.[17] This pain is transmitted via the pudendal nerve, a somatic nerve derived from the S2, S3, and S4 sacral nerve roots. In contrast to the visceral pain of the first stage of labor, the somatic pain experienced during delivery is intense and sharply localized.

NEURAL PATHWAYS OF PARTURITIONAL PAIN

The visceral pain of uterine contractions is transmitted to the T10 through L1 segments of the spinal cord by A-delta and C visceral afferent fibers that originate in the lateral wall and fornices of the uterus.[123] For many years, it was believed that the sensory supply of the body of the uterus was transmitted through the T11 and T12 spinal segments, and that nociceptive impulses from the lower uterine segment and the cervix were transmitted through sensory fibers that accompany the pelvic nerves (nervi erigentes) to the S2, S3, and S4 spinal segments.[132] However, Bonica, in a series of elegant experiments involving 240 parturients and 35 gynecologic patients over a period of 22 years,[133, 134] using a variety of discrete nerve blocks (i.e., paravertebral, segmental epidural, caudal epidural, and transsacral) of various nociceptive pathways, demonstrated conclusively that the lower uterine segment and the upper part of the cervix are in fact supplied by afferents that supply the body of the uterus, and accompany the sympathetic nerves, and not by any of the sacral nerves. The sequence of afferent nociceptive transmission from the uterus and cervix to the spinal cord is through the uterine and cervical plexuses, then sequentially through the inferior hypogastric (pelvic) plexus, the middle hypogastric plexus or nerve, and the superior hypogastric and aortic plexuses. From here, the nociceptive afferents then pass to the lumbar sympathetic chain and travel cephalad to the lower thoracic sympathetic chain, which they leave via the white rami communicantes associated with the T10 through L1 spinal nerves.[17, 135] Finally, they course through the associated posterior nerve roots to synapse with interneurons within the dorsal horn of the spinal cord (Figs. 1–14 and 1–15). Parasympathetic innervation of the uterus does not appear to have a role in uterocervical pain mediation.[122]

As mentioned previously, somatic pain results from distention of the pelvic floor, vagina, and perineum. Painful impulses are transmitted primarily through the pudendal nerve, which is derived from the anterior primary divisions of sacral nerves S2 to S4. In addition to innervating the vagina, the vulva, and the perineum, the pudendal nerve supplies motor fibers to various skeletal muscles of the pelvic floor and perineum.[136] The ilioinguinal nerve and the genital branch of the genitofemoral nerve provide peripheral innervation of the perineum anteriorly; the posterior femoral cutaneous nerve supplies lateral innervation.[136]

Berkley and colleagues,[137, 138] in a series of investigations, verified that nociceptive information from the uterus is transmitted via afferent fibers in the hypogastric nerves, whereas information concerning physiologic events involved in reproductive function is conveyed via afferent fibers of the pelvic nerve. It is likely that these two different types of nerve fibers are somehow coordinated during lifetime reproductive events.[137, 138]

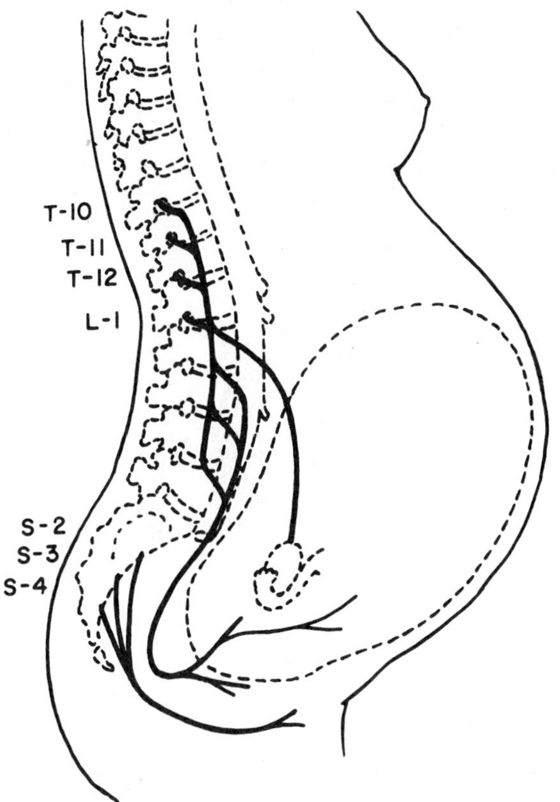

❖ **Figure 1–14** Schematic of the peripheral nociceptive pathways involved in the pain of childbirth. Note that the uterus, including the cervix, is supplied by sensory fibers that are associated with the sympathetic nerves supplied to the uterus. The course of the nociceptive fibers starting from the nerve endings in the uterus and cervix to the spinal cord pass through the uterine and cervical plexuses and then sequentially through the pelvic (inferior hypogastric) plexus, the middle hypogastric plexus or nerve, and the superior hypogastric plexus; from this structure they pass to the lumbar sympathetic chain through two major nerves that lie posterior to the common iliac arteries and also through lumbar splanchnic nerves. From the lumbar sympathetic chain they proceed cephalad through the lower thoracic chain and then leave it by coursing through the white rami communicates connected with T10, T11, T12, and L1 spinal nerves, and finally course through these nerves and their posterior roots to enter the spinal cord and make contact with dorsal horn neurons. Nociceptive fibers from the perineal structures course through the pudendal nerve and into the spinal cord through the posterior roots of S2, S3, and S4 spinal nerves. In addition, the lower lumbar and upper sacral segments supply nerves to pelvic structures that become involved in the pain of parturition. (From Bonica JJ: Labour pain. *In* Wall PD, Melzack R (eds): Textbook of Pain, 3rd ed. Edinburgh: Churchill Livingstone; 1994:619.)

Following transmission of nociceptive information from the uterus, cervix, and perineum to the dorsal horn, as with other acute pain states, this information is then relayed to other parts of the spinal cord, and

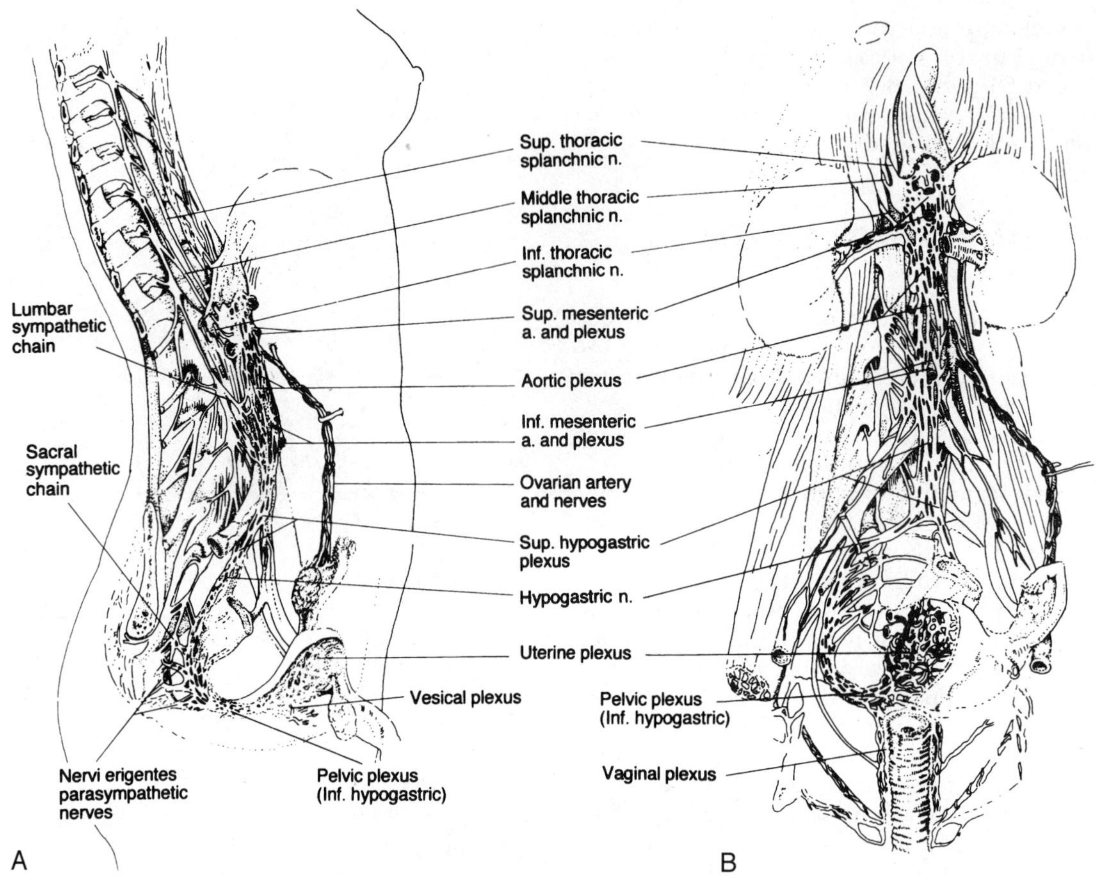

Figure 1–15 Gross anatomy of the nerve supply to the uterus. *A*, Lateral view; *B*, Anterior view. The uterus is shown in the nonpregnant state to permit the various nerves that supply it to be depicted. Note that the uterine and cervical plexuses are derived from the pelvic plexus, which contains parasympathetic and sympathetic efferents. The parasympathetic efferents have their cell bodies in the middle three sacral segments, and the parasympathetic afferents pass through these segments and progress cephalad through the neuraxis. The sympathetic efferents and afferents pass through the hypogastric nerve, which in turn is a continuation of the superior hypogastric and aortic plexuses. Note that fibers from the last two plexuses pass on to the lumbar sympathetic chain, the afferents of which mediate nociceptive impulses and accompany the sympathetic fibers through these structures. From the lumbar and lower thoracic sympathetic chain the nociceptive afferents pass to the T10, T11, T12, and L1 spinal nerves and reach the spinal cord via the posterior roots and rootlets. (From Bonica JJ: Principles and Practice of Obstetric Analgesia and Anesthesia. Philadelphia: FA Davis; 1967:110–111, as modified by Bonica JJ: The nature of pain in parturition. *In* Van Zundert A, Ostheimer GW (eds): Pain Relief and Anesthesia in Obstetrics. New York: Churchill Livingstone; 1996:40.)

then via the spinothalamic and other ascending pathways to the limbic system and higher centers of the brain,[17] where the multidimensional response to pain (i.e., sensory, affective, and evaluative dimensions), is determined. As mentioned previously (see Visceral Pain), the existence of a visceral nociceptive pathway in the dorsal columns has recently been verified.[101, 118–120]

It must be reemphasized here that the tissue damage sustained in the cervix and perineum during labor and delivery causes the responses to injury as described earlier under Acute and Chronic Pain Mechanisms. Severe pain, even when associated with a physiologic process such as parturition, has deleterious consequences if allowed to persist. Recent research into pain mechanisms has shown that the persistent pain and associated reflex responses that occur as a result of tissue injury can become maladaptive, leading to a variety of complications and abnormal states. As well as having the potential for physical injury, childbirth can be psychologically traumatic. Unrelieved pain may lead to long-standing psychologic and emotional problems.[123] Several cases of severe depression, anxiety, obsessive-compulsive behavior, phobic symptoms, and sexual problems following attempted "natural" childbirth have been reported.[139] There is also evidence to suggest that in some of these women, a variant of post-traumatic stress disorder may occur.[140, 141]

CLINICAL CHARACTERISTICS OF LABOR AND DELIVERY PAIN

The clinical characteristics of uterine contraction pain (i.e., first-stage labor pain) are distinct from those associated with delivery pain (i.e., second-stage labor

Table 1-2 CLINICAL CHARACTERISTICS OF LABOR PAIN

CONTRACTION PAIN	DELIVERY PAIN
Visceral	Somatic
Diffuse, poorly localized	Well localized, may follow distribution of somatic nerves
Dull, vague (may be colicky, cramping, squeezing)	Sharp, definite
Frequently referred; associated with internal factors	Not referred; associated with external factors
Delayed transmission	Rapid transmission
Related to intrauterine pressure	Related to perineal distention
Variable in intensity, often periodic, builds to peaks	Often constant, accompanied by urge to bear down
Often associated nausea, vomiting, sickening feeling	Nausea only with deep somatic pain
Evokes generalized autonomic response	Evokes circulatory changes secondary to intermittent Valsalva maneuvers
Very susceptible to central neural blockade	Less susceptible to central neural blockade

Modified from Brownridge P: The nature and consequences of childbirth pain. Eur J Obstet Gynecol Reprod Biol Suppl 1995;59:S10 with permission from Elsevier Science; and Siddall PJ, Cousins MJ: Introduction to pain mechanisms: implications for neural blockade. *In* Cousins MJ, Bridenbaugh PO (eds): Neural Blockade in Clinical Anesthesia and Management of Pain, 3rd ed. Philadelphia: Lippincott-Raven; 1998:690.

pain), suggesting use of distinct neural pathways (Table 1–2).

As described previously under Visceral Pain, peripheral visceral afferents branch considerably, overlap at the dorsal roots, and converge on the dorsal horn over a wide number of segments. They are also much fewer in number compared with somatic nociceptor fibers. These features explain why visceral pain is described clinically as being dull, vague, and very poorly localized. The concept of "referred pain," very often present during labor, may be explained in part by the convergence of visceral and somatic nociceptive afferents on the same dorsal horn neuron (see Fig. 1–12). The area of referral is generally segmental and superficial, that is, to muscle or skin, or both, innervated by the same spinal nerves as the affected viscus.[114] An important feature of referred pain is that the site of referral may additionally show hyperalgesia.[142] This is true for pain referred both to muscle and to skin. Central sensitization appears to be of major importance in hyperalgesia from somatic and visceral structures.[114, 117]

Thus, as expected, the visceral pain of uterine contractions has a delayed transmission, is diffuse in nature and poorly localized, and is commonly referred to the abdomen, lower back, and rectum—areas that correspond to the dermatomes supplied by the same spinal cord segments that receive nociceptive input from the uterus and cervix. Aching, cramping pain during the latent phase of labor is referred and limited to the T11 and T12 dermatomes (Fig. 1–16*A*). It becomes more severe in the active phase of the first stage of labor (cervix dilated 3–4 cm) with increasing intensity of uterine contractions, spreading to involve the T10 and L1 dermatomes (Fig. 1–16*B*) and becoming sharp and cramping in nature. Often, the pain is not referred to the entire dermatome but may be more severe in one or more areas within one or more dermatomes. Hyperalgesia is present in the entire extent of the involved dermatomes.

Low back pain is the result of nociceptive transmission in the T10 to L1 segments. Severe lumbar low back pain occurs in approximately 30% of women during the first stage of labor and appears to be associated with a history of menstrual pain (see under Other Factors, next).[143] The low back pain is probably the result of referred pain via the dorsal rami of nerve roots T10 to L1, the lateral branches of which travel caudally before becoming superficial and supplying the skin over the lower back and posterior pelvic rim.[123]

Descent of the fetal presenting part during the late first stage and second stage of labor produces sharp, well-localized somatic pain in the region innervated by the pudendal nerve, consistent with pain caused by stimulation of superficial somatic structures. Pain is perceived most acutely in the lower part of the sacrum, the perineum, vagina, rectum, and thighs (L2 to S1 spinal cord segments). Pressure on, and traction of, pain-sensitive structures in the pelvic cavity, including pressure on nerve roots of the lumbosacral plexus; stretching of ligaments, fascia, and muscles; traction on pelvic parietal peritoneum and uterine ligaments; and tension of the bladder, urethra, and rectum may be referred to the lower lumbar and sacral segments (see Fig. 1–16*A*); this mild pain may become moderate or severe (Fig. 1–16*C* and *D*) if there is undue pressure from the fetal presenting part.

OTHER FACTORS THAT INFLUENCE THE PAIN OF CHILDBIRTH

There is no doubt that labor pain is one of the most intense pains experienced, but the perception of pain varies strikingly between individuals—some women have extremely severe pain while others have almost none.[144–147] Apart from the expected influence of such factors as the intensity, duration, quality, and pattern of contractions on the amount of pain associated with labor and delivery, there are many other factors that are known to contribute to pain, albeit to varying degrees. These include physical, psychologic, emotional and motivational, ethnocultural, and neurohumoral factors[16, 145, 148–157] (Table 1–3), and they determine the incidence, intensity, duration, and quality of pain experienced by the individual woman during childbirth.

Physical Determinants

Factors identified as influencing the degree of labor pain experienced by the parturient include her age,

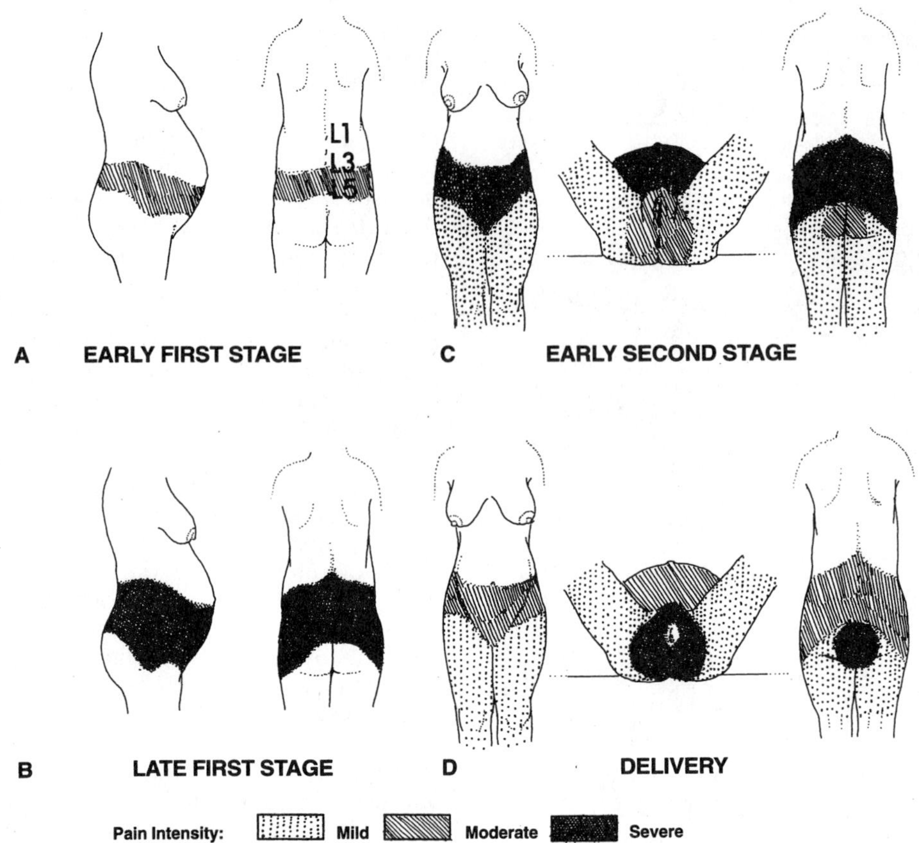

❖ **Figure 1–16** The intensity and distribution of parturition pain during the various phases of labor and delivery. *A,* In the early first stage, pain is referred to the T11 and T12 dermatomes. *B,* In the late first stage, however, the severe pain is also referred to the T10 and L1 dermatomes. *C,* In the early second stage, uterine contractions remain intense and produce severe pain in the T10 to L1 dermatomes. At the same time the presenting part exerts pressure on pelvic structures and thus causes moderate pain in the very low back and perineum and often produces mild pain in the thighs and legs. *D,* Intensity and distribution of pain during the later phase of the second stage and during actual delivery. The perineal component is the primary cause of pain, whereas uterine contractions produce moderate pain. (From Bonica JJ: Obstetric Analgesia and Anesthesia. World Federation of Societies of Anaesthesiologists. Seattle: University of Washington Press; 1980:46–47, as modified by Bonica JJ: The nature of pain in parturition. *In* Van Zundert A, Ostheimer GW (eds): Pain Relief and Anesthesia in Obstetrics. New York: Churchill Livingstone; 1996:41.)

Table 1–3 SUMMARY OF SOME OF THE FACTORS THAT MAY INFLUENCE THE PAIN OF CHILDBIRTH

PHYSICAL	PSYCHOLOGIC AND ETHNOCULTURAL	PROPOSED NEUROHUMORAL MECHANISMS
Age and parity	Attitude toward labor	Endogenous opioids
Physical condition	Fear and anxiety	Hormones
Size of infant/birth canal	Expectations of pain	Placental ± amniotic fluid substance
Abnormal fetal presentation	Prior experience of pain	Substance P
Stage of labor	Knowledge of childbirth	Nociceptin/ORL-1 receptor system
Speed and degree of cervical dilatation	Environment and support	Spinal cord noradrenergic-cholinergic system
Frequency of contractions	Confidence to cope with labor	
Maternal position in labor	Education and social class	
Menstrual history	Culture and beliefs	

ORL-1, opioid receptor–like-1 receptor.

parity, and physical condition, and the size of the infant in relation to the size of the birth canal.[17] Some studies have reported a negative incidence between age and pain, with younger women having more severe labor pain.[145, 152, 158] A large prospective study of more than 335,000 women found the highest frequency of epidural block among the youngest and the oldest of both nulliparous and parous women, implying to some extent a greater analgesic requirement for higher levels of pain.[159] However, other studies have not found any association between age and pain in labor.[151, 160–162] Primiparae appear to suffer more pain than multiparous women[13, 16, 145, 152, 158, 163–165]; however, a few studies have reported no difference related to parity.[151, 160, 161, 166] Interestingly, a recent investigation[167] found that very severe labor pain is common even in very experienced parturients, with a significant number of grand multiparae in this study reporting that they had received insufficient analgesia. There appears to be a differential pattern of the progression of labor pain, with nulliparae reporting more pain during early and active labor, and less pain during the second stage, than multiparae.[13, 14, 16, 145, 147, 149]

Other physical variables, such as the speed and degree of cervical dilatation and the frequency of contractions, have also been associated with pain.[145, 158, 162] It follows that a short first stage of labor with a rapidly dilating cervix should therefore involve more pain than a longer first stage.[168] However, in contrast, some studies have reported that longer labor is associated with higher pain levels,[165, 166] and others found no association.[145, 148, 151, 169] When the reports of individual women are studied,[11] increases and decreases in pain levels may be seen throughout labor. The combined influence of cervical dilatation and contraction frequency may be partially responsible for the intense pain experienced by some women during transitional labor.[170]

The parturient experiences more pain when there is dystocia caused by a contracted pelvis, a large fetus, or an abnormal presentation.[17] Melzack and associates[145] found that pain scores increased the heavier the primipara was per unit of height. Also, heavier mothers and those with larger fetuses had higher pain scores, although this observation is likely to be a function of the degree of "fit" between the fetus and the maternal passage.[170] However, other studies[148, 165] did not confirm an association between infant weight and pain. Position during labor also appears to influence the amount of pain experienced. Some evidence suggests that women feel less pain when they labor and deliver in an upright position.[171]

A history of severe menstrual pain is associated with high pain scores in labor.[16, 145, 149, 152] It has been suggested that excessive prostaglandin production, which produces greater intensity of uterine contractions,[154] is the common mechanism during menses and labor.[11] Research findings[172] that support this explanation demonstrate that the actual intensity of labor contractions is more important in the perception of pain than contraction duration.

Parturients exhibit a decreased tolerance of labor pain and increased pain behavior when they are suffering from loss of sleep, general fatigue, or other medical conditions.[17]

Psychologic Considerations

The influence of a variety of psychologic factors on a woman's perception of pain during labor is well known. These factors include attitude toward labor, fear and anxiety, expectations of pain, prior experience of pain, and knowledge of the process of pregnancy and parturition.

Fear, apprehension, and anxiety are commonly associated with increased pain perception[1, 152, 169, 173, 174] and may modify the experience of labor pain through psychologic and physiologic mechanisms.[169, 175–177] Significant elements of labor-related anxiety are fears of pain and suffering, loss of control, abandonment, self-injury, death, or injury to the fetus.[1, 13, 152, 178] A frequent cause of fear and anxiety is lack of knowledge of, or misinformation about, the process of labor and delivery. During the first stage of labor, fear of pain has a high correlation with pain levels, whereas in the second stage of labor, concerns about pain shift to concerns regarding the potential for self-injury during birth and the neonate's well-being.[162, 179–181] Anxiety about the pain of labor has been found to be a strong predictor of negative experiences during labor, lack of satisfaction with the birth, and poor emotional well-being postnatally.[174]

Anxiety may be precipitated or enhanced during the course of labor through the actions of individuals surrounding the parturient or by environmental factors, such as noise or unfamiliarity.[170] Several investigators have found that a positive attitude of the expectant father toward the pregnancy and labor plays an important role in decreasing the laboring parturient's apprehension and pain.[148, 151, 152] In other studies, women who had a supportive companion during labor had significantly lower postpartum depression scores[182] and higher self-esteem on day 1 as well as 6 weeks after delivery.[183] In contrast, Melzack[11] reported that the presence of the partner during labor appeared to increase the amount of pain reported by the parturient. He postulated that this could be either because affective pain scores were genuinely higher, or because the woman was attempting to impress the partner or express anger at him by deliberately choosing certain pain descriptors.

Excessive anxiety tends to magnify the perception of nociceptive stimuli at the cortical level.[170] A study examining labor experience, maternal mood, and cortisol and catecholamine levels found that women who were distressed and required analgesia had higher cortisol levels.[184] Those who described a more positive labor experience at 24 hours also had higher cortisol levels, suggesting that cortisol might have an amnestic or euphoric effect. No significant correlations were found between psychologic test scores and stress hormone levels.

Some data[165] suggest that prior experience of nongynecologic pain may be associated with decreased pain during labor, by affording the opportunity of developing coping skills. However, for most nulliparae, childbirth will be their first experience of significant physical pain. Nevertheless, when assessed retrospectively, labor pain was not an entirely negative experience, suggesting that coping with pain is a rewarding experience for some women.[144] Positive and negative feelings can coexist, underlining the multidimensional nature of the childbirth experience.[185]

The relationship of childbirth preparation to pain perception during labor is a complicated variable to assess. Although antenatal education seems to be associated with a positive experience of childbirth, it is difficult to measure its effect on pain. Studies usually suffer from selection bias; those women who attend classes have attitudes about childbirth issues that are different from nonattenders. Some research data indicate that women who attend classes report less pain throughout labor than do those who have had no preparation,[16] whereas other investigations[165, 169, 175, 177] have found no association. Ranta and colleagues[186] found that antenatal preparation for childbirth and efficient coping with labor discomfort do not diminish requirements for pain relief during labor. A woman's confidence in her ability to handle labor has been shown to be strongly related to decreased pain perception and decreased analgesia use during labor.[162, 177, 181, 187–191] Confidence is increased by antenatal education and by experience of labor. Thus, multiparous women express greater confidence to cope with labor than do nulliparous women.[147, 192]

A recent study[193] examined demographic, medical, and psychologic variables as predictors of childbirth pain. The sensory and affective dimensions of pain ("sensory pain" and "affective pain", respectively), are established by the choice of pain word descriptors as listed in the McGill Pain Questionnaire.[15] More sensory pain was reported by parturients with induced labor who had an unwanted pregnancy and unhelpful coaches. Parturients with long labors who had expectations that antenatal education would facilitate medication-free childbirth reported more affective pain. Women whose labor was induced for physician-anticipated complications, yet who were motivated to be medication-free, reported greater pain intensity. Women with less education experienced greater satisfaction. Variables determining pain intensity and pain attitude differ.[144] Pain intensity is influenced by anxiety during labor, expected pain, expected birth experience, midwife support, and duration of labor, whereas pain attitude is determined by pain intensity, anxiety, expected birth experience, physical well-being during pregnancy, and emergency cesarean delivery.[144]

Psychologic strategies of coping with labor pain, such as relaxation training, distraction, the use of "pleasant imagery," and "reversing the affect" of pain have been shown to be effective in modulation of the pain.[194] This study also found that the total number of strategies used in labor was inversely correlated with levels of labor pain.

Lower education and social class have been related to pain in some studies,[16, 148] but not in others.[151, 152, 160]

Cultural Aspects of Labor Pain

Ethnicity and culture affect the perception and expression of the pain and discomfort of childbirth. Researchers have reported strong associations of culture with pain responses, beliefs, and behaviors.[195] Observed differences in expression of pain among different racial and cultural groups are consequent to underlying attitudes toward the pain, rather than differences in the sensory experience.[17] For example, one study[179] found that pain levels during labor, measured using a visual analogue scale (VAS), in three groups of Arab women—Kuwaiti, Palestinian, and Bedouin—were the same, but there were significant differences in pain behavior. In Bedouin culture it is shameful and unacceptable for women to exhibit pain during labor, and accordingly, these women demonstrated complete absence of pain behavior, despite experiencing pain just as severe as the other two groups. Similarly, women from a Middle Eastern background gave higher pain ratings and showed more pain behaviors than did those from a Western background,[196] although both groups rated the pain of childbirth as high.

Neurohumoral Factors

Neurohumoral changes in pregnancy may modify the responses to pain.[155, 197] Many substances have been identified and implicated in nociception in parturients experiencing intense visceral pain during active labor; however, their current significance in the process of labor and delivery is incompletely understood. Some recent results of research into the role of putative neurotransmitters and neuromodulators in parturition are reviewed subsequently.

An increase in nociceptive threshold has been shown in women[156, 157] and in the rat,[155] perhaps as an endogenous defense against the pain of birth. On the basis of the observation that a rise in nociceptive threshold did not occur in rats administered opioid antagonists, Gintzler[155] suggested that the pregnancy-induced hypoalgesia observed in the rat was mediated by endogenous opioids, which are known to be released in response to nociception, and to have potent analgesic properties.[198] A further study in rats[199] implicated a spinal dynorphin/κ opioid receptor mechanism as responsible for the observed hypoalgesia. Moreover, it is likely that uterine distention and cervical stretching, which occur during the later stages of pregnancy and parturition, result in stimulation of afferent fibers in the pelvic and hypogastric nerves, thereby activating pregnancy-induced hypoalgesia via a spinal, probably κ, opioid system.[200, 201] Pregnancy-induced hypoalgesia may also be subject to hormonal control.[202, 203] Data from a recent investigation carried out by Dawson-Basoa and Gintzler[204] indicate that δ opioid receptor activity is a prerequisite for the manifestation of a substantial portion of gestational and hormone-simulated pregnancy analgesia, whereas the potent spinal μ opioid analgesia system does not participate. Estrogen and progesterone were also shown to modulate maternal antinociception of pregnancy.

Results of a recent study[205] suggest that, in the sow, nociceptive threshold increases during late pregnancy and during parturition; this change appears to be, at least in part, opioid mediated. Further evidence in support of this hypothesis comes from a study by Jayaram and colleagues.[206] These investigators found that SCH 32615, an inhibitor of an enkephalinase that degrades endogenous enkephalins, enhances pregnancy-induced analgesia in mice.

The placenta has been examined to determine its possible role in antinociception. The existence of an active hypoalgesic substance in the placenta has been postulated on the basis of the observation that ingestion of placenta and/or amniotic fluid by rats enhances pregnancy-induced hypoalgesia during parturition.[207–209] Tarapacki and associates[210] have shown that opioid-mediated analgesia induced by morphine injection in postpartum rats is enhanced by ingestion of amniotic fluid.

Substance P (SP) is one of a number of substances that may be implicated in modifying the response to pain. SP is a neuropeptide associated with nociception, and is widely distributed in the central and peripheral nervous systems, in blood, and in saliva.[211, 212] It is released in several species from afferent unmyelinated C fibers centrally[213, 214] or from peripheral sites,[215] but the relationship between these two sites is unknown. Increased progesterone during pregnancy is thought to increase sensitivity to analgesic agents,[216] and progesterone modifies deactivation of SP by an endopeptidase,[217] although the significance of this is unclear. Activation of opioid receptors is associated with decreased SP release.[44]

An investigation[218] of the effects of pregnancy and acute pain on SP-like immunoreactivity (SPLI) demonstrated that peripheral venous concentrations of SPLI were reduced in pregnancy, compared with the nonpregnant state. The presence of acute pain, whether it was labor pain or acute postoperative pain in nonpregnant subjects, had no significant effect on SPLI concentrations.[218]

As described previously (see Acute and Chronic Pain Mechanisms), animal data suggest a positive correlation between the EAAs aspartate and glutamate, NMDA receptor activation, NO, and increased nociception.[219–224] A study was performed to compare the cerebrospinal fluid (CSF) concentrations of aspartate, glutamate, and the NO metabolite, nitrate, in parturients in active labor to concentrations in parturients without pain who were awaiting elective cesarean section. As expected, aspartate was increased in those parturients experiencing severe visceral pain; however, contrary to data on somatic pain, a decrease in CSF nitrate in laboring parturients was found.[116] The mechanism behind this finding has not yet been determined. These investigators could detect no differences in putative excitatory (SP) or inhibitory (met-enkephalin) neuropeptides between laboring parturients and controls.[116] The SP results, in part, support those from previous work on peripheral venous SPLI concentrations.[218]

Additional information concerning the function of SP in pregnancy has been reported by Amira and colleagues.[225] SPLI is found in nerve fibers distributed throughout the genital tract in the rat; the uterus is the major source of SP. SPLI concentrations were used as a measure of changes in afferent innervation of the urogenital tract of rats during pregnancy and following parturition. Uterine hypertrophy was observed to cause an overall decrease in SPLI concentrations, but the amount of SPLI present per uterine horn increased nearly threefold by the end of pregnancy. There was a significant correlation between SPLI content and the number and total weight of fetuses. Substances such as NGF or hormonal factors may mediate hypertrophy of afferent innervation. Following parturition, a decrease in SPLI content of uterine horns occurred, perhaps as a result of neuropeptide release from afferent nerve endings brought about by the noxious events of parturition.[225]

The role of SP in pregnancy and parturition needs to be clarified by further study. The few investigations completed in this area to date have not yielded sufficient meaningful data to draw conclusions with any certainty. Currently, any explanation regarding its role in parturition is speculative.

In addition to the classic opioid receptors (μ, δ, and κ), cloning studies have revealed an atypical opioid receptor with 50% homology to μ, δ, and κ opioid receptors, termed ORL (opioid receptor-like)-1.[226–228] The ORL-1 receptor does not bind conventional opioid ligands but is found in central nervous system areas involved in pain perception.[229] An endogenous peptide ligand, nociceptin (orphanin FQ), has been isolated.[230, 231] There is debate about whether this ligand produces analgesia or hyperalgesia.[232, 233] Dawson-Basoa and Gintzler[234] have demonstrated that nociceptin, acting at the ORL-1 receptor, can negatively modulate the naturally occurring spinal analgesia associated with physiologic gestation. This may be due to antagonism of a spinal antinociceptive system that is activated by pregnancy. These investigators postulate the existence of a spinal physiologic mechanism, of which the nociceptin-ORL-1 system is a part, that determines sensitivity to nociceptive stimuli. Nociceptin may be involved in the etiology of extraordinarily painful pregnancy and labor.

Eisenach and coworkers[235] investigated the influence of descending inhibitory noradrenergic-cholinergic pathways on the diminishment of pain during labor by exploring the relationship between the known inhibitory neurotransmitters NE and ACh and pain-induced antinociception. Pain is known to increase spinal cord NE in animals, and spinally released NE induces ACh release to cause analgesia.[92, 93] In sheep, noxious stimulation was observed to increase NE and ACh concentrations in CSF in parallel, providing evidence in animals for activation of the spinal cord noradrenergic-cholinergic systems in response to pain. In contrast, no increase was observed in these neurotransmitters in women during painful labor compared

❖ Summary

Key Points

- Childbirth pain is more than a simple reflection of the physiologic processes of parturition; it is also the result of complex interactions of multiple physiologic and psychologic factors.
- Provision of optimal obstetric anesthesia care requires an understanding of the mechanisms of pain transmission during labor and delivery and the many factors that influence pain intensity, duration, distribution, and quality.
- Increased knowledge of the neuroanatomy, neurophysiology, and neuropharmacology of pain and continued research into the mechanisms of nociceptive processing may result in improved management of the pain of labor and delivery.

Key Reference

Siddall PJ, Cousins MJ: Introduction to pain mechanisms: implications for neural blockade. *In* Cousins MJ, Bridenbaugh PO (eds): Neural Blockade in Clinical Anesthesia and Management of Pain, 3rd ed. Philadelphia: Lippincott-Raven; 1998:675–713.

Case Stem

A primigravida at term is comfortable following initiation of epidural analgesia; however, in the late first stage, she becomes increasingly uncomfortable and complains of excruciating low back pain and rectal pressure. Discuss the timing of the onset of this pain, its presumed mechanisms, and its management. Compare and contrast the pain and anesthetic management of the first and second stages of labor.

with those without pain. A positive correlation was found, however, between CSF NE and ACh only in women with pain, supporting the hypothesis that these systems are linked in humans with pain.[235]

CONCLUSION

The amelioration of pain during labor is desirable, both for humanitarian reasons and to reduce maternal and perinatal morbidity and mortality. Childbirth pain is more than a simple reflection of the physiologic process of parturition. It is also the result of complex and subjective interactions of multiple physiologic and psychosocial factors on a woman's individual interpretation of labor stimuli,[170] producing the manifold physiologic, behavioral, and affective responses that characterize acute pain.[17]

An appreciation of the neurophysiology and neuropharmacology of pain enables the application of these principles toward an understanding of pain mechanisms in the parturient. In recent years, improved understanding of nociceptive processing has come about largely as the result of a greater understanding of afferent fiber physiology and synaptic processing in the dorsal horn of the spinal cord. This information may bring us closer to the development of the ideal management of the pain of labor and delivery. This may include the use of agents that are capable of altering neural transmission in such a way as to afford analgesia without motor, sensory, or sympathetic block.

References

1. Melzack R: Psychologic aspects of pain: implications for neural blockade. *In* Cousins MJ, Bridenbaugh PO (eds): Neural Blockade in Clinical Anesthesia and Management of Pain, 3rd ed. Philadelphia: Lippincott-Raven; 1998:781–792.
2. Morrison LMM, Wildsmith JAW, Ostheimer GW: History of pain relief in childbirth. *In* Van Zundert A, Ostheimer GW (eds): Pain Relief and Anesthesia in Obstetrics. New York: Churchill Livingstone; 1996:3–16.
3. Caton D: The history of obstetric anesthesia. *In* Chestnut DH (ed): Obstetric Anesthesia: Principles and Practice. St Louis: Mosby–Year Book; 1994:3–13.
4. Cohen J: Doctor James Young Simpson, Rabbi Abraham De Sola, and Genesis Chapter 3, verse 16. Obstet Gynecol 1996; 88:895–898.
5. Dick-Reade G: Childbirth Without Fear. New York: Harper; 1944.
6. Thorp JA, Hu DH, Albin RM, et al: The effect of intrapartum epidural analgesia on nulliparous labor: a randomized, controlled, prospective trial. Am J Obstet Gynecol 1993; 169:851–858.
7. Thorp JA, Parisi VM, Boylan PC, et al: The effect of continuous epidural analgesia on cesarean section for dystocia in nulliparous women. Am J Obstet Gynecol 1989; 161:670–675.
8. Halpern SH, Leighton BL, Ohlsson A, et al: Effect of epidural vs parenteral opioid analgesia on the progress of labor: a meta-analysis. JAMA 1998; 280:2105–2110.
9. Lieberman E: No free lunch on labor day: The risks and benefits of epidural analgesia during labor. J Nurse Midwifery 1999; 44:394–398.
10. Stolte K: A comparison of women's expectations of labor with the actual event. Birth 1987; 14:99–103.
11. Melzack R: The myth of painless childbirth. The John J Bonica Lecture. Pain 1984; 19:321–337.
12. Melzack R, Wall PD, Ty TC: Acute pain in an emergency clinic: latency of onset and descriptor patterns related to different injuries. Pain 1982; 14:33–43.
13. Gaston-Johansson F, Fridh G, Turner-Norvell K: Progression of labor pain in primiparas and multiparas. Nurs Res 1988; 37:86–90.
14. Lowe NK: Parity and pain during parturition. J Obstet Gynecol Neonatal Nurs 1987; 16:340–346.
15. Melzack R: The McGill Pain Questionnaire: major properties and scoring methods. Pain 1975; 1:277–299.
16. Melzack R, Taenzer P, Feldman P, et al: Labour is still painful after prepared childbirth training. Can Med Assoc J 1981; 125:357–363.
17. Bonica JJ: The nature of pain in parturition. *In* Van Zundert A, Ostheimer GW (eds): Pain Relief and Anesthesia in Obstetrics. New York: Churchill Livingstone; 1996:19–52.
18. Chestnut DH: Epidural analgesia and the incidence of cesarean section: time for another close look. Anesthesiology 1997; 87:472–476.
19. Chestnut DH: Does epidural analgesia during labor affect the incidence of cesarean delivery? Reg Anesth 1997; 22:495–499.
20. Bonica JJ: History of pain concepts and therapies. *In* Bonica JJ (ed): The Management of Pain. Philadelphia: Lea & Febiger; 1990:2–17.
21. Lundeberg T: Pain physiology and principles of treatment. Scand J Rehabil Med Suppl 1995; 32:13–41.
22. Beecher HK: Measurement of subjective responses. New York: Oxford University Press; 1959.
23. Szasz TS: Pain and pleasure. New York: Basic Books; 1957.

24. Melzack R, Wall PD: Pain mechanisms: a new theory. Science 1965; 150:971–979.
25. Wall PD: Inflammatory and neurogenic pain: new molecules, new mechanisms. Br J Anaesth 1995; 75:123–124.
26. Kanjhan R: Opioids and pain. Clin Exp Pharmacol Physiol 1995; 22:397–403.
27. Merskey H, Bogduk N: Classification of Chronic Pain: Descriptions of Chronic Pain Syndromes and Definitions of Pain Terms, 2nd ed. Seattle: IASP Press; 1994.
28. Woolf CJ: Recent advances in the pathophysiology of acute pain. Br J Anaesth 1989; 63:139–146.
29. Woolf CJ, Chong MS: Preemptive analgesia—treating postoperative pain by preventing the establishment of central sensitization. Anesth Analg 1993; 77:362–379.
30. Woolf CJ: Somatic pain—pathogenesis and prevention. Br J Anaesth 1995; 75:169–176.
31. Siddall PJ, Cousins MJ: Introduction to pain mechanisms: implications for neural blockade. *In* Cousins MJ, Bridenbaugh PO (eds): Neural Blockade in Clinical Anesthesia and Management of Pain, 3rd ed. Philadelphia: Lippincott-Raven; 1998:675–713.
32. Grubb BD: Peripheral and central mechanisms of pain. Br J Anaesth 1998; 81:8–11.
33. Meyer RA, Campbell JN, Raja SN: Peripheral neural mechanisms of nociception. *In* Wall PD, Melzack R (eds): Textbook of Pain, 3rd ed. Edinburgh: Churchill Livingstone; 1994: 13–44.
34. Dickenson AH: Spinal cord pharmacology of pain. Br J Anaesth 1995; 75:193–200.
35. Dray A: Inflammatory mediators of pain. Br J Anaesth 1995; 75:125–131.
36. Levine JD, Fields HL, Basbaum AI: Peptides and the primary afferent nociceptor. J Neurosci 1993; 13:2273–2286.
37. Dray A, Urban L, Dickenson A: Pharmacology of chronic pain. Trends Pharmacol Sci 1994; 15:190–197.
38. Perl ER: Sensitization of nociceptors and its relation to sensation. *In* Bonica JJ, Albe-Fessard D (eds): Advances in Pain Research and Therapy. New York: Raven Press; 1976:17–18.
39. Foster RW, Ramage AG: The action of some chemical irritants on somatosensory receptors of the cat. Neuropharmacology 1981; 20:191–198.
40. Fields HL: Pain. New York: McGraw-Hill; 1987.
41. McMahon S, Koltzenburg M: The changing role of primary afferent neurones in pain. Pain 1990; 43:269–272.
42. Schaible H-G, Schmidt RF: Direct observation of the sensitization of articular afferents during an experimental arthritis. *In* Dubner R, Gebhart GF, Bond MR (eds): Proceedings of the Vth World Congress on Pain. Amsterdam: Elsevier; 1988:44–50.
43. Czlonkowski A, Stein C, Herz A: Peripheral mechanisms of opioid antinociception in inflammation: involvement of cytokines. Eur J Pharmacol 1993; 242:229–235.
44. Stein C: Peripheral mechanisms of opioid analgesia. Anesth Analg 1993; 76:182–191.
45. Stein C: The control of pain in peripheral tissue by opioids. N Engl J Med 1995; 332:1685–1690.
46. Stein C, Millan MJ, Shippenberg TS, et al: Peripheral opioid receptors mediating antinociception in inflammation: evidence for involvement of mu, delta and kappa receptors. J Pharmacol Exp Ther 1989; 248:1269–1275.
47. Andreev N, Urban L, Dray A: Opioids suppress spontaneous activity of polymodal nociceptors in rat paw skin induced by ultraviolet irradiation. Neuroscience 1994; 58:793–798.
48. Taiwo YO, Levine JD: Kappa- and delta-opioids block sympathetically dependent hyperalgesia. J Neurosci 1991; 11:928–932.
49. Coggeshall RE, Zhou S, Carlton SM: Opioid receptors on peripheral sensory axons. Brain Res 1997; 764:126–132.
50. Dray A: Tasting the inflammatory soup: role of peripheral neurones. Pain Rev 1994; 1:153–171.
51. Rang HP, Bevan S, Dray A: Chemical activation of nociceptive peripheral neurones. Br Med Bull 1991; 47:534–548.
52. Rang HP, Bevan S, Dray A: Nociceptive peripheral neurons: cellular properties. *In* Wall PD, Melzack R (eds): Textbook of Pain, 3rd ed. Edinburgh: Churchill Livingstone; 1994:57–78.
53. Woolf CJ, Doubell TP: The pathophysiology of chronic pain—increased sensitivity to low threshold A beta-fibre inputs. Curr Opin Neurobiol 1994; 4:525–534.
54. Devor M: The pathophysiology of damaged peripheral nerves. *In* Wall PD, Melzack R (eds): Textbook of Pain, 3rd ed. Edinburgh: Churchill Livingstone; 1994:79–100.
55. Ollat H, Cesaro P: Pharmacology of neuropathic pain. Clin Neuropharmacol 1995; 18:391–404.
56. Lewin GR, Mendell LM: Nerve growth factor and nociception. Trends Neurosci 1993; 16:353–359.
57. Donnerer J, Schuligoi R, Stein C: Increased content and transport of substance P and calcitonin gene-related peptide in sensory nerves innervating inflamed tissue: evidence for a regulatory function of nerve growth factor in vivo. Neuroscience 1992; 49:693–698.
58. Bevan S, Geppetti P: Protons: small stimulants of capsaicin-sensitive sensory nerves. Trends Neurosci 1994; 17:509–512.
59. Devor M, Wall PD, Catalan N: Systemic lidocaine silences ectopic neuroma and DRG discharge without blocking nerve conduction. Pain 1992; 48:261–268.
60. Raja SN: Role of the sympathetic nervous system in acute pain and inflammation. Ann Med 1995; 27:241–246.
61. McMahon SB: Mechanisms of sympathetic pain. Br Med Bull 1991; 47:584–600.
62. Jänig W: The puzzle of "reflex sympathetic dystrophy": mechanisms, hypotheses, open questions. *In* Jänig W, Stanton-Hicks M (eds): Reflex Sympathetic Dystrophy: A Reappraisal. Seattle: IASP Press; 1996:1–24.
63. Jänig W, McLachlan EM: The role of modifications in noradrenergic peripheral pathways after nerve lesions in the generation of pain. *In* Fields HL, Liebeskind JC (eds): Pharmacological Approaches to the Treatment of Chronic Pain: New Concepts and Critical Issues. Seattle: IASP Press; 1994:101–128.
64. McLachlan EM, Jänig W, Devor M, Michaelis M: Peripheral nerve injury triggers noradrenergic sprouting within dorsal root ganglia. Nature 1993; 363:543–546.
65. Cervero F, Iggo A: The substantia gelatinosa of the spinal cord: a critical review. Brain 1980; 103:717–772.
66. Light AR, Perl ER: Spinal termination of functionally identified primary afferent neurons with slowly conducting myelinated fibers. J Comp Neurol 1979; 186:133–150.
67. Willis WD, Coggeshall RE: Sensory Mechanisms of the Spinal Cord. New York: Plenum Press; 1991.
68. Christensen BN, Perl ER: Spinal neurons specifically excited by noxious or thermal stimuli: marginal zone of the dorsal horn. J Neurophysiol 1970; 33:293–307.
69. Loh L, Nathan PW: Painful peripheral states and sympathetic blocks. J Neurol Neurosurg Psychiatry 1978; 41:664–671.
70. Siddall PJ, Cousins MJ: Spinal pain mechanisms. Spine 1997; 22:98–104.
71. Wilcox GL: Excitatory neurotransmitters and pain. *In* Bond MR, Charlton JE, Woolf CJ (eds): Proceedings of the VIth World Congress on Pain. Amsterdam: Elsevier; 1991:97–117.
72. Coggeshall RE, Carlton SM: Receptor localization in the mammalian dorsal horn and primary afferent neurons. Brain Res Brain Res Rev 1997; 24:28–66.
73. Coderre TJ: The role of excitatory amino acid receptors and intracellular messengers in persistent nociception after tissue injury in rats. Mol Neurobiol 1993; 7:229–246.
74. Price DD, Mao J, Mayer DJ: Central neural mechanisms of normal and abnormal pain states. *In* Fields HL, Liebeskind JC (eds): Pharmacological Approaches to the Treatment of Chronic Pain: New Concepts and Critical Issues. Seattle: IASP Press; 1994:61–84.
75. Dickenson AH: NMDA receptor antagonists as analgesics. *In* Fields HL, Liebeskind JC (eds): Pharmacological Approaches to the Treatment of Chronic Pain: New Concepts and Critical Issues. Seattle: IASP Press; 1994:173–187.
76. Davies SN, Lodge D: Evidence for involvement of *N*-methylaspartate receptors in "wind-up" of class 2 neurones in the dorsal horn of the rat. Brain Res 1987; 424:402–406.
77. Woolf CJ, Thompson SW: The induction and maintenance of central sensitization is dependent on *N*-methyl-D-aspartic acid receptor activation: implications for the treatment of post-injury pain hypersensitivity states. Pain 1991; 44:293–299.
78. Collingridge GL, Singer W: Excitatory amino acid receptors

and synaptic plasticity. Trends Pharmacol Sci 1990; 11:290–296.
79. Meller ST, Gebhart GF: Nitric oxide (NO) and nociceptive processing in the spinal cord. Pain 1993; 52:127–136.
80. Woolf CJ: Evidence for a central component of post-injury pain hypersensitivity. Nature 1983; 306:686–688.
81. Dubner R, Ruda MA: Activity-dependent neuronal plasticity following tissue injury and inflammation. Trends Neurosci 1992; 15:96–103.
82. Treede RD, Meyer RA, Raja SN, et al: Peripheral and central mechanisms of cutaneous hyperalgesia. Prog Neurobiol 1992; 38:397–421.
83. Woolf CJ: Generation of acute pain: central mechanisms. Br Med Bull 1991; 47:523–533.
84. Wall PD, Woolf CJ: Muscle but not cutaneous C-afferent input produces prolonged increases in the excitability of the flexion reflex in the rat. J Physiol 1984; 356:443–458.
85. Woolf CJ, Wall PD: Relative effectiveness of C primary afferent fibers of different origins in evoking a prolonged facilitation of the flexor reflex in the rat. J Neurosci 1986; 6:1433–1442.
86. Cook AJ, Woolf CJ, Wall PD, et al: Dynamic receptive field plasticity in rat spinal cord dorsal horn following C-primary afferent input. Nature 1987; 325:151–153.
87. Mendell LM: Physiological properties of unmyelinated fiber projection to the spinal cord. Exp Neurol 1966; 16:316–332.
88. Dickenson AH, Sullivan AF: Evidence for a role of the NMDA receptor in the frequency dependent potentiation of deep rat dorsal horn nociceptive neurones following C fibre stimulation. Neuropharmacology 1987; 26:1235–1238.
89. Lekan HA, Carlton SM, Coggeshall RE: Sprouting of A beta fibers into lamina II of the rat dorsal horn in peripheral neuropathy. Neurosci Lett 1996; 208:147–150.
90. Woolf CJ, Shortland P, Coggeshall RE: Peripheral nerve injury triggers central sprouting of myelinated afferents. Nature 1992; 355:75–78.
91. Yaksh TL, Reddy SV: Studies in the primate on the analgetic effects associated with intrathecal actions of opiates, alpha-adrenergic agonists and baclofen. Anesthesiology 1981; 54:451–467.
92. Gordh TJ, Jansson I, Hartvig P, et al: Interactions between noradrenergic and cholinergic mechanisms involved in spinal nociceptive processing. Acta Anaesthesiol Scand 1989; 33:39–47.
93. Detweiler DJ, Eisenach JC, Tong C, et al: A cholinergic interaction in alpha 2 adrenoceptor-mediated antinociception in sheep. J Pharmacol Exp Ther 1993; 265:536–542.
94. Klimscha W, Chiari A, Lorber C, et al: Additives in neuraxial anesthesia: opioids, alpha-2 adrenergic agonists, and neostigmine as a possible future drug for perioperative pain management. Acta Anaesthesiol Scand Suppl 1996; 109:176–178.
95. Hood DD, Eisenach JC, Tuttle R: Phase I safety assessment of intrathecal neostigmine methylsulfate in humans. Anesthesiology 1995; 82:331–343.
96. Meert TF, De Kock M: Potentiation of the analgesic properties of fentanyl-like opioids with alpha 2-adrenoceptor agonists in rats. Anesthesiology 1994; 81:677–688.
97. Lin Q, Peng YB, Willis WD: Role of GABA receptor subtypes in inhibition of primate spinothalamic tract neurons: difference between spinal and periaqueductal gray inhibition. J Neurophysiol 1996; 75:109–123.
98. Désarmenien M, Feltz P, Occhipinti G, et al: Coexistence of $GABA_A$ and $GABA_B$ receptors on Aδ and C primary afferents. Br J Pharmacol 1984; 81:327–333.
99. Willis WD: The Pain System: The Neural Basis of Nociceptive Transmission in the Mammalian Nervous System. Basel: Karger; 1985.
100. Kenshalo DRJ, Giesler GJJ, Leonard RB, et al: Responses of neurons in primate ventral posterior lateral nucleus to noxious stimuli. J Neurophysiol 1980; 43:1594–1614.
101. Willis WD, Westlund KN: Neuroanatomy of the pain system and of the pathways that modulate pain. J Clin Neurophysiol 1997; 14:2–31.
102. Davis KD, Wood ML, Crawley AP, et al: fMRI of human somatosensory and cingulate cortex during painful electrical nerve stimulation. Neuroreport 1995; 7:321–325.
103. Jones AK, Brown WD, Friston KJ, et al: Cortical and subcortical localization of response to pain in man using positron emission tomography. Proc R Soc Lond B Biol Sci 1991; 244:39–44.
104. Talbot JD, Marrett S, Evans AC, et al: Multiple representations of pain in human cerebral cortex. Science 1991; 251:1355–1358.
105. Wall PD: Pain mechanisms. Personal communication, 1998.
106. Chudler EH, Dong WK: The role of the basal ganglia in nociception and pain. Pain 1995; 60:3–38.
107. Stamford JA: Descending control of pain. Br J Anaesth 1995; 75:217–227.
108. Sawynok J, Reid A: Interactions of descending serotonergic systems with other neurotransmitters in the modulation of nociception. Behav Brain Res 1996; 73:63–68.
109. Reynolds DV: Surgery in the rat during electrical analgesia induced by focal brain stimulation. Science 1969; 164:444–445.
110. Sandkühler J: The organization and function of endogenous antinociceptive systems. Prog Neurobiol 1996; 50:49–81.
111. Munglani R, Hunt SP: Molecular biology of pain. Br J Anaesth 1995; 75:186–192.
112. Cameron AA, Khan IA, Westlund KN, et al: The efferent projections of the periaqueductal gray in the rat: a *Phaseolus vulgaris*–leucoagglutinin study. I. Ascending projections. J Comp Neurol 1995; 351:568–584.
113. Cameron AA, Khan IA, Westlund KN, et al: The efferent projections of the periaqueductal gray in the rat: a *Phaseolus vulgaris*–leucoagglutinin study. II. Descending projections. J Comp Neurol 1995; 351:585–601.
114. McMahon SB, Dmitrieva N, Koltzenburg M: Visceral pain. Br J Anaesth 1995; 75:132–144.
115. Jänig W: Neurobiology of visceral afferent neurons: neuroanatomy, functions, organ regulations and sensations. Biol Psychol 1996; 42:29–51.
116. Olofsson C, Ekblom A, Ekman-Ordeberg G, et al: Increased cerebrospinal fluid concentration of aspartate but decreased concentration of nitric oxide breakdown products in women experiencing visceral pain during active labour. Neuroreport 1997; 8:995–998.
117. Cervero F: Visceral pain: mechanisms of peripheral and central sensitization. Ann Med 1995; 27:235–239.
118. Al-Chaer ED, Lawand NB, Westlund KN, et al: Visceral nociceptive input into the ventral posterolateral nucleus of the thalamus: a new function for the dorsal column pathway. J Neurophysiol 1996; 76:2661–2674.
119. Al-Chaer ED, Lawand NB, Westlund KN, et al: Pelvic visceral input into the nucleus gracilis is largely mediated by the postsynaptic dorsal column pathway. J Neurophysiol 1996; 76:2675–2690.
120. Hirshberg RM, Al-Chaer ED, Lawand NB, et al: Is there a pathway in the posterior funiculus that signals visceral pain? Pain 1996; 67:291–305.
121. Moir C: The nature of the pain of labour. Br J Obstet Gynaecol 1939; 46:409–424.
122. Bonica JJ: Labour pain. *In* Wall PD, Melzack R (eds): Textbook of Pain, 3rd ed. Edinburgh: Churchill Livingstone; 1994:615–641.
123. Brownridge P: The nature and consequences of childbirth pain. Eur J Obstet Gynecol Reprod Biol Suppl 1995; 59:S9–15.
124. McMahon SB: Mechanisms of cutaneous, deep and visceral pain. *In* Wall PD, Melzack R (eds): Textbook of Pain, 3rd ed. Edinburgh: Churchill Livingstone; 1994:129–151.
125. Ness TJ, Gebhart GF: Visceral pain: a review of experimental studies. Pain 1990; 41:167–234.
126. Caldeyro-Barcia R, Poseiro JJ: Physiology of the uterine contraction. Clin Obstet Gynecol 1960; 3:386–408.
127. Javert CT, Hardy JD: Measurement of pain intensity in labor and its physiologic, neurologic and pharmacologic implications. Am J Obstet Gynecol 1950; 60:552–563.
128. Paul WM, Glickman BI, Cushner IM, et al: Clinical tone and pain threshold. Am J Obstet Gynecol 1956; 7:510–516.
129. Reynolds SRM: Innervation of the uterus: functional features. *In* Reynolds SRM (ed): Physiology of the Uterus. New York: Harper & Brothers; 1949:477–490.
130. Lees MH, Hill JD, Ochsner AJ, et al: Maternal placental and

myometrial blood flow of the rhesus monkey during uterine contractions. Am J Obstet Gynecol 1971; 110:68–81.

131. Danforth DN: Distribution and functional significance of the cervical musculature. Am J Obstet Gynecol 1954; 68:1261–1271.
132. Cleland JG: Paravertebral anaesthesia in obstetrics. Surg Gynaecol Obstet 1933; 57:51–62.
133. Bonica JJ: Current role of nerve blocks in the diagnosis and therapy of pain. *In* Bonica JJ (ed): Advances in Neurology. New York: Raven Press; 1974:445–453.
134. Bonica JJ: The nature of pain in parturition. Clin Obstet Gynecol 1975; 2:499–507.
135. Bonica JJ: Peripheral mechanisms and pathways of parturition pain. Br J Anaesth 1979; 51:3–9.
136. Cheek TG, Gutsche BB, Gaiser RR: The pain of childbirth and its effect on the mother and fetus. *In* Chestnut DH (ed): Obstetric Anesthesia: Principles and Practice. St Louis: Mosby–Year Book; 1994:314–329.
137. Berkley KJ, Robbins A, Sato Y: Afferent fibers supplying the uterus in the rat. J Neurophysiol 1988; 59:142–163.
138. Berkley KJ, Wood E: Responses to varying intensities of vaginal distension in the awake rat. Soc Neurosci Abst 1989; 15:979.
139. Stewart DE: Psychiatric symptoms following attempted natural childbirth. Can Med Assoc J 1982; 127:713–716.
140. Reynolds JL: Post-traumatic stress disorder after childbirth: the phenomenon of traumatic birth. Can Med Assoc J 1997; 156:831–835.
141. Fones C: Posttraumatic stress disorder occurring after painful childbirth. J Nerv Ment Dis 1996; 184:195–196.
142. Giamberardino MA, de Bigontina P, Martegiani C, et al: Effects of extracorporeal shock-wave lithotripsy on referred hyperalgesia from renal/ureteral calculosis. Pain 1994; 56:77–83.
143. Melzack R, Belanger E: Labour pain: correlations with menstrual pain and acute low-back pain before and during pregnancy. Pain 1989; 36:225–229.
144. Waldenström U, Bergman V, Vasell G: The complexity of labor pain: experiences of 278 women. J Psychosom Obstet Gynaecol 1996; 17:215–228.
145. Melzack R, Kinch R, Dobkin P, et al: Severity of labour pain: influence of physical as well as psychologic variables. Can Med Assoc J 1984; 130:579–584.
146. Lowe NK, Roberts JE: The convergence between in-labor report and postpartum recall of parturition pain. Res Nurs Health 1988; 11:11–21.
147. Lowe NK: Differences in first and second stage labor pain between nulliparous and multiparous women. J Psychosom Obstet Gynaecol 1992; 13:243–253.
148. Nettelbladt P, Fagerström CF, Uddenberg N: The significance of reported childbirth pain. J Psychosom Res 1976; 20:215–221.
149. Melzack R, Schaffelberg D: Low-back pain during labor. Am J Obstet Gynecol 1987; 156:901–905.
150. Scott-Palmer J, Skevington SM: Pain during childbirth and menstruation: a study of locus of control. J Psychosom Res 1981; 25:151–155.
151. Norr KL, Block CR, Charles A, et al: Explaining pain and enjoyment in childbirth. J Health Soc Behav 1977; 18:260–275.
152. Fridh G, Kopare T, Gaston-Johansson F, et al: Factors associated with more intense labor pain. Res Nurs Health 1988; 11:117–124.
153. Kohnen N: "Natural" childbirth among the Kankanaly-Igorot. Bull N Y Acad Med 1986; 62:768–777.
154. Marx JL: Dysmenorrhea: basic research leads to a rational therapy. Science 1979; 205:175–176.
155. Gintzler AR: Endorphin-mediated increases in pain threshold during pregnancy. Science 1980; 210:193–195.
156. Cogan R, Spinnato JA: Pain and discomfort thresholds in late pregnancy. Pain 1986; 27:63–68.
157. Whipple B, Josimovich JB, Komisaruk BR: Sensory thresholds during the antepartum, intrapartum and postpartum periods. Int J Nurs Stud 1990; 27:213–221.
158. Brown ST, Campbell D, Kurtz A: Characteristics of labor pain at two stages of cervical dilation. Pain 1989; 38:289–295.
159. Gerdin E, Cnattingius S: The use of obstetric analgesia in Sweden, 1983–1986. Br J Obstet Gynaecol 1990; 97:789–796.
160. Davenport-Slack B, Boylan CH: Psychological correlates of childbirth pain. Psychosom Med 1974; 36:215–223.
161. Cogan R, Henneborn W, Klopfer F: Predictors of pain during prepared childbirth. J Psychosom Res 1976; 20:523–533.
162. Lowe NK: Explaining the pain of active labor: the importance of maternal confidence. Res Nurs Health 1989; 12:237–245.
163. Ranta P, Spalding M, Kangas-Saarela T, et al: Maternal expectations and experiences of labour pain—options of 1091 Finnish parturients. Acta Anaesthesiol Scand 1995; 39:60–66.
164. Paech MJ: The King Edward Memorial Hospital 1,000 mother survey of methods of pain relief in labour. Anaesth Intensive Care 1991; 19:393–399.
165. Niven C, Gijsbers K: A study of labour pain using the McGill Pain Questionnaire. Soc Sci Med 1984; 19:1347–1351.
166. Bundsen P, Peterson LE, Selstam U: Pain relief during delivery: an evaluation of conventional methods. Acta Obstet Gynecol Scand 1982; 61:289–297.
167. Ranta P, Jouppila P, Jouppila R: The intensity of labor pain in grand multiparas. Acta Obstet Gynecol Scand 1996; 75:250–254.
168. Bonica JJ: Obstetric Analgesia and Anesthesia. World Federation of Societies of Anaesthesiologists. Seattle: University of Washington Press; 1980.
169. Reading AE, Cox DN: Psychosocial predictors of labor pain. Pain 1985; 22:309–315.
170. Lowe NK: The pain and discomfort of labor and birth. J Obstet Gynecol Neonatal Nurs 1996; 25:82–92.
171. Roberts J, Malasanos L, Mendez-Bauer C: Maternal positions in labor: analysis in relation to comfort and efficiency. Birth Defects 1981; 17:97–128.
172. Corli O, Grossi E, Roma G, et al: Correlation between subjective labour pain and uterine contractions: a clinical study. Pain 1986; 26:53–60.
173. Brown WA, Manning T, Grodin J: The relationship of antenatal and perinatal psychologic variables to the use of drugs in labor. Psychosom Med 1972; 34:119–127.
174. Green JM: Expectations and experiences of pain in labor: findings from a large prospective study. Birth 1993; 20:65–72.
175. Astbury J: Labour pain: the role of childbirth education, information and expectation. *In* Peck C, Wallace M (eds): Problems in Pain. London: Pergamon Press; 1980:245–252.
176. Connolly AM, Pancheri P, Lucchetti A, et al: Labor as a psychosomatic condition: a study on the influence of personality on self-reported anxiety and pain. *In* Carenza L, Pancheri P, Zichella L (eds): Clinical Psychoneuroendocrinology in Reproduction. London: Academic Press; 1978:369–379.
177. Lowe NK: Individual variation in childbirth pain. J Psychosom Obstet Gynaecol 1987; 7:183–192.
178. Green JM, Coupland VA, Kitzinger JV: Expectations, experiences, and psychological outcomes of childbirth: a prospective study of 825 women. Birth 1990; 17:15–24.
179. Harrison A: Childbirth in Kuwait: the experiences of three groups of Arab mothers. J Pain Symptom Manage 1991; 6:466–475.
180. Lowe NK: Critical predictors of sensory and affective pain during four phases of labor. J Psychosom Obstet Gynaecol 1991; 12:193–208.
181. Wuitchik M, Hesson K, Bakal DA: Perinatal predictors of pain and distress during labor. Birth 1990; 17:186–191.
182. Wolman WL, Chalmers B, Hofmeyr GJ, et al: Postpartum depression and companionship in the clinical birth environment: a randomized, controlled study. Am J Obstet Gynecol 1993; 168:1388–1393.
183. Hofmeyr GJ, Nikodem VC, Wolman WL, et al: Companionship to modify the clinical birth environment: effects on progress and perceptions of labour, and breastfeeding. Br J Obstet Gynaecol 1991; 98:756–764.
184. Mahomed K, Gülmezoglu AM, Nikodem VC, et al: Labor experience, maternal mood and cortisol and catecholamine levels in low-risk primiparous women. J Psychosom Obstet Gynaecol 1995; 16:181–186.
185. Waldenström U, Borg IM, Olsson B, et al: The childbirth experience: a study of 295 new mothers. Birth 1996; 23:144–153.

186. Ranta P, Spalding M, Kangas-Saarela T, et al: Maternal expectations and experiences of labour pain—options of 1091 Finnish parturients. Acta Anaesthesiol Scand 1995; 39:60–66.
187. Crowe K, von Baeyer C: Predictors of a positive childbirth experience. Birth 1989; 16:59–63.
188. Lowe NK: Maternal confidence in coping with labor: a self-efficacy concept. J Obstet Gynecol Neonatal Nurs 1991; 20:457–463.
189. Manning MM, Wright TL: Self-efficacy expectancies, outcome expectancies, and the persistence of pain control in childbirth. J Pers Soc Psychol 1983; 45:421–431.
190. Walker B, Erdman A: Childbirth education programs: the relationship between confidence and knowledge. Birth 1984; 11:103–108.
191. Wuitchik M, Bakal D, Lipshitz J: The clinical significance of pain and cognitive activity in latent labor. Obstet Gynecol 1989; 73:35–42.
192. Booth CL, Meltzoff AN: Expected and actual experience in labour and delivery and their relationship to maternal attachment. J Reprod Infant Psychol 1984; 2:79–91.
193. Dannenbring D, Stevens MJ, House AE: Predictors of childbirth pain and maternal satisfaction. J Behav Med 1997; 20:127–142.
194. Niven CA, Gijsbers K: Coping with labor pain. J Pain Symptom Manage 1996; 11:116–125.
195. Weber SE: Cultural aspects of pain in childbearing women. J Obstet Gynecol Neonatal Nurs 1996; 25:67–72.
196. Weisenberg M, Caspi Z: Cultural and educational influences on pain of childbirth. J Pain Symptom Manage 1989; 4:13–19.
197. Iwasaki H, Collins JG, Saito Y, et al: Naloxone-sensitive, pregnancy-induced changes in behavioral responses to colorectal distention: pregnancy-induced analgesia to visceral stimulation. Anesthesiology 1991; 74:927–933.
198. Dalayeun JF, Nores JM, Bergal S: Physiology of beta-endorphins: a close-up view and a review of the literature. Biomed Pharmacother 1993; 47:311–320.
199. Sander HW, Gintzler AR: Spinal cord mediation of the opioid analgesia of pregnancy. Brain Res 1987; 408:389–393.
200. Gintzler AR, Peters LC, Komisaruk BR: Attenuation of pregnancy-induced analgesia by hypogastric neurectomy in rats. Brain Res 1983; 277:186–188.
201. Gintzler AR, Komisaruk BR: Analgesia is produced by uterocervical mechanostimulation in rats: roles of afferent nerves and implications for analgesia of pregnancy and parturition. Brain Res 1991; 566:299–302.
202. Dawson-Basoa MB, Gintzler AR: 17-Beta-estradiol and progesterone modulate an intrinsic opioid analgesic system. Brain Res 1993; 601:241–245.
203. Dawson-Basoa ME, Gintzler AR: Estrogen and progesterone activate spinal kappa-opiate receptor analgesic mechanisms. Pain 1996; 64:608–615.
204. Dawson-Basoa M, Gintzler AR: Involvement of spinal cord delta opiate receptors in the antinociception of gestation and its hormonal simulation. Brain Res 1997; 757:37–42.
205. Jarvis S, McLean KA, Chirnside J, et al: Opioid-mediated changes in nociceptive threshold during pregnancy and parturition in the sow. Pain 1997; 72:153–159.
206. Jayaram A, Singh P, Carp H: SCH 32615, an enkephalinase inhibitor, enhances pregnancy-induced analgesia in mice. Anesth Analg 1995; 80:944–948.
207. Kristal MB, Thompson AC, Grishkat HL: Placenta ingestion enhances opiate analgesia in rats. Physiol Behav 1985; 35:481–486.
208. Kristal MB, Tarapacki JA, Barton D: Amniotic fluid ingestion enhances opioid-mediated but not nonopioid-mediated analgesia. Physiol Behav 1990; 47:79–81.
209. Kristal MB, Thompson AC, Abbott P, et al: Amniotic-fluid ingestion by parturient rats enhances pregnancy-mediated analgesia. Life Sci 1990; 46:693–698.
210. Tarapacki JA, Piech M, Kristal MB: Ingestion of amniotic fluid by postpartum rats enhances morphine antinociception without liability to maternal behavior. Physiol Behav 1995; 57:209–212.
211. Aimone LD: Neurochemistry and modulation of pain. *In* Sinatra RS, Hord AH, Ginsberg B, Preble LM (eds): Acute Pain: Mechanisms and Management. St Louis: Mosby–Year Book; 1992:29–43.
212. Pernow B: Substance P. Pharmacol Rev 1983; 35:85–141.
213. Basbaum AI: Mechanisms of substance P–mediated nociception and opioid-mediated antinociception. *In* Stanley T, Ashburn M (eds): Anesthesiology and Pain Management. Dordrecht: Kluwer Academic; 1994:1–19.
214. Hökfelt T, Johansson O, Ljungdahl A, et al: Peptidergic neurones. Nature 1980; 284:515–521.
215. Marshall KW, Chiu B, Inman RD: Substance P and arthritis: analysis of plasma and synovial fluid levels. Arthritis Rheum 1990; 33:87–90.
216. Jayaram A, Carp H: Progesterone-mediated potentiation of spinal sufentanil in rats. Anesth Analg 1993; 76:745–750.
217. Casey ML, Smith JW, Nagai K, et al: Progesterone-regulated cyclic modulation of membrane metalloendopeptidase (enkephalinase) in human endometrium. J Biol Chem 1991; 266:23041–23047.
218. Dalby PL, Ramanathan S, Rudy TE, et al: Plasma and saliva substance P levels: the effects of acute pain in pregnant and non-pregnant women. Pain 1997; 69:263–267.
219. Coderre TJ, Yashpal K: Intracellular messengers contributing to persistent nociception and hyperalgesia induced by L-glutamate and substance P in the rat formalin pain model. Eur J Neurosci 1994; 6:1328–1334.
220. Malmberg AB, Yaksh TL: Spinal nitric oxide synthesis inhibition blocks NMDA-induced thermal hyperalgesia and produces antinociception in the formalin test in rats. Pain 1993; 54:291–300.
221. Meller ST, Dykstra C, Gebhart GF: Production of endogenous nitric oxide and activation of soluble guanylate cyclase are required for *N*-methyl-D-aspartate-produced facilitation of the nociceptive tail-flick reflex. Eur J Pharmacol 1992; 214:93–96.
222. Meller ST, Pechman PS, Gebhart GF, et al: Nitric oxide mediates the thermal hyperalgesia produced in a model of neuropathic pain in the rat. Neuroscience 1992; 50:7–10.
223. Jones NM, Loiacono RE, Beart PM: Roles for nitric oxide as an intra- and interneuronal messenger at NMDA release-regulating receptors: evidence from studies of the NMDA-evoked release of [3H]noradrenaline and D-[3H]aspartate from rat hippocampal slices. J Neurochem 1995; 64:2057–2063.
224. Lawrence AJ, Jarrott B: Nitric oxide increases interstitial excitatory amino acid release in the rat dorsomedial medulla oblongata. Neurosci Lett 1993; 151:126–129.
225. Amira S, Morrison JFB, Rayfield KM: The effects of pregnancy and parturition on the substance P content of the rat uterus: uterine growth is accompanied by hypertrophy of its afferent innervation. Exp Physiol 1995; 80:645–650.
226. Darland T, Grandy DK: The orphanin FQ system: an emerging target for the management of pain? Br J Anaesth 1998; 81:29–37.
227. Mollereau C, Parmentier M, Mailleux P, et al: ORL1, a novel member of the opioid receptor family: cloning, functional expression and localization. FEBS Lett 1994; 341:33–38.
228. Wick MJ, Minnerath SR, Lin X, et al: Isolation of a novel cDNA encoding a putative membrane receptor with high homology to the cloned mu, delta, and kappa opioid receptors. Brain Res Mol Brain Res 1994; 27:37–44.
229. Harrison C, Smart D, Lambert DG: Stimulatory effects of opioids. Br J Anaesth 1998; 81:20–28.
230. Meunier JC, Mollereau C, Toll L, et al: Isolation and structure of the endogenous agonist of opioid receptor-like ORL1 receptor. Nature 1995; 377:532–535.
231. Reinscheid RK, Nothacker HP, Bourson A, et al: Orphanin FQ: a neuropeptide that activates an opioidlike G protein–coupled receptor. Science 1995; 270:792–794.
232. Meunier JC: Nociceptin/orphanin FQ and the opioid receptor-like ORL1 receptor. Eur J Pharmacol 1997; 340:1–15.
233. Henderson G, McKnight AT: The orphan opioid receptor and its endogenous ligand—nociceptin/orphanin FQ. Trends Pharmacol Sci 1997; 18:293–300.
234. Dawson-Basoa M, Gintzler AR: Nociceptin (Orphanin FQ) abolishes gestational and ovarian sex steroid–induced antinociception and induces hyperalgesia. Brain Res 1997; 750:48–52.
235. Eisenach JC, Detweiler DJ, Tong C, et al: Cerebrospinal fluid norepinephrine and acetylcholine concentrations during acute pain. Anesth Analg 1996; 82:621–626.

2

Physiologic Changes of Pregnancy

❖ ANDREW ROSS, MB, BS, FFA, RACS, FANZCA, GRAD DIPL HEALTH MED LAW, DIPL PSYCH

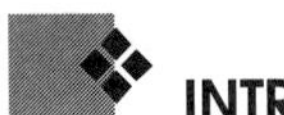

INTRODUCTION

As pregnancy develops there are many associated physiologic and anatomic changes that occur. These changes are complex and often expressed early in the pregnancy, well before the final stages of fetal development. Many changes are already well in place before the end of the first trimester. Hormonal, metabolic, and mechanical changes account for the majority of the physiologic alterations in pregnancy. The most significant changes are secondary to the effects of changes in hormone levels. Progesterone is the principal pregnancy hormone, the levels of which continue to rise through pregnancy. Initially released from the persisting corpus luteum of early pregnancy, placental progesterone comes to be the dominant pregnancy hormone by the end of the second month.[1] A fall in progesterone levels or at least an alteration in the estrogen-progesterone ratio is believed associated with the onset of labor in the third trimester. Much attention has been given to the anatomic influence of the enlarging uterus as it affects pulmonary and cardiovascular physiology. It may be that much of this has been overemphasized in terms of pure mechanical effect, with the changes that are induced being more under hormonal than anatomic influence.

METABOLIC CHANGES

Metabolic Rate

Metabolic demands increase in pregnancy in response to the growth and nutrition of the fetus, as well as the additional maternal cardiorespiratory demands imposed by the fetus and uteroplacental unit. The resting metabolic rate has been observed to increase steadily throughout pregnancy, in response to the demands of the developing fetus, and is maintained in the postpartum period with breast-feeding. The increase in metabolic rate shows large interindividual variation, with a range of increase of 8.6% to 35.4% from the nonpregnant baseline.[2] When expressed in relationship to actual body weight, no change was found. The actual maternal metabolic rate was significantly depressed by the second trimester owing to the increased efficiency of energy use at a time of high fetal energy demand.[3] The concept of "eating for two" may merely result in increased energy deposition as fat.[4] A total weight gain of about 12 kg occurs during pregnancy. Plasma volume and interstitial fluid volume increases account for half of this weight gain, the rest accounted for by the fetus, uterus, placenta, and amniotic fluid. Thus the weight gain that occurs is partly maternal and partly due to the enlarging fetus and uterus.

RESPIRATORY PHYSIOLOGY

Owing to the metabolic demands of the developing fetus, there is an increase in the respiratory minute volume and work of breathing in order to accommodate the increase in oxygen demand and the elimination of carbon dioxide. Because of the difficulties in performing clinical research on pregnant women, there has been scant investigation of the physiology of normal pregnancy using currently developed technology. Many of the quoted changes in existing studies are inconsistent, being based on older techniques that were applied to a limited number of subjects.

Respiratory Function in Pregnancy

There are significant anatomic changes that ultimately occur in pregnancy to accommodate the enlarging uterus. There has been much controversy regarding interpretation of lung volume changes in pregnancy, and much of this is probably due to variations in measurement technique as well as to individual patient changes in body habitus. Overall, vital capacity probably increases in pregnancy, but only by a few hundred milliliters, that is, less than 5%, and usually in the latter half of pregnancy, secondary to the rise in inspiratory capacity and tidal volume.[5] Minute volume increases, but a rise in tidal volume rather than respiratory rate accounts for the increase, the respiratory rate essentially remaining unchanged.[6] The increase in minute volume is approximately 40% above nonpregnant values although the exact amount varies with the research methods used.

Under the respiratory stimulus of progesterone, hyperventilation via an increase in tidal volume produces a decrease in $Paco_2$ to 28 to 34 mm Hg. The cost is an increase in oxygen consumption owing to the added work of breathing. A mild compensated respiratory alkalosis results, with a normal arterial pH of 7.44. This fall in $Paco_2$ is also seen in the second half of the normal menstrual cycle but then the pH remains unaltered. Significant changes in the work of breathing may be noted in the first trimester from as early as the 7th week of gestation, with an increase in both minute ventilation (24%) and oxygen consumption (10%).[7] The onset is ahead of the developmental demands of the fetus, and is attributed to the effects of progesterone.[8] This relative hyperventilation should be maintained if general anesthesia is performed. Some of the ventilatory increase is due to reduction in dead space ratio, rather than to an effect on the respiratory center.[9] Progesterone has a secondary protective action in raising the hypoxic ventilatory response.[10] Oxygen consumption continues to rise to 60% above resting levels by the third trimester. The effects of hyperventilation result in a lowered and left-shifted oxyhemoglobin dissociation curve. Maternal levels of 2,3-diphosphoglycerate increase by about 30% by midpregnancy to offset this effect.[11]

There is a small rise in the value of Pao_2 to 105 mm Hg owing to the rise in cardiac output exceeding the increased demand for oxygen, with an effective reduction in arteriovenous oxygen difference. Most women report subjective breathlessness as a nonspecific symptom at some stage of their pregnancy.

Anatomic and Mechanical Changes

Chest wall shape alters in pregnancy. By the third trimester, the lower ribs flare and the transverse diameter increases to accommodate the gravid uterus. These changes, however, are well established before significant uterine enlargement has occurred. The diaphragm rises but its excursion increases to maintain ventilation. Ventilation becomes more dependent on diaphragmatic than intercostal activity. The radiologic appearance is that of relatively increased markings, owing to a smaller lung volume in expiration, and increased pulmonary vessel prominence secondary to the increased pulmonary blood volume.

The general fluid retention and edema of pregnancy involves the upper respiratory tract with the potential for intubation difficulties at emergency general anesthesia. Development of preeclampsia further exacerbates this problem. The airway may be more prone to obstruction when loss of consciousness occurs at general anesthesia. A smaller endotracheal tube (e.g., 7.0 mm) should be used for intubation. Mucosal trauma at intubation is also more likely, and nasal intubation or instrumentation (e.g., for fiberoptic intubation) is not recommended because of the potential for epistaxis from the congested nasal mucosae. Pregnancy has been identified with an increased risk of failed intubation,[12] but the degree of absolute risk may depend on the experience of the anesthetist.[13, 14] Edema per se was not identified as a specific risk factor when adequately experienced staff were available for intubation.[15]

Although total lung capacity is largely unaltered, there are significant changes in many respiratory volumes and pulmonary capacities that serve to maintain overall function in the face of increased metabolic demand. Pulmonary capacities remain significantly unaltered in pregnancy (Table 2–1), with the exception of a 20% fall in functional residual capacity (FRC). There is a corresponding compensatory increase in inspiratory capacity. Expiratory reserve decreases to accommodate the increase in tidal volume. During pregnancy major changes in tidal volume, FRC, and residual volume (RV) occur, many by an early stage of pregnancy, that cannot be accounted for adequately by mechanical disturbance from the enlarging uterus. Total chest wall compliance as well as lung compliance fall in pregnancy as the uterus enlarges. Net airways resistance in pregnancy appears to remain unaltered, probably owing to the effects of the opposing actions of prostaglandins and progesterone.[16] Overall, the work of breathing rises with a 50% increase in oxygen consumption.[17] The closing volume has been observed to be greater than the FRC in the last month of pregnancy in a population in which many were hypertensive.[18] When the study was repeated in normotensive women, however, the changes in closing volume were much reduced and of no consequence. The unpredictability of change related to gestation is thought to be due to hormonal blood flow redistribution effects rather than to mechanical effects of the enlarged uterus.[19, 20]

A significant reduction in FRC and RV has been observed with a postural change to the supine position, with a reduction in FRC in the third trimester to half the predicted value but with no evidence of desaturation.[21] Despite this, the increased metabolic demand for oxygen and the reduced FRC mean that with a reduced oxygen reserve volume, hypoxia will develop more rapidly if ventilation or cardiac output becomes inadequate. Care must be taken to ensure an adequate period of preoxygenation before inducing general anesthesia in advanced pregnancy. A degree of head-up posture allows better oxygen reserve.[22] Uptake of inhalational agents under general anesthesia in the supine position is aided by the reduction in FRC.

Although pulmonary function is altered in pregnancy, it is not usually compromised. Overall mechanical efficiency is maintained, and disease states are usually well tolerated except in the extreme.[23] The use of magnesium sulfate in preeclampsia may potentially compromise pulmonary mechanics, as may the use of regional block for operative delivery in cases in which motor block is required.[24, 25] Mechanical hyperventilation under general anesthesia may physically impair

Table 2–1 CHANGES IN PULMONARY MECHANICS IN PREGNANCY

PARAMETER	CHANGE	AMOUNT
Tidal volume	Increased	40%
Rate	Unchanged	—
Minute volume	Increased	40%
Alveolar ventilation	Increased	40%
Inspiratory capacity	Increased	15%
Expiratory reserve volume	Decreased	15%
Forced vital capacity	Maintained	—
Total lung capacity	Decreased	5%
Inspiratory capacity	Increased	15%
Vital capacity	Minor increase	1-200 mL
Functional residual capacity	Decreased	20%
Residual volume	Decreased	15%

Values derived from references 5, 177–179.

venous return and reduce uterine blood flow. The lowering of $PaCO_2$ is insufficient to significantly impair uterine blood flow unless values are below 20 mm Hg.

Nocturnal hypoxemia may be found as a normal occurrence in 20% or more of women in the third trimester.[26] The exact mechanism is unclear, and probably involves changes in resting lung volumes rather than being due to possible effects of upper airway obstruction or to apneic episodes.

The pain of labor contractions may contribute significantly to oxygen consumption. Values of more than 3 mL/L of oxygen ventilation have been calculated, as opposed to 0.65 mL/L in healthy males. Extreme additional increases in ventilation of up to 300% may occur in response to the pain of advanced labor (Table 2–2). The additional hyperventilation decreases the $PaCO_2$ further. This may be ameliorated by effective epidural analgesia.[27]

This ventilatory pain response is further modified by the effects of parenteral narcotics. The additional effects of nitrous oxide and the potential for diffusion hypoxemia in labor must also be considered. Profound but short-lived periods of hypoxemia have been observed in seemingly normal labors, especially during the second stage, when effort and demand are greatest.[28, 29] The possible potentiating effects of neuraxially administered opioids have not been evaluated, but they may be of further significance with larger cumulative doses over long labors.

Upper airway obstruction and snoring become very common in pregnancy. The heightened respiratory drive was believed to provide some protection against this phenomenon, but there is no protection against hypoxic episodes secondary to sleep disorders or narcotic administration.[30]

Table 2–2 VENTILATORY VALUES WITH PAIN IN LABOR

Respiratory rate	Maximum 70 breaths/min
Tidal volume	Maximum 2 L
Minute ventilation	Maximum 30 L
$PaCO_2$	15–20 mm Hg
PaO_2	108 mm Hg

Effects of Exercise

Most women experience dyspnea at some stage in their pregnancy, and subjectively there is a reduced capacity for exercise. In uncomplicated pregnancy, cardiac output increases normally with exercise throughout the pregnancy. The augmented cardiac response to exercise during pregnancy is reduced by 2 months postpartum but some changes may persist for up to 7 months postpartum before resolution finally occurs. The rate of oxygen uptake and change in heart rate and stroke volume are increased in pregnancy, but there are no significant differences in maximal oxygen uptake or heart rate.[31] The pain of labor contractions may contribute significantly to oxygen consumption, with amelioration by effective epidural analgesia.[27]

Asthma and Pregnancy

Asthma is the most common respiratory condition seen in pregnancy. Approximately 1 in 15 women of childbearing age suffer from asthma to some degree. The course of asthma in pregnancy is extremely variable, but more often it worsens (42%) or remains static (40%) rather than improves (18%).[32] As noted earlier, progesterone has no effect in promoting bronchodilatation or reduction in airway reactivity. Airway responsiveness may improve in women who have asthma when they are pregnant, especially in those who are hyperresponsive, but the exact mechanism is unknown; however, it is not due to a smooth muscle relaxation effect as occurs in the gut, because pulmonary mechanics and spirometry remain unaltered from the prepregnant state.[33] Despite the immunosuppression of pregnancy, there seems to be no reduction in the need for anti-inflammatory therapy as part of asthma management.[34] Lack of control of asthma in pregnancy is associated with an increased incidence of prematurity, intrauterine growth retardation, and preeclampsia.[35]

Relative elevation of the normal pregnancy values of $PaCO_2$ (28–34 mm Hg) into the nonpregnant range must be treated with concern and vigilance, as it may represent developing respiratory failure. Peak expiratory flow is unaltered in normal pregnancy, so it can still serve as a useful monitor of progress. Gastroesophageal reflux, a common association of pregnancy, may be a potent trigger of asthma, especially at night.[36]

Approximately 10% of women with asthma have an exacerbation when in labor. β-Mimetic dosage and route of administration must be closely monitored to avoid potential problems such as tocolysis, fluid retention, hypokalemia, tachyarrhythmias, and pulmonary edema.[37] Elective epidural or combined spinal-epidural analgesia carefully titrated reduces stress, narcotic dosage, and the work of breathing. Adequate ventilation will be maintained if the motor component of the block is minimized. Care must be taken to avoid the potential respiratory depressant effects of neuraxially administered opioids. With care and titration, even the most difficult cases of respiratory compromise have been managed with regional techniques.[38]

CARDIOVASCULAR SYSTEM

Anatomic Changes

The heart is displaced upward and to the left by the enlarging uterus. The cardiac silhouette appears enlarged, secondary to the effects of the increased blood volume. The left atrial border straightens and the ventricles actually slightly enlarge. With the increase in cardiac output and dilutional anemia, systolic ejection murmurs are common, especially over the pulmonary area. The incidence of regurgitant murmurs increases by more than 20%, secondary to the volume loading and cardiac dilatation. A mild tachycardia results. Pleural effusions do not occur except in preeclampsia.[39] The combination of an effusion, pulmonary venodilatation, and cardiac enlargement may present a radiologic picture suggesting dilatational cardiac failure.

Cardiac Output

From the early stage of pregnancy, wide-ranging cardiovascular changes become apparent (Table 2–3). There is an increase in vascular capacitance and blood volume, an increase in cardiac output, a decrease in systemic vascular resistance, and specific regional redistribution of the high output state.

Cardiac output studies in the pregnant population have been, by nature, limited in availability and number. Small populations, variation in timing of the measurements and the methodology used, as well as the possible effects of aortocaval compression have all made precise interpretation difficult. At best, broad ranges of values may be obtained. There is an overall increase in total blood volume and cardiac output of approximately 30% to 50% to meet the increased demands of pregnancy and the increased blood flow to the uterus and other organs.

Plasma volume increases by about 40% (1200–1600 mL) by the third trimester. A physiologic anemia results as red cell mass increases to a lesser degree. Hematocrit falls until the 30th week of gestation and then slowly rises, as red cell production catches up. The mean arterial pressure commences to fall in the first trimester owing to hormonally induced vasodilatation and a reduction in plasma viscosity. The effects of the low-resistance uteroplacental bed also contribute to this decrease in later pregnancy.

There is a general increase in capacitance of the vascular system (especially in the venous system) to accommodate the increase in blood volume that occurs. Heart rate and stroke volume increase, producing a commensurate increase in cardiac output. Heart rate is one of the first cardiovascular parameters to change. An increase is seen within the first few weeks of pregnancy.[40, 41] The changes in heart rate are extremely difficult to quantify reliably, but there is general agreement of a rise of approximately 15 beats/min (20–30%) present from the 4th week.[42] The normal heart rate variability does not seem to be altered by pregnancy per se, but there is a reduction in the sympathetic component.[43] In disease states such as preeclampsia, there may be a reduction in the vagal component, as measured by heart rate variability.[44] Tachyarrhythmias become more common, under the influence of both hormonal and autonomic factors.[45] Plasma volume increases by 20% to 50%.[46] Cardiac output has been shown to increase from the 5th week, reaching its near maximal increase (40–45%) by 32 weeks, with

Table 2–3 CARDIOVASCULAR CHANGES IN PREGNANCY

PARAMETER	CHANGE	AMOUNT
Heart rate	Increased	20–30%
Stroke volume	Increased	20–50%
Cardiac output	Increased	30–50%
Contractility	Variable	±10%
Central venous pressure	Unchanged	—
Pulmonary capillary wedge pressure	Unchanged	—
Systemic vascular resistance	Decreased	20%
Systemic blood pressure	Slight decrease	Midtrimester 10–15 mm Hg, then rises
Pulmonary vascular resistance	Decreased	30%
Pulmonary artery pressure	Slight decrease	—

Values derived from references 43, 46, 49, and 107.

only a slight increment thereafter.[46, 47] Fifty percent of the cardiac output increase has occurred by the 8th week.[48] Stroke volume appears to peak by about 20 weeks, while the increase in heart rate continues to 32 weeks and beyond.[47] The effects are greater for multiple pregnancies owing to a relatively greater increase in heart rate rather than stroke volume. Cardiac catheter studies are limited but are consistent with other estimates.[49]

Mean arterial blood pressure falls owing to a fall in peripheral resistance from generalized vasodilatation and the development of the low-resistance uteroplacental unit, although the contribution of the latter has probably been overestimated. The mechanism producing vasodilatation remains controversial. Many substances affecting vasomotor tone have been implicated, including prostaglandins,[50] atrial natriuretic peptide (ANP),[51] and endothelium-derived nitric oxide.[52] Nitric oxide production may be selectively increased in uteroplacental beds in which increased flow is critical to maternal and fetal welfare. There is a decreased sensitivity to vasopressors, such as angiotensin II.[53] Interaction with components of the renin-angiotensin system results in an alteration in vasomotor responsiveness that varies with the phase of pregnancy.[54] Overall vasomotor response to angiotensin II is reduced, especially in the uteroplacental bed, perhaps by antagonism from increased prostaglandin production.[55]

Alteration in sensitivity to parenteral vasopressors, α-adrenergic agonists in particular, is unclear and conflicting results have been reported.[56, 57] The antihypertensive angiotensin-converting enzyme inhibitors may interfere with this balance and are contraindicated because of poor fetal outcome.[58] The precise mechanism of volume expansion remains controversial, and theories have been advanced involving activation of the renin-angiotensin mechanism, with resetting of the volume receptors, resulting in an overfill situation that requires progressive adjustment to maintain hemostasis as pregnancy develops.[59] Plasma volume increase involves activation of sodium (and water) retention via increased aldosterone production from the renin-angiotensin mechanism, in turn activated by placental estrogen, derived in part from the developing fetal adrenal gland. Progesterone is a potent natriuretic at the distal tubule level, but this effect is overcome by renin and aldosterone activation. Colloid oncotic pressure decreases in pregnancy, chiefly following a decrease in albumin levels. The precise etiology remains obscure. Albumin levels fall to a minimum immediately after delivery, often to values at which pulmonary edema might be expected.[60] Despite this, the incidence of pulmonary edema remains low for both cesarean and vaginal deliveries. Excess intravenous hydration may be poorly tolerated.

Left atrial size increases with the expansion in blood volume, and some degree of cardiac hypertrophy develops, with an increase in left ventricular mass.[41] The effect may not fully resolve for up to 6 months postpartum.[61] Myocardial contractility also increases.[62] The inotropic effects of estrogens are believed responsible for the increase in contractility, in a dose-related fashion.[63]

Blood Pressure

The changes in systolic blood pressure in normal pregnancy are minor, an initial fall occurring early in the first trimester. The diastolic fall is greater (as is the mean blood pressure fall), being maximal in the second trimester and returning to normal levels at term.[64] The maximal fall in diastolic pressure is 10 to 15 mm Hg. Difficulties have arisen with interpretation of the diastolic pressure value, but current opinion is that the phase 5 Korotkoff sound should be used for greatest accuracy.[65] Blood pressure measurement is also dependent both on patient posture (especially in the third trimester) and on the point of measurement. When the mother is lying in the lateral position, recumbent blood pressure has been found to be consistently lower than supine,[66] probably because of relief of aortic compression and increase in afterload. In this position, the dependent arm provides the most accurate and repeatable measurement.[67] This may be critical in the determination of hypotension (usually defined as a systolic drop of 30%, or an absolute value below 90 mm Hg) following regional anesthesia.[68]

Systemic vascular resistance, as influenced by both cardiac output and mean arterial pressure, also falls to a minimum in the second trimester, and then rises in the third, as does the mean blood pressure. However, because cardiac output remains elevated, systemic vascular resistance must remain decreased below prepregnancy levels to allow normalization of blood pressure. The mechanism of vasodilatation and fall in systemic vascular resistance remains unclear—it has been observed as early as 5 weeks' gestation.[64] Much theory has been attached to the effects of the uteroplacental unit acting as a low-resistance parallel circuit to reduce total peripheral resistance and act as a stimulus for volume expansion. The uteroplacental shunt does not seem to be as large as originally estimated, and the predominant effects are most likely secondary to circulating vasodilators, some of which may be derived from the fetoplacental unit.[69]

Supine Hypotension (Aortocaval Compression)

Posture itself may markedly influence blood pressure in pregnancy. Changes in cardiac output and blood pressure occur in the third trimester with gravidae lying in the supine position. Pregnant women are even more at risk because of reduced sensitivity to circulating vasopressors.[53] Although primarily a result of inferior vena caval occlusion and impairment of venous return by the gravid uterus,[70, 71] aortic compression also contributes to the supine hypotension syndrome in some. Flow to the uterus (and lower limbs) may be reduced by as much as 45% without systemic signs or evidence of aortic compression.[72] The degree depends on the efficiency of the collateral azygous and intervertebral venous plexuses. Approximately 1 in 10 pregnant women become symptomatic,[73] with pallor, sweating, nausea, and hypotension, accompanied by profound bradycardia and fall in cerebral blood flow resulting in unconsciousness if not corrected. The fetus is also affected.[73] The contractions of labor, raising the uterus off the vena cava, may provide some partial relief from the obstruction.[74]

Supine hypotension may occur in other than the conventional position—the upright and near-recumbent positions have also been associated with aortocaval compression.[75] Immediate relief may be effected by positioning in the left lateral position to relieve vena caval compression, although full right lateral tilt may be equally effective.[76] A wedge under the mother's right hip is usually sufficient to prevent symptoms, although extreme tilt may be required to effectively relieve the compression, especially in cases of multiple pregnancy or polyhydramnios. The Trendelenburg position may actually worsen aortocaval compression and impair ventilation, but leg wrapping may be an effective adjuvant at cesarean section.[77]

Sympathetic block owing to epidural or spinal anesthesia reduces the ability to compensate, especially if in a modified supine position. Hypotension may be extreme with extensive blocks, especially if the onset is rapid. Apart from posture and mechanical displacement of the gravid uterus, vasopressors may be required to correct hypotension from major regional blockade. The uteroplacental circulation is critically pressure dependent, and has no means of autoregulation. The uterine vasculature seems more sensitive to the effects of vasopressors than the systemic circulation,[78] and pure α-adrenergic agonists such as metaraminol are best avoided.[79] Ephedrine is the agent of choice, although pure α-adrenergic agents such as phenylephrine have been used with effect in a small dose (100 μg) in some studies in healthy pregnancy.[80, 81] Comparison with ephedrine in stressed physiology has been less favorable, with a demonstrated increase in uterine vascular resistance.[82, 83] Vasopressin is currently being evaluated. Prophylactic crystalloid loading is often ineffective.[84] Ephedrine or phenylephrine seem equally safe[81] when administered intravenously but not by prophylactic intramuscular injection.[85]

In cases requiring cardiopulmonary resuscitation in the third trimester, immediate delivery may be lifesaving as a means of absolutely relieving the compression and reducing the metabolic demand.[86, 87]

Electrocardiogram

The electrocardiogram may show accentuated left axis deviation and minor ST-T wave changes owing to anatomic displacement that are common by the third trimester. Additional changes may be seen at cesarean section under regional anesthesia, but are now thought to be benign, and secondary to imbalance between sympathetic and parasympathetic supply.[88] Similar nonspecific changes may be seen with β-adrenergic agents used for the suppression of premature labor.

Regional Blood Flow

The increase in cardiac output is chiefly directed at the organs of fetomaternal welfare, namely, the uterus and kidneys and also the skin. It is commonly quoted that the uterine blood flow is approximately 500 mL/min in pregnancy, the majority of which is fetoplacental—only 20% or so is estimated to be myometrial. There is very little reported measurement of the actual change in uterine blood flow in early pregnancy, and the studies quoted are old and unlikely to be repeated.[89, 90] The parameters of uterine blood flow seem linked to circulating levels of maternal hormones, at least in the first trimester. By term, the mean uterine arteriolar pressure is probably similar to the mean systemic arterial pressure. The filling of the placental intervillous space is pressure dependent, with no autoregulatory mechanism. Systemic arterial pressure and uterine tone (both resting and contractile) determine effective blood flow during labor. Care must be taken to maintain systemic pressure during major regional blockade both in normotensive and in hypertensive pregnancies.[91, 92]

Renal blood flow rises early in pregnancy, nearing maximum by the second trimester. The early renal vasodilatation of pregnancy may act like an arteriovenous shunt, and account for some of the early large increase in cardiac output. The kidneys become physically enlarged. There is an increase of 30% to 40% in renal blood flow and glomerular filtration rate that is maximal by midpregnancy, but declines in the third trimester toward prepregnant values.[93] The mechanism of this increase is unknown, but it is believed to be secondary to the generalized vasodilatation and volume expansion of early pregnancy. Active vasodilatation is involved, as primary volume expansion alone is not sufficient to explain the increase. The factors that initiate the gestational renal vasodilatation (and plasma volume expansion) are believed to be maternal, not fetoplacental in origin. The precise nature of the initiating factors has not yet been defined; no clear candidate has emerged as a specific renal vasodilator, but nitric oxide may be important in gestational vasodilatation.[94]

Skin blood flow markedly increases as part of general vasodilatation, but with the added purpose of assisting heat dissipation from fetal metabolism. Palmar erythema is often apparent, as is mucosal congestion of the upper airway and nasal passages. Snoring becomes common. Blood flow also increases to the enlarging breasts.

Pulmonary Blood Flow

Pulmonary blood flow increases by nearly 50%, but pulmonary pressures remain unaltered owing to the fall in pulmonary vascular resistance as part of the general vascular dilatation of the first trimester.[95] Most of the significant changes have resolved by 2 weeks postpartum, but full resolution may take 6 months.

Labor and Delivery

During labor and delivery cardiac output progressively rises. There are progressive increases in both stroke volume and heart rate, peaking with contractions. The rise in cardiac output between contractions varies from 12% to 31%, owing to an increase in stroke volume rather than heart rate.[43] The rise in cardiac output with contractions (approximately 15% on Doppler studies)[96] is complex, involving uterine contracture with squeezing of blood from the intervillous space, and reduction of the uteroplacental shunt, the sympathetic stimulation of pain, and possible relief of aortocaval compression as the contracting uterus lifts forward.[97] The volume contribution of the contraction has been estimated at 200 to 300 mL.[98] Systolic pressure increases in labor by about 35 mm Hg, and diastolic pressure by about 25 mm Hg.[96] Cesarean section also produces similar blood pressure rises with delivery.

Effective analgesia is known to significantly reduce the stress of labor and affect the circulating levels of catecholamines, mitigating the rise in blood pressure.[99] Epinephrine but not norepinephrine levels are significantly reduced.[100] Both epinephrine and norepinephrine decrease uterine contractility. Reduction in epinephrine levels has been shown to improve uterine contractility.[101] Excessively dramatic reductions in epinephrine levels with the profound analgesia that occurs with combined spinal-epidural analgesia have been postulated in the causation of acute hypertonus and fetal distress.[102] Cardiac output and uteroplacental perfusion (if normotension is maintained) is better maintained with regional rather than general anesthesia.[4] The effects of regional anesthesia on uteroplacental flow show some evidence for a small degree of autoregulation to offset small changes in maternal perfusion pressure.[103]

Postpartum Changes

Cardiac output peaks within 10 minutes of delivery,[4, 99] with the additional effect of relief of aortocaval compression,[104] and augmented venous return of parenteral oxytocics to offset any drop in output from blood loss. The cardiac output remains elevated (7 L/min) for about 24 hours after delivery, rapidly falling over the next 2 weeks, but not reaching prepregnancy levels until the sixth month.[48, 61] Left atrial size remains elevated for the first 48 hours owing to the increased venous return of the puerperium, with loss of the uteroplacental shunt.[105] Blood pressure falls mostly in the first 2 days.[106] Most cardiovascular parameters are well resolved by 2 weeks, but a mild degree of ventricular hypertrophy may persist for several months.[43]

RENAL FUNCTION

The urinary collecting system undergoes massive dilatation in pregnancy under the effect of progesterone and probably the secondary mechanical effects of compression on the distal ureters by the enlarging uterus. Compression may occur in the upright as well as supine posture. Ureteric and urinary stasis develops, with an increased incidence of urinary tract infection.

Renal plasma flow and glomerular filtration rate (GFR) both increase early in pregnancy as part of the rise in cardiac output. The increase in GFR precedes the expansion of blood volume, and is seen as an early marker of the phenomenon of generalized vasodilatation.[107] The rise in GFR of nearly 50% and the dilutional effect of the expanded plasma volume accounts for the fall in plasma creatinine and urea. Values for "normal" function in pregnancy are decreased below those of the nonpregnant state. Effective renal plasma flow (ERPF) increases by up to 80% by the second trimester[108] and then falls in the third trimester to about 50% above nonpregnant levels.[93] GFR increases less than the ERPF in early pregnancy, so that the filtration fraction (i.e., the GFR-ERPF ratio) actually decreases. The GFR rise is relatively maintained, and plasma creatinine rises slightly.[109] The filtration fraction rises to approach nonpregnant values in the third trimester because of the greater efficiency of the increased GFR, as well as the dilutional effect of the increased plasma volume.

Urea, creatinine, and uric acid clearance all rise, resulting in lowered "normal" levels in the pregnant state (Table 2–4). Nonpregnant values are effectively pathologic in the pregnant state. Glycosuria is common owing both to a reduction in tubular capacity for reabsorption and to the increased GFR.

Autoregulation of blood flow is maintained, even in the presence of renal vasodilatation. Orthostatic proteinuria commonly occurs, probably related to compression of the left renal vein by the enlarging uterus. The handling of sodium is maintained, but with a background of progressive accumulation of approximately 950 mmol/L of total body sodium over the duration of the pregnancy. Renal tubular handling of sodium loading is maintained, but plasma sodium levels fall by 4 to 5 mmol/L as part of the plasma volume expansion.

Osmolality falls by approximately 10 mOsm/kg because of the fall in sodium, and additional minor

Table 2–4 VALUES FOR RENAL FUNCTION

PARAMETER	PREGNANT	NONPREGNANT
Creatinine clearance	140–160 mL/min	90–110 mL/min
Urea	2.0–4.5 mmol/L	6–7 mmol/L
Creatinine	25–75 μmol/L	100 μmol/L
Uric acid	0.2	0.35
pH	7.44	7.40
Bicarbonate	18–22 mmol/L	23–26 mmol/L

Values derived from references 180 and 181.

alteration in plasma protein levels. Antidiuretic hormone threshold and thirst receptor sensitivities are both reduced in early pregnancy to potentiate this hypervolemia.[110] Protein excretion is increased, and the upper limit of normal in pregnancy is 300 mg/L. Uncomplicated pregnancy does not influence the course of most underlying renal disease if it is mild.[111]

Fluid Balance and Body Weight

Total body water increases by 7 to 8 L, and is the main source of weight increase. Plasma volume increases by 1.5 L, and extracellular volume increases by 6.5 L.[112] Lymphatic clearance is increased, and plasma oncotic pressure decreases in proportion to the fall in albumin, but the generalized edema is related to an alteration in capillary permeability. Owing to protein redistribution, tissue oncotic pressure decreases more than plasma oncotic pressure, contributing to the increase in plasma volume. There is a resting increase in lymphatic flow, which together with the reduction in oncotic pressure, reduces the safety margin in volume overload states.[113]

Acid-Base Balance

In normal pregnancy the changes of respiratory hyperventilation secondary to elevated progesterone levels produce a mild, compensated respiratory alkalemia with a pH of approximately 7.44. The venous pH rises from 7.35 to 7.38 because of the effect of increased cardiac output. The alkalemia occurs from early pregnancy. A partial renal compensation occurs with a fall in bicarbonate (and sodium) excretion. Normal plasma bicarbonate levels in pregnancy are reduced by 3 to 6 mmol/L. The alkalemia is exaggerated by hyperventilation in labor, and, with the further left shift of the oxyhemoglobin dissociation curve, may compromise fetal oxygenation.[114]

GASTROINTESTINAL FUNCTION

Gastric Emptying

Much controversy persists regarding the effects of pregnancy and labor on gastric emptying and gastric volume. The effects of increased progesterone levels may be seen in the first trimester with the development of esophageal reflux and symptoms of heartburn. The incidence increases with the period of gestation, as does the severity of symptoms: 22% in the first trimester, and more than 70% by the third trimester.[115] The reduction in tone is not directly related to progesterone levels. The incidence of reflux is higher than the incidence of symptoms, and all women at term must be considered at risk.[116] The etiology is complex and multifactorial and primarily involves reduced lower esophageal sphincter tone,[117] but also delayed intestinal transit time and duodenogastric reflux,[118] but only in the second and third trimesters.[119] Normalization of transit times occurs within 18 hours postpartum.[120] Intragastric pressure remains unchanged in pregnancy, with no mechanical effect exerted by the presence of the enlarged uterus. It was previously believed that gastric emptying was delayed in pregnancy, but recent studies have shown that there is no delay[121, 122] except in established labor, and then especially if prolonged.[123] All narcotics delay gastric emptying, but the effect is probably dose related. Epidural doses of fentanyl of less than 100 μg have been shown to have no effect on gastric function.[124] Acid secretion diminishes in the first and second trimester, and remains depressed with the immediate postpartum period.

"Morning sickness" of the first trimester is a common occurrence in early pregnancy, and usually disappears by the end of the first trimester, but may persist to a varying amount thereafter. This may occasionally progress to a syndrome of hyperemesis requiring hospitalization, parenteral rehydration, and possible parenteral nutrition. Associated mild hepatic dysfunction may occur. Elevated estrogen and progesterone levels are believed to be responsible for the delayed gastrointestinal transit time found in pregnancy. Arrhythmias of gastric motility secondary to elevated progesterone and estrogen levels are believed to be partly responsible for the nausea.[125] Thirty percent of women report constipation. Pregnancy has been associated with delay in gastric emptying, attributed to the effects of progesterone. Delay in gastric emptying is present from the end of the first trimester.

The issue is further complicated in labor, as pain and narcotics (including neuraxially administered narcotics) both delay emptying and promote emesis. The exact time of commencement remains controversial and persists into the puerperium for a variable period. The exact duration of risk remains uncertain, but is significantly reduced by the second day after delivery.[126] The volume of gastric secretion is believed to be increased secondary to the effects of high levels of placentally derived gastrin.[127]

The use of endotracheal intubation if general anesthesia is induced during this intrapartum period is mandatory, because of the ill-defined risk of aspiration of gastric contents.

Hepatic Function

Liver function is maintained in normal pregnancy, and the overall blood flow probably remains unchanged.[128] The general metabolic functions of the liver increase to cope with the demands of pregnancy. There is a threefold elevation of alkaline phosphatase (mainly placental in origin), and some reduction in sulfobromophthalein suggesting a mild degree of cholestasis. Bilirubin and transaminase levels remain within the normal range.[129] Plasma cholinesterase levels fall by nearly 30% by the first trimester and remain stable until delivery.[130] They fall again in the first week of the puerperium, and recover to normal by the first 6 weeks.[131] The prolongation is usually of no significance in the normal population, but those with atypical cholinesterase require careful monitoring. Nondepolarizing relaxants may also show some increased potency.[132, 133]

Total plasma proteins fall by about 20% by the second trimester. Plasma albumin levels fall sharply initially, and then plateau. It is this fall in albumin that is largely responsible for the fall in total proteins. The mechanism is unclear, as albumin synthesis is probably maintained.[134] The effect of drug binding is variable, because the fall in plasma concentration in the first half of pregnancy is offset by the rise in plasma volume in later pregnancy. The total circulating albumin remains unchanged. Plasma globulins increase but to a lesser degree than the fall in albumin, and the albumin-globulin ratio falls. Fibrinogen levels markedly increase, and there are rises in transferrin and specific binding proteins, for example, thyroid-binding globulin and corticosteroid-binding globulin.

Most plasma lipids, including triglycerides and cholesterol, rise progressively throughout pregnancy. A state of relative hyperlipidemia results.[135] Drug metabolism is variable. The extraction of hepatically cleared drugs remains unaltered, but protein binding, volume of distribution, fat solubility, renal clearance, and alteration in neurologic sensitivity all determine the clinical effect.

Gallbladder

Progesterone antagonizes the release of cholecystokinin and results in gallbladder dysfunction. Cholesterol secretion is increased and bile acid is decreased.[136] The incidence of biliary sludge and gallstones is increased in pregnancy.

ENDOCRINE FUNCTION

After fertilization, the corpus luteum is initially sustained by the secretion of human chorionic gonadotropin (hCG) from the developing placenta. Estrogen, progesterone, and relaxin are secreted. By the 6th to 8th week, placental function has developed as the primary source of progesterone and estrogen, with ovarian production no longer significant. The hCG levels peak in the first trimester, but estrogen, progesterone, and prolactin continue to rise until term, at which time falling levels are associated with the onset of labor.[137] Progesterone levels reach approximately 20 times the nonpregnant value. Human placental lactogen (HPL) levels rise throughout pregnancy, with effects on carbohydrate and protein metabolism similar to growth hormone. The main function of HPL is control of fetal growth and optimal utilization of fetal nutrients.[138] It is believed responsible for some of the acromegalic-like maternal changes sometimes seen that make anesthetic access difficult, as well as being a factor in maternal insulin resistance.

Diabetes

The hormonal and metabolic changes in pregnancy result in a diabetogenic state, and it is estimated that 4% of all pregnancies in the United States are now complicated by diabetes.[36] The vast majority of these women (88%) have gestational diabetes; only 4% of the total are insulin dependent. The primary fetal energy substrate is maternally derived glucose. During pregnancy, there is increased insulin production, and progressively increased resistance to its action. There is a further deterioration in the third trimester, the period of maximal fetal growth. Difficulties with control of insulin and an aging maternal population have now become factors in development of macrosomia and adverse fetal outcome.[139] Gestational diabetes may also develop from this hyperglycemia tendency in nondiabetic pregnant women—the actual incidence varies with the population and the diagnostic criteria applied to screening tests.[140] Unrecognized gestational diabetes carries special risks of macrosomia and difficult operative delivery.[141] All forms of diabetes carry associated risks of obesity, hypertension, and increased cesarean section rate.

Thyroid Function

Thyroid dysfunction may become apparent in the metabolic stress of pregnancy. The thyroid gland undergoes mild enlargement owing to a reactionary follicular hyperplasia. The enlargement increases iodine uptake and offsets iodine losses secondary to the increased renal clearance of iodine and the fetal transfer of iodine. Thyroid-binding globulin levels increase, as does total thyroxine (T_4) and triiodothyronine (T_3) levels, but free T_4 levels remain within normal values. T_4, T_3, and TSH (thyroid-stimulating hormone) (via the hypothalamic-pituitary-thyroid axis) functions are unchanged.[142]

Many of the features of pregnancy mimic hyperthyroidism apart from the expected weight gain. Hyperthyroidism may develop in pregnancy, although the immune suppression of pregnancy, under the influence of estrogen and progesterone, with fetal or maternal production of inhibitory cytokines, makes this less likely.[143, 144] Thyrotoxicosis, however, may be more likely to present postpartum, with the reversal of the physiologic immunosuppression of pregnancy.[145]

Parathyroid Function

Parathyroid function and calcium metabolism are critical to fetal growth and development. Serum calcium levels fall, but ionized calcium remains within the normal range, protecting calcium-dependent functions. Maternal parathyroid hormone levels progressively fall to 30% of prepregnancy values owing to inhibition by placentally produced peptide with parathyroid hormone activity.[146]

MUSCULOSKELETAL SYSTEM

Backache becomes increasingly common in the second half of pregnancy under the effects of progesterone and relaxin. The increased lordosis is necessary to accommodate the increasing size of the fetus within the abdominal cavity, and may increase the technical difficulty for epidural and spinal anesthesia. Ligamentous laxity in the widening of the pelvis and change in gait develop. The skin becomes thicker with increasing water retention. Nonspecific edema develops in over 40% of all pregnancies.[147, 148] Breast enlargement is a potential risk factor for difficult intubation in which conventional laryngoscopes are used—a shortened handle or offset blade may be of advantage.[149, 150] Backache during and following pregnancy remains a common problem, whether or not regional anesthesia has been used.[151, 152]

NEUROLOGIC CHANGES

Emotional changes are common in pregnancy. Diminished cognitive ability, often the subject of much conjecture and humor, has been demonstrated in at least one study, in which a specific memory loss related to recall was demonstrated in 81% of pregnant women.[153]

There is an increased sensitivity to centrally acting pharmacologic agents including opioids, sedatives, and general anesthetic agents. The minimal alveolar concentration (MAC) is reduced by about one third in most studies.[154, 155] Recovery usually occurs by the third day postpartum.[156] Care must be taken with the administration of sedative doses of agents, to avoid unexpected loss of consciousness. There is a similar reduction of about 30% in dose requirement for local anesthetics, for both epidural and spinal administration. Previously, anatomic and physiologic factors (reduced epidural space from venous distention and increased epidural pressures in labor) were viewed as the causes of this increased sensitivity. It is now believed to be progesterone mediated, since this reduction in dose requirement is present by the first trimester.[157]

Brain size has also been observed to be reduced, although the mechanism is not well understood.[158] There is evidence for sex differentiation in response to administered opioids, with female rats being more resistant to the antinociceptive properties of morphine. Whether this is due to hormonal or metabolic factors and its relevance to hormonal influences of pregnancy are yet to be elucidated.[159]

Increased toxicity to specific local anesthetics (i.e., bupivacaine and etidocaine) in pregnancy has been postulated.[160] This, however, has not been demonstrated on repeat investigation; differences are attributed to alteration in protein binding and free plasma levels rather than specific enhanced toxicity.[161]

The ligamentous relaxation of pregnancy, and postural adaptations to accommodate the growing fetus, may make regional anesthesia technically more difficult. Identification of landmarks may be difficult in the presence of generalized edema.

HEMATOLOGIC CHANGES

There is a dilutional anemia, despite an increase in red cell mass. The accepted normal lower level of hemoglobin in pregnancy is approximately 10.5 g/dL. Requirements for iron and folate are increased, and routine supplements are prescribed. A maximal rise in hemoglobin in response to treatment is approximately 0.8 g/dL per week.[162] Hemoglobin, hematocrit, and red cell count all fall. Erythrocyte volume actually increases as a consequence of the erythropoietic effect of placental chorionic somatomammotropin, progesterone, and prolactin.[69] Plasma volume ultimately increases by approximately 50%. The actual increase in volume correlates with fetal size.[163] Multiple pregnancy results in a further relative drop in hemoglobin owing to the greater plasma volume expansion.[164]

A progressive fall in hematocrit and blood viscosity occurs in the first and second trimesters. The fall in viscosity and hematocrit is due to the relative increase in plasma volume over hematocrit, producing a physiologic hemodilution. The reduction in viscosity contributes to the increase in cardiac output. This reduction peaks by the third trimester, with a slight increase in hematocrit and viscosity in the last 4 weeks. The plasma volume peaks at about 34 weeks. The rise in viscosity in the third trimester is due to the increase in high molecular weight proteins (e.g., fibrinogen and immunoglobulins) that outweighs the decrease in total protein and albumin with increasing gestation.[165]

Still greater reductions in blood viscosity and hematocrit levels will be found in populations with hemoglobinopathies or deficiency states. The subsequent intrapartum or postpartum blood loss that occurs varies with the mode of delivery, whether operative (forceps or cesarean section) or spontaneous vaginal delivery. There is some offset in the fall in hemoglobin that occurs as a result of the postpartum diuresis. The actual safe functional lower limit of hemoglobin in the postpartum period is still debated. Most transfusion services recommend a level of 7 g/dL for healthy nonpregnant patients. The functional level for an acute loss seems to be closer to 8 g/dL or greater to cope with the acute rise in metabolic demand in the postpartum period.

The changes in the coagulation system have been traditionally believed to be a physiologically protective adaptation for parturition and the risks of acute hemorrhage. There is a state of hypercoagulability, confirmed by thromboelastography.[166] Thrombosis leading to thromboembolism is one of the major causes of maternal mortality in the Western world. As discussed in Chapter 31, pregnancy increases the risk of thromboembolism sixfold, with cesarean section further increasing the risk 10- to 20-fold.

The platelet count remains unchanged throughout pregnancy, but with a small reduction in the third trimester with an increase in in vivo activity. The effective safe limit had been accepted as $100,000 \times 10^9/L$,[167] although this has been challenged in recent times, and counts as low as $69 \times 10^9/L$ have been postulated as acceptable in the absence of clinical bleeding.[168] The platelet count rises transiently postpartum as an acute reaction to activation of hemostasis at delivery.

There is a general increase in both absolute amounts and plasma levels of factors in both the intrinsic and extrinsic coagulation systems, especially factors XII, X, and VIII (Table 2–5). The exception is a fall in factor XI, which reaches its lowest value at term.[165] Factor VII, the main component of the extrinsic pathway, also increases. Within the final common pathway of coagulation, only factor X and fibrinogen are mark-

Table 2-5 COAGULATION FACTORS IN PREGNANCY

FACTOR	CHANGE
II	Unchanged
VII	Increased + + +
VIII, IX, X, XII	Increased
XI	Reduced
Fibrinogen	Increased + + +
Platelets	Stable

edly increased, the latter by the first trimester and doubling by term. The endogenous inhibitor of coagulation, antithrombin III, remains unchanged.[169] Fibrinolytic activity is impaired throughout pregnancy owing to a placentally derived plasminogen inhibitor. The coagulation and fibrinolytic systems are both further activated at delivery by placental separation with thromboplastin release.[170] Hemostatic systems return to the normal nonpregnant state by the end of the third or fourth week postpartum.[171]

Immunologic Changes

Total white blood cell count rises to about 9×10^9/L by the 30th week, with a further rise at delivery.[172] There is a relative neutrophilia, presumably owing to estrogen influence. The lymphocyte count is unchanged, with normal levels of circulating T and B cells.[173] Cell-mediated immunity is severely depressed by circulating factors, presumably estrogen mediated.[174, 175]

Human chorionic gonadotropin and prolactin are also associated with suppression of cellular immunity.[176] The success of the survival of the allografted fetoplacental unit probably depends on this depression of cellular immunity. Increased susceptibility to viral infections, such as hepatitis, herpes, rubella, and human papillomavirus, occurs as a result.

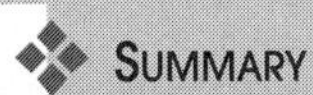

SUMMARY

Key Points

- Significant physiologic changes are well established by the end of the first trimester.
- Metabolic, cardiovascular, and respiratory changes are the most apparent, but no body system is unaffected.
- Decreased functional residual capacity (FRC), reduction in lower esophageal sphincter tone, and airway changes all increase the risk associated with general anesthesia.
- Compression of the inferior vena cava by the gravid uterus may produce profound hypotension; therefore, the patient in labor should avoid the supine position.
- Labor and delivery are the greatest stresses in pregnancy.

Key Reference

Sibai BM, Frangieh A: Maternal adaptation to pregnancy. Curr Opin Obstet Gynecol 1995; 7:420–426.

Case Stem

An obese multiparous patient at 26 weeks' gestation presents with abdominal pain following blunt trauma to the abdomen. On examination, she is tachypneic: BP = 100/70; heart rate = 98. Discuss the interpretation of these vital signs in light of her underlying pregnancy. Discuss the physiologic changes of pregnancy and their impact on the administration of anesthesia.

References

1. Steer PJ, Johnson MR: The genital system. *In* Chamberlain G, Pipkin FB (eds): Clinical Physiology in Obstetrics, 3rd ed. Oxford, England: Blackwell; 1998:308.
2. Prentice AM, Goldberg GR, Davies HL, et al: Energy-sparing adaptations in human pregnancy assessed by whole-body calorimetry. Br J Nutr 1989; 62:5.
3. Illingworth PJ, Jung RT, Howie PW, et al: Reduction in postprandial energy expenditure during pregnancy. Br Med J (Clin Res Ed) 1987; 294(G587):1573.
4. James CF, Banner T, Caton D: Cardiac output in women undergoing cesarean section with epidural or general anesthesia. Am J Obstet Gynecol 1989; 160(5 Pt 1):1178.
5. Puranik BM, Kaore SB, Kurhade GA, et al: A longitudinal study of pulmonary function tests during pregnancy. Indian J Physiol Pharmacol 1994; 38:129.
6. Knuttgen HG, Emerson K: Physiological response to pregnancy at rest and during exercise. J Appl Physiol 1974; 36:549.
7. Clapp JF, Seaward BL, Sleamaker RH, et al: Maternal physiologic adaptations to early human pregnancy. Am J Obstet Gynecol 1988; 159:1456.
8. Machida H: Influence of progesterone on arterial blood and CSF acid-base balance in women. J Appl Physiol 1981; 51:1433.
9. Takano N: Resting pulmonary ventilation and dead space ventilation during the menstrual cycle. Jpn Physiol 1982; 32:468.
10. Takano N: Changes of ventilation and ventilatory response to hypoxia during the menstrual cycle. Pflugers Arch 1984; 402:312.
11. McCullogh JC, Kelly AM: Investigation of pregnancy-related changes in red cell 2,3-diphosphoglycerate. Clin Chim Acta 1979; 98:235.
12. Samsoon GL, Young JR: Difficult tracheal intubation: a retrospective study. Anaesthesia 1987; 42:487.
13. Lyons G: Failed intubation: six years' experience in a teaching maternity unit. Anaesthesia 1985; 40:759.
14. Hawthorne L, Wilson R, Lyons G, et al: Failed intubation revisited: 17-yr experience in a teaching maternity unit. Br J Anaesth 1996; 76:680.
15. Rocke DA, Murray WB, Rout CC, et al: Relative risk analysis of factors associated with difficult intubation in obstetric anesthesia. Anesthesiology 1992; 77:67.
16. Milne JA, Mills RJ, Howie AD, et al: Large airway function during normal pregnancy. Br J Obstet Gynaecol 1977; 84:448.
17. Metcalfe J, Bissonnette JM: Gas exchange in pregnancy. *In* Fishman AP, Farhi LE, Tenney SM, et al (eds): Handbook of Physiology. Section 3: The Respiratory System. Bethesda, MD: American Physiological Society; 1987.
18. Bevan DR, Holdcroft A, Loh L, et al: Closing volume and pregnancy. Br Med J 1974; 1:13.
19. Garrard GS, Littler WA, Redman CW: Closing volume in pregnancy. Thorax 1978; 33:488.
20. Russell IF, Chambers WA: Closing volume in normal pregnancy. Br J Anaesth 1981; 53:1043.
21. Norregaard O, Schultz P, Ostergaard A, et al: Lung function

and postural changes during pregnancy. Resp Med 1989; 83:467.
22. Baraka AS, Hanna MT, Jabbour SI, et al: Preoxygenation of pregnant and nonpregnant women in the head-up versus supine position. Anesth Analg 1992; 75:757.
23. Boggess KA, Easterling TR, Raghu G: Management and outcome of pregnant women with interstitial and restrictive lung disease. Am J Obstet Gynecol 1995; 173:1007.
24. Herpolsheimer A, Brady K, Yancey MK, et al: Pulmonary function of preeclamptic women receiving intravenous magnesium sulfate seizure prophylaxis. Obstet Gynecol 1991; 78:241.
25. Conn DA, Moffatt AC, McCallum GDR, et al: Changes in pulmonary function tests during spinal anaesthesia for caesarean section. Int J Obstet Anaesth 1993; 2:12.
26. Bourne T, Ogilvy AJ, Vickers R, et al: Nocturnal hypoxaemia in late pregnancy. Br J Anaesth 1995; 75:678.
27. Ackerman DWE, Molnar JM, Juneja MM: Beneficial effect of epidural anesthesia on oxygen consumption in a parturient with adult respiratory distress syndrome. South Med J 1993; 86:361.
28. Zelcer J, Owers H, Paull JD: A controlled oximetric evaluation of inhalational, opioid and epidural analgesia in labour. Anaesth Intensive Care 1989; 17:418.
29. Reed PN, Colquhoun AD, Hanning CD: Maternal oxygenation during normal labour. Br J Anaesth 1989; 62:316.
30. Feinsilver SH, Hertz G: Respiration during sleep in pregnancy. Clin Chest Med 1992; 13:637.
31. Sady MA, Haydon BB, Sady SP, et al: Cardiovascular response to maximal cycle exercise during pregnancy and at two and seven months post partum. Am J Obstet Gynecol 1990; 162:1181.
32. Stenius-Aarniala B, Piirila P, Teramo K: Asthma and pregnancy: a prospective study of 198 pregnancies. Thorax 1988; 43:12.
33. Juniper EF, Daniel EE, Roberts RS, et al: Improvement in airway responsiveness and asthma severity during pregnancy: a prospective study. Am Rev Respir Dis 1989; 140:924.
34. Stenius-Aarniala BS, Hedman J, Teramo KA: Acute asthma during pregnancy. Thorax 1996; 51:411.
35. Fitzsimons R, Greenberger PA, Patterson R: Outcome of pregnancy in women requiring corticosteroids for severe asthma. J Allergy Clin Immunol 1986; 78:349.
36. Mason E, Rosene-Montella K, Powrie R: Medical problems during pregnancy. Med Clin North Am 1998; 82:249.
37. Crowhurst JA: Salbutamol, obstetrics and anaesthesia: a review and case discussion. Anaesth Intensive Care 1980; 8:39.
38. Ekblad U, Kanto J: Pregnancy outcome in an extremely small woman with muscular dystrophy and respiratory insufficiency. Acta Anaesthesiol Scand 1993; 37:228.
39. Wallis MG, McHugo JM, Carruthers DA, et al: The prevalence of pleural effusions in preeclampsia: an ultrasound study. Br J Obstet Gynaecol 1989; 96:431.
40. Capeless EL, Clapp JF: Cardiovascular changes in early phase of pregnancy. Am J Obstet Gynecol 1989; 161:1439.
41. Duvekot JJ, Cheriex EC, Pieters FAA, et al: Early-pregnancy changes in hemodynamics and volume hemostasis are consecutive adjustments triggered by a primary fall in systemic vascular tone. Am J Obstet Gynecol 1993; 169:1382.
42. Hytten FE, Leitch I: The Physiology of Human Pregnancy, 2nd ed. Oxford, England: Blackwell Scientific Publications; 1971.
43. Duvekot JJ, Peeters LL: Maternal cardiovascular hemodynamic adaptation to pregnancy. Obstet Gynecol Surv 1994; 49(12 suppl):S1.
44. Eneroth-Grimfors E, Westgren M, Ericson M, et al: Autonomic cardiovascular control in normal and pre-eclamptic pregnancy. Acta Obstet Gynecol Scand 1994; 73:680.
45. Widerhorn J, Widerhorn AL, Rahimtoola SH, et al: WPW syndrome during pregnancy: increased incidence of supraventricular arrhythmias. Am Heart J 1992; 123:796.
46. Mabie WC, DiSessa TG, Crocker LG, et al: A longitudinal study of cardiac output in normal human pregnancy. Am J Obstet Gynecol 1994; 170:849.
47. Hunter S, Robson SC: Adaptation of the maternal heart in pregnancy. Br Heart J 1992; 68:540.
48. Capeless EL, Clapp JR: When do cardiovascular parameters return to their preconception values? Am J Obstet Gynecol 1991; 161:883.
49. Clark SL, Cotton DB, Lee W, et al: Central hemodynamic assessment of normal term pregnancy. Am J Obstet Gynecol 1989; 161(6 Pt 1):1439.
50. Myatt L: Vasoactive factors in pregnancy. Maternal Fetal Med Rev 1992; 4:15.
51. Kaufman S, Deng Y, Thai W, et al: Influence of pregnancy on ANF release from isolated atria. Am J Physiol 1994; 266(5 Pt 2):1605.
52. Chu ZM, Beilin LJ: Mechanisms of vasodilatation in pregnancy: studies of the role of prostaglandins and nitric oxide in changes of vascular reactivity in the in situ blood perfused mesentery of pregnant rats. Br J Pharmacol 1993; 109(2):322.
53. Magness RR, Cox K, Rosenfeld CR, et al: Angiotensin II metabolic clearance rate and pressor responses in nonpregnant and pregnant women. Am J Obstet Gynecol 1994; 171:668.
54. Chu ZM, Beilin LJ: The role of angiotensin converting enzyme and nitric oxide in the enhanced systemic depressor responses to bradykinin in pregnant rats. Clin Exp Pharmacol Physiol 1995; 22:481.
55. Magness RR, Rosenfeld CR: Calcium modulation of endothelium-derived prostacyclin production in ovine pregnancy. Endocrinology 1993; 132:2445.
56. McLaughlin MK, Keve TM, Cooke R: Vascular catecholamine sensitivity during pregnancy in the ewe. Am J Obstet Gynecol 1989; 160:47.
57. Pan ZR, Lindheimer MD, Bailin J, et al: Regulation of blood pressure in pregnancy: pressor system blockade and stimulation. Am J Physiol 1990; 258(5 Pt 2):H1559.
58. Shotan A, Widerhorn J, Hurst A, et al: Risks of angiotensin-converting enzyme inhibition during pregnancy: experimental and clinical evidence, potential mechanisms, and recommendations for use. Am J Med 1994; 96:451.
59. Bayliss C, Davison JM: The urinary system. *In* Chamberlain G, Pipkin FB (eds): Clinical Physiology in Obstetrics, 3rd ed. Oxford, Blackwell Science; 1998:263.
60. Cotton DB, Gonik B, Spillman T, et al: Intrapartum to postpartum changes in colloid osmotic pressure. Am J Obstet Gynecol 1984; 149:174.
61. Robson SC, Hunter S, Moore M, et al: Haemodynamic changes during the puerperium: a Doppler and M-mode echocardiographic study. Br J Obstet Gynaecol 1987; 94:1028.
62. Rubler S, Damani PM, Pinto ER: Cardiac size and performance during pregnancy estimated with echocardiography. Am J Cardiol 1977; 40:534.
63. Slater AJ, Gude N, Clarke IJ: Haemodynamic changes and left ventricular performance during high-dose estrogen administration to male transsexuals. Br J Obstet Gynaecol 1986; 93:532.
64. Robson SC, Hunter S, Boys RJ: Serial study of factors influencing changes in cardiac output during human pregnancy. Am J Physiol 1989; 256(4 Pt 2):H1060.
65. Johenning AR, Barron WM: Indirect blood pressure measurement in pregnancy: Korotkoff phase 4 versus phase 5. Am J Obstet Gynecol 1992; 167:577.
66. Trower R, Walters WA: Brachial arterial blood pressure in the lateral recumbent position during pregnancy. Aust N Z J Obstet Gynaecol 1968; 8:146.
67. Kinsella SM, Spencer JA: Blood pressure measurement in the lateral position. Br J Obstet Gynaecol 1989; 96:1110.
68. Kinsella SM, Black AM: Reporting of 'hypotension' after epidural analgesia during labour: effect of choice of arm and timing of baseline readings. Anaesthesia 1998; 53:131.
69. Longo LD: Maternal blood volume and cardiac output during pregnancy: a hypothesis of endocrinologic control. Am J Physiol 1983; 245(5 Pt 1):R720.
70. Howard BK, Godson JH, Mengert WF: Supine hypotension in late pregnancy. Obstet Gynecol 1953; 1:371.
71. Kerr MG, Scott DB, Samuel E: Studies of the inferior vena cava in late pregnancy. BMJ 1964; 1:532.
72. Kinsella SM, Lee A, Spencer JA: Maternal and fetal effects of

the supine and pelvic tilt positions in late pregnancy. Eur J Obstet Gynecol Reprod Biol 1990; 36:11.
73. Pirhonen JP, Erkkola RU: Uterine and umbilical flow velocity waveforms in the supine hypotensive syndrome. Obstet Gynecol 1990; 76:176.
74. Ueland K, Hansen JM: Maternal cardiovascular dynamics. II. Posture and uterine contractions. Am J Obstet Gynecol 1969; 103:1.
75. Shneider KTM, Bollinger A, Huch A, et al: The oscillating "vena cava syndrome" during quiet standing—an unexpected observation in late pregnancy. Br J Obstet Gynaecol 1984; 91:700.
76. Clark SL, Cotton DB, Pivarnik JM, et al: Position change and central hemodynamic profile during normal third trimester pregnancy and post-partum. Am J Obstet Gynecol 1991; 164:883.
77. Bhagwanjee S, Rocke DA, Rout CC, et al: Prevention of hypotension following spinal anaesthesia for elective caesarean section by wrapping of the legs. Br J Anaesth 1990; 65:819.
78. Magness RR, Rosenfeld CR: Systemic and uterine responses to alpha-adrenergic stimulation in pregnant and nonpregnant ewes. Am J Obstet Gynecol 1986; 155:897.
79. Ralston DH, Shnider SM, DeLorimier AA: Effects of equipotent ephedrine, metaraminol, mephentermine, and methoxamine on uterine blood flow in the pregnant ewe. Anesthesiology 1974; 40:354.
80. Ramanathan S, Grant GJ: Vasopressor therapy for hypotension due to epidural anaesthesia for caesarean section. Acta Anaesthesiol Scand 1988; 32:559.
81. LaPorta RF, Arthur GR, Datta S: Phenylephrine in treating maternal hypotension due to spinal anaesthesia for caesarean delivery: effects on neonatal catecholamine concentrations, acid base status and Apgar scores. Acta Anaesthesiol Scand 1995; 39:901.
82. Sipes SL, Chestnut DH, Vincent RDJ, et al: Which vasopressor should be used to treat hypotension during magnesium sulfate infusion and epidural anesthesia? Anesthesiology 1992; 77:101.
83. McGrath JM, Chestnut D, Vincent RD, et al: Ephedrine remains the vasopressor of choice for treatment of hypotension during ritodrine infusion and epidural anesthesia. Anesthesiology 1994; 80:1073.
84. Rout CC, Rocke DA, Levin J, et al: A reevaluation of the role of crystalloid preload in the prevention of hypotension associated with spinal anesthesia for elective cesarean section. Anesthesiology 1993; 79:262.
85. Rout CC, Rocke DA, Brijball R, et al: Prophylactic intramuscular ephedrine prior to caesarean section. Anaesth Intensive Care 1992; 20:448.
86. Goodwin AP, Pearce AJ: The human wedge: a manoeuvre to relieve aortocaval compression during resuscitation in late pregnancy. Anaesthesia 1992; 47:433.
87. O'Connor RL, Sevarino FB: Cardiopulmonary arrest in the pregnant patient: a report of a successful resuscitation. J Clin Anesth 1994; 6:66.
88. McLintic AJ, Pringle SD, Lilley S, et al: Electrocardiographic changes during caesarean section under regional anaesthesia. Anesth Analg 1992; 74:51.
89. Assali NS, Rauramo L, Peltonen T: Uterine and fetal blood flow and oxygen consumption in early human pregnancy. Am J Obstet Gynecol 1960; 79:86.
90. Romney SL, Reid DE, Metcalfe J, et al: Oxygen utilization in the human fetus in utero. Am J Obstet Gynecol 1955; 70:791.
91. Jouppila R, Jouppila P, Hollmén A, et al: Epidural analgesia and placental blood flow during labour in pregnancies complicated by hypertension. Br J Obstet Gynaecol 1979; 86:969.
92. Baumann H, Alon E, Atanassoff P, et al: Effect of epidural anesthesia for cesarean delivery on maternal femoral arterial and venous, uteroplacental, and umbilical blood flow velocities and waveforms. Obstet Gynecol 1990; 75:194.
93. Conrad KP: Renal hemodynamics during pregnancy in chronically catheterized, conscious rats. Kidney Int 1984; 26:24.
94. Baylis C: Glomerular filtration and volume regulation in gravid animal models. Baillieres Clin Obstet Gynaecol 1994; 8:235.
95. Robson SC, Hunter S, Boys RJ, et al: Serial changes in pulmonary haemodynamics during human pregnancy: a non-invasive study using Doppler echocardiography. Clin Sci 1991; 80:113.
96. Robson SC, Dunlop W, Boys RJ, et al: Cardiac output during labour. BMJ (Clin Res Ed) 1987; 295:1169.
97. Lees MM, Scott DB, Slawson KB, et al: Haemodynamic changes during Caesarean section. J Obstet Gynaecol Br Commonw 1968; 75:546.
98. Hendricks CH: The hemodynamics of a uterine contraction. Am J Obstet Gynecol 1955; 76:969.
99. Ueland K, Hansen JM: Maternal cardiovascular dynamics. Part 3. Labor and delivery under local and caudal analgesia. Am J Obstet Gynecol 1969; 103:8.
100. Neumark J, Hammerle AF, Biegelmayer C: Effects of epidural analgesia on plasma catecholamines and cortisol in parturition. Acta Anaesthesiol Scand 1985; 29:555.
101. Segal S, Csavoy AN, Datta S: The tocolytic effect of catecholamines in the gravid rat uterus. Anesth Analg 1998; 87:864.
102. Albright GA, Forster RM: Does combined spinal-epidural analgesia with subarachnoid sufentanil increase the incidence of emergency cesarean delivery? Reg Anesth 1997; 22:400.
103. Albright GA, Jouppila R, Hollmén AI, et al: Epinephrine does not alter human intervillous blood flow during epidural anesthesia. Anesthesiology 1981; 54:131.
104. Camann WR, Ostheimer GW: Physiological adaptations during pregnancy. Int Anesthesiol Clin 1990; 28:2.
105. Robson SC, Hunter S, Dunlop W: Left atrial dimensions during early puerperium. Lancet 1987; 2:111.
106. Robson SC, Boys RJ, Hunter S, et al: Maternal hemodynamics after normal delivery and delivery complicated by postpartum hemorrhage. Obstet Gynecol 1989; 74:234.
107. Sibai BM, Frangieh A: Maternal adaptation to pregnancy. Curr Opin Obstet Gynecol 1995; 7:420.
108. Davison JM, Noble MC: Serial changes in 24-hour creatinine clearance during normal menstrual cycles and the first trimester of pregnancy. Br J Obstet Gynaecol 1981; 88:10.
109. Ezimokhai M, Davison JM, Philips PR, et al: Non-postural serial changes in renal function during the third trimester of normal human pregnancy. Br J Obstet Gynaecol 1981; 88:465.
110. Davison JM, Vallotton MB, Lindheimer MD: Plasma osmolality and urinary concentration and dilution during and after pregnancy: evidence that lateral recumbency inhibits maximal urinary concentrating ability. Br J Obstet Gynaecol 1981; 88:472.
111. Lindheimer MD, Katz AI: Gestation in women with kidney disease: prognosis and management. Baillieres Clin Obstet Gynaecol 1994; 8:387.
112. Theunissen IM, Parer JT: Fluid and electrolytes in pregnancy. Clin Obstet Gynecol 1994; 37:3.
113. Fadnes HO, Oian P: Transcapillary fluid balance and plasma volume regulation: a review. Obstet Gynecol Surv 1989; 44:769.
114. Huch A, Huch R, Schneider H, et al: Continuous transcutaneous monitoring of fetal oxygen tension during labour. Br J Obstet Gynaecol 1977; 84(suppl 1):1.
115. Marrero JM, Goggin PM, de Caestecker JS, et al: Determinants of pregnancy heartburn. Br J Obstet Gynaecol 1992; 99:731.
116. Hey VM, Cowley DJ, Ganguli PC, et al: Gastro-oesophageal reflux in late pregnancy. Anaesthesia 1977; 32:372.
117. Bainbridge ET, Nicholas SD, Newton JR, et al: Gastro-oesophageal reflux in pregnancy: altered function of the barrier to reflux in asymptomatic women during early pregnancy. Scand J Gastroenterol 1984; 19:85.
118. Okholm M, Jensen SM: Gastroosofageal refluks hos gravide. Ugeskr Laeger 1995; 157:1835.
119. Lawson M, Kern FJ, Everson GT: Gastrointestinal transit time in human pregnancy: prolongation in the second and third trimesters followed by postpartum normalization. Gastroenterology 1985; 89:996.

120. Whitehead EM, Smith M, Dean Y, et al: An evaluation of gastric emptying times in pregnancy and the puerperium. Anaesthesia 1993; 48:53.
121. Macfie AG, Magides AD, Richmond MN, et al: Gastric emptying in pregnancy. Br J Anaesth 1991; 67:54.
122. Sandhar BK, Elliott RH, Windram I, et al: Peripartum changes in gastric emptying. Anaesthesia 1992; 47:196.
123. Holdsworth JD: Relationship between stomach contents and analgesia in labour. Br J Anaesth 1978; 50:1145.
124. Porter JS, Bonello E, Reynolds F: The influence of epidural administration of fentanyl infusion on gastric emptying in labour. Anaesthesia 1997; 52:1151.
125. Walsh JW, Hasler WL, Nugent CE, et al: Progesterone and estrogen are potential mediators of gastric slow-wave dysrhythmias in nausea of pregnancy. Am J Physiol 1996; 270(3 Pt 1):G506.
126. Vanner RG, Goodman NW: Gastro-oesophageal reflux in pregnancy at term and after delivery. Anaesthesia 1989; 44:808.
127. Attia RR, Ebeid AM, Fischer JE, et al: Maternal fetal and placental gastrin concentrations. Anaesthesia 1982; 37:18.
128. Robson SC, Mutch E, Boys RJ, et al: Apparent liver blood flow during pregnancy: a serial study using indocyanine green clearance. Br J Obstet Gynaecol 1990; 97:720.
129. Sherlock S: The liver in pregnancy. *In* Philipp E, Setchell M, Ginsburg J (eds): Scientific Foundations of Obstetrics and Gynaecology, 4th ed. Oxford, England: Butterworth-Heinemann; 1991:230.
130. Evans RT, Wroe JM: Plasma cholinesterase changes during pregnancy: their interpretation as a cause of suxamethonium-induced apnoea. Anaesthesia 1980; 35:651.
131. de Peyster A, Willis WO, Liebhaber M: Cholinesterase activity in pregnant women and newborns. J Toxicol Clin Toxicol 1994; 32:683.
132. Camp CE, Tessem J, Adenwala J, et al: Vecuronium and prolonged neuromuscular blockade in postpartum patients. Anesthesiology 1987; 67:1006.
133. Puhringer FK, Sparr HJ, Mitterschiffthaler G, et al: Extended duration of action of rocuronium in postpartum patients. Anesth Analg 1997; 84:352.
134. Honger PE: Albumin metabolism in normal pregnancy. Scand J Clin Lab Invest 1968; 21:3.
135. Fahraeus L, Larsson-Cohn U, Wallentin L: Plasma lipoproteins including high density lipoprotein subfractions during normal pregnancy. Obstet Gynecol 1985; 66:468.
136. Kern FJ, Everson GT, DeMark B, et al: Biliary lipids, bile acids, and gallbladder function in the human female: effects of pregnancy and the ovulatory cycle. J Clin Invest 1981; 68:1229.
137. Ganong WF: The gonads: development and function of the reproductive system. *In* Ganong WF (ed): Review of Medical Physiology, 17th ed. East Norwalk, CT: Appleton & Lange; 1995:413.
138. Handwerger S: Clinical counterpoint: the physiology of placental lactogen in human pregnancy. Endocr Rev 1991; 12:329.
139. Fretts RC, Schmittdiel J, McLean FH, et al: Increased maternal age and the risk of fetal death. N Engl J Med 1995; 33:953.
140. Tallarigo L, Giampietro O, Penno G, et al: Relation of glucose tolerance to complications of pregnancy in nondiabetic women. N Engl J Med 1986; 315:989.
141. Adams KM, Li H, Nelson RL, et al: Sequelae of unrecognized gestational diabetes. Am J Obstet Gynecol 1998; 178:1321.
142. Mulder JE: Thyroid disease in women. Med Clin North Am 1998; 82:103.
143. Burrow GN: Thyroid function and hyperfunction during gestation. Endocr Rev 1993; 14:194.
144. Chiovato L, Lapi P, Fiore E, et al: Thyroid autoimmunity and female gender. J Endocrinol Invest 1993; 16:384.
145. Amino N, Mori H, Iwatani Y, et al: High prevalence of transient post-partum thyrotoxicosis and hypothyroidism. N Engl J Med 1982; 306:849.
146. Misra R, Anderson DC: Providing the fetus with calcium. BMJ 1990; 300:1220.
147. Thomson AM, Hytten FE, Billewicz WZ: The epidemiology of oedema during pregnancy. J Obstet Gynaecol Br Commonw 1967; 74:1.
148. Robertson EG: The natural history of oedema during pregnancy. J Obstet Gynaecol Br Commonw 1971; 78:520.
149. Datta S, Briwa J: Modified laryngoscope for endotracheal intubation of obese patients. Anesth Analg 1981; 60:120.
150. Kessell J: A laryngoscope for obstetrical use: an obstetrical laryngoscope. Anaesth Intensive Care 1977; 5:265.
151. Mantle MJ, Greenwood RM, Currey HL: Backache in pregnancy. Rheumatol Rehabil 1977; 16:95.
152. Russell R, Dundas R, Reynolds F: Long term backache after childbirth: prospective search for causative factors. Br Med J [Clin Res Ed] 1996; 312:1384.
153. Sharp K, Brindle PM, Brown MW, et al: Memory loss during pregnancy. Br J Obstet Gynaecol 1993; 100:209.
154. Datta S, Migliozzi RP, Flanagan HL, et al: Chronically administered progesterone decreases halothane requirements in rabbits. Anesth Analg 1989; 68:46.
155. Gin T, Chan MT: Decreased minimum alveolar concentration of isoflurane in pregnant humans. Anesthesiology 1994; 81:829.
156. Chan MT, Gin T: Postpartum changes in the minimum alveolar concentration of isoflurane. Anesthesiology 1995; 82:1360.
157. Datta S, Hurley RJ, Naulty JS, et al: Plasma and cerebrospinal fluid progesterone concentrations in pregnant and nonpregnant women. Anesth Analg 1986; 65:950.
158. Holdcroft A: Females and their variability [editorial]. Anaesthesia 1997; 52:931.
159. Cicero TJ, Nock B, Meyer ER: Gender-related differences in the antinociceptive properties of morphine. J Pharmacol Exp Ther 1996; 279:767.
160. Albright GA: Cardiac arrest following regional anesthesia with etidocaine or bupivacaine [editorial]. Anesthesiology 1979; 51:285.
161. Santos AC, Pedersen H, Harmon TW, et al: Does pregnancy alter the systemic toxicity of local anesthetics? Anesthesiology 1989; 70:991.
162. Nelson-Piercy C: Haematological problems. *In* Nelson-Piercy C (ed): Handbook of Obstetric Medicine. Oxford, England: Isis Medical Media; 1997:201.
163. Pirani BB, Campbell DM, MacGillivray I: Plasma volume in normal first pregnancy. J Obstet Gynaecol Br Commonw 1973; 80:884.
164. Rovinsky JJ, Jaffin H: Cardiovascular hemodynamics in pregnancy. II. Cardiac output and left ventricular work in multiple pregnancy. Am J Obstet Gynecol 1965; 93:1.
165. Forbes CD, Greer IA: Physiology of haemostasis and the effect of pregnancy. *In* Greer IA, Turpie AGG, Forbes CD (eds): Haemostasis and Thrombosis in Obstetrics and Gynaecology. London: Chapman & Hall; 1992.
166. Sharma SK, Philip J, Wiley J: Thromboelastographic changes in healthy parturients and postpartum women. Anesth Analg 1997; 85:94.
167. Rolbin SH, Abbott D, Musclow E, et al: Epidural anesthesia in pregnant patients with low platelet counts. Obstet Gynecol 1988; 71(6 Pt 1):918.
168. Beilin Y, Zahn J, Comerford M: Safe epidural analgesia in thirty parturients with platelet counts between 69,000 and 98,000 mm^3. Anesth Analg 1997; 85:385.
169. Hellgren M, Blomback M: Studies on blood coagulation and fibrinolysis in pregnancy, during delivery and in the puerperium. I. Normal condition. Gynecol Obstet Invest 1981; 12:141.
170. Gerbasi FR, Bottoms S, Farag A, et al: Changes in hemostasis activity during delivery and the immediate postpartum period. Am J Obstet Gynecol 1990; 162:1158.
171. Dahlman T, Hellgren M, Blomback M: Changes in blood coagulation and fibrinolysis in the normal puerperium. Gynecol Obstet Invest 1985; 20:37.
172. Cruickshank JM: The effects of parity on the leucocyte count in pregnant and nonpregnant women. Br Haematol 1970; 18:531.

173. Brain P, Marston RH, Gordon J: Immunological responses in pregnancy. BMJ 1972; 4:488.
174. Hill CA, Finn R, Denye V: Depression of cellular immunity in pregnancy due to a serum factor. BMJ 1973; 3:513.
175. Purtilo DT, Hallgren HM, Yunis EJ: Depressed maternal lymphocyte response to phytohaemagglutinin in human pregnancy. Lancet 1972; 1:769.
176. Karmali RA, Lauder I, Horrobin DF: Prolactin and the immune response. Lancet 1974; 2:106.
177. De Swiet M: The respiratory system. *In* Chamberlain G, Pipkin FB (eds): Clinical Physiology in Obstetrics, 3rd ed. Oxford, England: Blackwell Science; 1998:111.
178. Gazioglu K, Kaltreider NL, Rosen M, et al: Pulmonary function during pregnancy in normal women and in patients with cardiopulmonary disease. Thorax 1970; 25:445.
179. Alaily AB, Carrol KB: Pulmonary ventilation in pregnancy. Br J Obstet Gynaecol 1978; 85:518.
180. Nelson-Piercy C: Renal disease. *In* Nelson-Piercy C (ed): Handbook of Obstetric Medicine. Oxford, England: Isis Medical Media; 1997.
181. Syminds EM: The regulation of blood pressure and renal function in pregnancy; water and electrolyte balance. *In* Philipp E, Setchell M, Ginsburg J (eds): Scientific Foundations of Obstetrics and Gynaecology, 4th ed. Oxford, England: Butterworth-Heinemann; 1991:566.

3

Fetal Physiology

❖ RAMON MARTIN, MD, PHD

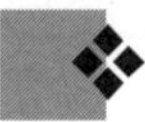

INTRODUCTION

Aside from providing analgesia to laboring parturients, the obstetric anesthesiologist must be ready to respond quickly to a wide range of clinical scenarios. In addition to assessment of the mother's physical condition, one must have an understanding of the associated clinical management issues, such as use of tocolytics, steroids, fetal malpresentation, premature rupture of membranes (PROM), chorioamnionitis, and so on, and the possible effects of any treatment on both mother and fetus. To communicate effectively with the patient and other care providers in labor and delivery, it is imperative to have an understanding of maternal and fetal physiology, and the impact on anesthetic management. This chapter summarizes the physiologic development of the fetal organ systems after an initial description of the nutritional requirements of the fetus. Maternal physiology is also covered in Chapter 2.

Normal gestation spans 38 to 40 weeks and is divided into an embryonic and a fetal period. The former spans weeks 3 through 8, during which most of the major organ systems are formed. The fetal period constitutes the rest of gestation and is a time mainly of maturation and growth of organs. The transition from fetus to neonate occurs at birth, during which a series of physiologic changes occur. This chapter focuses on the fetal period.

FETAL METABOLISM

The pivotal organ in maternal-fetal nutrient transfer is the placenta. The placenta has a variety of functions, including endocrine support of the pregnancy and transport of nutrients to the fetus against a concentration gradient. It produces several protein hormones, including human chorionic gonadotropin (hCG), human placental lactogen (HPL), and possibly human chorionic corticotropin (HCC). Both hCG and HPL are secreted primarily into the maternal circulation. At day 70 of gestation hCG reaches its maximum level then declines gradually,[1] but HPL rises slowly throughout gestation and disappears rapidly after delivery. HPL has a diabetogenic, glucose-sparing effect and also stimulates maternal lipolysis, causing an increase in maternal-serum free fatty acid levels.[2] Since the mother can then use larger amounts of free fatty acids as fuel, this frees maternal stores of glucose and amino acids for use by the fetus. Human chorionic gonadotropin stimulates the corpus luteum to produce progesterone during the first trimester, and may possibly direct steroid production by the fetal gonads[3] while increasing the catabolism of glycogen.[4] This may have a glucose-sparing effect in the placenta and make more glucose available for the fetus.

The progesterone produced by the placenta also has a diabetogenic, glucose-sparing effect in the mother. The primary role of estrogen is in stimulating uterine growth by increasing local DNA and protein synthesis. Another estrogen effect is to increase placental and uterine blood flow, thus increasing the transport of nutrients to the fetus.

Table 3–1 lists substances that cross the placenta as well as currently accepted transport mechanisms. In the case of glucose, both placental metabolism and facilitated diffusion contribute to the differences in concentration between maternal and fetal circulation.[5]

An active transport of amino acids is suggested by the fourfold higher concentration of amino acids in the fetal circulation compared with the maternal circulation.[6] In addition, amino acid concentrations in umbilical venous blood exceed those in umbilical arterial blood. Large proteins and polypeptides cross the placenta very slowly, probably by pinocytosis or through breaks in the membrane.[7] Free fatty acids exchange readily, although not as quickly as oxygen and carbon dioxide.[8] The diffusion of cholesterol and steroids is relatively slow and depends on their molecular configuration.

Water-soluble vitamins are found in higher concentrations in fetal blood than in maternal blood.[9] Although they are probably actively transported, their protein binding in fetal blood is also increased and might account for the large gradient. Fat-soluble vitamins readily cross the placenta by passive diffusion.

The concentration of water in both maternal and fetal circulations is affected by both hydrostatic and osmotic pressure differences. Changes in the concentration of any of the above-mentioned substances can affect the osmotic pressure gradient across the placenta and thereby influence water exchange. As a re-

Table 3-1 SUBSTANCES THAT CROSS THE PLACENTA AND CURRENTLY ACCEPTED MECHANISM OF TRANSPORT

TRANSPORT MECHANISM	SUBSTANCES TRANSPORTED
Passive diffusion	Oxygen Carbon dioxide Fatty acids Steroids Nucleosides Electrolytes Fat-soluble vitamins
Facilitated diffusion	Sugars
Active diffusion	Amino acids Some cations Water-soluble vitamins
Solvent drag	Electrolytes
Pinocytosis, breaks in membrane	Proteins

sult of carbon dioxide exchange, the osmotic water flux is also influenced by water shifts between erythrocytes and plasma, which can then affect the plasma concentration of numerous solutes.

Fetal and Placental Growth

Fetal growth and development have been defined in relation to growth curves that are constructed from large series of birthweights at varying weeks of gestation. Infants whose weights are between the 10th and 90th percentile for gestational age are termed appropriate for gestational age (AGA). When the birthweight is greater than the 90th percentile, infants are labeled large for gestational age (LGA), and conversely are labeled small for gestational age (SGA) when their birthweight falls below the 10th percentile.

Another classification denotes birthweight independent of gestational age:

Low birthweight infants (LBW) weigh less than 2500 g.

Very low birthweight infants (VLBW) weigh less than 1500 g.

Extremely low birthweight infants (ELBW) weigh less than 1000 g.

These terms do not necessarily imply abnormal growth (i.e., a fetus at 25 weeks' gestation would be classified as ELBW). Normal genetic variations may make a fetus SGA or LGA without underlying pathophysiology. Intrauterine growth retardation (IUGR), on the other hand, is the result of decreased fetal growth owing to an abnormality that either decreases transport of nutrients to the fetus or interrupts fetal use of nutrients.

IUGR may be classified as either asymmetric or symmetric. With the former, the development of the fetal trunk and limbs is below the mean, whereas fetal brain growth remains intact. This is usually due to a chronic decrease in the supply or utilization of nutrients. In cases of symmetric IUGR, both head and body development are decreased proportionately to weight. This can manifest as either a normal growth pattern or be the result of an injury that occurred early in gestation. With either type of IUGR, the fetus is more susceptible to any stress that decreases the supply of nutrients.

Fetal growth, as measured by changes in fetal body weight, increases gradually throughout pregnancy. Biochemical analyses of various organs have shown that fetal growth is proliferative up to the 25th week of gestation but becomes both hyperplastic and hypertrophic thereafter.[10] This pattern is similar to the growth pattern of the placenta. In early gestation, the placenta is larger than the fetus and probably has greater growth requirements. In later gestation, the rate of fetal growth exceeds that of the placenta. This is reflected by an increase in the ratio of fetal to placental weight. Because of this shift, the placenta must increase the amount of substrate per gram of placental tissue which is transferred into the fetal circulation to meet fetal growth needs.[11] This osmotic gain, in turn, affects fetal blood volume, venous return, cardiac output, and delivery of nutrients to fetal tissues.

There are several growth factors that may also play a role in fetal growth. The fetal blood concentration of somatomedin A has been correlated with birthweight. Somatomedin A has binding sites in the placenta and there is indirect evidence that it is synthesized in this organ. Somatomedin C, found in fetal erythrocytes, also has placental binding sites. It is found in increasing concentrations in the fetal pig placenta as gestation advances in the midst of decreased insulin binding. This suggests a possible role for somatomedin in placental growth.[12] Human placental lactogen has been shown to increase somatomedin production, suggesting that HPL may regulate placental growth through this mechanism.[13] In addition to the somatomedins, there are insulin-like growth factors (IGF-1 and IGF-2), about which little is known.

Individual Substrates

Carbohydrates. During pregnancy, fasting plasma glucose concentrations are somewhat lower than in the nonpregnant state, and they do not change significantly as pregnancy progresses. Fasting plasma insulin concentrations, however, rise slightly during pregnancy. In response to a standard glucose load, there is a rise in serum glucose during the first hour, with a return to fasting levels by 2 to 2½ hours. There is, though, a wide range in serum glucose values. In some patients there is only a small rise in serum glucose, whereas in others there is a secondary increase after the first peak. The resulting response for the former is probably rapid, causing an increase in diffusion from plasma to the extracellular space, as well as increased uptake by tissue. For the latter response, there is a corresponding secondary rise in plasma insulin. As pregnancy progresses, the time necessary to reach maximum glucose concentration increases. By 38 weeks of gestation, the mean time to peak plasma glucose is 55 minutes, compared with 34 minutes in the nonpregnant state. Return to fasting level, however, is still attained in 2 to 2½ hours.[14] The insulin response is characterized by a gradually increasing peak value throughout gestation as well as a delay in reaching this peak. By 2 hours, the insulin level is still above the fasting concentration.

The glomerular filtration rate (GFR) rises in pregnancy to about 50% above the prepregnancy level.[14] With the rise in postprandial glucose levels, this means an increase in the filtered load presented to the renal tubules. It has been shown that with elevated plasma glucose levels, tubular reabsorption increases, but with decreasing efficiency, which leads to glycosuria. In a study of urinary glucose excretion in 30 healthy pregnant women, it was found that 10 women excreted glucose in the normal, nonpregnant range of less than 100 mg/24 h.[15] The rest excreted more than 100 mg/24 h on some days. Of the latter group, 10 women excreted as much as 1000 mg/24 h. All patients had normal oral glucose tolerance tests. Evaluation of possible influencing variables (e.g., relationship to meals, time of day) showed no significant relationship. In addition to the glucose loss from glycosuria during pregnancy, there is also increased excretion of water-soluble vitamins as well as amino acids. In a well-nourished woman during pregnancy, this loss does not affect maternal-fetal nutritional balance. In women who have inadequate nutrient intake, defined as protein-calorie malnutrition (PCM), intermittent glycosuria could be another potentially significant source of nutritional loss.

The intravenous glucose tolerance test (IGTT) has been used in infants and neonates to calculate the rate of disappearance of glucose (K_G). In healthy full-term infants, the mean K_G starts at 1%/min and increases to 2%/min by 6 months (similar to the adult level). Infants of diabetic mothers have higher K_G values within the first 24 hours after birth, as do SGA infants or those with significant hypoglycemia. The K_G values for premature but AGA infants were less than those of full-term infants for the first 24 hours; however, there was a rapid increase in the K_G. In SGA infants, after the first 24 hours, the K_G decreased to a pattern similar to that of AGA infants.[16]

Amino Acids. As mentioned previously, the placenta has an active transport mechanism for amino acids, specifically the L-amino acids. Studies in rhesus monkeys, looking at the ratio of amino acid levels in cord and maternal blood (C/M ratio), showed that the cord levels were greater than those of the mother for all amino acids.[17] For lysine, taurine, and 3-methyl-histidine, the elevated C/M ratio is secondary to an increase in free amino acids in the fetus as well as reduced maternal levels. For the other amino acids, the elevated ratio is due entirely to a reduction in maternal serum levels. Taurine, alanine, lysine, and 3-methyl-histidine levels were elevated in full-term monkey fetuses as compared with 1-year-old animals. The serum levels of the other amino acids were either unchanged or decreased.

Ghadimi and Pecora[18] studied free amino acid levels at delivery in simultaneously drawn cord and maternal serum in humans during the second and third trimesters of pregnancy. As in the monkey, cord blood has a higher concentration of amino acids than maternal blood. The fetal-maternal ratios all favored the fetus, most showing a twofold greater concentration in the fetus. When maternal blood was analyzed 6 to 8 weeks postpartum, all amino acid concentrations were found to have increased from maternal levels at delivery. When the fetuses were stratified for gestational age (immature, <30 weeks; premature, 30–37 weeks; and full term, >37 weeks) the differences in C/M ratios were larger in the immature deliveries. Three diabetic mothers and their full-term infants were also included. Their C/M ratios did not differ from those of nondiabetic women with full-term deliveries. The amino acids in the Krebs-ornithine cycle (i.e., aspartic acid, glutamic acid, and ornithine) have higher ratios in the immature group than in the full-term group. This suggests an immaturity of the Krebs-ornithine cycle in early pregnancy, resulting in increased fetal concentrations of these amino acids.

These data indicate that the placenta concentrates amino acids in the fetal circulation. This system is probably best suited for periods of maternal nutritional deprivation.

Fatty Acid and Ketone Metabolism. The fetus needs fatty acids for structure (i.e., phospholipids) and storage. Although the fetus can synthesize some fatty acids, it cannot make essential fatty acids. Linoleic acid accounts for approximately 2.5% of fetal adipose tissue stores.[19] This indicates that fatty acids cross the placenta in sizable amounts. Studies in perfused human placentas have demonstrated fatty acid transfer and suggest that the flow to the fetus is determined by the free fatty acid concentration in the maternal serum. Elphick[20] infused 200 mL of a fat emulsion (10% Intralipid) over 1 hour into six pregnant women at 1 to 2 hours prior to delivery. The umbilical vein levels of all triglyceride fatty acids were higher than those in the umbilical artery, indicating placental transfer secondary to the establishment of a large maternal-fetal gradient of oleic and linoleic acids. There was a similar increase for free fatty acids. Maternal phospholipid levels were only slightly affected, with no significant umbilical venous-arterial difference. The profile of the venous-arterial cord levels for free fatty acids and triglycerides reflects the imprint of the infused fat emulsion.

During periods of maternal fasting, there is a reduction in both maternal and fetal serum glucose levels. The resulting maternal lipolysis and free fatty acid mobilization lead to increased ketone body formation. Because the fetus has limited ability to mobilize hepatic glycogen stores, increase gluconeogenesis, or extract free fatty acids from maternal serum, its serum ketone concentration also increases. This is the result of both placental transfer and endogenous production in the fetus. Under normal conditions in the human, measurements of arterial-venous differences show that the fetal brain extracts glucose, ketone bodies, and oxygen. This use is unique to the fetus. When one compares fractional extraction rates of ketone bodies by the brain in the neonate, infant, and adult, there is a gradual decrease with increasing age. This would explain why neonates are able to tolerate periods of hypoglycemia better than older infants.

Vitamins. Vitamin deficiency is a concern during pregnancy and is seen commonly in women who had inadequate nutrient intake that resulted in protein-calorie malnutrition. Baker[21] analyzed vitamin profiles of 174 women and their newborn infants at term: 133 of these women reported having taken supplemental vitamins during their pregnancy. There was a 1:2 to 1:5 ratio of serum vitamin levels between the mother and the neonate for all the women and infants studied. The exceptions were vitamins A, B_6, E, and β-carotene. Of the mothers found to be hypovitaminemic, serum levels of folate, thiamine, and vitamins B_{12}, C, and A were most depressed. In women not taking supplemental vitamins, the levels of nicotinate and vitamin B_6 were also depressed. In this latter group, the incidence of low serum folate and thiamine levels was 71% and 53%, respectively. The hypovitaminosis was also seen in the neonate. Based on these results, it is evident that most vitamins cross the placenta and accumulate in the fetus against a concentration gradient. The fat-soluble vitamins are the exception.

Baker[22] studied placental transfer in two groups of women (hypovitaminemic and normovitaminemic) who took no supplemental vitamins throughout gestation. In the hypovitaminemic group, the vitamin depletion in both maternal and fetal serum was the same as in the above-mentioned study; however, the placentas of these women had depressed levels of only vitamin B_{12} and folate when compared with placentas of normovitaminemic women. This suggests that the placenta not only is selective in the transport of vitamins but as a growing organ has its own vitamin requirements.

Trace Elements and Minerals. The need for iron supplementation during pregnancy is well established and has been reviewed.[23] Deficiency states of minerals and trace elements are rare. Dawson[24] measured maternal plasma levels in 244 pregnant adolescents. These women had not had any mineral supplements. The samples were drawn serially from the 10th week of pregnancy to term. Their serum concentrations of calcium, magnesium, iron, and zinc decreased progressively throughout pregnancy. Plasma copper levels rose slightly. All pregnancies in this series were uncomplicated. The role of the placenta in the maternal-fetal exchange of minerals and trace elements is still not clearly defined.

Effects of Maternal Nutritional Deprivation on the Fetus and Placenta

Studies in pregnant rats pair-fed 50% of the food normally consumed by nonpregnant controls showed no change in body composition of the mother. However, fetal mean body weights were significantly reduced.[25] When pregnant rats were restricted to 75% of their ad libitum intake, the mothers gained 9 g of net body weight, while the mean fetal weight remained within control values. With a decrease in the restriction to 50% of normal intake, the mothers lost 8% of the initial weight, with a decrease in mean fetal weight of 12%. At a 25% intake restriction, there was a 36% to 32% loss of initial body weight, with a 45% to 56% decrease in mean fetal weight. This was also associated with a 64% to 92% embryonic death rate.[26] These data suggest that there is no apparent effect on fetal growth in food-restricted rats unless the restriction is so severe that the mother cannot gain weight.

If nutrients are available and the mother increases her intake above normal, a portion of the excess goes to the fetus. When food intake is severely limited, however, the fetus is not favored over the mother. The maternal preference for nutrients is continued with refeeding. In pregnant guinea pigs, a low-protein diet resulted in a 10% to 12% reduction in maternal weight, 50% fetal mortality, and a 22% to 38% reduction in fetal birthweight.[27] Pigs fed a low-protein diet during pregnancy lost 17% of initial body weight, while the fetuses were 33% below control weight.[28] The same has been found in rhesus monkeys.[29, 30] When rats were restricted to 24% of normal intake for the first 5 days of pregnancy and then allowed to eat ad libitum for the remainder of the pregnancy, maternal and fetal weights were similar to those of controls. However, if refeeding was not permitted until the last 12 days of pregnancy, maternal net body weight increased 23%, while fetal body weight decreased 7% when compared with controls. When refeeding was begun during the last 10 days of gestation, maternal body weight increased by 21% and fetal body weight decreased by 12%.[31] This demonstrates that the mother is favored over the fetus when nutrients are available. These results also support the concept that nutrients go preferentially to the mother rather than the fetus during periods of starvation.

The Dutch famine that occurred during the winter of 1944–1945 demonstrated the effects of starvation on maternal weight gain. It has been estimated that the average daily intake during this time was approximately 1200 calories. When this occurred during the second and third trimesters, there was a 250-g decrease in mean fetal body weight (10% reduction). Rosso has estimated that the mean loss of weight for the mother was 1.5 kg of initial body weight, or less than 3%.[32] This is consistent with the experimental animal data described previously and suggests that with semistarvation, the mother maintains her own body stores rather than adapting to maintain fetal growth. If there are extra body stores, then she can maintain normal fetal growth even with inadequate food intake. However, if the stores are small, the amount of food intake becomes the critical factor in the maintenance of fetal growth.

The metabolic changes that the mother undergoes during starvation are still largely unknown. In pregnant rats that have been protein restricted, the rate of urea synthesis and the levels of hepatic enzymes involved in amino acid catabolism are reduced.[33, 34] Women on low-protein diets have reduced urea excretion, which suggests a similar mechanism to reduce amino acid catabolism,[35] although the reason for this is not clear. In humans as well as in experimental animal models, protein restriction beginning just after conception causes a significant reduction in the expected expansion of plasma volume.[36, 37] If blood volume is inadequate, uterine blood flow may be decreased, with subsequent compromise of fetal development. It has been shown that the volume of maternal plasma correlates with infant birthweight.[38]

The lack of normal plasma volume expansion and its consequent reduction in uterine blood flow may adversely influence nutrient transfer across the placenta. In addition, changes in placental morphology may reduce the size of the effective exchange area and thereby the rate of transfer for substances moved by simple or facilitated diffusion. A reduction in the metabolic activity of the trophoblast would influence active transport. Measurements of maternal cardiac output and regional blood flow have shown less expansion in cardiac output and placental blood flow for malnourished pregnant rats compared with controls, although the percentage of cardiac output distributed to the uterus was the same for both groups.[39] It was the lack of plasma volume expansion that accounted for the decreased placental blood flow and decreased nutrient supply.

The primary cause for the lack of weight gain in the nutritionally growth-retarded fetus is decreased placental transport. This is suggested by the frequent occurrence of hypoglycemia seen in nutritionally growth-retarded guinea pig fetuses. Plasma free fatty acids in these fetuses are also depressed, as is the arterial oxygen saturation.[40] In both guinea pig and human fetuses that suffer from nutritional IUGR, venous alanine concentrations are elevated owing to increased protein catabolism. Fetal serum ammonia levels are high because of inadequate clearing by the placenta, as well as a poorly developed fetal urea cycle. Fetal hepatic glycogen is reduced in the rat,[41] but not in the monkey[42] or guinea pig.[40] Triglyceride stores are also reduced with nutritional IUGR. Both glycogen and triglycerides are rapidly mobilizable energy stores for the neonate. Decreased glycogen storage probably accounts for the hypoglycemia that occurs frequently in human newborns who have experienced PCM during gestation.

Our understanding of fetal changes in response to maternal malnutrition is largely based on animal studies. A consistent feature seen with nutritional IUGR in both animal models and humans is an asymmetric effect on organ growth.[40] Length is not affected as much as the decrease in body weight. When compared with the reduction in total body weight, the decrease in brain weight is proportionally less and the decrease in lung, heart, and kidney weight is the same (Fig. 3–1).

In addition to a decrease in organ weight, there are also changes in morphology. The liver shows less cytosol, fewer mitochondria, and less endoplasmic reticulum. Hepatic enzyme function is also altered. Low levels of phosphoenolpyruvate carboxykinase suggest impairment of gluconeogenesis. Decreased activity of aminotransferase is consistent with reduced rates of peripheral amino acid metabolism.[40]

In the brain, the decrease in mass is associated with a fall in DNA, RNA, and protein content. In humans, most neurogenesis and some myelination have occurred by 26 weeks' gestation. If growth restriction starts after that time, brain mass at birth is reduced, but if postnatal nutrition is adequate,

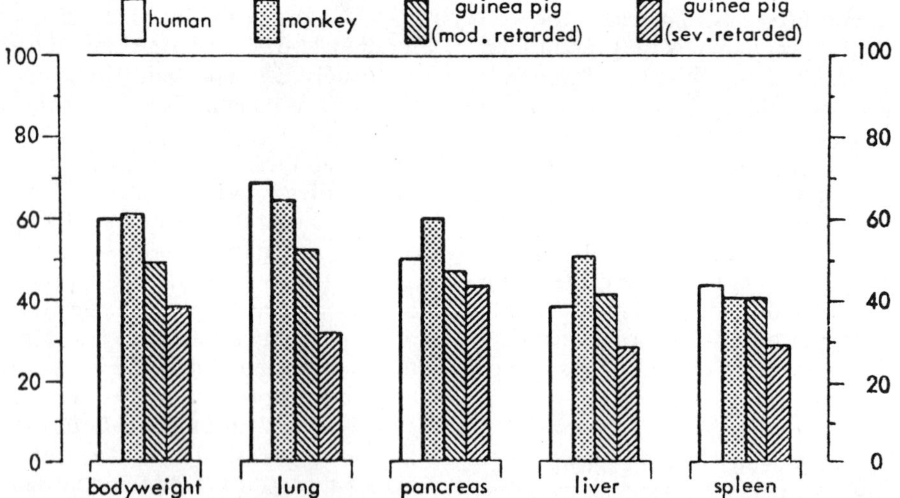

❖ **Figure 3–1** Comparative organ size in growth-retarded fetuses of humans, monkeys, and guinea pigs. (From LaFever HN, Jones CT, Rolph TP: Some of the consequences of intrauterine growth retardation. *In* Visser HKA (ed): Nutrition and Metabolism of the Fetus and Infant. The Hague, Netherlands: Martinus Nijhoff; 1979:47 With permission from Kluwer Academic Publishers.)

"catchup" growth compensates to produce a normal-sized brain.[43] Growth restriction before 26 weeks' gestation, however, leads to permanent stunting of brain growth and measurable neurologic damage.[44]

The skeletal system is affected by nutritional IUGR. In guinea pigs, there is delayed ossification, probably secondary to a decrease in factors that cause sulfate to be incorporated into cartilage.[40] These changes are caused primarily by decreased nutrient supply, although secondary changes in circulating levels of insulin have an effect as well.

There is clearly a relationship between maternal weight gain, fetal weight gain, and fetal outcome. A question yet to be answered is whether one can quantitate the relationship between the degree of maternal weight loss and the severity of fetal outcome.

FETAL CARDIOVASCULAR SYSTEM

Venous Flow from the Placenta to the Fetal Heart. Approximately 40% of fetal cardiac output goes to the placenta, with a similar amount returning to the right side of the heart via the umbilical vein (Fig. 3–2). The blood in the umbilical vein has the highest oxygen saturation in the fetal circulation, so its distribution is important for the delivery of oxygen to fetal tissues. Half of the umbilical venous blood enters the ductus venosus, which connects to the inferior vena cava. The rest enters the hepatoportal venous system.[45]

Streaming, which is the separation of blood with differing oxygenation saturations as it flows through a single vessel, is an important determinant of oxygen delivery to fetal tissues. This is seen when the more highly saturated umbilical venous blood passes through the ductus venosus into the inferior vena cava to meet the desaturated venous drainage from the lower trunk. In the liver, umbilical venous return is directed toward the left lobe and the portal venous return to the right lobe, so that there is a marked difference in oxygen saturation (higher in the left hepatic lobe than in the right lobe).[46, 47] Although both hepatic veins enter the inferior vena cava, the left hepatic vein streams preferentially with the blood flow from the ductus venosus,[47] whereas the right hepatic vein flow follows the same route as that from the abdominal vena cava.

There is preferential flow of the umbilical venous return to the left atrium because of the crista dividens, which splits the inferior vena cava blood flow into two streams. One stream includes the oxygenated blood from the umbilical vein that is directed toward the foramen ovale and into the left atrium; the other stream consists of deoxygenated blood from the lower extremities and portal vein that enters the right atrium. This results in a higher oxygen saturation in the left atrium than in the right atrium. Blood flow through the superior vena cava is also preferentially streamed along with blood flow through the coronary sinus via the tricuspid valve. The desaturated blood from the right side of the heart is directed toward the placenta for reoxygenation. The left side of the heart supplies oxygenated blood for the brain.

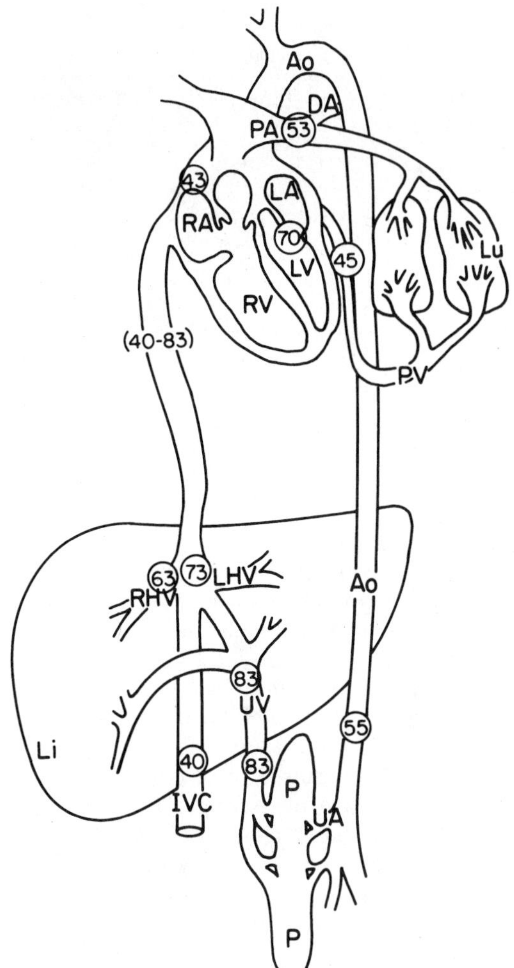

❖ **Figure 3–2** Normal fetal circulation with major blood flow patterns and oxygen saturation values (circled numbers indicate percent saturation). Ao, aorta; DA, ductus arteriosus; DV, ductus venosus; IVC, inferior vena cava; Li, liver; Lu, lung; P, placenta; PA, pulmonary artery; PV, pulmonary vein; RA and LA, right and left atria; RHV and LHV, right and left hepatic veins; RV and LV, right and left ventricles; SVC, superior vena cava; UA, umbilical artery; UV, umbilical vein.

Cardiac Output. Because of intracardiac and extracardiac shunts, the two ventricles do not work in series, as in adults. Therefore, they do not have the same stroke volume. The right ventricle ejects approximately two thirds of fetal cardiac output (300 mL/kg/min), and the left ventricle ejects about one third (150 mL/kg/min). Of the right ventricular output, only a small fraction (8%) flows through the pulmonary arteries. Most of the output crosses the ductus arteriosus and enters the descending aorta, allowing deoxygenated blood to return preferentially to the placenta. The left ventricular output enters the ascending aorta, and most of the output reaches the brain, upper thorax, and arms.[48–50]

This distribution of cardiac output to individual organs is shown in Table 3–2. Since blood flow to the organs below the diaphragm is derived from both ventricles, flow is expressed as a percentage of the combined ventricles.

Table 3-2 DISTRIBUTION OF CARDIAC OUTPUT IN FETAL LAMBS

ORGAN	BLOOD FLOW (mL/kg/min)	CARDIAC OUTPUT (%)
Heart	180	2
Brain	125	2
Upper body	25	16
Lungs	100	8
Gastrointestinal tract	70	5
Kidneys	150	2.5
Adrenals	200	0.1
Spleen	200	1.2
Liver	20	1.5
Lower body	25	20
Placenta	20	37

Myocardial Function. The fetal myocardium, relative to the adult myocardium, is immature in structure, function, and sympathetic innervation. Although the length of the fetal sarcomere is the same as that in the adult,[51] the diameter of the fetal sarcomere is smaller and the proportion of noncontractile mass to the number of myofibrils is less, 30% in the fetus versus 60% in adults.[52] Active tension generated is less than in the adult heart at all lengths of a muscle along a length-tension curve. Passive or resting tension is higher in fetal myocardium than in the adult, suggesting lower compliance for the fetus. A study of volume loading by infusion of blood or saline solution in fetal lambs showed that the right ventricle is unable to increase stroke work or output as much as the adult.[53] Cardiac output varies directly with heart rate, so an increase in rate from 180 to 250 beats/min increases cardiac output 15% to 20%. Conversely, a decrease in heart rate below basal levels causes a decrease in ventricular output. Histochemical staining of the sympathetic nervous system demonstrates delayed development. Compared with the adult, isolated fetal cardiac tissue has a lower response threshold to the inotropic effects of norepinephrine. This is presumed to be secondary to the incomplete development of the sympathetic nervous system.[52] As a result, the fetal heart appears to operate at or near peak performance normally.

Control of the Cardiovascular System

The cardiovascular system is controlled by a complex interrelationship between autoregulation, reflex effects, hormonal substrates, and the autonomic nervous system. Whereas many organs in adults are able to maintain fairly constant blood flow over a wide range of perfusion pressures, the placental circulation does not exhibit autoregulation.[54] As a result, blood flow changes directly with changes in arterial perfusion pressure. Papile and associates[55] demonstrated in fetal lambs that the cerebral circulation does autoregulate itself. The baroreflex has also been shown to exist in fetal animals. In adults, it functions to stabilize heart rate and blood pressure, but in the fetus it is relatively insensitive. Marked changes in blood pressure are required to produce minor responses, so that the function of the baroreflex is probably minimal in utero.[56]

The chemoreceptor reflex is governed by receptors in either the carotid body or in the central nervous system (CNS) and causes hypertension and mild tachycardia with increased respiratory activity. Chemoreceptors in the aorta cause bradycardia with a slight increase in blood pressure. The former are less sensitive than the latter so that bradycardia and hypertension are seen with hypoxia because of the overriding response of the aortic chemoreceptors.

The autonomic nervous system is fully developed in the fetus, as demonstrated by the presence of receptors and an acetylcholinesterase and its response to cholinergic or adrenergic agonists. The renin-angiotensin system is also important in regulating the normal fetal circulation and the response to hemorrhage. Angiotensin II exerts a tonic vasoconstriction on the peripheral vasculature to maintain systemic arterial blood pressure and umbilical blood flow.[57] Vasopressin, although detectable in the fetus, probably has little regulatory function. Stress (i.e., hypoxia) elicits an increase in vasopressin secretion and results in hypertension and bradycardia.[58] In the presence of decreased cardiac output, the renin-angiotensin system maintains the flow to the brain, heart, and placenta, while flow to the splanchnic bed decreases.[59] Circulating prostaglandins are present in high concentrations in the fetus[60, 61] and are produced by both the placenta and fetal vasculature. Prostaglandins (PGs) have diverse effects on the cardiovascular system. Infusions of PGE_1, PGE_2, PGF_2, and thromboxane constrict the umbilical-placental circulation,[62, 63] whereas prostacyclin has the opposite effect. PGE_1, PGE_2, PGI_2, and PGD_2 cause pulmonary vasodilation in the fetus, and PGF_2 produces vasoconstriction.[64, 65] Prostaglandins also relax smooth muscle in the ductus arteriosus, so that it remains patent in utero.[66, 67]

Fetal Heart Rate

The average fetal heart rate decreases from 155 beats/min at 20 weeks' gestation to 144 beats/min at 30 weeks' gestation and is 140 beats/min at term. The variability is 20 beats/min in a normal fetus. The sinoatrial (SA) and the atrioventricular (AV) nodes serve as intrinsic pacemakers, with the SA node setting the rate in the normal heart. Variability of the fetal heart rate is followed either beat to beat or over a longer period, and is an important prognostic variable. Control of the fetal heart rate is the result of a number of factors, both intrinsic and extrinsic.

The parasympathetic nervous system contributes to cardiac regulation through the vagus nerve. It has endings in both the SA and AV nodes. Stimulation of the vagus nerve results in bradycardia through a direct effect on the SA node. Blocking the vagus nerve results in an increase in heart rate of approximately 20 beats/min,[73] so the vagus nerve exerts a constant influence to decrease a higher intrinsic rate. In addition, the vagus nerve transmits impulses that result in beat-to-beat variability of the fetal heart rate.[74]

The sympathetic nervous system has nerve endings throughout the myocardium at term. Stimulation of the sympathetic nerves causes release of norepinephrine and an increase in heart rate and contractility, and therefore cardiac output. If the sympathetic nerves are blocked, there is an average decrease of 10 beats/min in the fetal heart rate.

The sympathetic and parasympathetic nervous systems are modulated by other factors. Chemoreceptors located in both the peripheral nervous system and the CNS exert their primary effect on the control of respiration, but they also have an effect on the circulation. With a decrease in arterial perfusion pressure or an increase in carbon dioxide content, a reflex tachycardia develops, leading to an increase in blood pressure.

Baroreceptors are located in the arch of the aorta and at the junction of the internal and external carotid arteries, and are sensitive to increases in blood pressure. When blood pressure rises, impulses are sent via the vagus nerve to decrease the heart rate and cardiac output.

Of the possible hormones that can contribute to heart rate control, three have an effect during periods of stress. Epinephrine and norepinephrine are secreted by the adrenal medulla during stress. Their effects are similar to those caused by sympathetic stimulation: an increase in heart rate, contractility, and blood pressure. The adrenal cortex produces aldosterone in reaction to hypotension. This increases blood volume by slowing renal sodium output, leading to water retention.

PLACENTAL RESPIRATORY GAS EXCHANGE AND FETAL OXYGENATION

Fetal Gas Exchange

Fetal gas exchange occurs via the placenta. Because the fetal lungs are nonfunctional, there are several shunts in the fetal circulation that allow oxygenated blood to pass from the placenta to the fetal systemic circulation. Streaming or laminar blood flow keeps oxygenated and deoxygenated blood separate in the venous system and assumes great importance in preferentially supplying oxygenated blood to organs such as the heart, brain, and adrenal glands during periods of hypoxia.

Although fetal viability is seen at earlier gestational ages, a significant amount of morbidity results from the underdevelopment of the respiratory system. After the embryonic period, the airways proliferate and branch from 8 to 16 weeks' gestation. Vascular channels appear from 17 to 27 weeks' gestation and approximate the potential air spaces. This is when effective gas exchange becomes possible. Surfactant appears and enhances adequate surface tension to keep alveoli open. Type I and II epithelial cells are also identified. From 28 to 35 weeks' gestation, the interstitial spaces thin and the peripheral air spaces develop. There is a gradual increase in the surface air for gas exchange. From 36 weeks' gestation and later, the number of alveoli rapidly increase and there is further differentiation of specific cell types.

The passage of oxygen from the atmosphere to the fetus can be described in a sequence of six steps. These steps alternate bulk transport of gases with diffusion across membranes. The first three steps are primarily maternal and the last three are fetal (Fig. 3–3).

Transport of oxygen starts from the atmosphere to the maternal alveoli through the large airways by the respiratory muscles, in exchange for carbon dioxide. The pressure of oxygen in the alveoli is regulated by several mechanisms that respond to changes in the levels of the partial pressures of oxygen (Po_2) and carbon dioxide (Pco_2), and the pH of maternal blood. Arterial Pco_2 in the pregnant woman is regulated at a lower level than in the nonpregnant woman, secondary to the effects of progesterone.[68]

With the second step, oxygen diffuses rapidly across the alveoli to maternal erythrocytes. The Po_2 of maternal arterial blood is slightly less than that in the alveoli because of shunting and inequality of ventilation and perfusion throughout the lung fields. In the pregnant woman, the gradient of oxygen in the arterioles and alveoli is dependent on position and widens when going from the upright to the supine position.

Maternal blood transports oxygen to the placenta in two forms, free and bound to hemoglobin. These two forms are in a reversible equilibrium.

In the diffusion of oxygen across the placenta, the oxygen uptake by the gravid uterus is greater than that by the fetus. This is because compared with the fetus,

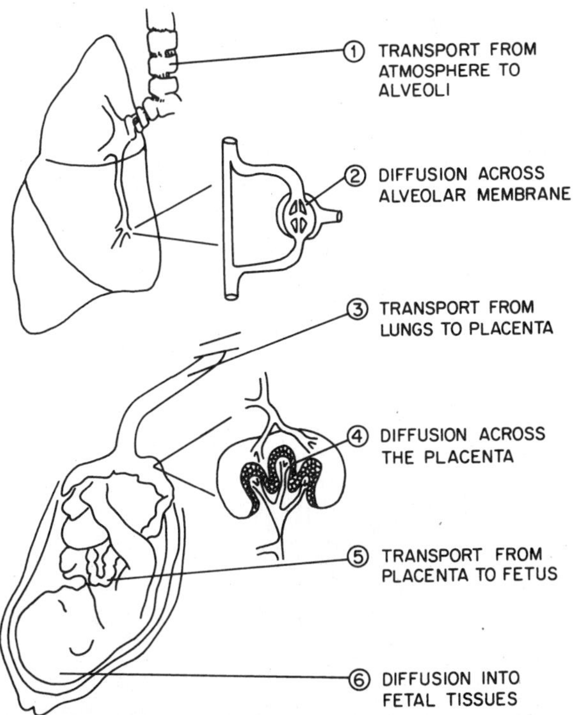

Figure 3–3 Six steps in the transport of oxygen from the atmosphere to the fetal tissues.

the placenta and the uterus extract oxygen and consume a relatively large fraction. In chronic sheep preparations, this has been calculated with the Fick principle: Uterine oxygen consumption is measured by the difference in oxygen content between the maternal arterial blood (A) and uterine venous blood (V). Multiplying the difference by uterine blood flow (F) yields uterine oxygen uptake:

$$(A - V)F = O_2 \text{ uptake by the gravid uterus}$$

In a sheep study the umbilical vein was observed to carry the highest concentrations of oxygenated blood delivered to the fetus, but this is low when compared with maternal Po_2. Attempts have been made to explain the low fetal Po_2 with either a concurrent or cross-current model of placental oxygen exchange, but the placenta is probably more complex. Nonetheless, the umbilical venous Po_2 depends on and is not higher than the venous Po_2 of the uterine circulation.[69] In addition, three other factors might contribute to the inefficiency of the exchange process:

Shunting, that is, the diversion of blood away from the exchange surface to perfuse the myometrium and endometrium.

Uneven perfusion—differences in the ratio of maternal-fetal blood flow—can vary in portions of the placenta.

Oxygen-diffusing capacity, which is the product of the quantity of oxygen transferred from maternal to fetal circulation divided by the mean Po_2 difference between maternal and fetal erythrocytes. It is the result of the permeability of the placental membrane to oxygen transport and the reaction rate of oxygen with hemoglobin.[70]

Uterine venous Po_2, a primary factor that determines umbilical venous Po_2, is in turn influenced by a number of other factors (Table 3–3). Chief among these are the oxygen saturation and the oxyhemoglobin dissociation curve of venous blood. The oxyhemoglobin dissociation curve is shifted by pH so that Po_2 is inversely related to pH (Bohr effect). As a result, maternal alkalosis shifts the curve to the left, decreasing oxygen delivery to the fetus. Other factors that can shift the curve are temperature, hemoglobinopathies, and the 2,3-diphosphoglycerate (2,3-DPG) content of erythrocytes. Oxygen saturation of uterine venous blood (Sv) is a function of four variables: maternal arterial oxygen saturation (Sa), oxygen capacity of maternal blood (O_2Cap), uterine blood flow (F), and the oxygen consumption rate (Vo_2) of the gravid uterus (including placental and fetal oxygen consumption). This can be formulated as:

$$\frac{Sv + Sa - Vo_2}{F\ (O_2Cap)}$$

which is an application of the Fick principle. Anemic, circulatory, or hypoxic hypoxia decreases uterine venous saturation, leading to a decrease in fetal oxygenation.

Although umbilical vein Po_2 is less than that in the maternal circulation, there are compensatory mechanisms to ensure adequate fetal oxygenation. Fetal erythrocyte hemoglobin has a high affinity for oxygen. The rate of perfusion of fetal organs, compared with adults, is high in relation to their oxygen requirements. Physiologically, the low level of Po_2 in fetal arterial blood is a part of the mechanism that keeps the ductus arteriosus open and the pulmonary vascular bed constricted.

Supplemental oxygen increases the Po_2 of maternal arterial blood, but causes only a small increase in fetal arterial Po_2. This is because of the differences in the oxyhemoglobin dissociation curves between mother and fetus (Fig. 3–4). Increasing the FIo_2 to 100% causes a rise in maternal Po_2 from 90 to 500 mm Hg, or an increase of 1 mmol for the arterial oxygen content.[71] Because there is no change in uterine blood flow, and presumably uterine oxygen consumption rate, uterine venous oxygen content also increases 1 mmol. The resulting increase in uterine venous Po_2 is 11.5 mm Hg. This is not to say that supplemental oxygen for the mother has no effect, because it probably is more important when the fetus is hypoxic.

As in the mother, carbon dioxide is one end product of fetal metabolism. Carbon dioxide from the fetus diffuses across the placenta from the umbilical circulation to the maternal side for transport to the lungs and excretion. The diffusion process requires that the Pco_2 of fetal blood be higher than that on the maternal side. In sheep, the umbilical venous blood is approximately 5 mm Hg higher than that in the maternal vein. As a result, perturbations in the maternal acid-base balance are quickly reflected in the fetus. Therefore, fetal respiratory alkalosis (low fetal Pco_2) is secondary to a low maternal Pco_2. Although fetal respiratory acidosis can be due to a high level of maternal Pco_2, decreased placental perfusion resulting in inadequate gas exchange can also play a role.

Table 3–3 Factors That Determine Uterine Venous Po_2

Oxyhemoglobin dissociation of maternal blood
Hemoglobin structure
Temperature
Erythrocyte pH (2,3-DPG)
Oxygen saturation in uterine venous blood
Arterial O_2 saturation
Uteroplacental blood flow
O_2 capacity
Placental and fetal O_2 consumption

2,3-DPG, 2,3-diphosphoglycerate.

Assessment of Fetal Lung Maturity

Because fetal chronologic age does not necessarily correlate with functional maturity, particularly the pulmonary system, methods of assessing fetal lung maturity are important adjuncts in clinical decision making.

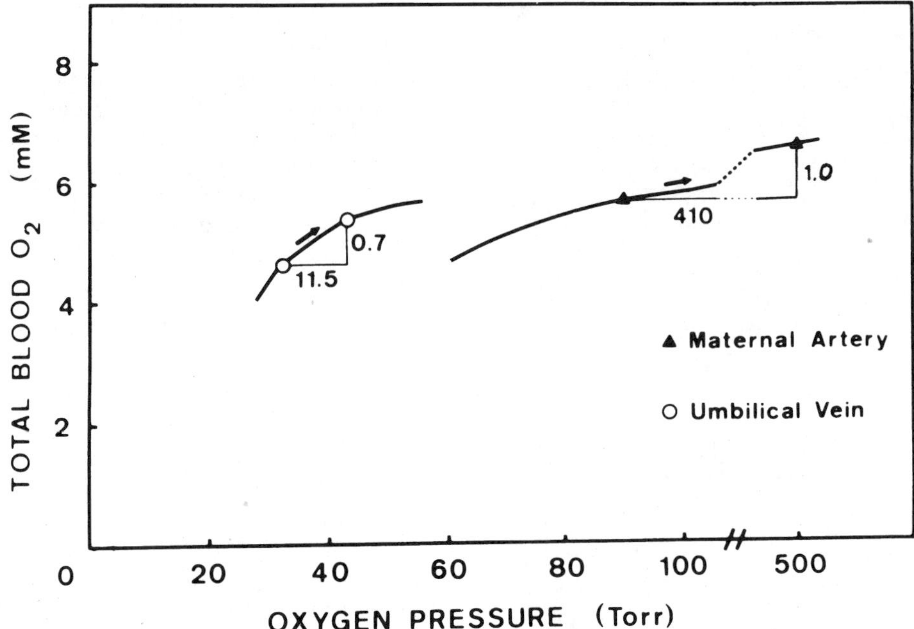

❖ **Figure 3–4** Relationship between oxygen content and Po_2 in maternal and fetal blood before and after maternal inhalation of 100% oxygen.

The majority of perinatal morbidity and mortality results from complications of premature delivery. The most frequently seen complication is the respiratory distress syndrome (RDS). This disorder is due to a deficiency of a surface-active agent (surfactant) that prevents alveolar collapse during expiration. Phospholipids, produced by fetal alveolar cells, are the major component of lung surfactant and are produced in sufficient amounts by 36 weeks' gestation. The most commonly used technique measures the lecithin-sphingomyelin (L/S) ratio. The concentration of lecithin, a component of surfactant, begins to rise in the amniotic fluid at 32 to 33 weeks' gestation and continues to rise until term. The concentration of sphingomyelin remains relatively constant, so that the ratio of the two provides an estimate of surfactant production that is not affected by variations in the volume of amniotic fluid. The risk of neonatal RDS when the L/S ratio is greater than 2 is less than 1%. If the ratio is less than 1.5, approximately 80% of neonates develop RDS.

Disaturated phosphatidylcholine (SPC) is the major component of fetal pulmonary surfactant. The technique that separates SPC from lecithin in amniotic fluid is complicated and the results can be altered by abnormalities in amniotic fluid production and excretion (i.e., oligohydramnios or polyhydramnios). A value greater than 500 μg/dL for SPC concentration in amniotic fluid is consistent with mature fetal lungs and a small risk for RDS. However, in diabetic gravidae, the SPC value should be 1000 μg/dL.

The disadvantage in measuring the L/S ratio includes a long turnaround time, the use of toxic reagents, a lack of technical expertise, and the inability to standardize the test. As a result, few hospitals are able to perform the test. Another test, the TDx fetal lung maturity test, is automated and avoids the technical involvement of sample preparation and measurement. The test relies on the fluorescence polarization of a dye added to a solution of amniotic fluid that is then compared with values on a standard curve to determine the relative concentration of surfactant and albumin. The determined values are expressed in milligrams of surfactant per gram of albumin. With a cutoff of 50 mg/g for maturity, the TDx test was equal in sensitivity (0.96) and more specific (0.88 vs. 0.83) when compared with the L/S ratio in one multicenter study.[72]

Fetal Breathing and Body Movements

Fetal breathing and body movements are important functions during fetal life. The development of skeletal and diaphragmatic muscle is dependent on these movements in utero. Fetal lung development is also dependent on diaphragmatic motion. This movement does have its cost, consuming 15% to 30% of available fetal oxygen supplies.[75] Therefore, absence of either movement or breathing can be a sign of hypoxia.[76, 77]

Fetal Breathing. Studies in lambs have demonstrated that breathing movements occur about 40% of the time during observation. This directly correlates with low voltage electroencephalogram activity and electro-ocular activity.[78] Flow in and out of the trachea to the lungs occurs in conjunction with diaphragmatic motion.[79] In ewes, the frequency of fetal breathing movements decreases from 39% to 7% when hypoxia is induced.[76] Gasping movements occur with asphyxia in dying fetal animal preparations.[80] Two to 3 days before the onset of labor, fetal breathing movements decrease.[81, 82] This is thought to be secondary to the rising concentration of PGE_2, which probably plays a

■ Table 3–4 FACTORS THAT ALTER FETAL BREATHING

DRUG/CONDITION	EFFECT
Hypoglycemia	Decrease
Glucose infusion	Increase
Ethanol	Decrease
Barbiturates	Decrease
Diazepam	Decrease
Catecholamines	Increase
Prostaglandin E_2	Decrease
Indomethacin	Increase

role in the onset of labor.[83] Infusing PGE_2[84] or inducing labor with adrenocorticotropic hormone (ACTH),[82] with a subsequent rise in PGE_2, is associated with a drop in fetal breathing movements from 40% to 15% of the time.

There are a number of other factors that can alter breathing activity (Table 3–4).[85–89] The time of day is very important, particularly during the last trimester. In addition to circadian rhythms, fetal breathing movements increase significantly 2 to 3 hours postprandially,[90] probably secondary to the increase in maternal blood glucose. After either an oral[91] or an intravenous glucose[92] load to the mother, fetal breathing movements increase.[93] A similar pattern is seen after meals. During the last 10 weeks of pregnancy, administration of carbon dioxide (5%) to healthy pregnant women results in increased breathing movements.[94] This is thought to represent maturation in the sensitivity of the fetal respiratory center. Maternal ingestion of drugs affects fetal breathing movements. After administration of ethanol[95] and methadone,[96] there is a marked decrease in breathing movements, whereas with maternal cigarette smoking,[97] there is a transient increase in the frequency of fetal breathing activity. During the 3 days prior to the onset of spontaneous labor, fetal breathing movements decrease and are absent during active labor.[98]

Fetal Body Movements. Fetal body movements are considered significant when the body rolls and the extremities stretch. Isolated limb movement is not of any consequence. During the last trimester, fetal body movements occur on average 3 to 16 minutes in each hour during a 24-hour period of observation.[99] The actual or mean number of fetal body movements ranges from 20 to 50 per hour, but up to 75-minute spans of no movement have been recorded in healthy fetuses. Unlike fetal breathing movements, body movements are not influenced by maternal plasma glucose concentration[100] and maternal alcohol ingestion,[95] and they do not decrease during the last 3 days prior to onset of spontaneous labor.[101] Fetal body movements, however, are closely related to fetal heart rate accelerations. Reports show that from 91% to 99.8% of fetal movements are associated with fetal heart rate accelerations.[102]

BIOPHYSICAL PROFILE

The biophysical profile involves evaluation of immediate biophysical activities (fetal movement, tone, breathing movements, and heart rate activity) as well as semiquantitative assessment of amniotic fluid. The biophysical parameters reflect acute CNS activity and when present correlate positively with the lack of depression (secondary to asphyxia) of the CNS. Amniotic fluid volume represents long-term or chronic fetal compromise. Major indications for referral for biophysical profile include suspected intrauterine growth retardation, hypertension, postdates gestation, and diabetes.

The biophysical evaluation of the fetus is done by ultrasound with the sole purpose of detecting changes in fetal activity owing to asphyxia. As previously mentioned, changes in fetal breathing movements, heart rate, and body movements are indicators of the state of fetal oxygenation. Superimposed on these factors are the nonrandom pattern of CNS output and the sleep state, with effects that might be mistaken for hypoxia. However, extending the period of observation to find a period of normal recovery for the latter conditions helps to differentiate asphyxia from normal variants.

The scoring of the fetal biophysical profile is an assessment of five variables (Table 3–5), four of which are monitored simultaneously by ultrasound. The variables are said to be normal or abnormal and are assigned a score of 2 for normal and 0 for abnormal. The nonstress test (NST) is monitored after the biophysical evaluation. When the test score is normal,

■ Table 3–5 BIOPHYSICAL PROFILE SCORING

VARIABLE	SCORE = 2	SCORE = 0
Fetal breathing movements	1 episode, 30-sec duration in 30 min	Absent
Gross body movement	3 discrete body/limb movements in 30 min	<2 episodes in 30 min
Fetal tone	1 episode of extension/flexion of hand, limb, or trunk	Absent or slow movement
Fetal heart rate	2 episodes of acceleration with fetal movement in 30 min	<2 episodes
Amniotic fluid volume	1 pocket 1 × 1 cm^2	No amniotic fluid or a pocket <1 × 1 cm^2

■ Table 3–6 INTERPRETATION AND MANAGEMENT OF BIOPHYSICAL PROFILE SCORE

SCORE	INTERPRETATION	RECOMMENDED MANAGEMENT
8–10	Normal infant	Repeat test in 1 week*
6	Suspect asphyxia	Repeat test in 4–6 h†
4	Suspect asphyxia	If >36 weeks, deliver
		If <36 weeks, repeat in 24 h
0–2	Probable asphyxia	Deliver

*Repeat test twice a week if diabetic or >42 weeks' gestation.
†Deliver if oligohydramnios is present.

conservative therapy is indicated, with some exceptions:

1. Postdates gestation with a favorable cervix.
2. Growth-retarded fetus with mature pulmonary indices and a favorable cervix.
3. Insulin-dependent diabetic woman at 37 weeks' or greater gestation with mature pulmonary indices.
4. Class A diabetic woman at term with a favorable cervix.
5. Women with medical disorders (e.g., asthma, preeclampsia, pregnancy induced hypertension) that might pose a threat to maternal and fetal health.

Table 3–6 lists recommendations for management of biophysical profile scores.

Several prospective studies, summarized in Table 3–7, have shown that the majority of women studied (>97%) have normal test results and delivery outcome. Perinatal mortality varies inversely with the last score before delivery. In 1981 and 1985, in large groups of patients, Manning and coworkers[107, 108] found that the gross perinatal mortality rate decreased from 11.7 to 7.4 per 1000 and the corrected value decreased from 5 to 1.9 per 1000. In Manitoba, since the use of this testing, the stillbirth rate has decreased by 30%. A stillbirth occurring within a week of a normal test result is defined as a false negative. This ranges from 0.41 to 1.01 per 1000 with a mean of 0.64 per 1000.

The false-negative rate, although small, directly reflects the negative predictive accuracy of the test. Manning and coworkers[103] calculated from a study of 19,221 pregnancies a negative predictive accuracy of 99.2%, or the probability of fetal death after a normal test result as 0.726 per 1000 patients.

Because the ideal testing method would result in no false-negative deaths, the biophysical profile is not perfect. The cause of the imperfection is the probability of change in the fetal status owing to a chronic condition or an acute variable. While more frequent testing of all patients would decrease the false-negative rate, this has not been attempted because of the increased workload. The proper selection of patients requiring more vigilant monitoring (e.g., an immature fetus with growth retardation, preeclampsia, diabetes) would render this more feasible.

Fetal Acid-Base Physiology

Fetal metabolism results in the production of carbonic and noncarbonic acids that require buffering. Carbonic acid is the hydration product of carbon dioxide, which in turn is the end product of the oxidative metabolism of glucose. Hemoglobin in the fetal erythrocyte buffers the carbonic acid and transports it to the placenta. Carbon dioxide is regenerated and diffuses quickly across the placenta. If maternal respiration and uteroplacental and umbilical blood flows are maintained, then large amounts of carbon dioxide can be eliminated rapidly. On a molar basis, the rate of fetal carbon dioxide production is basically equivalent to the oxygen consumption rate of the fetus.[109] The noncarbonic acids in the fetus include uric acid (from the metabolism of non–sulfur-containing amino acids), lactate, and keto acid (from the metabolism of carbohydrates and fatty acids). These noncarbonic acids are eliminated through the maternal kidneys, after diffusing slowly across the placenta. The maternal kidney regenerates bicarbonate from the excretion of the noncarbonic acids.

There are a number of other factors that affect acid-base balance in the fetus. These disrupt either the supply of oxygen or the removal of the carbonic and noncarbonic acids through the placenta. The maternal, fetal, and placental factors listed (Table 3–8) can result in either respiratory or metabolic perturbations of fetal acid-base balance. Fetal respiratory acidosis is secondary to decreased carbon dioxide elimination. This is most commonly due to either decreased minute ventilation or $\dot{V}/\dot{Q}$ mismatch, which results in maternal respiratory acidosis that is reflected in the fetus. As with primary fetal respiratory acidosis, rapidly reversing the cause in the mother restores fetal acid-base balance. Maternal respiratory alkalosis is caused by hyperventilation, which decreases the P_{CO_2}, increases the pH, and responds rapidly to reversal of the causes.

Fetal metabolic acidosis can be due to either primary fetal or secondary maternal metabolic acidosis. The decreased pH is from loss of bicarbonate and

■ Table 3–7 BIOPHYSICAL PROFILE AND PERINATAL MORTALITY

STUDY	NO. PATIENTS	NO. DEATHS	PERINATAL MORTALITY (%)
Manning[103]	19,221	141	1.9
Baskett[104]	5,034	32	3.1
Platt[105]	286	4	7.0
Schiffrin[106]	158	7	12.6

Table 3–8 FACTORS THAT AFFECT FETAL ACID-BASE BALANCE

Mother
Hypoxia
Hypoventilation
Altered hemoglobin
Metabolic acidosis
Decreased blood supply to placenta
Placenta
Infarction or separation
Insufficiency
Fetus
Obstruction of umbilical blood flow
Fetal anemia
Increased fixed acid production

is usually due to chronic metabolic disorders. With prolonged fetal respiratory acidosis, owing to cord compression or abruptio placentae the accumulation of noncarbonic acids can result in a mixed respiratory-metabolic acidosis.

Fetal Temperature Regulation

Fetal temperature parallels that of the mother. Heat is produced as a byproduct of metabolic processes that consume oxygen. Just as fetal oxygen consumption, which is approximately 6.8 to 8.0 mL/kg/min and twice that of the adult (3 to 4 mL/kg/min), fetal heat production is also large compared to the adult. This heat can be dissipated through either the umbilical circulation or the fetal skin. The former is the major source of heat loss. A decrease in uterine blood flow, as occurs during uterine contractions, might increase fetal temperature. This has not been shown directly; however, indirectly, the maternal and fetal temperature gradient does increase during labor.[110] Epidural anesthesia during labor has been associated with a small increased maternal temperature, but the mechanism has not been delineated and there is no evidence so far of a detrimental effect on the fetus.[111]

FETAL REACTION TO STRESS

During labor and delivery, the main causes of stress for the fetus are hypoxia and asphyxia. Fetal hypoxia is due to the mother breathing a hypoxic mixture of gases, which results in decreased oxygen tension. Asphyxia is secondary to a reduction of at least 50% in uterine blood flow. In addition to decreased oxygen tension there is also increased carbon dioxide tension, leading to both metabolic anad respiratory acidosis. With prolonged asphyxia, the fetus switches to anaerobic metabolism and produces a buildup of lactate. Metabolic acidosis subsequently develops. The fetal responses to hypoxia or asphyxia are as follows:

1. Bradycardia (owing to increased vagal activity) with hypertension.
2. Slight decrease in ventricular output.
3. Redistribution of blood from the splanchnic bed to the heart, brain, placenta, and adrenals.[112]
4. A decrease in fetal breathing movements (from 39% to 7% of the time).
5. Terminal gasping movements with asphyxia.
6. Increased circulating catecholamine levels in fetal sheep.
7. Increased α-adrenergic activity.

In chronically instrumented sheep, fetal oxygen consumption drops by as much as 60% of control values with hypoxia.[113] As described earlier, this is accompanied by fetal bradycardia, an increase in blood pressure, and progressive metabolic acidosis. Fetal sheep can tolerate this for approximately 1 hour; these changes are rapidly reversed with restoration of oxygenation.[114] Fetal cerebral[115] and myocardial[116] oxygen consumption have been shown to remain constant. When hypoxia is prolonged or proceeds to asphyxia, these compensatory mechanisms are lost.

TRANSITION FROM FETUS TO NEONATE

With labor and birth, the fetus becomes a neonate and undergoes a series of physiologic changes. Although these changes affect every major organ system, this section considers primarily the cardiovascular and respiratory systems.

With the separation of the placenta, the changes that occur include the following:

1. A decrease in blood flow through the inferior vena cava, with a resultant decrease in right atrial blood flow and pressure
2. An increase in pulmonary blood flow as pulmonary vascular resistance falls (secondary to lung expansion and vasodilation of the pulmonary vascular bed)
3. An increase in venous return to the left atrium as well as an increase in left atrial pressure

These changes produce a "series" flow pattern from the fetal "parallel" flow pattern.

Closure of Fetal Shunts. The ductus arteriosus closes in response to a rise in oxygen tension and decreased levels of circulating PGs. The latter effect is age dependent, so that premature infants have a decreased response to a rise in PO_2. Glucocorticoids, which are used in premature infants to accelerate fetal lung maturation, decrease this effect. The ductus venosus closes with the fall in partial venous and sinus pressures. Unlike the ductus arteriosus, the ductus venosus is not dependent on changes in PO_2 nor endogenous levels of catecholamines. The foramen ovale closes because the pressure in the left atrium rises above that in the right atrium. Anatomic closure of all three shunts, although begun at birth, is not completed until 24 hours to 3 months after birth.

Cardiac Output. Neonatal cardiac output is 600 to 850 mL/kg/min, a small increase over fetal cardiac output of 500 mL/kg/min. The left ventricular output increases 2 to 2.5 times that of the fetal left ventricular output, whereas the output from the right ventricle remains basically the same. Neonatal heart rate decreases from fetal levels, but it can vary from 140 beats/min in the awake infant to 90 to 120 beats/min in the sleeping infant.

Respiratory Changes. The intermittent, rhythmic respiratory movements of the fetus become continuous after birth and ensure gas exchange. A number of factors exert an effect, including changes in the physical environment (temperature, sound, and tactile stimulation), preconditioning changes during labor (increase in P_{CO_2} and a decrease in pH), and an increase in P_{O_2} secondary to the cardiovascular changes.

With a vaginal delivery, the compression of the head and thorax during the passage through the vaginal canal followed by the sudden expansion with the delivery of the trunk results in an elastic recoil of the thorax and active contraction of the respiratory muscles. This also stimulates the Hering-Breuer inflation reflex and Head's reflex. In the former, lung inflation results in inspiratory inhibition, causing a higher respiratory rate in the neonate which may be important in maintaining a higher functional residual capacity (FRC). Head's reflex results from an increase in inspiratory effort with rapid lung inflation.

Reabsorption of amniotic fluid from alveolar air spaces, along with an increase in lung volume, results in a rise in lung compliance with birth that gradually continues to rise in the hours after birth. In premature infants, both lung volume and compliance are decreased. This is further decreased in infants with RDS. Airway and pulmonary resistance, although initially high at birth, decrease with age as the diameter of the airways becomes larger. FRC increases quickly after birth as amniotic fluid is reabsorbed. Respiratory rate, initially 60 to 80 breaths/min gradually decreases to 30 to 40 breaths/min. Tidal volume is between 5 to 7 mL/kg body weight. Minute ventilation ranges from 150 to 250 mL/kg/min.

During labor and delivery, uterine contractions decrease uterine blood flow, which, in turn, can decrease fetal gas exchange. This can also be produced by cord compression or partial separation of the placenta, resulting in relative hypoxia and hypercapnia in neonates at birth. This is transient in most neonates because the start of regular breathing improves oxygenation.

❖ SUMMARY

Key Points

- Maternal metabolism, including fasting and ketonuria, may affect the fetus.
- Fetal heart rate monitoring and fetal scalp sampling are the main tools for monitoring the fetus during labor. Doppler ultrasonography is commonly used to estimate uterine blood flow.
- The fetus has no oxygen reservoir and cannot compensate for hypoxia. Although the fetal P_{O_2} level is low, the normal fetus is not hypoxic.
- Assessment of the premature fetus is important in predicting outcome during and after labor.

Key Reference

Battaglia FC: An Introduction to Fetal Physiology. New York; Academic Press; 1986.

Case Stem

A G2P1 patient at 32 weeks' gestation presents to labor and delivery in preterm labor. The membranes are intact despite regular contractions. Discuss the potential effects on the fetus of the obstetric and anesthetic management.

References

1. Grumbach MM, Kaplan SL, Sciarra JJ, et al: Chorionic growth hormone–prolactin (CGP): secretion, disposition, biological activity in man and postulated function as "growth hormone" of the second half of pregnancy. Ann N Y Acad Sci 1968; 148:501.
2. Kalikhoff RK, Kisselbah AH, Kim HK: Carbohydrate and lipid metabolism during normal pregnancy: relationship to gestational hormone action. Semin Perinatol 1978; 2:291.
3. Abramovich R, Baker TG, Neal P: Effect of human chorionic gonadotropin on testosterone secretion by the fetal human testis in organ culture. J Endocrinol 1974; 60:179.
4. Gabbe SG, Demers LM, Greep RO, et al: The effects of hypoxia on placental glycogen metabolism. Am J Obstet Gynecol 1972; 114:540.
5. Widdas WF: Inability of diffusion to account for placental glucose transfer in the sheep and consideration of the kinetics of a possible carrier transfer. J Physiol (Lond) 1952; 118:23.
6. Young M, Prenton MA: Maternal and fetal plasma amino acid concentrations during gestation and in retarded fetal growth. J Obstet Gynaecol Br Commonw 1969; 76:333.
7. Brambell FWR: Transport of proteins across the fetal membrane. Cold Spring Harbor Symp Quant Biol 1954; 19:71.
8. Robertson AF, Sprecher H: A review of human placental lipid metabolism and transport. Acta Paediatr Scand 1968; 57(suppl 183):1.
9. Snelling CE, Jackson SH: Blood studies of vitamin C during pregnancy, birth and early infancy. J Pediatr 1977; 14:447.
10. Widdowson EM, Grabb DE, Milveer RDG: Cellular development of some human organs before birth. Arch Dis Child 1972; 47:652.
11. Rosso P: Changes in transfer of nutrients across the placenta during normal gestation in the rat. Am J Obstet Gynecol 1975; 122:2761.
12. D'Ercole AJ, Foushee DB, Underwood LE: Somatomedin-C receptor ontogeny and levels in porcine fetal and human cord serum. J Clin Endocrinol Metab 1976; 43:1069.
13. Takano KT, Hizuka N, Shizuma N: The effects of growth hormone and fasting on the serum levels of somatomedin in rats and man determined by radioreceptor assay. Acta Endocrinol (Copenh) 1977; 85:189.
14. Davison JM: Changes in renal function and other aspects of

homeostasis in early pregnancy. J Obstet Gynaecol Br Commonw 1974; 81:1003.
15. Lind T, Hytten FE: The excretion of glucose during normal pregnancy. J Obstet Gynaecol Br Commonw 1972; 79:961.
16. Isles TE, Dickson M, Farquhar JW: Glucose tolerance and plasma insulin in newborn infants of normal and diabetic mothers. Pediatr Res 1968; 2:198.
17. Kerr GR, Waisman HA: Transplacental ratio of serum amino acids during pregnancy in Rhesus monkey. *In* Nyhan WL (ed): Amino Acids Metabolism and Genetic Variation. New York: McGraw-Hill; 1967:429.
18. Ghadimi H, Pecora P: Free amino acids of cord plasma as compared with maternal plasma during pregnancy. Pediatrics 1964; 30:500.
19. Widdowson EM, Southgate DAT, Hey EN: Body composition of the fetus and infant. *In* Visser HKA (ed): Nutrition and Metabolism of the Fetus and Infant. The Hague: Martinus Nijhoff; 1979:169.
20. Elphick MC: The passage of fat emulsion across the human placenta. Br J Obstet Gynaecol 1978; 85:610.
21. Baker H: Vitamin profile of 174 mothers and newborns at parturition. Am J Clin Nutr 1975; 28:56.
22. Baker H: Role of placenta in maternal-fetal vitamin transfer in humans. Am J Obstet Gynecol 1981; 141:792.
23. Pritchard JA: Anemias complicating pregnancy and the puerperium. *In* Maternal Nutrition and the Course of Pregnancy. Washington, DC: National Academy of Sciences; 1970.
24. Dawson EB: Plasma vitamins and trace metal changes during teenage pregnancy. Am J Obstet Gynecol 1969; 104:953.
25. Child CM: Some considerations concerning the nature and origin of physiological gradients. Biol Bull 1920; 39:147.
26. Eastman NJ, Jackson J: Weight relationships in pregnancy. 1. The bearing of maternal weight gain and pre-pregnancy weight on birth weight in full term pregnancies. Obstet Gynecol Surv 1968; 23:1003.
27. Young M, Widdowson E: The influence of diets deficient in energy or in protein on conceptus weight and the placental transfer of non-metabolizable amino acid in the guinea pig. Biol Neonate 1975; 27:184.
28. Pond WG, Stracham DN, Sinha YN, et al: Effect of protein deprivation of the swine during all or part of gestation on birth weight, postnatal growth rate, and nucleic acid content of the brain and muscle of progeny. J Nutr 1969; 99:61.
29. Riopelle AJ, Hill CW, Li SC: Protein deprivation in primates vs. fetal mortality and neonatal status of infant monkeys born of deprived mothers. Am J Clin Nutr 1975; 28:989.
30. Riopelle AJ: Weight gain of non-pregnant monkeys and pregnant monkeys fed low protein diets. Am J Clin Nutr 1975; 28:802.
31. Berg BN: Dietary restriction and reproduction in the rat. J Nutr 1965; 87:344.
32. Rosso P: Nutrition and maternal-fetal exchange. Am J Clin Nutr 1981; 34:744.
33. Beaton GH, Beare J, Ryu MH, et al: Protein metabolism in the pregnant rat. J Nutr 1954; 54:291.
34. Naismith DJ: Adaptations in the metabolism of protein during pregnancy and their nutritional implications. Nutr Rep Int 1973; 7:383.
35. Beydoun SN, Cuenca VG, Evans LP: Maternal nutrition. 1. The urinary urea nitrogen/total nitrogen as an index of protein nutrition. Am J Obstet Gynecol 1972; 114:198.
36. Blechner JN, Stenger VG, Prystowsky H: Uterine blood flow in women at term. Am J Obstet Gynecol 1974; 129:633.
37. Bruc NW: The distribution of blood flow to the reproductive organs of the rat near term. J Reprod Fertil 1976; 45:359.
38. Croall J, Sheriff S, Matthews J: Non-pregnant maternal plasma volume and fetal growth retardation. Br J Obstet Gynaecol 1978; 85:90.
39. Kava R, Rosso P: Mechanisms for fetal growth retardation in undernourished pregnant rats. Fed Proc 1979; 38:871.
40. LaFever HN, Jones CT, Rolph TP: Some of the consequences of intrauterine growth retardation, p. 43. *In* Visser HKA (ed): Nutrition and Metabolism of the Fetus and Infant. The Hague: Martinus Nijhoff; 1979.
41. Hehenauer L, Oh W: Body composition in experimental intrauterine growth retardation in the rat. J Nutr 1969; 99:23.
42. Myers RG, Hill DE, Holt AB, et al: Fetal growth retardation produced by experimental placental insufficiency in the Rhesus monkey. II. Chemical composition of the brain, liver, muscle and carcass. Biol Neonate 1971; 18:379.
43. Dobbing J: The influence of early nutrition on the development of myelination of the brain. Proc R Soc Lond [Biol] 1964; 159:503.
44. Fancourt R, Harvey DR, Norman AP, et al: Follow-up study of small for dates babies. BMJ 1976; 1:1435.
45. Edelstone DI, Rudolph AM, Heymann MA: Liver and ductus venosus flows in fetal lambs in utero. Circ Res 1978; 42:426.
46. Bristow J, Rudolph AM, Itskovitz J: A preparation for studying liver blood flow, oxygen consumption in the fetal lamb in utero. J Dev Physiol 1981; 3:255.
47. Bristow J, Rudolph AM, Itskovitz J: Hepatic oxygen and glucose metabolism in the fetal lamb. J Clin Invest 1983; 71:1.
48. Rudolph AM, Heymann MA: Circulatory changes during growth in the fetal lamb. Circ Res 1970; 26:289.
49. Peeters LLH, Sheldon RE, Jones MD Jr, et al: Blood flow to fetal organs as a function of arterial oxygen content. Am J Obstet Gynecol 1979; 135:637.
50. Peeters LLH, Sheldon RE, Jones MD Jr, et al: Redistribution of cardiac output and oxygen delivery in the hypoxic fetal lamb. Am J Obstet Gynecol 1979; 135:1071.
51. Sheldon CA, Friedman WF, Sybers HD: Scanning electron microscopy of fetal and neonatal lamb cardiac cells. J Mol Cell Cardiol 1976; 8:853.
52. McPherson RA, Kramer MF, Covell JW, et al: A comparison of the active stiffness of fetal and adult cardiac muscle. Pediatr Res 1976; 10:660.
53. Heymann MA, Rudolph AM: Effects of increasing preload on right ventricular output in fetal lambs in utero. Circulation 1973; 48:IV-37.
54. Berman W Jr, Goodlin RC, Heymann MA, et al: Pressure flow relationships in the umbilical and uterine circulations of the sheep. Circ Res 1976; 38:262.
55. Papile L, Rudolph AM, Heymann MA: Autoregulation of cerebral blood flow in the preterm fetal lamb. Pediatr Res 1985; 19:159.
56. Dawes GS, Johnston BM, Walker DW: Relationship of arterial pressure and heart rate in fetal newborn and adult sheep. J Physiol 1980; 309:405.
57. Iwamoto HS, Rudolph AM: Effects of angiotensin II on the blood flow and its distribution in fetal lambs. Circ Res 1982; 48:183.
58. Drummond WH, Rudolph AM, Keil LC, et al: Arginine vasopressin and prolactin after hemorrhage in the fetal lamb. Am J Physiol 1980; 238:E214.
59. Iwamoto HS, Rudolph AM, Keil LC, et al: Hemodynamic responses of the sheep fetus to vasopressin infusion. Circ Res 1979; 44:430.
60. Challis JRG, Patrick JE: The production of prostaglandins and thromboxanes in the feto-placental unit and their effects on the developing fetus. Semin Perinatol 1980; 4:23.
61. Mitchell MD, Flint AP, Bibby J, et al: Plasma concentrations of prostaglandins during late human pregnancy: influence of normal and preterm labor. J Clin Endocrinol Metab 1978; 46:947.
62. Novy MJ, Piasecki G, Jackson BT: Effect of prostaglandins E_2 and $F_{2\text{-alpha}}$ on umbilical blood flow and fetal hemodynamics. Prostaglandins 1974; 5:543.
63. Berman W Jr, Goodlin RC, Heymann MA, et al: Effects of pharmacologic agents on umbilical blood flow in fetal lambs in utero. Biol Neonate 1978; 33:225.
64. Cassin S: Role of prostaglandins and thromboxanes in the control of the pulmonary circulation in the fetus and newborn. Semin Perinatol 1980; 4:101.
65. Cassin S: Role of prostaglandins, thromboxanes and leukotrienes in the control of the pulmonary circulation in the fetus and newborn. Semin Perinatol 1987; 11:53.
66. Clyman RI: Ontogeny of the ductus arteriosus response to prostaglandins and inhibitors of their synthesis. Semin Perinatol 1980; 4:115.

67. Clyman RI: Ductus arteriosus: current theories of prenatal and postnatal regulation. Semin Perinatol 1987; 11:64.
68. Prowse CM, Gaensler EA: Respiratory and acid-base changes during pregnancy. Anesthesiology 1965; 26:381.
69. Rankin JHG, Meschia G, Makowski EL, et al: Relationship between uterine and umbilical venous Po_2 in sheep. Am J Physiol 1971; 220:1688.
70. Longo LD, Hill EP, Power GG: Theoretical analysis of factors affecting placental O_2 transfer. Am J Physiol 1972; 222:730.
71. Meschia G: Transfer of oxygen across the placenta. *In* Gluck L (ed): Intrauterine Asphyxia and the Developing Fetal Brain. Chicago: Year Book Medical Publishers; 1977:109.
72. Russell JC, Cooper CM, Ketchum CH, et al: Multicenter evaluation of TDx test for assessing fetal lung maturity. Clin Chem 1989; 35:1005.
73. Mendez-Bauer C, Poseirio JJ, Arellano-Hernandez G, et al: Effects of atropine on the heart rate of the human fetus during labor. Am J Obstet Gynecol 1963; 85:1033.
74. Vapaavouri EK, Shinebourne EA, Williams RL, et al: Development of cardiovascular responses to autonomic blockade in intact fetal and neonatal lambs. Biol Neonate 1973; 22:1977.
75. Rurak DW, Cooper CC, Taylor SM: Fetal oxygen consumption and Po_2 during hypercapnia in pregnant sheep. J Dev Physiol 1986; 8:447.
76. Boddy K, Dawes GS, Fisher R, et al: Foetal respiratory movements, electrocortical and cardiovascular responses to hypoxaemia and hypercapnia in sheep. J Physiol (Lond) 1974; 243:599.
77. Natale R, Clewlow F, Dawes GS: Measurement of fetal forelimb movements in lambs in utero. Am J Obstet Gynecol 1981; 140:545.
78. Dawes GS, Fox HE, Leduc BM, et al: Respiratory movements and rapid eye movements in the foetal lamb. J Physiol (Lond) 1972; 220:119.
79. Maloney JE, Adamson TM, Brodecky V, et al: Diaphragmatic activity and lung liquid flow in unanesthetized fetal sheep. J Appl Physiol 1975; 39:423.
80. Patrick JE, Falton KJ, Dawes GS: Breathing patterns before death in fetal lambs. Am J Obstet Gynecol 1976; 125:73.
81. Boddy K, Dawes GS: Fetal breathing. Br Med Bull 1975; 31:1.
82. Patrick J, Challis JRG, Cross J, et al: The relationship between fetal breathing movements and prostaglandin E_2 during ACTH-induced labour in sheep. J Dev Physiol 1987; 9:287.
83. Thorburn GD, Challis JRG: Control of parturition. Physiol Rev 1979; 59:863.
84. Kitterman JA, Liggins GC, Fewell JE, et al: Inhibition of breathing movements in fetal sheep by prostaglandins. J Appl Physiol 1983; 54:687.
85. Richardson B, Hohimer AR, Mueggler P, et al: Effects of glucose concentration on fetal breathing movements and electrocortical activity in fetal lambs. Am J Obstet Gynecol 1982; 142:678.
86. Patrick J, Richardson B, Hasen G, et al: Effects of maternal ethanol infusion on fetal cardiovascular and brain activity in lambs. Am J Obstet Gynecol 1985; 151:859.
87. Boddy K, Dawes GS, Fisher RL, et al: The effects of pentobarbitone and pethidine on foetal breathing movements in sheep. Br J Pharmacol 1976; 57:311.
88. Piercy WN, Day MA, Neims AH, et al: Alteration of ovine fetal respiratory-like activity by diazepam, caffeine and doxapram. Am J Obstet Gynecol 1977; 127:43.
89. Kitterman JA, Liggins GC, Clements JA, et al: Stimulation of breathing movements in fetal sheep by inhibitors of prostaglandin synthesis. J Dev Physiol 1979; 1:453.
90. Patrick J, Natale R, Richardson B: Pattern of human fetal breathing activity at 34 to 35 weeks' gestational age. Am J Obstet Gynecol 1978; 132:507.
91. Lewis PJ, Trudinger BJ, Mangey J: Effect of maternal glucose ingestion on fetal breathing and body movements in late pregnancy. Br J Obstet Gynecol 1979; 85:586.
92. Boddy K, Dawes GS, Robinson JS: Intrauterine fetal breathing movements. *In* Gluck L (ed): Modern Perinatal Medicine. Chicago: Year Book Medical Publishers; 1975:381.
93. Natale R, Patrick J, Richardson B: Effects of maternal venous plasma glucose concentrations on fetal breathing movements. Am J Obstet Gynecol 1978; 132:26.
94. Richie K: The fetal response to changes in the composition of maternal inspired air in human pregnancy. Semin Perinatol 1980; 4:295.
95. McLeod W, Brien J, Carmichael L, et al: Maternal glucose injections do not alter the suppression of fetal breathing following maternal ethanol ingestion. Am J Obstet Gynecol 1984; 148:634.
96. Richardson B, O'Grady JP, Olsen GD: Fetal breathing movements and the response to carbon dioxide in patients on methadone maintenance. Am J Obstet Gynecol 1984; 150:400.
97. Thaler JS, Goodman JDS, Dawes GS: The effect of maternal smoking on fetal breathing rate and activity patterns. Am J Obstet Gynecol 1980; 138:282.
98. Richardson B, Natale R, Patrick J: Human fetal breathing activity during induced labor at term. Am J Obstet Gynecol 1979; 133:247.
99. Manning FA, Platt LD, Siopos L: Fetal movements in human pregnancies. Obstet Gynecol 1979; 54:699.
100. Bocking A, Adamson L, Cousin A, et al: Effects of intravenous glucose injections on human fetal breathing movements and gross fetal body movements at 38 to 40 weeks' gestational age. Am J Obstet Gynecol 1982; 142:606.
101. Carmichael L, Cambell K, Patrick J: Fetal breathing, gross body movements and fetal heart rates before spontaneous labor at term. Am J Obstet Gynecol 1984; 148:675.
102. Timor-Tritsch IE, Dierker LJ, Zador I, et al: Fetal movements associated with fetal heart rate accelerations and decelerations. Am J Obstet Gynecol 1978; 131:276.
103. Manning FA, Morrison I, Harmon CR, et al: Fetal assessment by fetal BPS: experience in 19,221 referred high-risk pregnancies. II. The false negative rate by frequency and etiology. Am J Obstet Gynecol 1987; 157:880.
104. Baskett TF, Allen AC, Gray JH, et al: The biophysical profile score. Obstet Gynecol 1987; 70:357.
105. Platt LD, Eglington GS, Scorpios L, et al: Further experience with the fetal biophysical profile score. Obstet Gynecol 1983; 61:480.
106. Schiffrin BS, Guntes V, Gergely RC, et al: The role of real-time scanning in antenatal fetal surveillance. Am J Obstet Gynecol 1981; 140:525.
107. Manning FA, Baskett TF, Morrison I, et al: Fetal biophysical profile scoring: a prospective study in 1184 high-risk patients. Am J Obstet Gynecol 1981; 140:289.
108. Manning FA, Morrison I, Lange IR, et al: Fetal assessment based on fetal biophysical profile scoring: experience in 12,620 referred high-risk pregnancies. I. Perinatal mortality by frequency and etiology. Am J Obstet Gynecol 1985; 151:343.
109. Schiffrin BS: The rationale for antepartum fetal heart rate monitoring. J Reprod Med 1979; 23:213.
110. Peltonen R: The difference between fetal and maternal temperatures during delivery. Fifth European Congress of Perinatal Medicine, Uppsala, Sweden, 1976:188.
111. Power GG: Fetal thermoregulation: animal and human. *In* Poulin WW, Fox RA (eds): Fetal and Neonatal Physiology. Philadelphia: WB Saunders; 1998:477.
112. Cohn HE, Piasecki GJ, Jackson BT: Cardiovascular responses to hypoxemia and acidemia in fetal lambs. Am J Obstet Gynecol 1974; 129:817.
113. Parer JT: The effect of acute maternal hypoxia on fetal oxygenation and the umbilical circulation in the sheep. Eur J Obstet Gynecol Reprod Biol 1980; 10:125.
114. Mann LI: Effects in sheep of hypoxia on levels of lactate, pyruvate and glucose in blood of mother and fetus. Pediatr Res 1970; 4:46.
115. Jones MD, Sheldon RE, Peeters LL, et al: Fetal cerebral oxygen consumption at different levels of oxygenation. J Appl Physiol 1977; 43:1080.
116. Fisher DS, Heymann MA, Rudolph AM: Fetal myocardial oxygen and carbohydrate consumption during acutely induced hypoxemia. Am J Physiol 1982; 242:H657.

4

Uteroplacental Blood Flow

❖ Seppo Alahuhta, MD, PhD

ANATOMY AND HEMODYNAMIC CHANGES OF PREGNANCY

The maternal blood supply to the uterus is derived mainly from the uterine arteries, with a minor contribution from the ovarian arteries. The two uterine arteries follow tortuously the lateral margins of the uterus, giving rise to the arcuate arteries that encircle the uterus. The radial arteries branch from the arcuate arteries and discharge into the spiral arteries that enter the intervillous space. From the 150 spiral arteries blood spurts toward the chorionic plate of the placenta for nutrient exchange with fetal blood, which courses through the villi. Blood then drains through the venous openings in the decidual plate into the uterine veins. Fetal blood enters the placenta via the two umbilical arteries, which repeatedly divide into smaller vessels within the fetal villi. The fetal blood exchanges substances with the maternal blood and is then collected into a single umbilical vein.

The total uterine blood flow increases during pregnancy. It approaches 800 mL/min at term, accounting for 10% to 15% of the maternal cardiac output, 80% of which reaches the intervillous space for interfacing with the fetal circulation, while the remaining 20% supplies the uterine myometrium. The maternal cardiovascular system undergoes major anatomic and physiologic alterations during pregnancy in order to meet the increased demands on the uteroplacental circulation. Cardiac output and plasma volume increase in parallel, reaching a level 40% to 50% above the nonpregnant state in late pregnancy. This is associated with a decrease in uterine vascular resistance, which allows the increased perfusion and blood flow to meet the demands of the growing uterus, placenta, and fetus. The vascular bed of the uterus is believed to be almost maximally dilated under normal conditions, with little ability to dilate further. Placental blood flow, unlike cerebral blood flow, lacks an autoregulatory mechanism[1] and is thus dependent on perfusion pressure. Sensitivity to α-adrenergic agonists in the uterine circulation is, however, maintained. In fact, during pregnancy the uterine vessels are more sensitive to actions of α-adrenergic agonists than are the systemic vessels.[2] The vascular receptors, which control the intervillous blood flow, lie within the uterine, arcuate, radial, and basal arteries, whereas more distal parts of the uteroplacental arteries lack such vascular response elements.

DETERMINANTS OF UTEROPLACENTAL CIRCULATION

The uterine blood flow is dependent on perfusion pressure and vascular resistance according to the following formula:

$$\text{Uterine blood flow} = \frac{\text{Uterine arterial pressure} - \text{Uterine venous pressure}}{\text{Uterine vascular resistance}}$$

Hence, uterine blood flow is not maintained if there is a moderate decrease in perfusion pressure or an increase in vascular resistance.

Uterine arterial pressure depends on maternal arterial pressure. Systemic hypotension through any mechanism may potentially cause a decrease in uterine blood flow. This may occur as a result of sympathectomy during epidural or spinal anesthesia followed by hypotension. Aortocaval compression in an unmodified supine position may decrease uteroplacental flow through one or more of three mechanisms. Compression of the inferior vena cava by the gravid uterus obstructs the return of blood to the heart and, despite collateral venous circulation, the right atrial pressure consequently drops. The sequelae of this drop in pressure may be masked by the physiologic response to a decline in cardiac filling, that is, an increase in systemic vascular resistance and heart rate, and maternal arterial pressure is maintained.[3] Despite the minor maternal blood pressure and heart rate changes in the supine position, the intervillous blood flow may decrease.[4] If compensatory mechanisms fail, maternal cardiac output decreases and hypotension develops, threatening both maternal and fetal well-being. Impaired uterine arterial pressure in the supine position may also result from mechanical obstruction of the abdominal aorta and its branches by the gravid uterus.[5] As a result of the aortic obstruction, maternal blood flow to the uterus may severely deteriorate, as collateral blood supply to the uterus via the ovarian arteries and blood flow in the uterine arteries may be reduced. The degree of aortic obstruction is further increased if concomitant systemic hypotension renders the aorta collapsible.

Vena caval compression by the uterus is also associated with a pressure rise in the distal vena cava, which may lead to an increase in venous uterine pressure and a further reduction in uteroplacental perfusion. Uterine contractions cause repeated brief reductions in uterine blood flow as a result of increased uterine venous pressure. Uterine hypertonus from a tetanic contraction and intravenous oxytocin infusion may be accompanied by a decrease in uterine blood flow owing to increased uterine venous pressure.

Uterine blood flow may decrease as a result of increased uterine vascular resistance caused by endogenous and exogenous vasoconstrictors. Accordingly, excessive administration of vasopressors with predominantly α-adrenergic action or increased concentrations of endogenous vasoconstrictors (e.g., vasopressin and angiotensin II) secreted to correct hypotension may impair uterine blood flow.

METHODS FOR MEASURING UTEROPLACENTAL AND FETAL BLOOD FLOW

Until the late 1970s, almost all studies on placental blood flow during obstetric anesthesia in humans were performed using isotope techniques, such as the intravenous xenon-133 technique described by Rekonen and coworkers[6] in Finland in 1976. This radioisotope is freely diffusible and clears completely from the circulation on passage through the lungs. If the patient holds her breath for about 20 seconds after a rapid intravenous bolus injection of the agent, the tracer enters the systemic circulation as a bolus and reaches the placenta. Its clearance can then be registered by a scintillation detector placed over the placenta for 10 to 15 minutes. This quantitative technique measures the blood flow per unit volume of intervillous space. Both myometrial and intervillous blood flow can be calculated from a two-exponential curve. The method has been shown to be highly reproducible. Another noninvasive isotope technique using indium-113 was described by Nylund and colleagues[7] in Sweden in 1983. It is called placental functional scintigraphy and measures the total placental blood flow expressed as a uteroplacental blood flow index. It is a relative measure proportional to the uteroplacental blood flow expressed in milliliters per second. The method gives an erroneously low index of flow when the blood volume increases. Therefore, when cesarean section patients undergo functional placental scintigraphy, preloading in clinically adequate amounts before instituting the regional block must be avoided. The method has been validated in an animal model. Neither of the isotope techniques allows repeated measurements at short intervals, and the placenta must be on the anterior uterine wall. Furthermore, fetal circulation is not accessible with either method. Neither of these methods has gained widespread acceptance, however, owing to the use of radioactive markers in pregnant women, even though in the smallest possible amounts.

Over the last few years, the Doppler ultrasound technique has proved the most useful method for assessing the human uterine and fetal circulations during obstetric anesthesia. The basic principle underlying this method of examination is the Doppler effect. When an ultrasound wave from a fixed-frequency source hits a target that is moving relative to the source, the back-scattered signal has a different frequency compared with the emitted one. The change of frequency is directly proportional to the velocity of the moving target from which the wave is reflected. If an ultrasound beam is directed toward a blood vessel, the moving red blood cells act as reflectors causing a change in the reflected sound frequency.[8] The information provided by Doppler ultrasound studies of blood flow includes the volume blood flow and blood flow velocity waveforms. Volumetric flow measurement involves numerous sources of error. Consequently, the main interest in Doppler-based circulatory assessment focuses on a qualitative analysis of various indices derived from arterial blood flow velocity waveforms. The main Doppler indices are ratios based on the peak systolic (S) and end-diastolic (D) velocities and the averaged maximum flow velocity curve of the cardiac cycle (A). The following indices are predominantly used in obstetrics:

$$\text{Pulsatility index (PI)} = S - D/A$$

$$\text{Resistance index (RI)} = S - D/S$$

$$\text{S/D ratio} = S/D$$

The indices are without units and require measurements of relative rather than absolute velocities. Because these parameters are drawn from the same cardiac cycle, the ratios are independent of the angle between the ultrasound signal and the direction of blood flow.[9] There is a close correlation between the indices in normal pregnancies, but in situations in which diastolic flow is minimal or absent, the S/D ratio and the resistance index are less reliable than the pulsatility index. The Doppler flow velocity waveform recorded from a vascular bed of high resistance is associated with a low or even reversed flow in diastole. In contrast, low peripheral resistance results in high diastolic velocities.[10] Although the concept of peripheral resistance is frequently used to describe opposition to flow in arterial circulation, it is relevant in nonpulsatile flow conditions only. The flow of blood in an arterial system, however, is a pulsatile phenomenon, and the concept of vascular impedance should be used to characterize the peripheral hemodynamics. The shape of the arterial Doppler waveform is expected to be affected not only by the opposition to flow distal to the point of measurement but also by the performance of the cardiac pump, the heart rate, the compliance of the vessel wall, and blood flow viscosity.[11]

An in vitro model of circulation, which allowed independent control over volumetric flow, perfusion pressure, stroke volume, pulse rate, and peripheral resistance, showed the pulsatility index to be a flow- and pressure-independent proportional expression of peripheral resistance.[12] In experimental animals, increased ratios in the uterine and umbilical arteries have correlated with increased placental vascular resistance.[13] Both in vitro and clinical studies have shown that changes in heart rate affect the Doppler indices. Bradycardia increases diastolic duration and reduces end-diastolic velocity, leading to an increase in the ratios, while tachycardia results in opposite changes. The umbilical artery indices are not significantly influenced by the fetal heart rate, however, within the normal range of 120 to 160 beats/min.[14] Similarly, only extreme changes in the maternal heart rate give rise to abnormal flow indices for the uteroplacental vessels.[15] Flow rates through a given vessel also vary, depending on the viscosity of the perfusing fluid, although changes in viscosity contributed only 10% to the variability in the flow velocity waveforms obtained from the uteroplacental circulation[16] and no correlation was found between the Doppler indices for the umbilical artery and the fetal hematocrit values.[17] It may be concluded that increased downstream impedance is the major determinant of the increment in the indices. The shape of the flow velocity waveform in the umbilical artery is affected by the location of the measurement point.[18] Accordingly, the sampling site on the umbilical artery should be specified. In the uteroplacental circulation, the Doppler indices are lower in the placental than in the nonplacental uterine arteries, and each vessel should be analyzed individually.[19]

The validity of the technique has been tested with computer models.[20] There is a close correlation between the pulsatility index and peripheral vascular resistance in the brachial artery.[21, 22] The pulsatility index for the maternal femoral artery changes following epidural anesthesia with the femoral arterial resistance, calculated from leg blood flow and arterial pressure.[23] In laboratory animals, the vascular impedance spectra derived from measurements of blood flow velocity obtained by Doppler ultrasound and a surgically placed electromagnetic flow probe do not differ at rest and after vasodilatation.[24] The value of the method has been further increased by the development of color Doppler, which makes possible the localization of very small vessels and a rapid estimation of the direction of flow. The method does not allow discrimination between the placental and myometrial blood flows when the uterine vasculature is examined. The Doppler method is a noninvasive and reproducible way to detect relative changes in the uteroplacental and fetal circulations. Thanks to their high intraobserver repeatability,[25] index measurements can be used in serial studies of uterine and fetal hemodynamics and in assessing the impacts of various treatments.

Doppler methods are nowadays in routine use in the follow-up of at-risk pregnancies. Their main value is in focusing on umbilical arteries. Increased indices or absent end-diastolic velocities give an early warning signal for fetal asphyxia. Further Doppler studies dealing with fetal cerebral arteries, ductus venosus, and fetal cardiac performance give additional information about fetal condition.

REGIONAL ANESTHESIA AND UTEROPLACENTAL CIRCULATION

Obstetric regional anesthesia can affect the uteroplacental and fetal circulations in several ways. First, the extensive blockade of the sympathetic nerve outflow from the spinal cord with the consequent peripheral vasodilatation that invariably occurs with regional anesthesia tends to cause maternal hypotension, the most frequent complication of regional anesthesia in obstetrics, and to reduce uteroplacental perfusion. Furthermore, sympathectomy makes the parturient less able to compensate for other factors tending to cause hypotension, of which aortocaval compression is the most noteworthy. Second, local anesthetics in high concentrations may cause vasoconstriction in the uteroplacental and umbilical vessels.[26, 27] Thus, an unintentional intravenous injection of a local anesthetic may decrease uterine blood flow. Third, epinephrine added to local anesthetics may cause uterine vasoconstriction in a dose-dependent manner, at least after an intravascular injection.[28, 29] Finally, the vasopressors used in treating maternal hypotension secondary to regional anesthesia may reduce uterine blood flow, especially if they possess mainly α-adrenergic activity.[30]

On the other hand, regional anesthesia for labor pain relief may increase uterine blood flow. Vaginal delivery is associated with an increased release of maternal circulating catecholamines caused by pain, anxiety, and physical exertion.[31] This increase of maternal catecholamines causes uterine vasoconstriction through α-adrenergic stimulation, which may lead to moderate to severe asphyxia in the fetus owing to impaired uterine blood flow.[32] Epidural analgesia reduces maternal stress hormones significantly during labor.[33, 34] Thus, by alleviating the adverse effects of labor pain epidural analgesia could have a salutary effect on uterine blood flow. Indeed, a lumbar epidural block was associated with a significant improvement in intervillous blood flow in normal pregnancies,[35] while segmental epidural anesthesia caused no change.[36]

Several groups have examined the blood velocity waveforms in the uterine, umbilical, and fetal vessels during epidural labor analgesia in healthy parturients using the Doppler technique. These studies have confirmed the lack of any harmful effects of epidural analgesia on the uterine and umbilicoplacental circulation in parturients if maternal hypotension is avoided.[37, 38] Nor did epidural administration of a lipid-soluble opioid, sufentanil, change the uterine and umbilical artery blood velocity waveform indices during active labor.[39]

In preeclamptic women, intervillous blood flow increased significantly after lumbar epidural analgesia during labor.[40] The increase in uterine blood flow in preeclamptic pregnancies after regional block has also been demonstrated using Doppler velocimetry.[41] The increased blood velocity waveform indices of the uterine arteries decreased down to the level of normotensive controls after the institution of epidural analgesia in preeclamptic women. No change in uterine artery indices was found in parturients with chronic hypertension or in normal mothers. The umbilical artery ratios did not change in any group. These findings suggest that the sympathetic blockade induced by an epidural block is able to reduce the preeclamptic vasoconstriction of the uteroplacental circulation.

The effects of epidural anesthesia for cesarean section on uteroplacental and umbilical circulation have been studied extensively during the past few years. These studies suggest that epidural anesthesia induced slowly with bupivacaine, lidocaine, or chloroprocaine with or without epinephrine for cesarean section in women with full-term uncomplicated pregnancies does not involve any adverse effects on uterine blood flow, provided the maternal arterial pressure is maintained.[42–46] Ropivacaine, a new long-acting amide local anesthetic and a chemical congener of bupivacaine, has a vasoconstrictive effect when administered as an intradermal injection in small volumes.[47] Similar local vasoconstriction has been demonstrated for ropivacaine with regard to epidural blood flow.[48] Epidural 0.5% ropivacaine for cesarean section did not, however, compromise the uteroplacental circulation in healthy parturients with uncomplicated pregnancies.[49] The results correlate well with the fetal rating scales of these studies, including Apgar scores, umbilical cord acid-base status, and neurobehavioral adaptation scores, which indicate that newborns do extremely well after properly managed epidural cesarean delivery.

Spinal anesthesia for cesarean section is associated with more profound hemodynamic changes than epidural block. The incidence of hypotension was high in healthy parturients in spite of prophylactic preloading with either a colloid or a crystalloid.[50] The mean pulsatility index for the uterine arteries, however, did not change during spinal anesthesia, although some very high short-term individual PI values for the uterine artery were recorded. Another study reported elevated umbilical artery PI values after the induction of spinal anesthesia for cesarean section.[51] The authors concluded that the most likely explanation was a reduction in uteroplacental blood flow secondary to a reduction in maternal cardiac output, which decreased in 12 of 16 patients. Furthermore, the maximum change in maternal cardiac output and the umbilical artery pulsatility index correlated with umbilical artery pH at delivery, suggesting that changes in these variables predict the reduction in uteroplacental perfusion better than changes in arterial pressure. Spinal anesthesia for cesarean delivery induced with incremental injections of 0.5% bupivacaine via a spinal microcatheter was associated with greater maternal hemodynamic stability and no significant changes in umbilical artery PI values.[52]

Left uterine displacement and volume preloading have been recommended for the prevention of maternal hypotension during spinal anesthesia for cesarean section. Relief of aortocaval compression is easily achieved by left uterine displacement, using a wedge under the right hip rather than a mechanical displacer.[53] Recently, the role of preloading has been challenged and the need for prompt correction of hypotension with vasopressors emphasized.[54] Ephedrine has been recommended as the drug of choice for the treatment of maternal hypotension during obstetric anesthesia, based on evidence from animal trials, while pure α-adrenergic agonists, such as phenylephrine, have been considered contraindicated because of the risk of uterine vasoconstriction and reduced uteroplacental perfusion.[30] Prophylactic ephedrine infusion supplemented with small boluses was associated with no changes in the uteroplacental and fetal circulation, whereas the PI values for the uterine vasculature increased during phenylephrine infusion.[55] Umbilical artery PI values have been reported to remain unchanged after phenylephrine administration.[55, 56] Methoxamine, another pure α-adrenergic agonist, increased the PI values in the uteroplacental vessels, whereas no changes were observed after ephedrine administration during epidural anesthesia for cesarean section in healthy mothers.[57] However, the most marked increases in uteroplacental flow resistance were noted during hypotensive episodes. The gravidae who experienced an episode of hypotension had increased placental pH gradients at delivery. The authors concluded that the choice of the vasopressor seems to be of minor importance compared with the avoidance of hypotension in healthy women with uncomplicated pregnancies.

For fear of reduced placental blood flow owing to increased reactivity to vasoconstrictors, it has been recommended that local anesthetics containing epinephrine should be avoided in the case of hypertensive parturients. Indeed, in hypertensive mothers with signs of chronic fetal asphyxia, epidural bupivacaine with epinephrine for cesarean section caused an increase in the blood flow velocity waveform indices for the uterine arteries, while no changes in the Doppler ratios were observed after administration of bupivacaine alone.[58] The increase in vascular resistance in the uteroplacental circulation did not have detrimental effects on umbilical arterial and venous pH values or Apgar scores. Anyway, epinephrine in epidural local anesthetic solutions cannot be recommended for preeclamptic mothers. Spinal anesthesia for cesarean section in a patient with preeclampsia is considered contraindicated because of the risk of severe hypotension. However, reasonably stable maternal hemodynamic values were observed in preeclamptic women undergoing cesarean section under spinal anesthesia, as severe hypotension was seen in only 2 of 12 patients.[59] The hypotensive episodes were easily corrected with crystalloid infusion and small doses of intravenous ephedrine. Furthermore, the mean pulsatility index for the

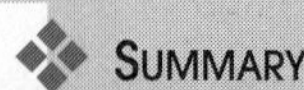

Summary

Key Points

- Uteroplacental blood flow is the major determinant of oxygen to the fetus.
- The vascular bed of the uterus is a dilated system of low resistance, and autoregulation does not occur.
- Uterine blood flow correlates directly with perfusion pressure and inversely with uterine vascular resistance.
- Measures to maintain uteroplacental blood flow during obstetric anesthesia include avoidance and prompt treatment of maternal hypotension, left uterine displacement, and prevention of uterine vasoconstriction.

Key References

Thaler I, Manor D, Itskovitz J, et al: Changes in uterine blood flow during human pregnancy. Am J Obstet Gynecol 1990; 162:121–125.

Moore J: Assessment of the placental circulation [editorial]. Br J Anaesth 1992; 67:671–673.

Case Stem

A primiparous patient in early labor requests labor analgesia for severe pain. Combined spinal-epidural (CSE) anesthesia is performed and 4 min following injection of 10 μg sufentanil, the fetal heart rate monitor demonstrates a tetanic contraction with fetal bradycardia. Explain the possible etiologies for this uterine hypertonus and subsequent fetal bradycardia. How would you treat this patient?

uterine artery did not change significantly, albeit high uterine artery PI values associated with severe maternal hypotension were noted on two occasions. The condition of the newborns was good as judged by the Apgar scores, which exceeded 7 in every infant at 5 minutes, and the mean umbilical artery pH value of 7.29 (range, 7.14–7.42). The results of this study with a small number of patients suggest that spinal anesthesia may be an alternative to epidural and general anesthesia for cesarean section also in preeclamptic patients, if time is of the essence.

References

1. Greiss JA Jr: Pressure-flow relationship in the gravid uterine vascular bed. Am J Obstet Gynecol 1966; 96:41–47.
2. Magness RR, Rosenfeld CR: Systemic and uterine responses to α-adrenergic stimulation in pregnant and nonpregnant ewes. Am J Obstet Gynecol 1986; 155:897–904.
3. Lees MM, Scott DB, Kerr MG, et al: The circulatory effects of recumbent postural change in late pregnancy. Clin Sci 1967; 32:453–465.
4. Kauppila A, Koskinen M, Puolakka J, et al: Decreased intervillous and unchanged myometrial blood flow in supine recumbency. Obstet Gynecol 1980; 55:203–205.
5. Bieniarz J, Crottogini JJ, Curuchet E, et al: Aortocaval compression by the uterus in late human pregnancy. Am J Obstet Gynecol 1968; 100:203–217.
6. Rekonen A, Luotola H, Pitkänen M, et al: Measurement of intervillous and myometrial blood flow by an intravenous ^{133}Xe method. Br J Obstet Gynaecol 1976; 83:723–728.
7. Nylund L, Lunell NO, Sarby B, et al: Functional placental scintigraphy. Acta Radiol Diagn 1983; 24:165–170.
8. Maulik D: Basic principles of Doppler ultrasound as applied in obstetrics. Clin Obstet Gynecol 1989; 32:628–644.
9. McParland P, Pearce JM: Doppler blood flow in pregnancy. Placenta 1989; 9:427–450.
10. Thompson RS, Trudinger BJ, Cook CM: A comparison of Doppler ultrasound waveform indices in the umbilical artery. I. Indices derived from the maximum velocity waveform. Ultrasound Med Biol 1986; 12:835–844.
11. Maulik D: Hemodynamic interpretation of the arterial Doppler waveform. Ultrasound Obstet Gynecol 1993; 3:219–227.
12. Legarth J, Thorup E: Characteristics of Doppler blood-velocity waveforms in a cardiovascular *in vitro* model. II. The influence of peripheral resistance, perfusion pressure and blood flow. Scand J Clin Lab Invest 1989; 49:459–464.
13. Morrow RJ, Adamson SL, Bull SB, et al: Effect of placental embolization on the umbilical arterial velocity waveform in fetal sheep. Am J Obstet Gynecol 1989; 161:1055–1060.
14. Kofinas AD, Espeland M, Swain M, et al: Correcting umbilical artery flow velocity waveforms for fetal heart rate is unnecessary. Am J Obstet Gynecol 1989; 160:704–707.
15. Mulders LGM, Jongsma HW, Wijn PFF, et al: The uterine artery blood flow velocity waveform: reproducibility and results in normal pregnancy. Early Hum Dev 1988; 17:55–70.
16. Steel SA, Pearce JMF, Nash G, et al: Maternal blood viscosity and uteroplacental blood flow velocity waveforms in normal and complicated pregnancies. Br J Obstet Gynaecol 1988; 95:747–752.
17. Legarth J, Lingman G, Stangenberg M, et al: Umbilical artery Doppler flow-velocity waveforms in rhesus-isoimmunized fetuses before and after fetal blood sampling or transfusion. J Clin Ultrasound 1994; 22:43–47.
18. Forouzan I, Cohen AW, Arger P: Measurement of systolic-diastolic ratio in the umbilical artery by continuous-wave and pulsed wave Doppler ultrasound: comparison at different sites. Obstet Gynecol 1991; 77:209–212.
19. Kofinas AD, Penry M, Greiss FC, et al: The effect of placental location on uterine artery flow velocity waveforms. Am J Obstet Gynecol 1988; 159:1504–1508.
20. Adamson SL, Morrow RJ, Bascom PA, et al: Effect of placental resistance, arterial diameter, and blood pressure on the uterine arterial velocity waveform: a computer modeling approach. Ultrasound Med Biol 1989; 15:437–442.
21. Legarth J, Nolsoe C: Doppler blood velocity waveforms and the relation to peripheral resistance in the brachial artery. J Ultrasound Med 1990; 9:449–453.
22. Fairlie FM, Walker JJ: Does the brachial artery Doppler flow velocity waveform reflect changes in downstream impedance? Am J Obstet Gynecol 1991; 165:1741–1744.
23. Kinsella SM, Lee A, Spencer JAD: Maternal peripheral arterial resistance changes following lumbar epidural anesthesia for Cesarean section: validation of Doppler ultrasound pulsatility index. J Maternal Fetal Invest 1991; 1:25–28.
24. Solomon S, Katz SD, Stevenson-Smith W, et al: Determination of vascular impedance in the peripheral circulation by transcutaneous pulsed Doppler ultrasound. Chest 1995; 108:515–521.
25. Räsänen J: Fetal heart and haemodynamics in risk pregnancies and their changes after maternal vasoactive agents. Acta Univ Oul [Series D] 1992; 247:49.
26. Greiss FC Jr, Still JG, Anderson SG: The effects of local anesthetic agents on the uterine vasculatures and myometrium. Am J Obstet Gynecol 1976; 124:889–899.
27. Monuszko E, Halevy S, Freese K, et al: Vasoactive actions of local anaesthetics on human isolated umbilical veins and arteries. Br J Pharmacol 1989; 97:319–328.
28. Wallis KL, Shnider SM, Hicks JS, et al: Epidural anesthesia in the normotensive pregnant ewe: effects on uterine blood flow and fetal acid-base status. Anesthesiology 1976; 44:481–487.
29. Hood DD, Dewan DM, James FM: Maternal and fetal effects of epinephrine in gravid ewes. Anesthesiology 1986; 64:610–613.

30. Ralston DH, Shnider SM, de Lorimier AA: Effects of equipotent ephedrine, metaraminol, mephentermine and methoxamine on uterine blood flow in the pregnant ewe. Anesthesiology 1974; 40:354–370.
31. Lederman RP, McCann DS, Work BA Jr, et al: Endogenous plasma epinephrine and norepinephrine in last trimester pregnancy and labor. Am J Obstet Gynecol 1977; 129:5–8.
32. Shnider SM, Wright RG, Levinson G, et al: Uterine blood flow and plasma norepinephrine changes during maternal stress in the pregnant ewe. Anesthesiology 1979; 50:524–527.
33. Jouppila R, Hollmén A, Jouppila P, et al: Segmental epidural analgesia and urinary excretion of catecholamines during labour. Acta Anaesthesiol Scand 1977; 21:50–54.
34. Shnider SM, Abboud TK, Artal R, et al: Maternal catecholamines decrease during labor after lumbar epidural anesthesia. Am J Obstet Gynecol 1983; 147:13–15.
35. Hollmén AI, Jouppila R, Jouppila P, et al: Effect of extradural analgesia using bupivacaine and 2-chloroprocaine on intervillous blood flow during normal labour. Br J Anaesth 1982; 54:837–842.
36. Jouppila R, Jouppila P, Hollmén A, et al: Effect of segmental extradural analgesia on placental blood flow during normal labour. Br J Anaesth 1978; 50:563–567.
37. Hughes AB, Devoe LD, Wakefield ML, et al: The effects of epidural anesthesia on the Doppler velocimetry of umbilical and uterine arteries in normal term labor. Obstet Gynecol 1990; 75:809–812.
38. Patton DE, Lee W, Miller J, et al: Maternal, uteroplacental, and fetoplacental hemodynamic and Doppler velocimetric changes during epidural anesthesia in normal labor. Obstet Gynecol 1991; 77:17–19.
39. Alahuhta S, Räsänen J, Jouppila P, et al: Epidural sufentanil and bupivacaine for labor analgesia and Doppler velocimetry of the umbilical and uterine arteries. Anesthesiology 1993; 78:231–236.
40. Jouppila P, Jouppila R, Hollmén A, et al: Lumbar epidural analgesia to improve intervillous blood flow during labor in severe preeclampsia. Obstet Gynecol 1982; 59:158–161.
41. Ramos-Santos E, Devoe LD, Wakefield ML, et al: The effects of epidural anesthesia on the Doppler velocimetry of umbilical and uterine arteries in normal and hypertensive patients during active term labor. Obstet Gynecol 1991; 77:20–26.
42. Veille JC, Youngström P, Kanaan C, et al: Human umbilical artery flow velocity waveforms before and after regional anesthesia for Cesarean section. Obstet Gynecol 1988; 72:890–893.
43. Morrow RJ, Rolbin SH, Ritchie JWK, et al: Epidural anaesthesia and blood flow velocity in mother and fetus. Can J Anaesth 1989; 36:519–522.
44. Turner GA, Newnham JP, Johnson C, et al: Effects of extradural anaesthesia on umbilical and uteroplacental arterial flow velocity waveforms. Br J Anaesth 1991; 67:306–309.
45. Alahuhta S, Räsänen J, Jouppila R, et al: Uteroplacental and fetal haemodynamics during extradural anaesthesia for Caesarean section. Br J Anaesth 1991; 66:319–323.
46. Alahuhta S, Räsänen J, Jouppila R, et al: Effects of extradural bupivacaine with adrenaline for Caesarean section on uteroplacental and fetal circulation. Br J Anaesth 1991; 67:678–682.
47. Cederholm I, Åkerman B, Evers H: Local analgesic and vascular effects of intradermal ropivacaine and bupivacaine in various concentrations with and without addition of adrenaline in man. Acta Anaesthesiol Scand 1994; 38:322–327.
48. Dahl JB, Simonsen L, Mogensen T, et al: The effect of 0.5% ropivacaine on epidural blood flow. Acta Anaesthesiol Scand 1990; 34:308–310.
49. Alahuhta S, Räsänen J, Jouppila P, et al: The effects of epidural ropivacaine and bupivacaine for Cesarean section on uteroplacental and fetal circulation. Anesthesiology 1995; 83:23–32.
50. Karinen J, Räsänen J, Alahuhta S, et al: Effect of crystalloid and colloid preloading on uteroplacental and maternal haemodynamic state during spinal anaesthesia for Caesarean section. Br J Anaesth 1995; 75:531–535.
51. Robson C, Boys RJ, Rodeck S, et al: Maternal and fetal haemodynamic effects of spinal and extradural anaesthesia for elective Caesarean section. Br J Anaesth 1992; 68:54–59.
52. Robson SC, Samsoon G, Boys RJ, et al: Incremental spinal anaesthesia for elective Caesarean section: maternal and fetal haemodynamic effects. Br J Anaesth 1993; 70:634–638.
53. Alahuhta S, Karinen J, Lumme R, et al: Uteroplacental haemodynamics during spinal anaesthesia for caesarean section with two types of uterine displacement. Int J Obstet Anesth 1994; 3:187–192.
54. Rocke DA, Rout CC: Volume preloading, spinal hypotension and Caesarean section [editorial]. Br J Anaesth 1995; 75:634–638.
55. Alahuhta S, Räsänen J, Jouppila P, et al: Ephedrine and phenylephrine for avoiding maternal hypotension due to spinal anaesthesia for caesarean section. Int J Obstet Anesth 1992; 1:129–134.
56. Thomas DG, Robson SC, Redfern N, et al: Randomized trial of bolus phenylephrine or ephedrine for maintenance of arterial pressure during spinal anaesthesia for Caesarean section. Br J Anaesth 1996; 76:61–65.
57. Wright PMC, Iftikhar M, Fitzpatrick KT, et al: Vasopressor therapy for hypotension during epidural anesthesia for cesarean section: effects on maternal and fetal flow velocity ratios. Anesth Analg 1992; 75:56–63.
58. Alahuhta S, Räsänen J, Jouppila P, et al: Uteroplacental and fetal circulation during extradural bupivacaine-adrenaline and bupivacaine for Caesarean section in hypertensive pregnancies with chronic fetal asphyxia Br J Anaesth 1993; 71:348–353.
59. Karinen J, Räsänen J, Alahuhta S, et al: Maternal and uteroplacental haemodynamic state in pre-eclamptic patients during spinal anaesthesia for Caesarean section. Br J Anaesth 1996; 76:616–620.

5

Intrapartum Fetal Assessment

❖ FRANK LAH, MBBS, FANZCA

❖ MICHAEL PEEK, MBBS, PhD, FRACOG

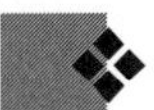

INTRODUCTION

Maternal morbidity and mortality have been impressively reduced during the 20th century owing to improvements in care. Attention has now been shifted to protecting the fetus by improvements in antepartum evaluation and surveillance and by appropriate intrapartum fetal monitoring.

Intrapartum asphyxia is a factor in over 90% of fetal deaths.[1] The incidence of fetuses surviving intrapartum asphyxia associated with motor and cognitive deficits at 1 year of age can be as high as 28%.[2] Deaths and morbidity related to intrapartum asphyxia are probably preventable.[3]

Antenatal evaluation and surveillance are clinically useful for predicting fetal compromise, particularly adverse events that are likely to occur during the course of labor, thereby allowing early intervention and reducing their incidence and severity. The anticipation that a fetus is at risk determines the sophistication of intrapartum fetal surveillance and the decision on whether labor should be allowed to progress.

ANTEPARTUM ASSESSMENT OF THE FETUS

MATERNAL CONDITIONS THAT PREDICT AN AT-RISK FETUS

- Pregnancy-induced hypertension
- Chronic hypertension
- Collagen-vascular diseases
- Diabetes mellitus
- Renal disease
- Anemia
- Hyperthyroidism
- Advanced maternal age
- Chronic heart disease
- Prolonged gestation >42 wk

Clinically the placenta is the primary site of pathology responsible for the most common forms of fetal risk.[4] The common factor in all the maternal conditions listed in the box is their propensity to produce uteroplacental insufficiency and therefore place the fetus at risk owing to poor nutritional status as evidenced by growth retardation and chronic hypoxia.

During the 9 months of pregnancy the placenta is effectively the fetal lung, gut, and kidney. It is also the partition between the maternal and fetal immune systems, a filter that allows the selective transport of maternal antibodies to the fetus and a protective barrier that excludes infections and other potentially harmful agents. It also produces large quantities of specific proteins and steroids that have transport and regulatory functions. Failure of adequate placental growth and function produces an at-risk fetus whose survival is compromised in utero.

The primary aim of antepartum evaluation and surveillance is to detect evidence of uteroplacental insufficiency as assessed by fetal size, growth, and well-being.

ASSESSMENT OF FETAL SIZE, GROWTH, AND WELL-BEING

- Abdominal examination
- Fetal movement counting
- Biophysical tests
  - Ultrasound
  - Doppler ultrasound
  - Cardiotocography
  - Contraction stress testing
  - Fetal biophysical profile
- Biochemical tests
  - Urinary and plasma estrogens
  - Human placental lactogen

Abdominal Examination

Abdominal examination is inexpensive and the most widely practiced method of estimating fetal size and growth. The measurement of fundal height (distance between the upper border of the pubic symphysis and the uterine fundus) is commonly used. Studies have shown quite good sensitivity and specificity of fundal height for predicting low birthweight for gestation. The ability to predict low birthweight is not the same as the ability to detect growth restriction. Fundal height is useful as a screening tool for assessing the need for further investigation.[5, 6]

Fetal Movement Counting

Reduction or cessation of fetal movements precedes fetal death by a day or more.[7] The basis of this assessment is that a malfunctioning placenta provides inadequate oxygenation and nutrition to the fetus. The fetus responds to this hostile environment by invoking adjustments that maximize the chance of survival. These include redistribution of blood flow (more to the brain and heart, less to the liver and kidneys) and limiting unnecessary movements.

The most commonly used method of counting fetal movements is to ask the mother to make a daily record of the time at which she has noticed 10 kicks. Not all late fetal deaths can be predicted by this method. In some at-risk fetuses, demise is not preceded by a reduction in fetal movements. In other fetuses in trouble, there may be insufficient time between the reduction of movements and fetal death to allow clinical action.

Screening by fetal movements has the advantage of daily monitoring and is a useful supplement to the other tests of fetal well-being.[8]

Biophysical Tests

Ultrasound

Ultrasound measurements are used to assess fetal age, fetal growth over a period of time, congenital abnormalities, amniotic fluid volume, and placental localization. Of these, analysis of the pattern of growth has helped uncover the underlying pathology that places the fetus at risk.[9]

Small-for-date fetuses can be divided into two groups. The first group has arrest of previously normal growth. This is thought to be associated with uteroplacental insufficiency. The second group has early departure from normal limits of growth that continues until delivery. This group includes fetuses that are inherently abnormal, those that have suffered a major insult during organogenesis, and those that are small because of genetic endowment.

Abdominal measurements are better than head measurements in determining intrauterine growth restriction, which is consistent with the "brain-sparing" effect seen in uteroplacental insufficiency. While there is a higher incidence of intrapartum fetal asphyxia and operative vaginal delivery in the uteroplacental insufficiency group, the perinatal mortality and the incidence of low Apgar scores are similarly high in both groups.

Doppler Ultrasound

This more sophisticated use of ultrasound allows the assessment of fetal breathing and the flow velocity waveforms of the arteries within the fetus and those surrounding the placenta to offer a broader profile on the pathophysiology of compromised pregnancies.[10]

Fetal Breathing. Fetal breathing is assessed by changing patterns in the umbilical vein flow velocity waveform.[11] Changes in intrathoracic pressure that occur with breathing alter these waveforms. A regular rhythmic pattern indicates fetal lung maturity. This noninvasive analysis is often used instead of the more invasive estimation of the lecithin/sphingomyelin ratio, which reflects the same degree of pulmonary surfactant production and therefore the same risk of hyaline membrane disease in the neonate at birth.[12]

When hypoxia is induced, fetal breathing movements decrease and when asphyxia ensues, gasping movements occur in dying fetal animal preparations. In the human fetus during active labor, fetal breathing movements are suspended.[13]

Arterial Flow Velocity Waveforms. Blood flow in the vessels surrounding the placenta is used to assess arteriolar resistance in the uteroplacental and the umbilical-placental circulations. The systolic/diastolic (S/D) ratio—that is, the ratio of the systolic flow velocity to the diastolic flow velocity—is commonly used. A reduction in this ratio with advancing gestational age occurs in the signal from the umbilical artery. In pathologic situations, such as a reduction in the placental tertiary stem villi, an increase in this ratio occurs, indicating an increasing resistance to flow in the umbilical-placental circulation.[14]

A normal range of umbilical artery flow velocity waveforms through the second half of pregnancy has been established. Deviations outside this range indicate compromised placental function with increased fetal risk (Fig. 5–1).

Directional ultrasound flowmeters are able to separate positive and negative components in the Doppler shift signals and thus discriminate between forward and reverse flow. With extreme pathologic changes within the placenta, the diastolic flow in the umbilical artery falls to zero or may reverse indicating the imminent demise of the fetus in utero. This change precedes fetal heart rate patterns that are preterminal (Fig. 5–2).[15, 16]

Fetal cerebral artery velocity waveforms indicate vasodilation when fetal hypoxia occurs. The middle cerebral artery pulsatility index is commonly used. This further refines the predictability of adverse perinatal outcomes in high-risk pregnancies.[17]

Cardiotocography

Cardiotocography (CTG) is a means of both antepartum and intrapartum fetal surveillance. Foremost, it provides an understanding of how fetal oxygenation affects the fetal heart rate.[18] Prior to labor it is used to measure inherent fetal heart rate changes and those associated with fetal movements. The normal fetal heart rate (FHR) pattern is characterized by a baseline rate of between 110 and 160 beats/min, and the presence of short-term variability (beat to beat) and long-term variability, which are transient accelerations or decelerations from the baseline (Fig. 5–3).

Short-term variability (beat to beat) is the normal irregularity of cardiac rhythm resulting from a continuous balancing interaction of the sympathetic (cardioacceleration) and the parasympathetic (cardiodeceleration) nervous systems. Short-term variability refers to variation in the FHR between successive intervals. It is difficult to interpret reliably with the naked eye. The average beat-to-beat variability is between 6 and 10 beats/min, with decreased variability being of particular significance because it may indicate the presence of chronic hypoxia and the accompanying fetal asphyxia. It is the baseline rate when there is no stress or stimulation to the fetus. It is therefore a measure of fetal reserve to handle the stress of labor.[19]

Long-term variability refers to fluctuations in the FHR over seconds. The frequency of long-term variations is usually between 2 and 6 cycles per minute. In the healthy fetus these are usually accelerations from the baseline; absence of accelerations and decelerations from the baseline indicate pathology associated with fetal hypoxia. There is no universally accepted technique for performing nonstress antepartum cardiotocography. Various durations and frequencies of monitoring are used. This variability can have a powerful influence on the predictive properties of CTG. Additional maneuvers, such as abdominal stimulation, sound stimulation, glucose infusions, postprandial repeat tests, and follow-up oxytocin challenge test for suspected abnormal records, have been suggested or used. None of these have been shown to improve the predictive value of CTG.

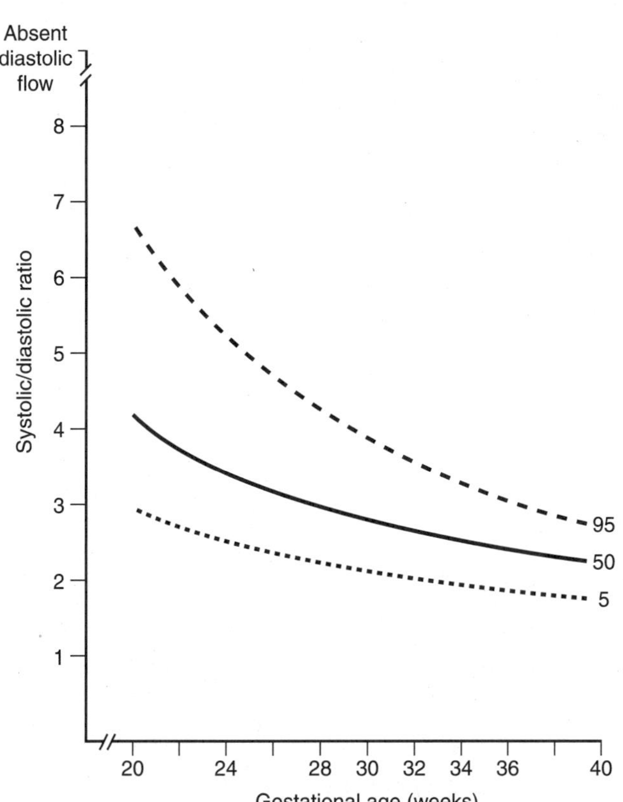

Figure 5–1 Normal range of umbilical artery flow velocity waveforms for systolic/diastolic ratios during the second half of pregnancy.

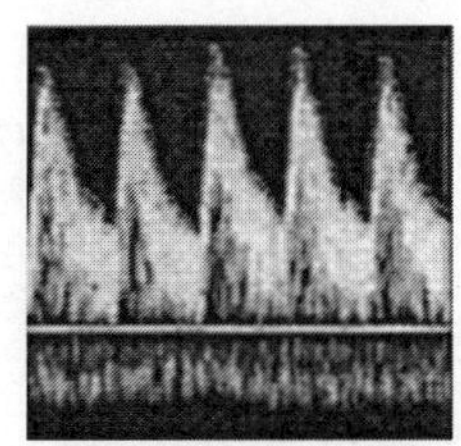

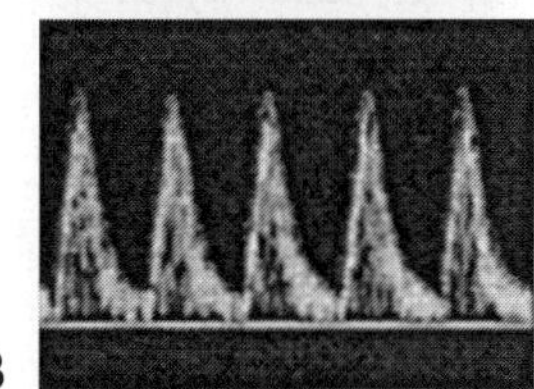

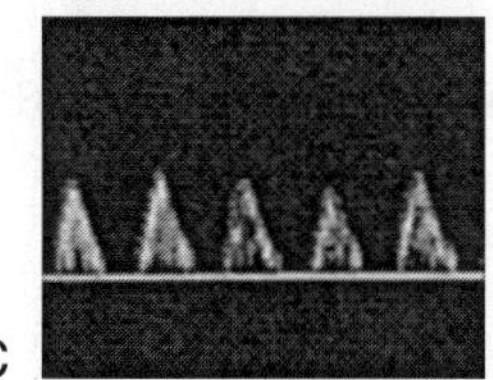

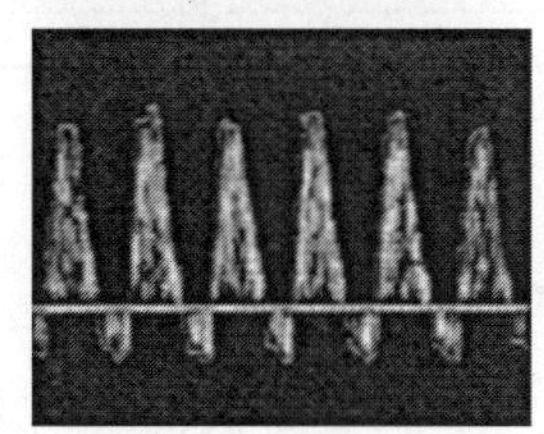

Figure 5–2 Umbilical artery flow velocity waveforms.

CTG is usually interpreted[20] as either reactive or nonreactive.

Reactive: An FHR between 110 and 160 beats/min, the presence of long-term accelerations, normal fetal heart variability, and the absence of decelerations. Fetal movements are also detected.

Nonreactive: FHR is within or outside the normal range, absence of long-term accelerations, poor or no fetal heart variability. No fetal movements are detected.

Many factors interfere with the interpretation of the CTG record, and the sophisticated equipment may occasionally malfunction. Fetal and maternal movements may produce artifacts, since ultrasound monitoring detects movements rather than sound. During fetal rest periods, which may be for an hour or longer, normal physiologic reduction in heart rate variability

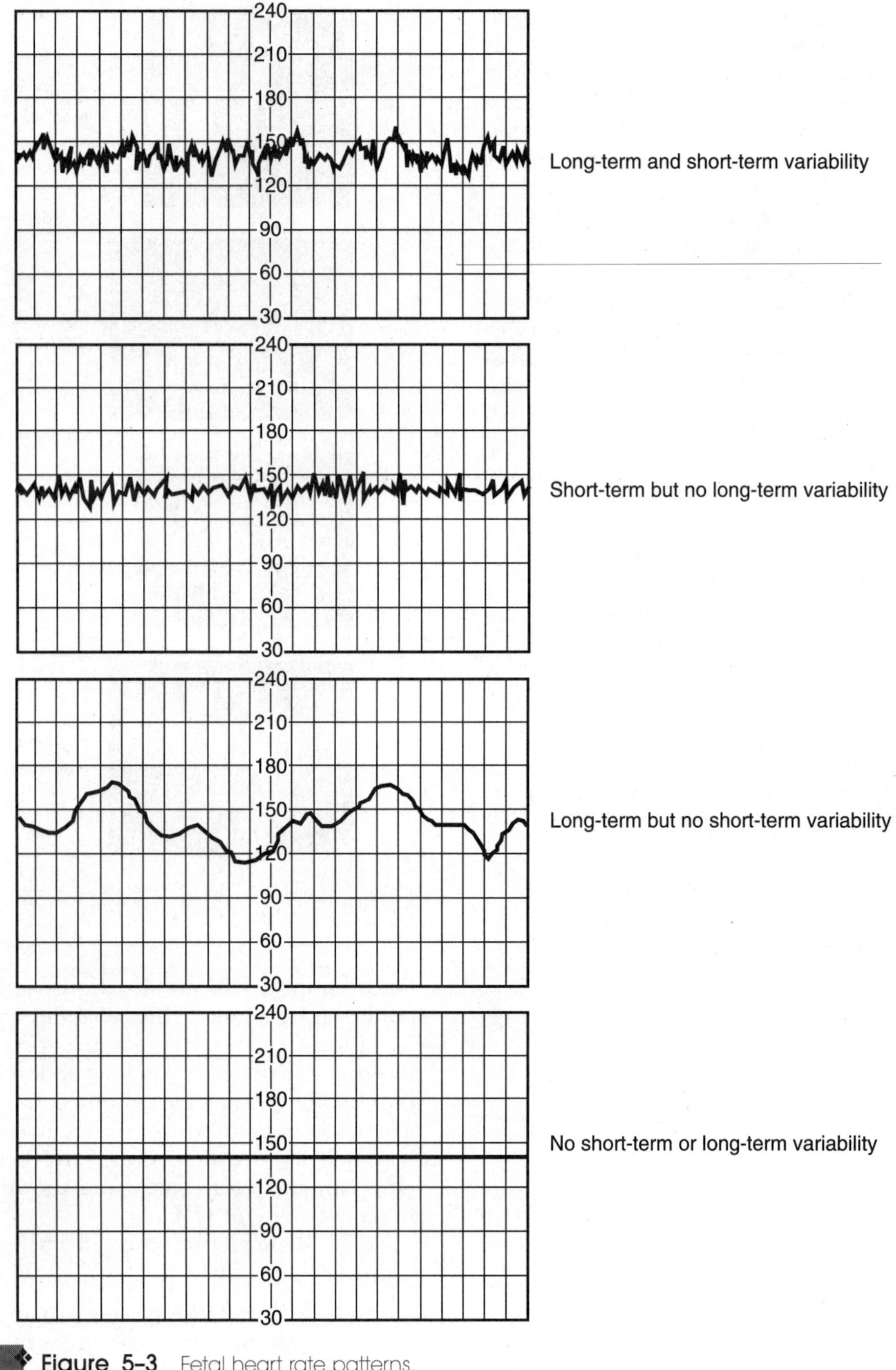

Figure 5–3 Fetal heart rate patterns.

may be confused with pathologic change. Medications taken by the mother are often transferred to the fetus, and particularly if they have a sedative effect on the fetal central nervous system may produce heart rate patterns that would be considered abnormal. Likewise the gestational age of the fetus has a strong influence on the frequency of false-positive nonreactive tests, abnormal patterns being more frequently described in the earlier preterm fetus. When all these factors are taken into consideration, as many as 20% of all records may be unsatisfactory for interpretation.

A reactive test is associated with a good fetal outcome within a week of the test in 99% of cases, while a nonreactive test is associated with a poor fetal outcome in 20% of cases.[21, 22] A nonreactive test therefore requires further evaluation. If pathology is suspected as the underlying cause, then further evaluation by contraction stress testing may be useful.

Contraction Stress Testing

The purpose of this test is to assess the fetal heart rate under labor-like conditions. The test is contraindicated in some pregnancies at risk, for example, when there has been antepartum bleeding, placenta previa, a history of preterm labor, or premature rupture of membranes. A positive response of persistent late deceleration after uterine contractions (stimulated by endogenous or exogenous oxytocin) is associated with a poor fetal outcome in 50% of cases.[21] The value of such a test is in establishing a trial of the induction of labor when this is indicated and then making the decision not to progress with labor at an early stage.

Fetal Biophysical Profile

This is a combination of five biophysical variables considered to be of prognostic significance: fetal movement, tone, reactivity, and breathing and amniotic fluid volume.[23] Combining these results into a score has reduced the frequency of false-positive and false-negative results compared with nonstress cardiotocography.[24] It also has the potential advantage of picking up congenital fetal abnormalities. It is now well documented that when all these biophysical tests are used, interpretation of results vary between different observers and even when an individual observer interprets the results at different times.[25–27]

Biochemical Tests

Estriol and human placental lactogen measurements are now of very limited value in the assessment of at-risk fetuses. They seem to lack the sensitivity to identify the majority of pregnancies destined to have an adverse outcome for the fetus.[8] Their value at best appears to be confirmatory when other tests suggest a fetus at risk.

CLINICAL METHODS OF FETAL MONITORING DURING LABOR

If an underlying fetoplacental pathology is detected during antepartum assessment, greater supervision of the fetus during the course of labor is required. The aim of monitoring the fetus during labor is to identify fetal problems which, if left uncorrected, might cause death, or short- or long-term morbidity after birth. Intrapartum monitoring should lead to appropriate interventions to avoid these adverse outcomes. Controversy persists as to what monitoring should be performed and the appropriate response to an abnormal result.

Intermittent Auscultation of the Fetal Heart

Intermittent auscultation of the fetal heart may be done with a fetal stethoscope or a portable ultrasound monitor. The fetal heart is auscultated for at least 30 seconds after a contraction. FHR above 160 or below 110 beats/min should be used as an indication for the need for continuous monitoring.[28] Intermittent techniques have the advantage of allowing the mother to move about freely during the course of labor. This has been shown to decrease the requirements for analgesics and to shorten the duration of labor.

Assessment of Amniotic Fluid

Passage of meconium is associated with an increased risk of intrapartum stillbirth, and of neonatal death and morbidity. Thick meconium recognized at the onset of labor carries the worst prognosis. It reflects events that have occurred prior to the onset of labor, and is usually a sign of impaired placental function that exposes the fetus to the risk of hypoxia during labor. It also reflects reduced amniotic fluid volume at onset of labor, which in itself is significant, as it may be associated with an increased risk of cord compression.

Passage of meconium for the first time after the onset of labor is not common but when it is associated with fetal heart rate abnormalities it warrants further investigation.

Continuous Assessment of the Fetal Heart

Continuous electronic fetal heart rate monitoring during labor is now most commonly achieved either externally by Doppler ultrasound or internally by electrocardiography. Ultrasound FHR monitors give a poorer impression of the fetal heart rate variability than that obtained with electrocardiographic surveillance. External monitoring is usually employed during early labor, particularly before the membranes have ruptured. Internal monitoring is preferred later in labor because it provides a more reliable trace and allows the mother greater freedom of movement. Uterine contractions are monitored by a tocodynamometer applied to the mother's abdomen over the uterus. The tocodynamometer detects pressure changes through the abdominal wall as the uterus contracts. The length and frequency of contractions, but not the absolute intensity of a contraction, can be recorded. To measure intensity an intrauterine catheter attached to a pressure transducer is necessary. This procedure is rarely done because of problems of placement and the potential problems of endometritis.

The relationship between fetal heart rate changes and uterine contractions can be graphically represented throughout the monitoring period. Although electronic FHR monitoring has no proven advantage over intermittent auscultation in low-risk pregnancies, it is strongly advisable when there is a risk of fetal hypoxia.[29]

INDICATIONS FOR CARDIOTOCOGRAPHY MONITORING DURING LABOR

Intrauterine growth retardation
Preterm labor
Postmaturity
Pregnancies complicated by medical problems
Meconium staining of the amniotic fluid
Use of uterine contraction stimulants
Abnormal auscultatory findings
Regional anesthesia

It is evident that each labor needs to be managed individually and has to be assessed at its starting point with the maternal wishes taken into consideration. It is probable that most impaired neurologic outcomes in fetuses at birth have their origin in the antepartum period, but it is impossible to determine what proportion of the insult is due to intrapartum events. If its reserve is diminished, the fetus is more likely to, and will more rapidly, decompensate during the time of uterine contractions, and earlier intervention is indicated.

Cardiotocography is not necessarily an absolute predictor of fetal asphyxia, but it can be used as a screening method with the use of adjunctive measures to predict the potential of birth asphyxia. The presence of accelerations of the fetal heart rate is the hallmark of fetal health[30] (Fig. 5–4). Good accelerations are characterized by amplitude of more than 10 beats/min from baseline and a total duration of more than 10 seconds at a level exceeding 5 beats/min from baseline.

Difficulty in interpreting accelerations occur after variable decelerations. The decelerative part of a variable deceleration may be very short and of limited amplitude, while the accelerative response (overshoot) may be of substantial duration and amplitude. This occurs at an end stage of fetal deterioration. Other characteristics of the FHR pattern, principally the loss of beat-to-beat variability with a smooth baseline, help to make the diagnosis of a pathologic tracing.

FHR changes that indicate fetal distress are changes in the baseline, periodic changes related to uterine contractions, and changes in the variability in the baseline rate. A baseline fetal heart rate between 110 and 100 beats/min is considered suspicious and if below 100 is considered pathologic. A baseline fetal heart rate above 160 beats/min is always pathologic.

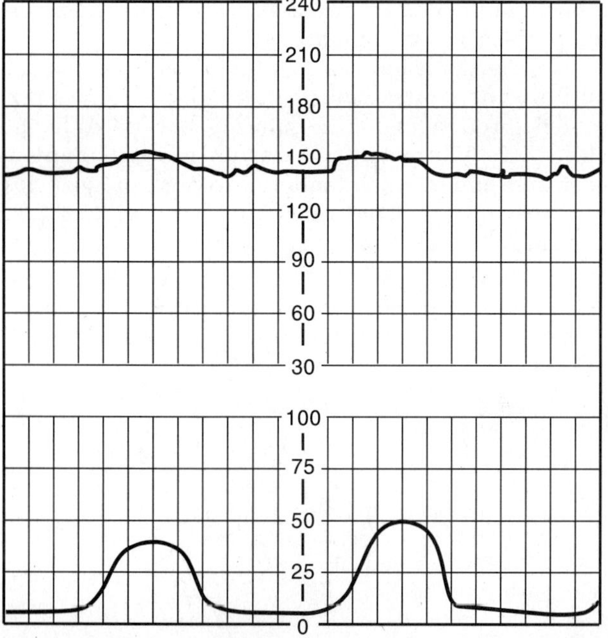

Figure 5–4 Fetal heart rate accelaration with uterine contractions.

CAUSES OF FETAL BASELINE BRADYCARDIA ON CARDIOTOCOGRAPHY

Cord compression
Placental abruption
Excessive uterine activity
Fetal cardiac arrhythmia
Postmaturity
Maternal medication
Maternal hypothermia
Maternal hypotension
Maternal convulsions
Recording of the maternal heart rate

CAUSES OF FETAL BASELINE TACHYCARDIA ON CARDIOTOCOGRAPHY

Fetal infection
Fetal anemia
Fetal hypoxia
Following prolonged decelerations
Fetal cardiac arrhythmia
Chorioamnionitis
Maternal fever
Maternal anxiety

Hon introduced the classification of early, variable, and late decelerations associated with uterine contractions. Each type has been connected to a specific pathophysiologic problem.[31] Early decelerations are attributed to head compression, variable decelerations are thought to be due to compression of the umbilical cord, and late decelerations are attributed to uteroplacental insufficiency. Early decelerations occur in a repetitive fashion, are uniform and symmetric, and occur simultaneously with uterine contractions. The nadir does not usually reach below 100 beats/min. This decelerative pattern was once thought to have little pathologic significance but the frequently disappointing condition of the infant at birth after a prolonged clinical course of this pattern has made observers look at the other features of the FHR pattern, such as baseline variability and the presence or absence of accelerations, before ignoring its pathologic significance.[28]

Variable decelerations are attributed to cord compression. They are baroreceptor mediated and reflect changes in blood pressure of the fetus owing to compression of the umbilical vein or arteries. Pure variable decelerations have the typical pattern of an initial acceleration, followed by rapid deceleration with a nadir between 60 and 80 beats/min, then a rapid return to baseline, and finally a secondary acceleration. Unfavorable characteristics of a variable deceleration pattern are loss of initial acceleration, slow return to baseline heart rate, loss of secondary acceleration, biphasic deceleration, loss of variability during deceleration, and a continuing of the baseline at a lower or higher level.

Late decelerations are repetitive and have a uniform shape with a slow onset (usually 30 seconds or more after the onset of the accompanying contraction) and a slow return to the baseline heart rate. The baseline heart rate is usually elevated, whereas beat-to-beat variability is decreased. Late decelerations are associated with a significant decrease in cerebral oxygenation.[32]

Variability is commonly defined by the width of distribution of heart rates. Variability is considered to be normal if the amplitude of the variability around the baseline is between 5 and 15 beats/min. An increase or decrease in the baseline heart rate is accompanied by a concomitant decrease or increase in variability. There is ample evidence that FHR variability is suppressed by factors that depress brain function. Increases in variability are often seen after increases in fetal activity but are also associated with baseline bradycardias and following variable decelerations. It is of particular comfort to the obstetrician that a normal FHR tracing reliably predicts the birth of an infant in good condition.[29] However, in the intrapartum period many traces do not fulfil the criteria of normality, particularly in the second stage of labor.

The problem with abnormal tracings is that their significance is very often unclear. They may indicate serious fetal distress finally resulting in preventable destruction of critical areas in the fetal brain or, on the contrary, they may indicate temporary changes in cardiovascular control which is part of the normal stress response of labor and is essentially benign. Acid-base sampling of fetal blood is therefore a useful adjunct.

Fetal Blood Acid-Base Sampling

Fetal blood sampling of the presenting part was introduced by Saling and Schneider[33] in 1962 and has become the final determinant of whether fetal asphyxia is present. A scalpel or stylet is passed through the cervical os to make a small incision on the presenting part of the fetus. A sample of blood is then collected in a capillary tube and analyzed to determine its acid-base status. On the basis of a large number of cases it is now accepted that a pH below 7.2 is pathologic.[33]

Fetal asphyxia results in both respiratory and metabolic acidemia. Both are the result of interference with placental gas exchange. Respiratory acidosis is attributable to an elevation of the plasma carbon dioxide tension, and metabolic acidosis is due to the accumulation of the products of anaerobic metabolism, mainly lactic acid, which occurs because of inadequate fetal oxygenation. In recent years greater interest has been focused on metabolic acidosis as a consequence of tissue hypoxia with lactate as the principal end product. Tissue lactate appears to be the final arbiter of the irreversibility of organ damage.[34, 35]

Intrapartum asphyxia damages the brain only if the brain experiences an episode of anoxia and if its available carbohydrate substrates as influenced by blood glucose are sufficient to produce a marked brain tissue acidosis. Prolonged intrapartum asphyxia produces a progressive systemic acidosis that ultimately impairs cardiovascular performance leading first to systemic hypotension and later to cardiovascular collapse. The very low fetal blood oxygen levels induced by asphyxia and poor cardiovascular performance result in significant reductions in cerebral blood flow. This eventually renders the brain anoxic, which is the precursor of the lactic acidosis causing brain injury or death.[36]

Fetuses' low serum glucose concentrations protect the brain during anoxia, resulting in less damaging brain patterns of injury. Elevations of fetal serum glucose concentrations (reflected by the elevation of maternal blood glucose level) at the time of cerebral anoxia markedly reduce the fetal brain's tolerance to anoxia and cause cerebral hemisphere patterns of brain injury.[37]

Animal studies using fetal sheep have shown that the initial response to hypoxia is an increase in the peripheral resistance, reducing the blood flow through the pulmonary, renal, and gastrointestinal circulations but increasing the blood flow to the brain, heart, and adrenal glands. The autonomic nervous system accounts for the redistribution of the cardiac output. This response is initiated through the arterial chemoreceptors,[38] circulating endogenous opiates, increased angiotensin activity, and the release of vasopressin.[39–41] This increased cerebral blood flow coupled with increased oxygen extraction from the blood maintains the oxygen supply to the brain. In fetal sheep studies cerebral oxygen was reduced and a progressive metabolic acidosis developed when oxygen saturation was below 30%. The threshold when electrocortical activity was suppressed and seizure activity began was a severe metabolic acidosis in which the base deficit is greater than 16 mmol/L. At this point progressive neuronal death occurs, with neurologic handicaps evidenced after birth.[42]

Total anoxia and cerebral ischemia are uncommon events in the human fetus. The more common insult, particularly during labor, is a degree of hypoxia present over a variable period of time. Such insults are associated with a period of fetal compensation. During this period the clinician can intervene before irreversible brain damage has occurred.

Fetal Pulse Oximetry

The measurement of arterial oxygen saturation has become an important monitoring tool in anesthesiology and critical care medicine. Attempts have been made to develop this technology for the continuous monitoring of fetal oxygenation during labor.[43] Reflectance pulse oximetry sensors have been developed so that the light-emitting diode and photodiode are integrated into one probe. Nellcor Inc. (Hayward, CA) has developed an integrated probe that is placed between the fetal cheek and the uterine wall. Thus far clinical investigations have shown a wide range of saturation values. Dildy and associates[44] showed a mean saturation in the early first stage of labor of 62% that dropped to an average 53% in the second stage. Other investigators have reported ranges of 11% to 80% in low-risk fetuses through the course of labor.[45] Poor signal quality is still the main technical problem.

McNamara and associates[46] showed a significant correlation between fetal oxygen saturation as measured by the oximeter probe and umbilical vein saturation. In another study fetal oxygen saturation increased when the mother was given supplemental oxygen; however, a large number of patients had be excluded because of poor signal quality.[47] Fetal pulse oximetry is therefore still undergoing further evaluation. Preliminary recommendations for its potential clinical use have been suggested in suspected cases of fetal hypoxia based on suspicious FHR monitoring. In most cases saturation values above 33% suggest fetal well-being.[45] Pulse oximetry may allow the differentiation between cases that need further evaluation (e.g., fetal blood sampling for the presence of acidosis) and those that do not.

CONSERVATIVE MANAGEMENT OF FETAL DISTRESS

The most common treatment for intrapartum fetal distress, diagnosed by persistent fetal heart rate abnormalities and confirmed by the presence of acidosis from fetal blood sampling, is prompt delivery. However, many FHR abnormalities resolve with simple conservative measures such as changes in maternal position (to relieve aortocaval or umbilical vessel compression), interruption of oxytocin administration to increase uteroplacental blood flow, and short-term maternal oxygen administration.

Intravenous or inhaled β-mimetics are useful for buying time when persistent FHR abnormalities indicate delivery. In a randomized controlled clinical trial involving 20 labors characterized by both ominous FHR changes and fetal scalp blood pH of less than 7.25, 10 of the 11 mothers treated with intravenous terbutaline showed improvement in the FHR pattern compared with none in the control group. At birth, the babies were less likely to be acidotic or to have low Apgar scores.[48] This short-term improvement is produced by the cessation of uterine contractions and could be useful in facilities where cesarean section is not immediately available, or to allow time to set up for regional anesthesia.

Amnioinfusion is another temporizing maneuver.[49] It is used to correct oligohydramnios and may be useful as a method of preventing or relieving umbilical cord compression during labor.[50] Saline or Ringer's lactate is infused through a catheter into the uterine cavity. The procedure significantly decreases the rate of persistent variable decelerations of the fetal heart.[49] It also improves more substantive outcomes such as a decrease in the rate of cesarean section and results in fewer neonates with birth asphyxia, low Apgar score, or low umbilical cord pH. In the presence of meconium it also reduces the incidence of meconium aspiration.[51]

Intrapartum asphyxia accounts for fetal as well as neonatal deaths. A recent report from the English *Confidential Inquiry into Stillbirths and Deaths in Infancy* reveals the incidence of intrapartum deaths as 0.31 per 1000 registrable births, 0.39 per 1000 in the first week and 0.04 per 1000 at 8 to 28 days. These figures have halved over the last 30 years. Much of the reduction has been attributed to the use of FHR monitoring.[52] The report from the *Confidential Inquiry* also made comment on the fact that 51% of the intrapartum deaths remained unexplained. The study's most adverse comment was related to the level of understanding and interpretation of FHR recordings.[3]

EFFECT OF ANESTHESIA ON THE FETUS

Painful labor can provoke a maternal stress response that is associated with a rise in maternal catecholamines, particularly epinephrine. The resulting acidosis and decrease in uteroplacental perfusion may be harmful, especially to the at-risk fetus. Analgesia is therefore appropriate for the mother but the risk versus benefit to the fetus should be taken into consideration before choosing a particular anesthetic technique. The nonpharmacologic techniques for pain relief in labor, learned and practiced during pregnancy, have much to offer in helping the mother prepare for childbirth and in reducing maternal anxiety levels. Maternal anxiety itself is a risk. Sjostrom and coworkers[53] have shown that mothers with high anxiety trait scores have significantly higher pulsatility index (PI) values in the umbilical-placental circulation and significantly lower PI values in the fetal middle cerebral artery, suggesting a change in blood distribution in favor of brain circulation in these fetuses.

Sedatives and anesthetic agents are generally associated with a reduction in baseline FHR variability and a low incidence of accelerations.[54] The effects of these agents may continue into the neonatal period, with increased need for supplemental oxygen and artificial ventilation at birth. Subtle and longer-term effects can be assessed with neurobehavioral assessments. The neonatal Neurologic and Adaptive Capacity Score (NACS) was specifically designed to detect most drug effects.[55] However, there has been little published information on drug effects for at-risk fetuses because of the number of confounding variables usually associated with delivery of these infants.

Drugs Decreasing Fetal Heart Rate Variability

- Central nervous system depressants
  - Volatile anesthetics
  - Barbiturates
  - Propofol
  - Tranquilizers, benzodiazepines, phenothiazines
  - Magnesium
- Local anesthetics
  - Lidocaine
  - Chloroprocaine
- Anticholingerics
- β-Sympathomimetics
- Narcotics

It is of interest that the local anesthetic bupivacaine has not been shown to affect FHR variability, which therefore makes it the agent of choice for epidural analgesia.[56]

Narcotics given to the mother have been associated with sinusoidal patterns[57] in FHR tracings. These are similar to the patterns seen with fetal anemia, severe acidosis, and anencephaly. The significance of this effect on the fetus has not been elucidated.

Effect on the Fetus of Conduction Blockade

Regional analgesia and anesthesia have mainly beneficial effects on the fetus but, if poorly managed, have the potential to cause serious harm.[58] During painful labor uteroplacental vasoconstriction occurs that is mediated by catecholamines and maternal hyperventilation, thereby reducing fetal oxygenation. These changes are without consequence in the normal healthy fetus, but they promote fetal asphyxia in the already compromised fetus.

Regional analgesia is the most effective means of providing pain relief in labor, having its predominant effect on uteroplacental and umbilical-placental perfusion. Jouppila and associates[59] using the radioactive xenon dilution technique suggested that in healthy pregnant women epidural anesthesia did not alter intervillous blood flow. However, Giles and colleagues[60] have shown a decrease in uteroplacental vascular resistance with preloading of crystalloid fluids and epidural anesthesia using flow velocity waveform analysis. Other studies[61, 62] have not shown a decrease in uteroplacental vascular resistance, arguing that the uteroplacental circulation is maximally dilated at term and no further decrease in resistance is possible. It is difficult to conceive that the adrenergic stimulus due to stress during labor and delivery does not increase uteroplacental vascular resistance. The prime benefit of epidural anesthesia in the normal healthy parturient is to restore the uteroplacental circulation to a nonstressed basal state.

In the parturient with toxemia who has a markedly compromised uteroplacental circulation, epidural anesthesia has an enormous beneficial effect by increasing intervillous blood flow by up to 77%.[63]

The umbilical-placental circulation is also affected by epidural anesthesia. Several authors have now shown a decrease in resistance to flow in the umbilical-placental circulation with epidural anesthesia.[60, 64] Giles also reported that fluid loading and epidural anesthesia were associated with a concomitant decrease in the uteroplacental and umbilical-placental vascular resistance.[60] This would indicate an improved matching of the two circulations with the likely improvement in nutriment and gas exchange. The mechanism for this change on the fetal side of the placental circulation is not understood. It appears, however, to be similar to a change that occurs in the lung.[65] Hypoxic pulmonary vascular resistance is decreased by improved ventilation to that segment of lung.[66] In this case the improvement in perfusion is prostaglandin mediated. These same prostaglandins are in abundant concentration on both sides of the placental circulation.

Regional anesthesia improves uteroplacental blood flow unless there is severe maternal hypotension associated with the technique, which then results in deterioration in the FHR tracing that resembles the late decelerative pattern of uteroplacental insufficiency.

One of the advances in epidural technique in the 1990s has been the combination of low doses of local anesthetics with short-acting narcotics. The analgesia produced is adequate from the maternal standpoint and at the same time it does not result in extensive sympathectomy. The risk of precipitating hypotension is therefore eliminated.

Hyperventilation in labor ceases when pain is relieved; hence, maternal P_{CO_2} rises. Although this reduces the transplacental carbon dioxide gradient, it also has the effect of reducing the affinity of maternal hemglobin for oxygen, thereby enhancing oxygen

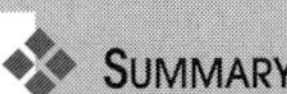

SUMMARY

Key Points

- Controversy exists regarding the clinical benefit of continuous versus intermittent fetal heart rate monitoring.
- The cardiotocograph recording is not an absolute predictor of fetal ashphyxia. A tracing of a normal fetal heart rate predicts fetal well-being; however, a tracing of an abnormal fetal heart rate is not necessarily predictive of fetal compromise. Late decelerations in the absence of fetal variability are highly suggestive of fetal compromise.
- Fetal pulse oximetry is still undergoing development and evaluation. Early evidence sugests that this may be a useful technology. In most cases, fetal saturation levels above 33% suggest fetal well-being.
- Many fetal heart rate abnormalities resolve after in utero resuscitative efforts, including the administration of oxygen, changes in maternal position, interruption of oxytocin administration, and the administration of a tocolytic agent.

Key Reference

Parer JT: Fetal heart rate. *In* Creasy RK, Resnik R (eds): Maternal-Fetal Medicine. Philadelphia: WB Saunders; 1989:332.

Case Stem

A 41-year-old primiparous woman being induced for post dates has a fetal heart rate tracing with a baseline in the 140s with variable decelerations and nonexistent beat-to-beat variability. The obstetrician requests an epidural for this patient. Discuss your management and whether anything can be done to assess fetal well-being.

transfer to the fetus. The improvement in uteroplacental blood flow and in oxygen transfer has a resuscitative effect on the fetus. This potential for resuscitation can occasionally be seen in an improvement in the beat-to-beat variability in the FHR seen with epidural analgesia. Further confirmation of this beneficial fetal effect has come from studies that show raised Po_2 values in neonates whose mothers had received epidural anesthesia.[67]

Ong and coworkers[68] reported that babies born with general anesthesia did worse in terms of Apgar score and the need for oxygen and artificial ventilation than babies born with regional blockade. Even with fetal distress diagnosed preoperatively, fetuses born with regional anesthesia for cesarean section were better off in terms of Apgar scores than those born with general anesthesia.[69]

All these findings would therefore appear to favor epidural analgesia for labor and operative deliveries.

References

1. Erkkolar R, Gronoos M, Punnonen R, Kikku P: Analysis of intrapartum fetal deaths: their decline with increasing fetal monitoring. Obstet Gynecol Scand 1984; 63:459–462.
2. Low J, Galbraith R, Muir D, et al: Motor and cognitive deficits after intrapartum fetal asphyxia in the mature fetus. Am J Obstet Gynecology 1988; 158:356–361.
3. Spencer J: Deaths related to intrapartum asphyxia [editorial]. BMJ 1998; 316:640.
4. Chard T: The human placenta. Clin Obstet Gynaecol September 1986; 13: Foreword.
5. Lindhard A, Nielsen P, Mouritsen L, et al: The implication of introducing the symphyseal-fundal height measurement: a prospective randomized controlled trial. Br J Obstet Gynaecol 1990; 97:675–680.
6. Bailey S, Sarmandal P, Grant J: A comparison of three methods of assessing inter-observer variation applied to the measurement of the symphysis-fundal height. Br J Obstet Gynaecol 1989; 96:1266–1271.
7. Grant A, Elbourne D, Valentin L, et al: Routine formal fetal movement counting and risk of antepartum late death in normally formed singletons. Lancet 1989; 2:345–349.
8. Thomsen S, Legarth J, Weber T, et al: Monitoring of normal pregnancies by daily fetal movement registration or hormone assessment: a random allocation study. Obstet Gynecol 1990; 10:189–193.
9. Harding K, Evans S, Newnham J: Screening for the small fetus: a study of the relative efficacies of ultrasound biometry and symphysiofundal height. Aust N Z J Obstet Gynaecol 1995; 35:160–164.
10. Marsal K: Role of doppler sonography in fetal maternal medicine [Current Opinions]. Obstet Gynaecol 1994; 6:36–34.
11. Trudinger B, Cook C: The fetal breath cycle. Early Hum Dev 1990; 21:181–191.
12. Marsal K, Gennser G, Lofgren O: Effects on fetal breathing movements of maternal challenges: crossover study on dynamic work, static work, passive movements, hyperventilation and hyperoxygenation. Acta Obstet Gynecol Scand 1979; 58:335–342.
13. Boylan P, Lewis P: Fetal breathing in labour. Obstet Gynecol 1980; 56:35–38.
14. Giles W, Trudinger B, Baird P: Fetal umbilical artery waveforms and placental resistance. Br J Obstet Gynaecol 1985; 92:31–38.
15. Trudinger B, Giles W, Cook C, et al: Foetal umbilical flow velocity waveforms and placental resistance: clinical significance Br J Obstet Gynaecol 1985; 92:23–30.
16. Trudinger B, Giles W, Cook C: Uteroplacental blood flow velocity-time waveforms in normal and complicated pregnancy. Br J Obstet Gynaecol 1985; 92:39–45.
17. Mari C, Deter R: Middle cerebral artery flow velocity waveforms in normal and small for gestational age fetuses. Am J Obstet Gynecol 1992; 166:1262–1270.
18. Schaffrin B: The rationale of antepartum fetal heart rate monitoring. J Reprod Med 1979; 23:213–219.
19. Freeman R, Gartie T: Fetal Heart Rate Monitoring. Baltimore: Williams & Wilkins; 1981; 176–180.
20. Keegan K, Paul R: Antepartum fetal heart rate testing. IV. The nonstress tests as the primary approach. Am J Obstet Gynecol 1980; 136:75–89.
21. Ott W: Antepartum biophysical evaluation of the fetus. Perinatal Neonatal 1978; 2:11–16.
22. Evertson L, Gauthier R, Collea J: Fetal demise following negative contraction stress test. Obstet Gynecol 1978;51:671–679.
23. Nageotte M, Towers C, Asrat T, et al: Perinatal outcome with the modified biophysical profile. Am J Obstet Gynecol 1994; 170:1672–1676.
24. Platt L, Walla C, Paul R, et al: A prospective trial of the fetal biophysical profile vs the nonstress test in the management of high-risk pregnancies. Am J Obstet Gynecol 1985; 153:624–633.
25. Trimbos J, Keirse M: Observer variability in assessment of antenatal tocograms. Br J Obstet Gynecol 1978; 85:900–906.
26. Thacker S, Berkelman J: Assessing the diagnostic accuracy and efficacy of selected antepartum fetal surveillance. Obstet Gynecol Surv 1986; 41:121–141.
27. Keirse M. Electronic monitoring: who needs a Trojan horse? Birth 1994; 21:111–113.
28. Morrison J, Chez B, Davis I, et al: Intrapartum fetal heart rate assessment: monitoring by auscultation or electronic means. Am J Obstet Gynecol 1993; 168:63–66.
29. Thacker S, Stroup D: Efficacy and safety of electronic fetal monitoring: an update, Obstet Gynecol 1995; 86:613–620.
30. Mantel R, Ververs I, Colenbrander G, et al: Automated antepartum baseline FHR determination and detection of accelerations and decelerations. *In* Van Geijin H (ed): A Critical Appraisal of Fetal Surveillance. Amsterdam: Excerpta Medica Elsevier; 1994:333–348.
31. Hon E: An Atlas of Fetal Heart Rate Patterns. New Haven, CT: Hary Press; 1968.
32. Aldrich C, D'Antona D, Spencer J, et al: Late fetal heart decelerations and changes in cerebral oxygenation during the first stage of labour. Br J Obstet Gynaecol 1995; 102:9–15.
33. Saling E, Schneider D: Biochemical supervision of the fetus during labour. J Obstet Gynaecol Br Commonw 1967; 74:799–805.
34. Eguiluz A, Lopez B, McPherson K, et al: The use of antepartum fetal blood lactate measurements for the early diagnosis of fetal distress. Am J Obstet Gynecol 1983; 147:949–954.
35. Fee S, Male K, Deddish R, et al: Severe acidosis and subsequent neurological status. Am J Obstet Gynecol 1990; 162:802–806.
36. Myers R, de Courten-Myers G: Metabolic principles of patterns of perinatal brain injury. *In* Crawford J (ed): Risks of Labour. New York: John Wiley & Sons; 1985:119–145.
37. Myers R, Wagner K, de Courten-Myers G: Brain metabolic and pathologic consequences of asphyxia: role played by serum glucose concentrations. *In* Milunski A (ed): Advances in Perinatal Medicine. New York: Plenum Medical; 1983:67–115.
38. Bartelds B, van Bel F, Teetel D, et al: Carotid not aortic chemoreceptors mediate the fetal cardiovascular response to acute hypoxemia in lambs. Paediatr Res 1993; 34:51–55.
39. LaGamma E, Itskovitz J, Rudloph A: Effects of naloxone on fetal circulatory responses to hypoxemia. Am J Obstet Gynecol 1982; 143:933–940.
40. Iwamoto H, Rudloph A: Effects of angiotension II on the blood flow and its distribution in fetal lambs. Cir Res 1981; 48:183–189.
41. Stark R, Wardlaw S, Daniel S, et al: Vasopressin secretion induced by hypoxia in sheep: development changes and relationships in beta endorphin release. Am J Obstet Gynecol 1982; 143:204–215.
42. Low J, Panagiotopoulos C, Derrick E: Newborn complications after intrapartum asphyxia with metabolic acidosis in the term fetus. Am J Obstet Gynecol 1994; 170:1081–1087.

43. Dildy G, Clark S, Loucks C: Preliminary experience with intrapartum fetal pulse oximetry in humans. Obstet Gynecol 1993; 81:630–634.
44. Dildy G, Van den Berg P, Katz M, et al: Intrapartum fetal pulse oximetry: fetal oxygen saturation trends during labor with normal neonatal outcome. Am J Obstet Gynecol 1994; 171:679–684.
45. Gardosi J, Schram C, Symonds M: Adaption of pulse oximetry for fetal monitoring during labor. Lancet 1991; 337:1265–1267.
46. McNamara H, Chung C, Lilford R, et al: Do fetal pulse oximetry readings at delivery correlate with cord oxygen saturation and acidaemia. Br J Obstet Gynaecol 1992; 99:735–738.
47. McNamara H, Johnson N: The effect on arteriolar oxygen saturation resulting from giving oxygen to the mother measured by pulse oximetry. Br J Obstet Gynaecol 1993; 100:446–449.
48. Magann E, Cleveland R, Dockery J, et al: Acute tocolysis for fetal distress: terbutaline versus magnesium sulphate. Aust N Z J Obstet Gynaecol 1993; 4:362–366.
49. Miyazaki F, Nevarez F: Saline aminofusion for relief of repetitive variable decelerations: a prospective randomized study. Am J Obstet Gynecol 1985; 153:301–306.
50. Chauhan S, Rutherford S, Hess L, et al: Prophylactic intrapartum amniofusion for patients with oligohydraminos: a prospective randomized study. J Reprod Med 1992; 37:817–820.
51. Dye T, Aubry R, Gross S, et al: Aminioinfusion and the intrauterine prevention of meconium aspiration. Am J Obstet Gynecol 1994; 171:1601–1605.
52. Maternal and Child Health Research Consortium: Confidential Inquiry into Stillbirths and Deaths in Infancy: 4th Annual Report. London: Department of Health; 1997.
53. Sjostrom K, Valentin L, Thelin T, et al: Maternal anxiety in late pregnancy and fetal hemodynamics. Eur J Obstet Gynecol Reprod Biol 1997; 74:149–155.
54. van Geijin H: Some reflections of fetal surveillance. *In* van Geijin H, Copray F (eds): Critical Appraisal of Fetal Surveillance. Amsterdam: Exerpta Medica Elsevier; 1994:659–674.
55. Amiel-Tison C, Barrier G, Shnider S, et al: The neonatal Neurologic and Adaptive Capacity Score. Anesthesiology 1982; 56:492–493.
56. Hood D, Parker R, Meis P: Epidural bupivacaine does not effect fetal heart tracing [abstract]. Anesthesiology 1993; 79:3A.
57. Epstein H, Waxman A, Gleichner N, et al: Meperidine induced sinusoidal fetal heart rate pattern and its reversal with naloxone. Obstet Gynecol 1982; 59:225–255.
58. Avard D, Nimrod C: Risks and benefits of obstetric epidural analgesia: a review. Birth 1985; 12:215–225.
59. Jouppila R, Jouppila P, Hollmen A, et al: Effect of segmental extradural analgesia on placental blood flow during normal labour. Br J Anaesth 1978; 50:563–567.
60. Giles W, Lah F, Trudinger B: The effect of epidural anesthesia for caesarean section on maternal uterine and fetal umbilical artery blood flow velocity waveforms. Br J Obstet Gynaecol 1987; 94:55–59.
61. Morrow R, Rolbin S, Ritchie J, et al: Epidural anaesthesia and blood flow velocity in mother and fetus. Can J Anaesth 1989; 36:519–522.
62. Valli J, Pirhonen J, Aantaa R, et al: The effect of regional anesthesia for caesarean section on maternal and fetal blood flow velocities measured by Doppler ultrasound. Acta Anaesthesiol Scand 1994; 38:165–169.
63. Jouppila P, Jouppila R, Hollmen A, et al: Lumbar epidural analgesia to improve intervillous blood flow during labour in severe pre-eclampsia. Obstet Gynecol 1982; 59:158–161.
64. Marx G, Shashikant P, Berman J, et al: Umbilical blood flow velocity waveforms in different maternal positions and epidural analgesia. Obstet Gynecol 1986; 68:61–64.
65. Grover R: The fascination of the hypoxic lung. Anesthesiology 1985; 63:580–582.
66. Marshall B, Marshall C: A model for hypoxic constriction of the pulmonary circulation. J Appl Physiol 1988; 64:68–77.
67. Swanstrom S, Bratteby L: Metabolic effects of obstetric regional analgesia and of asphyxia in the newborn infant during the first two hours after birth. III. Adjustment of arterial blood gases and acid-base balance. Acta Paediatr Scand 1981; 70:811–818.
68. Ong B, Cohen M, Palahniuk R: Anaesthesia for cesarean section: effect on neonates. Anaesth Analg 1989; 68:270–275.
69. Marx G, Luykx W, Cohen S: Fetal-neonatal status following caesarean section for fetal distress. Br J Anaesth 1984; 56:1009–1013.

6

Pharmacology of Local Anesthetics

❖ GORDON LYONS, FRCA

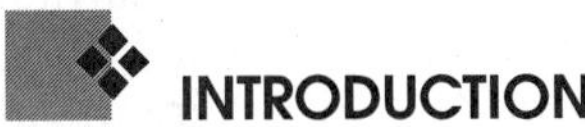

INTRODUCTION

Any comprehensive consideration of local anesthetics would occupy a sizable volume, and for this reason this chapter is selective. Topical issues such as single enantiomer local anesthetics and motor sparing are examined together with molecular expression and the possibility of deriving therapeutic ratios for epidural anesthetics. Topics are viewed from the standpoint of the practicing anesthesiologist with emphasis on their clinical significance. Readers who require more information are directed to De Jong's authoritative text.[1]

Background

Whether it was Bier and Hildebrand in Kiel, in 1898, or Corning, accidentally, in New York, in 1885, who deserve credit for the first intrathecal injection of a local anesthetic (cocaine), regional anesthesia has achieved its first centenary. International standards did not exist in the 19th century, and inability to match the needle to the syringe resulted in the formation of a significant external puddle of Bier's cerebrospinal fluid (CSF). Corning advanced his needle with the syringe attached, so that while incompatibility did not defeat him, he failed to recognize the difference between epidural and intrathecal injection. Cocaine is a crystalline substance that was dissolved before injection, sometimes in tap water.[2] Dissatisfaction with the aftereffects of dural puncture led to Parisians Cathelin and Sicard independently investigating the sacral approach to the epidural space, and Stoeckel, in Germany, in 1909, used the technique for vaginal delivery.[3] Cocaine was toxic, addictive, short-lived, and difficult to sterilize and in 1903 Fourneau developed amylocaine, and a year later Einhorn produced procaine, which has stood the test of time. These developments followed the discovery that cocaine was a benzoic acid ester.[1] Pages described the lumbar approach to the epidural space in 1921 and Aburel, in 1936, described an epidural catheter. Because epidural anesthesia has a higher dosing requirement than intrathecally administered drugs, the vision as well as the proper needle and catheter were not enough to establish the technique. It also required the development of a local anesthetic with a reasonable duration that could be given in appropriate volume without toxicity. As a result, Aburel's contribution was overlooked and the credit given to Curbelo, who pioneered continuous blockade in the 1940s, the decade that saw Lofgren synthesize lignocaine from a series of aniline derivatives. Mass production of sterile disposable and reusable needles and catheters was associated with an explosion in use of the technique in the 1960s. Sweden's preeminence in local anesthetics was established when the piperidine ring of cocaine was linked with the xylidine fraction of lignocaine. Mepivacaine and bupivacaine were produced from pipecolyl xylidine (PPX) derivatives (Fig. 6–1). The latest developments make use of the chiral nature of local anesthetics so that only a single enantiomer is represented, as in ropivacaine and levobupivacaine.[1]

Presently in the United Kingdom, only bupivacaine and ropivacaine are approved for epidural use, and only bupivacaine for intrathecal use. Although lidocaine is used for both epidural and intrathecal anesthesia, the hyperbaric 5% version is unavailable. Chloroprocaine is available in the United States and a number of European countries, and some countries can boast a larger range of intrathecal agents. It is unlikely that the availability of new drugs will be as "patchy" in the future because the European Union has assumed responsibility for licensing drugs throughout Europe. Licensing authorities in Europe and the United States are cooperating to reduce duplication, bureaucracy, and expense. All this should improve the time it takes to get a new drug into global clinical practice.

To appreciate the significance of these developments, some understanding of the molecular foundation of local anesthetics is required, and this will make better sense if we first consider the way that local anesthetics work.

Mepivacaine — NHCO — N—CH_3

Lidocaine — CH_3, CH_3 — NHCOCH_2 — N(C_2H_5)(C_2H_5)

Bupivacaine — NHCO — N—C_4H_9

❖ **Figure 6–1** The xylidine ring of lidocaine on the left was combined with the piperidine ring of cocaine to produce the pipecolyl xylidine derivatives, mepivacaine and bupivacaine. The two methyl groups of the xylidine faction contribute to the stability of the molecule. (From Tucker GT, Mather LE: Properties, absorption and disposition of local anesthetic agents. *In* Cousins MJ, Bridenbaugh PO (eds): Neural Blockade in Clinical Anesthesia and Management of Pain, 2nd ed. Philadelphia: JB Lippincott; 1988:51.)

MECHANISM AND STRUCTURE OF LOCAL ANESTHETICS

Ion Channels and Action Potentials

Local anesthetics work by blocking the transmission of the action potential as it progresses along the nerve fiber membrane. They progressively decrease the rate of rise and the amplitude of the action potential, elevate the firing threshold, and lengthen the refractory period. As a result, conduction velocity slows until conduction eventually ceases. The depolarization of the nerve fiber membrane that produces the action potential is due to a flux of positively charged sodium ions moving from the extracellular fluid into the nerve fiber. The nerve membrane consists of a double thickness of phospholipid, with hydrophobic lipid tails in the center and hydrophilic polar ends facing outward. Charged ions are unable to penetrate this barrier. There is evidence for the existence of channels in the nerve membrane, specific for a single ion, such as sodium, potassium, and calcium (Fig. 6–2). The sodium and potassium channels open and close in response to electrical and chemical switches, and through them pass the ion fluxes that initiate and propagate the action potential.

At rest, the membrane has a potential of −70 mV, but when an impulse arrives and increases the resting potential to the firing threshold at −55 mV, the sodium ion influx begins, rapidly raising the membrane potential to +40 mV. Once the firing threshold is reached, the action potential becomes independent of the strength of the stimulus. Because the extracellular concentration of sodium ions is vastly greater than the intracellular concentration, and because the sodium ions are positively charged, this movement occurs along a concentration gradient and an electrical gradient. This is followed immediately by the opening of potassium ion channels, and intracellular potassium moves out along the concentration gradient but against the electrical gradient, into the extracellular fluid (Fig. 6–3).

Sodium ion channels soon close and potassium efflux increases, bringing the potential back toward resting. After the passage of the action potential, the ion channels are inactive for a short refractory period. This ensures that depolarization occurs only in a forward direction.

The extracellular sodium and intracellular potassium concentrations are maintained by the sodium-potassium pump, which expels sodium out of the nerve fiber into the extracellular fluid. Relative to the ion channel flux, this mechanism is slow and is not blocked by local anesthetics at therapeutic concentrations.

Current in unmyelinated nerve fibers is propagated along the surface of the membrane at a much slower rate than in myelinated fibers. In the latter the ion channels are concentrated at the nodes of Ranvier, and are capable of generating action potentials strong enough to skip to the next node. This is known as *saltatory conduction.* The internodal distance is proportional to the diameter of the fiber, so fatter fibers have faster speeds of conduction.

Mechanism of Local Anesthesia Block

Local anesthetics interfere with the action potential by blocking the sodium ion flux. The uncharged lipophilic local anesthetic base penetrates the nerve membrane, but not through the ion channel. One theory for the mechanism of conduction block by local anesthetics is that the distribution of drug molecules in the lipid bilayer of the nerve fiber membrane produces sufficient expansion to close the sodium ion channels. Some local anesthetic passes through the nerve fiber membrane to reach the axoplasm and dissociates. The charged hydrophilic moiety enters the internal open-

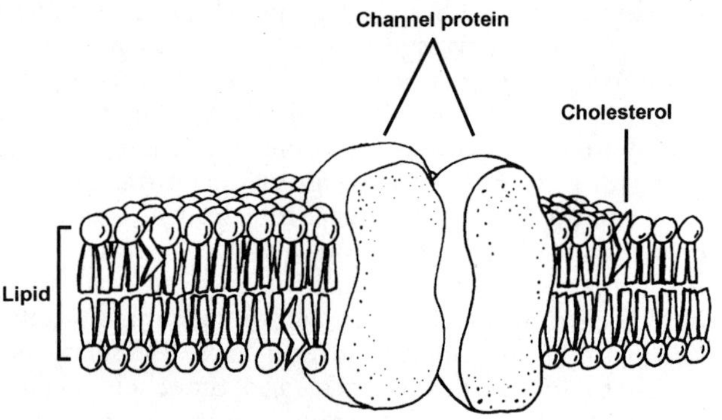

❖ **Figure 6–2** The nerve membrane consists of a double thickness of phospholipid with hydrophobic tails in the center, and hydrophilic polar ends facing outward. Ions are unable to penetrate this barrier. The presence of cholesterol increases the degree of order in the membrane. Ion movement across the membrane occurs through ion-specific channels. (From Covino BG: Mechanism of impulse block. *In* McClure JH, Wildsmith JAW (eds): Conduction Blockade for Postoperative Analgesia. London, England: Edward Arnold; 1991:28.)

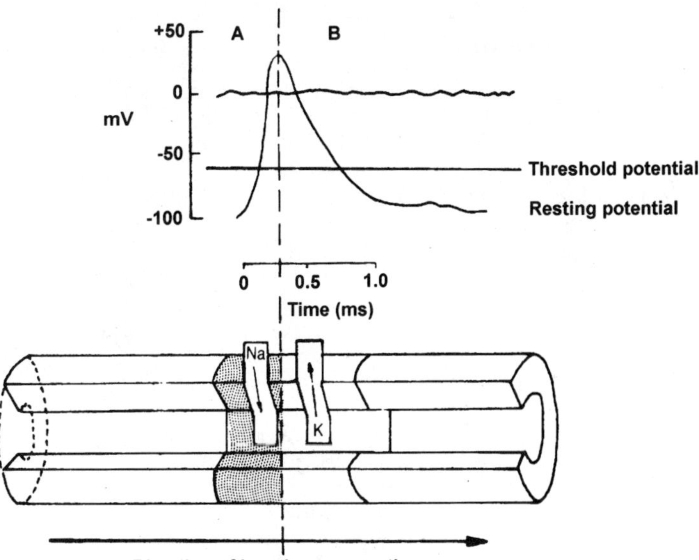

Figure 6–3 At rest the membrane has a potential of −70 mV. The arrival of an impulse triggers depolarization *(A)*, increasing the resting potential to the firing threshold at −55 mV. Rapid influx of sodium ions begins, raising the membrane potential to +40 mV. Depolarization soon follows *(B)*, as potassium ions move out of the fiber. The closure of sodium channels brings the potential back toward resting. A short refractory period ensures that depolarization occurs only in a forward direction. (From Covino BG: Mechanism of impulse block. *In* McClure JH, Wildsmith JAW (eds): Conduction Blockade for Postoperative Analgesia. London, England: Edward Arnold; 1991:30.)

ing of the sodium channel, and interacts with receptors to block ion flux (Fig. 6–4). For lidocaine and bupivacaine it has been estimated that 90% of conduction blockade is due to the cation inside the sodium channel, and 10% is due to the lipophilic base in the membrane.[4] Before cation-receptor blockade can occur, the channel has to open. The stimulus to open the channel is the arrival of an action potential, and repeated action potentials are required to allow sufficient local anesthetic to enter the ion channels. The terms used to describe this kind of blockade are *use-dependent* or *frequency-dependent* block. The external application of local anesthetic to the nerve fiber membrane can block sodium current by binding to the closed sodium channel and this is known as *tonic* block.

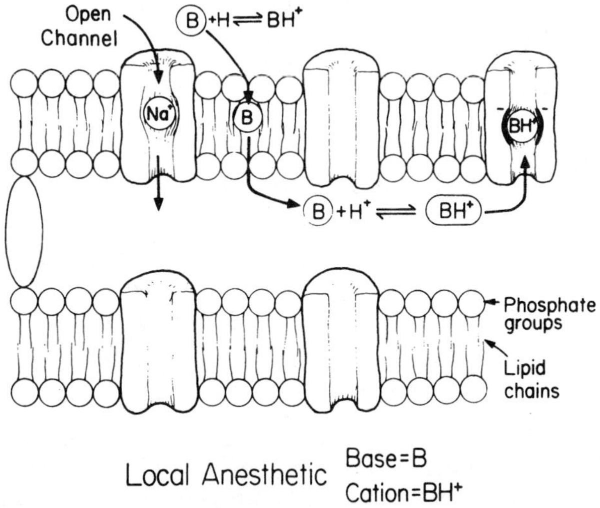

Figure 6–4 The uncharged lipophilic local anesthetic base penetrates the nerve membrane, but not through the sodium channel. The molecule dissociates within the axoplasm, and the hydrophilic cation enters the sodium channel by the internal opening. Within the sodium channel, the cation combines with receptors to block ion flux. (From DiFazio CA: Mixtures. *In* Prithvi Raj P (ed): Clinical Practice of Regional Anesthesia. New York: Churchill Livingstone; 1991:156.)

Stereoselectivity of sodium channels occurs because receptors are chiral amino acids with stereoselective properties.[5] R enantiomers are better at blocking sodium flux than S enantiomers and this should confer on R enantiomers, in general, greater potency than their S counterparts.[6] In support of this, when molar concentrations are considered, levobupivacaine, the S(−) enantiomer of bupivacaine, is 13% less potent than racemic bupivacaine when given epidurally to women in labor.[7] Frequency-dependent block is also applicable to cardiac muscle fibers, and so is stereoselectivity. Consequently the R(+) enantiomer of bupivacaine produces not only a denser frequency-dependent block than the S(−) enantiomer but also a greater reduction in the rate of cardiac muscle action potential depolarization and duration.[8] Stereoselectivity and frequency-dependent block are important issues when cardiotoxicity is considered.

The site of action for central neural blockade is generally considered to be the spinal nerve root. It is now recognized that local anesthetic can diffuse from the nerve root into the dorsal horn of the cord. Modern patch clamping techniques, using whole cell pipettes on dorsal horn neurons of rats, show that lidocaine, mepivacaine, and bupivacaine produce both tonic and frequency-dependent block of sodium channels, and tonic block in potassium channels.[9] While this contributes to our understanding, as yet there is no clinical application.

Molecular Structure

To be effective, local anesthetics require certain physical and structural properties. Lipophilicity is required for penetration of the nerve membrane, but to block the sodium channel flux from within, local anesthetics must have a polar structure. In addition, to add to the complexity, there must be a means of maintaining a

Stereoisomerism: Terminology

Isomers	Two compounds or ions that contain the same number of atoms of the same elements, but in different structural arrangements.
Enantiomers	Pairs of isomers that have a mirror image relationship.
Chiral	Describes a molecule that is not superimposable on its mirror image.
(+)	Indicates that an enantiomer rotates polarized light to the right (clockwise or dextrorotatory).
(−)	Indicates that an enantiomer rotates polarized light to the left (anticlockwise or levorotatory).
Rectus (right) *Sinister (left)*	Describes the configuration of four ligands around the stereogenic carbon atom. If the atomic number count from high to low around the carbon atom is in a clockwise direction, the term R is used, and S for anticlockwise.

The two naming systems are independent of each other. Prilocaine exists as S(+) and R(−), and bupivacaine as S(−) and R(+).[10]

balance between these two properties. The chiral nature of some local anesthetic molecules gives rise to stereoselective properties and enantiomeric differences. The necessary terminology is defined in the box Stereoisomerism: Terminology.

Amide and Ester Links. The chemical structure of local anesthetics links an aromatic lipophilic head to a polar hydrophilic tail, which tends to confer a chiral structure, along with the physical properties mentioned (Fig. 6–5). The nature of the linkage is either ester (–COOH) or amide ($–NH_2$). The hydrophilic tail imparts solubility in water, and the lipophilic head is important for tissue penetration. Because neural tissue is lipid-rich, lipid solubility can have a bearing on duration of action and correlates well with in vitro potency. Bupivacaine, which is more lipid soluble than lidocaine, has a slower onset and longer duration of action. In general terms, amide-linked local anesthetics are less potent, but more sensitive to the production of frequency-dependent block than ester-linked anesthetics.[11] The latter are hydrolyzed by esterases, whereas amide links require a more complex process of decay, and some drug is excreted with little change. The linkage is sufficiently flexible to assist molding to receptors.[1]

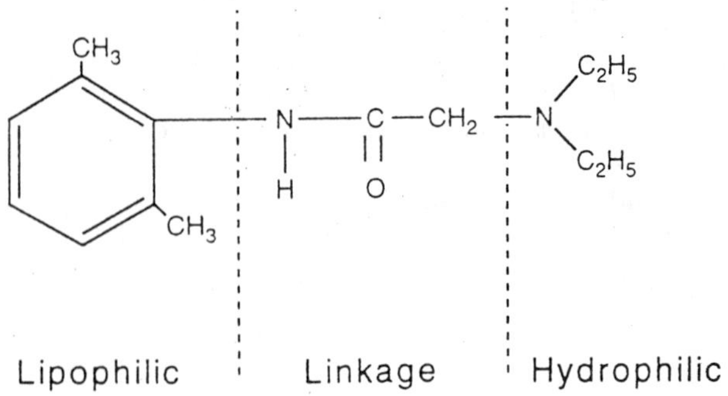

Figure 6–5 Local anesthetics have an aromatic lipophilic head linked to a polar hydrophilic tail. The latter imparts solubility in water, and the lipophilic head is important for tissue penetration. The linkage has a degree of flexibility, which aids molding to receptors. The nature of the linkage determines the mechanism of breakdown. (From Sidebotham DA, Schug SA: Stereochemistry in anaesthesia. Clin Exp Pharmacol Physiol 1997; 24:126–130.)

Pipecolyl Xylidines. Bupivacaine, mepivacaine, and ropivacaine come from a family of molecules known as the pipecolyl xylidines, which combine the piperidine ring of cocaine with xylidine from lignocaine (PPX derivatives). Substitution of methyl, butyl, and propyl groups on the piperidine ring give rise, respectively, to mepivacaine, bupivacaine, and ropivacaine. The piperidine ring is the hydrophilic tail and the xylidine ring is the lipophilic head. Two methyl groups on the xylidine ring confer great stability (see Fig. 6–1). This has relevance for the clinical anesthesiologist. Chloroprocaine does not have this structure and at different times in its history has been combined with methylparaben, metabisulfite, and ethylenediaminetetraacetic acid to improve stability. Imputations of toxicity have been made against all three.[12, 13] All PPX molecules are chiral, and commercial preparations of mepivacaine and bupivacaine are racemic mixtures made up of equal quantities of dextro- and levorotatory forms. Ropivacaine and levobupivacaine are single S(−) enantiomers (Fig. 6–6).

Local anesthetics are tertiary amines, weakly basic, and relatively insoluble. They combine readily with acids to make stable salts that are soluble in water. Ionization yields a quaternary amine cation (NH_4^+) which may dissociate further into uncharged tertiary amine base and hydrogen ion, the significance of which is discussed in Dissociation subsection (p.85).

Molecular Expression and Units

Lidocaine, bupivacaine, and ropivacaine are salts of hydrochloric acid. In solution they exist as hydrochlorides, but in crystalline form they are hydrochloride monohydrates. Lignocaine is expressed as a hydrochloride monohydrate with molecular weight 288, but lidocaine is expressed as an anhydrous hydrochloride with molecular weight 270. Lidocaine base has a molecular weight of 234. If we compare a 2% solution of each, lignocaine contains 20 mg/mL of lidocaine hydrochloride monohydrate and lidocaine contains 20 mg/mL of lidocaine hydrochloride. The ampule of lignocaine contains more inactive molecules than lidocaine, and when the active moiety alone is considered, lignocaine has 6% less than lidocaine. If the potencies of the two are compared, lidocaine should prove marginally more potent than lignocaine.[1]

Ropivacaine and racemic bupivacaine are expressed as hydrochlorides. The commercial prepara-

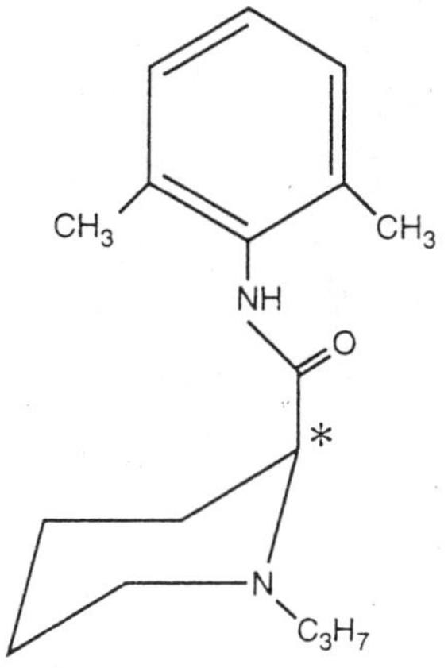

A S-(-)-Ropivacaine

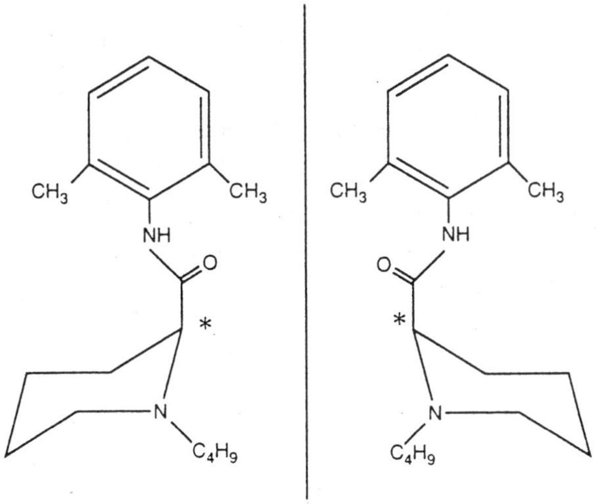

B S-(-)-Bupivacaine R-(+)-Bupivacaine

❖ **Figure 6–6** *A*, The combination of the hydrophilic piperidine ring of cocaine and the lipophilic xylidine ring of lidocaine gives rise to the pipecolyl xylidine group of local anesthetics, which are chiral in nature. Substitution of a propyl group on the piperidine ring gives rise to propivacaine. The S(−)enantiomer is known as ropivacaine, and is the only form available. *B*, Substitution by a butyl group gives rise to bupivacaine. The chirality of this molecule is clearly shown by the diagrammatic representation of levo- and dexbupivacaine, the S(−) and R(−)enantiomers. (From Sidebotham DA, Schug SA: Stereochemistry in anaesthesia. Clin Exp Pharmacol Physiol 1997; 24:126–130.)

tion of the 0.25% concentration of the latter is equivalent to 2.64 mg/mL of the crystalline hydrochloride monohydrate, to give 2.5 mg/mL of bupivacaine hydrochloride, and this explains the labeling information. Levobupivacaine is recently registered, and is bound by Directive 91/507 of the European Economic Community, part 2, section A, clause 3.3, which stipulates that formulations of hydrates and salts must be expressed as milligrams of active moiety. Levobupivacaine 0.25% contains 2.5 mg/mL free base, which means that ampule for ampule levobupivacaine has 11% more active moiety than racemic bupivacaine. The commercial preparations of each have very similar potencies, but if the differences in molecular expression are taken into account, levobupivacaine is 13% less potent than racemic bupivacaine.[7] It is unlikely that the manufacturer will produce more than one formulation, so the European directive will probably prevail worldwide.

Drug concentrations are generally given in units of milligrams per milliliters but it is not commonly indicated whether this applies to hydrate, salt, or base. For this reason the Système Internationale d'Unités (SI system) in use in many countries (but not the U.S.) recommends the use of molar concentrations. By expressing concentration in terms of the molecular weight of the base, the problem is bypassed.

Physical Properties and Clinical Practice

Molecular structure and physical properties, which include lipid solubility, dissociation, and protein binding, all contribute to the way that local anesthetics function.

Lipid Solubility. The solubility of local anesthetics in lipid is measured by comparing solubility in a nonpolar solvent, such as alcohol or *n*-heptane with solubility in water. Different methods not only give rise to different results but also to different orders of rank. Lipophilicity is the property that promotes spread of the local anesthetic through tissues and uptake in the nerve fiber membrane. Lipid solubility may influence potency, duration of action, and time to onset of block (latency).[1] To the clinical anesthesiologist, these data appear confusing because in vitro experiments on devascularized nerve fibers, sheathed or unsheathed, can give rise to conclusions that do not fit comfortably with clinical experience and observation. The epidural space contains fat and vessels, and in vivo, myelinated nerves have a rich blood supply. A molecule with an affinity for lipid does not distinguish between neural lipid and adiposity, and the effect of vascularity is to remove drug from all sites. Not only is clinical practice different from the laboratory, but different sites of administration may yield different results. In an attempt to bypass tissue factors, Langerman and colleagues studied intrathecal local anesthetics in mice and rabbits, and found correlations between potency and duration, and lipid solubility.[14, 15] Table 6–1 shows a compilation of data derived from clinical practice. Lipid solubility correlates poorly with onset of action, but duration and potency accord quite well.

Dissociation. Significant lipophilicity ensures excellent tissue and nerve membrane penetration, but if lipophilicity dominates, the ionic phase may prove inadequate and ion channel blockade may be ineffective. The ideal local anesthetic should exist as a lipophilic, tertiary amine base until it reaches the axoplasm, and then dissociate totally to yield charged quaternary amine. In reality, the best compromise that can be achieved is a pH-dependent balance between uncharged tertiary amine base and charged quaternary amine. The factor that decides the nature of the balance is the coefficient pK_a, which defines the pH at

Table 6–1 RANKING OF LOCAL ANESTHETICS USED IN LABOR*

	ONSET	DURATION	LIPID SOLUBILITY (*n* - HEPTANE / WATER)	RANKED POTENCY†
Chloroprocaine	Very fast	Short	0.05	2
Lignocaine	Fast	Moderate	1	1
Etidocaine	Fast	Long	39	—
Bupivacaine	Moderate	Long	10	4
Ropivacaine	Moderate	Long	3	3

*Table shows local anesthetics ranked in terms of onset, duration, lipid solubility, and epidural potency measured in labor, using compiled data. While there seems to be little correlation between lipid solubility and onset, there is accord with duration and potency. Data compiled from references 14, 57, 59, 60, 87–91.

†Ranked potency is from 1 (low) to 4 (high). EC_{50} (effective concentration in 50% of population), epidural pain relief in labor.

which the concentrations of charged and uncharged moiety are equal. Each local anesthetic has its own value for pK_a. Bupivacaine and ropivacaine both share a pK_a of 8.1, and the ratio of charged to uncharged moiety is determined by the difference between this and the ambient pH. Laboratory studies with sheathed nerves show that an increase in ambient pH is associated with increased conduction blockade, but for unsheathed nerves the results are not impressive or even reversed. A more alkaline pH discourages ionization, leaving uncharged base to penetrate the sheath, but without the sheath, diffusibility is no longer required, and blockade suffers for want of ionized moiety. A more acidic pH encourages ionization.[4]

Addition of Bicarbonate and Epinephrine. The pH of an ampule of bupivacaine 0.5% is 5.4 to 6.0,[16] considerably more acidic than the pK_a. At this pH, one estimate is that less than 5% of drug is un-ionized, when the more desirable situation would be a greater concentration of uncharged tertiary amine base.[17] The addition of bicarbonate to increase pH should, in theory, aid tissue penetration and improve blockade. Capogna and coworkers added 1 mEq of bicarbonate to 10 mL of local anesthetic before epidural injection. This raised the pH to 6.65. The alkalinized local anesthetic produced a regional blockade that was 2 to 3 minutes quicker and rose one dermatome higher than untreated bupivacaine.[18] Ideally, the bicarbonate breaks down to carbon dioxide and water within the axoplasm, lowering the pH and promoting cation production and ion channel blockade. The lipophobic cations are unable to diffuse out through the nerve fiber membrane, a phenomenon known as *ion trapping*. Not all studies show clinical advantages from alkalinization,[17, 19] perhaps because the bicarbonate breaks down long before the nerve fiber is breached.[20] Even minute volumes of 8.4% sodium bicarbonate are sufficient to cause precipitation when added to bupivacaine, and the stability of alkalinized solutions requires that they be used within 6 hours. Epinephrine-containing solutions are buffered to a lower pH to protect the catecholamine from oxidation and require a greater amount of alkali to elevate pH.[16] For stability, both agents need to be added fresh and the solution used immediately. Stabilizing agents such as cyclodextrins may allow extension of the shelf life of pH-adjusted local anesthetics, but their use is experimental.[21] Lidocaine hydrocarbonate is available in Canada, but not elsewhere, perhaps because the results are unimpressive.[17, 22]

Protein Binding and Placental Transfer. Before a local anesthetic can bind to protein it has to enter the bloodstream. Consequently, differences in protein binding are of little direct relevance to therapeutic activity but can influence distribution, elimination, and toxicity. Most local anesthetics bind to α_1-acid glycoprotein rather than albumin, and the large molecules formed remain within the circulation. Bupivacaine and ropivacaine are 85% to 95% bound, but lidocaine is 65% bound,[5] and is a free, unbound drug that is available for transfer, biotransformation, excretion, and toxicity (Fig. 6–7). Stereoselective binding differences are seen with bupivacaine enantiomers, but the relevance of this is uncertain.[23] There is a limit to the amount of plasma protein, so binding has a ceiling, and once this is reached, free drug increases rapidly with significant potential for toxicity. The concentration of α_1-acid glycoprotein is reduced in pregnancy, and this is one source of the concern that pregnant women are more susceptible to local anesthetic toxicity. Another potential problem is interaction with other protein-bound drugs. Displacement from binding sites can increase the concentration of free drug, and this has implications for toxicity and placental transfer.[24]

Unbound free drug moves across the placenta by passive diffusion, and the rate of transfer is proportional to lipophilicity. Polar and protein-bound molecules are unable to cross the placenta. Uptake of local anesthetic into the fetal circulation is not the sole reason for placental clearance, since some drug accumulates in the placenta. Once in the fetal circulation, binding to fetal α_1-acid glycoprotein occurs, but because fetal levels of this protein are much lower than maternal levels at term, total plasma concentration of local anesthetic is lower on the fetal side. Free drug transfers to the fetal circulation until equilibrium is reached, and the rate of transfer is proportional to the degree of protein binding on the fetal side. The phenomenon of ion trapping also occurs in the fetal circulation when acidosis promotes greater dissocia-

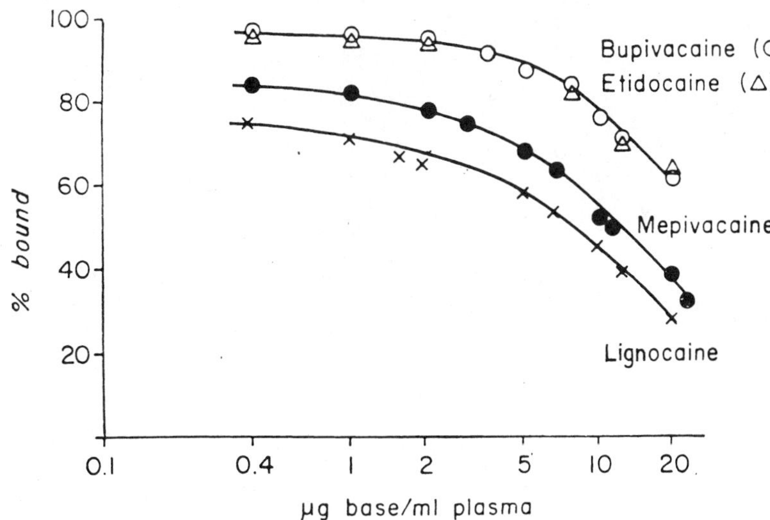

❖ **Figure 6–7** Bupivacaine is almost 100% protein bound. With increasing plasma concentration, the ability of protein to buffer diminishes, and the free drug fraction dominates. (From Tucker GT, Mather LE: Pharmacokinetics of local anaesthetic agents. Br J Anaesth 1975; 47:215.)

tion than on the maternal side. The polar molecules are unable to diffuse further.[25] Johnson and colleagues using their in vivo perfused rabbit placenta model showed that declining fetal pH increased the transfer of bupivacaine, lidocaine, and 2-chloroprocaine from mother to fetus. Equilibration of free, unbound drug as ionization increased on the fetal side was the probable explanation for this phenomenon.[26]

Clinical concerns relate to proteinuric hypertension (preeclampsia) and maternal hypoproteinemia, reducing the therapeutic ratio in the mother and increasing transfer to the fetus. The acidotic fetus has a greater potential for accumulation of local anesthetic. To what extent is this a real concern? Epidural anesthesia for cesarean section involves administration of large doses of local anesthetic and provides the greatest opportunity for undesirable effects. Rolbin and coworkers, in a retrospective study, found fewer Apgar scores of 3 or less at 5 minutes in singletons of less than or equal to 32 weeks' gestation, many compromised, when epidural anesthesia was compared with general anesthesia.[27] Choice of technique remains a clinical decision.

PHARMACOKINETICS

The movement of injected local anesthetic can be followed from the point of injection to elimination. Drug concentrations are measured in sequential blood samples and plotted against time to give a dynamic picture of the balance between systemic absorption and removal from the bloodstream, as drug is lost by sequestration into organs, biotransformation, and excretion. Systemic absorption gives an opportunity for systemic toxicity, and this provides much of the rationale for analyses of this nature. Central nervous system and cardiac effects are a product of the drug concentrations presented to these organs; therefore arterial samples are preferred for analyses.[28] The invasive nature of widespread and repeated sampling, together with the potential for toxic effects, means that much of the experimental work is conducted on animals. A favorite model is the chronically instrumented sheep.[29]

The peak and slope of declining local anesthetic is analyzed in sections, which allows for calculations of slope and area under the curve (Fig. 6–8). Some plots are subjected to complex mathematics. A description of the fate of a bolus of local anesthetic takes on the appearance of a number of symbols with values attached. A typical plot shows an exponential decay with an initial rapid phase, dilution and fan distribution, followed by a slower phase of distribution. The exponential curve can be treated mathematically as two slopes, the first with a rapid rate constant (α) and the second slower distribution in the β slope. The latter may be referred to as steady state. Each slope has its own half-life. A guide to the terminology of pharmacokinetics is provided in the following sections.

Volume of Distribution. The volume of distribution is calculated following the immediate dilution of a bolus of drug from the time when concentration peaks through its decay as it diffuses out of the circulation. Rapid dilution followed by rapid diffusion is desirable because it limits the exposure of the heart and brain to circulating drug. The dilution phase of lidocaine lasts 1.5 minutes.[1] Protein binding, by buffering free drug, and lipid solubility, by promoting organ uptake, both increase the initial volume of dilution (V_1). The second phase of distribution (V_2) marks the uptake of drug into organs and tissues, at a slower rate of decay. Steady state occurs when arrival and removal are balanced (V_{dss}). Volume of distribution is expressed in liters or in liters per kilogram of water. The uptake in some organs exceeds the solubility of drug in water, and therefore the volume of distribution can equal a volume of water that exceeds physiologic possibility.

Half-Life. The change of concentration with time can be calculated from the slopes that make up the plot. The time taken for the concentration to decay by 50% is the half-life (t), and for lidocaine it is 1.6

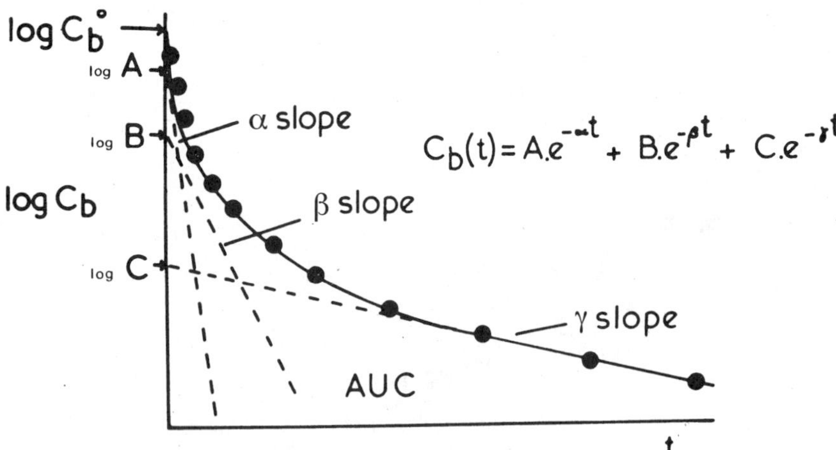

❖ **Figure 6–8** The profile of an intravenous injection. The blood concentration decays with time. Three slopes are fitted to this curve (α, β, γ), and each has its own half-life (tα, tβ, tγ). Clearance is calculated by dividing the dose by the area under the curve. (From Tucker GT, Mather LE: Pharmacokinetics of local anaesthetic agents. Br J Anaesth 1975; 47:217.)

hours.[1] Each exponential function of the plot has its own half-life (tα,tβ).

Clearance. Clearance (Cl) is a measure of elimination, and is defined as the volume of drug cleared per minute or hour. It is calculated by dividing dose by the area under the curve. Chloroprocaine, which undergoes hydrolysis by plasma cholinesterase, is rapidly cleared, but amide-linked local anesthetics are subject to oxidative metabolism in the liver, and clearance is much slower. Hepatic extraction is proportional to the rate at which the liver is supplied with drug. Small quantities of chloroprocaine are excreted unchanged in the urine.

The pharmacokinetic model is useful in anticipating the pattern of behavior of a new drug, but once introduced into practice, theoretic predictions take second place to clinical experience. The model can provide information on the fate of an accidental intravenous injection, an epidural bolus, and an epidural infusion. The two situations with greatest potential for toxic effects are accidental intravenous injection and epidural infusion by way of accumulation. For the former, the initial volume of distribution and opportunities for buffering are important safety features, and if arrhythmias occur, rapid diffusion out of the circulation is desirable to aid reversibility of cardiac receptor binding. The cardiac effects of lidocaine, which is 65% protein bound, are easier to reverse than those of bupivacaine, which is 95% protein bound, and has a slower rate of decay. Absorption following an epidural bolus is biphasic, with an initial rapid phase, followed by a slower phase (Fig. 6–9). For ropivacaine, the half-life of the rapid phase is 14 minutes, and 4.2 hours for the slower phase, which probably represents absorption from lipid and correlates with duration of action.[30] Intrinsic vasoactivity may have a bearing on the rate of systemic absorption, and this is considered later. The biphasic nature of absorption is common to all local anesthetics administered epidurally. For epidural bolus injections and infusions, slow absorption prolongs duration of drug action, potentially reducing the total dose required.[31] If increments are given during the course of an epidural infusion, and if at the end of labor, a terminal anesthetic bolus is required for cesarean section, blood concentration is likely to be high. In these circumstances a large steady state volume of distribution and brisk clearance are beneficial.

Intrinsic Vasoactivity. All local anesthetics produce vasodilatation at high concentrations, perhaps by a direct effect on smooth muscle.[32] When given subcutaneously to piglets at anesthetic concentrations, laser Doppler assessment showed that bupivacaine dilates, while ropivacaine constricts, cutaneous blood flow. The addition of epinephrine to slow the absorption of ropivacaine was considered superfluous.[33] Bupivacaine, when given to volunteers by the intradermal route, is shorter-acting than ropivacaine, and duration of action for both is extended by the addition of epinephrine.[34] At high concentrations, again by the intradermal route, both enantiomers of bupivacaine produce vasodilatation, but when concentration is re-

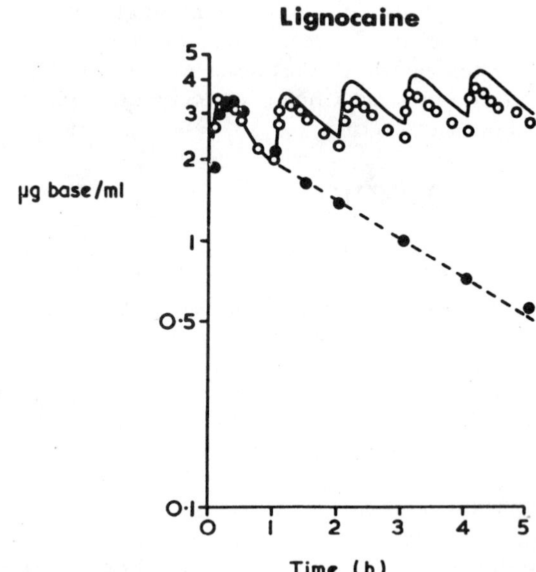

❖ **Figure 6–9** Plasma concentration of lidocaine after single epidural dose (●) and multiple doses (○). (From Tucker GT, Cooper S, Littlewood D, et al: Observed and predicted accumulation of local anaesthetic agents during continuous extradural analgesia. Br J Anaesth 1977; 49:239.)

duced, a vasoconstrictor effect is observed with levobupivacaine but not with dexbupivacaine.[32] Vasoconstriction is a property common to L-enantiomers at low concentration.[31] When applied to spinal pia mater in dogs, ropivacaine produces arteriolar vasoconstriction in a concentration-dependent manner, and bupivacaine produces vasodilatation.[35] When given intravenously to dogs, ropivacaine at a dose of 4 mg/kg produces generalized pial vasoconstriction.[36] While differing vasoactivity brings about clinically significant differences between ropivacaine, racemic bupivacaine, levobupivacaine, and dexbupivacaine when given cutaneously, evidence that this will be important for epidural administration is not available.

Pharmacokinetic evidence supports greater intravenous clearance for ropivacaine compared with bupivacaine, but profiles after epidural administration are similar. McClure feels that the differences between bupivacaine and ropivacaine are not clinically significant.[5] In labor and after prolonged epidural infusion, plasma concentrations of both drugs are at a safe level.[12, 37] Differences also exist between the racemate and enantiomers of bupivacaine,[31, 38–40] but the clinical significance of these findings is uncertain. Lidocaine, however, when given with epinephrine to provide anesthesia for cesarean section, can produce plasma levels that exceed those considered toxic in animals.[28] None of the local anesthetics in common use have an ideal pharmacokinetic profile. The various methods of administration have conflicting requirements, and the ideal may be an impossible goal. Of greater importance is that, whatever the mode of administration, clinical practice demonstrates that for local anesthetics used in the labor suite, therapeutic efficacy can be achieved unaccompanied by toxic effects. The influence of potency on accidental intravenous injection has yet to be discussed.

Toxicity

Much has been written on this topic. From the clinical point of view, concern revolves almost exclusively around intravenous injection, which has been responsible for deaths of pregnant women in the United States,[41] and children in Great Britain.[42] Therapeutic doses of local anesthetic appropriately administered are not a source of systemic morbidity or mortality, but have long been implicated in local neurotoxicity.[43] The clinical manifestations of sudden high blood levels of local anesthetic are seizures, cardiac arrhythmia, and collapse. These are considered in turn.

Seizures. In low doses local anesthetics have a stabilizing effect on the central nervous system, but at high doses particularly when suddenly presented, they cause seizures. Central nervous system toxicity is related to potency. Among the first clinical manifestations of circulating local anesthetic are numbness and tingling in the face, a noticeable taste, ringing in the ears, dizziness, and other subjective sensations. Lidocaine, 1 mg/kg, given intravenously on induction of anesthesia had 100% specificity and 95% sensitivity for these symptoms.[44] When these symptoms appear during or immediately after a bolus injection of local anesthetic, there should be a very high index of suspicion. The dose of lidocaine given by infusion over 20 minutes has to reach 7 mg/kg before humans convulse, and less is required if a bolus is used. The corresponding plasma level is in the region of 22 μg/mL.[1] The symptoms are premonitory and serve as one end point in toxicity studies on volunteers.[45]

Animal studies tend to take two forms. Fixed doses (in mg/kg) are given to prepared animals, and the survivors counted, or the dose required to achieve an end point such as convulsion or death is measured. One measure used for comparisons between local anesthetics is the dose required to produce convulsions in 50% (CD_{50}) and 100% (CD_{100}), respectively, of the population under study. In sheep, CD_{100} of bupivacaine is approximately half that of ropivacaine, and a quarter that of lidocaine,[1] and in rabbits, CD_{50} of racemic bupivacaine is two thirds that of levobupivacaine.[6] When convulsions occur in the labor suite, the onset is sudden and upsetting, but the gap between CD_{50} and lethal dose (LD_{50}) ranges from three times CD_{50} for lidocaine, to twice CD_{50} for racemic bupivacaine and levobupivacaine.[6] This margin of safety, the ratio between convulsant dose and that producing cardiovascular collapse, is another index used for comparison.[46] Dogs infused with either bupivacaine or ropivacaine failed to show a difference in the convulsant dose, but the margin of safety was greater for ropivacaine.[47] A point to note is that cardiovascular collapse is not always preceded by a convulsion. Collapse can be the first manifestation of cardiotoxicity, and it can take a number of forms.

Cardiotoxicity. Cardiac action potentials consist of sodium currents, and interference in the working of sodium channels in cardiac muscle impairs contractility and excitability. The effects of local anesthetics on cardiac sodium channels relate to dose and potency,[8] but even when these are taken into account, bupivacaine is four times more toxic than lidocaine. The additional difference is attributed to slower release of bupivacaine from binding sites within the cardiac sodium channels.[5] The cardiac myocyte is very susceptible to local anesthetic, and is subject to frequency-dependent block. Association and dissociation kinetics determine the dwell time of local anesthetic in the sodium channel. Bupivacaine binds 10 times longer than lidocaine, which has a reputation for "fast-in, fast-out", and has greater potassium channel[48] and perhaps greater calcium channel blocking properties than lidocaine.[1] Long dwell time leads to prolonged resuscitation, with all its implications.[5] The rate of increase in the cardiac potential is dependent on sodium ion flux, and slows in the presence of local anesthetic, with lengthening of PR and QRS intervals.[49] This predisposes to reentrant phenomena and arrhythmias.[5] Hypoxia and acidosis increase these effects, especially in the fetus. Ventricular arrhythmias, hypotension, and respiratory arrest, leading to death, are all seen as independent terminal events in animals.[47]

Cardiac sodium channel blockade is not the only mechanism of cardiotoxicity. The myocyte takes up local anesthetic according to lipophilicity, and contractility is directly impaired. There is evidence of interference with mitochondrial function that may be proportional to lipid solubility.[50] Cardiovascular collapse can also occur secondary to an effect on the central nervous system.[1]

Toxicity studies in humans are performed on healthy volunteers. Local anesthetic is infused intravenously at 10 mg/min until 150 to 250 mg are given, or symptoms appear. Outcome measures are the number surviving the entire infusion, the incidence and nature of electrocardiographic (ECG) irregularities, and the incidence and nature of changes in heart rate, blood pressure, and cardiac parameters measured by echocardiography or by thoracic bioimpedance. Finally, plasma drug concentrations are measured when symptoms appear, changes occur, or the study is completed.

Ropivacaine and Levobupivacaine. Animal studies suggest that bupivacaine might be more arrhythmogenic than lidocaine and ropivacaine.[47] Studies have been conducted in vitro and in vivo, on cloned human ventricle, guinea pigs, rabbits, sheep, dogs, and pigs. The general findings have been that ropivacaine has less effect on the cardiac action potential,[5] gives quicker recovery of potassium channels,[48] and requires higher doses to produce convulsions and collapse[49] than racemic bupivacaine.

In humans, ropivacaine is associated with higher-tolerated plasma levels, fewer central nervous effects, shorter recovery of symptoms, less widening of QRS complexes, and less interference with cardiac performance, when compared with racemic bupivacaine.[45, 51] Onset of central nervous symptoms is at free plasma concentration of approximately 0.6 μg/mL of ropivacaine, compared with 0.3 μg/mL of bupivacaine.[51] By general consensus, ropivacaine is less toxic than bupivacaine.

More than 25 years ago, Aberg reported that levobupivacaine had higher CD_{50} and LD_{50} than both dexbupivacaine and racemate.[6] Enantiomer-selective central nervous and cardiac effects have been observed in human cardiac muscle, guinea pigs, mice, rats, and rabbits. Levobupivacaine consistently produces less central nervous and cardiac effects, with quicker recovery, than racemic bupivacaine.[48, 49, 52–55]

Gristwood and colleagues have reported on a human volunteer study. They found that higher doses of levobupivacaine were tolerated and produced less ECG change, and less change in myocardial contractility index and stroke index, as measured by thoracic bioimpedance, when compared with racemic bupivacaine.[56] There is therefore sufficient evidence to justify claims that levobupivacaine is less toxic than racemic bupivacaine.

A single comparison of the effects of levobupivacaine with those of ropivacaine and bupivacaine on guinea pig and human myocytes showed that bupivacaine produced the worst results in terms of contractility and excitability, while ropivacaine was marginally the best.[54] Before attempts to establish a hierarchy in terms of toxicity, the clinician needs to appreciate that a conclusive advantage of one agent over another in the laboratory does not guarantee that the advantage will be maintained in the clinical setting. The influence of potency needs to be considered.

Toxicity and Potency. Penetration of nerve fibers by local anesthetic, to block sodium channels, is influenced by lipid solubility, which determines potency. Because the uptake of local anesthetic by cardiac muscle, and subsequent sodium channel blockade, are among causes of cardiotoxicity, potency has a direct bearing. Comparative assessments of toxicity between bupivacaine and ropivacaine, and bupivacaine and levobupivacaine, have been conducted in the laboratory using similar doses for all drugs. This assumes equivalent potency. In the clinical setting, variations in the potency of individual local anesthetics are adjusted for by corresponding variations in the dose, and when accidental intravenous injection occurs, the heart is presented with the contents of the syringe. At cesarean section the syringe might contain 100 to 150 mg of bupivacaine or 300 to 400 mg of lidocaine with epinephrine. At anesthetic concentrations, the epidural potency ratio of bupivacaine to lidocaine is 4:1,[57] and if this is not recognized in the design of laboratory studies, the relevance of the result to clinical practice is open to question. If potency differences were to exist between bupivacaine, ropivacaine and levobupivacaine, the toxicity table established in the laboratory would not necessarily hold good in clinical practice.

The minimum local analgesic concentration (MLAC) of an epidural local anesthetic in labor is the effective concentration in 50% of the study population (EC_{50}) and is a clinical index of potency. Because the absolute values are influenced by local demographic and obstetric factors,[58, 59] differences in MLAC are often expressed as percentages of the potency of racemic bupivacaine. Epidural ropivacaine is 60% as potent as bupivacaine and requires a 67% upward dose adjustment to achieve equivalence.[60, 61] When molar concentrations of levobupivacaine are considered, it is 13% less potent than the racemate. The difference in molecular expression between the racemate and its levo form means that they are interchangeable in clinical practice, but the advantage of reduced toxicity is offset by the difference in potency, albeit a small one.[7] At present, there is no means of incorporating this information into the toxicity table, but clinicians should be reluctant to accept toxicity claims that are not qualified by potency data.

Therapeutic Ratio. Relative safety is assessed using the therapeutic ratio, that is, the margin between the effective dose and the toxic dose (Fig. 6–10). For local anesthetics, MLAC and the EC_{50} provide a midpoint on the slope for efficacy, but there are objections to using efficacy indices against toxicity indices such as CD_{50} and LD_{50}. The clinical data are subject to variations within patients, obstetric practices, and pharmacologic units, while the laboratory data provide a range of end points, all of which would have their own significance. A future development might be to establish

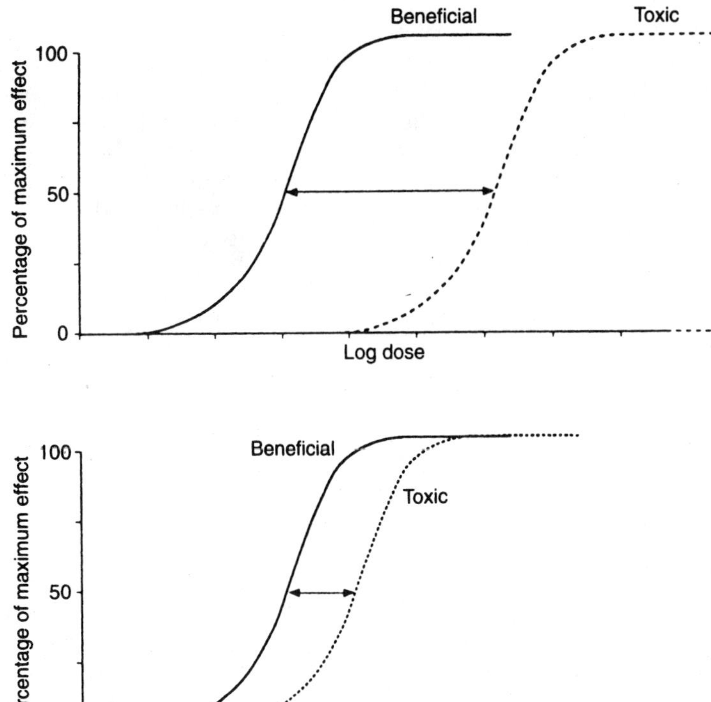

❖ **Figure 6–10** Dose-response curves for a drug with a wide safety margin *(top)* and one with a narrow safety margin *(bottom)*. For each drug the first curve illustrates the therapeutic effect, and the second curve the toxic effect. The wider the separation between the two curves, the safer the drug. (From Ferner RE: Forensic Pharmacology. Oxford, England: Oxford University Press; 1996:26.)

a convention that overcomes the objections, and provides for toxicity comparisons with allowance for potency differences. The issue for clinicians would then be transparent. Given the current information, there is no guarantee that differences between the therapeutic ratios of the new local anesthetics and bupivacaine would reach statistical significance.

Pregnancy. In the United States[41] bupivacaine toxicity became apparent in pregnant women, whereas in Great Britain,[42] children undergoing intravenous regional anesthesia were the victims. Interest in the United States has focused on whether pregnancy predisposes to cardiotoxicity, citing reduced protein binding in pregnancy with increased free drug, and possibly a progesterone effect on the myocardium. Santos and colleagues failed to detect any differences in toxic effects between pregnant and nonpregnant ewes exposed to bupivacaine, levobupivacaine, and ropivacaine. They challenge the findings of previously published in vitro studies that reported a predisposition, and are skeptical about its existence.[46] Central neuraxial blocks in pregnant women tend to be more extensive, for a given dose, than in nonpregnant women.[62] Some of the differences between pregnant and nonpregnant animals that are seen in toxicity studies could be explained by larger block and also by the greater difficulty in performing adequate resuscitation in pregnancy. In vitro comparisons of nerves removed from pregnant and nonpregnant rats do not demonstrate a difference.[63]

Neurotoxicity. It was first suggested more than 60 years ago that high concentrations of local anesthetic could produce axonal damage.[43] More recently, lidocaine has been implicated in cauda equina syndrome[64] and lower limb dysesthesia.[65] Problems have occurred only after intrathecal administration, and it is likely that damage is a product of local anesthetic concentration and time,[64] and neither hyperosmolarity[65, 66] nor antioxidants are responsible. Neurotoxicity may be related to potency but not to whether anesthetics are amide or ester linked.[67] Clinical evidence does not support the potency claim. Three mechanisms have been suggested. First, there is evidence of disruption of Schwann cells, even at clinical concentrations, and greater disruption with increasing concentration. Second, in the axon, irreversible block is associated with degeneration; and interference with blood supply leading to nerve ischemia is a third possibility.[67] High concentrations of anesthetic act like a metabolic poison, inactivate the sodium-potassium pump, and eventually stop axonal transport, which is the internal cytoplasmic flow that replaces, renews, and supports cell functions.[1] Effects on mitochondria might lead to energy failure within the axon, high cytoplasmic calcium levels, and cell death.[50, 68] The intracellular effect of lidocaine is greater than that of bupivacaine,[24] and reflects the clinical impression that bupivacaine is benign. The relationship of neurotoxicity to cardiotoxicity has not been established, and the next era of local anesthetic development might see interest in this area.

Differential Nerve Block and Motor Sparing

Clinical interest in differential nerve block relates to a desire for mobile, pain-free women in labor. Motor sparing and walking in labor are not necessarily associated with beneficial effects,[69] but clearly do improve satisfaction.[70] Reducing the amount of local anesthetic given should increase safety. The traditional explanation for differential nerve block is that the larger the nerve fiber, the higher the concentration required for blockade.[71] The index used for comparisons is based on the lowest concentration required to block two nodes of Ranvier (Cm) in the laboratory.[72] Large, fast, myelinated fibers are recognized to have the highest Cm, but texts are not in agreement as to whether B sympathetic or C pain fibers require the least Cm.[71, 73] The clinician's approach to conflicting data is to consider the lessons of clinical practice. Motor sparing requires that A-alpha motor fibers are unblocked. If pain relief in labor requires blockade of both A-delta and C pain fibers, then blockade of B sympathetic fibers should accompany all effective blocks. Breen and colleagues found that 92% of women receiving a bupivacaine/epinephrine/fentanyl cocktail were comfortable, 68% walked, 17% had evidence of motor block, and 9% had postural hypotension.[74] This suggests that unmyelinated C fibers are blocked first, and that many women do not have complete B fiber block. If this is true, then it also suggests that the pain of the first stage of labor is conducted mainly through C fibers. Capogna and colleagues have shown that as labor progresses, the concentration of epidural local anesthetic needs to be increased.[75] Perhaps the explanation for this is the recruitment ofA-delta fibers as the fetal head descends. In the laboratory, myelinated fibers can appear more sensitive to local anesthetics than unmyelinated fibers, a discrepancy that is attributed to absence of normal physiologic activity.[76] This refers chiefly to the contribution of the circulation.

It is possible to achieve conduction blockade at concentrations less than Cm, but the local anesthetic must be spread over a number of nodes. As the length of fiber available to the local anesthetic increases, so the concentration required to block it is reduced. The rate of rise and the amplitude of the action potential diminish progressively until depolarization fails to reach threshold. This phenomenon is known as *decremental block*.[70]

Modern ideas no longer support the theory that differential nerve block is a product of fiber size and conduction velocity, and it is possible that Cm differences relate to artifacts of in vitro techniques. One alternative explanation is that there is a difference in ion channel kinetics between motor and sensory nerves. Another is that spinal local anesthetics may not work on nerve roots, but work at the point where dorsal root axons enter the dorsal horn. This is an area of transition where Schwann cells are replaced by oligodendrocytes, making them more vulnerable to the action of local anesthetics. Sensory and motor fibers have different destinations and so begin to segregate. The hypothesis is that the anatomic configuration of this makes the bundle of sensory fibers more accessible to block than the motor nerves.[77] There is evidence that bupivacaine and ropivacaine block C fibers first, whereas mepivacaine and etidocaine block A fibers preferentially.[73] This can be explained by the ion channel hypothesis.

Assessment of Block. Complaints of pain during cesarean section have sometimes led to litigation.[78] One explanation for pain during surgery might be that blocks are inadequately assessed.[79] Common methods of checking a nerve block involve the use of a thermal test (often ice), pinprick, and touch. To ensure comfort during cesarean delivery, anesthesia must be established to the level of the T5 dermatome.[80] Touch seems to correspond well with anesthesia, and provides the lowest dermatomal level of the sensory modalities tested. Pinprick is frequently two dermatomes higher.[81] The differential between cold and pinprick can vary from 2 to 6 dermatomes. Cold provides the nearest indication of the height of sympathetic blockade.[82]

More recently, block height has been assessed using the cutaneous application of electric current. Frequencies of 2000, 250, and 5 Hz have been found to correlate with A-beta, A-delta, and C fiber function, and with touch, pinprick, and cold. The duration of surgical anesthesia correlated with elevated A-beta fiber threshold.[83] At present, cutaneous current perception threshold measurement is a research tool that allows quantitative assessment of block, but not all users are able to show a correlation with traditional methods of assessment.[84] At this time, its place is unclear.

Opioids as Local Anesthetics

Pethidine/meperidine, fentanyl, and sufentanil are phenylpiperidines, a group of opioids that are thought to have intrinsic local anesthetic action. Pethidine/meperidine has been used as the sole intrathecal agent for cesarean delivery, but the effects of the other opioids are not so clear. An in vitro study on rat dorsal root axons found that pethidine/meperidine blocked conduction in 61% of axons and reduced conduction velocity in the remainder, but fentanyl and sufentanil failed to affect conduction velocity to any detectable degree.[85] The mechanism of opioid action in epidural and intrathecal analgesia is not wholly understood, but it seems that the only one that behaves like a local anesthetic is pethidine/meperidine.

FURTHER DEVELOPMENTS

A derivative of lidocaine, *N*-β-phenylethyl lidocaine quaternary ammonium bromide appears to be more potent at blocking sodium channels than lidocaine with a greatly extended duration of action, particularly for afferent fibers.[86] Longer duration of action will be beneficial for obstetric use only if the differential between sensory and motor components is considerable. An agent that blocks only afferent fibers would be advantageous. Neurotoxicity issues may lead to the development of specific local anesthetics for intrathecal use, and the same could become true for opioids.

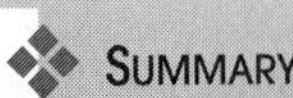

SUMMARY

Key Points

- Bupivacaine is associated with greater toxicity than lidocaine because of its predisposition to ventricular arrhythmias when injected intravascularly.
- Single levo formulations of amide local anesthetics (ropivacaine and levobupivacaine) have less potential to produce cardiotoxicity than does racemic bupivacaine.
- Local anesthetics are weak bases. Alkalinization of local anesthetics produces an increase in the uncharged base and thus speeds the onset of block.
- 2-Chloroprocaine is rapidly hydrolyzed by plasma pseudocholinesterases. Because of its speed of onset and fetal safety, it is often chosen for emergency cesarean sections.

Key References

Santos AC, Arthur GR, Lehning EJ, Finster M: Comparative pharmacokinetics of ropivacaine and bupivacaine in nonpregnant and pregnant ewes. Anesth Analg 1997; 85:87–93.

Covino BG, Vassallo HG: Local anesthetics: mechanisms of action and clinical use. New York: Grune & Stratton; 1976.

Case Stem

A parturient is sent to you for preanesthetic evaluation at 28 weeks' gestation because of an allergy to procaine hydrochloride (Novocain). What will you ask this patient and what are your options in treating a parturient with a documented ester allergy? How would you treat an anaphylactic reaction?

There are clearly problems related to the mixing of local anesthetics with additives, which might be overcome by more stable formulations. PPX derivatives have been popular for 30 years, and for the forseeable future, their position is secure.

Increasing internationalism will eventually bring about standardization of formulations, licensing, and units. Europe is likely to lead in this area because of its greater experience across borders.

References

1. De Jong RH: Local Anesthetics. St Louis: Mosby; 1994.
2. Lee JA, Atkinson RS, Watt MJ (eds): Lumbar Puncture and Spinal Analgesia, 5th ed. Edinburgh: Churchill Livingstone; 1985:8.
3. Wildsmith JAW: The history and development of local anaesthesia. *In* Wildsmith JAW, Armitage EN (eds): Principles and Practice of Regional Anaesthesia. Edinburgh: Churchill Livingstone; 1987:5.
4. Covino BG: Mechanism of impulse block. *In* McClure JH, Wildsmith JAW (eds): Conduction Blockade for Postoperative Analgesia. London, England: Edward Arnold; 1991:26–54.
5. McClure JH: Ropivacaine. Br J Anaesth 1996; 76:300–307.
6. Aberg G: Toxicological and local anaesthetic effects of optically active isomers of two local anaesthetic compounds. Acta Pharmacol Toxicol 1972; 31:273–286.
7. Lyons G, Columb MO, Wilson RC, et al: Epidural pain relief in labour: relative potencies of bupivacaine and levobupivacaine. Br J Anaesth 1998; 81:280P–281P.
8. Vanhoutte F, Vereecke J, Verbeke N, et al: Stereoselective effects of the enantiomers of bupivacaine on the electrophysiological properties of the guinea pig papillary muscle. Br J Pharmacol 1991; 103:1275–1281.
9. Olschewski A, Hempelmann G, Vogel W, et al: Blockade of Na^+ and K^+ currents by local anesthetics in the dorsal neurons of the spinal cord. Anesthesiology 1998; 88:172–179.
10. Sidebotham DA, Schug SA: Stereochemistry in anaesthesia. Clin Exp Pharmacol Physiol 1997; 24:126–130.
11. Wildsmith JAW, Brown DT, Paul D, et al: Structure-activity relationships in differential nerve block at high and low frequency stimulation. Br J Anaesth 1989; 63:444–452.
12. Hughes S: Chloroprocaine and obstetric anesthesia. *In* Gatt SP (ed): Hypertextbook of Regional Anaesthesia for Obstetrics—An International Perspective. Sydney: Pybus; 1996.
13. Sklar EML, Quencer RM, Green BA, et al: Complications of epidural anesthesia: MR appearances of abnormalities. Radiology 1991; 181:549–554.
14. Langerman L, Bansinath M, Grant GJ: The partition coefficient as a predictor of local anesthetic potency for spinal anesthesia: evaluation of five local anesthetics in a mouse model. Anesth Analg 1994; 79:490–495.
15. Langerman L, Golomb E, Grant G, et al: Duration of spinal anaesthesia is determined by the partition coefficient of local anaesthetic. Br J Anaesth 1994; 72:456–459.
16. Bonhomme L, Benhamou D, Martre H, et al: Chemical stability of bupivacaine and epinephrine in pH adjusted solutions. Anesthesiology 1987; 67:A279.
17. Morison DH: Alkalinisation of local anaesthetics. Can J Anaesth 1995; 42:1076–1079.
18. Capogna G, Celleno D, Laudano D, et al: Alkalinisation of local anesthetics: which block, which local anesthetic? Reg Anesth 1995; 20:369–377.
19. Gaggero G, Meyer O, Van Gessel E, et al: Alkalinisation of lidocaine 2% does not influence the quality of epidural anaesthesia for elective Caesarean section. Can J Anaesth 1995; 42:1080–1084.
20. Covino BG: Clinical pharmacology of local anesthetic agents. *In* Cousins MJ, Bridenbaugh PO (eds): Neural Blockade in Clinical Anesthesia and Management of Pain, 2nd ed. Philadelphia: JB Lippincott; 1988:119–120.
21. Miyoshi M, Imoto T, Hiji Y: Alkalinizing water soluble local anesthetic solutions by addition of cyclodextrin. Reg Anesth 1998; 23:176–181.
22. Moir DD, Slater PJ, Thorburn J, et al: Extradural analgesia in obstetrics: a controlled trial of carbonated lignocaine and bupivacaine hydrochloride with or without adrenaline. Br J Anaesth 1976; 48:129–134.
23. Mazoit JX, Cao LS, Samii K: Binding of bupivacaine to human serum proteins, isolated albumin and isolated alpha-1-acid glycoprotein: differences between the two enantiomers are partly due to cooperativity. J Pharmacol Exp Ther 1996; 276:109–115.
24. Johnson RF, Herman N, Arney TL, et al: Bupivacaine transfer across the human term placenta: a study using the dual perfused model. Anesthesiology 1995; 82:459–468.
25. Reynolds F: Principles of placental drug transfer: its measurement and interpretation. *In* Reynolds F (ed): Effects on the Baby of Maternal Analgesia and Anaesthesia. London: WB Saunders; 1993.
26. Johnson RF, Herman N, Johnson HV, et al: Effects of fetal pH on local anesthetic transfer across the placenta. Anesthesiology 1996; 85:608–615.
27. Rolbin SH, Cohen MM, Levinton CM, et al: The premature infant for cesarean delivery. Anesth Analg 1994; 78:912–917.
28. Downing JW, Johnson HV, Gonzalez HF, et al: The pharmacokinetics of epidural lidocaine and bupivacaine during cesarean section. Anesth Analg 1997; 84:527–532.
29. Santos AC: The effects of levobupivacaine, bupivacaine and ropivacaine on uterine blood flow [abstract]. Reg Anesth 1998; 23(suppl):45.
30. Emanuelsson B-MK, Persson J, Alm C, et al: Systemic

absorption and block after epidural injection of ropivacaine in healthy volunteers. Anesthesiology 1997; 87:1309–1317.
31. Reynolds F: Does the left hand know what the right is doing? An appraisal of single enantiomer local anesthetics. Int J Obstet Anesth 1997; 6:257–269.
32. Aps C, Reynolds F: An intradermal study of the local anesthetic and vascular effects of the isomers of bupivacaine. Br J Clin Pharmacol 1978; 6:63–68.
33. Kopacz DJ, Carpenter RL, Mackey DC: Effect of ropivacaine on cutaneous capillary blood flow in pigs. Anesthesiology 1989; 71:69–74.
34. Cederholm I, Akerman B, Evers H: Local analgesic and vascular effects of intradermal ropivacaine and bupivacaine in various concentrations with and without adrenaline in man. Acta Anaesthesiol Scand 1994; 38:322–327.
35. Ishiyama T, Dohi S, Iida H, et al: The effects of topical and intravenous ropivacaine on canine pial microcirculation. Anesth Analg 1997; 85:75–81.
36. Iida H, Watanabe Y, Dohi S, et al: Direct effects of ropivacaine and bupivacaine on spinal pial vessels in canine: assessment with closed spinal window technique. Anesthesiology 1997; 87:75–81.
37. Emanuelsson B-M, Zaric D, Nydahl P-A, et al: Pharmacokinetics of ropivacaine and bupivacaine during 21 hours of continuous epidural infusion in healthy male volunteers. Reg Anesth 1995; 81:1163–1168.
38. Faccenda KA, Morrison LMM: The pharmacokinetics of levobupivacaine and racemic bupivacaine following extradural administration [abstract]. Reg Anesth 1998; 23(suppl):52.
39. Rutten AJ, Mather LE, McClean CF: Cardiovascular effects and regional clearances of iv bupivacaine in sheep: enantiomeric analysis. Br J Anaesth 1991; 67:247–256.
40. Mather LE, Rutten AJ, Plummer JL: Pharmacokinetics of bupivacaine enantiomers in sheep: influence of dosage regimen and study design. J Pharmacokin Biopharmacokin 1994; 6:481–498.
41. Albright GA: Cardiac arrest following regional anesthesia with etidocaine or bupivacaine. Anesthesiology 1979; 51:286–287.
42. Heath M: Deaths after intravenous regional anaesthesia. BMJ 1982; 285:913–914.
43. Ferguson FR: Discussion on the neurological sequelae of spinal anaesthesia. Proc R Soc Med 1937; XXX:1020–1024.
44. Michels AM, Lyons G, Hopkins PM: Lignocaine test dose to detect intravenous injection. Anaesthesia 1995; 50:211–213.
45. Scott DB, Lee A, Fagan D, et al: Acute toxicity of ropivacaine compared with that of bupivacaine. Anesth Analg 1989; 69:563–569.
46. Santos AC, Richard AG, Wlody D, et al: Comparative systemic toxicity of ropivacaine and bupivacaine in nonpregnant and pregnant ewes. Anesthesiology 1995; 82:734–737.
47. Feldman HS, Arthur GR, Covino BG: Comparative systemic toxicity of convulsant and supraconvulsant doses of intravenous ropivacaine, bupivacaine and lidocaine, in the conscious dog. Anesth Analg 1998; 69:794–801.
48. Valenzuela C, Delpon E, Franqueza L, et al: Effects of ropivacaine on a potassium channel (hKv 1.5) cloned from human ventricle. Anesthesiology 1997; 86:718–728.
49. Harding DP, Collier PA, Huckle RM, et al: Comparison of the cardiotoxic effects of bupivacaine, levobupivacaine and ropivacaine: an in vitro study in guinea pigs and human cardiac muscle [abstract]. Reg Anesth 1998; 23S:6.
50. Sztark F, Malgat M, Dabadie P, et al: Comparison of the effects of bupivacaine and ropivacaine on heart cell mitochondrial bioenergetics. Anesthesiology 1998; 88:1340–1349.
51. Knudsen K, Suurkula MB, Blomberg S, et al: Central nervous and cardiovascular effects of iv infusions of ropivacaine, bupivacaine and placebo in volunteers. Br J Anaesth 1997; 78:507–514.
52. Luduena FP, Bogado EF, Tullar BF: Optical isomers of mepivacaine and bupivacaine. Arch Int Pharmacodyn 1972; 200:359–369.
53. Denson DD, Behbehani MM, Gregg RV: Enantiomer specific effects of an intravenously administered arrhythmogenic dose of bupivacaine on neurons of the nucleus tractus solitarius and the cardiovascular system in the anesthetized rat. Reg Anesth 1992; 17:311–316.
54. Mazoit JX, Boico O, Samii K: Myocardial uptake of bupivacaine. II. Pharmacokinetics and pharmacodynamics of bupivacaine enantiomers in the isolated perfused rabbit heart. Anesth Analg 1993; 77:477–482.
55. Graf BM, Bosnjak ME, Stowe DF: Stereospecific effect of bupivacaine isomers on atrioventricular conduction in the isolated perfused guinea pig heart. Anesthesiology 1997; 86:410–419.
56. Gristwood R, Bardsley H, Baker H, et al: Reduced cardiotoxicity of levobupivacaine compared with racemic bupivacaine (Marcaine): new clinical evidence. Exp Opin Invest Drugs 1994; 3:1209–1212.
57. Columb MO, Lyons G: Determination of the minimum local analgesic concentrations of epidural bupivacaine and lidocaine in labor. Anesth Analg 1995; 81:833–837.
58. Columb MO, Lyons G, Polley LS, et al: Minimum local analgesic concentration of bupivacaine in labor: a metanalysis. Presented at the 29th Annual Meeting of Society for Obstetic Anesthesia and Perinatology, April, Bermuda, 1997:125.
59. Columb MO, Lyons G, Polley LS: Minimum local analgesic concentration of bupivacaine in labor; factors. Presented at the 29th Annual Meeting of SOAP, 1997:124.
60. Capogna G, Celleno D, Fusco P, et al: Relative potencies of bupivacaine and ropivacaine for labour analgesia. Br J Anaesth 1999; 82:371–373.
61. Polley LS, Columb MO, Naughton NN, et al : Relative analgesic potencies of ropivacaine and bupivacaine for epidural analgesia in labor [abstract]. Anesth Analg 1998; 86:2S384.
62. Hirabayashi Y, Shimizu R, Saitoh K, et al: Acid-base state of cerebrospinal fluid during pregnancy and its effect on spread of spinal anaesthesia. Br J Anaesth 1996; 77:352–355.
63. Dietz FB, Jaffe RA: Pregnancy does not increase susceptibility to bupivacaine in spinal root axons. Anesthesiology 1997; 87:610–616.
64. Drasner K, Rigler ML, Sessler DI, et al : Cauda equina syndrome following intended epidural anesthesia. Anesthesiology 1992; 77:582–585.
65. Hampl KF, Schneider MC, Thorin D, et al: Hyperosmolarity does not contribute to transient radicular irritation after spinal anesthesia with hyperbaric 5% lidocaine. Reg Anesth 1995; 20:363–368.
66. Lambert LA, Lambert DH, Strichartz GR: Irreversible conduction block in isolated nerve by high concentrations of local anesthetics. Anesthesiology 1994; 80:1082–1093.
67. Kalichman MW: Physiologic mechanisms by which local anesthetics may cause injury to nerve and spinal cord. Reg Anesth 1993; 18:448–452.
68. Johnson MC, Uhl CB, Sachz JA, et al: Lidocaine more neurotoxic than bupivacaine with a different mechanism of cytoplasmic calcium elevation [abstract]. Reg Anesth 1998; 23:S30.
69. Bloom SL, McIntire DD, Kelly MA, et al: Lack of effect of walking on labor and delivery. N Engl J Med 1998; 339:76–79.
70. Murphy JD, Henderson K, Bowden MI: Bupivacaine versus bupivacaine plus fentanyl for epidural analgesia: effect on maternal satisfaction. BMJ 1991; 302:564–567.
71. Strichartz GR: Neural physiology and local anesthetic action. *In* Cousins MJ, Bridenbaugh PO (eds): Neural Blockade in Clinical Anesthesia and Management of Pain, 2nd ed. Philadelphia: JB Lippincott; 1988:36.
72. Fink BR: Towards the mathematization of spinal anesthesia. Reg Anesth 1992; 17:263–273.
73. Wildsmith JAW, Brown DT, Paul D, et al: Structure-activity relationships in differential nerve block at high and low frequency stimulation. Br J Anaesth 1989; 63:444–452.
74. Breen TW, Shapiro T, Glass B, et al: Epidural anesthesia for labor in an ambulatory parturient. Anesth Analg 1993; 77:919–924.
75. Capogna G, Celleno D, Lyons G, et al: Minimum local analgesic concentration of epidural bupivacaine increases with progression of labour. Br J Anaesth 1998; 80:11–13.
76. Jaffe RA, Rowe MA: Differential nerve block: direct measurements on individual myelinated and unmyelinated dorsal root axons. Anesthesiology 1996; 84:1455–1464.

77. Dietz FB, Jaffe RA: Bupivacaine preferentially blocks ventral root axons in rats. Anesthesiology 1997; 86:172–180.
78. Aitkenhead AR: The pattern of litigation against anaesthetists. Br J Anaesth 1994; 73:10–21.
79. Bourne TM: A survey of how British obstetric anaesthetists test regional anaesthesia before caesarean section. Anaesthesia 1997; 52:901–903.
80. Russell IF: Levels of anaesthesia and intraoperative pain at caesarean section under regional block. Int J Obstet Anesth 1995; 4:71–77.
81. Rocco AG, Raymond SA, Murray E, et al: Differential spread of blockade of touch, cold, and pinprick during spinal anesthesia. Anesth Analg 1985; 64:917–923.
82. Greene NM: Physiology of Spinal Anesthesia. London: Bailliere; 1958:8.
83. Liu S, Kopacz DJ, Carpenter RL: Quantitative assessment of differential sensory nerve block after lidocaine spinal anesthesia. Anesthesiology 1995; 82:60–63.
84. Tay B, Wallace MS, Irving G: Quantitative assessment of differential sensory blockade after lumbar epidural lidocaine. Anesth Analg 1997; 84:1071–1075.
85. Jaffe RA, Rowe MA: A comparison of the local anesthetic effects of meperidine, fentanyl, and sufentanil on dorsal root axons. Anesth Analg 1996; 83:776–781.
86. Wang GK, Quan C, Vladimirov M, et al: Quaternary ammonium derivative of lidocaine as a long acting local anesthetic. Anesthesiology 1995; 83:1293–1301.
87. Difazio CA: Adjuvant techniques to improve the success of regional anesthesia: mixtures. *In* Raj PP (ed): Clinical Practice of Regional Anesthesia. New York: Churchill Livingstone; 1991:154–160.
88. Cousins MJ, Bromage PR: Epidural neural blockade. *In* Cousins MJ, Bridenbaugh PO (eds): Neural Blockade in Clinical Anesthesia and Management of Pain, 2nd ed. Philadelphia: JB Lippincott; 1988:253–260.
89. Covino BG: General considerations, toxicity and complications of local anaesthesia. *In* Nimmo WS, Smith G (eds): Anaesthesia, Vol II. Oxford: Blackwell Scientific; 1989:1011–1033.
90. Columb MO, Lyons G, Naughton NN, et al: Determination of the minimum local analgesic concentration of epidural chloroprocaine in labor. Int J Obstet Anesth 1997; 6:39–42.
91. Santos AC: Local anesthetics. *In* Chestnut DH (ed): Obstetric Anesthesia: Principles and Practice. St Louis: CV Mosby; 1994:203.

7

Perinatal Pharmacology of Local Anesthetics and Opioids

❖ RUDOLF STIENSTRA, MD, PHD

❖ ANTON G. L. BURM, MSC, PHD

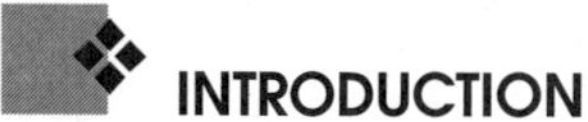

INTRODUCTION

In this chapter, the fetal and neonatal consequences of local anesthetics and opioids administered to the mother are discussed. For fetal transfer to occur, a drug given to the mother has to be transported to the placenta. Maternal pharmacokinetic principles governing the appearance and time profile of the maternal drug plasma concentration are described. The placenta is a unique interface between the maternal and fetal circulation. A brief description of the anatomy and physiology of the placenta is provided.

Placental transfer is the process by which a drug is transferred from mother to fetus as well as from fetus to mother. Factors affecting placental transfer are discussed in detail. The fetal circulation differs from the circulation after birth, and as a consequence, fetal pharmacokinetics are different. Fetal circulation is discussed together with other factors involving fetal pharmacokinetics, followed by a description of fetal pharmacodynamics. Finally, attention is given to the most frequently used local anesthetics and opioids.

Local anesthetics and opioids are frequently administered to women during labor and at cesarean section. Central neuraxis blockade, including epidural and spinal analgesia, is popular as a means of pain relief during labor and delivery because of its efficacy and safety for both mother and child. Most mothers, obstetricians, and anesthesiologists prefer regional to general anesthesia for cesarean section for a number of reasons. Regional anesthesia is efficient and safe. It avoids the necessity of a rapid-sequence induction and the possible hazards associated with endotracheal intubation in pregnant women at term. Regional anesthesia allows the mother to stay awake during the procedure and experience the birth of her child.

From a clinical point of view, the perinatal pharmacology of local anesthetics and opioids has two important features: first, the amount of drug ultimately present in the fetus at the time of birth and its pharmacodynamic consequences for the newborn; and second, fetal systemic toxicity as a result of sudden, unintended high fetal plasma levels. The amount of drug that accumulates in the fetus is determined by maternal pharmacokinetics, by placental transfer, and by fetal pharmacokinetics. Depending on its physicochemical characteristics, a drug present in the maternal circulation may reach the fetus by passing the placenta. Most anesthetic drugs easily cross the placenta by simple passive diffusion according to the concentration gradient for free, un-ionized drug. As long as the placental interface between mother and fetus is intact, fetal drug clearance may be achieved by placental transfer from fetus to mother once the maternal concentration of the drug has declined sufficiently and the direction of the concentration gradient of free, unionized drug reverses from fetus to mother. However, at birth the connection between mother and neonate is severed, and the newborn is on its own regarding the elimination of drugs.

ANATOMIC AND PHYSIOLOGIC CONSIDERATIONS

The placenta is a complex organ with a number of functions aimed at keeping an optimal relation between mother and fetus. It produces hormones to sustain pregnancy, it protects the fetus from the maternal immune system, and it allows for the active and passive transport of nutrients and metabolites in both directions.

The uterine and ovarian arteries anastomose, from which blood vessels penetrate into the myometrium of the uterus. These blood vessels form the arcuate arteries, from which the radial arteries originate and then divide into the spiral arteries. Trophoblast cells invade the myometrium of the uterus and the spiral arteries, destroying the tunica media containing muscle and elastic fibers.[1, 2] The destruction of the vessel wall of the spiral artery makes the placental circulation a low-resistance circuit devoid of the ability to maintain flow by vasodilatation. As a consequence, placental flow is directly dependent on the pressure in the supplying uterine and ovarian arteries.

The functional unit of the placenta is the cotyledon.[3] Human placenta contains 10 to 40 cotyledons,[3] divided by septa formed by cytotrophoblast and maternal decidual tissue. The maternal side is formed by the basal plate, and the fetal side originates from the chorionic plate. Through the chorionic plate the placental villi enter the cotyledon. Fetal blood enters the placenta through the umbilical arteries. These arteries divide into the chorionic arteries, from which vertical branches originate that enter the placental villi. These branches divide as they continue down the villi to form arterioles and capillaries. The capillaries fuse to form venules, which in turn fuse to form veins, which ultimately form the umbilical vein, returning blood to the fetus. Maternal blood from the spiral arteries enters the cotyledon through holes in the basal plate and circulates in the space between the placental villi, the intervillous space. By way of holes in the basal plate at the side of the cotyledon maternal blood leaves the cotyledon again, to return to venous plexuses in the basal decidua, from where it continues via the uterine veins to the inferior vena cava. Adjacent cotyledons are separated by septa originating from the basal plate and projecting toward, but never reaching, the chorionic plate; near the chorionic plate the intervillous spaces of adjacent cotyledons therefore communicate with each other, allowing maternal blood to go from one cotyledon to another.

In a simplified view, the cotyledon may be seen as a chamber. The walls rising from the floor do not reach completely to the roof, but leave an open space between the roof and the top of the walls. The villi hang from the roof like a giant tree with numerous branches filling the room. Fetal blood flows through blood vessels inside the villi. The space in the room between the tree branches is the intervillous space. Maternal blood sprays with a certain force upward into the chamber through a central hole in the floor, engulfing the fetal tree hanging down from the roof and leaving the chamber again via holes in the floor at the side of the chamber and spilling over the top of the walls into adjacent chambers. Exchange between maternal and fetal blood takes place in the cotyledon, the most important site being the terminal villi, where fetal and maternal blood are separated only by the basal lamina and a thin layer of syncytiotrophoblast cells.[4, 5]

MATERNAL PHARMACOKINETICS

A primary determinant of the fetal exposure to local anesthetics and opioids is the maternal drug serum or plasma concentration-time profile. This in turn is dependent on the pharmacokinetics of the agents in the mother. Since local anesthetics and opioids used in obstetric practice are often administered via the epidural or subarachnoid route, a consideration of the pharmacokinetics should include both the systemic absorption, that is, the uptake into the systemic circulation, and the systemic disposition, that is, the tissue distribution and elimination. A complicating factor in this consideration is that most local anesthetics, including bupivacaine (but not lidocaine and ropivacaine), are currently available as racemates, consisting of equal amounts of the S- and R-enantiomers, and there is increasing evidence that enantiomers have different pharmacokinetics.[6–8] However, most pharmacokinetic studies have been based on the measurement of mixed enantiomers. Furthermore, formal pharmacokinetic analyses, discriminating between systemic absorption and systemic disposition, have been conducted only in volunteers and surgical patients.[9–13] Therefore, the findings in these populations are described first.

Systemic Absorption

Systemic absorption of local anesthetics and opioids has two major implications. First, by decreasing the amount of drug that is available for the intended action, systemic absorption limits the duration of action and as such it is a primary determinant of the dose rate. Second, by giving rise to systemic blood concentrations, it may give rise to systemic effects. Consequently, opioids could cause a dual analgesic effect by affecting both spinal and supraspinal opioid receptors and may potentially cause systemic side effects, including respiratory depression. The systemic absorption of local anesthetics is of some concern, because of their central nervous system and cardiovascular toxicity.

Systemic absorption occurs by uptake of drug into blood vessels within the epidural and subarachnoid space and subsequent transfer to the systemic circulation via the azygos vein, which drains into the superior vena cava. Studies with lidocaine and bupivacaine have suggested that the uptake after subarachnoid administration occurs in part into epidural veins after transfer from the subarachnoid to the epidural space.[11] The primary factors influencing the systemic absorption rate are local perfusion and binding of drug to tissues at and near the site of administration.[14] These in turn are dependent on the physicochemical and vasoactive properties of the agents. Unfortunately, systemic absorption rates cannot be derived directly from the blood or plasma concentration-time profiles after epidural or subarachnoid injection, because systemic absorption, distribution to and from the tissues in the body, and elimination are overlapping processes. However, systemic absorption rates can be estimated using a stable-isotope method, which entails simultaneous administration of a regular local anesthetic or opioid via the epidural or subarachnoid route and a deuterium-labeled (nonradioactive) analogue via the intravenous route. This method has been used to examine the systemic absorption kinetics of lidocaine, ropivacaine, and bupivacaine after epidural administration.[10, 12] Although the study with bupivacaine was based on measurements of mixed enantiomers, the results are still interpretable, because a recent study suggested that the systemic absorption of this agent after epidural administration is not enantioselective.[8] The studies demonstrated that the systemic absorption of lidocaine, ropivacaine, and bupivacaine after epidural administration is biphasic, that is, a rapid initial absorption phase is followed by a much slower secondary absorption phase (Table 7–1). The rapid initial absorption rate is most likely caused by the high concentration gradient that exists between the drug in the injected solution and in the blood and may be enhanced by profound vasodilatation, as has been observed with epidural administration of bupivacaine, although not with ropivacaine.[15] It is also possible that bulk uptake of local anesthetic solution plays a role in this phase. The rapid initial absorption rate is responsible for peak drug concentrations. Initial absorption rates and the times at which peak concentrations are reached appear to be broadly comparable between the investigated local anesthetics. The secondary absorption phase is likely to be dependent on tissue-blood partitioning after the local anesthetic has been taken up into local tissues, in particular epidural fat. The secondary absorption rate varies considerably with the agent and appears to be related to the lipophilicity of the agent. The slower secondary absorption rate explains the longer duration of action of ropivacaine and bupivacaine compared with lidocaine.

Initial absorption rates after subarachnoid administration are considerably slower than those after epidural administration (Table 7–1). In fact, the slowing of the initial absorption rate is such that with lidocaine a biphasic absorption no longer exists. The slowing of the initial absorption rate after subarachnoid compared with epidural administration is most likely due to immediate dilution of the solution by cerebrospinal fluid and poorer perfusion of the subarachnoid space. Secondary absorption rates after subarachnoid administration are similar to those after epidural administration, which suggests that secondary absorption occurs from a common site, most likely from epidural fat, even after subarachnoid administration. Systemic absorption profiles of epidurally or subarachnoidally administered opioids have been poorly defined. One study examined the absorption of alfentanil after epidural administration to surgical patients and demonstrated a monophasic and relatively slow absorption in most patients (Table 7–1).[13] The lack of a rapid initial absorption phase with this agent is most likely related to its physicochemical properties. In contrast to local anesthetics and other opioids, alfentanil has a low pK_a and consequently exists mainly in the un-ionized form. This would be expected to promote rapid uptake into local tissues. Although absorption rates of other opioids have not been investigated, inspection of blood concentration-time profiles after epidural administration suggests a biphasic absorption pattern of both fentanyl and sufentanil, which would be in keeping with their physicochemical properties.

Systemic Disposition

When administered intravenously or after uptake into the systemic circulation after extravascular administration, local anesthetics and opioids are rapidly distributed to the body tissues. Agents that are currently used in obstetrics are generally lipophilic in nature and as such can readily cross biologic membranes, including the blood-brain barrier and the placenta. Consequently, tissue distribution is likely to be highly dependent on tissue perfusion, and distribution is likely to involve the total volume of body fluid. In addition, local anesthetics and opioids show significant, although widely varying, degrees of tissue binding. This may not be obvious when considering the volumes of distribution (Table 7–2). The reason is that local anesthetics and opioids bind to significant degrees to

Table 7–1 Systemic Absorption Kinetics of Lidocaine, Ropivacaine, Bupivacaine,* and Alfentanil After Epidural and Subarachnoid Administration in Surgical Patients

Parameter	Epidural Lidocaine	Epidural Bupivacaine	Epidural Ropivacaine	Epidural Alfentanil	Subarachnoid Lidocaine	Subarachnoid Bupivacaine
F_1	0.38	0.28	0.52	—	—	0.35
$t_{1/2a1}$ (h)	0.16	0.12	0.23	—	—	0.83
F_2	0.58	0.66	0.48	—	—	0.61
$t_{1/2a2}$ (h)	1.36	6.03	4.20	1.53	1.18	6.80
F (F_1 + F_2)	0.96	0.94	0.98	1.00	1.03	0.96

*Bupivacaine data are based on measurements of mixed enantiomers.

F_1 and F_2, fractions of the dose characterizing the fast and slow absorption phases; $t_{1/2a1}$ and $t_{1/2a2}$, half-lives characterizing the fast and slow absorption phases; F, estimated total fraction of the dose that is ultimately absorbed into the general circulation (values of F do not differ significantly from 1, indicating 100% systemic availability).

Data from references 10–13.

Table 7-2 Representative Pharmacokinetic Data, Characterizing the Disposition of Commonly Used Amide-Type Local Anesthetics and Opioids Following Intravenous Administration in Volunteers*

	V_{ss} (L)	Cl (L/min)	$t_{1/2}$ (h)
Local Anesthetics			
Lignocaine	76	0.80	1.6
Ropivacaine	42	0.50	1.9
S(−)-bupivacaine	54	0.32	2.6
R(+)-bupivacaine	84	0.40	3.5
Opioids			
Morphine	224	1.03	2.9
Meperidine	305	1.02	3.7
Fentanyl	257	0.96	3.7
Alfentanil	35	0.34	1.6
Sufentanil	196	1.20	3.1

*Except for sufentanil data, which are from healthy surgical patients.

V_{ss}, volume of distribution at steady state; Cl, total plasma clearance; $t_{1/2}$, terminal (elimination) half-life.

Data are specified with respect to plasma concentrations. Data for bupivacaine enantiomers were obtained after intravenous administration of the racemate.

Data from references 7, 16–22.

blood constituents, in particular proteins. A high degree of blood binding therefore masks extensive tissue binding. For example, the steady-state volume of distribution of ropivacaine, based on total plasma concentrations is approximately 40 L, whereas the corresponding volume based on unbound plasma concentrations exceeds 700 L, which is far in excess of the volume of body fluid.[17] With bupivacaine the tissue distribution appears to be enantioselective: The volume of distribution of the R-enantiomer exceeds that of the S-enantiomer by approximately 50%. This can be largely explained by the difference in the degree of protein binding of the enantiomers. Volumes of distribution, based on unbound plasma concentrations, are about 1500 L for both enantiomers, again reflecting a high degree of tissue binding, which does not appear to be enantioselective.[7]

Local anesthetics and opioids are mainly removed from the body by biotransformation. In adults renal excretion of unchanged drug accounts for only small fractions of the administered doses. Ester-type local anesthetics undergo very rapid hydrolysis by plasma cholinesterases and red cell esterases in the blood, in addition to esterases in the liver. However, ester-type agents are not routinely used in obstetrics today and therefore are not considered in detail here. Biotransformation of the amide-type local anesthetics and the opioids occurs predominantly in the liver. Clearance rates of lidocaine, morphine, meperidine, fentanyl, and sufentanil are relatively high (Table 7–2). The clearance of these agents is likely to be highly dependent on hepatic blood flow. Clearance rates of ropivacaine, bupivacaine, and alfentanil are lower. With these agents the clearance is more likely to be primarily dependent on the intrinsic activity of the enzymes involved in the biotransformation and the degree of plasma protein binding. With bupivacaine total plasma clearance is enantioselective, being higher for the R-enantiomer than for the S-enantiomer. This again can be largely explained by differences in the degree of plasma protein binding of the enantiomers. Half-lives vary from 1.6 to 3.5 hours with local anesthetics and from 1.6 to 3.7 hours with opioids (Table 7–2). These figures apply after intravenous administration. Half-lives after epidural or subarachnoid administration may be considerably prolonged, as has been demonstrated with bupivacaine. The reason for this prolongation is that the systemic absorption rate is much slower than the elimination rate observed after intravenous administration, so that after epidural or subarachnoid administration the systemic absorption rate limits elimination of drug from the body.

Influence of Pregnancy

The pharmacokinetic considerations just described are based on studies in healthy volunteers or surgical patients. Although the general principles also apply to pregnant women, the pharmacokinetics in these subjects could be altered. For example, engorgement of vertebral veins and the hyperdynamic circulation might be expected to enhance the systemic absorption of epidurally administered local anesthetics and opioids. This could explain why peak plasma concentrations of meperidine after epidural administration are higher in pregnant women than in nonpregnant women.[23] However, a study comparing serum concentrations of bupivacaine following epidural administration of this agent to nonpregnant women and pregnant women at term showed grossly similar serum concentration-time profiles, with peak concentrations reached at approximately the same times after injection and comparable half-lives.[24]

Cardiovascular changes and changes in plasma protein binding and in enzyme activities may affect the distribution and elimination of local anesthetics and opioids. Plasma cholinesterase activity is markedly decreased in pregnant women at term, but it is still sufficient to effectively hydrolyze chloroprocaine.[25] Plasma concentrations of α_1-acid glycoprotein, which plays an important role in the binding of local anesthetics and opioids, are decreased in pregnant women with about a 30% reduction at term.[26, 27] Consequently, the degree of protein binding may be decreased and this may be expected to result in larger volumes of distribution and a higher clearance of drugs with a small hepatic extraction ratio, such as bupivacaine and alfentanil. However, the clearance of bupivacaine in pregnant women at term tends to be somewhat depressed.[24] This can be best explained in terms of hepatic enzyme inhibition.

Studies in animals demonstrated that pregnancy is associated with an increased volume of distribution and an increased clearance of lidocaine, but with an unaltered or decreased volume of distribution and a decreased clearance of ropivacaine.[28, 29] The contradictory findings with respect to the changes in the volumes of distribution could not be explained readily, but may be related to alterations in cardiovascular profiles and to changes in protein binding and tissue binding during pregnancy. The apparently contradictory findings with respect to the clearance rate of lidocaine and ropivacaine can be explained by considering the factors that influence the clearance of these agents. Thus, the clearance of lidocaine, which has a large hepatic extraction ratio, would be predicted to be highly dependent on liver blood flow, which may be enhanced during pregnancy. In contrast, the clearance of ropivacaine, which has a lower hepatic extraction ratio, is more likely to depend on hepatic enzyme activity, which may be inhibited in pregnancy.

It is difficult, however, to extrapolate the findings from animal studies to humans. For example, whereas the clearance rate of lidocaine in pregnant ewes is markedly increased, the clearance rate of lidocaine in pregnant women appears to be little affected.[30] Studies comparing the pharmacokinetics of meperidine and alfentanil in pregnant and nonpregnant women showed that pregnancy did not affect the volumes of distribution, clearances, or half-lives of these agents.[31, 32]

Plasma Levels of Local Anesthetics and Opioids

Within the clinically used dose range, concentrations of local anesthetics and opioids are likely to be proportional to the administered dose. Following single epidural injections the rapid initial absorption of epidurally administered local anesthetics and most opioids is reflected in a rapid rise of the blood concentrations. Peak blood concentrations of lidocaine, bupivacaine, and ropivacaine are generally reached after 10 to 30 minutes and are roughly 1 μg/mL per 100-mg dose for lidocaine and half as much for bupivacaine and ropivacaine.[14] Peak concentrations in venous blood are reached later and are generally lower than those in arterial blood. Corresponding plasma concentrations are generally higher as a result of plasma protein binding.

Blood or plasma concentration-time data of the opioids after epidural administration are relatively scarce. A study in volunteers examined venous plasma concentrations after epidural administration of two consecutive bolus doses of fentanyl (30 μg and 100 μg), alfentanil (300 μg and 1000 μg), and sufentanil (3 μg and 10 μg).[33] The mean peak plasma concentration after the first and second bolus doses of fentanyl were 0.19 ng/mL and 0.36 ng/mL, respectively, and were reached after approximately 15 minutes, on average. With alfentanil the mean peak concentration after the first bolus dose was 5.4 ng/mL and was reached in 60 minutes whereas the mean peak concentration after the second bolus dose was 26.1 ng/mL and was reached after 15 minutes. Sufentanil concentrations after the first bolus dose were undetectable in many cases and mean peak concentrations after the second bolus dose were 0.035 ng/mL and were reached in approximately 5 minutes. The concentrations measured after the second, larger, bolus doses of all three agents approached the minimum effective analgesic concentration (MEAC). The mean peak plasma concentration after epidural administration of fentanyl (100 μg) to patients recovering from abdominal aortic surgery was 0.29 ng/mL and was reached after 16 minutes.[34] This is in keeping with the aforementioned observations in volunteers. However, peak plasma concentrations during the first stage of labor in pregnant patients given an 80-μg epidural bolus dose of fentanyl in combination with 0.3% bupivacaine were as high as 1.01 ng/mL, on average, and were reached in 5 to 20 minutes.[35] These concentrations were higher than those after intramuscular administration in the same study and exceed the MEAC. Similar observations have been reported for meperidine (dose 100 mg) in pregnant patients with a mean peak plasma concentration of approximately 650 ng/mL, which was reached in about 10 minutes.[30] However, in another study smaller doses of meperidine were associated with plasma concentrations that were below the MEAC, but still epidural meperidine was effective in relieving labor pain in most patients.[36]

Plasma concentrations after subarachnoid administration of local anesthetics increase much slower than after epidural administration, reflecting a slower absorption from the subarachnoid space.[11] Because of this and because of the low subarachnoid dose requirements, the plasma concentrations reached are of little concern. Plasma concentrations of morphine and meperidine after subarachnoid injection of 3-mg and 10-mg doses were very low (mean 4.5 and 36 ng/mL, respectively) and were reached in 5 to 10 minutes.[37] In contrast, the mean peak plasma concentration of sufentanil after subarachnoid administration of a 15-μg bolus dose (0.15 ng/mL) was reached after approximately 40 minutes.[38] In another study, however, the mean peak plasma concentration (0.54 ng/mL) after a subarachnoid dose of sufentanil was reached in 6.6 minutes on average.[39] This suggests a very rapid uptake of sufentanil from the subarachnoid space, which may be related to the high dose (150 μg) given in this study. However, plasma concentrations during the first hour after subarachnoid injection were lower than those after epidural administration of the same dose, whereas after 1 hour they were higher after subarachnoid administration, suggesting a slower initial absorption from the subarachnoid space.

Repeated epidural injections or continuous epidural infusion of local anesthetics result in either systemic or local accumulation. Systemic accumulation is likely to be more pronounced with lidocaine than with bupivacaine or ropivacaine, whereas the reverse is likely to be the case for local accumulation, even though dosing intervals are longer with bupivacaine and ropivacaine than with lidocaine.[14] Plasma concentrations of local anesthetics measured on repeated epidural administration appear to correspond closely to those predicted on the basis of pharmacokinetic data obtained after single injections.[40] During continuous epidural infusion one would predict a slower initial rise of the plasma concentrations compared with intravenous infusion, but ultimately concentrations should reach a steady state, similar to that during intravenous infusion, provided that epidural administration does not affect the systemic disposition. In keeping with this, continuous epidural infusion of fentanyl (100 μg/h) given to patients after knee surgery resulted in plasma concentrations of 1.7 ± 0.4 ng/mL after 18 hours, which was similar to that produced by an intravenous infusion of fentanyl at the same rate (1.8 ± 0.4 ng/mL).[41] Plasma concentrations in pregnant women, receiving an epidural bolus dose of 30 μg/kg of alfentanil followed by an epidural infusion of 30 μg/kg/h for normal vaginal delivery, were 21 to 48 ng/mL at the time of birth.[32]

Inadvertent intravenous injections of epidural doses of local anesthetics are commonly feared because this is the most common cause of toxicity. Although epidural doses used in obstetrics are smaller than those used in surgical patients, accidental injection of a full epidural dose is a serious threat to both the mother and fetus. In such event it is therefore advisable to proceed with delivery as soon as possible. Alternatively, there is a theoretic advantage in delaying delivery until significant back transfer from fetus to mother has occurred.[14] The same considerations may apply in the event of accidental intravenous injections of opioids. The enhanced plasma concentrations are likely to produce effective analgesia but also cause profound respiratory depression in the mother and newborn.

PLACENTAL TRANSFER

Most anesthetic drugs and gases are transferred across the placenta by simple passive diffusion determined by a concentration gradient of free, un-ionized drug. Given a concentration gradient, the flux is directly related to the surface area available for diffusion and inversely related to the thickness of the surface through which diffusion takes place. Other factors unique to a specific drug, such as molecular weight, molecular shape, and lipid solubility affect the rate of diffusion as well. The relationship between these factors is known as Fick's law and described by the following equation:

$$Q/t = K \cdot A \cdot ([M] - [F])/D$$

where Q/t is flux, K is a diffusion constant specific for a given drug, A is the surface area available for diffusion, [M] is the concentration of free, un-ionized drug at the maternal side of the placenta, [F] is the concentration of free, un-ionized drug at the fetal side of the placenta, and D is the thickness of the surface through which diffusion takes place.

Lipophilic drugs transfer more easily than hydrophilic drugs and permeability of the placenta is inversely related to molecular weight: For lipophilic drugs, the limit is a molecular weight of ± 600 Da, whereas for hydrophilic drugs the limit is ± 100 Da.[42]

Obviously, in order to be transferred from mother to fetus, a given drug has to reach the placenta first. Consequently, the route of administration to the mother, absorption from the site of administration, distribution, elimination from maternal plasma, and the percentage of maternal cardiac output directed to the placenta are key factors in determining the amount of drug that is transferred to the fetus. Likewise, fetal factors such as cardiac output, uptake of drug by fetal tissues, and the amount of free, un-ionized drug at the fetal side of the placental barrier affect redistribution of the drug from fetus to mother. Thus, the amount of drug that is ultimately present in the neonate at the time of delivery depends on many maternal and fetal variables.

In the human fetus, a concentration-time profile of a drug given to the mother cannot be obtained easily; although blood may be sampled from the fetal scalp, almost all estimates regarding placental transfer of local anesthetics and opioids in in vivo studies have been based on single measurements of the concentrations of drug in arterial and venous umbilical cord blood samples and maternal samples, taken simultaneously at birth. By dividing the umbilical vein (UV) concentration by the maternal vein (MV) concentration, the UV/MV ratio, a rough estimate of placental transfer, is obtained. However, the UV/MV ratio may vary as a result of a number of factors, such as maternal and fetal pH differences, differences in fetal and maternal protein binding, vascular shunts on either side of the placenta, and sampling before equilibrium between maternal and fetal tissues has been reached.[43] Even in case of rapid equilibration between maternal and fetal blood, the fetal concentration lags behind the maternal concentration. Depending on the time at which the samples are taken relative to the time, route, and duration of administration of drug to the mother, the UV/MV ratio may yield falsely high or low values for placental transfer.[44] Similarly, in case of continuous administration of a local anesthetic or opioid to the mother, as for instance in continuous epidural analgesia, the UV/MV ratio would vary with time until maternal plasma levels have stabilized and equilibrium between maternal and fetal tissues has been established.

In animal and human cotyledon perfusion models placental transfer may be expressed as placental clearance:

$$Clx = UF \cdot ([Fv] - [Fa])/[M]$$

where Clx is the placental clearance of drug X, UF is umbilical flow, and [Fv], [Fa], and [M] are the concentrations of drug X in the umbilical vein, umbilical artery, and maternal arterial blood, respectively. Although this method of expressing placental transfer is far more accurate than the UV/MV ratio, it is obviously much more laborious and presently not suitable for human in vivo studies.

Because only free, un-ionized drug is capable of diffusion, the degree of protein binding and the degree of ionization are important factors. The effects of protein binding on placental transfer are complex. At first glance, it would seem that protein binding inhibits placental transfer by lowering the fraction of free, unionized drug. The UV/MV ratio for lidocaine reported in the literature averages 0.58 with a range of 0.2 to 1.0, whereas the UV/MV ratio for bupivacaine, which has higher protein binding than lidocaine, averages 0.29 with a range of 0.15 to 0.86.[43] In a rabbit placenta model comparing placental transfer of lidocaine, bupivacaine, and pethidine, bupivacaine had the highest protein binding and the lowest transfer rate.[45] Tucker, on the other hand, has suggested that protein binding does not notably impair placental transfer, because protein-bound drugs dissociate from protein virtually immediately.[46]

Studies in the dual-perfused, human cotyledon model[47] have shown that increasing maternal protein binding capacity reduces placental transfer of bupivacaine[48, 49] and the highly protein-bound sufentanil,[50] but not lidocaine.[49] These studies indicate that protein binding has an inhibitory effect on placental transfer. Free, un-ionized drug is in equilibrium with free, ionized drug, which in turn is in equilibrium with protein-bound drug. The protein binding capacity of fetal or neonatal plasma is reduced compared with adult plasma,[51–53] owing to decreased levels of α_1-acid glycoprotein in the fetus and newborn.[54, 55] Since only free, un-ionized drug is available for transplacental equilibration, a reduced protein binding capacity at the fetal side of the placenta leads to a lower total (free plus protein-bound) drug concentration compared with the maternal side, and this would explain the inverse relation between protein binding of a drug and the UV/MV ratio.

It thus seems that the effects of protein binding on placental transfer are twofold: Protein binding itself has an impeding effect on placental transfer, and owing to a decreased protein binding capacity of fetal plasma, highly protein-bound drugs have a lower UV/MV ratio. The degree of ionization is an important determinant of placental transfer. As mentioned earlier, only the free, un-ionized drug rapidly crosses the placenta, equilibrating between maternal and fetal plasma. The degree of ionization of a drug is determined by its pK_a and by pH. The pK_a of a drug represents the pH at which 50% of the drug is ionized and 50% is un-ionized. For a base, the fraction of ionized to un-ionized drug is given by the Henderson-Hasselbalch equation:

$$pK_a = pH + \log([\text{cation}]/[\text{base}])$$

where [cation] and [base] represent the concentrations of ionized and un-ionized drug. This formula can be written as:

$$\log([\text{base}]/[\text{cation}]) = pH - pK_a$$

From this formula, the fraction of un-ionized drug can be calculated as:

$$Fn = 10^{pH - pKa} / (1 + 10^{pH - pKa})$$

where Fn represents the fraction of un-ionized drug.

Most opioids and all local anesthetics are weak bases, with pK_a ranging from 7.7 to 8.9. The lower the pK_a, the weaker the base, and the higher the percentage of un-ionized drug at the physiologic pH of 7.4. Thus, lidocaine has a pK_a of 7.9 and bupivacaine has a pK_a of 8.1. This means that at a pH of 7.4, a greater fraction of lidocaine is in the un-ionized form and available for placental transfer. Apart from other factors, the fraction of un-ionized drug corresponds directly with placental transfer. Because the pK_a of local anesthetics and opioids is inversely related to the un-ionized fraction at a physiologic pH of 7.4, the pK_a is inversely related to placental transfer. Table 7–3 shows the pK_a values and the ionized percentages of commonly used local anesthetics and opioids.

Differences in pH cause differences in the ionized to un-ionized ratio. In the case of local anesthetics and opioids, a decrease in pH results in an increase of the ionized portion. This is important, since the pH in fetal blood tends to be lower than maternal pH. Consequently, at the fetal side of the placental barrier a weak base has a larger ionized to un-ionized ratio as compared with the maternal side. Normal fetal pH ranges from 7.30 to 7.35. As long as the difference between maternal and fetal pH remains small, the

Table 7–3 Physicochemical Properties of Commonly Used Local Anesthetics and Opioids

Agent	Molecular Weight	pK_a	% Ionized at pH 7.4	Partition Coefficient*	Serum Protein Binding (%)
Local Anesthetics					
Chloroprocaine	271	9.30	99	9	—
Lidocaine	234	8.19	86	43	70
Ropivacaine	262	8.16	85	115	95
Bupivacaine	288	8.21	87	346	95 (96/93)†
Opioids					
Morphine	285	7.90	76	1	35
Meperidine	253	8.70	95	21	70
Fentanyl	336	8.43	91	955	84
Alfentanil	417	6.50	11	129	92
Sufentanil	387	8.01	80	1748	93

*Octanol/buffer or octanol/water (pH = 7.4).
†Plasma protein binding of individual enantiomers (S-enantiomer/R-enantiomer).
Data from references 7, 56–60.

slightly higher ionized-un-ionized ratio of weak bases in the fetus has no clinical consequences. However, if fetal acidosis develops and the gap between maternal and fetal pH widens, progressively more drug is in the ionized form in fetal blood. Because only un-ionized drug is capable of passive diffusion, a higher fraction of ionized drug at the fetal side of the placenta may result in "trapping" of the local anesthetic, causing an increased fetal-maternal total drug ratio. An elevated fetal-maternal concentration of lidocaine and mepivacaine has been reported in acidotic newborns, and it has been suggested that ion trapping caused this.[61] Subsequent studies using animal models demonstrated that fetal acidosis increases the fetal-maternal ratio of lidocaine,[62] bupivacaine,[63, 64] and meperidine.[64] Studies in human placenta models confirmed that an increase in the maternal to fetal pH difference results in an increased fetal-maternal ratio of lidocaine, 2-chloroprocaine,[49] bupivacaine,[48, 49] and sufentanil.[50, 65] Whereas the phenomenon of ion trapping in itself explains the increase in the fetal-maternal drug ratio, the latter studies using human placenta perfusion models clearly demonstrated that a widening in the maternal to fetal pH difference also resulted in an increased placental transfer. Thus, fetal acidosis results in an increase in the fetal-maternal drug ratio of local anesthetics and the commonly used opioids, partly by the mechanism of ion trapping, partly by an increase in placental transfer.

FETAL PHARMACOKINETICS

Drugs administered to the mother enter the fetal circulation via the placenta. The fetal circulation is shown in Figure 7–1. The umbilical vein carries blood away from the placenta to the systemic fetal circulation. A large portion of the umbilical venous blood passes first through the liver; a smaller portion enters the inferior vena cava through the ductus venosus, where the umbilical venous blood is mixed with venous blood from the lower limbs and viscera. The inferior vena cava enters the right atrium together with the superior vena cava. For the most part, blood from the right atrium enters the left atrium through the oval foramen. A small portion of the blood in the right atrium enters the truncus pulmonalis via the right ventricle, but because the pulmonary vascular resistance is very high ante partum, this blood flows predominantly to the aorta descendens via the ductus arteriosus Botalli. Blood from the left atrium enters the aorta via the left ventricle. From the aorta, blood is supplied to the brain and other fetal tissues. Finally, the umbilical arteries originating from the abdominal aorta carry blood to the placenta.

Fetal distribution and absorption of drugs transferred via the placenta result from typical features of the fetal circulation. A large portion of the umbilical venous blood passes through the liver, where drug may be absorbed by liver cells. The fetal heart is the next organ receiving umbilical vein blood with a relatively high concentration of drug. A large portion of the output of the left ventricle goes to the fetal brain. Absorption of drug by fetal brain tissue is comparable with placental transfer: Passing the blood-brain barrier is largely determined by lipid solubility and the fraction of free, un-ionized drug. The blood-brain barrier in the fetus is not yet fully developed and consequently has an increased permeability,[66] probably allowing for increased transfer of local anesthetics and opioids as compared with adults. As a consequence, fetal liver, heart, and brain are the main organs that are relatively overexposed to drugs that enter the fetal circulation by placental transfer.

Fetal excretion is accomplished largely by reversed placental transfer and by renal excretion, reversed placental transfer being the predominant mechanism. The placenta receives a large portion of the fetal cardiac output, allowing for a large volume of fetal blood flowing through the placenta per minute. When maternal plasma drug concentrations decrease in accordance with maternal drug elimination, reversed transfer from the fetus to the mother becomes enhanced. As long as there is no asphyxia and fetal cardiac output remains adequate, fetal plasma drug levels continuously equilibrate with maternal plasma levels via placental exchange of free, un-ionized drug. If maternal plasma levels remain within the therapeutic range, the occurrence of high, toxic plasma levels in the fetus is extremely unlikely.

In cases of fetal asphyxia, increased accumulation of local anesthetics and opioids in fetal tissues may result by several mechanisms. Asphyxia causes changes in the fetal circulation, resulting in redistribution in favor of the heart, the brain, and the placenta.[67] As discussed previously, acidosis increases placental transfer of local anesthetics and opioids. Acidosis decreases protein binding,[68, 69] thereby increasing the free fraction of drug. Hypercapnia results in an increase in cerebral blood flow and an increase in permeability of the blood-brain barrier. The overall consequence of these changes is an increased amount of drug available for uptake in the fetal brain and heart. Indeed, animal experiments have shown that the uptake of lidocaine by fetal heart, brain, and liver is increased by asphyxia[70–72] and that the signs of local anesthetic toxicity in asphyxiated animals develop at lower plasma concentrations when compared with nonasphyxiated animals.

While the placental connection is intact, transfer from fetus to mother is the predominant mechanism of drug elimination. However, once the neonate is on its own, other mechanisms come into play. Fetal and neonatal elimination half-lives of local anesthetics and opioids are prolonged compared with adults. This may be partly explained by the immaturity of some hepatic enzyme systems in the fetus and newborn involved in the biotransformation of local anesthetics and opioids, partly by a larger volume of distribution. For instance, the elimination half-life of mepivacaine in the neonate is prolonged approximately five times, at least partly because of immaturity of the hepatic ring hydroxylation enzyme system.[73, 74] On the other hand, biotransformation of lidocaine and bupivacaine occurs by dealkylation in the liver at approximately the same rate as

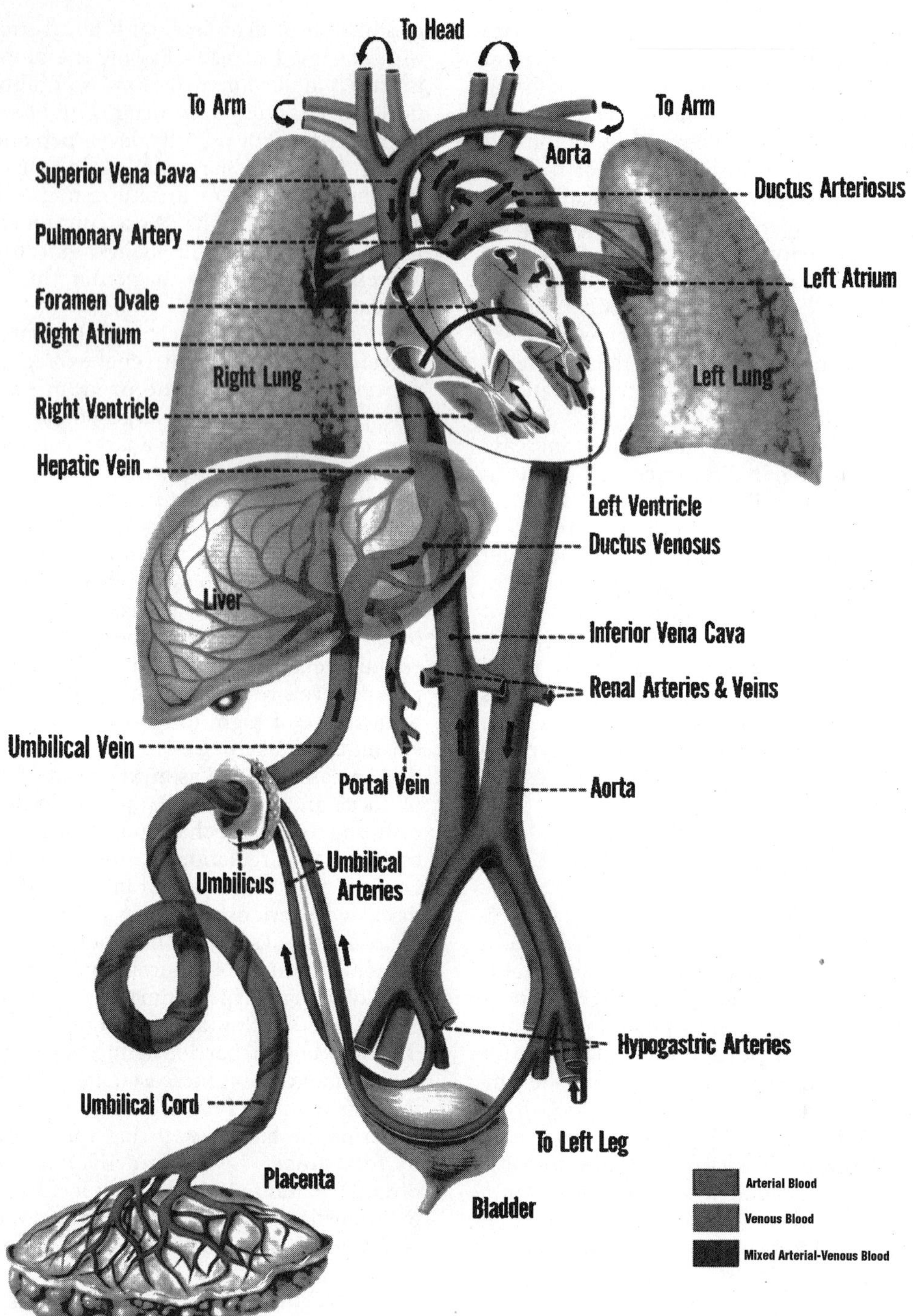

Figure 7–1 Fetal circulation. Arrows indicate the course of blood. (From Bissonnette JM: Placental transfer of anesthetics and related drugs and effects. *In* Bonica JJ, McDonald JS (eds): Principles and Practice of Obstetric Analgesia and Anesthesia, 2nd ed. Baltimore: Williams & Wilkins; 1995:233.)

in the adult, indicating that the prolonged elimination half-life of these drugs in the fetus and neonate is caused mainly by the larger volume of distribution.[74] 2-Chloroprocaine is rapidly metabolized by plasma cholinesterases, but small fractions may be transferred to the fetus[25]; although the elimination half-life in the fetus and neonate is prolonged, metabolization still occurs within 1 minute and accumulation is less likely to occur.[74, 75]

Renal excretion is an important pathway for drug elimination in the neonate. Because tubular reabsorption is decreased, 20% of an administered lidocaine dose is excreted unchanged in the urine as compared with 3% to 5% in the adult.[74] Renal excretion of unchanged bupivacaine has also been shown to be higher in neonates as compared with their mothers.[76]

PHARMACODYNAMIC CONSEQUENCES

Local anesthetics and opioids given to the mother during labor and delivery or for cesarean section are present in the neonate. Neonatal assessment by the Early Neonatal Neurobehavioral Scale (ENNS),[79] the Brazelton Neonatal Behavioral Assessment Scale (BNBAS),[77] or the Neurologic and Adaptive Capacity Score (NACS)[78] may reveal subtle changes as the result of local anesthetic effects present in the newborn. The use of epidural lidocaine was reported to be associated with decreased muscle tone in the neonate, described as "floppy but alert,"[79] but later studies failed to confirm this.[80–85] In recent years, the doses used for epidural analgesia have gradually decreased, and there is now general consensus that within the dose range presently en vogue and under normal circumstances the effects of the local anesthetic on the neonate have little or no clinical significance.

Opioids, whether given intravenously or epidurally, rapidly cross the placenta and may cause neonatal depression, manifesting itself as respiratory depression, hypotonia, poor primary reflexes, and poor adjustment to repeated stimuli. Traditionally, the use of intravenous or intramuscular meperidine (pethidine) for maternal pain relief has been very popular in the obstetric community, probably on the unproven assumption that meperidine causes less respiratory depression than morphine. Meperidine causes neonatal depression, the effects being maximal when delivery is 2 to 3 hours after intramuscular administration to the mother.[86] Despite the advent of newer opioids, the use of meperidine is still widespread. Nevertheless, the last decade has shown a sharp increase in the use of regional techniques for obstetric analgesia. In most institutions, analgesia for labor and delivery pain is frequently obtained by epidural or combined spinal-epidural analgesia. Central neuraxis blockade is obtained either by local anesthetic alone or by a combination of local anesthetic and opioid, the lipophilic opioids fentanyl and sufentanil being the most widely used. Because the dosage of opioid in these regimens is reduced, the likelihood of opioid-induced neonatal depression is minimal. Systemic local anesthetic toxicity in the fetus follows the same pattern as in the adult. Central nervous system and/or cardiotoxic manifestations may result from sudden, high plasma levels of drug. Inadvertent intravenous injection of a large dose of local anesthetic in the mother causes a high plasma level and concomitant massive placental transfer. In the past, perinatal deaths have been associated with accidental fetal injection of local anesthetic during attempted paracervical block.[43] As in the adult, the fetus may suffer from convulsions and cardiovascular depression. As long as the placental interface is intact and fetal cardiac output remains adequate, the fetal plasma concentration follows the maternal drug concentration-time profile and declines fairly rapidly. If fetal circulatory collapse occurs, the fetus may sustain severe damage or fetal death may ensue.

The sensitivity of the fetus and newborn for local anesthetic toxicity is probably similar to that of adults. In sheep, the plasma concentrations associated with systemic toxicity in fetal, newborn, and adult animals are comparable.[87–89] It has been reported that convulsions as a result of inadvertent fetal injection of mepivacaine during attempted maternal caudal anesthesia stopped as soon as the plasma concentration of mepivacaine fell below the threshold level for convulsions, as seen in the adult.[90]

It would thus seem that the effects of local anesthetics on the fetus and newborn are minimal, provided toxic plasma levels in the mother are avoided; as outlined earlier, fetal acidosis may enhance accumulation of local anesthetic in the fetus and decrease the plasma concentration at which systemic toxicity occurs.

LOCAL ANESTHETICS

2-Chloroprocaine. From a pharmacokinetic point of view, 2-chloroprocaine would be the next to ideal local anesthetic for use in obstetrics. In maternal plasma, it is rapidly hydrolyzed by plasma cholinesterases, limiting the amount of drug available for placental transfer. Although transfer does occur and fetal metabolism of 2-chloroprocaine is prolonged, it is still rapid and consequently fetal accumulation of the drug virtually does not occur. In the 1980s, the use of 2-chloroprocaine was associated with possible neurotoxicity.[91–94] The neurotoxic effects have been attributed to a low pH and the preservative sodium bisulfite.[95] Currently available formulations of 2-chloroprocaine do not contain these preservatives.

Lidocaine. The use of lidocaine in obstetric anesthesia was challenged by a study indicating adverse neurologic effects in the newborn,[79] but this finding was not substantiated in numerous later studies.[80–85] UV/MV ratios reported in the literature average approximately 0.4 to 0.6,[85, 96–99] the variation being caused by factors outlined previously and by differences in methodology. Nevertheless, the UV/MV ratio for lidocaine is consistently higher than that for bupivacaine, partly because of its lower protein binding and partly because of a lower pK_a and hence a higher placental transfer. This has been confirmed in studies comparing lidocaine and bupivacaine transfer using human placenta.[49, 100]

Bupivacaine. Bupivacaine is presently the most widely used local anesthetic in obstetric anesthesia and analgesia. UV/MV ratios average approximately 0.25 to 0.30 in single-dose studies[76, 101, 102] and 0.30 to 0.50 in continuous infusion studies.[85, 103–107] There is evidence that bupivacaine is absorbed by placental tissue,[48, 100] reducing fetal exposure. Although the placental transfer of bupivacaine is less than that of lidocaine, the amount of drug that will ultimately be present in the neonate is also affected by the duration of placental exposure. Given enough time, a steady state will ensue, and fetal tissues become saturated. The fact that neonates may excrete bupivacaine in their urine for 3 days after delivery[76] indicates that fetal tissues may absorb a substantial amount of bupivacaine, despite a low UV/MV ratio.

Ropivacaine. Ropivacaine is a new local anesthetic, structurally closely related to bupivacaine. In in vitro[108, 109] and clinical[110–114] studies, ropivacaine displays a greater separation between sensory and motor blockade than bupivacaine. Moreover, ropivacaine has a lower cardiovascular and central nervous system toxicity compared with bupivacaine.[115] In ewes, pregnancy enhances the toxicity of bupivacaine[116] but not of ropivacaine.[117] This profile makes ropivacaine an attractive alternative for bupivacaine, especially in obstetrics.

The UV/MV ratios for ropivacaine and bupivacaine have been determined in a study comparing both drugs for cesarean section.[118] The ratio of free, unbound drug at the time of delivery was 0.72 for ropivacaine and 0.69 for bupivacaine. In accordance with the lower lipid solubility and lesser degree of protein binding of ropivacaine, the concentration of free, unbound ropivacaine was about twice that of bupivacaine in both maternal and umbilical blood, but the concentrations were far below those associated with systemic toxicity. A meta-analysis comprising six labor studies comparing ropivacaine and bupivacaine showed marginally but significantly better NACS 24 hours post partum for the neonates whose mothers had received ropivacaine.[119]

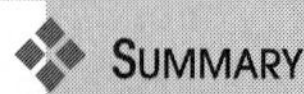

Summary

Key Points

- Only free, un-ionized drug is capable of diffusion. Protein binding has an inhibitory effect on placental transfer.
- With the exception of 2-chloroprocaine, all local anesthetics and opioids cross the placenta.
- Fetal excretion of local anesthetics and opioids is largely by reversed placental transfer.
- Fetal asphyxia may be associated with an increased accumulation of local anesthetics and opioids in fetal tissues.

Key Reference

Ralston DHR, Shnider SM: The fetal and neonatal effects of regional anesthesia in obstetrics. Anesthesiology 1978; 48:34–64.

Case Stem

A 22-year-old G1P0 receives an epidural top-up with 50 mg of bupivacaine. Thirty seconds later she complains of tinnitus and a dry mouth. Seconds later, she becomes unresponsive and has generalized convulsions lasting 15 sec and resolving spontaneously. Ventilation by face mask is instituted, but the parturient resumes spontaneous breathing. Aspiration of the epidural catheter reveals blood. Discuss the immediate actions to be taken and the implications for mother and fetus.

Fentanyl and Sufentanil. Fentanyl and sufentanil are used in obstetric analgesia and anesthesia, alone or in combination with a local anesthetic. In a number of studies, the efficacy and safety of epidural fentanyl or sufentanil for both mother and child have been established.[120] Like local anesthetics, sufentanil binds predominantly to α_1-acid glycoprotein. Maternal protein binding for sufentanil is approximately 93%, of which 83% is bound to α_1-acid glycoprotein.[60] In the neonate, α_1-acid glycoprotein levels are decreased[54, 55]; consequently, protein binding of sufentanil is decreased to approximately 79%.[120] By contrast, fentanyl binds to both α_1-acid glycoprotein and albumin. Maternal protein binding of fentanyl is approximately 84%, of which 44% is bound to α_1-acid glycoprotein.[60] In the neonate, protein binding of fentanyl is 87%.[120] Fetal and neonatal levels of albumin are slightly higher than maternal albumin levels and fetal albumin has a similar binding affinity.[121] This may explain the fact that contrary to sufentanil, protein binding of fentanyl in the neonate is similar to maternal protein binding.

Opinions as to which opioid is preferable as an adjunct to an epidurally administered local anesthetic to the mother vary and data are scarce. Sufentanil accumulates in placental tissue,[50, 65] and as a consequence, the placenta may act as a buffer against rapid changes in sufentanil concentrations. Also, placental uptake has been shown to slow the initial transfer of sufentanil, and based on this finding sufentanil has been suggested as the opioid of choice when delivery is expected within 45 minutes.[65]

Loftus and coworkers[122] compared the addition of either fentanyl or sufentanil to epidural bupivacaine for pain relief during labor and delivery. These authors found a UV/MV ratio of 0.37 for fentanyl and 0.81 for sufentanil. However, although fentanyl and sufentanil were administered in a ratio of 5.7:1, maternal plasma concentrations showed a ratio of 27:1 (fentanyl vs. sufentanil). This indicates that maternal tissue uptake and clearance of sufentanil is greater than that of fentanyl, which would result in less fetal exposure to sufentanil. Although of little clinical significance, these authors also found a lower NACS at 24 hours in the fentanyl group.

In another study comparing the addition of fentanyl or sufentanil to epidural bupivacaine in a ratio of 2:1 (fentanyl vs. sufentanil), no differences were found in neonatal Apgar scores, but maternal pain relief was better in the sufentanil group.[123] Epidural sufentanil, up to a maximum of 30 μg, has been shown not to affect the NACS,[124] and this study is often cited with respect to the maximum allowable sufentanil dose. However, a number of studies using higher doses without apparent adverse effects have been published,[120] and in a study using epidural sufentanil doses ranging from 15 to 150 μg, no neonatal effects as determined by BNBAS were found.[125] Similarly, the safety of epidural fentanyl has been well established.[120, 126]

It thus seems that, based on the available literature, both fentanyl and sufentanil are suitable for maternal epidural administration with regard to neonatal safety. Because of the scarcity of data, no convincing evidence supports the preference of one opioid over the other for maternal epidural administration.

References

1. Brosens I, Robertson WB, Dixon HG: The physiological response of the vessels of the placental bed to normal pregnancy. J Pathol Bacteriol 1967; 93:569–579.
2. Pijnenborg R, Bland JM, Robertson WB, et al: Uteroplacental arterial changes related to interstitial trophoblast migration in early human pregnancy. Placenta 1983; 4:387–414.
3. Boyd JD, Hamilton WJ: The Human Placenta. Cambridge, England: W. Heffer & Sons; 1970.
4. Kaufmann P, Sen DK, Schweikhart G: Classification of human placental villi. I. Histology. Cell Tissue Res 1979; 200:409–423.
5. Sen DK, Kaufmann P, Schweikhart G: Classification of human placental villi. II. Morphometry. Cell Tissue Res 1979; 200:425–434.
6. Mather LE: Disposition of mepivacaine and bupivacaine enantiomers in sheep. Br J Anaesth 1991; 67:239–246.
7. Burm AGL, Van der Meer AD, Van Kleef JW, et al: Pharmacokinetics of the enantiomers of bupivacaine following intravenous administration of the racemate. Br J Clin Pharmacol 1994; 38:125–129.
8. Groen K, Mantel M, Zeijlmans PWM, et al: Pharmacokinetics of the enantiomers of bupivacaine and mepivacaine following epidural administration of the racemates. Anesth Analg 1998; 86:361–366.
9. Tucker GT, Mather LE: Pharmacokinetics of local anaesthetic agents. Br J Anaesth 1975; 47:213–224.
10. Burm AGL, Vermeulen NPE, Van Kleef JW, et al: Pharmacokinetics of lignocaine and bupivacaine in surgical patients following epidural administration: simultaneous investigation of absorption and disposition kinetics using stable isotopes. Clin Pharmacokinet 1987; 13:191–203.
11. Burm AGL, Van Kleef JW, Vermeulen NPE, et al: Pharmacokinetics of lidocaine and bupivacaine following subarachnoid administration in surgical patients: simultaneous investigation of absorption and disposition kinetics using stable isotopes. Anesthesiology 1988; 69:584–592.
12. Emanuelsson B-MK, Persson J, Alm C, et al: Systemic absorption and block after epidural injection of ropivacaine in healthy volunteers. Anesthesiology 1997; 87:1309–1317.
13. Burm AGL, Haak-van der Lely F, Van Kleef JW, et al: Pharmacokinetics of alfentanil after epidural administration: investigation of systemic absorption kinetics with a stable isotope method. Anesthesiology 1994; 81:308–315.
14. Tucker GT, Mather LE: Properties, absorption, and disposition of local anesthetic agents. *In* Cousins MJ, Bridenbaugh PO (eds): Neural Blockade in Clinical Anesthesia and Management of Pain, 3rd ed. Philadelphia: Lippincott-Raven; 1998:55–95.
15. Dahl JB, Simonsen L, Mogensen T, et al: The effect of 0.5% ropivacaine on epidural blood flow. Acta Anaesthesiol Scand 1990; 34:308–310.
16. Tucker GT, Mather LE: Clinical pharmacokinetics of local anaesthetics. Clin Pharmacokinet 1979; 4:241–278.
17. Lee A, Fagan D, Lamont M, et al: Disposition kinetics of ropivacaine in humans. Anesth Analg 1989; 69:736–738.
18. Stanski DR, Greenblatt DJ, Lowenstein E: Kinetics of intravenous and intramuscular morphine. Clin Pharmacol Ther 1978; 24:52–59.
19. Mather LE, Tucker GT, Pflug AE, et al: Meperidine kinetics in man: intravenous injections in surgical patients and volunteers. Clin Pharmacol Ther 1975; 17:21–30.
20. McClain DA, Hug CC: Intravenous fentanyl kinetics. Clin Pharmacol Ther 1980; 28:106–114.
21. Bower S, Hull CJ: Comparative pharmacokinetics of fentanyl and alfentanil. Br J Anaesth 1982; 54:871–877.
22. Sear JW: Sufentanil disposition in patients undergoing renal transplantation: influence of choice of kinetic model. Br J Anaesth 1989; 63:60–67.
23. Husemeyer RP, Cummings AJ, Rosankiewicz JR, et al: A study of pethidine kinetics and analgesia in women in labour following intravenous, intramuscular and epidural administration. Br J Clin Pharmacol 1982; 13:171–176.
24. Pihlajamaki KK, Kanto J, Lindberg L, et al: Extradural administration of bupivacaine: pharmacokinetics and metabolism in pregnant and non-pregnant women. Br J Anaesth 1990; 64:556–562.
25. Kuhnert BR, Kuhnert PM, Prochaska AL, et al: Plasma levels of 2-chloroprocaine in obstetric patients and their neonates after epidural anesthesia. Anesthesiology 1980; 53:21–25.
26. Wood M: Plasma drug binding: implications for anesthesiologists. Anesth Analg 1986; 65:786–804.
27. Notarianni LJ: Plasma protein binding of drugs in pregnancy and in neonates. Clin Pharmacokinet 1990; 18:20–36.
28. Santos AC, Pedersen H, Morishima HO, et al: Pharmacokinetics of lidocaine in nonpregnant and pregnant ewes. Anesth Analg 1988; 67:1154–1158.
29. Santos AC, Pedersen H, Sallusto JA, et al: Pharmacokinetics of ropivacaine in nonpregnant and pregnant ewes. Anesth Analg 1990; 70:262–266.
30. Kanto J: Obstetric analgesia: clinical pharmacokinetic considerations. Clin Pharmacokinet 1986; 11:283–298.
31. Kuhnert BR, Kuhnert PM, Prochaska AL, et al: Meperidine disposition in mother, neonate and non-pregnant females. Clin Pharmacol Ther 1980; 27:486–491.
32. Gepts E, Heytens L, Camu F: Pharmacokinetics and placental transfer of intravenous and epidural alfentanil in parturient women. Anesth Analg 1986: 65:1155–1160.
33. Coda BA, Brown MC, Schaffer R, et al: Pharmacology of epidural fentanyl, alfentanil and sufentanil in volunteers. Anesthesiology 1994; 81:1149–1161.
34. Rostaing S, Bonnet F, Levron JC, et al: Effect of epidural clonidine on analgesia and pharmacokinetics of epidural fentanyl in postoperative patients. Anesthesiology 1991; 75:420–425.
35. Justins DM, Knott C, Luthman J, et al: Epidural versus intramuscular fentanyl: analgesia and pharmacokinetics in labour. Anaesthesia 1983; 38:937–942.
36. Skjöldebrand A, Garle M, Gustafsson LL, et al: Extradural pethidine with and without adrenaline during labour: wide variation in effect. Br J Anaesth 1982; 54:415–420.
37. Sjöström S, Tamsen A, Persson MP, et al: Pharmacokinetics of intrathecal morphine and meperidine in humans. Anesthesiology 1987; 67:889–895.
38. Hansdottir V, Hedner T, Woestenborghs R, et al: The CSF and plasma pharmacokinetics of sufentanil after intrathecal administration. Anesthesiology 1991; 74:264–269.
39. Ionescu TI, Taverne RH, Houweling PL, et al: Pharmacokinetic study of extradural and intrathecal sufentanil anaesthesia for major surgery. Br J Anaesth 1991; 66:458–464.
40. Tucker GT, Cooper S, Littlewood D, et al: Observed and predicted accumulation of local anaesthetic agents during continuous extradural analgesia. Br J Anaesth 1977; 49:237–242.
41. Loper KA, Ready LB, Downey M, et al: Epidural and intravenous fentanyl infusions are clinically equivalent after knee surgery. Anesth Analg 1990; 70:72–75.
42. Thornburg KL, Burry KJ, Adas AK, et al: Permeability of placenta to inulin. Am J Obstet Gynecol 1988; 158:1165–1169.
43. Ralston DHR, Shnider SM: The fetal and neonatal effects of regional anesthesia in obstetrics. Anesthesiology 1978; 48:34–64.
44. Anderson DF, Phernetton TM, Rankin JHG: Prediction of fetal drug concentrations. Am J Obstet Gynecol 1980; 137:735–738.
45. Hamshaw-Thomas A, Rogerson N, Reynolds F: Transfer of

bupivacaine, lignocaine and pethidine across the rabbit placenta: influence of maternal protein binding and fetal flow. Placenta 1984; 5:61–70.
46. Tucker GT: Plasma binding and disposition of local anesthetics. Int Anesthesiol Clin 1975; 13:33–59.
47. Schneider H, Panigel M, Dancis J: Transfer across the perfused human placenta of antipyrine, sodium, and leucine. Am J Obstet Gynecol 1972; 114:822–828.
48. Johnson RF, Herman N, Arney TL, et al: Bupivacaine transfer across the human term placenta: a study using the dual perfused human placental model. Anesthesiology 1995; 82:459–468.
49. Johnson RF, Herman NL, Johnson HV, et al: Effects of fetal pH on local anesthetic transfer across the human placenta. Anesthesiology 1996; 85:608–615.
50. Johnson RF, Herman NL, Arney TL, et al: The placental transfer of sufentanil: effects of fetal pH, protein binding, and sufentanil concentration. Anesth Analg 1997; 84:1262–1268.
51. Tucker GT, Boyes RN, Bridenbaugh PO, et al: Binding of anilide-type local anesthetics in human plasma. II. Implications in vivo, with special reference to transplacental distribution. Anesthesiology 1970; 33:304–314.
52. Mather LE, Long GJ, Thomas J: The binding of bupivacaine to maternal and foetal plasma proteins. J Pharm Pharmacol 1971; 23:359–364.
53. Ehrnebo M, Agurell S, Jalling B, et al: Age differences in drug binding by plasma proteins: studies on human foetuses, neonates and adults. Eur J Clin Pharmacol 1971; 3:189–193.
54. Wood M, Wood AJ: Changes in plasma drug binding and alpha 1-acid glycoprotein in mother and newborn infant. Clin Pharmacol Ther 1981; 29:522–526.
55. Lerman J, Strong HA, LeDez KM, et al: Effects of age on the serum concentration of alpha 1-acid glycoprotein and the binding of lidocaine in pediatric patients. Clin Pharmacol Ther 1989; 46:219–225.
56. Strichartz GR, Sanchez V, Arthur GR, et al: Fundamental properties of local anesthetics. II. Measured octanol: buffer partition coefficients and pK_a values of clinically used drugs. Anesth Analg 1990; 71:158–170.
57. Arthur GR, Covino BG: Pharmacokinetics of local anaesthetics. Baillieres Clin Anaesthesiol 1991; 5:635–658.
58. Meuldermans WEG, Hurkmans RMA, Heykants JJP: Plasma protein binding and distribution of fentanyl, sufentanil, alfentanil and lofentanil in blood. Arch Int Pharmacodyn Ther 1982; 257:4–19.
59. Mather LE: Clinical pharmacokinetics of fentanyl and its newer derivatives. Clin Pharmacokinet 1983; 8:422–446.
60. Bovill JG: Pharmacokinetics of opioids. *In* Bowdle TA, Horita A, Kharash ED (eds): The Pharmacologic Basis of Anesthesiology. New York: Churchill Livingstone; 1994:37–81.
61. Brown WU, Bell GC, Alper MH: Acidosis, local anesthetics, and the newborn. Obstet Gynecol 1976; 48:27–30.
62. Biehl D, Shnider SM, Levinson G, et al: Placental transfer of lidocaine: effects of fetal acidosis. Anesthesiology 1978; 48:409–412.
63. Pickering B, Biehl D, Meatherall R: The effect of foetal acidosis on bupivacaine levels in utero. Can Anaesth Soc J 1981; 28:544–549.
64. Gaylard DG, Carson RJ, Reynolds F: Effect of umbilical perfusate pH and controlled maternal hypotension on placental drug transfer in the rabbit. Anesth Analg 1990; 71:42–48.
65. Krishna BR, Zakowski MI, Grant GJ: Sufentanil transfer in the human placenta during in vitro perfusion. Can J Anaesth 1997; 44:996–1001.
66. Himwich WA: Physiology of the neonatal central nervous system. *In* Stave U (ed): Physiology of the Perinatal Period. New York: Appleton-Century-Crofts; 1970:725–728.
67. Cohn HE, Sacks EJ, Heymann MA, et al: Cardiovascular responses to hypoxemia and acidemia in fetal lambs. Am J Obstet Gynecol 1974; 120:817–824.
68. Burney RG, DiFazio CA, Foster JA: Effects of pH on protein binding of lidocaine. Anesth Analg 1978; 57:478–480.
69. McNamara PJ, Slaughter RL, Pieper JA, et al: Factors influencing serum protein binding of lidocaine in humans. Anesth Analg 1981; 60:395–400.
70. Morishima HO, Covino BG: Toxicity and distribution of lidocaine in nonasphyxiated and asphyxiated baboon fetuses. Anesthesiology 1981; 54:182–186.
71. O'Brien WF, Cefalo RC, Grissom MP, et al: The influence of asphyxia on fetal lidocaine toxicity. Am J Obstet Gynecol 1982; 142:205–208.
72. Morishima HO, Santos AC, Pedersen H, et al: Effect of lidocaine on the asphyxial responses in the mature fetal lamb. Anesthesiology 1987; 66:502–507.
73. Meffin P, Long GJ, Thomas J: Clearance and metabolism of mepivacaine in the human neonate. Clin Pharmacol Ther 1973; 14:218–225.
74. Woods AM, DiFazio CA: Pharmacology of local anesthetics and related drugs. *In* Bonica JJ, McDonald JS (eds): Principles and Practice of Obstetric Anesthesia, 2nd ed. Baltimore: Williams & Wilkins; 1995:312–314.
75. O'Brien JE, Abbey V, Hinsvark O, et al: Metabolism and measurement of 2-chloroprocaine, an ester type local anesthetic. J Pharm Sci 1979; 68:75–78.
76. Kuhnert PM, Kuhnert BR, Stitts JM, et al: The use of a selected ion monitoring technique to study the disposition of bupivacaine in mother, fetus, and neonate following epidural anesthesia for cesarean section. Anesthesiology 1981; 55:611–617.
77. Brazelton TB: Neonatal behavioral assessment scale. Clinics in Developmental Medicine, no. 50. Spastics International Medical Publications. London: William Heinemann Medical Books; 1973.
78. Amiel-Tison C, Barrier G, Shnider SM, et al: A new neurologic and adaptive capacity scoring system for evaluating obstetric medications in full-term newborns. Anesthesiology 1982; 56:340–350.
79. Scanlon JW, Brown WU, Weiss JB, et al: Neurobehavioral responses of newborn infants after maternal epidural anesthesia. Anesthesiology 1974; 40:121–128.
80. Abboud TK, Khoo SS, Miller F, et al: Maternal, fetal, and neonatal responses after epidural anesthesia with bupivacaine, 2-chloroprocaine, or lidocaine. Anesth Analg 1982; 61:638–644.
81. Abboud TK, Sarkis F, Blikian A, et al: Lack of adverse neonatal effects of lidocaine. Anesth Analg 1983; 62:473–475.
82. Abboud TK, Kim KC, Noueihed R, et al: Epidural bupivacaine, chloroprocaine, or lidocaine for cesarean section—maternal and neonatal effects. Anesth Analg 1983; 62:914–919.
83. Kuhnert BR, Harrison MJ, Linn PL, et al: Effects of maternal epidural anesthesia on neonatal behavior. Anesth Analg 1984; 63:301–308.
84. Kileff ME, James FM III, Dewan DM, et al: Neonatal neurobehavioral responses after epidural anesthesia for cesarean section using lidocaine and bupivacaine. Anesth Analg 1984; 63:413–417.
85. Abboud TK, Afrasiabi A, Sarkis F, et al: Continuous infusion epidural analgesia in parturients receiving bupivacaine, chloroprocaine, or lidocaine—maternal, fetal, and neonatal effects. Anesth Analg 1984; 63:421–428.
86. Belfrage P, Boreus LO, Hartvig P, et al: Neonatal depression after obstetrical analgesia with pethidine: the role of the injection-delivery time interval and of the plasma concentrations of pethidine and norpethidine. Acta Obstet Gynecol Scand 1981; 60:43–49.
87. Teramo K, Benowitz N, Heymann MA, et al: Gestational differences in lidocaine toxicity in the fetal lamb. Anesthesiology 1976; 44:125–130.
88. Morishima HO, Pedersen H, Finster M, et al: Toxicity in adult, newborn and fetal sheep. Anesthesiology 1981; 55:57–61.
89. Morishima HO, Pedersen H, Finster M, et al: Etidocaine toxicity in the adult, newborn and fetal sheep. Anesthesiology 1983; 58:342–346.
90. Finster M, Poppers PJ, Sinclair JC, et al: Accidental intoxication of the fetus with local anesthetic drug during caudal anesthesia. Am J Obstet Gynecol 1965; 92:922–924.

91. Reisner LS, Hochman BN, Plumer MH: Persistent neurologic deficit and adhesive arachnoiditis following intrathecal 2-chloroprocaine injection. Anesth Analg 1980; 59:452–454.
92. Moore DC, Spierdijk J, Van Kleef JW, et al: Chloroprocaine neurotoxicity: four additional cases. Anesth Analg 1982; 61:155–159.
93. Barsa J, Batra M, Fink BR, et al: A comparative in vivo study of local neurotoxicity of lidocaine, bupivacaine, 2-chloroprocaine, and a mixture of 2-chloroprocaine and bupivacaine. Anesth Analg 1982; 61:961–967.
94. Kalichman MW, Powell HC, Reisner LS, et al: The role of 2-chloroprocaine and sodium bisulfite in rat sciatic nerve edema. J Neuropathol Exp Neurol 1986; 45:566–575.
95. Gissen AJ, Datta S, Lambert D: The chloroprocaine controversy. II. Is chloroprocaine neurotoxic? Reg Anesth 1984; 9:135.
96. Zador G, Englesson S, Nilsson B: Low dose intermittent epidural anaesthesia with lidocaine for vaginal delivery. Acta Obstet Gynecol Scand 1974; 34:3–16.
97. Zador G, Willdeck-Lund G, Nilsson B: Continuous drip lumbar epidural anaesthesia with lidocaine for vaginal delivery. Acta Obstet Gynecol Scand 1974; 34:31–40.
98. Brown WU, Bell GC, Lurie AO, et al: Newborn blood levels of lidocaine and mepivacaine in the first postnatal day following maternal epidural anesthesia. Anesthesiology 1975; 42:698–707.
99. Ramanathan J: Continuous epidural lidocaine infusion in preeclampsia: maternal and neonatal effects. Reg Anesth 1987; 12:95–96.
100. Ala-Kokko TI, Pienimaki P, Herva R, et al: Transfer of lidocaine and bupivacaine across isolated perfused human placenta. Pharmacol Toxicol 1995; 77:142–148.
101. Hyman MD, Shnider SM: Maternal and neonatal blood concentrations of bupivacaine associated with obstetrical conduction anesthesia. Anesthesiology 1971; 34:81–86.
102. McGuinness GA, Merkow AJ, Kennedy RL, et al: Epidural anesthesia with bupivacaine for cesarean section. Anesthesiology 1978; 49:270–273.
103. Matouskova A, Hanson B: Continuous mini-infusion of bupivacaine into the epidural space during labor. II. Blood concentration of bupivacaine. Acta Obstet Gynecol Scand Suppl 1979; 83:31–41.
104. Evans KRL, Carrie LES: Continuous epidural infusion of bupivacaine in labor: a simple method. Anaesthesia 1979; 34:310–315.
105. Clark MJ: Continuous mini-infusion of 0.125 percent bupivacaine into the epidural space during labor. J Am Osteopath Assoc 1982; 81:484–491.
106. Rosenblatt R: Continuous epidural infusion for obstetric analgesia. Reg Anesth 1983; 8:10–15.
107. Denson DD, Knapp RM, Turner P, et al: Serum bupivacaine concentrations in term parturients following continuous epidural analgesia for labor and delivery. Ther Drug Monit 1984; 6:393–398.
108. Rosenberg PH, Heinonen E: Differential sensitivity of A and C nerve fibres to long-acting amide local anaesthetics. Br J Anaesth 1983; 55:163–167.
109. Bader AM, Datta S, Flanagan H, et al: Comparison of bupivacaine- and ropivacaine-induced conduction in blockade in the isolated rabbit vagus nerve. Anesth Analg 1989; 68:724–727.
110. Brockway MS, Bannister J, McClure JH, et al: Comparison of extradural ropivacaine and bupivacaine. Br J Anaesth 1991; 66:31–37.
111. Morrison LMM, Emanuelsson B-M, McClure JH, et al: Efficacy and kinetics of extradural ropivacaine: comparison with bupivacaine. Br J Anaesth 1994; 72:164–169.
112. Kerkkamp HEM, Gielen MJM, Edström H: Comparison of 0.75% ropivacaine with epinephrine and 0.75% bupivacaine with epinephrine in lumbar epidural anesthesia. Reg Anesth 1990; 15:204–207.
113. Brown DL, Carpenter RL, Thompson GE: Comparison of 0.5% ropivacaine 0.5% bupivacaine for epidural anesthesia in patients undergoing lower-extremity surgery. Anesthesiology 1990; 72:633–636.
114. Zaric D, Nydahl PA, Adel SO, et al: The effect of continuous epidural infusion of ropivacaine (0.1%, 0.2% and 0.3%) on nerve conduction velocity and postural control in volunteers. Acta Anaesthesiol Scand 1996; 40:342–349.
115. McClure JH: Ropivacaine. Br J Anaesth 1996; 76:300–307.
116. Morishima HO, Pedersen H, Finster M, et al: Bupivacaine toxicity in pregnant and non-pregnant ewes. Anesthesiology 1985; 63:134–139.
117. Santos AC, Arthur GR, Pedersen H, et al: Systemic toxicity of ropivacaine during ovine pregnancy. Anesthesiology 1991; 75:137–141.
118. Datta S, Camann W, Bader A, et al: Clinical effects and maternal and fetal plasma concentrations of epidural ropivacaine versus bupivacaine for cesarean section. Anesthesiology 1995; 82:1346–1352.
119. Writer DR, Stienstra R, Eddleston JM, et al: Neonatal outcome and mode of delivery after epidural labour analgesia with ropivacaine and bupivacaine: a prospective meta-analysis. Br J Anaesth 1998; 81:713–717.
120. Helbo-Hansen HS: Neonatal effects of maternally administered fentanyl, alfentanil and sufentanil. *In* Bogod DG (ed): Obstetric Anaesthesia. Baillière's Clinical Anaesthesiology, Vol 9. London: Baillière Tindall; 1995:675–689.
121. Hill MD, Abramson FP: The significance of plasma protein binding on the fetal/maternal distribution of drugs at steady-state. Clin Pharmacokinet 1988; 14:156–170.
122. Loftus JR, Hill H, Cohen SE: Placental transfer and neonatal effects of epidural sufentanil and fentanyl administered with bupivacaine during labor. Anesthesiology 1995; 83:300–308.
123. Cohen S, Amar D, Pantuck CB, et al: Epidural analgesia for labour and delivery: fentanyl or sufentanil? Can J Anaesth 1996; 43:341–346.
124. Vertommen JD, VanderMeulen E, Van Aken H, et al: The effects of the addition of sufentanil to 0.125% bupivacaine on the quality of analgesia during labor and on the incidence of instrumental deliveries. Anesthesiology 1991; 74:809–814.
125. Steinberg RB, Dunn SM, Dixon DE, et al: Comparison of sufentanil, bupivacaine, and their combination for epidural analgesia in obstetrics. Reg Anesth 1992; 17:131–138.
126. Bader AM, Fragneto R, Terui K, et al: Maternal and neonatal fentanyl and bupivacaine concentrations after epidural infusion during labor. Anesth Analg 1995; 81:829–832.

8

The Effects of Drugs Used in Pregnancy

❖ Marco A. E. Marcus, MD, PhD

❖ Hans-Fritz Gramke, MD

❖ Wiebke Gogarten, MD

❖ Hugo Van Aken, MD, FRCA, FANZCA, PhD

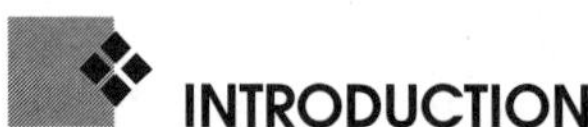

INTRODUCTION

Many different drugs are administered during pregnancy. In spite of this, only a few randomized trials exist that document the safety of these drugs to the mother and fetus. Many of these drugs are of interest in obstetric anesthesia. These drugs can be arbitrarily divided into drugs for induction of general anesthesia, those for induction of regional anesthesia, those for procurement of analgesia, those for treatment of asthma, and antihypertensives.

GENERAL ANESTHETICS

Although regional anesthesia is regarded as the preferred choice for cesarean section, there are still situations in which general anesthesia is indicated, such as when regional anesthesia is contraindicated.

Propofol

Propofol (2,3-diisopropylphenol) is not water-soluble and therefore is used as an aqueous emulsion for intravenous administration. It is suitable for both induction and maintenance of general anesthesia. Because of its pharmacokinetic profile, it has excellent recovery characteristics.[1]

Propofol is conjugated in the liver, to produce inactive metabolites. The neonatal elimination of propofol is slower than that in the mother.[2] The use of propofol in obstetric anesthesia is still controversial. Lower neonatal Apgar scores have been reported after induction of general anesthesia for cesarean section with propofol,[3] but these results have not been confirmed in subsequent studies.[4, 5] Gin and associates[1] concluded that Apgar scores were higher as a consequence of shorter incision-to-delivery times but did not find a correlation of Apgar score with umbilical blood levels of propofol.

Transplacental passage of propofol is expected to be rapid because it is a lipid-soluble, largely un-ionized drug with a low molecular weight. There is probably no significant placental metabolism of propofol.[1]

Propofol does not adversely affect uterine blood flow in pregnant ewes[6]; however, hypotension, largely caused by a direct vasodilatory effect, is a potential side effect of propofol and can cause a decrease of uteroplacental flow. In a recent study, the effect of propofol on uterine smooth muscle was investigated. A significant reduction in uterine muscle tone was found, but only at concentrations much higher than those commonly used during cesarean section.[7] Perioperative blood loss does not seem to be made worse by propofol.[4]

Thiopental (Thiopentone)

Many studies have investigated the maternal and neonatal effects of thiopental (also called thiopentone), and many clinicians prefer to use it for intravenous induction of general anesthesia in the parturient. Thiopental is a barbituric acid derivative with hypnotic and anticonvulsant properties. It is characterized by high lipid solubility and protein binding. The degradation of thiopental involves hepatic oxidation into inactive water-soluble metabolites.

Although the hepatic metabolic capacity in neonates is not fully developed, and despite a rapid placental transfer,[8] Apgar scores and neurobehavioral scores reported after elective cesarean section at term are satisfactory.[8–10] With a single intravenous dose of thiopental of up to 4 mg/kg body weight, umbilical arterial levels are much lower than umbilical venous levels.

Blood coming from the placenta passes through the liver or reaches the inferior vena cava through the ductus venosus. Therefore, most of the thiopental is diluted by blood from the lower extremities and the viscera. On the other hand, redistribution in the mother causes a swift decline of drug concentration in maternal blood. This can explain the lack of neonatal depression after a single induction dose of thiopental.[11]

Administration of thiopental for induction of general anesthesia can cause an initial decline of maternal blood pressure,[12] which may reduce uteroplacental flow. In vitro studies of human intramyometrial arterial flow revealed a nonspecific inhibition of the response to norepinephrine and vasopressin with high concentrations of thiopental. Thiopental did not seem to interfere with vascular relaxation induced by prostacyclin[13]; however, because of the high protein binding of thiopental in vivo, a major direct vascular effect during anesthesia for cesarean section is unlikely. There is no evidence that placental perfusion is directly impaired by thiopental.

Ketamine

In 1964, the phencyclidine derivative ketamine was introduced. It causes fewer psychomimetic effects than phencyclidine itself, but a high incidence of "bad dreams" is very common in patients anesthetized with ketamine as a sole anesthetic.[12, 14] The incidence of nightmares can be reduced by the concomitant use of benzodiazepines.[14]

Ketamine is an enantiomeric mixture, but the recently isolated S-ketamine seems to cause a decrease in side effects. Ketamine is more lipid-soluble and less protein-bound than thiopental. The drug is metabolized in the liver, and some of the metabolites (e.g., norketamine) have anesthetic activity.[15]

Ketamine produces an increase in maternal blood pressure and heart rate, owing to central stimulation of the sympathetic nervous system.[12] Furthermore, ketamine is a potent bronchodilator. These characteristics make it especially suitable for patients with asthma or hypovolemia, such as in emergency cesarean section with major blood loss prior to surgery.[16] On the other hand, ketamine is contraindicated in patients with hypertension.

Placental transfer of ketamine is rapid. At high doses, low Apgar scores and neonatal muscular hypertonicity have been described.[17] However, Apgar scores were satisfactory in studies using clinically recommended doses of up to 1.2 mg/kg for intravenous induction.[16, 18]

Benzodiazepines

In obstetrics, benzodiazepines may be used as sedatives or as anticonvulsants. Diazepam and midazolam are the two most frequently used benzodiazepines. The pharmacologic effects of benzodiazepines have been attributed to an increase in the quantity or facilitation of effectiveness of the inhibitory neurotransmitters γ-aminobutyric acid (GABA) and glycine.[19]

Diazepam has a long half-life. Used in large doses, its principal adverse effects on the fetus are hypotonia, lethargy, feeding problems, and hypothermia ("floppy infant syndrome"). After maternal diazepam administration, glucuronidation can be decreased and serum bilirubin increased in the neonate.[20] In the mother, it can cause a cyclical return of drowsiness because of enterohepatic recirculation.[19]

The umbilical-to-maternal ratio of *midazolam* appears to be lower compared to that of diazepam, suggesting an increased placental transfer of the latter.[8] Midazolam has a rapid onset and a short duration of action; therefore, the use of midazolam is preferred over that of diazepam.

Volatile Anesthetics

To reduce the incidence of recall and awareness of intraoperative events, most clinicians use low concentrations of a potent volatile anesthetic combined with nitrous oxide for maintenance of general anesthesia. This technique also allows the use of a higher inspired oxygen concentration. There has been much clinical experience with isoflurane, enflurane, and halothane, but information on the newer volatile anesthetics sevoflurane and desflurane in obstetric anesthesia is limited.

Sevoflurane is not pungent or irritating to the airways. Fast inhalation induction with sevoflurane is possible because of its low blood-gas partition coefficient. However, intravenous rapid sequence induction is recommended for cesarean section because of the increased risk of aspiration in late pregnancy. Nevertheless, in the case of emergency cesarean section, when intravenous access is impossible, inhalation induction with sevoflurane has been described with good outcome for both mother and child.[21]

Volatile anesthetics are highly lipid-soluble and cross the placenta freely. The blood-gas partition coefficients are lower in neonates than in adults, and therefore volatile anesthetics should be rapidly eliminated once respiration has been established.[22] Several studies investigating isoflurane, enflurane, and halothane have shown no evidence of neonatal depression when used in low concentrations. Neonates were evaluated by Apgar score, blood gas tension, and neurobehavioral scores.[22–24] Animal studies suggest an increase in uterine blood flow during anesthesia with volatile anesthetics.[24]

Halothane has the disadvantage of sensitizing the myocardium to the dysrhythmogenic effects of catecholamines.[23] β-Adrenergic therapy for preterm labor can also cause arrhythmias, which may be potentiated by halothane. Available data on sevoflurane and desflurane do not show any important differences, compared with other halogenated agents, in terms of maternal and neonatal effects,[25–27] but further evaluation is required.

Another concern secondary to the use of halogenated volatile anesthetics in obstetric surgery is a decrease in uterine muscle tone with increased uterine blood loss.[23] This only occurs at higher concentrations.[24, 25, 27] The uterus still responds appropriately to oxytocin stimulation.[24] However, because of the potential for uterine atony, many anesthesiologists discontinue the use of these agents after delivery of the newborn.

REGIONAL ANESTHETICS

In recent years, regional anesthesia has become very popular in obstetrics. It provides excellent analgesia while reducing the risk of the serious complications associated with general anesthesia (e.g., failed intubation, aspiration of gastric fluids). Sympatholytic effects of regional anesthesia may lead to hypotension. Because maternal arterial blood pressure is one of the main determinants of uteroplacental hemodynamics, fluid preloading prior to induction of the block is recommended to prevent hypotension. Crystalloid solutions such as Ringer's lactate are often used for this purpose; however, some have suggested that colloid solutions may be better. Hydroxyethyl starch can significantly increase uterine blood flow, cardiac output, total oxygen delivery capacity, and uterine arterial oxygen delivery in pregnant ewes.[28] The same beneficial effects can be found in women undergoing cesarean section under regional anesthesia.[29] The importance of preventing hypotension was illustrated in a study that measured Doppler indices of the uterine artery and umbilical artery during epidural anesthesia for cesarean section.[30] Acute hypotension was accompanied by increases in uteroplacental Doppler ratios, indicating increased resistance to flow. Furthermore, these increases persisted despite vasopressor treatment and normalization of blood pressure. Uteroplacental Doppler indices remained unchanged in parturients who did not develop hypotension during epidural anesthesia. Transient hypotension ($<$2 min) may lead to a lower pH in umbilical cord blood, but has not been shown to have adverse consequences in normal term pregnancies.[31] In preeclampsia, uteroplacental circulation is already compromised; therefore, it is more crucial that maternal hypotension be avoided.[32]

Drugs used for regional anesthesia in obstetrics are local anesthetics with or without the addition of opioids. Three popular amide-type local anesthetics are lidocaine, bupivacaine, and, more recently, ropivacaine.

Lidocaine (Lignocaine)

Lidocaine, also known as lignocaine, is a weak base with a pK_a of 7.8. Protein binding is 56% (chiefly to α_1-acid glycoprotein, an acute phase protein that is more concentrated in maternal than in fetal plasma). Lidocaine is metabolized by hepatic enzymes into two pharmacologically active metabolites: monoethylglycinexylidide and glycinexylidide. The neonate is also able to metabolize lidocaine.[33] Lidocaine is available as hydrochloride and hydrocarbonate solutions. There seems to be no obvious advantage of one over the other.[34, 35] Both lidocaine solutions have comparable transplacental transfer (fetal-to-maternal concentration ratio $\approx$0.50). Their use is regarded as safe for cesarean section in normal-term pregnancy.[35] The placental transfer of lidocaine is increased by fetal acidemia. The ionic form of lidocaine does not cross the placenta in significant amounts, in contrast to the nonionic form, which is highly diffusable. The larger the difference between the (acidotic) fetal pH and the pK_a of lidocaine, the larger the proportion of ionized agent on the fetal side. The ionized form cannot diffuse back and may become trapped on the fetal side.[36] This enhanced transfer of lidocaine is limited by maternal protein binding of the drug.[36] Other factors that may play a role are decreased local anesthetic clearance by the fetus and changes in tissue distribution. Therefore, in clinical situations in which the fetus is likely to be acidotic, all efforts must be taken to minimize the dose of local anesthetic.

The neonatal effects of epidural lidocaine are mild. It is now clear that lidocaine does not seem to compromise the neurobehavioral status of the newborn when used for epidural anesthesia in healthy term patients.[37, 38] An effect of epidural lidocaine on the fetal heart rate pattern could not be shown in healthy term parturients.[39]

Bupivacaine

Bupivacaine is one of the long-acting amide-type local anesthetics. Its pK_a is 8.1 and it shows more protein-binding than lidocaine. Passive diffusion rather than active drug transport is probably the mechanism of placental transfer of bupivacaine (fetal-to-maternal concentration ratio $\approx$0.3).[40] Passage seems to be influenced by the maternal and fetal plasma protein binding, the fetal pH, and placental uptake.[41] The placental transfer of bupivacaine is enhanced by fetal acidosis. The main mechanism for this phenomenon is ion-trapping due to decreased fetal pH.[36] In a study using the dual-perfused placenta model, Johnson and colleagues[41] illustrated the influence of protein binding on the placental transfer. Increased maternal protein binding leads to less fetal transfer. Their experiments also showed an ability of the placenta to accumulate bupivacaine. In human placenta, the amount of placental transfer of bupivacaine is less than that of lidocaine. This was explained by placental bupivacaine binding because of its higher lipophilicity.[42]

Cardiovascular collapse after accidental intravascular injection of bupivacaine has been reported. Since many of these cases have occurred in obstetric patients, this has led to the question of whether cardiotoxicity of bupivacaine is increased in pregnancy.[43] Current evidence suggests that this is not the case. Previous work, however, suggested that lower doses of bupivacaine seem to be needed to produce cardiovascular collapse in pregnant ewes compared with non-pregnant sheep.[44] Two factors may play a role in these findings. First, the proportion of protein-bound bupivacaine is lower in pregnant than in non-pregnant sheep. Second, the concentration of free drug is similar, suggesting a gestational increase in the availability of free bupivacaine.[43] Additionally, the myocardium in the late stages of pregnancy is more sensitive to cardiodepressant effects.[44] In a more recent animal study, this increase of systemic toxicity of bupivacaine during gestation could not be reproduced.[45] The use of a test dose can minimize the risk of intravascular injection and is therefore strongly recommended. To reduce cardiotoxic effects, bupivacaine 0.75% is no longer used in obstetrics.

Drug effects on the fetal heart have a minor, if any, influence on immediate fetal outcome. Prolonged decelerations following bupivacaine use in epidural anesthesia for labor have been reported.[46] The cause of these prolonged decelerations is not clearly understood; uterine hypertonus might play a role.[46] Direct drug effects, maternal hypotension, and constriction of uterine or umbilical vessels are other possible factors in the genesis of this phenomenon.[39] Factors associated with labor and delivery may also account for the increased incidence of fetal heart rate changes after epidural labor analgesia.[39]

Bupivacaine has been used for epidural labor analgesia and cesarean section without any adverse effects on the neurobehavioral score of the newborn.[37, 40, 47] Epidural bupivacaine does not have any detrimental effects on the uteroplacental circulation, provided that long hypotensive periods are avoided (see earlier discussion).[48, 49]

Ropivacaine

A more recently introduced long-acting local anesthetic of the amide type is ropivacaine. Like other local anesthetics, it is a weak base (pK_a 8.1). Its physiochemical properties are similar to those of bupivacaine, except for a lower lipid solubility. Protein binding of ropivacaine is also lower compared with bupivacaine. In comparison to bupivacaine, systemic toxicity of ropivacaine is not enhanced during pregnancy, and higher doses are needed to provoke signs of central nervous system or cardiovascular toxicity.[45, 50] Consequently, ropivacaine, if equipotent, is less cardiotoxic than bupivacaine and thus may have an increased margin of safety.[51] The transplacental passage of the drug is similar to that of bupivacaine (fetal-to-maternal concentration ratio, ≈0.3).[52] Several studies[50, 52, 53] could not show any adverse effects in the neonate during and after epidural anesthesia with ropivacaine for elective cesarean section, even when high doses (up to 25 mL ropivacaine 0.75%) were used.[53] Epidural ropivacaine probably does not compromise the uteroplacental circulation in healthy pregnant women with uncomplicated pregnancies. The pulsatility index of the maternal uterine artery increased significantly on the nonplacental side, but Doppler indices of the fetal renal and middle cerebral artery remained unchanged.[54] In pregnant ewes, uterine blood flow does not decrease during intravenous administration of ropivacaine.[49]

ANALGESICS

The use of pain-relieving drugs during pregnancy is common.

Acetylsalicylic Acid

Although acetylsalicylic acid in high doses is teratogenic in animals, it has not been proved teratogenic in humans. These agents block prostaglandin synthesis when given in analgesic doses. They are highly bound to plasma proteins but are lipophilic. Therefore, placental transfer of the free fraction is high but the concentration in the fetus is below the maternal concentration. Elimination in the fetus is slow. Inhibition of prostaglandin synthesis may prolong labor and delivery through a blockade of uterine contractions.[55] Acetylsalicylic acid blocks thrombocyte aggregation with a possible increase in blood loss during delivery. The incidence of bleeding after delivery is also higher.

Nonsteroidal Anti-inflammatory Agents

There is concern that the use of nonsteroidal anti-inflammatory drugs late in pregnancy can induce premature closure of the ductus Botalli.[56] Nonsteroidal anti-inflammatory drugs (e.g., diclofenac) block prostaglandin synthesis and are, therefore, relatively contraindicated during pregnancy.

Paracetamol

Paracetamol does not block prostaglandin synthesis and is not teratogenic. Of the weak analgesics, paracetamol should be the first-line drug.

Opioids

The opioids are more potent than simple analgesics. Short-term opioids are excellent analgesics. Although a wide variety of opioids is now available, only a few are used currently in obstetrics. The ones in common use are morphine, meperidine (pethidine), fentanyl, sufentanil, and tramadol. Several studies are currently being conducted to determine the place of remifentanil and alfentanil for analgesia in obstetrics.

All opioids cause a variety of side effects in the mother, including respiratory depression, orthostatic hypotension, nausea, vomiting, and delay of gastric motility. All opioids are rapidly transferred across the placenta and are capable of producing neonatal respiratory depression and changes in the neurobehavior of the child. To diminish the usual side effects observed with systemically and intramuscularly administered opioids, alternative ways of administration have been sought. Spinal and epidural delivery of opioids was introduced in 1979 and has been widely accepted in obstetric analgesia.

Morphine

Intravenous *morphine* has too many undesirable effects to be of routine use in modern obstetric practice. Its hypotensive effects in the mother and its slow onset of action makes titration difficult. Infants are highly susceptible to the respiratory depressant effect of intravenously administered morphine.

Several studies describe the administration of intrathecal morphine during parturition.[57–60] Intrathecal morphine, a highly ionized, water-soluble opioid, produces analgesia of long duration but slow onset. The slow onset of action, plus a high incidence of side effects such as nausea, vomiting, and pruritus and the potential for delayed respiratory depression limit the usefulness of intrathecal morphine for labor analgesia especially at a dose of greater than 0.2 mg. It also is not the drug commonly used for epidural analgesia in the laboring patient. Its onset of action is 20 to 45 minutes after epidural administration.[61] It causes a high incidence of maternal side effects such as nausea (53%), urinary retention (43%), and somnolence (43%).[59] Morphine is hydrophilic and might cause late respiratory depression, which is dangerous when the patient is not adequately monitored. Because of these side effects, interest has turned to the more lipophilic opioids like meperidine (pethidine), fentanyl, sufentanil, and, lately, tramadol.

Meperidine

Meperidine (pethidine) is one of the opioids most frequently used in obstetrics. Usual doses are 50 to 100 mg intramuscularly and 25 to 50 mg intravenously. Peak analgesic action occurs 40 to 50 minutes after intramuscular administration and 5 to 10 minutes after intravenous administration. The duration of action is 3 to 4 hours.[17] When given intravenously, maternal and fetal blood concentrations rise rapidly after 90 seconds.[62] Maternally administered meperidine may produce neonatal respiratory depression, as evidenced by delay in sustained respiration, decreased Apgar scores,[63] lower oxygen saturation,[64] decreased minute ventilation,[65] respiratory acidosis,[66] and abnormal neurobehavior after birth.[67] Fetal exposure to meperidine is highest 2 to 3 hours after intramuscular maternal drug administration.[68] The concentration of normeperidine, an active metabolite of meperidine, rises steadily in fetal blood. Fetal changes attributed to meperidine persist for 72 hours after birth. The use of meperidine in complicated pregnancies was studied by Rhien et al.[69] They compared a group of 214 infants whose mothers received meperidine with 401 infants whose mothers did not receive meperidine. All deliveries (the control and treatment groups) were complicated with meconium-stained amniotic fluid. This study failed to identify additional neonatal risks if meperidine was used.[69]

Fentanyl

Fentanyl has been administered intravenously as a labor analgesic. Doses of 50 to 100 μg per hour as needed (PRN) were given to women in labor. No major side effects were seen, apart from mild sedation. Umbilical blood fentanyl concentration never exceeded 0.4 ng/mL.[70] In a study in which fentanyl was compared with meperidine, moderate to severe pain was recorded in both groups during active labor. No mother in the fentanyl group suffered side effects, compared with 20% in the meperidine group. In the meperidine group, 13% of the babies required naloxone at birth, compared with 2% in the fentanyl group.[71] In gravid ewes, Craft et al.[72] showed a rapid rise and decline of fetal fentanyl blood concentrations (appearance after 1 minute and peak at 5 minutes) after maternal intravenous injection of 50 to 100 μg fentanyl.[72] In humans, the ratio of umbilical vein concentration to maternal artery concentration is 0.31.[73]

Intrathecal injection of a more lipid-soluble opioid leads to rapid relief of labor pain with fewer side effects, but the duration of analgesia is relatively short.[74, 75] Intrathecal *fentanyl* 25 μg has a rapid onset of analgesia but lasts only 60 to 90 minutes.[76] In a retrospective study with patients receiving intrathecal fentanyl 25 to 30 μg, plus 0.25 to 0.3 mg morphine and 6 to 8 mg lidocaine, Rust et al.[77] reported excellent pain relief without any respiratory depression. However, a significant proportion of patients experienced pruritus and urinary retention.[77] In several studies, epidural fentanyl in combination with low doses of bupivacaine improved the quality of analgesia and reduced the severity of motor blockade and the incidence of hypotension.[78, 79] However, several side effects are reported after the use of epidural fentanyl. In the mother, 100 μg of epidural fentanyl may cause late respiratory depression.[80, 81] Neonates can also suffer from respiratory depression. In a study by Noble et al.,[82] two neonates had to be given naloxone after the mother received epidural fentanyl, whereas in a study by Carrie et al.,[83] one neonate had to be intubated. These results were contradicted in a study from Preston et al.,[84] however, in which Apgar scores and neurobehavior and adaptive capacity scores were normal and neonatal blood levels at delivery were below the level expected to cause respiratory depression. Similar conclusions were derived from a study in pregnant ewes, in which the placental passage and uterine effects of epidural fentanyl were investigated.[85] This study showed that an epidural injection of 50 μg fentanyl has minimal effect on maternal or fetal cardiovascular and acid-base status, uterine tone, and uterine blood flow. It also demonstrated only minimal placental passage of fentanyl to the fetus.

Continuous epidural infusions containing a combination of low concentrations of local anesthetics and opioids have become increasingly popular in labor analgesia. Bader and colleagues[86] examined the potential for fetal drug accumulation after a continuous (up to 15 hours) epidural infusion of 0.125% bupivacaine with 2 μg/mL fentanyl. They concluded that the concentrations of both drugs remained low and that none of the neonates showed any significant accumulation of drug or adverse effects, as demonstrated by umbilical blood gases and neurobehavioral scores.

Sufentanil

Because of its potency, sufentanil was never popular for systemic administration for labor pain relief. In pregnant sheep, Vertommen and associates[87] showed that after a maternal injection of 50 μg, a mean peak level of sufentanil was detected in maternal plasma at 1 minute (1.28 ng/mL). A mean peak plasma level of 0.037 ng/mL in the fetus was obtained 3 minutes after injection. Fetal sufentanil levels decreased in parallel with maternal levels, as evidenced by a constant maternal-to-fetal ratio of 5.5 for 15 to 60 minutes after the injection of sufentanil.[87] From a theoretical standpoint, *sufentanil* is an ideal drug for intrathecal use. Its high lipophilicity limits its rostral spread in the cerebrospinal fluid and speeds its onset of action. D'Angelo and associates[88] compared 10 μg intrathecal sufentanil with 12 mg bupivacaine administered epidurally and found a faster onset of analgesia with intrathecal sufentanil. However, the incidence of hypotension was comparable in both groups and intrathecal sufentanil spread cephalad rapidly. These observations were confirmed by Grieco and coworkers[89] and Cohen and associates,[90] who additionally showed a relatively short mean duration of action (123 minutes). When 2.5 mg intrathecal bupivacaine was added to 10 μg intrathecal sufentanil, it significantly prolonged labor analgesia (from 114 minutes in the sufentanil group to 148 minutes in the combined sufentanil/bupivacaine group) without adverse maternal or fetal side effects.[91] The analgesic effects of epidural sufentanil have also been investigated in several studies. The addition of sufentanil to bupivacaine 0.25% did not improve the quality of analgesia, but the duration was prolonged.[92] Van Steenberghe and associates[93] combined 7.5 μg and 15 μg sufentanil with bupivacaine 0.125% plus epinephrine (adrenaline) during labor in 107 women and found superior analgesia with faster onset and longer duration compared with local anesthetic alone. The hourly bupivacaine requirements were significantly reduced and "top-up" injections were required less frequently. The authors also found that the addition of sufentanil allowed relief of any residual pain resulting from an incomplete sensory block. Although 1-minute Apgar scores were significantly lower in the group that received 15 μg sufentanil, at 5 minutes after birth, there were no differences between the three groups.[93] Vertommen and coworkers[94] showed, in a study of 695 women, that the addition of sufentanil to bupivacaine 0.125% not only improved analgesia but also reduced the incidence of instrumental deliveries. The addition of up to 30 μg sufentanil did not cause neonatal respiratory depression.[94, 95] In conclusion, the risk of neonatal respiratory depression by sufentanil is minimal. In chronically instrumented pregnant sheep, no fetal plasma sufentanil could be detected after the maternal administration of 50 μg sufentanil.[87] Palot et al.[96] compared the placental transfer of fentanyl and sufentanil after continuous epidural administration in laboring women and found a significantly higher transfer of fentanyl than of sufentanil.[96] Loftus et al.[97] contradicted these results and found that fetal-to-maternal ratios were higher for sufentanil than for fentanyl. However, because of its greater potency, less epidural sufentanil is needed, so maternal and fetal concentrations were lower.

One potential disadvantage of epidural opioids is their effect on gastric emptying.[98–100] Geddes et al.[100] added fentanyl 100 μg to epidural bupivacaine 0.5% after cesarean section and demonstrated a statistically significant delay in gastric emptying after surgery, as did Ewah et al.[98] and Wright et al.[99] The addition of smaller doses of opioids does not delay gastric emptying, however. Zimmerman et al.[101] demonstrated that a bolus of 50 μg epidural fentanyl followed by an infusion delivering fentanyl at 20 μg/h does not delay gastric emptying in laboring women 2 hours after epidural analgesia is initiated. Other side effects from epidural opioids are pruritus (1.3%) and nausea and vomiting (1%).[102] Thus, the addition of small doses of opioids for epidural use carries fewer side effects compared with systemic and spinal opioids.

Although some older studies that used high local anesthetic concentrations showed prolongation of labor and a higher incidence of instrumental deliveries, epidural anesthesia with a combination of opioids and low local anesthetic concentrations "normalized" the duration of labor and delivery.[103, 104]

Butorphanol and Nalbuphine

The few studies that have been done with *butorphanol* and *nalbuphine*, two agonist-antagonist analgesics, have demonstrated no advantages over other opioids.

Tramadol

Tramadol is a centrally acting weak agonist.[105] It is reported that, in therapeutic doses, fewer side effects will occur and, especially, less respiratory depression than with other opioids.[106] Bitsch and colleagues[107] reported that 50 mg tramadol administered intramuscularly was effective in relieving labor pain in more than 60% of patients; analgesia began about 10 minutes after injection and lasted for as long as 45 minutes. Viegas and associates[108] compared intramuscular tramadol 50 mg and 100 mg with intramuscular meperidine 75 mg for relief of labor pain. They found that the pain relief was similar with meperidine and 100 mg tramadol, but that the meperidine group suffered more side effects.[108]

Remifentanil

Remifentanil is a new ultrashort-acting anilidopiperidine with a μ-specific opioid action. Kan and coworkers[109] studied the placental transfer of remifentanil and the neonatal effects when it was administered as an intravenous infusion for additional analgesia during cesarean section under epidural anesthesia. Nineteen parturients received 0.1 μg/kg/min remifentanil intravenously. The umbilical vein-to-maternal artery ratio was 0.88. These results indicate that remifentanil crosses the placenta but appears to be rapidly metabolized, redistributed, or both. Maternal sedation and respiratory changes occur, but without adverse neonatal or maternal effects. In chronically instrumented pregnant sheep, Gogarten and associates[110] concluded that intravenous administration of remifentanil has no effect on maternal and fetal cardiovascular and acid-base status.

With these unique properties, remifentanil could be of particular use for fetal and maternal analgesia during fetal surgery. In a study by Marcus et al.,[111] three patients received an intravenous infusion with continuous remifentanil 0.08 to 0.15 μg/kg/min for intrauterine microendoscopic procedures. Maternal analgesia was always satisfactory and fetuses did not move. The saturation never dropped below 95%. Mean fetal heart rate declined after the remifentanil infusion was started and quickly returned to normal after the infusion was stopped. Mean maternal heart rate did not change significantly.

ANTIHYPERTENSIVES

Antihypertensive therapy is necessary when the blood pressure is over 110 diastolic or over 180 systolic or both.[112] Prolonged episodes of hypertension can lead to placental insufficiency and intrauterine growth retardation. Whether antihypertensive therapy prevents this intrauterine growth retardation is controversial.

Magnesium Sulfate

Magnesium sulfate is frequently used for the prevention and treatment of eclamptic convulsions. It also has antihypertensive properties and increases uterine blood flow.[113] Its mode of action is still largely unknown. Eclamptic convulsions may be caused by periods of cerebral arterial vasospasm. Zaret proposed that magnesium sulfate may prevent vasospasm by acting like a competitive calcium antagonist.[115] Magnesium sulfate acts as a muscle relaxant by competing with calcium at the presynaptic membrane of the neuromuscular end plate so that calcium-dependent acetylcholine release decreases. Owing to this mechanism, the duration of action of muscle relaxants can be prolonged in patients who are given magnesium sulfate.[116]

Because of its muscle-relaxing effect, magnesium sulfate is also used in the treatment of preterm labor.[117] Several studies have indicated that magnesium sulfate decreases the total biophysical profile score. Magnesium sulfate may decrease fetal heart rate variability and breathing.[118, 119] However, one study by Gray et al.[117] showed that intravenous magnesium sulfate did not significantly alter the biophysical profile in 25 healthy preterm fetuses.

Methyldopa

A drug of first choice for the oral treatment of nonsevere hypertension in pregnancy is methyldopa. It is not suitable for acute therapy of severe preeclampsia because of its slow onset of action (4–6 hours). Methyldopa is a centrally acting antihypertensive. Possible cardiovascular side effects in the mother are a decreased heart rate and retention of sodium and water.[120] Maternal cerebral hemodynamics are also influenced by antihypertensive treatment with methyldopa. "α-Methyl-dopa reduces middle cerebral artery flow velocities suggesting a dilatation of the cerebral arteries."[121] During an average duration of treatment of 24 days, there were no negative effects on fetal hemodynamics.[122] Methyldopa reduces peripheral resistance in placental and umbilical vessels.

Occasionally, hypotension, hypoglycemia, reduced head circumference, and a Parkinson-like tremor have been observed in neonates after administration of methyldopa during pregnancy.[120] There is complete transfer of methyldopa to the fetus.

Adverse effects in the mother may be sedation and depression after the use of methyldopa.

Hydralazine

Hydralazine is a widely used drug for the management of severe hypertension in pregnancy.[123] It is a direct-acting vasodilator. Peripheral vascular resistance decreases and is accompanied by a reflex tachycardia, which leads to an increase in cardiac output.[120] Hydralazine can cause abrupt falls in perfusion pressure, resulting in fetal compromise. This problem may be reduced by adequate hydration prior to administration of hydralazine.[123] Hydralazine does not significantly increase or decrease uteroplacental blood flow.[124]

Of major concern are the common side effects of hydralazine—headache, dizziness, and paresthesias—which can disguise prodromal signs of eclampsia, thereby interfering with correct diagnosis.[120]

Labetalol

Labetalol is a combined α- and β-adrenoreceptor blocking drug, which is commonly used for the treatment of pregnancy-induced hypertension.[125] It is effective in lowering maternal blood pressure in patients with preeclampsia. It does not seem to influence either uteroplacental or fetal hemodynamics when given intravenously.[125] Oral treatment with labetalol does not have any effect on intrauterine growth or birthweight. Occasionally, a mild reduction of neonatal blood pressure during the first 24 hours after delivery is observed.[126]

Beta-Blocking Drugs

Beta-blocking drugs produce few side effects in the mother. On the other hand, a decrease of the fetal basal heart rate (without reaching the pathologic range) can occur.

Beta-blocking agents cause bronchoconstriction and are contraindicated in patients with asthma.

Beta-blocking agents should be avoided in pregnancies with severe intrauterine growth retardation because an increase in perinatal mortality rate has been observed.[120] It is possible that the fetus exposed to these drugs is not able to react adequately to additional hypoxia and stress.

Calcium Antagonists

Nifedipine produces a rapid and smooth decrease in blood pressure. The peripheral vascular resistance decreases and a baroreceptor-mediated compensating tachycardia occurs. Nifedipine can also normalize enhanced erythrocyte aggregation in preeclampsia.[120] The maternal cerebral circulation is influenced by nifedipine. Flow velocities in the middle cerebral artery decrease following administration of nifedipine, suggesting cerebral vasodilatation.[121] There is no reduction of uteroplacental blood flow.[127] If nifedipine is used together with magnesium sulfate, severe hypotension and fetal distress can result.[118]

Angiotensin-Converting Enzyme Inhibitors

Angiotensin-converting enzyme inhibitors are contraindicated during pregnancy because their use led to a higher incidence of stillbirths in animal experiments. In addition, severe fetal hypotension and acute renal failure in the neonate have been described in association with angiotensin-converting enzyme inhibitors.[120, 128]

ANTIASTHMATIC MEDICATION

Approximately 1% of all parturients suffer from asthma. The different groups of anti-asthmatic medications are discussed.

Inhaled Corticosteroids

Asthma is associated with inflammation of the airway mucosa in nearly all cases.[129, 130] This airway inflammation seems to be associated with increased bronchial responsiveness. Inhaled corticosteroids have no effect on airway smooth muscle, but they effectively reduce bronchial hyperreactivity and the symptoms of asthma.[130] Besides their anti-inflammatory effect, they seem to increase the effectiveness of β_2-agonists by inducing formation of new β-receptors.[129] During pregnancy, several endocrinologic changes take place. For example, elevations in free plasma cortisol and possible tissue refractoriness to corticosteroids may be observed.[129]

There are concerns about the potential adverse effects of oral or high-dose inhaled corticosteroids, such as adrenal suppression, weight gain, hypertension, diabetes, cataract, and osteoporosis in the mother and impaired growth in the fetus. Patients with severe asthma or systemic corticosteroid treatment during pregnancy seem to have a higher incidence of mild preeclampsia.[131] The effects on fetal bone development are unknown. It is not clear whether suppression of the hypothalamic-pituitary-adrenal axis can also be caused by inhaled corticosteroids in moderate doses.[129, 132]

Theophylline

Theophylline has been the most widely prescribed drug in pregnant women with asthma. The risk of congenital malformations does not seem to be increased with theophylline treatment during pregnancy.[129] High doses of theophylline can cause jitteriness, tachycardia, and vomiting. Life-threatening complications have been observed with severe toxic serum levels, such as seizures and cardiac dysrhythmias. The therapeutic range for theophylline is rather narrow. The serum concentration of theophylline should be maintained between 8 and 12 μg/mL during pregnancy.[129] Theophylline serum concentration can be influenced by other drugs. For example, cimetidine and erythromycin significantly increase the serum levels of theophylline. Compared with β_2-agonists, theophylline is a weak bronchodilator. Its long duration of action makes it especially suitable for the treatment of nocturnal asthma.

Inhaled β_2-Agonists

β_2-Agonists cause a rapid relaxation of bronchial smooth muscles and a rapid relief of acute bronchospasm. They are used in all degrees of asthma during

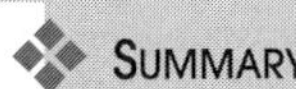

SUMMARY

Key Points

- Opioids, given by any route, can significantly delay gastric emptying.
- Maternally administered meperidine can produce neonatal respiratory depression, decreased Apgar scores, lower oxygen saturation, respiratory acidosis, and abnormal neurobehavior after birth. Fetal exposure to meperidine is highest 2 to 3 hours after intramuscular maternal drug administration.
- Ketamine is especially suitable for induction of general anesthesia in parturients with major hemorrhage and in parturients with severe asthma. Apgar scores were satisfactory in studies that used doses up to 1.2 mg/kg for intravenous induction.
- Passive tissue diffusion, rather than active drug transport, is probably the mechanism for placental transfer of bupivacaine. This transfer is influenced by the maternal and fetal plasma protein binding, the fetal pH, and placental uptake.

Key Reference

Bernstein K, Gisselsson L, Jacobsson L, et al: Influence of two different anaesthetic agents on the newborn and the correlation between foetal oxygenation and induction-delivery time in elective caesarean section. Acta Anaesthesiol Scand 1985; 29:157–160.

Case Stem

A 24-year-old parturient in active labor has been given two intramuscular injections of meperidine and is now requesting epidural analgesia. She is receiving intravenous oxytocin for stimulation of labor and magnesium sulfate for preeclampsia. Discuss the various agents and techniques that can be used to provide analgesia, and outline the possible interactions with the previously administered agents.

pregnancy. β_2-Agonists are very useful in the treatment of acute exacerbations of asthma, but they do not reduce airway hyperresponsiveness.[129]

CONCLUSION

This chapter describes the actions of some drugs encountered in pregnancy, labor, and delivery. Although this overview is far from complete, it should render the choice of commonly used drugs easier.

References

1. Gin T, Gregory MA, Chan K, et al: Maternal levels of propofol at cesarean section. Anaesth Intensive Care 1990; 18:180–184.
2. Gin T, Yau G, Chan K, et al: Disposition of propofol infusions for caesarean section. Can J Anaesth 1991; 38:31–36.
3. Celleno D, Capogna G, Tomassetti M, et al: Neurobehavioural effects of propofol on the neonate following elective caesarean section. Br J Anaesth 1989; 62:649–654.
4. Abboud TK, Zhu J, Richardson M, et al: Intravenous propofol vs thiamylal-isoflurane for caesarean section, comparative maternal and neonatal effects. Acta Anaesthesiol Scand 1995; 39:205–209.
5. Gregory MA, Gin T, Yau G, et al: Propofol infusion anaesthesia for caesarean section. Can J Anaesth 1990; 37:514–520.
6. Alon E, Ball RH, Gillie MH, et al: Effects of propofol and thiopental on maternal and fetal cardiovascular and acid-base variables in the pregnant ewe. Anesthesiology 1993; 78:562–576.
7. Shin YK, Kim YD, Collea JV: The effect of propofol on isolated human pregnant uterine muscle. Anesthesiology 1998; 89:105–109.
8. Bach V, Carl P, Ravlo O, et al: A randomized comparison between midazolam and thiopental for elective cesarean section anesthesia: III. Placental transfer and elimination in neonates. Anesth Analg 1989; 68:238–242.
9. Gin T, O'Meara ME, Kan AF, et al: Plasma catecholamines and neonatal condition after induction of anaesthesia with propofol or thiopentone at caesarean section. Br J Anaesth 1993; 70:311–316.
10. Yau G, Gin T, Ewart MC, et al: Propofol for induction and maintenance of anaesthesia at caesarean section: A comparison with thiopentone/enflurane. Anaesthesia 1991; 46:20–23.
11. Shnider SM, Levinson G: Anesthesia for cesarean section. *In* Shnider SM, Levinson G (eds): Anesthesia for Obstetrics, 3rd ed. Baltimore: Williams & Wilkins; 1993:211–245.
12. Krissel J, Dick WF, Leyser KH, et al: Thiopentone, thiopentone/ketamine, and ketamine for induction of anaesthesia in cesarean section. Eur J Anaesthesiol 1994; 11:115–122.
13. Allen J, Svane D, Petersen LK, et al: Effects of thiopentone and chlormethiazole on human myometrial arteries from term pregnant women. Br J Anaesth 1992; 68:256–260.
14. Adams HA, Hempelmann G: 20 Jahre Ketamin: Ein Überblick. Anaesthesist 1990; 39:71–76.
15. Reves JG, Glass PSA, Lubarsky DA: Nonbarbiturate intravenous anesthetics. *In* Miller RD (ed): Anesthesia, 4th ed, volume 1. New York: Churchill-Livingstone; 1994:260.
16. Bernstein K, Gisselsson L, Jacobsson L, et al: Influence of two different anaesthetic agents on the newborn and the correlation between foetal oxygenation and induction-delivery time in elective caesarean section. Acta Anaesthesiol Scand 1985; 29:157–160.
17. Shnider SM, Levinson G: Anesthesia for obstetrics. *In* Miller RD (ed): Anesthesia, 4th ed, volume 2. New York: Churchill-Livingstone; 1994:2031–2076.
18. Dich-Nielsen J, Holasek J: Ketamine as induction agent for caesarean section. Acta Anaesthesiol Scand 1982; 26:139–142.
19. Levinson G, Shnider SM: Systemic medication for labor and delivery. *In* Shnider SM, Levinson G (eds): Anesthesia for Obstetrics, 3rd ed. Baltimore: Williams & Wilkins; 1993:115–133.
20. Spielman H, Steinhof R (eds): Taschenbuch der Arzneimittelverordnung in Schwangerschaft und Stillperiode. Stuttgart: Gustav Fischer Verlag; 1989.
21. Schaut DJ, Khona R, Gross JB: Sevoflurane inhalation induction for emergency cesarean section in a parturient with no intravenous access. Anesthesiology 1997; 86:1392–1394.
22. Dwyer R, Fee JPH, Moore J: Uptake of halothane and isoflurane by mother and baby during caesarean section. Br J Anaesth 1995; 74:379–383.
23. Abboud TK, D'Onofrio L, Reyes A, et al: Isoflurane or halothane for cesarean section: Comparative maternal and neonatal effects. Acta Anaesthesiol Scand 1989; 33:578–581.
24. Warren TM, Datta S, Ostheimer GW, et al: Comparison of the maternal and neonatal effects of halothane, enflurane, and isoflurane for cesarean delivery. Anesth Analg 1983; 62:516–520.
25. Gambling DR, Sharma SK, White PF, et al: Use of sevoflurane during elective cesarean birth: A comparison with isoflurane and spinal anesthesia. Anesth Analg 1995; 81:90–95.
26. Abboud TK, Zhu J, Richardson M, et al: Desflurane: A new volatile anesthetic for cesarean section. Acta Anaesthesiol Scand 1995; 39:723–726.
27. Tatekawa S, Asada A, Nishikawa K, et al: Comparison of sevoflurane with isoflurane anesthesia for use in elective cesarean section. Anesthesiology 1993; 79:A1018.
28. Marcus MAE, Vertommen JD, Van Aken H: Hydroxyethyl starch versus lactated Ringer's solution in the chronic maternal-fetal sheep preparation: A pharmacodynamic and pharmacokinetic study. Anesth Analg 1995; 80:949–954.
29. Marcus MAE, Gogarten W, Buerkle H, et al: Are indexes the right way to interpret acute changes in uterine blood flow during epidural anesthesia in the parturient: Pain therapy & regional anesthesia, London, XVI. ESRA Congress, Sept. 17–20, 1997.
30. Wright PMC, Iftikhar M, Fitzpatrick KT, et al: Vasopressor therapy for hypotension during epidural anesthesia for cesarean section: Effects on maternal and fetal flow velocity ratios. Anesth Analg 1992; 75:56–63.
31. Philipson EH, Kuhnert B, Pimentel R, et al: Transient maternal hypotension following epidural anesthesia. Anesth Analg 1989; 69:604–607.
32. Karinen J, Räsänen J, Alahuhta S, et al: Maternal and uteroplacental haemodynamic state in pre-eclamptic patients during spinal anaesthesia for caesarean section. Br J Anaesth 1996; 76:616–620.
33. Kuhnert BR: Human perinatal pharmacology: Recent controversies. *In* Reynolds F (ed): Effects on the Baby of Maternal Analgesia and Anaesthesia. London: WB Saunders; 1993:46–66.
34. Cole CP, McMorland GH, Axelson JE, et al: Epidural blockade for cesarean section comparing lidocaine hydrocarbonate and lidocaine hydrochloride. Anesthesiology 1985; 62:348–350.
35. Guay J, Gaudreault P, Boulanger A, et al: Lidocaine hydrocarbonate and lidocaine hydrochloride for cesarean section: Transplacental passage and neonatal effects. Acta Anaesthesiol Scand 1992; 36:722–727.
36. Johnson RF, Herman NL, Johnson V, et al: Effects of fetal pH on local anesthetic transfer across the human placenta. Anesthesiology 1996; 85:608–615.
37. Abboud TK, Kim KC, Noueihed R, et al: Epidural bupivacaine, chloroprocaine, or lidocaine for cesarean section: Maternal and neonatal effects. Anesth Analg 1983; 62:914–919.
38. Abboud TK, Sarkis F, Blikian A, et al: Lack of adverse neonatal neurobehavioral effects of lidocaine. Anesth Analg 1983; 62:473–475.
39. Loftus JR, Holbrook H, Cohen S: Fetal heart rate after epidural lidocaine and bupivacaine for elective cesarean section. Anesthesiology 1991; 75:406–412.
40. Abboud TK, Afrasiabi A, Sarkis F, et al: Continuous infusion

epidural analgesia in parturients receiving bupivacaine, chloroprocaine, or lidocaine: Maternal, fetal, and neonatal effects. Anesth Analg 1984; 63:421–428.
41. Johnson RF, Herman N, Arney TL, et al: Bupivacaine transfer across the human term placenta. Anesthesiology 1995; 82:459–468.
42. Ala-Kokko TI, Pienimäki P, Herva R, et al: Transfer of lidocaine and bupivacaine across the isolated perfused placenta. Pharmacol Toxicol 1995; 77:142–148.
43. Santos AC, Pedersen H, Harmon TW, et al: Does pregnancy alter the systemic toxicity of local anesthetics? Anesthesiology 1989; 70:991–995.
44. Morishima HO, Pedersen H, Finster M, et al: Bupivacaine toxicity in pregnant and nonpregnant ewes. Anesthesiology 1985; 63:134–139.
45. Santos AC, Arthur GR, Wlody D, et al: Comparative systemic toxicity of ropivacaine and bupivacaine in nonpregnant and pregnant ewes. Anesthesiology 1995; 82:734–740.
46. Steiger RM, Nageotte MP: Effect of uterine contractility and maternal hypotension on prolonged decelerations after bupivacaine epidural anesthesia. Am J Obstet Gynecol 1990; 163:808–812.
47. Abboud TK, Khoo SS, Miller F, et al: Maternal, fetal, and neonatal responses after epidural anesthesia with bupivacaine, 2-chloroprocaine, or lidocaine. Anesth Analg 1982; 61:638–644.
48. Alahuhta S, Räsänen J, Jouppila P, et al: Uteroplacental and fetal circulation during extradural bupivacaine-adrenaline and bupivacaine for caesarean section in hypertensive pregnancies with chronic fetal asphyxia. Br J Anaesth 1993; 71:348–353.
49. Santos AC, Arthur GR, Roberts DJ, et al: Effect of ropivacaine and bupivacaine on uterine blood flow in pregnant ewes. Anesth Analg 1992; 74:62–67.
50. Datta S, Camann W, Bader A, et al: Clinical effects and maternal and fetal plasma concentrations of epidural ropivacaine versus bupivacaine for cesarean section. Anesthesiology 1995; 82:1346–1352.
51. Santos AC, Arthur GR, Pedersen H, et al: Systemic toxicity of ropivacaine during ovine pregnancy. Anesthesiology 1991; 75:137–141.
52. Morton CPJ, Bloomfield S, Magnusson A, et al: Ropivacaine 0.75% for extradural anaesthesia in elective caesarean section: An open clinical and pharmacokinetic study in mother and neonate. Br J Anaesth 1997; 79:3–8.
53. Irestedt L, Emanuelsson BM, Ekblom A, et al: Ropivacaine 7.5 mg/ml for elective caesarean section: A clinical and pharmacokinetic comparison of 150 mg and 187.5 mg. Acta Anaesthesiol Scand 1997; 41:1149–1156.
54. Alahuhta S, Räsänen J, Jouppila P, et al: The effects of epidural ropivacaine and bupivacaine for cesarean section on uteroplacental and fetal circulation. Anesthesiology 1995; 83:23–32.
55. Lewis RB, Sculman JD: Influence of acetylsalicylic acid, an inhibitor of prostaglandin synthesis, on the duration of human gestation and labour. Lancet 1973; 11:1159–1161.
56. Levin DL, Mills LJ, Weinberg AG: Hemodynamic, pulmonary vascular, and myocardial abnormalities secondary to pharmacologic constriction of the fetal ductus arteriosus. A possible mechanism for persistent pulmonary hypertension and transient tricuspic incompetence in new-born infants. Circulation 1979; 60:360–364.
57. Scott PV, Bowen FE, Cartwright P, et al: Intrathecal morphine as a sole analgesic during labour. Anesthesiology 1981; 54:136–140.
58. Baraka A, Noueihid RD, Haji S: Intrathecal injection of morphine for obstetric analgesia. Anesthesiology 1981; 54:136–140.
59. Abboud TK, Shnider SM, Daily A: Intrathecal administration of hyperbaric morphine for the relief of pain in labour. Br J Anaesth 1984; 56:1351–1359.
60. Leighton BL, DeSimone CA, Norris MC, et al: Intrathecal narcotics for labor revisited: The combination of fentanyl and morphine intrathecally provides rapid onset of profound, prolonged analgesia. Anesth Analg 1989; 69:122–125.
61. Hughes SC, Rosen MA, Shnider SM, et al: Maternal and neonatal effects of epidural morphine for labor and delivery. Anesth Analg 1984; 63:318–324.
62. Crawford JS, Rudofsky S: The placental transmission of pethidine. Br J Anaesth 1965; 37:929–933.
63. Shnider SM, Moya F: Effects of meperidine on the newborn infant. Am J Obstet Gynecol 1964; 89:1009–1011.
64. Taylor ES, von Fumetti HH, Essig LL: The effects of demerol and trichloroethylene on arterial oxygen saturation in the newborn. Am J Obstet Gynecol 1955; 69:348.
65. Roberts H, Kane KM, Percival N: Effects of some analgesic drugs used in childbirth. Lancet 1957; 1:128–130.
66. Koch G, Wandel H: Effect of meperidine on the postnatal adjustment of respiration and acid-base balance. Acta Obstet Gynecol Scand 1968; 47:27–37.
67. Brackbill Y, Kane J, Maniello RL: Obstetric meperidine usage and assessment of neonatal status. Anesthesiology 1974; 40:116–120.
68. Savonna-Ventura C, Sammut M, Sammut C: Meperidine blood concentrations at time of birth. Int J Gynecol Obstet 1991; 36:103–107.
69. Rhien A, Rhien F, Wiedemann B, et al: Pethidine-Anwendung bei Geburten mit mekoniumhaltigem Fruchtwasser: Einfluss auf fetal Outcome und respiratorische Störungen. Z Geburtsh Neonatol 1995; 199:103–106.
70. Rayburn W, Rathke A, Leuschen MP, et al: Fentanyl citrate analgesia during labor. Am J Obstet Gynecol 1989; 161:202–206.
71. Rayburn W, Smith CV, Parriott JE, et al: Randomized comparison of meperidine and fentanyl during labor. Obstet Gynecol 1989; 74:604–607.
72. Craft JR, Coaldrake LA, Bolan JC, et al: Placental passage and uterine effects of fentanyl. Anesth Analg 1983; 62:894–898.
73. Esthaphenous FG: Opioids in Anesthesia. Boston: Butterworth Publishers; 1984:104–108.
74. Leight CH, Evans DE, Durkin WJ: Intrathecal sufentanil for labor analgesia: Results of a pilot study. Anesthesiology 1990; 73:A980.
75. Honet JE, Arkoosh VA, Norris MC, et al: Comparison among intrathecal fentanyl, meperidine, and sufentanil for labor analgesia. Anesth Analg 1992; 75:734–739.
76. Zakowsky MI, Goldstein MJ, Ramanathan S, et al: Intrathecal fentanyl for labor analgesia. Anesthesiology 1991; 75:A840.
77. Rust LA, Waring RW, Hall GL, et al: Intrathecal narcotics for obstetric analgesia in a community hospital. Am J Obstet Gynecol 1994; 170:1643–1648.
78. Cohen SE, Tan S, Albright GA, et al: Epidural fentanyl/bupivacaine mixtures for obstetric analgesia. Anesthesiology 1987; 67:403–407.
79. Celleno D, Capogna G: Epidural fentanyl plus bupivacaine 0.125 per cent for labour: Analgesic effects. Can J Anaesth 1988; 35:375–378.
80. Brockway MS, Noble DW, Sharwood-Smith GH, et al: Profound respiratory depression after extradural fentanyl. Br J Anaesth 1990; 64:243–245.
81. Wang CY: Respiratory depression after extradural fentanyl. Br J Anaesth 1992; 69:544.
82. Noble DW, Morrison LM, Brockway MS, et al: Adrenaline, fentanyl, or adrenaline and fentanyl as adjuncts to bupivacaine for extradural anaesthesia in elective caesarean section. Br J Anaesth 1991; 66:645–650.
83. Carrie LES, O'Sullivan GM, Seegobin R: FORUM epidural fentanyl in labour. Anaesthesia 1981; 36:965–969.
84. Preston MD, Rosen M, Daniels M, et al: Epidural fentanyl with lidocaine for cesarean section [abstract]. Anesthesiology 1987; 67:A442.
85. Craft JB, Robichaux AG, Kim H, et al: The maternal and fetal cardiovascular effects of epidural fentanyl in the sheep model. Am J Obstet Gynecol 1984; 148:1098–1104.
86. Bader A, Fragneto R, Terui K, et al: Maternal and neonatal fentanyl and bupivacaine concentrations after epidural infusions during labor. Anesth Analg 1995; 81:829–832.
87. Vertommen JD, Marcus MAE, Van Aken H: The effects of intravenous and epidural sufentanil in the chronic maternal-fetal sheep preparation. Anesth Analg 1995; 80:71–75.
88. D'Angelo R, Anderson MT, Philip J, et al: Intrathecal

sufentanil compared to epidural bupivacaine for labor analgesia. Anesthesiology 1994; 80:1209–1215.

89. Grieco W, Norris M, Leighton BL, et al: Intrathecal sufentanil analgesia: The effects of adding morphine or epinephrine. Anesth Analg 1993; 77:1149–1154.
90. Cohen S, Amar D, Pantuck CB, et al: Postcesarean delivery epidural patient-controlled analgesia. Anesthesiology 1993; 78:486–491.
91. Campbell DC, Camann WR, Datta S: The addition of bupivacaine to intrathecal sufentanil for labor analgesia. Anesth Analg 1995; 81:305–309.
92. Jorrot JC, Lirzin JD, Daillard P, et al: A combination of sufentanil and 0.25% bupivacaine administered epidurally for obstetrical analgesia: Comparison with fentanyl and placebo. Ann Fr Anesth Reanim 1989; 8:321–325.
93. Van Steenberghe A, Debroux HC, Noorduin LH: Extradural bupivacaine with sufentanil for vaginal delivery. Br J Anaesth 1987; 59:1518–1522.
94. Vertommen JD, Vandermeulen E, Van Aken H, et al: The effects of the addition of sufentanil to 0.125% bupivacaine on the quality of analgesia during labor and on the incidence of instrumental deliveries. Anesthesiology 1991; 74:809–814.
95. Van Aken H, Kick O, WeiBauer W: Geburtshilfliche Periduralanästhesie mit Sufentanil. Anaesthesist 1994; 43:667–670.
96. Palot M, Visseaux H, Botmans C, et al: Placental transfer and neonatal distribution of fentanyl, alfentanil, and sufentanil after continuous epidural administration for labor. Anesthesiology 1992; 77:A991.
97. Loftus JR, Hill H, Cohen SE: Placental transfer and neonatal effects of epidural sufentanil and fentanyl administration with bupivacaine during labor. Anesthesiology 1995; 83:300–308.
98. Ewah B, Yau K, King M: Effect of epidural opioids on gastric emptying in labour. Int J Obstet Anesth 1993; 2:125–128.
99. Wright PMC, Allen RW, Moore J, et al: Gastric emptying during lumbar extradural analgesia in labour: Effect of fentanyl supplementation. Br J Anaesth 1992; 68:248–251.
100. Geddes SM, Thorbum J, Logan RW: Gastric emptying following caesarean section and the effect of epidural fentanyl. Anaesthesia 1991; 46:1016–1018.
101. Zimmerman DL, Breen TW, Fick G: Adding fentanyl 0.0002% to epidural bupivacaine 0.125% does not delay gastric emptying in laboring parturients. Anesth Analg 1996; 82:612–616.
102. Norris MC, Grieco WM, Borkowski M, et al: Complications of labor analgesia: Epidural versus combined spinal epidural techniques. Anesth Analg 1994; 79:529–537.
103. Newton ER, Schroeder BC, Knape KG, et al: Epidural analgesia and uterine function. Obstet Gynecol 1995; 85:749–755.
104. Chestnut DH, Vincent DR Jr, Mcgrath JM, et al: Does early administration of epidural analgesia affect obstetric outcome in nulliparous women who are receiving intravenous oxytocin? Anesthesiology 1994; 80:1193–1200.
105. Arend L, Arnim von B, Nijsen J: Tramadol and pentazocin in a double blind crossover comparison. Arzneim Forsch Drug Res 1978; 28(1a):199–208.
106. Cossmann M, Wilsman KM: Application of tramadol injection (TRAMAL®) in acute pain: Open trial to assess the acute effect and safety after a single parenteral administration. Therapeut News 1988; 130(36):633–636.
107. Bitsch M, Emmrich J, Hary J: Obstetric analgesia with tramadol. Fortschr Med 1980; 16:632–634.
108. Viegas OAC, Khaw B, Ratnam SS: Tramadol in labour pain in primiparous patients. A prospective comparative clinical trial. Eur J Obstet Gynecol Reprod Biol 1993; 49:131–135.
109. Kan RE, Hughes SC, Rosen MA, et al: Intravenous remifentanil: Placental transfer, maternal and neonatal effects. Anesthesiology 1998; 88:1167–1174.
110. Gogarten W, Van Aken H, Brodner G, et al: Hemodynamic effects and placental transfer after continuous intravenous application of remifentanil in the chronic maternal-fetal sheep preparation. Anesth Analg 1999, in press.
111. Marcus MAE, Gogarten W, Van Aken H, et al: Remifentanil for fetal intrauterine microendoscopic procedures. Anesth Analg Feb 1999, p S257.
112. Kyank H: Praeeklampsie und Eklampsie. *In* Kyank H, Gulzow MG (eds): Erkrankungen in der Schwangerschaft. Leipzig: Thieme, 1979:229–244.
113. Kyank H, Birnbaum H: Chronische hypertonie. *In* Kyank H, Gulzow MG (eds): Erkrankungen in der Schwangerschaft. Leipzig: Thieme, 1979:136–149.
114. Flowers CE: Discussionsbemerkungen. Am J Obstet Gynecol 1975; 123:549.
115. Zaret GM: Possible treatment of pre-eclampsia with calcium channel blocking agents. Med Hypotheses 1983; 12:303–319.
116. Sadeh M: Action of magnesium sulfate in the treatment of preeclampsia-eclampsia. Stroke 1989; 20:1273–1275.
117. Gray SE, Rodis JF, Lettieri L, et al: Effects of intravenous magnesium sulfate on the biophysical profile of the healthy preterm fetus. Am J Obstet Gynecol 1994; 170:1131–1135.
118. Rey E, LeLorier J, Burgess E, et al: Report of the Canadian Hypertension Society Consensus Conference: 3. Pharmacologic treatment of hypertensive disorders in pregnancy. Can Med Assoc J 1997; 157(9):1245–1254.
119. Carlan SJ, O'Brien WF: The effect of magnesium sulfate on the biophysical profile of normal term fetuses. Obstet Gynecol 1991; 77:681–684.
120. Rath W: Die Behandlung hypertensiver Schwangerschaftserkrankungen-allgemeine MassBnahmen und orale Langzeittherapie. Z Geburtsh Neonatol 1997; 201:240–246.
121. Serra-Serra V, Kyle PM, Chandran R, et al: The effect of nifedipine and methyldopa on maternal cerebral circulation. Br J Obstet Gynaecol 1997; 104:532–537.
122. Montan S, Anandakumar C, Arulkumaran S, et al: Effects of methyldopa on uteroplacental and fetal hemodynamics in pregnancy-induced hypertension. Am J Obstet Gynecol 1993; 168:152–156.
123. Steyn DW, Odendaal HJ: Dihydralazine or ketanserin for severe hypertension in pregnancy? Preliminary results. Eur J Obstet Gynecol Reprod Biol 1997; 75:155–159.
124. Lunell NO, Lewander R, Nylund L, et al: Acute effect of dihydralazine on uteroplacental blood flow in hypertension during pregnancy. Gynecol Obstet Invest 1983; 16:274–282.
125. Jouppila P, Kirkinen P, Koivula A, et al: Labetalol does not alter the placental and fetal blood flow or maternal prostanoids in pre-eclampsia. Br J Obstet Gynaecol 1986; 93:543–547.
126. Pickles CJ, Symonds EM, Pipkin FB: The fetal outcome in a randomized double-blind controlled trial of labetalol versus placebo in pregnancy-induced hypertension. Br J Obstet Gynaecol 1989; 96:38–43.
127. Lindow SW, Davies N, Davey DA, et al: The effect of sublingual nifedipine on uteroplacental blood flow in hypertensive pregnancy. Br J Obstet Gynaecol 1988; 95:1276–1281.
128. Rosa FW, Bosco LA, Graham CF, et al: Neonatal anuria with maternal angiotensin-converting enzyme inhibition. Obstet Gynecol 1989; 74:371–374.
129. Dombrowski MP: Pharmacologic therapy of asthma during pregnancy. Obstet Gynecol Clin North Am 1997; 24:559–574.
130. Haahtela T, Järvinen M, Kava T, et al: Comparison of a β_2-agonist, terbutaline, with an inhaled corticosteroid, budesonide, in newly detected asthma. N Engl J Med 1991; 325:388–392.
131. Stenius-Aarniala B, Piirilä P, Teramo K: Asthma and pregnancy: A prospective study of 198 pregnancies. Thorax 1988; 43:12–18.
132. Tabachnik E, Zadik Z: Diurnal cortisol secretion during therapy with inhaled beclomethasone dipropionate in children with asthma. J Pediatr 1991; 118:294–297.

9

Functional Anatomy of Central Blockade in Obstetrics

KENNETH KARDASH, MD, FRCPC

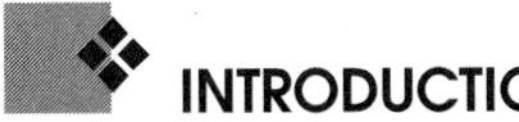

INTRODUCTION

A detailed knowledge of pertinent spinal anatomy is essential for the anesthesiologist wishing successful needle placement. This knowledge is also important in order to understand the patterns and limits of distribution of injected agents. This has applications in controlling the spread of analgesia and anesthesia as well as correcting abnormal spread. Unless otherwise specified in this chapter, the term *epidural* refers to the lumbar epidural space.

SPINAL ANATOMY

Vertebral Surface Landmarks

Knowledge of segmental differences in spinal anatomy is prerequisite to the safe performance of central neuraxial blockade. For this knowledge to be safely applied, accurate surface anatomic landmarks of various vertebral levels are needed. The most useful of these are presented in Figure 9–1. A very commonly used and important landmark, Tuffier's line is made by joining the tops of the iliac crests. This intercristal line usually crosses the spine at the level of the L4 spinous process. Since the spinal cord terminates at or above the L1 to L2 intervertebral disk in most adults, lumbar neuraxial blockade is usually performed no more than two interspaces above Tuffier's line, to avoid possible cord trauma. However, there is a normal distribution among individual patients in both the termination of the cord and the anatomic level of the intercristal line (Fig. 9–2).[1] In addition, in pregnancy the weight of the gravid uterus increases lumbar lordosis and rotates the pelvis anteriorly, so that the intercristal line tends to be higher than the L4 spinous process.[2] Because of these considerations, caution should be exercised in performing spinal anesthesia more than one interspace above this landmark in obstetric patients.

For anesthesiologists who choose to undertake epidural puncture in the thoracic region, it should be noted that the landmark for the T7 vertebra in Figure 9–1 is based on the scapular position when the arms are hanging freely by the sides.

Vertebral Column

The human spine consists at birth of 33 vertebrae categorized into 5 segments: 7 cervical, 12 thoracic, 5 lumbar, 5 sacral, and 4 coccygeal. With age, the coccygeal vertebrae fuse completely and the sacral nearly so. When lying supine, the spinal column has four curves of importance in regard to the spread of injected drugs, particularly in the subarachnoid space: the cervical lordosis, the lumbar lordosis, and the anterior concavity of the thoracic and sacrococcygeal elements, respectively. Normally, the supine lumbar spine slopes downward from a high point at the L4 vertebra to a nadir at vertebra T8. The thoracic spine then slopes upward from this point at an angle of 23 degrees. Although pregnancy causes an exaggeration of the normal lumbar lordosis in the standing position, this effect disappears when the patient lies supine. The combined effect of the weight of the uterus and the increased laxity of spinal ligaments[3] in late pregnancy causes changes in both the lumbar lordosis and thoracic kyphosis when supine (Fig. 9–3).[4] The spine's apex moves down to the L5 vertebra and its low point is displaced upward to the T6 to T7 vertebral level. The upslope of the thoracic kyphosis is reduced to 16 degrees. These changes may contribute to the enhanced cephalad spread of hyperbaric spinal anesthetics in pregnancy.

Each vertebra consists of an anterior load-bearing body connected to a posterior laminar arch to form

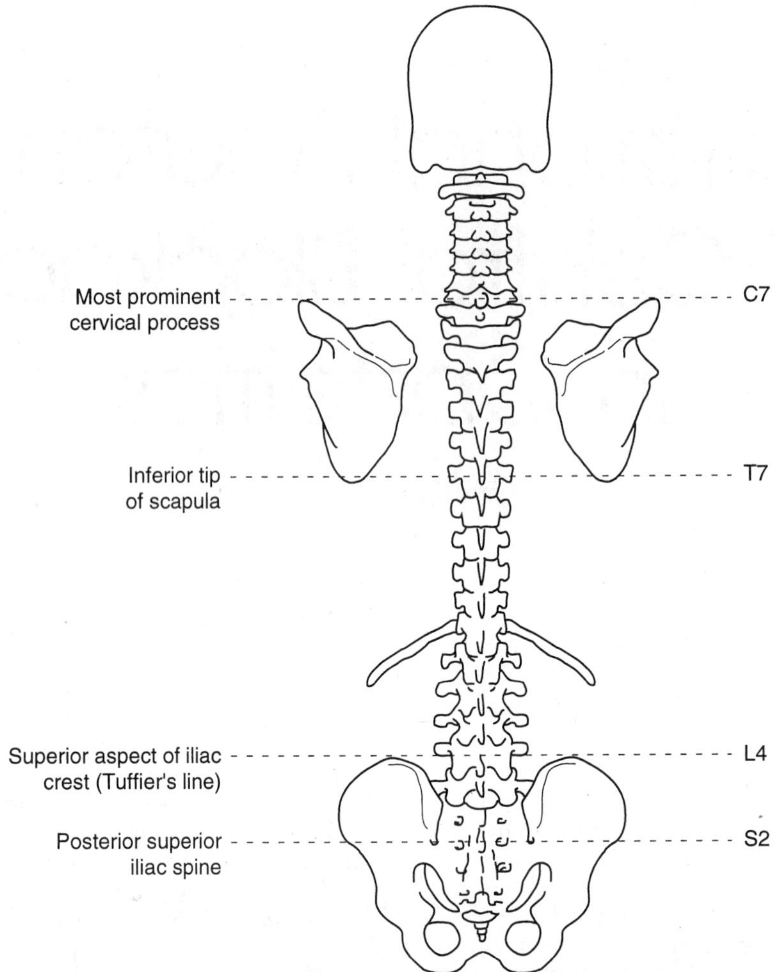

❖ **Figure 9–1** Surface landmarks of vertebral segments. Scapular position is with arms hanging by sides.

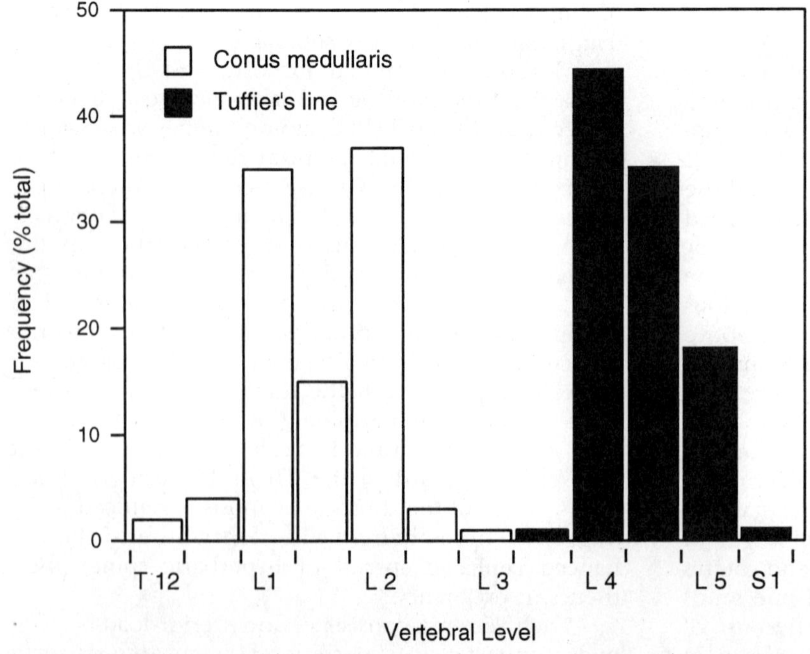

❖ **Figure 9–2** Frequency distribution of vertebral level where the spinal cord terminates and where Tuffier's line (between iliac crests) crosses the spine. Spaces between vertebral levels represent disk spaces. (Data from Hogan QH: Tuffier's line: the normal distribution of anatomic parameters [letter]. Anesth Analg 1994; 78:194.)

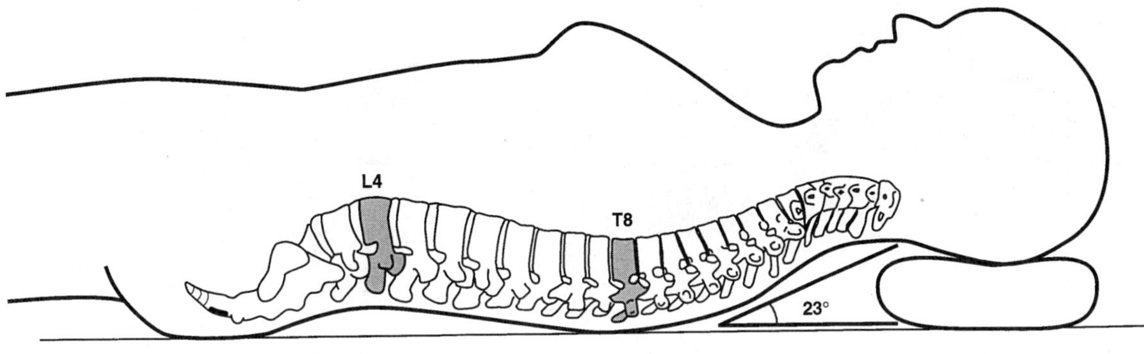

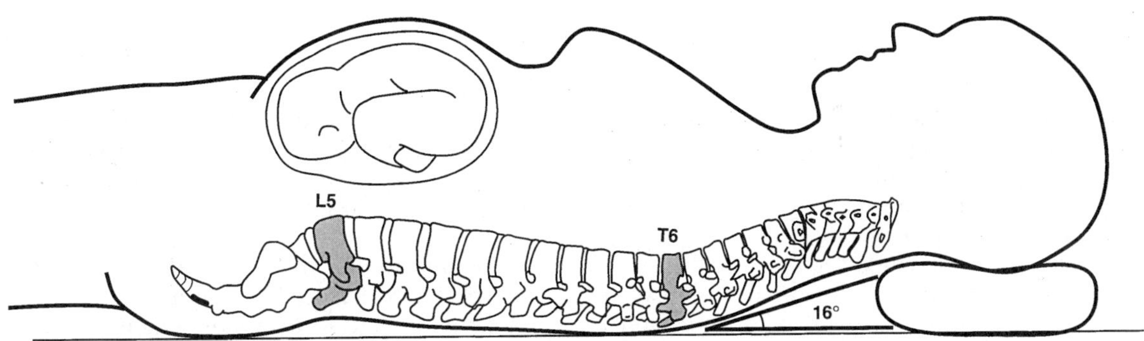

Figure 9–3 Spinal configuration in the supine position in the nonpregnant female *(top)* and in late pregnancy *(bottom)*. The apex of the lumbar lordosis is moved caudad and the thoracic kyphosis reduced in the parturient. Median high and low points of the two curves are shaded. (Data from Hirabayashi Y, Shimizu R, Fukuda H, et al: Anatomical configuration of the spinal column in the supine position. II. Comparison of pregnant and non-pregnant women. Br J Anaesth 1995; 75:6–8.)

the spinal canal (Fig. 9–4). These two components are joined by bony pedicles at the upper half of the vertebral body. Intervertebral foramina, formed between adjacent pedicles and allowing for the passage of spinal nerves and vessels, are thus created at the lower half of each vertebral body. Because the spinal canal has a triangular, posterior-pointing configuration, the posterior epidural space is always widest in the midline. The pedicles bear superior and inferior facets to articulate with adjacent laminar arches. Transverse processes for muscle attachments project from the pedicles anteriorly in the cervical and lumbar regions, and posteriorly in the thoracic region. The laminar arch slopes downward and posteriorly; thus the underlying epidural space is always widest at the inferior laminar edge (Fig. 9–5). Spinous processes angle downward at varying degrees from the midline of the lamina, overlapping most in the midthoracic region and becoming almost

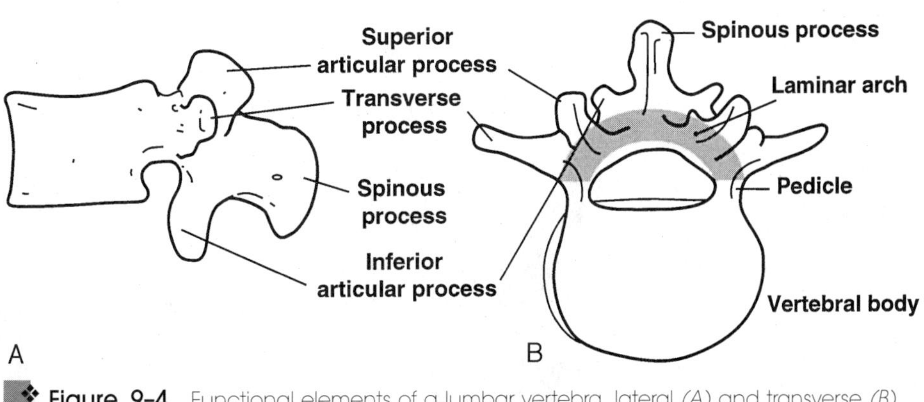

Figure 9–4 Functional elements of a lumbar vertebra, lateral *(A)* and transverse *(B)* aspects.

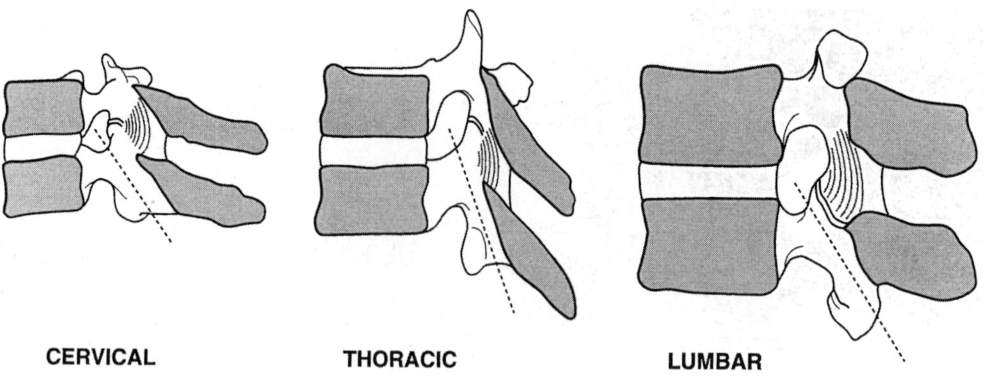

Figure 9–5 Downward-posterior sloping of vertebral lamina is consistent throughout the spine. As the bony posterior wall of the epidural space, this tends to make the epidural space widest at the inferior edge of the lamina, adjacent to the caudal surface of the attached spinous process.

horizontal in the lumbar segments. The space between adjacent laminae is always greater than that between adjacent spinous processes; this is the anatomic basis for paramedian access to the spinal canal. In the lumbar region, the spinous processes extend in a nearly horizontal direction. Their caudad tips overlie the middle of the interlaminar space. Their cephalad tips overlie the middle of the lamina to which they are connected, a landmark for the paramedian technique. In the midthoracic region, the marked downslope of the spinous processes brings their caudad tips even with the middle of the laminar arch of the vertebra below (Fig. 9–6).

In the sacrum, the vertebral bodies and laminae undergo bony fusion by adulthood. The fusion remains incomplete to a variable extent in the midline

Thoracic

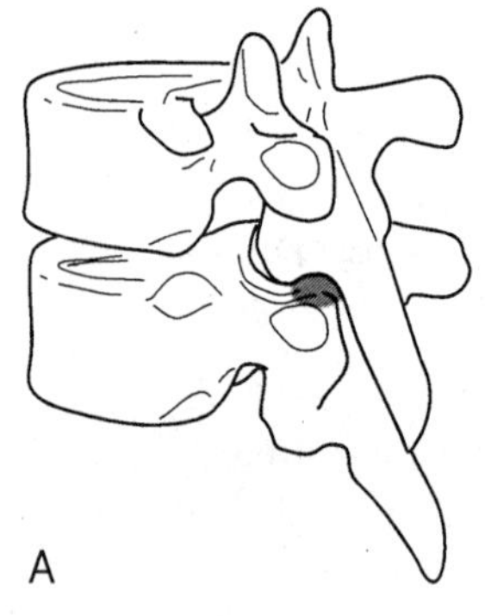

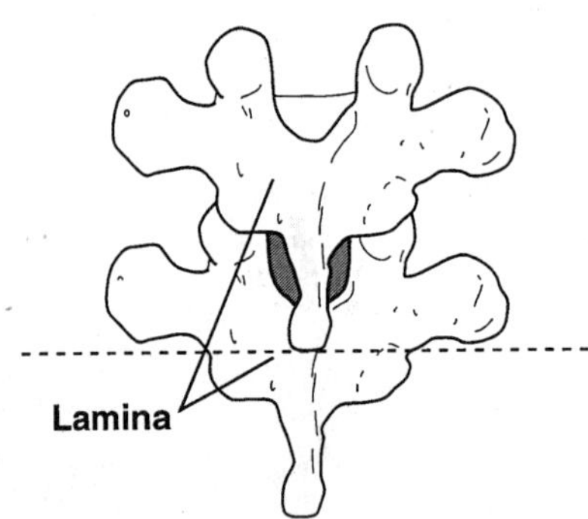

Lumbar

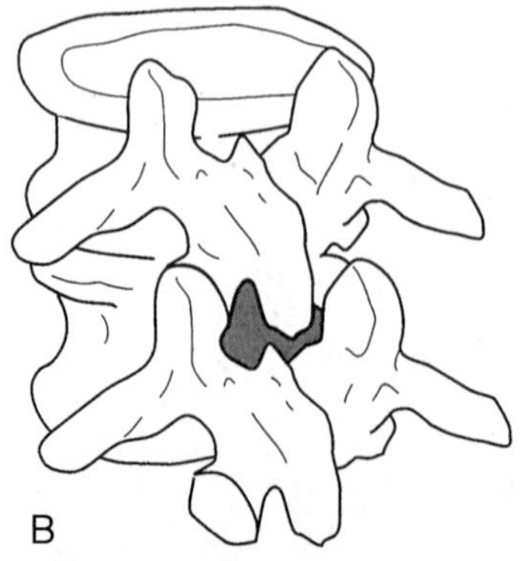

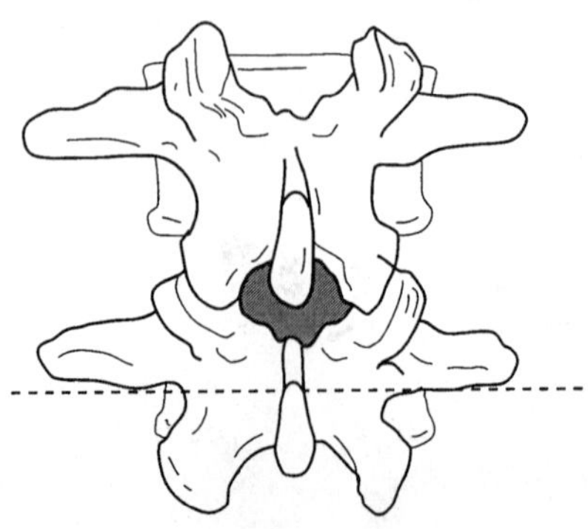

Figure 9–6 The interlaminar space and its relationship to the spinous processes, left posterior oblique (*A* and *B*, *left side of figure*) and posterior (*A* and *B*, *right side of figure*) views. Note that the interlaminar space is wider than the space between adjacent spinous processes, the basis for the paramedian approach. At the midthoracic level (*A*, *right side*) the spinous process of each vertebra overlaps the lamina of the vertebra below. At the lumbar level (*B*, *right side*) the cephalad tip of the spinous process is in line with the lamina of the same vertebra (see also Fig. 9–15).

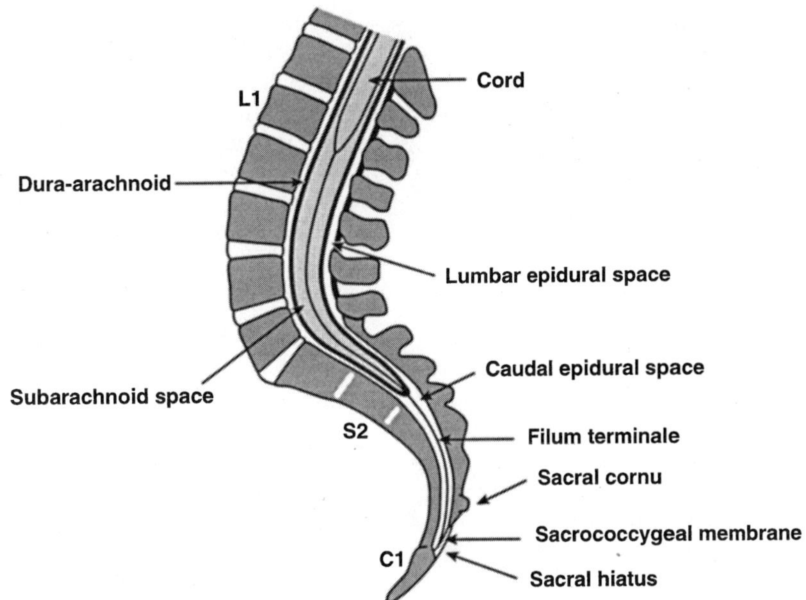

❖ **Figure 9–7** Termination of the spinal cord, dural sac, and epidural space. The cord is anchored by the filum terminale, formed from the pia mater then invested by dura. It is attached to the sacrococcygeal membrane, the inferior boundary of the epidural space.

at the caudad end, creating the sacral hiatus. Covered by the sacrococcygeal membrane, the sacral hiatus serves as the inferior terminus of the epidural space and the entry site for caudal epidural injection. The adjacent sacral cornua, which serve as landmarks for this approach, are vestiges of the inferior articular facets of the fifth sacral vertebra (Fig. 9–7).

Spinal Ligaments

The spinal vertebrae are held together and strengthened by a system of ligaments. The vertebral bodies and disks are connected by thick anterior and thin posterior longitudinal ligaments. Often giving rise to confusion because it is named in relation to the vertebral bodies it binds, the posterior longitudinal ligament lies at the *anterior* boundary of the epidural space.

The following ligaments, of relevance to the anesthesiologist, are traversed in sequence during a midline approach to central blockade (Fig. 9–8).

Supraspinous Ligament. The supraspinous ligament is a broad, tough fibrous cord that connects the tips of the spinous processes. In the cervical spine it becomes the ligamentum nuchae and anchors to the external occipital protuberance. At the lumbar level, it becomes progressively thicker in a caudal direction.

Interspinous Ligament. If a scrupulously midline approach is followed, the needle passes the length of this weblike connection between adjacent spinous processes. The interspinous ligament fuses with the supraspinous ligament posteriorly and the ligamentum flavum anteriorly. Like the supraspinous ligament, this ligament becomes thicker caudally. Below the L4 to L5 vertebral level, however, it becomes somewhat less defined.[5] The fibrous nature of the tissue imparts a more clicking sensation as the advancing needle cuts through collagen fibers, as opposed to the parting of elastic tissue in the ligamentum flavum.[6]

Ligamentum Flavum. The Latin word *flavum* means yellow, referring to the color imparted to the

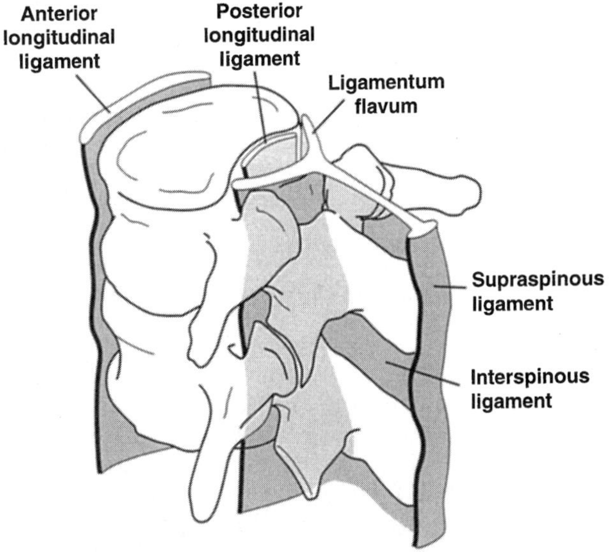

❖ **Figure 9–8** Spinal ligaments. Each half of the ligamentum flavum thickens as it approaches the midline, where it may fuse with the other half. Because it is V-shaped, needles in the midline or paramedian plane will pass somewhat obliquely through its fibers, increasing the perceived thickness. Note that the posterior longitudinal ligament forms the anterior boundary of the epidural space.

ligament by its elastin content. The ligamentum flavum connects the bony laminae of adjacent vertebrae, thus providing a soft tissue continuation of the posterior wall of the spinal canal. Although referred to as a single ligament, it is really composed of two halves, running along each lamina on either side of the spinous process. They join the interior portion of the lamina above to the exterior surface of the one below. The two halves fuse variably in the midline, where tiny nutrient vessels must pass. The thickness of the ligament increases steadily with each segment caudally, achieving 3 to 5 mm at the lumbar level. In the lumbar region the two halves meet at an angle of 70 to 80 degrees in the midline.[7] This acute angulation ensures that a midline or paramedian needle approach passes through a depth of ligament greater than its thickness (see Fig. 9–8). The ligamenta flava are the last structure through which an advancing needle must pass before entering the epidural space and their 80% elastin content[6] transmits a tactile sensation of gripping tightness as they are breached.

Dura

At the foramen magnum where the spinal cord exits the base of the skull, the cerebral dura splits into an outer layer continuous with the vertebral periosteum, and into the inner dura or *theca,* which hangs as a cylindrical sac down to its termination at the S2 vertebral level. It is a tough fibroelastic sheath whose collagen fibers run mostly in a longitudinal direction in humans to support the vertical load of the spinal fluid and tissue within.[8] A Quincke-tipped needle bevel turned parallel to the spinal axis is thus less likely to transect the supporting fibers, and the resulting puncture hole is smaller than with a perpendicular approach.[9] In vivo, this seems to lower the incidence of postdural puncture headache.[10–12] The dura becomes progressively thinner as it descends in the spinal canal, measuring 0.3 to 1.0 mm in thickness at the lumbar level.[13] Throughout its course, the dura seems strong enough to resist puncture by an epidural catheter unless it is first nicked by a needle.[14] Thickest in the posterior midline, it thins laterally as it stretches as a cuff or sleeve over the nerve roots before ultimately blending with the epineurium of the spinal nerves where their anterior and posterior roots combine into a single nerve trunk. It is this dural cuff, pierced by arachnoid granulations, lymphatics, and blood vessels, that likely provides the first site of penetration of epidural drugs to the central nervous system (CNS) (Fig. 9–9). The lateral extent of this dural cuff varies with the vertebral level, gradually moving from just outside the intervertebral foramen at the cervical level to being completely within the spinal canal in the lumbosacral region.[15]

The dural sac is anchored caudally to the coccygeal periosteum; it is intermittently tethered posteriorly to the laminae and anteriorly to the posterior longitudinal ligament as well. This can result in the dura tensing and stretching slightly cephalad during spinal flexion.[16] It has been postulated that puncturing the dura when tensed with exaggerated spinal flexion may give rise to larger puncture holes.[17] Cineradiographic studies[18] have demonstrated that the dural sac is not a passive structure of fixed dimensions. It expands or contracts almost immediately in response to changes in epidural pressure or CNS blood volume, acting as a reservoir for the translocation of spinal fluid between the cranium and spinal canal. Thus, the dura is compressed during a cough or Valsalva maneuver and contracts in response to cerebral vasoconstriction during hyperventilation. When fluid is injected into the epidural space, the dura is transiently compressed, acting as a buffer to increases in epidural pressure.[19, 20]

Arachnoid

The arachnoid mater is a thin, filmy membrane closely applied to the inner surface of the dura throughout the CNS. It consists of several loosely bound layers of epithelial cells with tight junctions between them to contain the cerebrospinal fluid (CSF) on its inner aspect. Unlike the dura, it serves as more than an inert, protective barrier. Its cells are metabolically active in transporting CSF and debris out of the subarachnoid space by a process of transmembrane vacuolization (see Fig. 9–9).[21] This clearance function is localized in the arachnoid granulations, or villi; these outpouchings of arachnoid penetrate the dura to varying degrees. The arachnoid granulations range in size from microscopic to as large as 3 mm in diameter, and are concentrated in the dural cuffs of the lumbosacral region. Here, the thinned dura stretched over the spinal nerve roots is easily penetrated by the villi that come into contact with veins and lymphatics draining out the intervertebral foramina. Through these granulations, the arachnoid has direct contact with the epidural space and drugs injected there.

Subdural Space

Because the arachnoid is applied so closely to the inner surface of the dura, puncturing the dura is usually synonymous with entering the subarachnoid space. However, it is possible to inject or pass a catheter between the dura and arachnoid. This plane has traditionally been described as the subdural space, a potential space containing only scant serous fluid, allowing the two membranes to slide alongside each other. More recently it has been proposed that the arachnoid is actually adherent to the dura, and the subdural space is created by delamination of arachnoid cell layers.[22] Radiologists have long known that this space can be entered approximately 13% of the time during subarachnoid injection for myelography.[23] For the delivery of anesthesia, inadvertent subdural injection of the small volumes used for spinal anesthetics would simply result in a failed block; this scenario may be the most common explanation for failed spinal blocks.[24, 25] Inadvertent subdural injection of drug volumes intended for the epidural space spreads the anesthetic agent further owing to the smaller volume of the space available, resulting in an unexpectedly higher spread

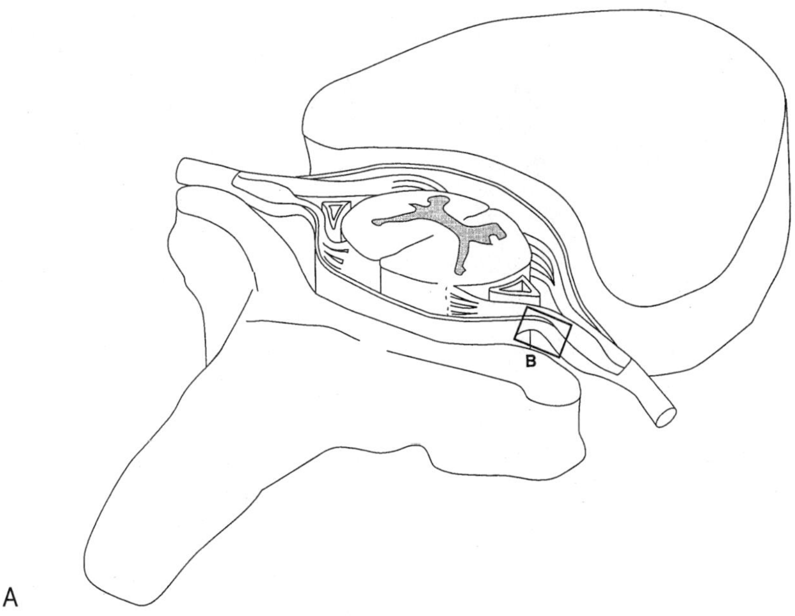

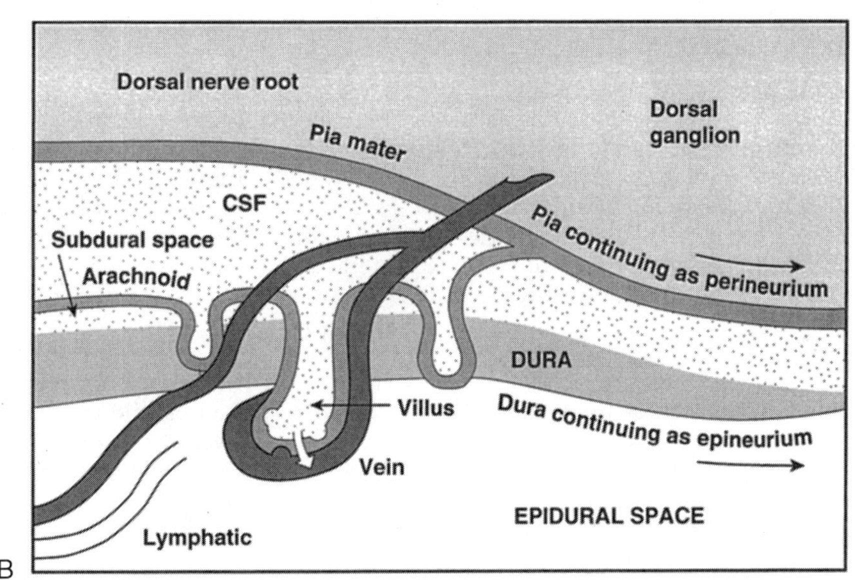

❖ **Figure 9–9** The dural cuff region. *A,* The dura thins as it approaches and then invests the dorsal and ventral nerve roots, eventually becoming continuous with the spinal nerve perineurium. *B,* Enlarged view of dural cuff overlying the dorsal root ganglion. It is here that arachnoid villi or granulations occur most densely. The villi serve not only as points of entry for epidural drugs but also for elimination of cerebrospinal fluid (CSF) and debris by transmembrane vacuolization across the arachnoid membrane *(white arrow).*

of anesthesia.[26–31] Subdural anesthesia has been characterized as differing from subarachnoid anesthesia in its relative sparing of motor function and the more gradual onset of sympathetic and sensory block.[31] However, cases of abrupt onset have been reported.[27]

Unlike the epidural space, the subdural space continues beyond the foramen magnum in continuity with the cranial cavity. Subdural injectate tends to rise slowly to this level.[32] In studying subdural injections undertaken deliberately for pain relief, Mehta and Maher[33] found the subdural space to be widest in the cervical region and in its lateral aspect where the dural cuffs extend beyond the termination of the arachnoid. This extension is reported to be greatest over the dorsal nerve root (Fig. 9–10).[34] This dorsolateral distribution may explain reports of unilateral subdural anesthesia.[27, 30] It has also been postulated to explain relative sparing of motor and sympathetic function owing to preferential exposure of the dorsal root ganglia versus the ventral nerve roots.[26, 28]

Several clinical factors have been identified that increase the likelihood of subdural injection. Rotating

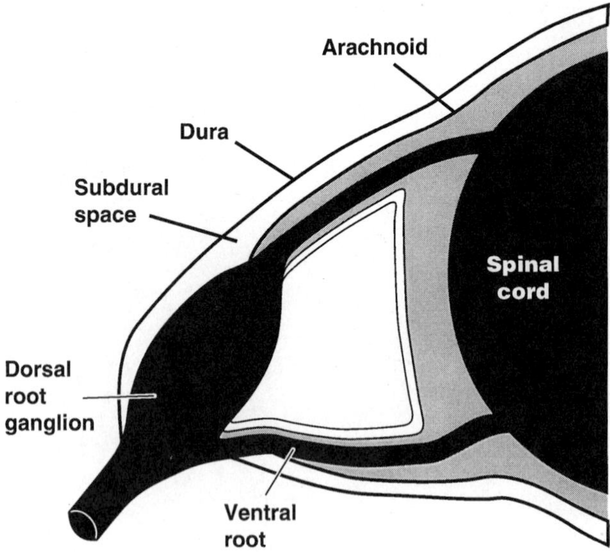

Figure 9–10 Lateral extent of the subdural space. The arachnoid and dura do not fuse uniformly with the nerve roots. The subdural space is more extensive over the dorsal roots. This may explain the frequent motor sparing seen in inadvertent subdural block.

the bevel of a needle after entering the epidural space may bring the needle tip into the subdural space.[33] Recent subarachnoid puncture may cause leakage of CSF into the subdural space, expanding it and making its subsequent entry more likely.[23, 25] This risk is relevant when an epidural catheter is inserted into the same interspace as an inadvertent dural puncture.[29]

Pia Mater

The pia mater is a thin membrane of tight-junction epithelial cells. It covers the surface of the brain, spinal cord, and nerves, ultimately joining the arachnoid to become continuous with the perineurium of the spinal nerves.[35] It supports and invests the rich vascularity of the spinal cord and nerve roots as these vessels penetrate into nerve tissue. The pia also provides a structural function by forming the lateral denticulate ligaments, which anchor the cord to the dura, and the filum terminale, which extends from the termination of the cord to the coccygeal periosteum.

Subarachnoid Space

Bounded by the arachnoid and pia mater, the subarachnoid space surrounds the entire CNS and is filled with cerebrospinal fluid. Its only other contents are connective tissue trabeculae and blood vessels. CSF at 37°C has a mean specific gravity of 1.006, ranging from 1.003 to 1.009. In attempting to predict the spread of local anesthetics injected into this fluid, at least 25 clinical factors have been implicated.[36] The most important of these are the dose, site of injection, baricity, and patient position.[37] Yet none of these factors explains the greater than 50% interindividual variability in distribution of anesthesia,[38] and patient characteristics are notoriously unpredictable.[39] It has recently become clear that the overwhelmingly important variable in the spread of spinal anesthesia is the individual spinal CSF volume.[38] This amount is highly variable, ranging threefold between subjects in one study,[40] but consistent within each individual.[41] On average, the total CSF volume in the spinal canal seems to be approximately 100 mL. The volume of CSF in the lumbar cistern, that portion of the subarachnoid space below the termination of the cord that contains the cauda equina, averages 50 mL. These levels are reduced in pregnancy,[40, 42] suggesting a tendency for increased spread of spinal anesthesia. The reduced CSF volume in pregnancy may be a result of epidural venous distention, transmission of increased abdominal pressure, or both.

Another recent finding with profound implications for the spread of spinal anesthesia is the demonstration of pulsatile flow in the CSF, increasing in amplitude in a cranial direction.[43] This too may be enhanced in pregnancy.[24] In addition to subarachnoid injections, this phenomenon may also explain the tendency for cranial spread of subdural injections.[33]

Microanatomy of the subarachnoid space may also have an impact on the distribution of spinal anesthetics.[44] In addition to the lateral denticulate ligaments, the cord is also suspended by a posterior midline septum that is continuous at the lumbar level in 28% of patients.[45] This septum, and saccular cysts originating from it,[24] may explain rare reports of unilateral spinal blockade (Fig. 9–11).[46]

Spinal Cord and Nerves

The spinal cord extends down from the foramen magnum to terminate as the conus medullaris, usually at the L1 to L2 vertebral level. About 45 cm long, it averages approximately 10 mm in lateral width and 6 to 7 mm in depth. It enlarges by up to 50% at the origin of the cervical and lumbosacral nerves serving the limbs, being largest at the C6 and T12 vertebral levels. These cervical and lumbar enlargements of the cord and surrounding dural sac leave room for a relatively smaller epidural space at these levels.

Each of the 31 pairs of spinal nerves originates from the cord as ventral and dorsal nerve roots. These roots are in turn formed from a number of filamentous, longitudinally arranged rootlets at each segmental level. Since there are eight cervical nerves and only seven cervical vertebrae, each spinal nerve exits the intervertebral foramen above its corresponding vertebra until the C7 level, and from the C8 vertebral level downward each exits from the foramen below. As the cord ends at the beginning of the lumbar spine, the lumbosacral nerves hang together as the cauda equina in the terminal portion of the dural sac. Because these lumbosacral nerves are bathed for relatively longer distances in CSF, they are the most susceptible to spinal anesthetics. The spinal nerve roots vary in size in relation to the population of neurons they carry, being

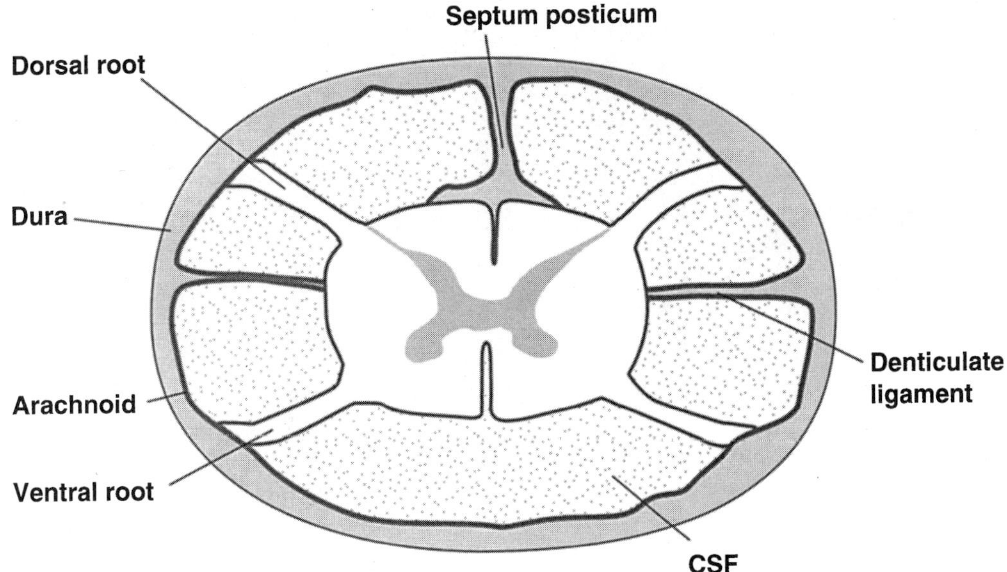

❖ **Figure 9–11** Ligamentous microanatomy of the subarachnoid space. In addition to support from the segmental denticulate ligaments, the septum posticum may extend continuously for variable distances and occasionally give rise to saccular cysts. Such structures may explain rare cases of asymmetric subarachnoid blockade. CSF, cerebrospinal fluid.

largest at the C8 and S1 vertebral segments.[47, 48] These segments are the most resistant to epidural blockade.[49]

Spinal Arteries

The blood supply of the spinal cord is provided by two posterior arteries and a single midline anterior artery. All three originate with cranial vessels and run the length of the pial surface of the cord. The posterior arteries are branches of the posterior inferior cerebellar arteries and run along the posterior surface of the cord medial to the spinal nerve roots. The single anterior spinal artery is formed at the level of the medulla in the brain stem from terminal branches of the two vertebral arteries. It runs along the surface of the anterior median fissure of the cord, sending penetrating branches deep into the central sulcus as well as circumferential vessels to the anterolateral portions. The anterior spinal artery provides the primary blood supply for the anterolateral two thirds of the cord, with the paired posterior spinal arteries nourishing the posterior third, and with anastomoses between all three (Fig. 9–12).

Although the spinal arteries anatomically run the entire length of the cord, they are really composite vessels formed by contributions at multiple segmental levels. At each intervertebral foramen, a segmental spinal artery originating from the subclavian, aortic, or iliac level enters anterior to the spinal nerve and pierces the dura to supply primarily the nerve root region and adjacent portion of the cord. These segmental arteries are enlarged into feeder, or radicular, arteries at multiple levels along the spine that anastomose with either the anterior or posterior system. The largest and best described of these is the radicularis magna, or artery of Adamkiewicz, which anastomoses with the anterior spinal artery at the level of the lumbosacral cord enlargement. Arising from the aorta as a branch of an intercostal artery, it enters on the left in 78% of patients, and between vertebrae T8 and L3 in 85% (Fig. 9–13).[50]

The blood supply of the spinal cord and nerves is thus best understood as not three longitudinal top-to-bottom conduits, but rather a segmental reinforcement of anterior and posterior systems correlated with the metabolic activity of that level. This is important when considering the risk of ischemia. The poorest vascularization of the cord occurs at the T4 vertebral level, but the cord is thinnest at this level and thus supply is balanced with demand. The cervicodorsal and lumbosacral enlargements have the highest vascularity, but the lumbosacral area is especially dependent on the single artery of Adamkiewiecz. In general, the cord is most vulnerable to ischemia in its anterior and central regions, given the larger territory served by the single anterior artery and the pattern of blood flow from peripheral to central. Thus the clinical presentation of the anterior spinal artery syndrome, which can occur with global hypoperfusion or local trauma to the radicularis magna artery, involves predominantly a painless motor deficit because the anterolateral motor columns of the cord are most affected.

Epidural Space

Boundaries, Depth, and Size

The epidural space comprises the contents of the spinal canal exterior to the dural sac. It extends from the foramen magnum superiorly to the sacrococcygeal ligament inferiorly. The space is open laterally at each

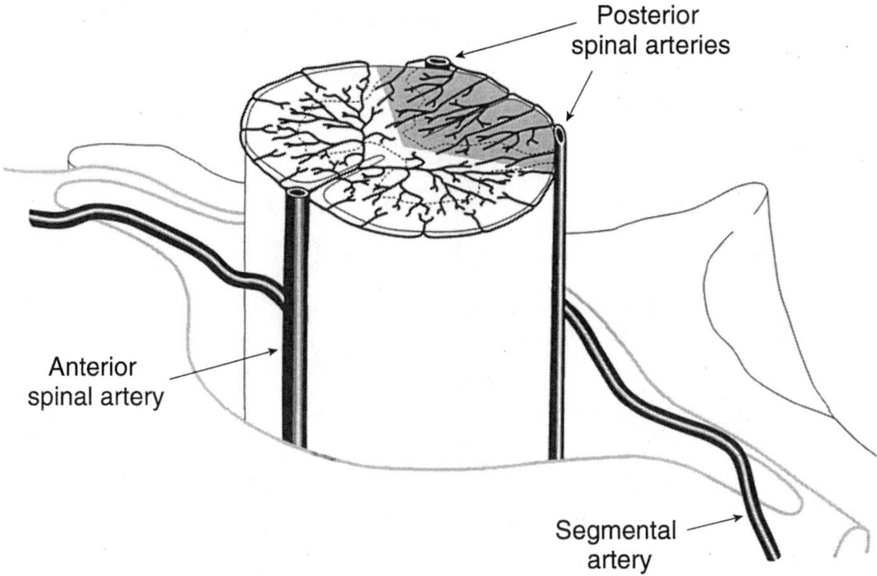

❖ **Figure 9–12** Arterial supply of the spinal cord. Note the paired posterior arteries supplying the dorsal one third of the cord, comprising largely sensory pathways. The single anterior spinal artery serves the ventral two thirds of the cord, including motor columns. Segmental feeder arteries and circumferential anastomosis provide collateral flow.

of the 58 intervertebral foramina, and freely communicates with adjacent body cavities. These openings and the adjacent pedicles serve as the lateral limit of the space. Posteriorly, the lamina and connecting ligamenta flava form a continuous but undulating boundary; anteriorly, the space is limited by the posterior longitudinal ligament and vertebral column.

The distance from skin to midline entry of the lumbar epidural space has been studied clinically,[51–57] sonographically,[58, 59] and with magnetic resonance imaging (MRI).[60] On average, it measures 5 cm at the lumbar level in obstetric patients; this is remarkably consistent between studies. The distance does not seem significantly different from nonpregnant patients.[56, 57] Depth tends to increase slightly in a caudal direction, being on average 0.5 cm greater at the L5 than the L1 vertebral level.[52, 61] Individual distances range from 3 to 9 cm, with the distance in 50% less than 5 cm and in 80% less than 6 cm (Fig. 9–14). Some 16% of obstetric patients have their epidural space less than 4 cm beneath the skin, increasing the risk of inadvertent dural puncture even with the needle used for skin analgesia.[54] Data from all these studies assume midline penetration. Given the posterior-pointing V shape of the posterior lumbar epidural space, veering off to the lateral limit of the interlaminar space could add at least 1 cm to this distance.[62] Required depth of penetration may also be increased in the lateral position[63] and in the presence of edema.[53] Although depth of the epidural space correlates loosely with body mass and other parameters,[51–53] attempts to predict depth of insertion have not been clinically useful.[55]

The width of the posterior epidural space, or ligamentum flavum–dura distance, varies greatly depending on the spinal level and even within each

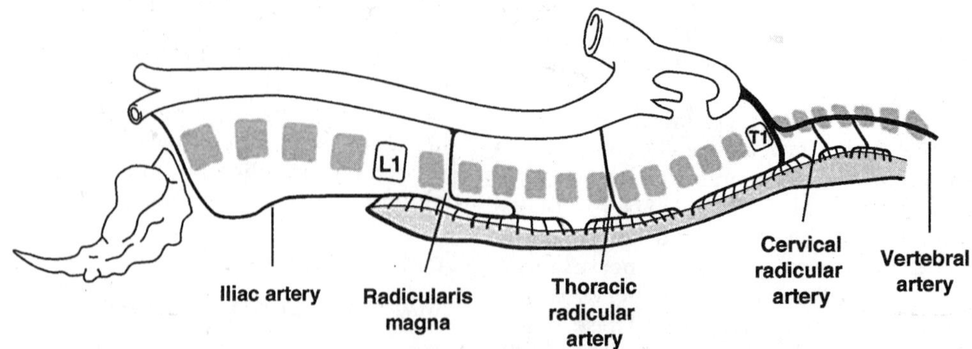

❖ **Figure 9–13** Main levels of anastomosis with the spinal arterial supply. The most vulnerable is the anterior spinal artery territory of the lumbosacral enlargement, dependent on the single radicularis magna, or artery of Adamkiewicz.

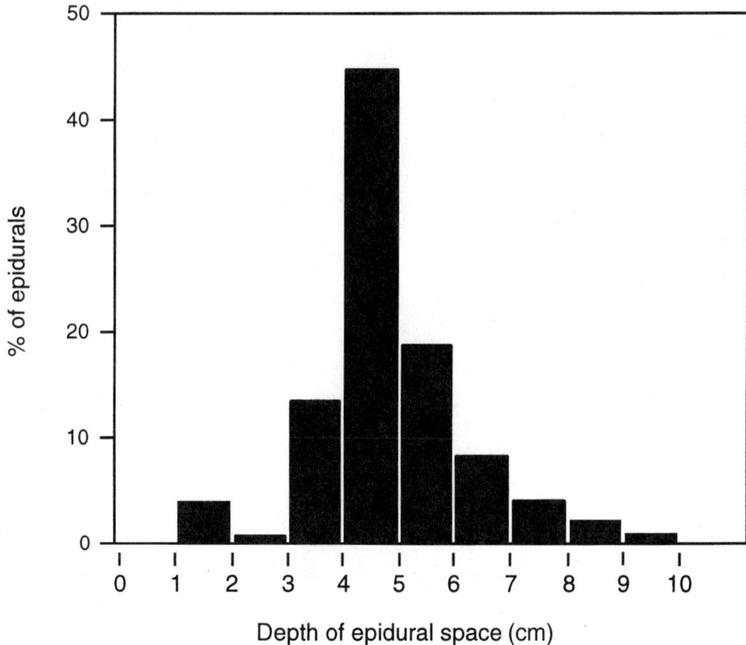

❖ **Figure 9–14** Distribution of skin to lumbar epidural space distance measured clinically in 4011 obstetric cases. (Data from Harrison GR, Clowes NWB: The depth of the lumbar epidural space from the skin. Anaesthesia 1985; 40:685–687; and Sutton DN, Linter SPK: Depth of epidural space and dural puncture. Anaesthesia 1991; 46:97–98.)

interspace (see Epidural Space Topography). It does not seem significantly altered in pregnancy, however.[42, 57, 64] For most of the cervical level, the space is nonexistent, as the dura lies directly opposed to the spinal canal.[13, 62] A 1- to 2-mm space opens at about the C7 vertebra, but flexing the neck slides the cervical enlargement of the spinal cord cephalad, widening the C7 to T1 vertebral space to 3 to 4 mm.[65] The space widens progressively down the spine, measuring 3 to 5 mm at the midthoracic level and reaching a maximum at the L3 to L4 interspace where it may be as wide as 25 mm but averages 6 to 7 mm.[57, 60, 62, 64] The dural sac usually terminates at the S2 vertebral level and the epidural space occupies a volume varying from 12 to 65 mL in the remainder of the sacral canal.[66] To fill the entire epidural space to the foramen magnum required 118 mL of contrast dye in one study.[67]

Epidural Pressures and Spread of Anesthesia

On entering the cervical or thoracic epidural space, there is an ambient subatmospheric pressure that can serve to identify the space. This is the basis for the hanging drop technique. However, below the thoracic level the epidural pressure may well be positive, particularly in the sitting position or with pregnancy.[68] Deep inspirations or the vacuum effect created by the advancing needle tenting the dura can create negative pressure in the lumbar epidural space,[69, 70] but the utility of the hanging drop as a marker for initial contact with the epidural space is lost. During labor, the baseline pressure becomes more positive, and each contraction can add a further 8 to 10 cm H_2O of pressure.[71]

All the aforementioned observations relate to the continuity of the epidural space with the adjacent body cavity with the change of pressure taking place via the intervertebral foramina. Thus cervicothoracic segments transmit interpleural pressures, in the range of −5 to −10 cm H_2O. Lumbosacral pressures take on resting abdominal pressure. The changes with pregnancy and labor reflect abdominal pressure changes, and are not necessarily related to epidural venous pressure.[19, 40]

As a result of the epidural pressure gradient between lumbar and thoracic levels, solutions injected in the lumbar region tend to spread more cephalad than caudad. Distribution around a thoracic injection site is more symmetric.[72] This tendency is more important than positional effects. Sitting or lying decubitus may favor spread in the dependent direction, but this effect is on the order of 1 or 2 segments and not clinically significant.[73, 74] The preferential cephalad spread of lumbar injections has practical importance in the conduct of an epidural blood patch. Patching should be undertaken at or below the lowest interspace suspected of resulting in dural puncture, particularly if low volumes are used.[75, 76]

Epidural Space Topography

Despite its obvious importance to the conduct of anesthesia, the precise configuration of the epidural space has been controversial, even after extensive study. The subtle and delicate features of this potential space are often distorted by the very techniques used to examine it. The act of opening the epidural space even in surgical dissection causes the contents to fall away from the vertebral wall,[77] and the elastic ligamentum flavum retracts when cut.[7] Postmortem studies are prone to tissue distortion, especially from preservatives.[13, 78, 79] Attempts to visualize the epidural space by injecting radiographic contrast,[80–83] resin for later dissection,[84, 85] or air for epidurography[86, 87] can result in artifact from the injection itself. Cryomicrotome studies by Hogan[78] have allowed detailed examination of tissue in situ with apparently minimal disruption from the living state. Recent advances in MRI have even allowed detailed observations in living, pregnant patients without the risk of ionizing radiation.[42, 60] These latter techniques have made significant contributions to understanding the functional anatomy of this area.

It has been well demonstrated that the epidural space is not continuous. In its undisturbed state, most of the epidural space is obliterated by the dura resting directly against the adjacent spinal canal. Catheters and injected solutions usually pass freely between them, however, as the dura and canal wall are only occasionally adherent.[62] Intermittently the epidural space opens up as compartments of various widths, depending on the vertebral region and even on the level within each vertebral segment (Fig. 9–15). These epidural compartments are categorized as anterior, lateral, and posterior in relation to the dural sac. Of these, the posterior compartment is of most direct significance to the anesthesiologist, as it is the route of

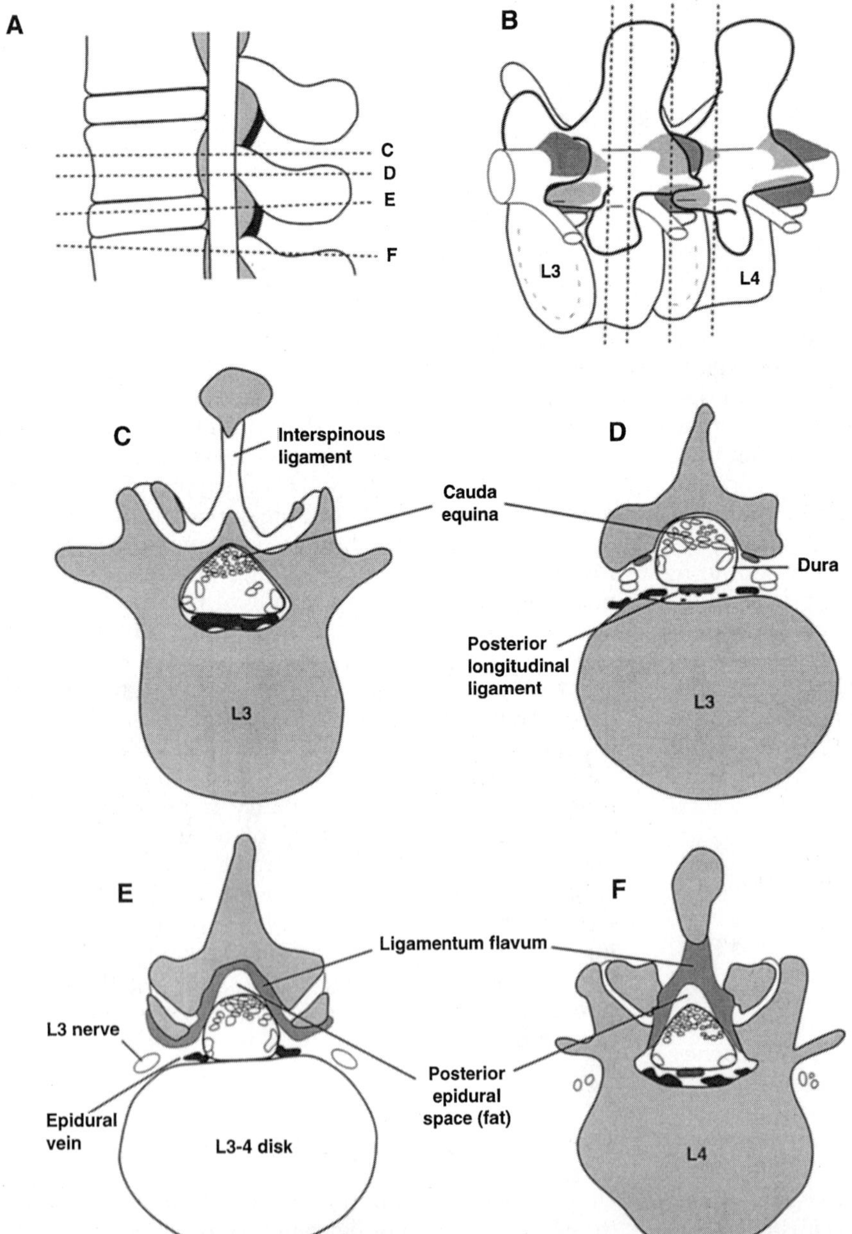

❖ **Figure 9–15** Topographic anatomy of the L3 to L4 epidural space based on cryomicrotome sectioning. Sawtooth outline of the posterior space is demonstrated in midline *(A)* and lateral oblique *(B)* views. Transverse sections are shown in *C* through *F*. Note that the V-shaped posterior epidural space widens only at the intervertebral level, where the epidural fat pad separates the dura from the ligamentum flavum. In the lumbar region, the anterior epidural space is nonexistent, as the dura and posterior longitudinal ligament are fused. (From Hogan QH: Lumbar epidural anatomy: a new look by cryomicrotome section. Anesthesiology 1991; 75:767–775.)

needle insertion to the spinal canal. In the sagittal plane it has a sawtooth appearance,[60, 78, 82] varying between collapse of the epidural space at the level of the pedicles to its maximum width at the caudal edge of each lamina. As shown in Figure 9–15*A*, this sawtooth feature is a result of the downward and posterior slant of the laminar arches, which form the posterosuperior roof of each of these outpouchings. Entering the epidural space at the L3 to L4 level in the midline following a course parallel to the caudal surface of the L3 spinous process would thus provide access to the segment of the epidural space at its widest point. In cross section, the posterior compartment has a triangular form with the deepest dimension in the midline. A needle entering the space off midline is much more likely to encounter dura, as the V-shaped lamina and ligamenta flava approach and then contact the dura in the lateral parts of the epidural space.

The anterior epidural space is largely devoid of contents except for the epidural veins, which lie anterolaterally beneath a lateral membranous extension of the posterior longitudinal ligament. The dura usually adheres to this ligament, although a space can be created between them with forceful injection.[85] In the lumbar region, they are effectively fused.[88]

Contents of the Epidural Space

Nerve Roots. The lateral epidural space contains the exiting nerve roots and their accompanying vasculature, padded with fat. There is scant fibrous tissue in this compartment, with only intermittent adhesions of the nerve roots to the membranous extension of the posterior longitudinal ligament. The concept of a fibrous "operculum"[89] or psoas fascia[90] barrier at the intervertebral foramina has not been supported by modern histologic studies,[78, 91] even in the aged.[92] There is thus no barrier to diffusion at the intervertebral foramina; the epidural space communicates freely with adjacent paravertebral tissue spaces.[40]

Fat. Epidural fat, found mostly in the posterior and lateral aspects of the epidural space, is semiliquid and lobulated. It differs from fat stores elsewhere in the body by being virtually devoid of fibrous tissue.[91, 93] Because of this lack of fibrous infrastructure, the fat lobules slide freely alongside each other with only intermittent adhesions to the spinal canal or dura, none of which provide significant anatomic barriers to spread of epidural injectate. The midline fat pad in the posterior epidural space has a minute vascular

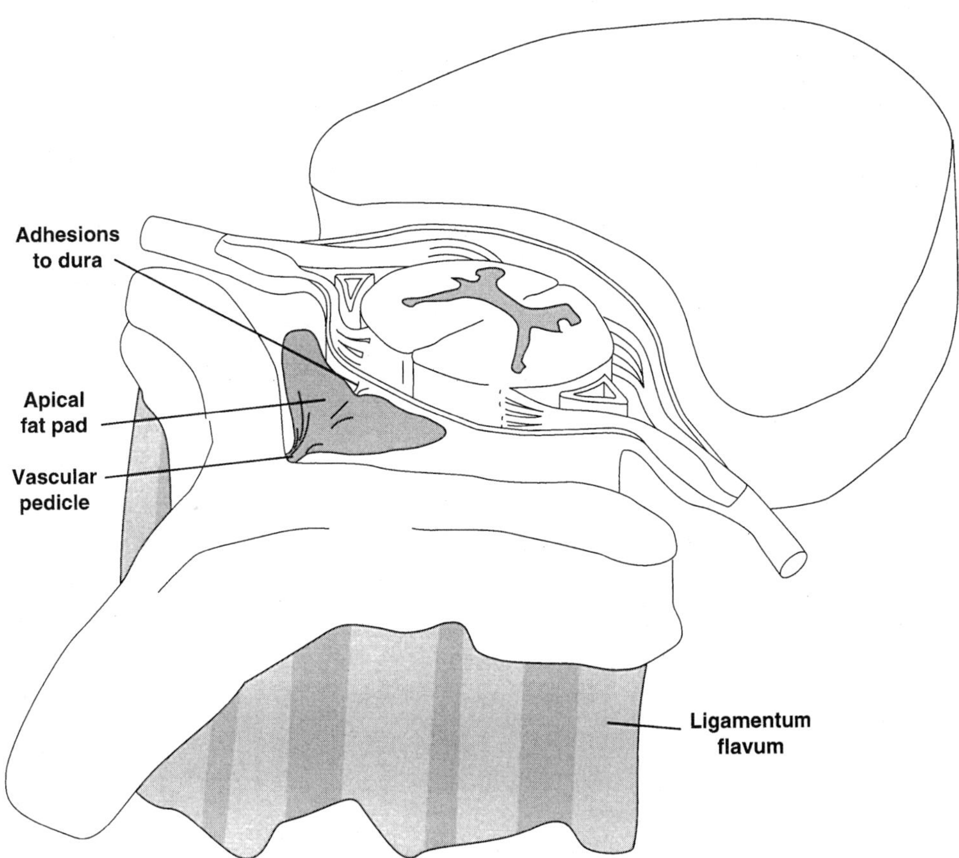

Figure 9–16 The apical epidural fat pad supported by its midline vascular pedicle. This pad creates an artifactual midline filling defect in contrast studies. Adhesions to the dura in the midline can also create a folding of the dura, the plica mediana dorsalis, when the epidural space is opened or injected (see also Fig. 9–19).

pedicle arising from the midline joining of the two limbs of the ligamentum flavum. When compressed by contrast injection or epiduroscopic insufflation, it is this midline fat pad that creates an artifact[78] previously interpreted as a midline fibrous septum (Fig. 9–16).[83] Adhesions between the midline fat pad and the dura may likewise create an artifactual midline protrusion of the dura termed the plica mediana dorsalis. This midline fold is caused by compression from epidural injectate.[94, 95] Neither of these artifacts seems to constitute a clinically significant barrier to the spread of injected solutions (see Fig. 9–19).[83, 96]

Epidural fat has a significant pharmacodynamic role in competing with nerve tissue for the binding of epidural local anesthetics, depending on their lipophilicity.[97] Below the L4 to L5 interspace, the fat content of the spinal canal increases, particularly in the anterior epidural space. This may be part of the reason for the typical resistance of L5 and S1 nerve roots to epidural blockade, and the difficulty in achieving cephalad spread of caudal epidural anesthesia.[78]

Lymphatics. Lymphatic vessels in the epidural space are concentrated around the dural cuff regions and empty anteriorly from the intervertebral foramina into paravertebral lymphatic channels. They invest the arachnoid granulations and carry away any particulate material that may appear in the CSF or epidural space.[98]

Epidural Veins. The venous drainage of the spinal canal undergoes changes during pregnancy that have fundamental effects on the anatomy and physiology of the epidural space. Epidural veins drain blood from the vertebral canal and its contents through a highly anastomotic, valveless system known as the internal vertebral venous plexus. It is in continuity with the cranial sinuses cephalad and the inferior vena cava via anastomoses in the sacral canal caudally. In 1940, Oscar Batson[99] showed that the vertebral venous plexus could carry metastases to the brain from the pelvis without involving the inferior vena cava; for this reason, it is sometimes referred to as Batson's plexus.

At each intervertebral foramen, the epidural veins absorb cerebrospinal fluid from the arachnoid granulations in the dural cuff and join the respective vertebral, posterior intercostal, lumbar, and lateral sacral veins. Thus the system communicates segmentally and at each end with the caval system. However, there is a crucial anastomosis with the azygos venous system, which runs in the right side of the mediastinum before emptying into the superior vena cava. In pregnancy, chronic inferior vena caval obstruction produced by the weight of the gravid uterus increases flow and venous pressure through this vertebral venous-azygos anastomosis, and significantly distends the epidural veins. This venous engorgement reduces available volume for distribution in both the epidural and subarachnoid space, and has long been a putative mechanism for the increased spread of neuraxial blockade in pregnancy.[36, 100, 101] Recent studies by Hirabayashi and coworkers[42] using MRI in supine pregnant women have confirmed epidural venous distention at the expense of the dural area. Hogan and colleagues,[40] however, using MRI in an abdominal compression model, have suggested that part of this effect may be from direct compression of soft tissue through the intervertebral foramina.

As well as affecting spread of injectate, epidural venous engorgement increases the risk of intravascular injection during pregnancy in two ways. First, the enlarged veins are more difficult to avoid with needle or catheter.[2] Second, the increased flow through the vertebral plexus emptying directly into the central circulation via the azygos vein results in more abrupt increases in systemic blood levels after intravascular injection compared with nonpregnant patients. In the parturient, these changes are further exacerbated with each uterine contraction as a result of a 300- to 500-mL autotransfusion effect,[102] producing an 8 to 10 cm H_2O rise in epidural venous distending pressure.[71] This distention is only partially relieved with position changes, hence the common practice of timing entry of an epidural needle or catheter between contractions.

In attempting to avoid injecting into epidural veins, clear understanding of their anatomic location is desirable. Figure 9–17 illustrates how the epidural plexus is arranged into two anterolateral columns, each divided into medial and lateral compartments that are often fused. Note that these columns are located in the anterior epidural space, covered by a thin membrane that extends laterally from the posterior longitudinal ligament.[62] The columns run medial to the pedicles and bulge laterally at the intervertebral foramina. The posterior epidural space, where midline epidural needles are aimed, is usually filled with fat and devoid of veins. This has been confirmed in a series of 1200 epidural venograms,[103] yet the image of veins in the posterior epidural space is perpetuated by drawings in many anatomy textbooks.[104, 105] Even under the conditions of increased epidural venous flow in supine pregnant patients, Hirabayashi and associates[42] could find no evidence of such posterior epidural veins. These anatomic findings suggest that epidural venous cannulation is related to needle or catheter placement that is too deep and lateral.

Cardiovascular Significance of the Epidural Veins. The epidural veins are intimately involved in the cardiovascular consequences of the supine position in pregnancy and labor. The supine hypotensive syndrome refers to symptomatic maternal hypotension resulting from partial or complete occlusion of the inferior vena cava by the weight of the gravid uterus. The cava is compressed against the right side of the vertebral column. The decrease in venous return, only partially offset by collateral flow through the epidural veins discussed earlier, leads to lowered ventricular preload and a 25% to 50% decrease in cardiac output. Although occurring in less than 10% of unanesthetized parturients,[106] the incidence of clinical supine hypotensive syndrome increases markedly with the lower-body sympathectomy and vasodilatation produced by central

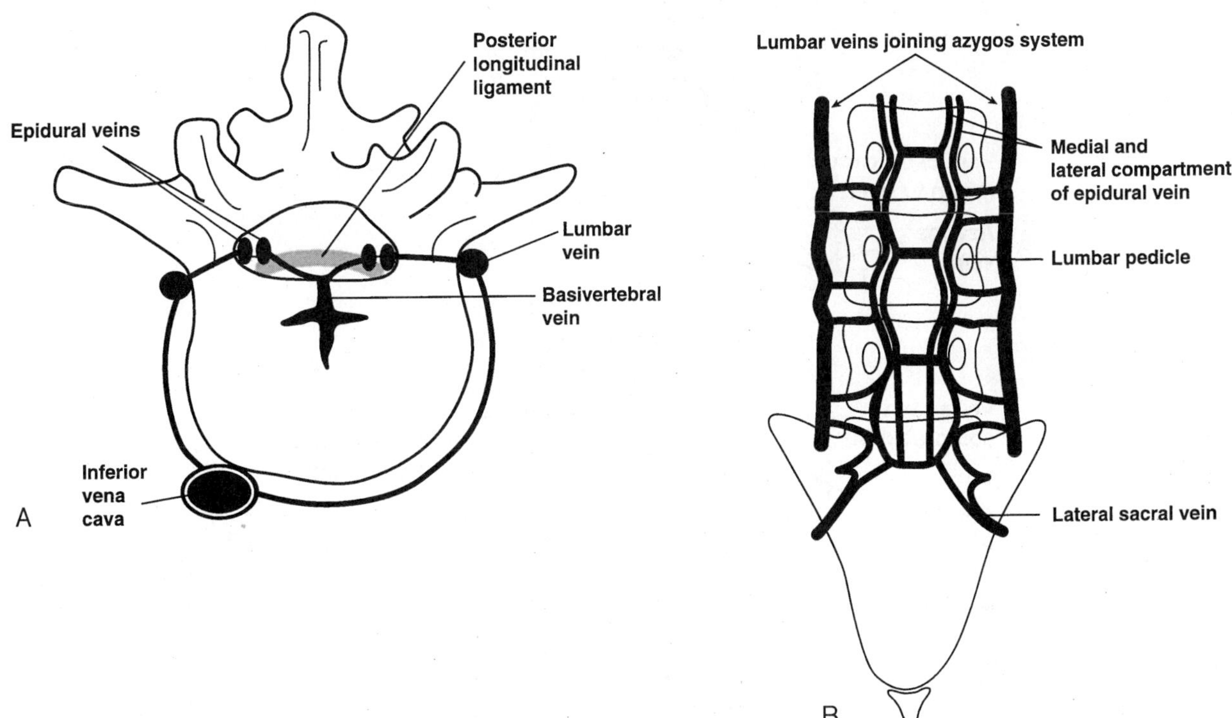

❖ **Figure 9–17** The lumbar epidural veins. Transverse *(A)* and posterior *(B)* views. Note the anterolateral location of the veins, which may be divided into medial and lateral components. There are no veins in the posterior epidural compartment. The epidural veins anastomose with the basivertebral drainage of the vertebral bodies, and the lumbar veins which join the azygos system. (Data from Gershater R, St. Louis EL: Lumbar epidural venography: review of 1200 cases. Radiology 1979; 131:409–421.)

blockade. The dangers of this syndrome, and its prevention by tilting the patient to the left, have long been championed.[107, 108]

Less commonly appreciated are the effects of uterine contraction while in the supine position. During contractions before the head is well engaged in the pelvis, the tightening uterus levers against the pelvic brim and can produce both aortic and caval compression. In about one third of unanesthetized parturients, this results in leg and placental hypoperfusion known as the Poseiro effect.[109] Because of simultaneous autotransfusion of uterine blood during contractions into the maternal circulation via epidural venous plexus collaterals, maternal cardiac output and arm blood pressure may be preserved. The need for vigilant lateral tilting, and fetal heart rate monitoring, is thus further apparent (Fig. 9–18), especially following regional analgesia and anesthesia.

ANATOMIC CONSIDERATIONS OF EPIDURAL CATHETER PLACEMENT

Catheter Type and Depth of Insertion. Catheters for continuous epidural drug administration should ideally be positioned in the midline of the posterior epidural space. Excessive insertion lengths may lead to intravenous, subdural, or subarachnoid cannulation; misdirection; coiling; or exit out an intervertebral foramen. Textbooks recommend inserting the tip of the catheter no more than 1 to 2 cm[110] or 2 to 3 cm[111] into the epidural space. Presumably this refers to single lumen, open-end catheters. D'Angelo and coworkers, however, found that 12.5% of such catheters inserted 2 cm would be dislodged during labor. They recommend 6-cm insertion for all but precipitous labor. If necessary, the catheter could be withdrawn and satisfactory analgesia obtained in 91% of cases.[112] Open-end catheters are prone to obstruction,[113] tend to produce a higher incidence of paresthesia on insertion, and result in 2 to 3 times the rate of unsatisfactory blocks than do closed-end types.[114–116] The poor spread of anesthesia seems related to the longitudinal streaming effect produced by the terminal opening.[117] To overcome this problem, multiorifice, closed-end catheters which are commonly used have a series of three holes separated by 120 degrees to allow more uniform spread. The most proximal of these orifices may lay 1.2 to 1.9 cm away from the catheter tip. In the first prospective study of optimal insertion depth for such catheters, Beilin and associates[118] found that insertion 5 cm into the epidural space produced the best compromise between secure placement and complicated cannulation (Table 9–1). Interestingly, they noted that paresthesias seem to be associated with where the needle position directs the initial entry of the catheter, not with the subsequent length of advancement.

Volume Dilatation of the Epidural Space. A common clinical practice is to inject air or local anesthetic

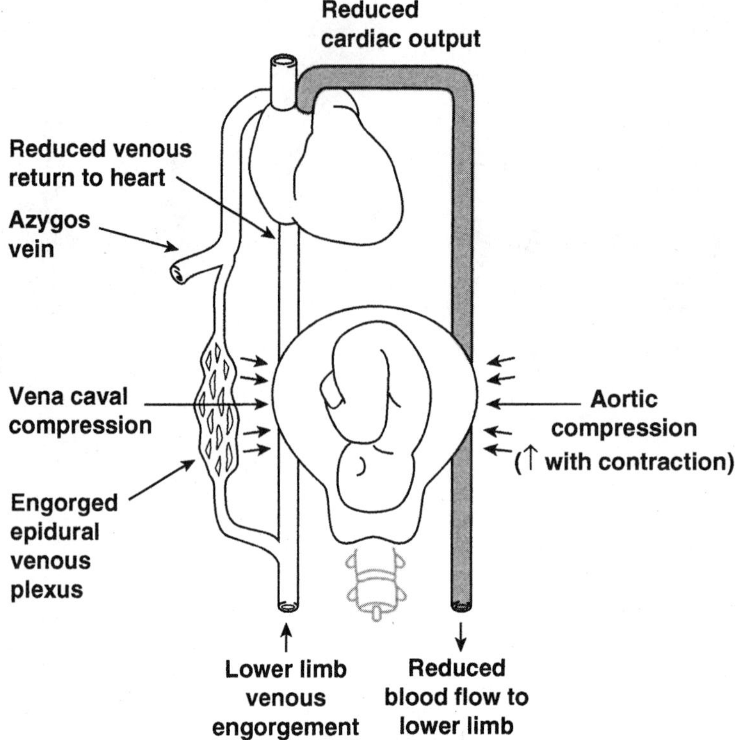

❖ **Figure 9-18** Aortocaval compression in late pregnancy. Caval compression leads to decreased maternal preload and possibly the supine hypotension syndrome, while distending the epidural veins with collateral flow through the azygos system. Aortic and iliac artery compression, increased with contractions (Poseiro effect), leads to maternal lower body and placental hypoperfusion. This latter effect may not be apparent in measurements of arm blood pressure because of simultaneous autotransfusion from the contracting uterus.

through the epidural needle before passing the catheter. Ostensibly, this is meant to dilate the potential space beyond the needle tip and lower the incidence of dural puncture, venous cannulation, or paresthesia from striking a spinal nerve fiber.[119] Using 3-mL volumes of local anesthetic or saline, Rolbin and associates showed no difference in these end points when compared with "dry" insertion as judged by an independent observer.[120] Although Verniquet showed a significant reduction in inadvertent venous cannulation by preinjecting 10 mL of local anesthetic,[121] this volume could prove problematic if dural or venous puncture were not recognized. Philip studied the injection of 10 mL of air.[122] Paresthesias were reduced from 49% to 29% and vessel cannulation declined from 5.8% to 1.6%. However, deliberate injection of air into the epidural space may lead to air embolism,[123] loculated bubbles impeding spread of local anesthetic and consequent patchy analgesia,[124, 125] or direct spinal nerve fiber compression.[126]

Needle Bevel Direction. Traditionally the epidural needle bevel is oriented cephalad, as recommended by Bromage.[127] When compared in a double-blind fashion by Muñoz and associates, the caudad orientation increased the incidence of paresthesia on catheter insertion from 20% to 40%, with a significant increase in intensity of the paresthesia.[128] Level of sensory block, however, was no different between groups. A paramedian versus midline needle introduction has been suggested by one author to improve the chances of midline catheter placement. This is based on epiduroscopic observations that the more tangential entry to the epidural space afforded by the paramedian approach resulted in less lateral deflection of the catheter when it made contact with the dura.[129]

Table 9-1 PERCENTAGE OF COMPLICATIONS WITH MULTIORIFICE CATHETERS (N = 100) AT VARIOUS DEPTHS OF INSERTION INTO THE EPIDURAL SPACE

	INSERTION DEPTH (CM)		
	3	5	7
Paresthesia	29	38	36
Intravenous cannulation	3	3	21*
Subarachnoid cannulation	0	0	0
Incomplete analgesia	31	6*	33

*$P < 0.05$ compared with other two groups.

Data from Beilin Y, Bernstein HH, Zucker-Pinchoff B: The optimal distance that a multiorifice epidural catheter should be threaded into the epidural space. Anesth Analg 1995; 81:301–304.

Catheter Migration. Movement of epidural catheters after placement is surprisingly common, with displacements of at least 0.5 cm occurring in 36% to 54% of patients.[61, 130, 131] The direction of this migration tends to be outward, particularly in the obese.[131] Duration of labor has not been shown to be a factor, and only one study has shown an association between migration and clinical inadequacy of block.[61] This may be because the majority of migrations are less than 2 cm. Even this amount may be significant, however, with multiorifice catheters inserted less than 4 cm into the epidural space. Migration has been noted even when the catheter is secured with a transparent adhesive dressing,[61, 131] which had earlier been proposed as a solution to this problem.[132] Such dressings may have their greatest value in allowing monitoring of catheter position at the skin.

Incomplete Blockade. Achieving effective epidural blockade seems to be more challenging in obstetric than nonpregnant patients.[133] While technique and dosing varies from study to study, inability to make the parturient comfortable with the initial epidural intervention varies from 6.3%[118] to 33%[114] in obstetric series. This failure most often takes the form of an asymmetric onset of effect. One hypothetic explanation for this is misdirection of catheters by the engorged epidural veins in pregnancy.

Catheters may exit through an intervertebral foramen if threaded too far[134, 135] or even as little as 3 cm[136] into the epidural space. This presents usually as total failure of analgesia, but sensory examination usually reveals unilateral block of one or several adjacent segments. Collier believes this phenomenon is almost unique to obstetrics.[133] Paresthesia from the nerve of the foramen involved is an unreliable sign of foraminal exit.[137] Withdrawing the catheter back into the spinal canal is not always successful; the escaped catheter may create a persistent channeling effect leading solution out via its former path.[133]

Even with the catheter tip well within the epidural space, marked asymmetry of blockade can occur. This ranges from missed segments of analgesia to completely unilateral blockade. When unilateral analgesia does occur, it is usually on the right; the preponderance has been reported as 80% of cases.[138, 139] The reason for this is not known. Radiographic contrast studies have suggested that such cases are due to lateral

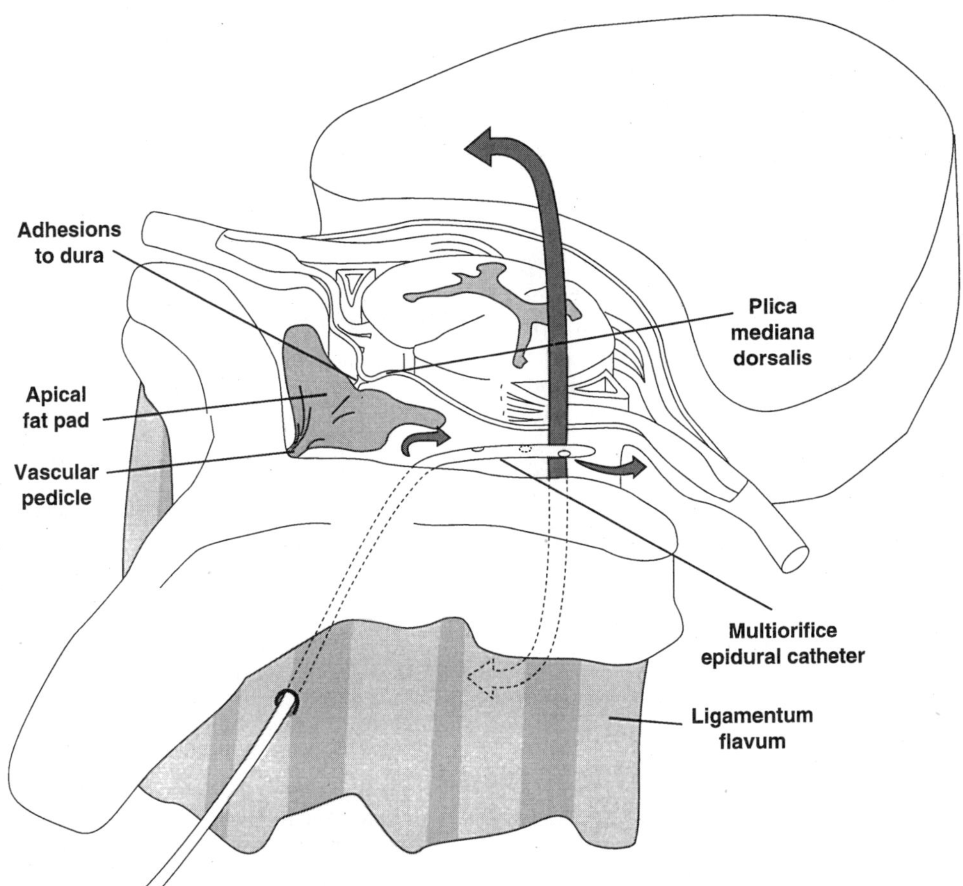

❖ **Figure 9–19** Putative mechanism for asymmetric epidural blocks. With the catheter tip in the anterolateral reaches of the epidural space, and midline obstruction to injectate spread by the midline fat pad and folding dura, unilateral analgesia or missed segments on the contralateral side may occur. Such midline barriers are rarely extensive longitudinally, however. Catheter withdrawal and increased volume of injectate can usually achieve spread to the contralateral side.

❖ SUMMARY

Key Points

- The epidural space differs between vertebral segments and is discontinuous circumferentially and longitudinally.
- The posterior lumbar epidural compartment is widest in the midline at the caudal edge of the spinous process.
- To minimize complications and replacement, multiorifice epidural catheters should enter at the midline and be threaded 3 to 5 cm into the epidural space.
- Anatomic barriers may occasionally cause abnormal spread of spinal anesthesia, even if cerebrospinal fluid is aspirated.

Key Reference

Hogan QH: Lumbar epidural anatomy: a new look by cryomicrotome section. Anesthesiology 1991; 75:767–775.

Case Stem

A 25-year-old GP0 requests epidural analgesia for active labor. A catheter is inserted 5 cm beyond the needle tip after using a midline approach just cephalad to the L3 spinous process. After administration of a total dose of 10 mL of bupivacaine 0.25%, a left-sided unilateral block from the T10 to L4 vertebral level is noted. Discuss the possible causes and management.

placement of the catheter or anatomic barriers to diffusion.[133–135, 140, 141] However, clinical spread of block does not always correlate with contrast spread in the epidural space.[142–145] Narang and Linter found an association between depth of the epidural space and unilateral blocks.[146] They hypothesized that lateral entry into the epidural space was increasingly likely because of magnification of needle angulation errors, and epidural anatomy was not to blame. Also, as previously discussed, anatomic barriers may be artifactually created by the force of the injectate itself, and overcome with increased volume or longitudinal spread. In any case, persistent dosing, with or without incremental withdrawal of the catheter, improves symmetry of blockade in the majority of such instances (Fig. 9–19).[112, 138, 139]

Disruption of the epidural space makes subsequent incomplete blockade more likely. Even mild scoliosis can restrict the spread of solutions to the concave side of the spinal curvature.[133] Distortion of the epidural space after corrective spinal surgery may leave only the subarachnoid route available for reliable anesthetic spread.[147] Epiduroscopy has demonstrated inflammatory adhesions after catheterization of the epidural space that interfered with subsequent cannulation.[148] This has been supported by the clinical finding of a higher incidence of unilateral epidural analgesia with successive blocks.[149] Unsatisfactory blockade may occur in up to 40% of patients with a previous epidural blood patch.[150] It is unclear whether this is attributable to effects of the blood patch or antecedent dural puncture. Failure of an epidural block to provide adequate pain relief is discussed in further detail in Chapter 36.

Increased Spread of Central Blocks During Pregnancy. Pregnancy has long been associated with decreased dose requirements for both subarachnoid[101] and epidural[151, 152] anesthesia. Traditionally, this has been attributed to physical changes related directly or indirectly to the weight of the gravid uterus. These include reduction of spinal CSF volume by distention of epidural veins[36, 42, 100] or direct transmission of raised intra-abdominal pressure,[40] changes in spinal curvature leading to more cephalad spread,[4] or enhanced CSF pulsatile flow during dural compression.[24] It has been further hypothesized that epidural venous pulsations during uterine contraction result in accentuated spread in laboring patients, but this has been shown to be clinically insignificant.[153]

All these physical models do not account for the similarly increased sensitivity seen in early pregnancy[154] and the postpartum period.[155] Furthermore, the approximately one-third reduction in dose requirement for central blockade in pregnancy[100] is remarkably similar to that for general anesthesia.[156] This suggestion of an increased neuronal sensitivity was confirmed in isolated rabbit nerve studies by Datta and colleagues.[157] The effect has been attributed to increased levels of free plasma progesterone in the cerebrospinal fluid as well as in plasma,[155] but the exact mechanism has yet to be elucidated.

References

1. Hogan QH: Tuffier's line: the normal distribution of anatomic parameters [letter]. Anesth Analg 1994; 78:194.
2. Brown DL: Spinal, epidural and caudal anesthesia: anatomy, physiology and technique. *In* Chestnut DH (ed): Obstetric Anesthesia: Principles and Practice. St Louis: CV Mosby; 1994:182.
3. Calguneri M, Bird HA, Wright V: Change in joint laxity occurring during pregnancy. Ann Rheum Dis 1982; 41:126–128.
4. Hirabayashi Y, Shimizu R, Fukuda H, et al: Anatomical configuration of the spinal column in the supine position. II. Comparison of pregnant and non-pregnant women. Br J Anaesth 1995; 75:6–8.
5. Bromage PR: Epidural Analgesia. Philadelphia: WB Saunders; 1978:8–9.
6. Hogan Q: Spinal anatomy. *In* Hahn M, McQuillan PM, Sheplock GJ (eds): Regional Anesthesia: An Atlas of Anatomy and Technique. St Louis: CV Mosby; 1996:205–212.
7. Zarzur E: Anatomic studies of the human lumbar ligamentum flavum. Anesth Analg 1984; 63:499–502.
8. Patin DJ, Eckstein EC, Harum K: Anatomic and biomechanical properties of human lumbar dura mater. Anesth Analg 1993; 76:535–540.
9. Dittman M, Schafer HG, Ulrich J, et al: Anatomic reevaluation of lumbar dura mater with regard to postspinal headache: effect of dural puncture. Anaesthesia 1988; 43:635–637.
10. Mihic DN: Postspinal headache and relationship of needle bevel to longitudinal dural fibers. Reg Anesth 1985; 10:76–81.
11. Norris MC, Leighton B, DeSimone CA, et al: Needle bevel

direction and headache after inadvertent dural puncture. Anesthesiology 1989; 70:729–731.
12. Lybecker H, Moller JT, May O, et al: Incidence and prediction of postdural puncture headache: a prospective study of 1,021 spinal anesthesias. Anesth Analg 1990; 70:389–394.
13. Cheng PA: The anatomical and clinical aspects of epidural anesthesia. I. Anesth Analg 1963; 42:398–406.
14. Hardy PAJ: Can epidural catheters penetrate dura mater? An anatomical study. Anaesthesia 1986; 41:1146–1147.
15. Bromage PR: Epidural Analgesia. Philadelphia: WB Saunders; 1978:22–23.
16. Bromage PR: Epidural Analgesia. Philadelphia: WB Saunders; 1978:14.
17. Rosser BH, Schneider M: The unflexed back and a low incidence of severe spinal headache. Anesthesiology 1956; 17:288–292.
18. Martins AN, Wiley JK, Myers PW: Dynamics of the cerebrospinal fluid and the spinal dura mater. J Neurol Neurosurg Psychiatry 1972; 35:468–473.
19. Shah JL: Influence of cerebrospinal fluid on epidural pressure. Anaesthesia 1981; 36:627–631.
20. Hirabayashi Y, Shimizu R, Matsuda I, et al: Effect of extradural compliance and resistance on spread of extradural analgesia. Br J Anaesth 1990; 65:508–513.
21. Tripathi RC: Ultrastructure of the arachnoid mater in relation to outflow of cerebrospinal fluid. Lancet 1973; 2:8.
22. Shantha TR: Subdural space: What is it? Does it exist? [abstract]. Reg Anesth 1992; 17(3S):85.
23. Schultz EH, Brogdon BG: The problem of subdural placement in myelography. Radiology 1962; 79:91–95.
24. Hogan Q: Anatomy of spinal anesthesia: some old and new findings. Reg Anesth 1998; 23:340–343.
25. Sechzer PH: Subdural space in spinal anesthesia. Anesthesiology 1963; 24:869–870.
26. Boys JE, Norman PF: Accidental subdural analgesia. Br J Anaesth 1975; 47:111–113.
27. Manchanda VN, Murad SHN, Shilyansky G, et al: Unusual clinical course of subdural local anesthetic injection. Anesth Analg 1983; 62:1124–1126.
28. Pearson A: A rare complication of extradural analgesia. Anaesthesia 1984; 39:460–463.
29. Stevens RA, Stanton-Hicks MDA: Subdural injection of local anaesthetic: a complication of epidural anaesthesia. Anesthesiology 1985; 63:323–326.
30. Brindle Smith G, Barton FL, Watt JH: Extensive spread of local anaesthetic solution following subdural insertion of an epidural catheter during labour. Anaesthesia 1984; 39:355–358.
31. Collier C: Total spinal or massive subdural block? Anaesth Intensive Care 1982; 10:92–93.
32. Jones MD, Newton TH: Inadvertent extra-arachnoid injections in myelography. Radiology 1963; 80:818–822.
33. Mehta M, Maher R: Injection into the extra-arachnoid subdural space. Anaesthesia 1977; 32:760–766.
34. Shapiro R: Myelography, 3rd ed. Chicago: Year Book Medical Publishers; 1975:124–126.
35. Shantha TR, Evans JA: The relationship of epidural anesthesia to neural membranes and arachnoid villi. Anesthesiology 1972; 37:543–557.
36. Greene NM: Distribution of local anesthetic solutions within the subarachnoid space. Anesth Analg 1985; 64:715–730.
37. Stienstra R, Greene NM: Factors affecting the subarachnoid spread of local anesthetic solutions. Reg Anesth 1991; 16:1–6.
38. Carpenter RL, Hogan QH, Liu SS, et al: Lumbosacral cerebrospinal fluid volume is the primary determinant of sensory block extent and duration during spinal anesthesia. Anesthesiology 1998; 89:24–29.
39. Norris MC: Patient variables and the subarachnoid spread of hyperbaric bupivacaine in the term parturient. Anesthesiology 1990; 72:478–482.
40. Hogan QH, Prost R, Kulier A, et al: Magnetic resonance imaging of cerebrospinal fluid volume and the influence of body habitus and abdominal pressure. Anesthesiology 1996; 84:1341–1349.
41. Taivainen TR, Tuominen MK, Kuulasmaa KA, et al: A prospective study on reproducibility of the spread of spinal anesthesia using plain 0.5% bupivacaine. Reg Anesth 1990; 15:12–14.
42. Hirabayashi Y, Shimizu R, Fukada H, et al: Soft tissue anatomy within the vertebral canal in pregnant women. Br J Anaesth 1996; 77:153–156.
43. Enzmann DR, Pelc NJ: Normal flow patterns of intracranial and spinal cerebrospinal fluid defined with phase-contrast cine MR imaging. Radiology 1991; 178:467–474.
44. Nauta HJ, Dolan E, Yasargil MG: Microsurgical anatomy of the spinal subarachnoid space. Surg Neurol 1983; 19:431–437.
45. Di Chiro G, Timins EL: Spinal myelography and the septum posticum. Radiology 1974; 111:319–327.
46. Armstrong PJ: Unilateral subarachnoid anaesthesia. Anaesthesia 1989; 44:918–919.
47. Bromage PR: Epidural Analgesia. Philadelphia: WB Saunders; 1978:33.
48. Hogan Q: Size of human lower thoracic and lumbosacral nerve roots. Anesthesiology 1996; 85:37–42.
49. Galindo A, Hernandez J, Benavides O, et al: Quality of spinal extradural anaesthesia: the influence of spinal nerve root diameter. Br J Anaesth 1975; 47:41–47.
50. Crock HV, Yoshizawa H: The Blood Supply of the Vertebral Column and Spinal Cord in Man. New York: Springer-Verlag; 1979.
51. Palmer SK, Abram SE, Maitra AM, et al: Distance from the skin to the lumbar epidural space in an obstetric population. Anesth Analg 1983; 62:944–946.
52. Harrison GR, Clowes NWB: The depth of the lumbar epidural space from the skin. Anaesthesia 1985; 40:685–687.
53. Meiklejohn BH: Distance from skin to the lumbar epidural space in an obstetric population. Reg Anesth 1990; 15:134–136.
54. Sutton DN, Linter SPK: Depth of epidural space and dural puncture. Anaesthesia 1991; 46:97–98.
55. Segal S, Beach M, Eappen S: A multivariate model to predict the distance from skin to the epidural space in an obstetric population. Reg Anesth 1996; 21:451–455.
56. Rosenberg H, Keykhak MM: Distance to the epidural space in obstetric patients [letter]. Anesth Analg 1984; 63:538–546.
57. Bevacqua BR, Haas T, Brand F: A clinical measure of the posterior epidural space depth. Reg Anesth 1996; 21:456–460.
58. Cork RC, Kryc JJ, Vaughn RW: Ultrasonic localization of the lumbar epidural space. Anesthesiology 1980; 52:513–516.
59. Currie JM: Measurement of the depth to the extradural space using ultrasound. Br J Anaesth 1984; 56:345–347.
60. Westbrook JL, Renowden SA, Carrie LES: Study of the anatomy of the extradural region using magnetic resonance imaging. Br J Anaesth 1993; 71:495–498.
61. Crosby ET: Epidural catheter migration during labour: an hypothesis for inadequate analgesia. Can J Anaesth 1990; 37:789–793.
62. Hogan QH: Epidural anatomy: new observations. Can J Anaesth 1998; 45(issue 5,pt ii):R40–R44.
63. Hamza J, Smida M, Benhamou D, et al: Parturient's posture during epidural puncture affects the distance from skin to epidural space. J Clin Anesth 1995; 7:1–4.
64. Nickalls RWD, Kokri MS: The width of the posterior epidural space in obstetric patients [letter]. Anaesthesia 1986; 41:432–433.
65. Bromage PR: Epidural Analgesia. Philadelphia: WB Saunders; 1978:14.
66. Trotter M: Variations of the sacral canal: their significance in the administration of caudal analgesia. Anesth Analg 1947; 26:192–202.
67. Farr RE: Sacral anesthesia: some practical and experimental points. Arch Surg 1926; 12:715.
68. Usubiaga JE, Moya F, Usubiaga LE: Effect of thoracic and abdominal pressure changes on the epidural space pressure. Br J Anaesth 1967; 39:612–618.
69. Bryce-Smith R: Pressures in the extradural space. Anaesthesia 1950; 5:213.
70. Eaton LM: Observations on the negative pressure in the epidural space. Mayo Clin Proc 1939; 14:566.

71. Bromage PR: Epidural Analgesia. Philadelphia: WB Saunders; 1978:518.
72. Bromage PR: Epidural Analgesia. Philadelphia: WB Saunders; 1978:133–134.
73. Merry AF, Cross JA, Mayadeo SV, et al: Posture and the spread of extradural analgesia in labour. Br J Anaesth 1983; 55:303–306.
74. Datta S, Alper MH, Ostheimer GW, et al: Effects of maternal position on epidural anesthesia for cesarean section, acid-base status, and bupivacaine concentrations at delivery. Anesthesiology 1979; 50:205–209.
75. Beards SC, Jackson A, Griffiths AG, et al: Magnetic resonance imaging of extradural blood patches: appearances from 30 min to 18 h. Br J Anaesth 1993; 71:182–188.
76. Szeinfeld M, Ihmeidan IH, Moser MM, et al: Epidural blood patch: evaluation of the volume and spread of blood injected into the epidural space. Anesthesiology 1986; 64:820–822.
77. Luyendijk W: The plica mediana dorsalis of the dura mater and its relation to lumbar peridurography (canalography). Radiology 1976; 11:147–149.
78. Hogan QH: Lumbar epidural anatomy: a new look by cryomicrotome section. Anesthesiology 1991; 75:767–775.
79. Parkin IG, Harrison GR: The topographical anatomy of the lumbar epidural space. J Anat 1985; 141:211–217.
80. Luyendijk W, van Voorthuisen AE: Contrast examination of the spinal epidural space. Acta Radiol (Diagn) 1966; 5:1051–1066.
81. Hatten HP: Lumbar epidurography with metrizamide. Radiology 1980; 137:129–136.
82. Reynolds AF, Roberts PA, Pollay M, et al: Quantitative anatomy of the thoracolumbar epidural space. Neurosurgery 1985; 17:905–907.
83. Savolaine ER, Pandya JB, Greenblatt SH, et al: Anatomy of the human lumbar epidural space: new insights using CT-epidurography. Anesthesiology 1988; 68:217–220.
84. Husemeyer RP, Wite DC: Topography of the lumbar epidural space. Anaesthesia 1980; 35:7–11.
85. Harrison GR, Parkin IG, Shah JL: Resin injection studies of the lumbar extradural space. Br J Anaesth 1985; 57:333–336.
86. Blomberg R: The dorsomedian connective tissue band in the lumbar epidural space of humans: an anatomical study using epiduroscopy in autopsy cases. Anesth Analg 1986; 65:747–752.
87. Blomberg R, Olson SS: The lumbar epidural space in patients examined with epiduroscopy. Anesth Analg 1989; 68:157–160.
88. Blikra G: Intradural herniated lumbar disc. J Neurosurg 1969: 31:676–679.
89. Forestier J: Le trou de conjugaison vertebral et l'espace epidural. Paris: Jouve et Cie; 1922:105.
90. Rauschning W: Normal and pathologic anatomy of the lumbar root canals. Spine 1987; 10:1008–1019.
91. Hogan Q, Lynch K, Lacitis I: Histologic features of epidural soft tissue and its relation to the dura and canal wall [abstract]. Reg Anesth 1993; 18(suppl):54.
92. Hogan QH: Epidural anatomy examined by cryomicrotome section: influence of age, vertebral level, and disease. Reg Anesth 1996; 21:395–406.
93. Ramsey HJ: Comparative morphology of fat in the epidural space. Am J Anat 1959; 105:219–232.
94. Blomberg RG: Anatomy of the epidural space [letter]. Anesthesiology 1988; 69:797.
95. Huson A, Luyendijk W, Tielbeek A, et al: CT-epidurography and the anatomy of the human lumbar epidural space [letter]. Anesthesiology 1988; 69:797.
96. Asato F, Hirakawa N, Oda M, et al: A median epidural septum is not a common cause of unilateral epidural blockade. Anesth Analg 1990; 71:427–429.
97. Rosenberg PH, Kytta J, Alila A: Absorption of bupivacaine, etidocaine, lignocaine and ropivacaine into n-heptane, rat sciatic nerve and human extradural and subcutaneous fat. Br J Anaesth 1986; 58:310–314.
98. Brierley JB, Field FJ: The connexions of the spinal subarachnoid space with the lymphatic system. J Anat 1948; 82:153.
99. Batson OV: The function of the vertebral veins and their role in the spread of metastases. Ann Surg 1940; 112:138.
100. Bromage PR: Epidural Analgesia. Philadelphia: WB Saunders; 1978:141.
101. Barclay DL, Renegar OJ, Nelson EW: The influence of inferior vena cava compression on the level of spinal anesthesia. Am J Obstet Gynecol 1968; 101:792–800.
102. Hendricks CH: The hemodynamics of uterine contraction. Am J Obstet Gynecol 1958; 76:969.
103. Gershater R, St. Louis EL: Lumbar epidural venography: review of 1200 cases. Radiology 1979; 131:409–421.
104. Clemente CD (ed): Gray's Anatomy, 30th ed. Philadelphia: Lea & Febiger; 1985:830.
105. Agur AMR: Grant's Atlas of Anatomy. Baltimore: Williams & Wilkins; 1991:229.
106. Bienarz J, Crottogini JJ, Curuchet E, et al: Aortocaval compression by the uterus in late human pregnancy. Am J Obstet Gynecol 1968; 100:203–217.
107. Scott DB: Inferior vena caval occlusion in late pregnancy and its importance in anaesthesia. Br J Anaesth 1968; 40:120–128.
108. Crawford JS: Time and lateral tilt at Caesarean section. Br J Anaesth 1972; 44:477–484.
109. Bromage PR: Epidural Analgesia. Philadelphia: WB Saunders; 1978:521.
110. Shnider SM, Levinson G, Ralston DH: Regional anesthesia for labor and delivery. *In* Shnider SM, Levinson G (eds): Anesthesia for Obstetrics, 3rd ed. Baltimore: Williams & Wilkins; 1993:135–153.
111. Brown DL: Spinal, epidural and caudal anesthesia. *In* Miller RD (ed): Anesthesia, 4th ed. New York: Churchill Livingstone; 1994:1522–1525.
112. D'Angelo R, Berkebile BL, Gerancher JC: Prospective examination of epidural catheter insertion. Anesthesiology 1996; 84:88–93.
113. Scott DB, Wilson J: Insertion of epidural catheters. Anaesthesia 1983; 38:1108–1109.
114. Michael S, Richmond MN, Birks RJS: A comparison between open-end (single-hole) and closed-end (three lateral holes) epidural catheters. Anaesthesia 1989; 44:578–580.
115. Segal S, Eappen S, Datta S: Superiority of multiorifice over single-orifice epidural catheters for labor analgesia and cesarean delivery. J Clin Anesth 1997; 9:109–112.
116. Collier CB, Gatt SP: Epidural catheters for obstetrics: terminal hole or lateral eyes? Reg Anesth 1994; 19:378–385.
117. Magides AD, Richmond MN: Lumbar epidurography in multi-orifice and single orifice epidural catheters [abstract]. Reg Anesth 1992; 17(3S):180.
118. Beilin Y, Bernstein HH, Zucker-Pinchoff B: The optimal distance that a multiorifice epidural catheter should be threaded into the epidural space. Anesth Analg 1995; 81:301–304.
119. Bromage PR: Epidural Analgesia. Philadelphia: WB Saunders; 1978:218.
120. Rolbin SH, Halpern SH, Braude BH, et al: Fluid through the epidural needle does not reduce complications of epidural catheter insertion. Can J Anaesth 1990; 37:337–340.
121. Verniquet AJW: Vessel puncture with epidural catheters. Anaesthesia 1980; 35:660–662.
122. Philip BK: Effect of epidural air injection on catheter complications. Reg Anesth 1985; 10:21–23.
123. Naulty SJ, Ostheimer GW, Datta S, et al: Incidence of venous air embolism during epidural catheter insertion. Anesthesiology 1982; 57:410–412.
124. Dalens B, Bazin JE, Haberer JP: Epidural bubbles as a cause of incomplete analgesia during epidural anesthesia. Anesth Analg 1987; 66:679–683.
125. Boezaart AP, Levendig B: Epidural air-filled bubbles and unblocked segments [letter]. Can J Anaesth 1989; 36:603–604.
126. Kennedy TM, Ullman DA, Harte FA, et al: Lumbar root compression secondary to epidural air. Anesth Analg 1988; 66:1184–1186.
127. Bromage PR: Epidural Analgesia. Philadelphia: WB Saunders; 1978:192.
128. Muñoz HR, Dagnino JA, Allende M, et al: Direction of catheter insertion and incidence of paresthesias and failure rate in continuous epidural anesthesia: a comparison of cephalad and caudad catheter insertion. Reg Anesth 1993; 18:331–334.

129. Blomberg RG: Technical advantages of the paramedian approach for lumbar epidural puncture and catheter introduction: a study using epiduroscopy in autopsy subjects. Anaesthesia 1992; 47:610–612.
130. Phillips DC, Macdonald R: Epidural catheter migration during labour. Anaesthesia 1987; 42:661–663.
131. Bishton IM, Martin PH, Vernon JM, et al: Factors influencing epidural catheter migration. Anaesthesia 1992; 47:610–612.
132. Duffy BL: Securing epidural catheters. Can Anaesth Soc J 1982; 29:636–637.
133. Collier CB: Why obstetric epidurals fail: a study of epidurograms. Int J Obstet Anesth 1996; 5:19–31.
134. Sanchez R, Acuna L, Rocha F: An analysis of the radiological visualization of the catheters placed in the epidural space. Br J Anaesth 1967; 39:485–489.
135. Bridenbaugh LD, Moore DC, Bagdi P, et al: The position of plastic tubing in continuous-block techniques: an x-ray study of 552 patients. Anesthesiology 1968; 29:1047–1049.
136. Boezaart AP: Computerized axial tomo-epidurographic and radiographic documentation of unilateral epidural analgesia. Can J Anaesth 1989; 36:697–700.
137. Hehre FW, Sayig JM, Lowman RM: Etiologic aspects of failure of continuous lumbar peridural anesthesia. Anesth Analg 1960; 39:511–517.
138. Ducrow M: The occurrence of unblocked segments during continuous lumbar epidural analgesia for pain relief in labour. Br J Anaesth 1971; 43:1172–1173.
139. Beilin Y, Zahn J, Bernstein HH, et al: Treatment of incomplete analgesia after placement of an epidural catheter and administration of local anesthetic for women in labor. Anesthesiology 1998; 88:1502–1506.
140. Usubiaga JE, Reis A, Usubiaga LE: Epidural misplacement of catheters and mechanisms of unilateral blockade. Anesthesiology 1970; 32:158–161.
141. Asato F, Goto F: Radiographic findings of unilateral epidural block. Anesth Analg 1996; 83:519–522.
142. Shanks CA: Four cases of unilateral analgesia. Br J Anaesth 1968; 40:999–1002.
143. Gielen MJM, Slappendel R, Merx JL: Asymmetric onset of sympathetic blockade in epidural anaesthesia shows no relation to epidural catheter position. Acta Anaesthesiol Scand 1991; 35:81–84.
144. Burn JM, Guyer PB, Langdon L: The spread of solutions injected into the epidural space. Br J Anaesth 1973; 45:338–345.
145. Bromage PR: Epidural Analgesia. Philadelphia: WB Saunders; 1978:131.
146. Narang VPS, Linter SPK: Failure of extradural blockade in obstetrics: a new hypothesis. Br J Anaesth 1988; 60:402–404.
147. Kardash K, King BW, Datta SD: Spinal anaesthesia for Caesarean section after Harrington instrumentation. Can J Anaesth 1993; 40:667–669.
148. Igarashi T, Hirabayashi Y, Shimizu R, et al: Inflammatory changes after extradural anaesthesia may affect the spread of local anaesthetic within the extradural space. Br J Anaesth 1996; 77:347–351.
149. Withington DE, Weeks SK: Repeat extradural analgesia and unilateral block. Can J Anaesth 1994; 41:568–571.
150. Ong BY, Graham CR, Ringaert KRA, et al: Impaired epidural analgesia after dural puncture with and without subsequent blood patch. Anesth Analg 1990; 70:76–79.
151. Bromage PR: Spread of analgesic solutions in the epidural space and their site of action: a statistical study. Br J Anaesth 1962; 24:161.
152. Hehre FW, Moyes AZ, Senfield RM, et al: Continuous lumbar epidural anesthesia in obstetrics. II. Use of minimal amounts of local anesthetics during labor. Anesth Analg 1965; 44:89–93.
153. Sivakumaran C, Ramanathan S, Chalon J, et al: Uterine contractions and the spread of local anesthetics in the epidural space. Anesth Analg 1982; 61:127–129.
154. Fagareus L, Urban BJ, Bromage PR: Spread of epidural analgesia in early pregnancy. Anesthesiology 1983; 58:184–187.
155. Datta SD, Hurley RJ, Naulty S, et al: Plasma and cerebrospinal fluid progesterone concentrations in pregnant and nonpregnant women. Anesth Analg 1986; 65:950–954.
156. Palahniuk RJ, Shnider SM, Eger EI: Pregnancy decreases requirements for inhaled anesthetic agents. Anesthesiology 1974; 41:82–83.
157. Datta S, Flanagan HL, Lambert DH, et al: Differential sensitivities of mammalian nerve fibers in pregnancy. Anesth Analg 1983; 62:1070–1072.

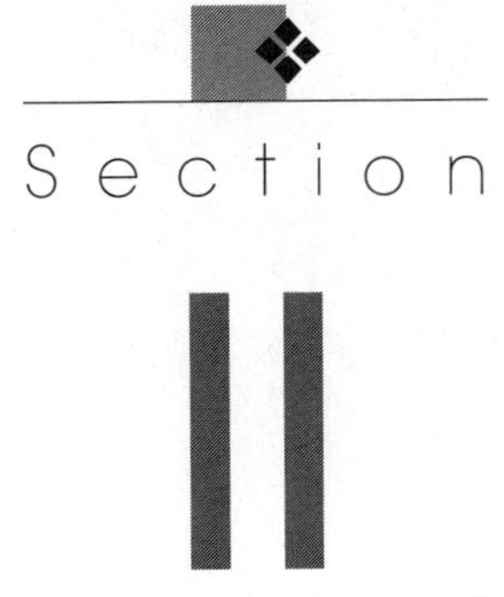

ANALGESIA FOR LABOR

10

Epidural Analgesia for Labor

❖ JOHN PAULL, FANZCA, Dip Ed

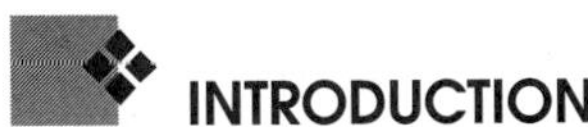

INTRODUCTION

The relief of pain in labor has been an objective pursued by mothers and their medical and midwife attendants for centuries. The first major step toward current techniques of pain relief was made in 1942 when Hingson and Edwards[1] proposed the use of continuous caudal epidural local anesthetic infusion as a technique for maternal pain relief. The efficacy of their technique was diminished by the relatively brief duration of effect of the local anesthetics then available, the development of maternal drug toxicity, and the anatomic fact that the nerves principally responsible for pain transmission in labor were 10 segments further up the spinal canal than the point of entry of the caudal epidural catheter.

Since then, the evolution of analgesic techniques has been dependent on a number of personalities and technical and pharmacologic factors. Those who have made advances have asked the questions, "What is the anesthesiologist's role? Is it that of a technically skilled expert who initiates a sophisticated pain relief technique and then leaves it to others to manage, or is it that of a specialist who manages the whole spectrum of obstetric analgesic requirements?" Fortunately they have universally answered in the affirmative to the second possibility and have thereby steadily improved analgesic services.

The principal pioneers involved have devoted their professional lives to the promotion of regional analgesic techniques in labor and to teaching others to perform and to critically assess and improve those techniques. Technical advances in needles, catheters, and drugs have all contributed to the increased availability and safety of epidural techniques. Advances in the understanding of neural pathways and pain receptors and their diverse pharmacology have opened up new prospects for modifying pain sensation with non-opioid and non-local anesthetic drugs.

The evolution of obstetric epidural analgesia has occurred over half a century. We have seen the use of silver, malleable epidural needles for continuous pain relief, using lidocaine solutions, progress to sophisticated catheters for delivering drugs designed to give prolonged pain relief, with minimal motor block. Adjuvants such as opioids and other drugs have allowed the anesthesiologist to reduce the doses and concentrations of local anesthetic to the point where women now expect good pain relief with little or no motor block.

The realization that total loss of sensation was not a necessary accompaniment of labor analgesia and that the mother relieved of pain did not need to be confined to bed were philosophical changes generated by Brownridge[2] and others.

The wider use of epidural blockade in postoperative pain relief has meant that more anesthesiologists now have the procedural skills necessary for safe maternal pain relief. Forty years ago, obstetric epidural pain relief could only be provided by a small subset of anesthesiologists, trained by the pioneers. The days when the obstetrician needed to be skilled in spinal and epidural anesthesia as well as obstetric management have almost passed.

Problems still exist in the provision of epidural pain relief for mothers having their delivery in smaller centers. These problems arise because of the sporadic nature of obstetric pain relief requirements, a matter that affects the administrative mechanisms for assigning an anesthesiologist to exclusive labor ward analgesia duties when remuneration is on a case-by-case basis.

Finally, active educational programs for expecting mothers and their partners have increased the demand for better pain relief in labor, something that epidural analgesia provides safely and effectively. Despite this safety and efficacy, unrealistic parental expectations or inappropriate behavior or practice by the anesthesiologist have resulted in medicolegal storm clouds appearing on the horizon from time to time. Occasional court cases remind mothers, midwives, and anesthesiologists that risk management is a fact of life demanding our diligent attention.

ANATOMY

Understanding the process of perception of labor pain is dependent on understanding the neural pathways involved. Although briefly discussed here, this subject is thoroughly reviewed in Chapter 1. Cleland[3] first described these pathways in 1933. In general, first-stage pain is transmitted by sympathetic fibers originating in the uterine muscle, passing downward to the area of the broad ligament and thence laterally to the pelvic wall. The fibers travel medially and pass through the relatively ill-defined inferior, middle, and superior hypogastric plexuses. Through these plexuses, the fibers enter the lumbar sympathetic chain and, passing in the white rami of the T10 to L1 spinal nerves, ultimately enter their dorsal roots and pass into the cord. The localization of this visceral pain is poor, and its somatic referral tends to produce an aching sensation in the cutaneous distribution of the T10 to L1 spinal nerves, that is, in the lower abdomen and the small of the back. The pain is usually synchronous with the contractions and its intensity tends to reflect the strength of the uterine contraction.

During the latter third of the first stage, when cervical dilation becomes more rapid, stimulation of the sacral parasympathetic innervation of the cervix tends to result in lower sacral pain. It sometimes radiates down the backs of the thighs and frequently has a most unpleasant subjective component. Despite assertions by some that the parasympathetic component of cervical pain is of no importance, the fact that many women vomit when full dilation of the cervix is achieved suggests otherwise.[4]

The pressure of the presenting part on pelvic structures during this period, including the rectum, ureters, bladder, and the pelvic somatic nerves, can result in a spectrum of pain that is particularly distressing for the mother and her partner.

During the second, or expulsive, stage of labor, the perineal somatic innervation becomes significant. The posterior two thirds of the perineum and the clitoral area are innervated by the pudendal nerve and its branches originating in sacral segments 2, 3, and 4. The anterior third of the vulva is innervated by the genital branch of the genitofemoral nerve, originating from L1.

The practical implication of these anatomic realities is that neither a lumbar nor a sacral epidural block alone is sufficient to anesthetize the whole of the perineal area, a fact often overlooked by anesthesiologists and obstetricians.

In the third stage of labor, the pain associated with the expulsion of the placenta is often not consciously registered by the mother if placental expulsion follows soon after the delivery of the infant. The emotional overload of the events surrounding the birth effectively displaces appreciation of pain from the sensorium. However, if placental expulsion is delayed, or if the placenta must be removed manually by the obstetrician, then pain relief may be required. In the latter case, both perineal and uterine nerves are involved in the pain transmission, and steps must be taken to block both if the procedure is to be performed without distress or discomfort.

PHYSIOLOGIC CHANGES IN LABOR

Labor is a physically demanding event that stresses the mother physiologically and forces her to call on her cardiac, respiratory, renal, and hepatic reserves. The mother in whom these reserves are already diminished, whether by congenital abnormalities, disease, or drug therapy, may be stressed to the point that organ failure becomes a reality.

Although regional blockade can do much to reduce the stresses experienced in labor, especially those resulting from the physiologic responses to pain, the blockade in itself creates a different set of stresses, albeit usually of a lesser magnitude. Complications of the regional block process, on the other hand, may create stresses of a much greater magnitude and may in themselves be life-threatening.

To identify and understand the pregnancy- and labor-induced stresses experienced by the laboring woman, it is essential that the anesthesiologist providing obstetric pain relief have an understanding of these physiologic changes.

Cardiovascular Changes

The hormonally induced changes in the vasculature of the uterus, the breasts, and the skin associated with pregnancy lead to an increased vascular capacitance and a lowering of peripheral resistance.[5] The normal hemodynamic response to this is activation of the mechanisms to increase intravascular volume and a 30% to 50% increase in cardiac output to maintain perfusion pressures and organ blood flow.[6] This increase in cardiac output is achieved at the expense of the mother's functional cardiac reserve, which is correspondingly reduced. This leaves her less well able to cope with additional cardiac stressors that may arise in pregnancy, such as hypertension and hemorrhage, or preexisting valvular or myocardial disease.

On the other hand, the fall in hemoglobin concentration that occurs during pregnancy is associated with an increase in total hemoglobin content.[7] In effect, the mother has initiated two physiologically beneficial processes. Firstly, she has reduced her hematocrit and blood viscosity, effectively improving tissue perfusion and oxygen delivery with a minimal increase in cardiac work. Secondly, she has implemented a process of hypervolemic hemodilution, reducing hemoglobin loss at delivery, despite potentially significant blood loss.

The anesthesiologist providing epidural analgesia must be aware of these cardiovascular and hemodynamic changes to ensure that the physical signs seen in the pregnant woman are not misinterpreted.

Because the uterine circulation is effectively a low-resistance shunt, uterine blood flow is highly pressure dependent. Falls in maternal blood pressure, however induced, or falls in venous return leading to increases in peripheral vascular resistance may compromise uterine perfusion and hence oxygen transfer to the fetus.

In clinical practice, this situation can arise if the pregnant woman in the third trimester is allowed to remain supine for any length of time. The compression of the vena cava by the gravid uterus leads to a rise in lower limb venous pressure, increased blood sequestration in the lower half of the body, and a fall in venous return, which is reflected as a fall in cardiac output. In turn, vasoconstrictive compensatory mechanisms assist in maintaining systemic blood pressure at the expense of blood flow. In many women, a gradual rise in pulse rate and a minimal fall in blood pressure are seen for some minutes. Then, an abrupt fall in pulse rate, nausea and vomiting, and impaired consciousness rapidly supervene together with a profound fall in blood pressure. This mechanism is clearly a marked vagal response to a progressive fall in perfusion. The fetus may show signs of distress with a fall in heart rate at any stage during this process.

Turning the mother on her side is the appropriate prevention and treatment, and, if maternal bradycardia persists, 0.6 mg of atropine given intravenously will rapidly restore the circulation and reverse the adverse phenomena described. If the mother must lie on her back, for example for an examination, the onset of the supine hypotensive syndrome can be delayed or avoided by tilting her pelvis with a sandbag or wedge under the right hip, or by physically displacing the uterus to the left, or by allowing her to flex her hips and knees. This last maneuver flattens the lumbar curve and tends to reduce the pressure on the vena cava by reducing abdominal wall tension and increasing the anteroposterior depth of the lower abdomen.

Aortic compression may occur in association with caval compression or independently. The classic syndrome of aortic compression manifests itself as an unusually high maternal arm blood pressure measurement associated with fetal bradycardia in a supine pregnant woman. The treatment is the same as for caval compression.

An additional effect of caval compression, of significance to the anesthesiologist, is that the venous blood, hindered in its flow through the vena cava, takes alternative routes through the azygos system and the epidural venous plexus. The increase in epidural venous plexus volume effectively reduces the volume of the epidural space and potentially increases the spread of epidurally injected local anesthetic.

It is also important for the anesthesiologist to recognize that epidural anesthesia, with its associated partial sympathetic blockade, may significantly impair the ability of the pregnant woman to activate the normal physiologic response to caval occlusion, leading to an increased frequency and severity of the supine hypotensive syndrome in the mother with an epidural block who lies on her back.

Fetal "distress" associated with the maternal supine position is well documented.[8, 9] The problem may be compounded during labor or at cesarean section (CS), particularly if regional analgesia is in use.

Further stresses on the maternal cardiovascular system can arise from factors such as multiple pregnancy, in which case the usual uterine blood flow of 500 to 700 mL/min at term may be increased significantly, or from preeclampsia. In preeclampsia, peripheral vascular resistance may be significantly increased, elevating cardiac work and oxygen consumption. The impaired organ perfusion may result in abnormal biochemistry that affects the myocardial milieu. The increased vascular tone and frequently associated hypovolemia pose special problems for the anesthesiologist, who must recognize that epidurally induced partial sympathectomy may result in profound falls in maternal blood pressure.

Respiratory Changes

As is the case for the cardiovascular system, pregnancy diminishes functional reserve. The increased metabolism of pregnancy increases oxygen requirements and the quantity of carbon dioxide to be excreted. This means that respiratory work is increased and there will be a consequent reduction in functional respiratory reserve. Depending on whether the mother is erect or supine, respiratory work may be significantly increased in pregnancy. For example, in the supine position, chest wall compliance falls because of the increased abdominal mass due to the size of the uterus, liquor, and fetus, and respiratory work increases. In the erect position this effect is not so apparent.

Normally this is of little consequence when an epidural anesthetic is given in labor, but if the block unexpectedly extends cranially, respiratory function may be impaired, especially if some degree of intercostal motor block results. The anesthesiologist must then administer oxygen by mask and assess whether ventilatory assistance is required.

DRUGS

Ropivacaine has been advocated for CS owing to a decreased risk of cardiotoxicity compared with bupivacaine and has also become more popular to provide labor analgesia.[10] Isolated human placental perfusion studies show that the placental transfer of ropivacaine and bupivacaine is similar. The transfer rates are limited by the protein binding of the two drugs, which in both cases is high.[11] Ropivacaine used for epidural analgesia in labor has an analgesic potency of 0.57 compared with bupivacaine.[12]

Opioids are often administered to supplement the epidural local anesthetics. The use of opioid and local anesthetic mixtures means that lower doses and concentrations of both classes of drugs can be used, reducing the toxicity and side effects of each.[13] The use of epidural fentanyl in aliquots of 10 to 30 μg does not appear to affect the fetus or breast-feeding success on day 1 post partum.[14, 15]

Hydromorphone has been used as an epidural local anesthetic supplement, based on its supposed greater neuraxial specificity, more rapid onset, and reduced side effects when compared with morphine. Sinatra et al.[16] reported the onset of satisfactory analgesia in 89% of 622 laboring women within 15 minutes of the epidural administration of 8 to 12 mL of 0.5% bupivacaine and adrenaline 1:200,000 with hydromorphone 100 μg in 5 mL of normal saline.[16] Mild to moderate pruritus was present in 1.6% of the mothers, and 1.1% required treatment for this complication.

Claes et al.[17] suggest that the addition of clonidine to a bupivacaine-epinephrine-sufentanil mixture improved the quality and duration of analgesia as compared with solutions containing no clonidine. The frequency of side effects in the clonidine groups was comparable, with the exception of hypotension and sedation. Hypotension was easily treated by fluids or ephedrine and caused no fetal distress. The level of sedation was mild, and all parturients were easily aroused by verbal commands.

Interest in midazolam as an activator of γ-aminobutyric acid A/benzodiazepine dorsal horn receptors, which subsequently activate the opioid delta receptors to produce a different antinociceptive effect, suggests that this drug or its congeners may also have a future role to play in labor analgesia.[18]

TECHNIQUE

Regardless of the type of epidural analgesic delivery planned for a mother's labor, the initiation of the epidural has a number of constant features. Consent for the procedure must be obtained from the mother following an adequate explanation of the procedure and its risks. The operator must have the appropriate technical skills or be supervised by someone who has. The location for the procedure must have suction, equipment for administering oxygen, and sufficient resuscitative drugs as might be required to deal with intravascular injection of local anesthetic, or accidental high or total spinal anesthesia. If the fetus is at risk, fetal monitoring equipment should also be utilized.

A secure intravenous line must be in place, with a cannula of sufficient size to facilitate rapid transfusion if hemorrhage should occur during delivery.

The mother's blood pressure should be measured, and if a noninvasive blood pressure device is being used, a manual sphygmomanometer should be available to validate the measurement of the noninvasive equipment, if necessary.

The epidural may be inserted with the mother lying on her side, or sitting, particularly if she is obese or has a multiple pregnancy or polyhydramnios. Vasovagal syncope is perhaps a little more common if the mother is sitting, but can also occur in the lateral position. It needs to be distinguished from an adverse drug-related response.

Today, sterile epidural kits of various types and degrees of complexity are relatively freely available. A work area of adequate size on a trolley or table is helpful, and an assistant able to position the mother is invaluable.

The insertion site should be identified prior to cleansing and disinfecting of the area. An area of the back sufficient to allow the anesthesiologist to touch the mother without rendering the gloved hands unsterile is washed with an appropriate antiseptic solution. The minimum draping required is a sterile towel covering the area of the bed or trolley immediately adjacent to the mother's back, but some practitioners prefer to use drapes to completely cover the remainder of the patient. The disadvantage of this is that important skeletal landmarks may be obscured, such as the position of the hips and shoulders and the curvature of the spine. In addition, it is frequently the case that the uppermost drape, unsterile on its patient surface after being deployed, slides down over the insertion site, making it unsterile. Recently, clear plastic drapes have become available. These drapes allow excellent visibility while providing a large sterile field.

After anesthetizing the skin and interspinal ligament, the anesthesiologist inserts the epidural needle, usually at L3–L4 plus or minus one interspace. It is difficult to justify the use of large-bore (16-gauge) needles, when smaller epidural needles (18-gauge) are available. The use of smaller 18-gauge epidural needles will save the mother considerable discomfort and, if a dural puncture does occur, will reduce the frequency of post–dural puncture headache (PDPH), which is related to the size of the puncturing needle.

Test Dose

After defining the epidural space by loss of resistance or the hanging drop method, the anesthesiologist is faced with a choice, to inject a test dose or not. It has been suggested that the test dose is used to determine whether the needle tip is in the subarachnoid space, in which case a dense, rapid-onset block should ensue. If the needle tip is in an epidural vein, tachycardia or systemic symptoms of local anesthetic toxicity, such as tingling of the lips or light-headedness, will alert the anesthesiologist to the intravascular position of the needle. Most anesthesiologists do not administer a test dose via the needle, but rather test the catheter.

The safest philosophy of dosing an epidural catheter is to administer every dose incrementally, regarding every increment as a test dose, and assuming the worst for each administration, until time proves otherwise. Many anesthesiologists continue to believe that an epidural test dose adds safety to the procedure by increasing the likelihood of detection of an intravascular catheter. Unfortunately, test-dosing with lidocaine 1.5%, 3 mL with adrenaline 5 μg/mL may result in sufficient motor block as to prevent ambulation in labor.[19]

The second matter that must be dealt with is to decide whether to inject the initial dose of local anesthetic drug through the needle or through the catheter. Cousins[20] suggested that the injection of the initial dose of the drug incrementally through the needle results in a lower incidence of missed segments and unsatisfactory blocks. Cohen et al.[21] have suggested that the administration of local anesthetic by gravity, via the needle during the initiation of epidural analgesia, produces a better block than the administration of local anesthetic via the epidural catheter. Theoretically, the filling of the epidural space with local anesthetic solution might be expected to facilitate the insertion of the epidural catheter and reduce the frequency of radicular pain associated with catheter insertion, although this has not been reported. Many anesthesiologists, however, prefer to administer all the medications through the catheter, so that in the event of an emergency CS, they know that the catheter is functioning.

Following the insertion of the initial dose of local anesthetic, the mother is returned to the lateral position, if she has been sitting, or turned to the opposite side if the lateral position has been used. If air has been used in determining epidural entry with the mother in the left lateral position, then the air will rise to the upper side of the epidural space when the local anesthetic is injected. If the mother is not turned to the opposite side, segmental block failure on the upper side, in this case the right side, may occur.

The mother's blood pressure should be measured at frequent intervals until her hemodynamic status has stabilized.

Many anesthesiologists use a solution of bupivacaine 2.5 mg/mL to establish the block quickly and effectively and to gain the mother's confidence. At that point, the continuous infusion can be started using either a dilute local anesthetic alone or local anesthetic and narcotic mixture. At present, fentanyl (1–4 μg/mL) appears to be the drug most frequently used, but sufentanil and pethidine are also used by some.[22]

PATIENT-CONTROLLED EPIDURAL ANALGESIA VERSUS CONTINUOUS EPIDURAL INFUSION

Initially, epidural analgesia was provided by intermittent catheter "top-ups." This tended to produce peaks and troughs of analgesic effect depending on the availability of the anesthesiologist or the alertness of the midwife or labor nurse and their action threshold for maternal pain. As better infusion devices and drugs have become available, it has become possible to provide continuous epidural infusion of local anesthetic at a rate sufficient to maintain analgesia in the majority of women, without deleterious side effects. Ultimately it was realized that pregnant women, given a modicum of instruction, could modulate their own epidural analgesia and patient-controlled epidural analgesia (PCEA) was born. Gambling et al.,[23] in 1988, reported the first comparison of PCEA and continuous infusion epidural analgesia in a nullipara and reported greater maternal satisfaction with the PCEA technique.

In part because of the costs involved in providing PCEA devices in the delivery suite, debates continue to rage concerning the relative efficacy and economy of continuous and PCEA administration of epidural local anesthetic. Factors considered by the protagonists include efficacy, total drug use, and anesthesia care provider time needed to maintain a satisfactory level of block.

Harke et al.[24] have demonstrated that PCEA and continuous epidural infusion are equally effective in producing labor analgesia and that the use of PCEA does not necessarily reduce the total quantity of drug used, as some had hoped, nor does it necessarily reduce the time required by the anesthesia care provider to ensure that a satisfactory block is maintained.

More recently, nonelectronic, disposable plastic, spring-operated PCEA devices have become available, and the use of these may avoid the significant capital costs associated with electronic PCEA devices, making PCEA more widely available.

When PCEA is used, a loading dose of local anesthetic is required to establish adequate pain relief. Russell et al.[25] have shown, however, that it is not necessary to give the mother a loading dose of epidural narcotic as well. Before proceeding to PCEA, the majority of anesthesiologists will establish a block with 8 to 10 mL of 0.25% bupivacaine to achieve rapid and adequate pain relief and gain the mother's confidence. They would also hope to demonstrate that the catheter was correctly situated and that all of the required area was blocked.

When all of those criteria are achieved, the PCEA with a low concentration of bupivacaine with fentanyl can be initiated.

Some anesthesiologists prefer to add sufentanil to the 0.125% bupivacaine because it appears that this drug may improve the quality of analgesia as compared with fentanyl, and perhaps reduces the incidence of instrumental delivery when epinephrine is also added to the solution.[26]

The size of the bolus administered during PCEA must of course be adjusted depending on the effect achieved in each individual case. Most commonly, a bolus dose of 3 to 6 mL would be prescribed initially. The rate of administration of the bolus will depend, to some degree, on the characteristics of the PCEA pump being used and on the resistance offered by the catheter and the epidural filter. It is reasonable to set the pump to deliver the bolus dose over 3 to 5 minutes, to reduce the incidence of pump over-pressure alarms.

The lockout interval must also be set by the anesthesiologist. Most plastic disposable PCEA devices have a 4 mL maximum dose and a 15-minute lockout built into them. This cannot be altered. When electromechanical devices are used, a lockout of 10 to 20 minutes has been reported as the most satisfactory. This time is dependent on the pharmacokinetics of the drugs being injected. Increasing experience of the anesthesiologist and the labor room nurse will allow them to tailor the PCEA settings to their particular clientele.

In most reported studies, background infusion of drugs has not improved maternal satisfaction.

COMPLICATIONS OF EPIDURAL ANALGESIA

Hypotension

Because the injection of local anesthetic epidurally effectively may produce a limited sympathectomy, it is not surprising that maternal hypotension is one of the most common complications of epidural analgesia.

As mentioned earlier, the uterine circulation is effectively a low-resistance shunt, and uterine blood flow is heavily pressure dependent. Falls in maternal blood pressure, however induced, may compromise uterine perfusion and hence oxygen transfer to the fetus.

Maternal hypotension and its complications can be minimized or avoided in many cases if the anesthesiologist appropriately assesses the mother's fluid and cardiovascular status before proceeding and immediately treats hypotension.

Many authorities agree that a fluid load of 750 to 1000 mL of lactated Ringer's solution should be administered prior to initiation of conventional epidural analgesia. If the mother has preeclampsia or eclampsia and is edematous, administration of colloid or a reduced volume of crystalloid may be appropriate.

Administering only as much local anesthetic as is required to relieve maternal pain will also reduce the extent of the sympathetic block and hence reduce the risk of hypotension. In other words, the dose should be titrated so the minimum dose necessary to achieve sensory analgesia is used.

If hypotension occurs and persists despite apparently adequate intravenous fluids and the assurance that the mother is lying in a lateral position, then intravenous ephedrine (5–30 mg) should be administered. If maternal bradycardia is observed, atropine (0.6–1.2 mg) intravenously will block any untoward vagal overactivity that may be contributing to the hypotension. If profound hypotension follows institution of a labor epidural, further investigation should be made to determine whether an accidental intrathecal injection has occurred.

Dural Puncture Management

If a dural puncture occurs during the insertion of an epidural needle, the natural response is to withdraw the needle and start again at another space. The better response is for the practitioner to remind himself or herself that the purpose of the exercise is to provide the mother with analgesia, not to put a catheter in her epidural space. Under these circumstances, it is appropriate to inject intrathecally a small dose of bupivacaine or ropivacaine, or of fentanyl or sufentanil, and then to either thread the epidural catheter intrathecally or to withdraw the needle and reinsert it at another interspace. The mother's pain will be significantly, if not completely, relieved and the next step can be considered without the distressed mother, or her partner, or the midwives placing pressure on the anesthesiologist.

It is acknowledged that while dural puncture is an uncommon complication of epidural analgesia it has the potential for disrupting the normal postpartum experience. The low-pressure headache that follows dural puncture in the majority of cases is disabling and distressing.[27] The use of epidural blood patch (EBP) techniques to minimize the distress caused by PDPH was originally suggested by Gormley[28] in 1960, was implemented by DiGiovanni and Dunbar[29] in 1970, and is now well established.

A controversial subject was whether it was appropriate to attempt a period of conservative management prior to using the blood patch, to reduce the need for another invasive procedure. It was also thought by many practitioners that the success rate of EBP increased if its use was delayed for a period after the dural puncture had occurred.

Some anesthesiologists advocate a 24- to 48-hour period of bed rest, intravenous fluids, and simple analgesics (with or without caffeine supplements) to try to provide a noninvasive resolution of the headache. If this management fails, EBP is implemented.

Colonna-Romano and Shapiro[30] have demonstrated that prophylactic EBP has an 80% success rate in preventing PDPH and advocate its routine use. Lowenwirt et al.[31] confirm that prophylactic EBP is effective management. In their experience, the early use of EBP resulted in fewer headaches and a lower frequency of the dural puncture complications such as diplopia, photophobia, and tinnitus. In those mothers receiving prophylactic blood patch, the autologous blood was injected through the epidural catheter 5 hours or more after the last analgesic drug dose. The catheter was then removed. Mothers in the control group had a blood patch applied, at their request, after conservative treatment had failed.

The volume of blood that should be used when performing EBP is another issue. Palahniuk and Cumming[32] failed to reliably prevent PDPH by the injection of 5 to 10 mL of autologous blood, whereas Crawford[33] suggested that 20 mL was the appropriate volume, unless the patient complained of pain in the back or leg, in which case the injection was stopped. Szeinfeld et al.,[34] using labeled red cells, showed that 12 to 15 mL was effective, with an average segmental spread of one segment per 1.6 mL of blood. They also showed that preferential cephalad spread occurred, with the caudal spread terminating in most cases at S1 or S2.

Rarely, EBP results in significant transfer of blood to the intrathecal space through the dural hole. Patients with this complication may suffer neck stiffness and photophobia for 24 hours.

Intravascular Injection

As mentioned earlier, a useful aphorism for the anesthesiologist is "Every epidural injection is intravascular, until proved otherwise." With that in mind, another aphorism falls into place, "Every dose should be a test dose." The anesthesiologist who proceeds with epidural injections with these thoughts in mind is unlikely to experience the untoward sequelae of an unintentional intravascular injection.

Many techniques have been proposed for facilitating the recognition of epidural intravascular injection. The use of preservative-free epinephrine in a concentration of 1:200,000 is popular. Gogarten et al.[35] suggested that isoproterenol may be a more logical choice, since tachycardia is the end point being looked for. Isoproterenol is a potent β_2-mimetic and might be expected to give a clearer indication of intravascular injection. However, as might be expected, visual analogue pain scores were higher for patients receiving a local anesthetic containing isoproterenol, and the duration of action of the local anesthetic was shorter as compared with epinephrine-containing epidural solutions.

The anesthesiologist should immediately stop injecting the drug if the mother experiences symptoms of intravascular local anesthetic injection or a rise in heart rate when epinephrine-containing solutions are being used. The mother should be observed for further signs of local anesthetic toxicity and an assistant should marshal the resuscitation equipment, which should always be nearby. The mother should receive oxygen by face mask and should be reassured, if appropriate, that the injection into a vein has been detected and stopped. The fetal heart rate should be checked and the obstetrician notified. Once these matters have been dealt with, the anesthesiologist should proceed with placement of another epidural injection at another site, if the mother is willing.

Accidental Intrathecal Blockade

In approximately 0.2% to 4% of epidural insertions, dural puncture occurs. In the majority of cases, the puncture is recognized by the anesthesiologist and appropriate action is taken. In a small percentage of cases, the puncture is not recognized and intrathecal injection of local anesthetic occurs, either through the needle or through the catheter. In rare cases, it has been suggested that the epidural catheter has migrated into the intrathecal space after originally being sited in the epidural space.

Whatever the circumstances, the injection of a quantity of local anesthetic intrathecally results in the rapid onset of a dense sensory and motor blockade of a magnitude related to the quantity and concentration of local anesthetic injected and to other maternal factors. In the least serious situation, the mother experiences unexpectedly rapid and complete pain relief, with some motor paralysis. In the worst case, local anesthetic ascends intrathecally to the brain stem, on the way leading to a rapidly increasing motor block, a progressive respiratory paralysis, total autonomic blockade, and, ultimately, unconsciousness.

This complication is not, as some have suggested, an indication for immediate CS. It is, however, an indication for immediate maternal life support. Having protected the airway, supported ventilation and oxygenation, and corrected any hypotension by fluid or vasopressor administration and lateral tilt, the anesthesiologist should find that the mother becomes hemodynamically stable and the labor progresses painlessly and often quite satisfactorily. Ongoing fetal compromise as determined by the obstetrician should be the indication for surgical intervention. After approximately 1 hour, respiratory efforts, consciousness, and circulatory control will return and the mother can be extubated, hopefully none the worse for her harrowing experience. She and her partner will of course need a detailed explanation of what has occurred.

Inadequate or Absent Blockade

Occasionally, with a frequency inversely related to the anesthesiologist's skill and experience, a mother who has apparently been given an epidural injection will not experience adequate pain relief. Several mechanisms may cause this.

Failed Block

If absolutely no block has resulted, two possible causes need to be considered. First, the local anesthetic has been injected into an area other than the epidural or intrathecal space. Second, the injected solution was not local anesthetic.

In performing an epidural injection, it is possible, on occasion, to enter an area that offers a loss of resistance but is not the epidural space. One potential space lies immediately superficial to the vertebral lamina and sometimes can be very difficult to distinguish from the epidural space. One warning sign is the fact that despite an apparent loss of resistance, air returns into the syringe after pressure on the plunger is released. If a liquid, either the anesthetic solution or saline, is injected, another warning sign is that the pressure required to inject the fluid is greater than normal and rises steadily as the injection proceeds. Often, a quantity of lightly blood-stained fluid returns into the syringe when the pressure on the plunger is released.

The nature of this problem is finally revealed if the epidural needle is advanced 1 or 2 mm. Bone is encountered, indicating that the needle has touched a lamina. This problem is more common if the needle tip strays from the midline as it is advanced. Because the interlaminar space is diamond-shaped, with the long axis running across the interlaminar space, the further the needle tip moves from the midline, the more likely it is that a lamina will be encountered.

Another potential space sometimes located by the inexperienced practitioner is the paraligamentous space associated with the tissues adjacent to the interspinous ligament. Injection into this space produces exactly the same phenomena noted previously in the case of the perilaminar space.

Occasionally, some women have such diffuse and lax interspinous ligaments and ligamenta flava that it is difficult to tell whether the advancing needle has entered the epidural space. Again, injection of liquid into the ligaments results in the phenomena described previously.

If saline rather than local anesthetic has been injected into the epidural space, the analgesia will be inadequate. If liquid other than saline has been injected, the anesthesiologist should immediately try to identify the injected solution, dilute it if appropriate, consult a senior colleague for advice, and inform the medical malpractice insurance provider. Obsessive attention to reading ampule and vial labels is the answer to this problem.

Atypical Block

Two sorts of atypical block can be observed when epidural analgesia is attempted. In the first case, air is used for the loss of resistance, sometimes in large amounts, and the mother is usually on her side for the procedure. If, after injection of the local anesthetic, the mother is left in this position, a unilateral segmental block will often ensue. Injected air has risen to the upper part of the epidural space, preventing local anesthetic access to the nerves and roots in that area. The L1 dermatome on the right side is the segment most often unblocked. Reducing the amount of injected air to only 1 or 2 mL or using saline as the loss of resistance medium and ensuring that the mother is turned to the opposite side after the local anesthetic is injected will reduce the frequency of this troublesome complication.

A second type of atypical block is much rarer but it can prove most puzzling. After apparently uncomplicated insertion of an epidural catheter, the injection of local anesthetic produces a high and unilateral block, often to upper thoracic levels and occasionally resulting in unilateral Horner's syndrome, with a minimal block on the opposite side. Investigations suggest that this outcome occurs when a subdural injection has been made. The subdural space is a potential space, usually not identified during epidural or intrathecal needle insertion. It appears to have a well-defined midline dorsal septum and a very limited capacity for injected fluid. These features explain the physical findings.[36]

Very occasionally, an epidural catheter will appear to travel into a paravertebral space, resulting in dense analgesia in one unilateral segment and minimal analgesia elsewhere. Withdrawing the catheter so that only 3 cm lie in the epidural space and reinjecting a dose of local anesthetic may resolve this rare problem.

In general, it can be said that it is never wise to inject any solution epidurally if pain results. One should check the solution, reposition the needle or the catheter, and choose an alternative analgesic strategy if the problem cannot be resolved.

Persistent Neurologic Deficit

Persistent neurologic deficit occurs in approximately 1 in 20,000 obstetric epidural administrations. Temporary deficit is more common, apparently occurring as often as 1 per 800 obstetric epidural administrations.[37–39] However, postpartum neurologic deficits, both temporary and permanent, have been reported in women who never received an epidural. The complication is rare, but the natural tendency to always blame the anesthesiologist should be resisted. The physician's best ally if the patient develops this complication is an anesthesiologist who has spent a lifetime in obstetric epidural administration. That anesthesiologist will have an understanding of the likely causes far better than a neurologist or obstetrician, and his or her assistance should be sought in analyzing possible causes of the problem, investigating it, and developing a prognosis. Constant communication with the mother and her partner and meticulous record-keeping will go a long way toward keeping the problem out of the courts. The medical malpractice insurance provider should be notified.

Epidural Hematoma

The factors that result in an epidural hematoma are not well understood. It seems likely that the production of an epidural hematoma is a relatively common event, but the production of a clinically significant hematoma is very rare. The fact that anesthesiologists routinely create epidural hematomas while treating PDPH without any significant long-term complications suggests that the harmful epidural hematoma is different from the "normal" and the therapeutic epidural hematoma. The harmful epidural hematoma causes neurologic complications by diminishing cord blood flow to the point where the cord circulation is jeopardized. To do this, the spinal canal pressure must rise to a point at which it approaches or exceeds mean arterial pressure. This suggests that the intraspinal hemorrhage must be arterial rather than venous. Arterial bleeding during an epidural insertion appears to be a very rare phenomenon, and this perhaps explains why harmful epidural hematoma is so rare. Taking aspirin does not appear to increase the risk for epidural hematoma.[40]

The conditions or circumstances that increase the risk of epidural hematoma formation include prior heparinization, preexisting coagulopathy (as, for example, that occurring in eclampsia or preeclampsia), thrombocytopenia from any cause, and the use of low molecular weight heparin prior to the insertion of the epidural.

The classic clinical features that raise the suspicion of epidural hematoma are segmental pain and paresis continuing after the epidural block is expected to have worn off. Consultation with a neurologist and a neurosurgeon must be arranged urgently, and, if possible, a magnetic resonance image (MRI) of the spine should be obtained as soon as possible. Anecdotal evidence suggests that if definitive treatment is delayed beyond 16 hours, neurologic recovery becomes increasingly unlikely. If the MRI demonstrates the presence of an epidural hematoma, then decompression laminectomy should be performed as soon as possible.

Thrombocytopenia and Epidural Analgesia

The most common cause of thrombocytopenia in pregnancy is preeclampsia. The severity of the preeclampsia or eclampsia usually determines the extent of the fall in the platelet count.

Although infection with human immunodeficiency virus (HIV) may cause a fall in the platelet count in both the early infective stage and the later and more advanced, complex stage of the disease related to acquired immunodeficiency syndrome, a study by Gershon et al.[41] has shown that HIV-positive pregnant women do not usually experience a fall in their platelet count. Zidovudine, used to ameliorate the maternal HIV infection's effect on the fetus, does not appear to affect the platelet count either, despite its known side effect of depression of bone marrow function.

EPIDURAL ANALGESIA AND THE DURATION OF LABOR

The effect of epidural analgesia on labor duration and the effects of the variants of epidural and combined spinal and epidural analgesia (CSEA) have been the subject of many investigations. In a comparison of the various studies, confounding factors appear frequently. Racial, ethnic, and community views on the desirability of epidural analgesia are often ignored. Augmentation of labor and even the definition of the onset of labor are often confusing factors. Parity is usually taken into consideration, but maternal expectations and prenatal education are often not mentioned. They will clearly have significant effects on the mother's desire for a normal delivery or wish to resolve a difficult labor with forceps delivery or CS. Delivery management overseen by midwives and that overseen by obstetricians may well result in different outcomes.

Retrospective studies have suggested that epidural analgesia does have an effect on the outcome of labor, increasing cesarean delivery rates, and the frequency of dystocia.[42] Retrospective studies, however, are always subject to potential selection bias, and controlled randomized studies are relatively few. Thorp et al.,[43] in 1993, using a randomized allocation of narcotic and epidural analgesia in nulliparous women, showed that the frequency of prolonged first- and second-stage labor, requirement for oxytocin augmentation, and need for cesarean delivery were all increased in those women who received an epidural block.

Thorp et al.[42] also demonstrated that women receiving epidural analgesia before 5 cm of cervical dilatation had an incidence of fetal malposition late in labor of 21.8%, compared with a frequency of 5.1% in those women receiving their epidural after 5 cm of cervical dilatation. Similarly, the frequency of CS for dystocia was 28% if the epidural analgesia was started at or before 3 cm of cervical dilatation, 16% if placed at 4 cm dilatation, and 11% if placed at 5 cm dilatation or greater. Critics have suggested that those women requiring early epidurals are those with a greater propensity to cervical dystocia and the epidural timing is a reflection of that propensity rather than the cause.

McGrady,[44] in an editorial, has pointed out that in the Thorp study the investigators were not blinded for the analgesic method. The investigators themselves decided what constituted an arrest of first- and second-stage labor and there were no written guidelines for the management of labor or for oxytocin use.

Many studies, nonrandomized and uncontrolled, have shown an association between epidural analgesia in labor and increased instrumental deliveries and CS. None have established a causal relationship. The study by Studd[45] is an example of a well-conducted trial.

Bailey and Howard[46] have shown that increasing epidural rates do not necessarily result in increasing forceps rates. If there were a causal relationship, then it would be expected that studies would have shown a prolongation of labor by now.

The major problem is that studies of epidural analgesia can never be effectively randomized and still stay within current ethical guidelines. Women who request epidural analgesia in labor are those who are more likely to have longer, more painful labors and may well be more likely to require intervention at delivery, forceps delivery, or CS.

It has been shown that active management of labor does decrease the need for CS and forceps delivery. In the study by Turner et al.,[47] the epidural rate was 31% and the CS rate was 5.6%. It is clear that induction rates influence instrumental and CS delivery rates. Women whose labors are induced have more painful labors and higher interference rates and need more analgesia.

Chestnut et al.[48] have demonstrated that epidural analgesia instituted early does not necessarily result in prolonged labor or increase operative delivery either in women laboring spontaneously or in those receiving oxytocin.

As long ago as 1981, Thorburn and Moir[49] showed that increased motor block increases forceps rates. As epidural bupivacaine concentration increased, so did forceps rates. As a result of this study, generations of anesthesiologists have been attempting to reduce drug concentrations. They have supplemented local anesthetic with narcotics and reduced the dose of drugs to the minimum necessary. Vertommen et al.,[50] in a randomized, prospective, double-blind, multicenter study showed that in 695 women receiving epidural analgesia, the addition of sufentanil to 0.125% bupivacaine significantly reduced the incidence of instrumental deliveries from 36% to 24%. Other studies have failed to confirm these findings, but this is understandable, considering the large number of confounding factors present in obstetric management.

If epidural blocks do modify the length and nature of the first and second stages of labor, we do not know for certain how this might be effected. Goodfellow et al.[51] have shown that in the second stage of labor, Ferguson's reflex[52] is inhibited and oxytocin release is reduced by epidural analgesia. Bates et al.[53] have also shown that uterine activity is reduced in the second stage in the presence of epidural analgesia.

It has been assumed that pelvic floor relaxation consequent to epidural analgesia encourages malrotation of the head and lessens maternal expulsive efforts. In the first stage of labor, epidurals do not appear to affect uterine contractility, but they may slow cervical dilatation.[54] Cheek et al.[55] have demonstrated yet another confounding factor. A fluid load of 1000 mL of saline prior to epidural analgesia also decreases uterine activity.

McGrady[44] has suggested that there is no firm evidence that epidural analgesia contributes to rising CS rates. Anesthesiologists should resist attempts by obstetricians to blame them for this phenomenon.

Perhaps the last word for now on this topic was

put forward by Zhang et al.[56] in a review of original studies published in English from 1965 to 1997. They suggest that epidural analgesia increases the risk of oxytocin augmentation twofold. Clinical trials studied suggest that epidural analgesia did not increase the risk for cesarean delivery either overall or for dystocia, nor did it significantly increase the risk for instrumental vaginal delivery. They conclude that epidural analgesia with low-dose bupivacaine may increase the risk for oxytocin augmentation but not that for cesarean delivery.

EPIDURAL ANALGESIA AND INSTRUMENTAL DELIVERY

A significant number of women in labor may require an instrumental delivery. In many cases in which an epidural has been used, the obstetrician will be able to demonstrate that perineal analgesia has developed during the time that an epidural infusion has been running. In such a case, no additional analgesia is required and the instrumental delivery can proceed without maternal discomfort.

If perineal analgesia cannot be demonstrated, the anesthesiologist and obstetrician have several options. The obstetrician may elect to administer a pudendal block. This is probably the least satisfactory solution. The anesthesiologist may elect to administer an epidural bolus of local anesthetic. Many would use 10 to 15 mL of 2% lidocaine with 1:200,000 epinephrine, or chloroprocaine, as these will provide a fast-acting dense perineal analgesia. An anesthesiologist familiar with the caudal epidural technique might elect to administer 10 mL of the same solution caudally and if successful this would also provide satisfactory analgesia. The final option would be to administer a small dose, 1.5 to 2 mL, of 2% heavy lidocaine intrathecally at a space one or two segments lower than the site of the epidural catheter insertion and with the mother in the sitting position. The advantage of this would be the speed with which a dense perineal block is achieved.

COMBINED SPINAL AND EPIDURAL ANALGESIA VERSUS EPIDURAL ANALGESIA

To some practitioners, the use of CSEA in labor appears to be "a solution in search of a problem."[57] The creation of a dural puncture to provide analgesia that can usually be provided by epidural analgesia is a controversial matter.

Pan et al.[58] have demonstrated that there is no difference in the obstetric outcome when spontaneously laboring nulliparae are given epidural analgesia or CSEA in labor before 5 cm cervical dilatation. Some workers, however, are enthusiastic about the apparent benefits of the CSEA technique. When sufentanil 5 to 10 μg is administered intrathecally, rapid and effective relief of labor pain is achieved. This analgesia lasts 1 to 2 hours, and at the end of that time, or when the mother requests further analgesia, a low-concentration local anesthetic and opioid infusion via the epidural catheter is instituted.[59] Concerns about the potential for the intrathecal spread of epidurally administered drugs have meant that workers have been particularly cautious about this new, but possibly valuable, technique.

CONCLUSION

Epidural analgesia in labor aims to provide high-quality pain relief of rapid onset and prolonged duration, while minimizing both maternal side effects, particularly impairment of mobility, and impact on the fetus or on the outcome of labor. In conjunction with pharmacologic research on spinal analgesics (local anesthetics, opioids, and other drug classes), refinement of new or established drug delivery techniques has allowed progress toward more reliable and improved

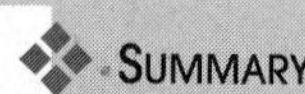

Summary

Key Points

- Neuraxial techniques provide the most effective means of achieving intrapartum analgesia.
- Although epidural analgesia is a safe and effective technique, it is associated with side effects and complications, including hypotension, accidental intrathecal or intravascular injection, and post–dural puncture headache.
- A preanesthetic evaluation must occur prior to placement of an epidural block, and resuscitative equipment must be readily available.
- Administration of a test dose via the catheter will increase the likelihood of recognition of intravascular and intrathecal catheters. Every dose of local anesthetic should be administered incrementally.

Key Reference

Beilin Y, Leibowitz AB, Bernstein HH, Abramovitz SE: Controversies of labor epidural analgesia. Anesth Analg 1999; 89:969–978.

Case Stem

A 22-year-old primiparous patient who had wanted "natural" childbirth requests epidural labor analgesia at 5 cm. She had received an injection of meperidine (pethidine) 2 hours previously, and did not achieve adequate pain relief. Her husband, who is an attorney, tells you that prior to labor she clearly stated that she did not want an epidural and he feels that because of pain and the previously administered opioid, she is not thinking clearly and therefore should not receive an epidural. The patient affirms that she wants an epidural. Before he will allow you to proceed, the husband wants a list of the side effects and their frequency at your institution. How would you proceed?

pain relief at all stages of labor and childbirth. It has also reduced individual drug doses with reduction of unwanted effects and facilitated greater safety and enhancement of maternal satisfaction. Patient-controlled epidural analgesia in labor has been in use for almost a decade, although it is only now at a stage where its role is well defined and utility can be increased. Combined spinal and epidural analgesia is a more recent refinement that appears promising but awaits further investigation.

References

1. Hingson RA, Edwards WB: Continuous caudal analgesia: an analysis of the first ten thousand confinements thus managed with the report of the authors' first thousand cases. JAMA 1943; 123:538–546.
2. Brownridge P: A three-year survey of an obstetric epidural service with top-up doses administered by midwives. Anaesth Intensive Care 1982; 10:298–308.
3. Cleland JGP: Paravertebral anesthesia in obstetrics. Surg Gynecol Obstet 1933; 57:51–62.
4. Brownridge P, Cohen SE, Ward EM: Neural blockade for obstetrics and gynecologic surgery. *In* Cousins MJ, Bridenbaugh PO (eds): Neural Blockade in Clinical Anesthesia and Management of Pain, 3rd ed. Philadelphia: Lippincott-Raven; 1998: 559.
5. Clark SL, Cotton DB, Pivarnik JM, et al: Position change and central hemodynamic profile during normal third-trimester pregnancy and post partum. Am J Obstet Gynecol 1991; 164:883–887.
6. Lees MM, Scott DB, Kerr MG: Haemodynamic changes associated with labour. J Obstet Gynaecol Br Commonw 1970; 77:29–36.
7. Holly RG: Anemia in pregnancy. Obstet Gynecol 1955; 5:562–568.
8. Bieniarz J, Crottogini JJ, Curuchet E, et al: Aortocaval compression by the uterus in late human pregnancy. Am J Obstet Gynecol 1968; 100:203–217.
9. Eckstein KL, Marx GF: Aortocaval compression and uterine displacement. Anesthesiology 1974; 40:92–96.
10. Arsiradam NM, Maliti Z, Rocke DA: Ropivacaine 7.5 mg/ml for epidural anesthesia in elective Cesarean section: a comparison with 5 mg/ml bupivacaine. Anesth Analg 1998; 86:S361.
11. Johnson RF, Olenick M, Minzter B, et al: A comparison of the placental transfer of ropivacaine versus bupivacaine: effect of maternal protein binding. Anesth Analg 1998; 86:S376.
12. Polley LS, Columb MO, Naughton NN, et al: Relative analgesic potencies of ropivacaine and bupivacaine for epidural analgesia in labor. Anesth Analg 1998; 86:S384.
13. Collis RE, Baxandall ML, Srikantharajah ID, et al: Combined spinal-epidural analgesia with ability to walk throughout labour. Lancet 1993; 341:767–768.
14. Armand S, Jasson J, Talfre M-L, Amiel-Tison C. *In* Reynolds F (ed): Effects on the Baby of Maternal Analgesia and Anaesthesia. Philadelphia: WB Saunders; 1993: 54–56.
15. Beilin Y, Andres LA, Comerford MD, Salemo JL: Epidural analgesia with and without fentanyl during labor does not impact on breast feeding. Anesth Analg 1988; 86:S363.
16. Sinatra RS, Eige S, Sevarino FB, et al: Continuous epidural infusion of hydromorphone plus bupivacaine 0.05% during labor and delivery: safety and analgesic efficacy. Anesth Analg 1998; 86:S388.
17. Claes B, Soetens M, Van Zundert A, Datta S: Clonidine added to bupivacaine-epinephrine-sufentanil improves epidural analgesia during childbirth. Reg Anesth Pain Med 1998; 23:540–547.
18. Goodchild CS, Guo Z, Musgreave A, Gent JP: Antinociception by intrathecal midazolam involves endogenous neurotransmitters acting at spinal cord delta opioid receptors. Br J Anaesth 1996; 77:758–763.
19. Roccaforte JD, Susser L, Lax J, et al: Should a test dose of lidocaine with epinephrine be used with the "Walking Epidural" technique? Anesth Analg 1998; 86:S385.
20. Cousins MJ: Epidural neural blockade. *In* Cousins MJ, Bridenbaugh PO (eds): Neural Blockade in Clinical Anesthesia and Management of Pain. Philadelphia: Lippincott-Raven; 1980: 241.
21. Cohen S, Pantuck CB, Pantuck EJ, et al: Epidural block for Cesarean section (C/S): comparison of epidural catheter injection of local anesthetic with gravity flow technique. Anesth Analg 1998; 86:S364.
22. Crowhurst JA, Simmons SW: Patient-controlled analgesia in pregnancy. Int Anesthesiol Clin 1994; 32:45–67.
23. Gambling DR, Yu P, Cole C, et al: A comparative study of patient controlled epidural analgesia (PCEA) and continuous infusion epidural analgesia (CIEA) during labor. Can J Anaesth 1988; 35:249–254.
24. Harke S, Mandell G, Ramanathan S: Patient controlled epidural analgesia versus continuous infusion for labor pain relief. Anesth Analg 1998; 86:S371.
25. Russell R, Groves P, Reynolds F: Is opioid loading necessary before opioid/local anaesthetic epidural infusions? A randomized double blind study in labour. Int J Obstet Anaesth 1993; 2:78–84.
26. Vertommen D, Vandermeulen E, Van Aken H, et al: The effects of the addition of sufentanil to 0.125% bupivacaine on the quality of analgesia during labor and on the incidence of instrumental deliveries. Anesthesiology 1991; 74:809–814.
27. Brownridge P: The management of headache following accidental dural puncture in obstetric patients. Anaesth Intensive Care 1983; 11:4–15.
28. Gormley JB: Treatment of post spinal headache. Anesthesiology 1960; 21:565–566.
29. DiGiovanni AJ, Dunbar BS: Epidural injection of autologous blood for post lumbar puncture headache. Anesth Analg 1970; 49:268–270.
30. Colonna-Romano P, Shapiro BE: Unintentional dural puncture and prophylactic epidural blood patch in obstetrics. Anesth Analg 1989; 69:522–523.
31. Lowenwirt I, Cohen S, Zephyr J, et al: Can prophylactic epidural blood patch reduce the incidence and severity of postpartum dural puncture headache in obstetrics? Anesth Analg 1998; 86:S378.
32. Palahniuk RJ, Cumming M: Prophylactic blood patch does not prevent post lumbar puncture headache. Can Anaesth Soc J 1979; 26:132–133.
33. Crawford JS: Experiences with epidural blood patch. Anaesthesia 1980; 35:513–515.
34. Szeinfeld M, Ihmeidan IH, Moser MM, et al: Epidural blood patch: evaluation of the volume and spread of blood injected into the epidural space. Anesthesiology 1986; 64:820–822.
35. Gogarten W, Van Aken H, Buerkle H, et al: The effects of the addition of isoproterenol to 0.125% bupivacaine on the quality and duration of epidural analgesia during labor in the parturient. Anesth Analg 1988; 86:S369.
36. McMenemin IM, Sissons GR, Brownridge P: Accidental subdural catheterization: radiological evidence of a possible mechanism for spinal cord damage. Br J Anaesth 1992; 69:417–419.
37. Dawkins CJM: An analysis of the complications of extradural and caudal block. Anaesthesia 1969; 24:554–558.
38. Kane RB: Neurological deficits following epidural or spinal anesthesia. Anesth Analg 1981; 60:150–156.
39. Usubiaga JE: Neurological complications following epidural anesthesia. Int Anesthesiol Clin 1975; 13:1.
40. Paull JD: Aspirin and epidurals: The anaesthetist's dilemma. Int J Obstet Anaesth 1994; 3:1–2.
41. Gershon RY, Dolak J, Board E, et al: Platelets and the HIV-infected parturient. Anesth Analg 1988; 86:S368.
42. Thorp JA, Eckert LO, Ang MS, et al: Epidural analgesia and cesarean section for dystocia: risk factors in nulliparas. Am J Perinatol 1991; 8:402–410.
43. Thorp JA, Hu DH, Albin RM, et al: The effect of intrapartum epidural analgesia on nulliparous labor: a randomized, controlled, prospective trial. Am J Obstet Gynecol 1993; 169:851–858.
44. McGrady EM: Extradural analgesia: does it affect progress and outcome in labour? [Editorial.] Br J Anaesth 1997; 78:115–117.

45. Studd JWW: The effect of lumbar epidural analgesia on the rate of cervical dilatation and the outcome of labour of spontaneous onset. Br J Obstet Gynaecol 1980; 87:1015–1021.
46. Bailey PW, Howard FA: Epidural analgesia and forceps delivery: laying a bogey. Anaesthesia 1983; 38:282–285.
47. Turner MJ, Brassil M, Gordon H: Active management of labor associated with a decrease in the cesarean section rate in nulliparas. Obstet Gynecol 1988; 71:150–154.
48. Chestnut DH, Vincent RD, McGrath JM, et al: Does early administration of epidural analgesia affect obstetric outcome in nulliparous women who are receiving intravenous syntocinon? Anesthesiology 1994; 80:1193–1200.
49. Thorburn J, Moir DD: Extradural analgesia: the influence of volume and concentration of bupivacaine on mode of delivery, analgesia efficacy and motor block. Br J Anaesth 1981; 53:933–939.
50. Vertommen JD, Vandermeulen E, Van Aken H, et al: The effects of the addition of sufentanil to 0.125% bupivacaine on the quality of analgesia during labor and on the incidence of instrumental deliveries. Anesthesiology 1991; 74:809–814.
51. Goodfellow CF, Hull MGR, Swaab DF, et al: Oxytocin deficiency at delivery with epidural analgesia. Br J Obstet Gynaecol 1983; 90:214–219.
52. Ferguson JKW: A study of the motility of the intact uterus at term. Surg Gynecol Obstet 1941; 73:359–366.
53. Bates RG, Helm CW, Duncan A, Edmonds DK: Uterine activity in the second stage of labour and the effect of epidural analgesia. Br J Obstet Gynaecol 1985; 92:1246–1250.
54. Newton ER, Schroeder BC, Knape KG, Bennett BL: Epidural analgesia and uterine function. Obstet Gynecol 1995; 85:749–755.
55. Cheek TG, Samuels P, Miller F, et al: Normal saline i.v. fluid load decreases uterine activity in active labour. Br J Anaesth 1996; 77:632–635.
56. Zhang J, Klebanoff MA, DerSimonian R: Epidural analgesia in association with duration of labor and mode of delivery: a quantitative review. Am J Obstet Gynecol 1999; 180:970–977.
57. Paech M: New epidural techniques for labour analgesia: patient-controlled epidural analgesia and combined spinal-epidural analgesia. Baillieres Clin Obstet Gynaecol 1998; 12:377–395.
58. Pan PH, Moore C, Fragneto R, et al: Do obstetric outcomes differ between early combined spinal-epidural and epidural anesthesia in spontaneously laboring nulliparous parturients? Anesth Analg 1998; 86:S382.
59. Norris MC, Arkoosh VA: Spinal opioid analgesia for labor. Int Anesthesiol Clin 1994; 32:64–81.

11

The Combined Spinal-Epidural Technique

❖ Narinder Rawal, MD, PhD
❖ Björn Holmström, MD, PhD
❖ André Van Zundert, MD, PhD
❖ John A. Crowhurst, D(Obst), RCOG, FANZCA

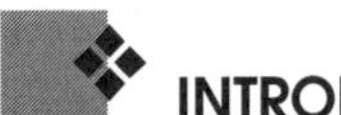

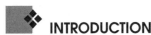

INTRODUCTION

In the last two decades there has been considerable revival of interest in and use of regional anesthesia techniques for surgery and pain management. New drugs, new needle designs, and developments in catheter technology have contributed to improve the quality and safety of regional anesthesia. Several modifications of blockade techniques have been described to improve the efficacy and safety of brachial plexus, femoral, sciatic, and other peripheral nerve blocks. New regional anesthesia techniques such as interpleural, intra-articular and combined spinal-epidural (CSE) anesthesia and analgesia have been introduced in recent years.

The CSE technique has attained widespread popularity for patients undergoing major surgery below the umbilical level who require prolonged and effective postoperative analgesia. Epiduroscopy and spinaloscopy, as well as the newer radiologic imaging techniques, have revealed new insights into the anatomic structures in the lumbar-epidural and subarachnoid areas, thus improving the performance and safety of central regional blocks. The CSE technique is now well established in many institutions. This chapter includes the history, clinical experience, advantages, and potential problems, and points out some future perspectives of the CSE technique.

History

During the last century several workers used different equipment and techniques to achieve the goal of combining the advantages of both subarachnoid and epidural anesthesia (Table 11–1). In the 1920s the two major central blocks for surgery under the umbilical level were subarachnoid anesthesia and sacral (caudal-epidural) block. Lumbar-epidural block was unknown at that time. In 1923 Rodzinski, a Polish surgeon, published his 2 years' experience with sacrolumbar anesthesia for abdominal and lower extremity surgery.[1] The technique consisted of injection of 3 to 4 mL of 1% procaine hydrochloride (Novocain) intrathecally followed by 30 to 40 mL of 1% procaine hydrochloride in the caudal-epidural space. In 1937 Soresi, a New York surgeon, reported use of what he called "episubdural block."[2] The aim was to overcome two disadvantages of the two existing techniques for central regional block, namely the short duration of the subarachnoid block and the slow onset of the epidural block. To accomplish this, he first injected a dose of procaine hydrochloride epidurally and then, by advancing the fine needle, punctured the dura mater and administered an intrathecal dose of procaine hydrochloride with the assumption that the initially rapid but shorter-acting intrathecal block would gradually be taken over by the longer-acting epidural block. Soresi provided episubdural anesthesia to over 200 patients with analgesia lasting 24 to 48 hours.

The first report on the combination of subarachnoid block with continuous epidural catheter technique was published in 1979 by Curelaru.[3] He used a double interspace CSE technique in 150 patients undergoing upper and lower abdominal, urologic, and lower extremity surgery. The technique consisted of introducing the epidural catheter followed by a sub-

Table 11–1 Historical Development of Combined Spinal-Epidural Technique

Technique	First Published Report: Author	Year	Surgery/Indication	Reference
Single Segment (one skin puncture)				
Same needle, lumbar approach	Soresi	1937	General surgery	2
Needle-through-needle	Coates, Mumtaz et al	1982	Orthopedic surgery	5, 6
Needle-through-needle	Carrie and O'Sullivan	1984	Cesarean section	7
Needle-through-needle, sequential technique	Rawal	1986	Cesarean section	8
Needle-through-needle	Abouleish et al	1991	Labor analgesia	24
Needle-beside-needle, double barrel	Torrieri and Aldrete	1988	Miscellaneous surgery below the umbilicus	9
Needle-beside-needle, double barrel	Eldor	1988	Miscellaneous surgery below the umbilicus	10
Needle-beside-needle	Turner	1992	Miscellaneous surgery below the umbilicus	11
Needle beside catheter	van Dijk et al	1994	Miscellaneous surgery below the umbilicus	12
Epidural and subarachnoid catheters	Vercauteren et al	1993	"High-risk patients"	13
Double Segment (two separate skin punctures)				
Sacral block followed by subarachnoid block	Rodzinski	1923	Miscellaneous surgery below the umbilicus	1
Epidural block followed by spinal block	Curelaru	1979	General surgery	3
	Brownridge	1981	Cesarean section	4
Epidural and subarachnoid catheters	Møiniche et al	1994	General surgery	15

arachnoid block in an adjacent lumbar interspace (Fig. 11–1). In 1981 Brownridge reported successful use of a double segment CSE technique in nearly 200 parturients undergoing cesarean section. In about 90% of the patients, the subarachnoid block alone was adequate for cesarean section.[4] The epidural catheter was available to extend the block if necessary and to provide postoperative analgesia.

A modification of the combined subarachnoid-epidural technique was reported by Coates[5] and by Mumtaz and associates[6] for orthopedic surgery and by Carrie and O'Sullivan[7] for cesarean section. These investigators described a single-space, "needle-through-needle" technique in which the epidural needle served as an introducer for a long, fine-gauge spinal needle (Fig. 11–2*A* and *B*). In 1986 Rawal described a sequential, single-segment CSE technique for cesarean section.[8] In this two-stage technique the epidural catheter was not just a reserve catheter, it served as a conduit for local anesthetic to gradually raise the level of an intentionally low subarachnoid block.

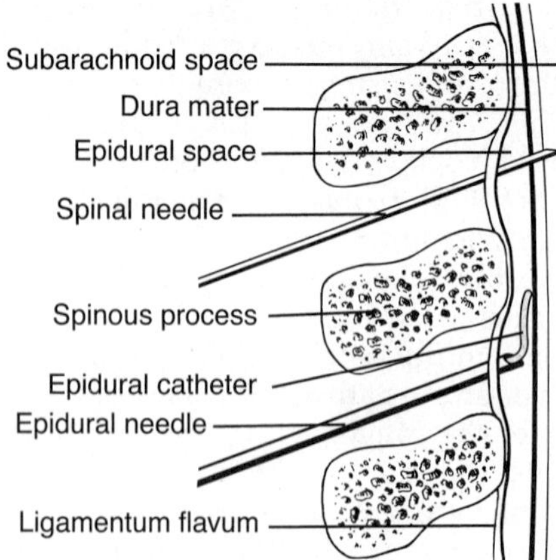

Figure 11–1 Double segment combined spinal-epidural (CSE) technique. The spinal needle and the epidural needle are introduced in separate interspaces in the lumbar area. Either the spinal or the epidural needle can be introduced first.

Torrieri and Aldrete[9] as well as Eldor[10] have reported modifications of the CSE technique using specially designed needles, with the spinal needle (or a spinal needle introducer) welded to the epidural needle (Fig. 11–3). This allows the anesthesiologist to first perform the epidural catheter insertion (thus making it possible to give an epidural test dose) and then perform the subarachnoid block in the same interspace. Other authors have used the Tuohy needle inserted into the epidural space as a guide and introduced the spinal needle alongside the Tuohy needle in the same interspace.[11, 12] A combination of epidural and spinal catheters was described for surgical anesthesia in high-risk patients by Vercauteren and colleagues.[13]

CLINICAL EXPERIENCE WITH THE COMBINED SPINAL-EPIDURAL TECHNIQUE

The CSE technique has been used for general surgery,[3, 14–16] orthopedic and trauma surgery of the lower limb,[5, 17–19] urologic surgery,[20] gynecologic surgery (including cesarean section),[4, 7, 21–23] management of labor pain,[24–28] and postoperative pain.[13, 17, 29–31] CSE blocks have also been used as research tools for controlled comparison between different epidural and subarachnoid techniques.[17, 18, 27, 32–48] Furthermore, the

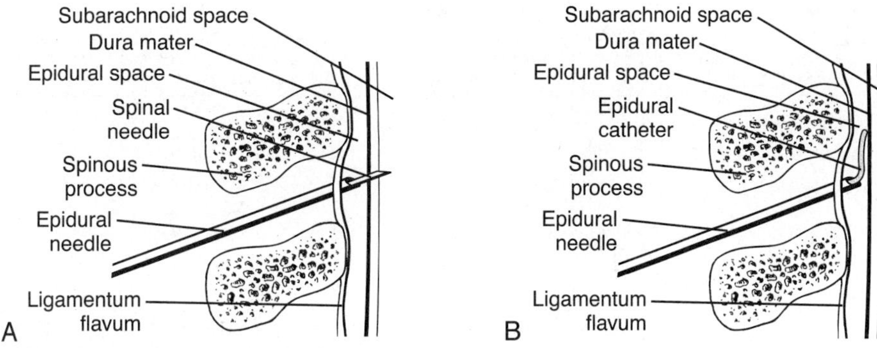

Figure 11–2 *A,* Needle-through-needle technique, stage 1: the spinal needle is introduced through the epidural needle and punctures the dura mater. *B,* Stage 2: after the spinal needle is withdrawn, the epidural catheter is introduced and secured in place.

technique has been used successfully in all age groups including preterm neonates[49] and infants,[50] the very old,[17, 51] and other high-risk patients.[13, 23, 28]

Currently the CSE technique is mainly used for major orthopedic surgery, where severe postoperative pain may be anticipated, for cesarean section and assisted vaginal delivery, and for analgesia and other indications in labor.[16, 52–54]

Combined Spinal-Epidural Block for Surgical Anesthesia

CSE Block for General Surgery. Epidural postoperative analgesia after major general surgery has become very popular in recent years. When appropriate (e.g., surgery below the umbilical plane) the surgical procedure may be performed under epidural anesthesia alone. However, because it is well recognized that epidural block does not always provide acceptable surgical conditions, several authors have reported use of the CSE technique for general surgery.[3, 14, 16, 20, 23] The subarachnoid part of the block provides rapid and efficient surgical anesthesia and the epidural catheter can be used if needed during surgery, but most commonly for postoperative pain relief. For high-risk patients the CSE technique can also facilitate careful titration of anesthetic spread of the block. If a sequential technique is used, initiating surgical anesthesia with a reduced dose of subarachnoid local anesthetic produces a limited sensory block. The desired level of sensory block is then achieved by incremental epidural injections of local anesthetics alone or in combination with opioids (Table 11–2). This method of CSE block extension can even be achieved by epidural injection of saline alone.[55–57]

CSE Block for Orthopedic Surgery. Almost without exception, major orthopedic surgery requires ef-

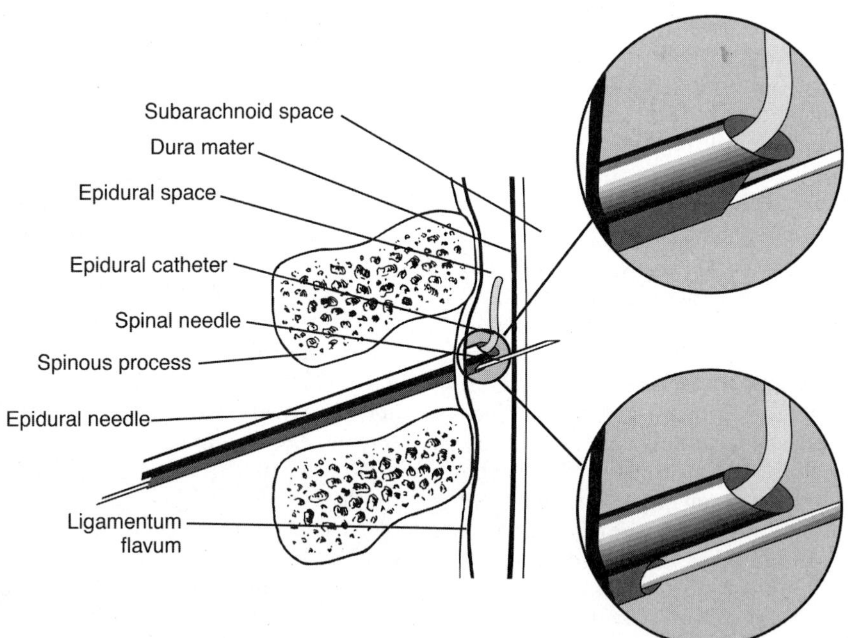

Figure 11–3 Single-segment needle-beside-needle technique. Introduction of the spinal needle beside the formerly introduced epidural needle. It is emphasized that in recent years many different needle-tip designs have been introduced.

Table 11-2 Suggested Drug Doses and Mixtures for Combined Spinal-Epidural (CSE) Anesthesia*

Procedure	Administration	Local Anesthetic	Opioid	Notes
Standard CSE for Cesarean Section				
	Intrathecal injection	BUP 0.5%–0.75%, 7.5–15.0 mg	FEN, 20–25 μg *or* SUF, 3–5 μg *or* MO, 0.1–0.2 mg	Epinephrine, 2–5 μg, may be added
	Epidural top-up†	BUP 0.25%–0.5%, 10–40 mg	FEN, 20–25 μg *or* SUF, 5–10 μg	
Sequential CSE for Cesarean Section				
	Intrathecal injection	BUP 0.5% hyperbaric, 5.0–12.5 mg	FEN, 20–25 μg *or* SUF, 3–5 μg	Epinephrine, 2–5 μg, may be added
	Epidural top-up†	BUP 0.2%–0.5%, 10–50 mg	FEN, 20–25 μg *or* SUF, 5–10 μg	
Standard CSE for Nonobstetric Surgery				
	Intrathecal injection	BUP 0.5%, 12.5–20.0 mg	MO, 0.1–0.3 mg	Epinephrine, 2–5 μg, may be added
	Epidural top-up†	BUP 0.5%, 20–30 mg *or* MEPI 2%, 40–80 mg	FEN, 25 μg *or* SUF, 25 μg	

*Doses and recommendations in this table are based on studies cited in the text and on the authors' clinical experience in more than 8000 administrations.

†Epidural dose administered *after* intrathecal injection; 10 mL of saline injected epidurally within 10 min following intrathecal injection often increases cranial spread of subarachnoid block (see text).

BUP, bupivacaine; MEPI, mepivacaine; MO, morphine sulfate (preservative-free); FEN, fentanyl; SUF, sufentanil.

fective prolonged postoperative pain management. Hence orthopedic surgery has become another important indication for CSE technique. Clinical studies have demonstrated that the CSE technique provides excellent surgical conditions as quickly as with a "single-shot" subarachnoid block, and better conditions than with epidural block alone.[17, 58] When CSE block was compared with either epidural or subarachnoid block for hip or knee arthroplasty, CSE anesthesia was superior to epidural anesthesia. With the CSE technique, surgical anesthesia was rapidly established, saving 15 to 20 minutes compared with epidural anesthesia. Furthermore, the epidural catheter provided the possibility to supplement insufficient subarachnoid anesthesia. In Holmström and coworkers' study, 0.2 mg and 0.4 mg of intrathecally administered morphine was equally as effective for postoperative pain relief as was 4.0 mg of epidural morphine.[17]

CSE Block for Outpatient Surgery. To perform surgery on an outpatient basis is an increasing challenge for anesthesiologists. Using the potential advantages of the CSE technique, it can be well used for such procedures. Urmey and coworkers used the CSE technique to investigate the appropriate dose of intrathecal isobaric 2% lidocaine for outpatient arthroscopy.[18] In all 90 patients the technique provided excellent anesthesia. The patients receiving a reduced dose (40 mg), however, had significantly shorter-duration anesthesia, which allowed quicker discharge than for the patients receiving 60 or 80 mg of intrathecal lidocaine.[18] Norris suggested use of a CSE technique with intrathecal sufentanil alone for outpatient shock wave lithotripsy, saving the epidural catheter for patients with inadequate analgesia.[20]

CSE Block for Cesarean Section. Worldwide, cesarean section is the major surgical procedure most frequently performed under regional anesthesia. Moir reports that "the delivery of the infant into the arms of a conscious and pain-free mother is one of the most exciting and rewarding moments in medicine".[59] To achieve this, the technique chosen for regional anesthesia for cesarean section needs to be efficient, safe, reliable, and often, rapidly induced. Several factors are responsible for the increasing popularity of regional anesthesia for cesarean section. Many advantages of regional over general anesthesia have been identified.[60] Safe, effective prophylaxis against maternal hypotension,[61] and improved surveillance techniques and equipment, such as needles and catheters, have contributed to regional anesthesia's popularity.[38] However, both epidural and subarachnoid anesthesia still have drawbacks, making these techniques potentially unreliable as the sole methods of anesthesia for cesarean section.

It is generally recognized that a sensory block of the T4 to S5 vertebral segment is necessary for adequate anesthesia during cesarean section, even though it has been shown that satisfactory analgesia can be achieved with less extensive motor block.[62] Extensive sensory block may be associated with a relatively high incidence of hypotension[63, 64] and risk of local anesthetic toxicity if such a block requires large doses of drugs.[65–67] Furthermore, despite these large doses epidural block may be inadequate in up to 25% of patients, mainly because of difficulty in blocking sacral nerve roots or because the block is not high enough.[60, 65, 68] Subarachnoid anesthesia is more reliable than epidural anesthesia because of its more intense motor and sensory block, but the upper level of a subarachnoid block may be very variable and the technique may be hazardous for the fetus if uncontrolled maternal hypotension develops.[69–73] Since subarachnoid block is usually a single-shot technique, there is little possibility of improving an inadequate block or providing extended postoperative pain relief without using an intrathecal opiate such as morphine. The use of intrathecal morphine can be hazardous in high-risk or elderly patients, but in low doses (<0.2 mg) it is considered safe in obstetric and low-risk populations.[74]

When regional anesthesia became popular for both analgesia and anesthesia in obstetrics during the 1970s and 1980s, epidural block was the technique of choice. Subarachnoid block was associated with disturbing side effects such as maternal hypotension and postdural puncture headache (PDPH). Increased knowledge of placental physiology and better maternal blood pressure control, along with the reintroduction of fine gauge, noncutting (pencil-point) spinal needles, has generated an increased interest in the subarachnoid route for cesarean section anesthesia.[38]

Following the first reports by Brownridge and by Carrie and O'Sullivan on their experience with CSE block for cesarean section,[4, 7] several authors have compared the CSE technique with other central blocks, in both controlled studies and in large patient series.[21, 22, 30, 75, 76] To achieve the desirable T4 to S5 segment sensory block for surgical anesthesia, the CSE technique can be used with different approaches.

Standard CSE Block. The "standard" CSE technique for cesarean section reported by several authors is to use the subarachnoid part of the block for surgery, and only use the epidural catheter during surgery in the few cases in which the subarachnoid block is deficient. Postoperatively, the epidural catheter is used for pain control.

Vucevic and Russell used the CSE technique to test two different volumes of subarachnoid plain bupivacaine, 15 mg (12 mL 0.125% solution vs. 3 mL 0.5% solution) in 40 women, scheduled for elective cesarean section.[77] This resulted in a significant difference in the upper level of the subarachnoid block between the two groups during the 30-minute period the patients maintained their initial lateral position. When the patients were turned supine with a right tilt, this difference disappeared, but owing to the insufficient spread in the 3-mL group, 5 patients (25%) required supplemental epidural lidocaine before surgery. Notable is that all patients demonstrated a significant rise in block level when turned 30 minutes after subarachnoid injection.[77]

Today most authors advocate use of hyperbaric bupivacaine 0.5% or 0.75% in a dose ranging from 10 to 15 mg injected intrathecally with the patient either sitting or in the lateral position. Furthermore, several obstetric anesthesiologists also combine the subarachnoid bupivacaine with fentanyl, 15 to 25 μg or sufentanil, 5 to 10 μg (Table 11–2). Studies currently in progress suggest that if sequential CSE or block extension technique is used within 5 to 10 minutes of the intrathecal injection, the bupivacaine dose can be reduced to less than 10 mg (J. A. Crowhurst, personal observations; R. Stienstra, personal communication, 1999).[78]

In a recent randomized, blinded study Davies and colleagues compared CSE block with epidural block for cesarean section.[79] The time to a T4 sensory block and to start of surgery was significantly shorter with the CSE technique, even though the epidural technique consisted of epidural injection of pH-adjusted lidocaine with added fentanyl for optimal onset of block. One of the study end points was maternal satisfaction with the anesthesia technique, and interestingly parturients receiving CSE blocks were less anxious and more satisfied during both placement of the block and induction of surgical anesthesia. Furthermore the patients having CSE blocks experienced less pain, especially during needle and catheter insertion and during delivery of the fetus.[79]

Sequential CSE Technique. In a controlled study a sequential CSE technique was compared with epidural block for cesarean section.[21] In the patients in the sequential CSE group a reduced dose of hyperbaric bupivacaine was injected intrathecally, followed by epidural injection of bupivacaine if needed (Table 11–2). All patients receiving sequential CSE block had good to excellent analgesia, compared with only 74% receiving epidural block. The muscular relaxation was also better following sequential CSE block. The total dose of bupivacaine for a T4 block was three times larger in patients receiving only epidural block. The maternal and fetal blood bupivacaine levels were correspondingly about three times higher in the epidural group. In addition, the incidence of maternal hypotension was higher in patients receiving only epidural block. Apgar scores, umbilical cord blood gases, and neurobehavioral evaluation did not show any differences between the two groups of neonates. Thus the investigators concluded that sequential CSE block was superior to epidural block alone for cesarean section and that CSE block combined the reliability of subarachnoid block and the flexibility of epidural block while minimizing their drawbacks.[21] Similar results were obtained by Randalls and coworkers, who compared four different intrathecal drug doses with CSE block for cesarean section.[78]

Although the sequential CSE technique takes somewhat longer than the standard CSE technique, the use of minimal doses of local anesthetics has been shown to reduce the frequency and severity of maternal hypotension when compared with epidural or spinal techniques.[34, 80, 81] Decreased frequency and severity of hypotension during CSE block is presumably due to less extensive and slower onset of the supplemental low-dose epidural block, which allows more time for compensatory mechanisms to be effective.

In summary, for cesarean section the CSE technique can reduce or eliminate most of the disadvantages of subarachnoid or epidural anesthesia alone, while preserving their respective advantages. The CSE block offers the speed of onset, efficacy, and minimal toxicity of a subarachnoid block combined with the potential of improving an inadequate block or prolonging the duration of anesthesia with epidural supplements, and extending the analgesia well into the postoperative period.

Combined Spinal-Epidural Analgesia in Labor

In several centers low-dose CSE analgesia has begun to replace traditional epidural techniques. While there remains some concern about dural puncture, the CSE technique offers many advantages in the parturient. Few obstetric anesthesiologists advocate the use of CSE analgesia for all labors, but many indications are beginning to be recognized. These include women who are in severe pain when regional anesthesia is requested; the oxytocin-augmented labor; malpresentation in late first-stage labor; obstructed labor; second-stage fetal distress; and women whose epidural blocks in previous labors were unsatisfactory. The latter group often includes the obese and patients in whom there is some spinal anatomic abnormality. Indeed, in many units, requests for regional anesthesia are not received until severe pain is present. The difficulty in predicting the duration of first-stage of labor and occasional late request for epidural analgesia may result in delivery before the requested epidural block has become established. In these circumstances the low-dose subarachnoid injection affords relief within 2 to 3 minutes.[26]

Injecting local anesthetics,[82] opioids,[25, 27] or combination of drugs[25, 26, 35, 36, 44, 47, 83–86] intrathecally provides rapid onset analgesia. Intrathecal opioids are being used increasingly by obstetric anesthesiologists to provide labor analgesia; the commonest opioids used are sufentanil[25, 27, 48, 83, 87–91] and fentanyl.[44, 87, 92] Morphine[24, 89] and meperidine[87] are less popular in the context of labor analgesia. However, one of the main limitations of intrathecal opioids such as sufentanil and fentanyl is the short duration of analgesic effect, which would require additional dural puncture(s). Therefore intrathecal opioids would most appropriately be used with the CSE technique.[27] When the CSE technique is employed, the epidural catheter can be used if labor continues beyond the duration of the subarachnoid block or to improve analgesia if the subarachnoid block is inadequate (Table 11–3). Figure 11–4 shows the rapidity of onset of analgesia with a low-dose mixture CSE block compared with a "high-dose" (10 mL bupivacaine 0.25% alone) epidural block. With CSE, the initial intrathecal dose of bupivacaine, 2.5 mg, and fentanyl, 25 μg, is extremely efficacious, removing most severe pain in less than 5 minutes. This intrathecal dose can be a low-dose mixture of local anesthetic and opioid, or sufentanil alone (10–15 μg). Sufentanil has been reported to cause acute fetal bradycardia, but recent studies which suggest the median effective dose (ED_{50}) of intrathecal sufentanil to be less than 3 μg have failed to demonstrate any fetal problems.[93, 94]

Thus, injecting low-dose local anesthetics and/or opioids or their combination intrathecally can avoid the problem of delivery before epidural analgesia has become established. In other urgent second-stage labor situations, this rapid-onset analgesia makes it possible for an assisted delivery to proceed without the delay seen when epidural block alone is administered. Low-dose CSE block in these situations offers a further advantage in that if vaginal delivery fails, the epidural catheter can then be used to induce anesthesia for abdominal delivery. Similarly, the epidural catheter can be used later if labor continues beyond the duration of the initial subarachnoid block; for continuation of labor; for perineal repairs; for removal of placental products; or for postnatal analgesia.

Other CSE Advantages. Epidural techniques have a small failure rate, owing in part to the "blind" nature of the method. Identification of the epidural space by loss of resistance to saline or air is the most reliable method by which the epidural space is identified. However, this method is not objective in itself and confirmation of correct epidural placement of needle and/or catheter can be made only by injection of an initial dose of local anesthetics alone, or local anesthetics with epinephrine and/or opioid, and allowing sufficient time for the signs of epidural blockade to appear. To date there are no definitive comparative studies comparing failure rates of low-dose CSE and epidural techniques. With the CSE technique, epidural catheter failure or misplacement is still possible, but the initial analgesia provided by the intrathecal injection can assist in placing or replacing an unreliable epidural

Table 11-3 Suggested Drug Doses and Mixtures for the Combined Spinal-Epidural Technique in Labor*

Administration	Local Anesthetic	Opioid
Intrathecal injection	BUP 0.1%–0.25% isobaric, 1.0–2.5 mg	FEN, 20–25 μg *or* SUF, 3–10 μg
Epidural top-ups	BUP 0.1–0.125%, 10–15 mg for 1st-stage labor. During 2nd stage of labor or for assisted delivery (e.g., lift-out forceps), this dose will usually be sufficient. For other operative deliveries, the doses should be titrated to surgical requirements using BUP 0.5% *or* LIDO 2% *or* chloroprocaine 3%.	FEN, 20–25 μg *or* SUF, 5–10 μg

Doses and recommendations in this table are based on studies cited in the text and on the authors' clinical experience in more than 10,000 administrations.

BUP, bupivacaine; LIDO, lidocaine; FEN, fentanyl; SUF, sufentanil.

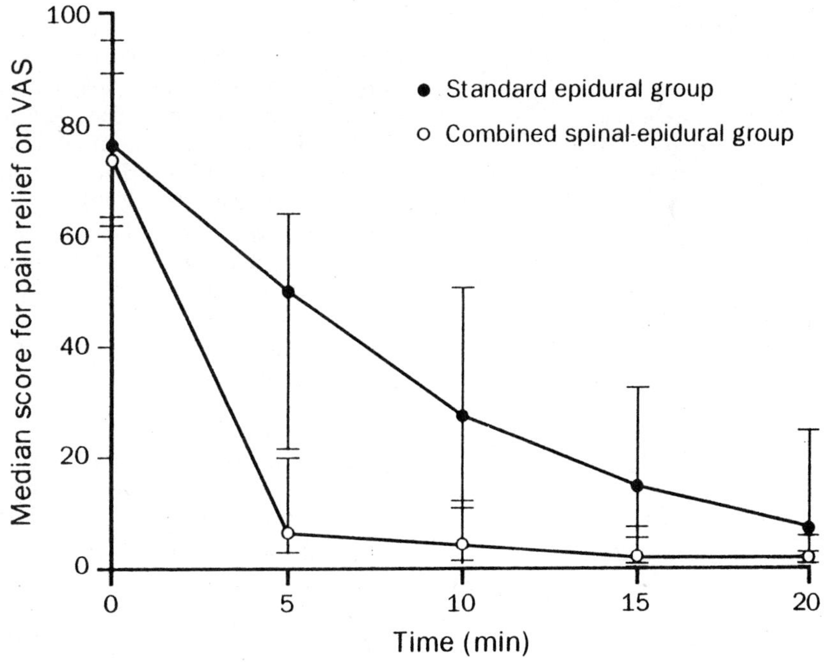

❖ **Figure 11–4** Median pain relief scores (visual analogue scale, VAS) during first 20 min after establishment of block. Note that in the epidural group there are, even after 10 min, several patients still experiencing pain with a VAS rating above 5. Error bars indicate IQR (interquartile range). 0 = best outcome. (From Collis RE, Davies DWL, Aveling W: Randomised comparison of combined spinal-epidural and standard epidural analgesia in labour. Lancet 1995; 345:1413–1416. ©The Lancet, 1995.)

catheter. Initial intrathecal drug placement improves reliability too, in that very small doses of drugs placed in the cerebrospinal fluid (CSF) are distributed more evenly than larger doses placed in the epidural space, where epidural fat, epineurium sheaths, other tissues, and epidural veins may greatly reduce drug availability. Rapidity of onset and reliability of technique improve quality of analgesia. Although finely tuned, selective blockade can be achieved slowly with low-dose epidural mixtures, the initial quality of rapid-onset CSE analgesia has been reported as increasing maternal satisfaction.[79] Satisfaction data are very "soft," however, and are confused with satisfaction related to the ability to ambulate. However, to date, large studies comparing low-dose epidural analgesia with CSE analgesia in this context are not available.

Ambulation with CSE Analgesia. For labor pain the CSE technique offers the possibility of combining rapid-onset intrathecal analgesia with the flexibility of epidural analgesia. This approach, using low-dose local anesthetic and/or opioid, can provide a very selective sensory block with minimal motor blockade, allowing parturients to ambulate during labor.[37] The neurologic features of low-dose local anesthetic and opioid CSE analgesia versus epidural block alone for the parturient in the first 20 to 30 minutes after the initial dose are shown in Table 11–4. In one study of 300 parturients

Table 11–4 NEUROLOGIC FEATURES OF REGIONAL LABOR ANALGESIA

	LOW-DOSE CSE BLOCK (INTRATHECAL DOSE)	LOW-DOSE EPIDURAL BLOCK (NO TEST DOSE)
Motor Block		
Lumbar plexus grade 0–1*	No	Yes
Sacral plexus (pelvic floor to S2–S4 nerve roots)	No	Yes
Sensory Block		
Proprioception	No	No
Sympathetic Block	Minimal	Yes
Analgesia		
VAS pain score	0–2	4–6

*Bromage Scale.
CSE, combined spinal-epidural analgesia; VAS, visual analogue scale.

receiving a combination of intrathecal bupivacaine and fentanyl, the CSE technique provided analgesia yet allowed most mothers to walk throughout labor.[26] While it is unclear whether ambulation in labor reduces its duration, it has been suggested that analgesic requirements are reduced by ambulation, and that women appreciate the opportunity to ambulate even for short periods during labor.

Traditionally, motor blockade is assessed clinically using the Bromage Scale or related scales. These scales attempt to quantify power of muscle groups of the leg, foot, and anterior, medial, and lateral thigh. (Knee flexors and hip extensors [hamstrings] are rarely assessed in clinical practice.) Changes in power in such muscle groups give a good indication of motor blockade of the lumbar spinal nerve roots, but not the sacral nerve roots. Weakness in the L1 to L5 lumbar roots is easily detected and graded by the clinical tests shown in Table 11–5. To enable ambulation, all muscle groups innervated by the L5 to S1 nerve roots should have normal or near-normal power.

Minimal motor block of abdominal muscles—not categorized on the Bromage Scale—suggests there should be improved maternal muscle strength for pushing in the second stage of labor, another advantage of low-dose regional blockade. However, afferent blockade of sacral nerves S2 to S5 is still present and coordination of pushing with contractions continues to be a controversial aspect of these blocks. Nevertheless, low-dose CSE can be fine-tuned to allow many parturients to be aware of contractions, which are painless. (The use of an external tocograph can also assist mothers to coordinate pushing efforts.) One feature of motor-sparing low-dose CSE analgesia seen when a block is maintained for many hours is that CSE preserves motor power longer than epidural block alone. Undoubtedly, this is due to lower total dosage over time (Fig. 11–5).

Present-day low-dose neuraxial blockade has all but eliminated motor and proprioceptive block of muscle groups of the leg, thigh, and foot, but pelvic floor muscles are still blocked with minute intrathecal and/or epidural doses of local anesthetics and/or opioids. (J. A. Crowhurst, personal observations, 1999). Studies of the nature and significance of pelvic sacral neuronal blockade are not yet available. While a discussion of the controversial subject of regional blockade and mode of delivery is beyond the scope of this chapter, it cannot be denied that lower sacral nerve roots continue to be affected by low-dose CSE techniques. Despite a lack of clear evidence that *low-dose* regional anesthesia prolongs labor, it is widely acknowledged that labors conducted with regional anesthesia are longer and are more likely to result in an operative delivery if the regional anesthesia is administered before 4 cm of cervical dilatation.[95, 96] Until a method of analgesia is developed that eliminates pelvic sacral nerve block, thus preserving pelvic floor tone, this debate will continue. Perhaps elimination of local anesthetic drugs completely will be the definitive answer to this problem.

Many workers have established that proprioceptive (dorsal column) functions can be selectively preserved with low-dose CSE and epidural analgesic blockade. In addition to lack of motor block, proprioception, especially joint-position sense, is required for safe coordinated activities such as walking. Recent studies have demonstrated that the CSE technique of Morgan and associates[26] provides a block with minimal (lumbar and S1 nerve roots) motor blockade, and truly selective sensory blockade in that dorsal column (proprioceptive) functions are preserved, thus making ambulation possible.[97–99] To achieve this, however, it is necessary to omit the traditional epidural test dose.[98, 100]

There is little doubt that the ability to walk, or at least to get out of bed during labor, contributes greatly to maternal satisfaction, but decreased cesarean section rates have not been elucidated, despite two recent attempts to do so.[96, 101] Morgan concludes that, to date, "there is as yet no conclusive study which shows that maintaining the upright position in labor reduces the incidence of forceps delivery. . . . Advantages *seem* to be less pain and shorter labours."[102]

To be pain-free and able to walk in labor is extremely popular with many women, but safe ambulation with low-dose CSE analgesia requires

- No postural hypotension or symptoms
- Minimal or no motor block
- Minimal or no proprioceptive block
- Monitoring facilities, including the fetus
- A cooperative, understanding parturient
- Presenting part of fetus engaged and well applied to cervix

Ambulating with low-dose CSE or epidural block can be hazardous, so it is prudent to take the following precautions:

- Avoid postural hypotension.
- Avoid aortocaval compression and Valsalva straining.
- Monitor motor block.
- Provide a suitable environment, for example, shoes, safe floors, no cables, and the like.
- Avoid epidural catheter displacement; ensure good fixation of catheter to skin.
- Simplify intravenous therapy by use of a heplock intravenous cannula and disconnect the intravenous line or have the parturient ambulate with an IV pole on wheels.

Table 11–5 CLINICAL TESTS OF MOTOR NERVE AND MUSCLE GROUPS

MOTOR FUNCTION	TESTED NERVE ROOTS
Hip flexion	L1–L3
Straight leg raise	L1–L4
Knee extension	L2–L4
Ankle dorsiflexion	L4–L5
Great toe dorsiflexion	L5
Ankle and forefoot plantarflexion	L5–S1*
Foot eversion	L5–S1*
Pelvic floor and sphincters	S2–S4

*Blocked only by the subarachnoid route.

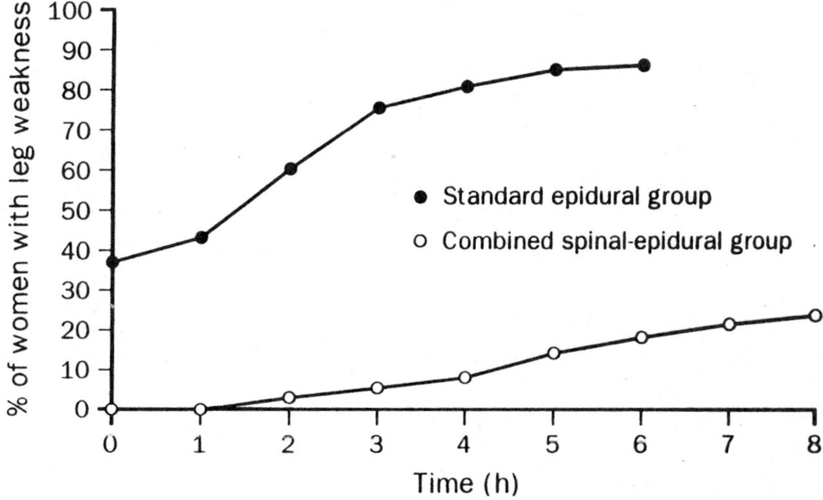

❖ **Figure 11–5** Frequency of leg weakness, as shown by inability to sustain straight-leg raise. (From Collis RE, Davies DWL, Aveling W: Randomised comparison of combined spinal-epidural and standard epidural analgesia in labour. Lancet 1995; 345:1413–1416. ©The Lancet, 1995.)

- Provide suitable (remote, cordless) fetal monitoring.

Epidural maintenance of analgesia is readily achieved with a low-dose mixture of local anesthetic and opioid. Bupivacaine/fentanyl or bupivacaine/sufentanil have been the most studied combinations, but recently interest has turned to ropivacaine, which in higher doses appears to spare motor nerves more than bupivacaine. This is yet to be confirmed, however, because at higher doses (concentrations of >0.1%), ropivacaine is only 40% as potent as bupivacaine, and most studies to date have not compared equipotent doses. Epidural dose requirement studies of both opioid and local anesthetics indicate that the doses given in Table 11–3 provide satisfactory analgesia in 95% of patients. At present 0.1% bupivacaine with fentanyl, 2 μg/mL, is a most popular combination in Great Britain. (Some situations, however, do require higher epidural top-up doses. Examples include persistent fetal occipito-posterior position, as well as transverse vertex, deflexed fetal head, and other potentially obstructing presentations in late first-stage and second-stage labor.)

COMBINED SPINAL-EPIDURAL TECHNIQUES

There are several options for performing the CSE block. In the early years CSE blocks were performed with multiple-use extra long 25- to 30- gauge spinal needles which were introduced through standard Tuohy needles. In recent years special CSE needle sets have been introduced. At present there are more than a dozen medical equipment companies that distribute specialized CSE needle sets worldwide.

Needle-Through-Needle Technique. Probably the most popular technique for CSE block is the single-segment "needle-through-needle" technique. With the patient in the sitting or lateral decubitus position, an appropriate epidural needle is inserted at the desired intervertebral space (below the L2 nerve root) and the epidural space is identified in the usual manner. Next an extra long 24–27-gauge (or smaller diameter) spinal needle is introduced through the epidural needle and advanced until the tip of the spinal needle is felt to penetrate the dura (the dural "click"). When the stylet is removed, correct intrathecal placement of the spinal needle is confirmed by free flow (or aspiration) of CSF, and the appropriate dose of local anesthetic and/or opioid is injected. If loss of resistance to air is employed to identify the epidural space, any clear fluid coming out of the spinal needle will be CSF. The loss of resistance felt when the epidural space is entered can be regarded as a sign similar to the dural puncture "click" felt with the needle-through-needle technique when the spinal needle enters the subarachnoid space. Because the dural click is not in itself an objective sign, the free flow of CSF from the spinal needle hub is needed to confirm correct placement. During the injection into the subarachnoid space, the parturient is asked to report feelings of warmth under the buttocks and thighs. If this symptom is not reported within 30 seconds, the dose has most probably not been delivered intrathecally. This routine enables one to detect proper intrathecal placement while the spinal needle is still in place. A further, almost immediate sign of correct subarachnoid placement is to ask the patient to contract her pelvic floor muscles. Loss of muscular contraction is further confirmation of subarachnoid injection. Most pregnant women are well aware of their pelvic floor because of frequent exercises that are practiced during pregnancy.

It should be emphasized that at this stage the

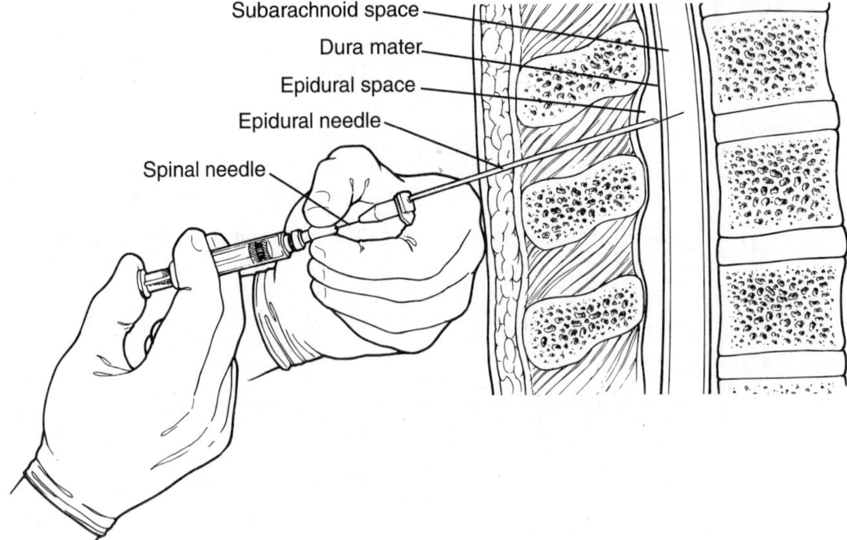

Figure 11–6 To prevent dislocation of the spinal needle tip when using the needle-through-needle CSE technique, this steadying grip may be helpful. The back of the hand rests against the back of the patient, while the fingers "lock" the two needle hubs during the injection through the spinal needle.

spinal needle is held in place only by the dura mater; therefore, there is a risk of needle displacement during syringe connection or during injection of local anesthetic. This is a critical stage in the needle-through-needle technique.[103] The problem can be overcome by steadying the spinal needle using the grip shown in Figure 11–6. Spinal needle displacement may not be a problem with the newer special CSE kits in which the hub of the spinal needle locks into the hub of the Tuohy needle (Fig. 11–7).[104]

After the spinal needle is withdrawn, a catheter is introduced about 4 to 5 cm into the epidural space through the Tuohy needle. Epidural catheter position is confirmed by negative aspiration of blood or CSF, or by the administration of an epidural test dose such as lidocaine plus epinephrine. This is followed by injection of about 1 mL of saline into the epidural catheter to test its patency. The catheter is secured firmly with tape and is now available for use.

Sequential CSE Technique. Sympathetic block–induced, precipitous maternal hypotension remains one of the most common problems associated with subarachnoid block for cesarean section. Despite prophylactic measures, such as fluid preloading, prophylactic vasopressors (ephedrine), elastic support stockings, and lateral tilt, it may be difficult to maintain normal blood pressure. Maternal hypotension may lead to maternal cerebral hypoperfusion, and parasympathetic imbalance may trigger nausea and vomiting. Uncorrected,

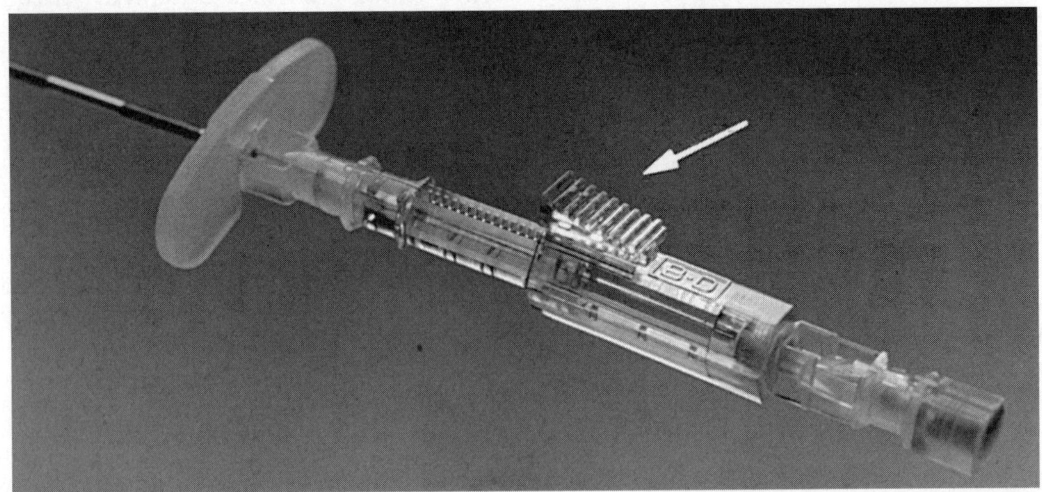

Figure 11–7 The Adjustable Durasafe CSE needle system (courtesy of Becton-Dickinson, Franklin Lake, NJ) contains a locking mechanism *(arrow)* between the two needle hubs.

maternal hypotension may result in fetal hypoxemia and acidosis owing to uteroplacental hypoperfusion.[72, 73] To reduce the incidence and severity of hypotension, a two-stage sequential CSE technique has been described.[8, 21] This technique is quite similar to that described previously, but the main differences are

1. The block is performed with the patient in the sitting position.
2. The dose of intrathecal hyperbaric bupivacaine is intentionally kept low (5–10 mg of hyperbaric 0.5% bupivacaine solution) because the aim is to achieve only an S5 to T8 to T9 block.
3. The patient is then placed supine with a left lateral tilt.
4. Within 10 minutes the sensory block is extended to the T4 nerve root by injecting fractionated doses of local anesthetic (0.25% bupivacaine) solution or normal saline into the epidural catheter (1.0–1.5 mL for every unblocked segment is often sufficient) (Fig. 11–8).

In patients undergoing cesarean section, intrathecal dose reduction of hyperbaric bupivacaine from 12.5 to 7.5 mg resulted in less hypotension and quicker recovery.[81] When compared with single-shot subarachnoid block with 12.5 mg of hyperbaric bupivacaine, 7.5 mg of hyperbaric bupivacaine injected intrathecally using the CSE technique resulted in significantly slower onset of maternal hypotension.[34] In another study four different intrathecal doses of hyperbaric bupivacaine (2.5 mg, 5 mg, 7.5 mg, and 10 mg) were compared in patients undergoing cesarean section under sequential CSE block. The authors demonstrated that 5 mg of intrathecal bupivacaine combined with appropriate-dose epidural lidocaine provided adequate surgical anesthesia. Higher doses of intrathecal bupivacaine were associated with adverse effects of high subarachnoid block, such as nausea, vomiting, and dyspnea.[76]

The sequential CSE technique may be particularly advantageous in high-risk parturients in whom gentler onset of sympathetic blockade is desirable. This is important in patients with preeclampsia, pheochromocytoma, some cardiac diseases, or other conditions (such as small stature) in which the use of subarachnoid block alone may be hazardous or difficult to control. This may also be the case with other high-risk patients in the nonobstetric population, as, for instance, the very old orthopedic patient. Traditionally such patients are managed with slow epidural blockade that requires much higher total dosages than sequential CSE. By careful positioning of the patient before induction of subarachnoid anesthetic and by allowing titration with small incremental epidural doses to the precise level of anesthesia desired, the sequential CSE technique may enhance the safety of the central regional block.

Double-Barrel or Double-Segment CSE Technique. During induction of CSE block using a needle-through-needle technique it may occasionally be difficult to thread a catheter into the epidural space after the subarachnoid injection. If some minutes are spent in replacing the epidural needle, the subarachnoid block may become "fixed" in the dependent area. If difficulty is experienced threading the catheter, its insertion should be abandoned or attempted at another level. However, subarachnoid anesthesia may obscure a paresthesia during epidural catheter insertion. Moreover, it may be difficult to verify the position of the epidural catheter because of difficulty in identifying unintentional subarachnoid or subdural injections in the presence of the existing spinal block.

These problems may be overcome if the epidural catheter is introduced before the subarachnoid injection. Placement of the epidural catheter before subarachnoid injection can be accomplished by the use of the one of the single-segment "double-barreled" needles, such as E-SP (NeuroDelivery Inc, Tempe, AZ) and Eldor (CSEN, Jerusalem, Israel) needles or by using the separate spaces technique described by Brownridge.[4] Yet another approach is to insert the spinal needle in the same lumbar segment adjacent to the epidural needle already in place.[12]

However, prior placement of an epidural catheter does not necessarily guarantee an increased success rate. A Swedish survey from 1993 showed that depart-

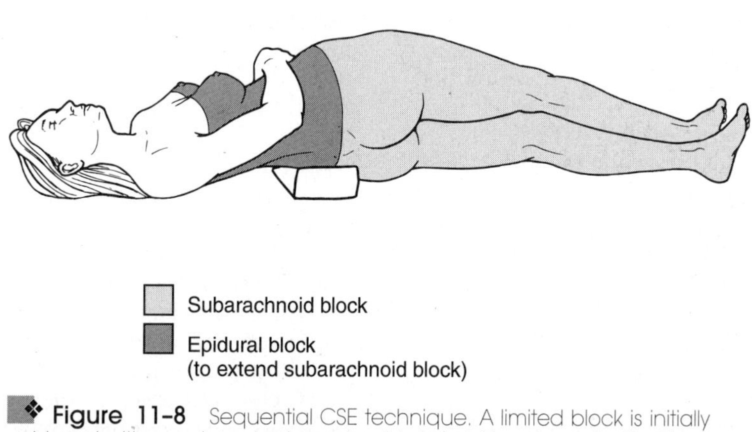

❖ **Figure 11–8** Sequential CSE technique. A limited block is initially achieved with a reduced subarachnoid dose of local anesthetic. The block is then gradually extended by incremental doses of local anesthetic injected through the epidural catheter.

ments using the double interspace technique for CSE (epidural first, then subarachnoid injection) reported more epidural catheter penetrations through the dura than departments using a single interspace CSE technique.[53] Norris and colleagues also noted an increased incidence of unintended dural puncture during conventional epidural technique for labor analgesia when compared with CSE block using the needle-through-needle method.[105] Since epidural catheter migration can occur over time, only a recently injected epidural test dose holds significance. In our opinion an epidural test dose prior to spinal block is of little use if the epidural catheter is to be activated after surgery. Furthermore, if an epidural test dose is administered before the subarachnoid injection, a portion of this test dose may appear in the hub of the spinal needle and create confusion. Finally, the direction of epidural catheter passage is unpredictable. Radiologic and video epiduroscopic studies have shown that epidural catheters may take unpredictable paths.[106–108] A catheter may even tie itself in a knot.[109] It is hence conceivable that a prior-positioned epidural catheter may divert the spinal needle.

Whether the epidural catheter is introduced before or after the subarachnoid injection and irrespective of the CSE technique used, it should be remembered that accidental subdural catheter placement can occur and that this is more common than generally believed[110] (see Chapter 9). This may account for such phenomena as delayed-onset block, profound and extensive blockade, Horner's syndrome, and for unexplained headaches, total spinal blocks, and neurologic sequelae. The commonly used safeguards, aspiration and test dose, may be unreliable because they cannot detect subdural placement.[110]

So far, there is no controlled study that has compared morbidity after single versus double interspace techniques, nor has morbidity been compared between needle-through-needle and double-barrel needle techniques. Compared with introducing needles into two interspaces, the single interspace technique may be expected to cause considerably less discomfort, trauma, and morbidity from interspinous tissue penetration including backache, epidural venous puncture, hematoma, infection, and technical difficulties.[111, 112]

In conclusion, it is obvious that either CSE sequence has its advantages and disadvantages. However, if the patient is experiencing severe pain, for example, is well into labor, when the block is being administered, the better option is to perform the subarachnoid injection first to achieve rapid analgesia, and then to place the epidural catheter in a calmer, more cooperative patient.[37]

Two-Catheter CSE Technique. Reports on the use of continuous intrathecal combined with epidural catheter techniques have been published.[13, 29] In one study the double-catheter technique was combined with general anesthesia for abdominal surgery. The intrathecal and epidural catheters were inserted at different levels.[29] Vercauteren and colleagues have described a double-catheter technique through a single interspace. The main advantages claimed were the possibility of testing the correct position of the epidural catheter before injecting drugs intrathecally, and of titrating the intrathecal dose of local anesthetic to the desired dermatomal level. Because of the requirement of a large-diameter spinal needle (22 gauge), the risk of catheter penetration may be high. Knotting of the catheters is also a theoretic risk.[13]

CONTROVERSIAL ASPECTS OF THE COMBINED SPINAL-EPIDURAL TECHNIQUE

The only major difference between a CSE block and a conventional epidural block with a catheter is, from a technical point of view, the deliberate puncture of the dura mater with the fine spinal needle during CSE administration. The resulting dural hole may constitute a theoretic risk with the CSE technique, irrespective of whether it is performed with the needle-through-needle method, a single-segment/double-barrel, or a double-segment technique.

Four major concerns about risks with CSE have been expressed in the literature. First, the risk of epidural catheter migration through the dural hole has been suggested, especially with the needle-through-needle CSE technique.[113, 114] Second, the potential risk of increased drug leakage through the dural hole has been the concern of others.[31] Unexpectedly high sensory blocks, or "total spinals," when spinal anesthesia has been performed after failed epidural anesthesia[115, 116] or following injection of local anesthetics through an epidural catheter, inserted after an unintended dural puncture with the Tuohy needle, constitute clinical concerns of a leakage mechanism.[117, 118] Third, case reports of infectious complications after CSE blocks have implied an increased risk of spread of infectious agents through the dural hole.[119–121] Furthermore, a fourth concern, contamination of CSF with metal particles from damaged spinal needle tips during the needle-through-needle CSE technique, has been suggested.[122]

Risk of Catheter Migration Through the Dural Hole. Epidural catheter migration into the subarachnoid space is potentially very serious because failure to recognize catheter misplacement and injection of a usual epidural dose could result in total subarachnoid anesthesia if appropriate testing is omitted. However, the infrequency with which this complication has been reported indicates that the risk does not constitute a major problem in clinical practice.[123] At our respective institutions, we have not seen any late epidural catheter migration in more than 16,000 patients since 1992. When testing an epidural catheter in this context, extensive subarachnoid block is unlikely if only small increments of low-dose solutions are used.

However, at the time of performing CSE block we have seen odd cases of epidural catheter penetration into the subarachnoid space. Aspiration of CSF has confirmed such intrathecal placement. Dural damage by the Tuohy needle could not be ruled out in either case. A similar case report was published by Robbins and coworkers.[124] At Queen Charlotte's Hospital in London where CSE blocks have been used for vaginal and cesarean deliveries in over 10,000 cases since 1992, no catheter migrations were noted during a 3-year period[82] or subsequently. In the Swedish survey four cases of epidural catheter penetration were detected among the 2381 CSE blocks reported. All catheter migrations occurred while the blocks were being performed and they were all identified by spontaneous CSF flow or by aspiration test.[53]

In an experimental study on pieces of isolated human dura, Rawal and coworkers reported that it was virtually impossible to force an 18-gauge epidural catheter through dural holes made by 26- or 27-gauge needles.[21] With epiduroscopy and video recording in the human epidural space, the dynamic events during CSE block may be examined with the dura left intact. In a cadaveric model we performed an epiduroscopic study of epidural catheter migration during CSE administration (Fig. 11–9). After visualization of the Tuohy needle tip in the epidural space, a CSE block was performed with a single dural puncture by the spinal needle, followed by insertion of an epidural catheter into the epidural space. With the aim to simulate a difficult CSE block (in which multiple dural puncture attempts may be performed), four additional holes were made with the spinal needle before the epidural catheter was inserted. Lastly, a dural puncture was made with the Tuohy needle, and the insertion of an epidural catheter was recorded. In every subject the anatomic structures and experimental steps described were video recorded at one or several lumbar levels. It was impossible to force a 16- or 18-gauge epidural catheter through the dural hole after a single dural puncture with a 25-gauge spinal needle. Even when five holes were made with a 25-gauge spinal needle in the same area of the dura, epidural catheter penetration into the subarachnoid space occurred in only 1 out of 20 recordings (5%). After intentional dural puncture with a Tuohy needle, epidural catheter penetration into the subarachnoid space occurred in 45% of cases.[106]

It must be emphasized that the possibility of subarachnoid or intravenous placement exists with *any* epidural catheter and that the danger of a massive intrathecal dose is not unique to the CSE technique. Total spinal blocks are an acknowledged complication of "top-ups" of previously normally functioning epidural catheters.[107, 108, 118, 125, 126] Such catheters that have functioned normally with previous injections have also been documented to perforate epidural blood

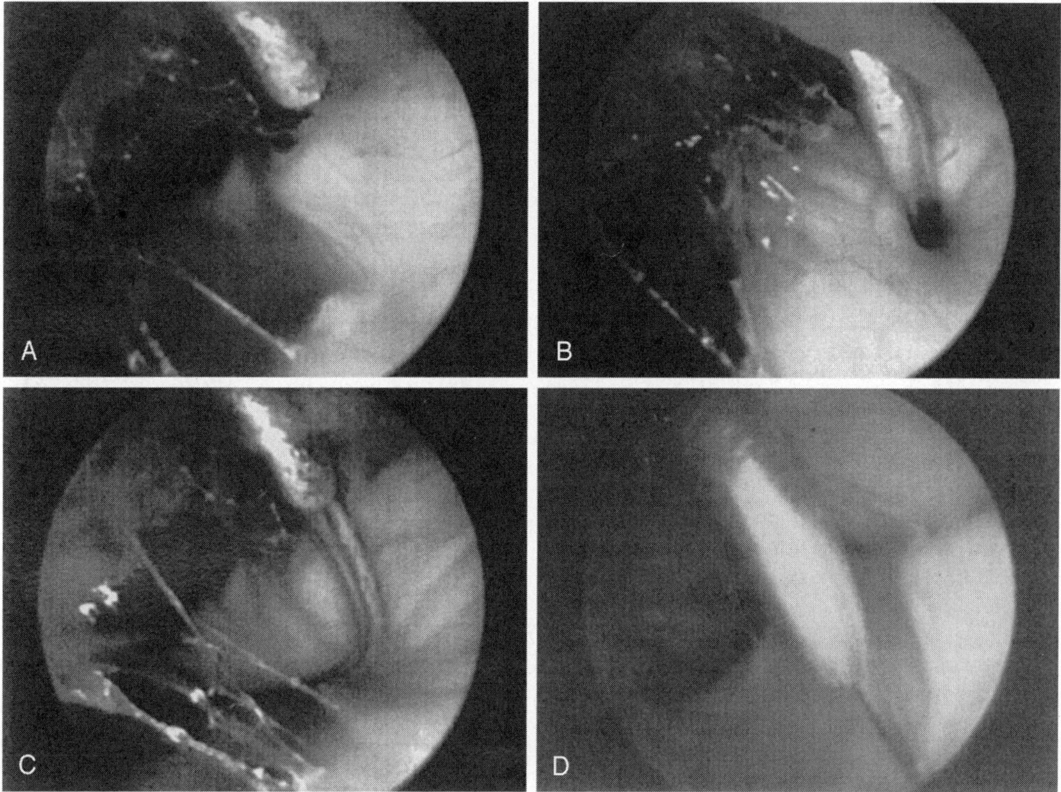

❖ **Figure 11–9** Epiduroscopy view of epidural space and CSE needles. *A,* The Tuohy needle enters the epidural space through the ligamentum flavum *(top).* At right and bottom of picture is the dura mater. *B,* The tip of the epidural catheter enters the epidural space through the tip of the Tuohy needle and immediately impacts the dura. *C,* The fine spinal needle punctures the dura in front of the Tuohy needle tip. *D,* The epidural catheter takes a straight cephalad route in the epidural space. Note the fragile connective tissue filaments between the dura mater *(bottom)* and ligamentum flavum *(top and left).*

vessels.[127, 128] With regular continuous epidural technique Ready and Wild reported three catheter migrations in 12,000 doses of epidural opioids. All were easily detected by using an aspiration test.[129] The risk of catheter migration can be expected to be greater if there is a hole in the dura. Therefore it is important that the routine for epidural top-up doses should be clearly defined at all institutions where the CSE technique is practiced. This routine is not different from that of standard epidural technique and consists of confirmation of the catheter position by aspiration test as well as frequent assessment of the block following injection of **fractionated doses**. Continuous epidural infusion of low-concentration local anesthetic may be safer than high-concentration bolus injection. Every reinjection should be considered a "test dose," especially in the parturient.[130] If motor blockade of the distal L5 to S1 nerve roots is noticed after low-dose top-ups or within 45 to 60 minutes of continuous low-dose infusion, intrathecal catheter siting is likely. The core bundles of these nerve roots can be blocked only by low doses of local anesthetics injected intrathecally.[131]

Rotation of the Epidural Needle. It has been advocated that the Tuohy needle be rotated 90 to 180 degrees between subarachnoid injection and epidural catheter insertion so that the site of dural puncture is at some distance from the point at which the catheter impinges.[8, 132, 133] Presumably this would decrease the risk of catheter migration into the subarachnoid space. This may not be a good idea, however. It has been reported that rotation of the epidural needle may cause dural tear or puncture, or relieve an obstruction to CSF flow.[105, 134–137] In one report a complication rate of 3% increased to 17% when rotation of the epidural needle was introduced.[136] All of us have stopped this practice since 1988.

Controlling Upper Level of Block. The difficulty in controlling the upper level of subarachnoid block and consequent fear of inadequate analgesia appears to have prompted the use of relatively large subarachnoid doses of local anesthetic for cesarean section. With the CSE technique the presence of an epidural catheter permits the anesthesiologist to use smaller doses for subarachnoid block, thereby decreasing the incidence and severity of maternal hypotension.[21, 34] Single-shot intrathecal doses of bupivacaine in the range of 7.5 to 10.0 mg have been shown to provide effective anesthesia for most patients undergoing cesarean section.[21, 138, 139] These doses are considerably less than those reported by others.[67, 140] When additional doses of epidural local anesthetic have been necessary to extend the spinal block, some authors have reported rapid extension of the subarachnoid block after relatively small doses of epidural catheter top-ups.[21, 138]

The mechanism of this phenomenon is unknown, but the following hypotheses have been proposed:

- Continuing spread of initial subarachnoid block (unrelated to epidural injection).[141]
- Existence of "subclinical" analgesia at a higher level that is enhanced and becomes evident by perineural or transdural spread of epidural local anesthetic.[142]
- Leakage of epidural local anesthetic through the dural hole into the subarachnoid space.[143–146]
- Change in epidural pressure. The pressure becomes atmospheric, which may result in better spread of local anesthetic through an effect on volume and circulation of CSF.[138]
- Compression of the theca by the epidurally injected volume of local anesthetic (or even saline) solution resulting in a "squeezing" of CSF and more extensive spread of subarachnoid local anesthetic.[21, 55, 147–149]

Transdural Drug Transport. Theoretically a dural puncture may allow dangerously large quantities of subsequently administered epidural drugs to reach the subarachnoid space.[143] The possibility of this hazard is supported by reports of high or total spinal block during epidural anesthesia after unintentional and unidentified dural perforation with the epidural needle.[117, 150, 151] Experimental studies have shown that transdural leakage of CSF may occur after dural punctures and that the flow rate through the dural hole depends on the diameter and shape of the spinal needle.[152–154] However, these studies were all performed with dural preparations in laboratory settings and focused on CSF leakage from subarachnoid to epidural space as a possible explanation for the difference in PDPH rate after dural puncture with different types of spinal needles.[152–154] Although leakage of epidural local anesthetic into the subarachnoid space is theoretically possible, the rapidity with which block extension occurs suggests some other mechanism. Furthermore, our knowledge of pressures within the epidural and subarachnoid spaces and of the role of CSF leakage in PDPH suggests that the flow of fluids is more likely to be away from the subarachnoid space rather than toward it.

Data from clinical studies of the CSE technique did not demonstrate any clinically important additional increase in spread of sensory block.[17, 34] These results suggest that there is no substantial passage of epidurally injected drugs through the dural opening left by the spinal needle. However, Myint and associates reported a case of cardiorespiratory arrest in a patient who had received CSE block for cesarean section.[31] The complication occurred 40 minutes after diamorphine was administered in the epidural catheter to provide postoperative analgesia. Respiratory arrest was believed to be a complication of epidural diamorphine, rather than the CSE technique.[31] It is emphasized that epidural diamorphine has caused respiratory depression and death even when the dura is not breached.[155]

Results of experimental studies demonstrate that the amount of any leakage through the perforated dura depends on the size of the dural hole.[143, 146, 154, 156] Bernards and coworkers tried to maintain the physiologic properties of the meninges in experiments with monkey dura preparations with reference to the CSE technique.[143] The authors used bicarbonate-buffered "mock" CSF solution and bubbled a mixture of oxygen and carbon dioxide through the test chambers. The results were presented as total drug flux, thus including both passive diffusion and active leakage of drug. The drug flux resulting from the puncture of a 27-gauge pencil-point needle was 1.8% of the drug flux through a Tuohy needle puncture.[143] Westbrook and coworkers, studying the forces needed to puncture bovine dura preparations and the subsequent CSF leakage, reported a corresponding relationship between leakage after a 27-gauge pencil-point and a Tuohy needle puncture (2.6%).[154] The net amount of epidural drug in the subarachnoid space can be expected to increase considerably if a small volume of concentrated solution is injected close to the dural hole made by a large-bore needle.[143]

In our recent experiments in fresh cadavers, we evaluated the potential leakage in comparison to a standard leakage level of 3%. The 3% level chosen was based on pharmacokinetic studies of morphine and meperidine suggesting the fraction of drug to cross the dura to be about 3% to 4%,[157] and clinical data indicating that equipotent intrathecal morphine dose is about 3% of the corresponding epidural dose.[158]

When comparing doses of drugs administered intrathecally or epidurally, a considerably larger ratio for equipotency is reported for local anesthetics than for morphine or meperidine. For instance, 12.5 to 20.0 mg of intrathecal bupivacaine produces a similar block to that of 75 to 120 mg of bupivacaine injected epidurally, giving a ratio of about 1:5 to 1:8 or equal to 15% to 20%.[159] Consequently it was decided to set a lowest level of clinical importance at 3%. Radioactive iodinated serum albumin (^{125}I-RISA) was used as "drug" and the CSF sample was analyzed for the amount of radioactivity using a well-type scintillation detector in a sampler changer, calibrated for the ^{125}I photon energy. The intrathecal injection of a 3% ^{125}I-RISA dose resulted in CSF activity 7 times higher than the leakage through a dural hole made by a 27-gauge spinal needle. Thus the results show that the leakage after a dural puncture with a 27-gauge pencil-point needle is well below this 3% level, and hence the leakage after a 27-gauge pencil-point needle puncture may not be of clinical importance. The leakage through a dural hole made by a Tuohy needle resulted in CSF activity of ^{125}I-RISA more than 12 times higher than in the 3% group, offering a reasonable explanation for the reported extensive sensory blocks following epidural administration of local anesthetics after an unintended dural puncture with the Tuohy needle.

Hence our results confirm that the leakage through a dural hole clearly depends on the diameter of the puncturing needle. The relationship between the values in the "Tuohy" and the "CSE" groups in our study (1.8%) corresponds well with the earlier reports on drug leakage through dural holes made by different-sized needles.[143, 154] Consequently, a dural puncture with the 18-gauge Tuohy needle causes a leakage large enough to possibly cause a clinical effect, which indicates that caution must prevail when an epidural block is performed directly after an unintended dural puncture with an epidural needle in an adjacent lumbar interspace. Our experimental design stresses the sole mechanical impact of the dural hole on any drug leakage from the epidural into the subarachnoid space, possibly even more than in vivo, in which there is a counteracting CSF pressure.

In a clinical study Suzuki and associates investigated the influence of a dural puncture made by a 26-gauge spinal needle on the spread of 2% mepivacaine (18 mL) administered through an epidural catheter.[160] The authors were able to demonstrate a difference in sacral spread by two additionally blocked dermatomes after 15 minutes. However, the cephalad spread ranged between the T2 and T11 dermatomes in both groups, which must be considered of greater clinical importance than the extended sacral spread. Furthermore, the total number of blocked dermatomes in the two groups was not reported.

Pressure Changes in the Epidural and Subarachnoid Spaces. Far more important than any drug leakage during CSE block seems to be the influence on spread of intrathecal block by the changes in epidural and, subsequent, CSF pressures induced by injections of drug solutions or saline into the epidural space.

Blumgart and colleagues suggested that increased epidural pressure may lead to an increase in cephalad spread of the subarachnoid block.[55] The same increase in cephalad spread was noted with either 10 mL of saline or 10 mL of local anesthetic solution injected epidurally. No increase in cephalad spread was recorded in a control group who received no epidural injection.[55] Based on these results Felsby and Juelsgaard in a review of the CSE technique suggested epidural saline as a method of prolonging the subarachnoid block.[161] Stienstra and associates, however, demonstrated a dual effect, with an epidural injection of 10 mL of local anesthetic solution causing a larger increase in cephalad spread of the subarachnoid block than did the same volume of epidurally administered saline. Both injections did cause a greater cephalad spread than the control group not receiving any epidural injection at all.[56] In a study with patients scheduled for orthopedic surgery, Mardirosoff and coworkers could not demonstrate any increase in block level following an epidural dose of 10 mL of saline administered 20 minutes after intrathecal injection of 15 mg of hyperbaric bupivacaine, if the intrathecal dose had been administered with the patient in the sitting position and the patient had been turned supine after 2 minutes.[57] In another group the patients were left sitting for 5 minutes after an intrathecal injection of 12.5 mg of hyperbaric bupivacaine. In this group an epidural dose of 10 mL of 0.2% bupivacaine with 1:500,000 epinephrine administered 7 minutes after the intrathecal dose did not result in any increase of sensory block level, compared with the test group not receiving any epidural injection at all.[57] Takiguchi and colleagues investigated the effect of an epidural dose of 10 mL of saline in nonobstetric patients undergoing surgical procedures under CSE anesthesia.[149] If the intrathecal dose of 7.5 to 9.0 mg (2.5–3.0 mL) of 0.3% hyperbaric dibucaine did not result in anesthetic block level appropriate for surgery in 10 minutes, 10 mL of saline was administered through the epidural catheter. Within 5 minutes a significant cephalad extension of the block was demonstrated in the test group, but not in the control group not receiving any epidural injection. This study was further complemented with myelography in two volunteers receiving repeated doses of 5 mL of saline through an epidural catheter. It could be demonstrated that epidural injections of 5-mL volumes do compress the lumbosacral theca. The thecal diameter diminished to approximately 40% after the first epidural injection of saline and to 25% after the second injection.[149]

Thus it seems clear that epidural administration of drugs affects the theca and its contents and that the magnitude of this influence on the spread of an earlier-induced subarachnoid block depends on the time interval between the injections and the volume of the epidural injectate (Fig. 11–10). These data are also consistent with the general belief that alterations in the contents of the spinal canal can influence the spread of local anesthetic. In late pregnancy, for example, increased vertebral venous volume leads to a reciprocal decrease in thecal CSF volume. This is believed to be the principal reason for the decreased dose requirement of spinal local anesthetics in parturients.[117, 147, 150, 151, 162, 163] Inferior venal caval compression has been shown to increase the cephalad spread of subarachnoid block in both pregnant and nonpregnant patients,[163, 164] and an epidural bolus injection of 10 mL of local anesthetic solution transiently increases CSF pressure by up to 12 mm Hg.[165] Furthermore, in a recent study using magnetic resonance imaging, Carpenter and colleagues concluded that the variability in lumbosacral CSF volume between individual patients is the determining factor for the variability in spread and duration of subarachnoid sensory blockade.[166]

In summary, caution is necessary when large volumes of drugs are injected over short periods, as epidural pressure may become positive. Both during CSE anesthesia and after Tuohy needle dural puncture, even greater safety may be achieved by using low-concentration epidural solutions. Again, it is reasonable to administer such injections in small increments or to use low-rate infusions rather than to inject large volumes over short periods.

Risk of Meningitis. As a CSE block is performed, the dura mater is perforated by the spinal needle. This breach of the protective barrier of the central nervous system involves an increased risk of spread of infectious agents. Case reports of meningitis associated with the

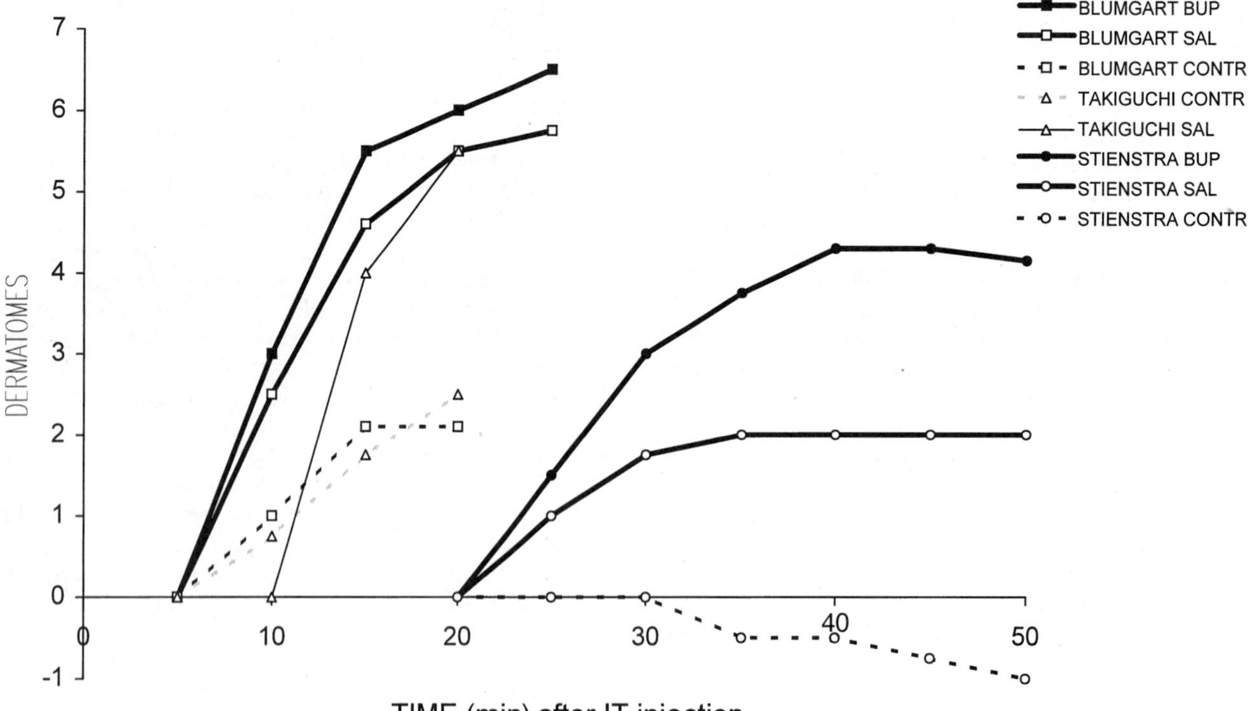

Figure 11–10 Extension of subarachnoid sensory block by epidural administration of 10 mL of bupivacaine (BUP) (-■-, -●-) or 10 mL of saline (SAL) (-□-, -△-, -○-). In the control (CONTR) groups (--□--, --△--, --○--) no epidural injections were given. IT, intrathecal. The change in additional cranial spread of block is presented with the mean number of dermatomes as reported by Blumgart et al,[55] Stienstra et al[56] and Takiguchi et al.[149]

use of the CSE technique were recently published.[120, 121, 167–169] However, in five of the reported cases there were some difficulties in performing a CSE block with the needle-through-needle technique. Furthermore, rare cases of bacterial meningitis have also been reported following traditional spinal or epidural blocks.[170–174]

When more than one skin puncture is performed and especially when epidural analgesia is prolonged after surgery, one has to bear in mind that the breach of the dura is a potential risk and as with all regional anesthesia methods, aseptic technique must be meticulous.[175]

The common practice of extemporaneous, "at the bedside" mixing of drug solutions for epidural and subarachnoid administration must be mentioned too when considering sequelae, such as meningitis and spinal epidural abscess formation.[119, 176] Ideally, but perhaps not realistically in all practices, such mixing should be carried out in a properly equipped and staffed pharmacy or pharmaceutical manufacturing laboratory.[177] To minimize the transmission of infection when extemporaneous mixing is carried out, strict aseptic precautions should be employed. Such precautions should include the use of sterile packaged ampules and the use of appropriate sterile 0.2-μm filters to remove shards of glass and other extraneous material.[178] With standard spinal blocks introducer needles have been used to prevent the introduction into the CSF of foreign particulate matter, including epidermal cells and detritus, which may attach to the spinal needle if the latter is allowed to contact the skin.[179] In the needle-through-needle technique, the Tuohy needle is the introducer that prevents spinal needle–skin contact.

Proponents of the CSE technique were reassured that the frequency of meningitis after a lumbar puncture is no greater than in the ordinary population.[180]

CSE Block and Decreased Risk of Postdural Puncture Headache. It is interesting to note that even for traditional spinal block, needles have been placed in the epidural space as introducers for very fine spinal needles (26–32 gauge) in an effort to reduce the risk of PDPH.[181–183] However, a high incidence of PDPH remains a major concern in the parturient, which may be as high as 10% to 15% even when 25- to 26-gauge spinal needles are used.[184, 185] It is an important cause of postoperative morbidity. There are no data from controlled studies regarding the frequency of PDPH associated with the CSE technique. However, several workers have commented on the very low incidence or lack of PDPH following CSE block (Table 11–6).[18, 21, 24, 37, 76, 112, 138, 139, 186–191] Dennison reported only two cases of PDPH in 400 patients (0.5%) who received CSE for cesarean section,[139] and Brownridge reported experience of "well over 1000 patients without one single case of PDPH."[186] In another report based on experience with 300 cesarean section patients, Kumar reported two cases of mild headache, and in both cases multiple spinal punctures were attempted because of technical difficulties.[138] Interestingly, in one CSE study where the single space needle-through-needle technique was compared with the separate spaces technique, only one PDPH was noted, which occurred in the group using the separate spaces technique.[112] A retrospective review of the use of the CSE needle-through-needle technique in over 1000 patients at Queen Charlotte's Hospital in London indicated a PDPH incidence of 0.13% in patients in whom the 27-gauge Whitacre spinal needle was passed not more than twice.[190] From 1995 through 1997, PDPH incidence at Queen Charlotte's Hospital has remained consistently below 0.5% in a further 3500 CSE administrations (J. A. Crowhurst, F. Plaat, unpublished data, 1999). These reports suggest that the risk of PDPH in parturients, particularly if spinal or epidural opioids are used as part of the technique, is very low or nonexistent. This is noteworthy because the risk of PDPH is considerably higher in this group of patients even when fine pencil-point needles are used.[192] The possible reasons for this lowered risk of PDPH may include

Table 11–6 INCIDENCE OF POSTDURAL PUNCTURE HEADACHE (PDPH) FOLLOWING CONTINUOUS SPINAL-EPIDURAL BLOCK

SURGERY/PROCEDURE	NO. OF PATIENTS	PDPH (%)	SPINAL NEEDLE SIZE/TYPE		REFERENCE
Cesarean section	400	0.5	—	—	Dennison[139]
Cesarean section	100	0	26 G	Q	Rawal et al[21]
Cesarean section	>1000	0	26 G	—	Brownridge*[186]
Cesarean section	150	1.3	26 G	W	Westbrook et al[187]
Cesarean section	100	1	26 G	—	Lyons et al[112]
Cesarean section	300	0.7	26 G	Q	Kumar[138]
Cesarean section	80	0	26 G	—	Fan et al[76]
Cesarean section	163	0	29 G	Q	Carrie[188]
Orthopedic surgery	90	0	27 G	W	Urmey et al[18]
Labor and delivery	62	2.5	26 G	—	Abouleish et al[24]
Labor and delivery	1080	0.28	26 G	GM	Birnbach et al[189]
Labor and delivery	300	2.3	27 G	W	Collis et al[37]
Labor and delivery	6000	0.13	27 G	W	Cox et al[190]
Obstetric patients	219	0.9	25–27 G	W	Newman et al[191]

*Spinal and epidural blocks performed at two lumbar interspaces.
Q, Quincke; W, Whitacre; GM, Gertie Marx; G, gauge.

- The technique allows the use of very fine diameter spinal needles.
- The Tuohy needle in the epidural space serves as an introducer and allows a meticulous puncture of the dura. Multiple attempts at identifying the subarachnoid space can thus be avoided.
- The risk of CSF leakage through the dura is decreased because of the increased pressure in the epidural space that results from administration of epidural local anesthetic and opioid solutions. This can be expected to splint the dura against the arachnoid membrane.[82]
- With a single-segment CSE technique the spinal needle is deflected somewhat as it exits through the Tuohy needle; thus the spinal needle approaches the dura at an angle. The holes in the dura and subarachnoid are less likely to overlap, thereby reducing the risk of CSF leakage.[82]
- Epidural or intrathecal opioids may have a prophylactic effect against PDPH. This is controversial. Reports claiming[186, 193, 194] and denying[195] the prophylactic effects of spinal opioids have been published. Epidural morphine has been successfully used to treat established PDPH.[196]

Norris and coworkers compared epidural block versus CSE block for labor analgesia and concluded that intentional dural puncture with a small-gauge pencil-point needle during the induction of CSE block does not increase the risk of PDPH when compared with epidural analgesia.[105] Furthermore, patients who had epidural analgesia were significantly more likely to suffer an unintended dural puncture with the epidural needle than those who received CSE block.

Epidural Test Doses. Since the introduction of low-dose local anesthetic and/or low-dose opioid combination epidurals for labor analgesia, many combinations of local anesthetics and adjuvants (such as epinephrine) have been suggested as "test doses" to confirm correct placement of the catheter in the epidural space.[197] It has long been a tradition to verify epidural placement by administering a test dose such that if the catheter was intrathecally, subdurally, intravascularly, or otherwise misplaced, the effects of the test dose would be readily apparent.[198] Unfortunately a positive test dose may be indicated, at best, by no analgesia; or, at worst, by a dense and possibly high spinal block, or undesirable systemic hemodynamic effects in mother and fetus. In addition, traditional test doses frequently fail to detect subdural catheter placement.[110]

These concerns have urged some obstetric anesthesiologists to advocate that when low-dose mixtures of opioids and/or local anesthetics are used, as in the CSE analgesia technique, or for epidural analgesia alone, epidural test doses are unnecessary.[199] Furthermore, a traditional epidural test dose causes unwanted loss of motor and proprioceptive functions, the preservation of both of which are necessary to permit safe ambulation and optimal muscle power for spontaneous vaginal delivery of the fetus.[98, 100]

The case against traditional test doses is strengthened further by the demonstration that when low-dose local anesthetics, or low-dose mixtures of local anesthetic and opioid, are administered via a catheter intravascularly or intrathecally, serious sequelae are avoided. At best, intravascular injection results in minimal analgesia, and minimal effects in mother and fetus. If the administration is intrathecal (or subdural), the worst scenario is an increasing degree of slow-onset motor blockade, with minimal loss of sympathetic tone.[131]

The omission of a traditional epidural test dose (15 mg of bupivacaine or 45 mg of lidocaine with or without epinephrine) is a radical departure from traditional thinking and practice of epidural analgesia in labor. Nevertheless, it would appear that if motor functions are to be preserved, and if a truly selective sensory block with safe ambulation and minimal sympathetic block are desired, then traditional epidural test doses should be omitted, especially for the laboring patient. Based on the CSE experience with over 9000 labors at Queen Charlotte's Hospital alone, it can be argued that such omission is safe.[199] Many anesthesiologists continue to perform a test dose if the parturient subsequently requires the administration of a dense block for operative delivery.

Patient safety requirements depend on the available presence in the delivery suite of skilled, vigilant staff, including anesthesiologists, and ongoing clinical observations and monitoring of the parturient and her fetus. Such requirements are already in place in many obstetric units, and are widely accepted as minimal standards of anesthesia care in obstetric units where regional analgesia services are provided.[200]

Failure Rate. In one study of cesarean section patients the technical aspects of the needle-through-needle versus the double interspace technique were compared. A high technical failure rate (13%) has been noted with the former technique. This is mainly due to difficulty in establishing a subarachnoid block.[112] No other study has reported such high technical failure rates.[17, 21, 67, 73, 78] Indeed the spinal block is easier to perform because the Tuohy needle serves as an introducer. Because the Tuohy introducer needle is in the epidural space, the spinal needle does not have to go through ligamentous and other tissues; it has to penetrate only the meninges. Furthermore, the dural click marking successful entry into the subarachnoid space is most distinct with the needle-through-needle technique, and lack of tissue penetration by fine-gauge spinal needles is more likely to avoid needle bending or damage.[201] Many anesthesiologists perform CSE blocks using long spinal needles (11–12 cm) of varying diameters that are introduced through 16- or 18-gauge regular Tuohy needles.

As mentioned earlier, there is a risk of spinal needle displacement at the time of syringe connection, aspiration of CSF, or injection of local anesthetic. Special devices to fix the spinal needle in place while it is in the Tuohy needle have been described (see Fig. 11–7).[103, 202] In a study of 150 cesarean section patients using Portex (Keene, NH) CSE needles, the failure rate was 0.67%.[187] This is considerably lower than the failure rate for spinal block reported in the recent literature.[187, 203] Commenting on the technical aspects of CSE administration, the authors concluded that the combined technique was readily learned by both senior and trainee anesthesiologists, with a high percentage of technically perfect blocks and a low incidence of PDPH.[187] It has been commented by some that combining spinal and epidural blocks appears cumbersome. However, in experienced hands the entire procedure takes less than about 4 to 6 minutes.[9, 17, 25] It is estimated that when either epidural or spinal anesthesia is used alone for cesarean section, an alternative technique is required in approximately 4% of parturients. Lyons has reported that the use of CSE blocks reduced the need for rescue with general anesthesia to 1 in 900 cesarean sections.[204] The failure rate may also be influenced by which spinal needle is used when performing the CSE block.

A well-known problem with fine-gauge spinal needles is the greater risk of placement failure, and the subsequent inadequate subarachnoid block. The results of Carpenter and colleagues' study using magnetic resonance imaging indicate that one of the determinant factors for intrathecal drug spread is the individual CSF volume.[166] Other authors have suggested that speed of intrathecal injection and patient posture is of importance.[205, 206] As the definitive end point for successful dural puncture is free flow of CSF at the spinal needle hub, the flow rate through the spinal needle used is of crucial importance. Both clinical and experimental studies have investigated the flow rates and patterns of flow through spinal needles of different length, types, sizes, and brands.[205, 207–209] The results are summarized in Table 11–7. Abouleish and coworkers, testing several "normal length" spinal needles, concluded that "needles of the same gauge (outer diameter) do not necessarily have the same flow rate" and that "the flow rates through pencil-tip needles tend to be higher than those of corresponding Quincke needles."[207] In a clinical study Patel and associates compared the flow rates through the 120-mm-long spinal needles, commonly used for the needle-through-needle CSE technique. The tested 120-mm 27-gauge Becton-Dickinson needle (Becton-Dickinson, Franklin Lakes, NJ) had flow characteristics superior to the 120-mm 26-gauge Spinocan needle (B. Braun, Melsungen AG, Germany).[208]

In conclusion, these studies demonstrate that flow characteristics are different with every individual brand, type, and size of spinal needle, and that slow flow rate through the long fine-gauge spinal needle may mask or delay confirmation of successful placement of the needle tip.

Another potential problem with fine-gauge spinal needles is the risk of needle deviation or tip damage during insertion through ligaments. Kinking, "barbing" of the needle tip, and even needle fracture have been reported when these needles are so inserted.[210, 211] Different laboratory models have been used to quantify and compare path deflection from the axis of insertion of different, commonly used spinal needles.[212, 213] In a model with porcine muscle preparations Sitzman and Uncles could demonstrate that 24-gauge Quincke-type spinal needles deflected up to 3.4 mm at a depth of 60 mm, whereas the tip deflection of an already bent needle was 10-fold. The magnitude of deflection with pencil-point needles (27-gauge Whitacre and 25-gauge Sprotte) was significantly less, but it is conceivable that using 18- or 16-gauge Tuohy epidural needle introducers for the fine spinal needle improves the safety and efficacy of subarachnoid spinal needle tip placement and should be advocated in clinical practice.[201, 213]

Table 11–7 CEREBROSPINAL FLUID (CSF) FLOW THROUGH DIFFERENT SPINAL NEEDLES*

NEEDLE TYPE AND SIZE (G)	NEEDLE LENGTH (MM)	TIME TO FIRST CSF DROP IN NEEDLE HUB (SEC)
Sprotte 22	90	<1
Sprotte 25	90	1–2
Sprotte 27	90	2
B-D Whitacre 27†		
Sitting patient position	120	9.4
Lateral patient position	120	12.3
Spinocan 27‡		
Sitting patient position	120	20.7
Lateral patient position	120	46.8
Quincke 22	120	20
Gertie Marx 24	120	35
Whitacre 25	120	55
Whitacre 27	120	65
Sprotte 27	120	160

*Mean flow through spinal needles of different brands and sizes, based on the reports in references 207–209.
†Becton-Dickinson, Franklin Lakes, NJ.
‡B. Braun, Melsungen AG, Germany.
G, gauge.

Optimal Design of CSE Needle Combinations. The distance from the tip of the epidural needle to the posterior wall of the dural sac in the midline varies considerably between patients (0.3–1.05 cm).[103, 214] Further, the anteroposterior diameter of the dural sac varies considerably during extension and flexion of the spinal column. At the L3 to L4 segment the diameter increases from a range of 9 to 20 mm in extension and to a range of 11 to 25 mm in flexion.[182] Additionally, this is only valid when the epidural puncture is performed in the midline. This is because the dural sac is triangular with its base resting on the vertebral body and the triangle top pointing posteriorly to the ligamentum flavum.[215] Although successful subarachnoid injection of local anesthetic is possible, the point of dural contact by the spinal needle clearly depends on the direction of the spinal needle (Fig. 11–11).[80] In some special CSE kits, the hub of the spinal needle locks into the hub of the Tuohy needle

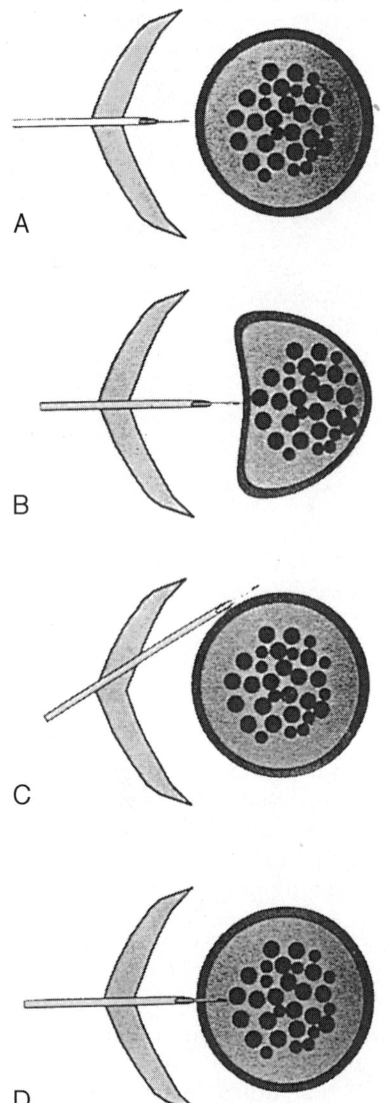

❖ **Figure 11–11** *A–C*, Various possibilities for CSE block failure owing to incorrect technique. *A*, Length of spinal needle protruding from the tip of the epidural needle is too short (or epidural needle is not introduced far enough into epidural space). *B*, Tip of spinal needle "tents" the dura but fails to pierce it (possibly a greater risk with "pencil-point" needles, especially if spinal needle protrusion out of the epidural needle is not long enough). *C*, Malposition of epidural needle. *D*, Correct position of epidural and spinal needles.

and a fixed length of spinal needle protrudes from the tip of the Tuohy needle. This length of protrusion may vary from 10 mm to 16 mm, depending on manufacturer. In one study in which different sets were compared, a failure rate of 15% with one CSE set led the authors to conclude that the length of protrusion should be more than 13 mm.[111] The Becton-Dickinson Durasafe CSE kit has a protrusion of 15 mm of the 27-gauge pencil-point spinal needle beyond the tip of the Tuohy-Weiss epidural needle. Vandermeersch considers a protrusion of at least 17 mm optimal; he also recommends selection of separate long spinal needles of sufficient length for maximal flexibility rather than needles with locking hubs and fixed protrusion.[80] In a study testing a new interlocking device, Hoffman and coworkers concluded that there is a need for spinal needles that extend further than those currently available.[104] The type of spinal needle may also influence the success rate of the CSE block, and because of needle design, the length of protrusion for pencil-point needles should be greater than that for Quincke-point needles (see Fig. 11–11).[216]

It has to be pointed out that as a safety precaution, the anesthesiologist performing the block should test the spinal and epidural needle compliance or "matching" in vitro before beginning the clinical procedure.

Special CSE Administration Equipment. In order to overcome potential problems, several modifications of the CSE technique or needle design have been reported. Disposable CSE sets have been commercially available since 1986. A great variety of CSE needles or needle modifications are available on the market. The same is true for epidural catheters. Equipment companies are launching "improved" CSE systems as well as producing custom-made CSE kits. However, it is difficult to confirm the claims of superior performance of needles and catheters because there are very few systematic cooperative studies. The 17-nation European survey showed that the type of needles used for CSE varied greatly. Special CSE sets were used by 31% of respondents; the remainder used their own combinations of epidural needles and extra long spinal needles. CSE sets were particularly popular in Belgium, Iceland, and Italy. The majority of spinal needles were pencil-point type. However, Quincke needles were also used by many. Almost all epidural needles were Tuohy types.[52] In the technical modification described by Eldor, a fine spinal needle is introduced alongside the outer wall of the epidural needle after a Tuohy needle is placed in the epidural space.[10] These workers have modified and improved their needle further.[217] The Eldor needle also allows the CSE block to be performed in reverse order (i.e., the spinal block is performed after the epidural catheter is in place). An almost identical needle is the "T-A pair" needle, composed of an 18-gauge epidural and a 22-gauge spinal needle welded together. The distal ends of the needles make a common tip (see Fig. 11–1). The epidural needle points cephalad and permits the passage of a 20-gauge epidural catheter, while the bevel of the spinal needle points caudad and allows the passage of a 26-gauge or finer spinal needle.[9] The E-SP needle (NeuroDelivery Inc, Tempe, AZ) is conceptually similar to the Eldor and Torrieri-Aldrete pair needles, the main difference being that the needle wall configuration is "over-under" rather than parallel. In the E-SP needle it is also possible to introduce the epidural catheter prior to spinal block. The different trajectories of spinal needle and epidural catheter in these newer CSE kits may be expected to reduce the risk of catheter migration because the dural puncture is physically separated from the Tuohy needle tip.

In the Espocan CSE set (B. Braun, Melsungen AG, Germany) the epidural and spinal needles have also been modified to reduce the risk of catheter penetration through the dura (Fig. 11–12). A "back eye" at the epidural needle curve near its bevel permits the passage of the spinal needle. The point of dural contact by the epidural catheter is thus at some distance from the dural hole. The dural click may be appreciated better if the epidural needle has a back eye opening. With the needle-through-needle CSE technique, the tip of the spinal needle may scrape against the inner wall of the Tuohy needle and concern has been expressed about possible metal particles being carried into the epidural or subarachnoid spaces.[122] However, in an elegant and convincing study, Herman and colleagues could not find any evidence of additional metal particles produced by the needle-through-needle technique.[218] The damage to fine spinal needle tips that is caused by bone contact during needle insertion has been clearly demonstrated by Rosenberg and coworkers, using fluorescence microscopy.[219] The risk of damage to the bevel of a spinal needle may be eliminated by the Espocan system, which contains a spinal needle with a plastic sleeve that keeps it centrally in the epidural needle and guides it through the back eye in the curve of the epidural needle tip. The spinal needle enters this hole easily and can be introduced into the dura without coming into contact with the internal wall of the epidural needle.

An example of an adjustable interlocking device has been presented by Becton-Dickinson. The interlocking piece between the two needle hubs secures the spinal needle position during injection of the subarachnoid drug (see Fig. 11–7). This device has recently been tested by Hoffman and collaborators.[104] The authors have concluded that the lockable needle provides safe and stable conditions during subarachnoid injection and a high rate of success in reaching the subarachnoid space, but there is also an inability to feel the dural click in 26% of cases. Other manufacturers are developing similar hub-locking systems.

CSE Technique Versus Continuous Spinal Technique. One of the main problems with single-injection spinal anesthesia is dose selection. In nonpregnant patients most anesthesiologists err on the side of giving a larger rather than a smaller dose because the risk of a failed spinal block owing to inadequate sensory level is far greater than the risk of a total spinal block. The converse is true of spinal anesthesia in parturients. A 1- to 2-mg difference in dosage may make the difference between effective surgical block and difficulty in breathing.[220] There is disagreement about the effective and safe bupivacaine dose for single-injection spinal anesthesia for cesarean section. Doses ranging from 9 mg[221] to 15 mg[222] have been recommended. Norris reported respiratory problems requiring intubation in 1% of single-shot spinal anesthetics using higher doses of bupivacaine.[223] The ideal approach to spinal anesthesia in obstetric and high-risk patients is the use of a continuous technique that allows dose titration to effect. However, continuous spinal anesthetic technique is undergoing reevaluation following the controversy regarding the role of spinal microcatheters in causing neurologic sequelae. Finucane favored the CSE technique as an excellent alternative to the continuous spinal technique because "one does not have to commit to a large initial subarachnoid dose of local anesthetic, supplementation may be administered epidurally, and opioids may be administered in this fashion for postoperative pain relief."[220]

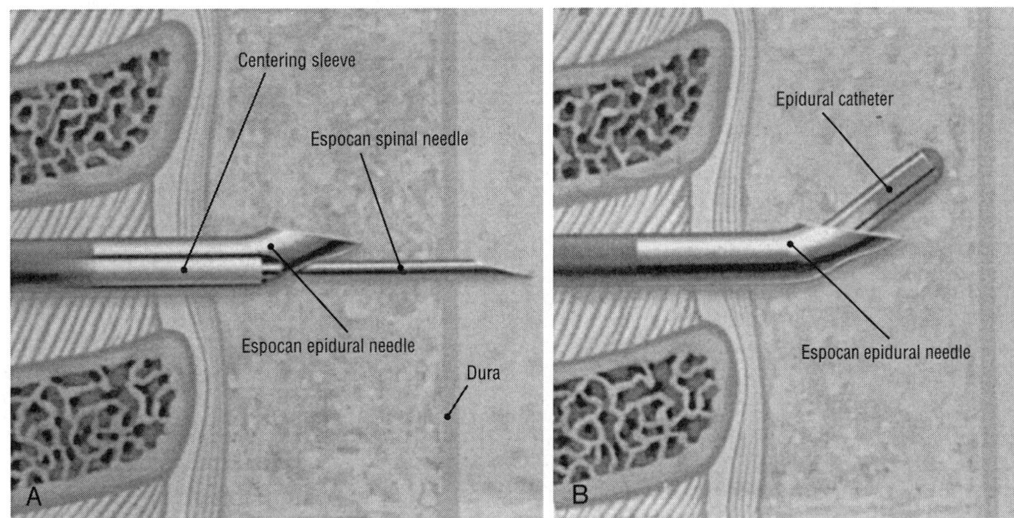

❖ **Figure 11–12** Espocan CSE system (B. Braun, Melsungen AG, Germany). *A*, The spinal needle is kept in the center, along the axis of the epidural needle, by the plastic sleeve. This facilitates the spinal needle tip's entrance into the epidural space through the "back eye" hole of the epidural needle. *B*, The epidural catheter enters the epidural space through the "regular" epidural needle eye and takes a curved course in the epidural space. (Courtesy of H. Otto, B. Braun, Melsungen AG, Germany.)

Summary

Key Points

- CSE is now widely recognized as a technique of neuraxial blockade that provides greater flexibility and reliability than what can be achieved with either spinal or epidural alone.
- Selective neural blockade is readily achieved with CSE and produces a pain-free parturient who can ambulate.
- Single-spaced, needle-through-needle CSE technique is quickly becoming the most popular method of neuraxial analgesia for labor worldwide.
- Small doses of lipid-soluble intrathecal opioids provide excellent analgesia for the first stage of labor. The addition of 1.25 to 2.5 mg of bupivacaine to the opioid improves the quality of analgesia for the second stage of labor.

Key Reference

Rawal N, Van Zundert A, Holmström B, Crowhurst JA: Combined spinal epidural technique. Reg Anesth 1997; 22:406–423.

Case Stem

A 40-year-old primiparous patient in labor requests analgesia. When you arrive in her room, she tells you that she has looked up "epidural" on the Internet and, based on her research, requests a "walking epidural." What options can you give this patient? Discuss the advantages and disadvantages of CSE for labor.

References

1. Rodzinski R: Uber eine neue Betäbungsmetode der unteren Körpergebiete: Sakrolumbalanästhesie. Zentralbl Chir 1923; 50:1249–1251.
2. Soresi A: Episubdural anesthesia. Anesth Analg 1937; 16:306–310.
3. Curelaru I: Long duration subarachnoid anaesthesia with continuous epidural block. Prakt Anästh 1979; 14:71–78.
4. Brownridge P: Epidural and subarachnoid analgesia for elective caesarean section [letter]. Anaesthesia 1981; 36:70.
5. Coates M: Combined subarachnoid and epidural techniques: a single space technique for surgery of the hip and lower limb [letter]. Anaesthesia 1982; 37:89.
6. Mumtaz MH, Daz M, Kuz M: Combined subarachnoid and epidural techniques [letter]. Anaesthesia 1982; 37:90.
7. Carrie LES, O'Sullivan G: Subarachnoid bupivacaine 0.5% for Caesarean section. Eur J Anaesth 1984; 1:275–283.
8. Rawal N: Single segment combined spinal epidural block for cesarean section. Can Anaesth Soc J 1986; 33:254–255.
9. Torrieri A, Aldrete JA: The TA pair needle [letter]. Acta Anaesthesiol Belg 1988; 39:65–66.
10. Eldor J: Combined spinal-epidural needle [abstract]. Reg Anesth 1988; 15:89.
11. Turner MA: Combined spinal/epidural anaesthesia for Caesarean section—single-space double-barrel technique [letter]. Anaesthesia 1992; 47:814.
12. van Dijk B, Wagemans MFM, Spoelder EM, et al: The different spinal needles and their effect and complications. *In* Proceedings of the SAVA/SASA Congress, Bloomfontein, South Africa, March 12–18, 1994.
13. Vercauteren MP, Geernaert K, Vandeput DM, et al: Combined continuous spinal-epidural anaesthesia with a single interspace, double-catheter technique. Anaesthesia 1993; 48:1002–1004.
14. Nakatsuka M, Long SP, Shy DG: Spinal anesthesia combined with epidural anesthesia for peripheral vascular emergency with dual catheters [abstract]. Anesth Analg 1994; 78:S309.
15. Møiniche S, Dahl JB, Rosenberg J, et al: Colonic resection with early discharge after combined subarachnoid-epidural analgesia, preoperative glucocorticoids, and early postoperative mobilization and feeding in a pulmonary high-risk patient. Reg Anesth 1994; 19:352–356.
16. Vandermeersch E: Combined spinal-epidural anaesthesia. Curr Opin Anaesthesiol 1996; 9:391–394.
17. Holmström B, Laugaland K, Rawal N, et al: Combined spinal epidural block versus spinal and epidural block for orthopedic surgery. Can J Anaesth 1993; 40:601–606.
18. Urmey WF, Stanton J, Peterson M, et al: Combined spinal-epidural anesthesia for outpatient surgery: Dose-response characteristics of intrathecal isobaric lidocaine using a 27-gauge Whitacre needle. Anesthesiology 1995; 83:528–534.
19. Wilhelm S, Standl T, Burmeister M, et al: Comparison of continuous spinal with combined spinal-epidural anesthesia using plain bupivacaine 0.5% in trauma patients. Anesth Analg 1997; 85:69–74.
20. Norris MC: Combined spinal-epidural anesthesia for urological and lower extremity vascular procedures. Tech Reg Anesth Pain Manage 1997; 1:131–136.
21. Rawal N, Schollin J, Wesström G: Epidural versus combined spinal epidural block for Caesarean section. Acta Anaesthesiol Scand 1988; 32:61–66.
22. Abouleish E, Rawal N, Fallon K, et al: Combined intrathecal morphine and bupivacaine for cesarean section. Anesth Analg 1988; 67:370–374.
23. Cherng YG, Wang YP, Liu CC, et al: Combined spinal and epidural anesthesia for abdominal hysterectomy in a patient with myotonic dystrophy. Reg Anesth 1994; 19:69–72.
24. Abouleish E, Rawal N, Shaw J, et al: Intrathecal morphine 0.2 mg versus epidural bupivacaine 0.125% or their combination: effect on parturients. Anesthesiology 1991; 74:711–716.
25. Camann WR, Minzter BH, Denney RA, et al: Intrathecal sufentanil for labor analgesia: effects of added epinephrine. Anesthesiology 1993; 78:870–874.
26. Collis RE, Baxandall ML, Srikantharajah ID, et al: Combined spinal epidural analgesia with ability to walk throughout labour. Lancet 1993; 1:767–768.
27. D'Angelo R, Anderson M, Philip J, et al: Intrathecal sufentanil compared to epidural bupivacaine for labor analgesia. Anesthesiology 1994; 80:1209–1215.
28. D'Angelo R, Gerancher JC: Combined spinal epidural analgesia in a parturient with severe myasthenia gravis. Reg Anesth Pain Med 1998; 23:201–203.
29. Dahl JB, Rosenberg J, Dirkes WE, et al: Prevention of postoperative pain by balanced analgesia. Br J Anaesth 1990; 64:518–520.
30. Roulson CJ, Bennett J, Shaw M, et al: Effect of extradural diamorphine on analgesia after caesarean section under subarachnoid block. Br J Anaesth 1993; 71:810–813.
31. Myint Y, Bailey PW, Milne BR: Cardiorespiratory arrest following combined spinal epidural anaesthesia for caesarean section. Anaesthesia 1993; 48:684–686.
32. Dirkes WE, Rosenberg J, Lund C, et al: The effect of subarachnoid lidocaine and combined subarachnoid lidocaine and epidural bupivacaine on electrical sensory thresholds. Reg Anesth 1991; 16:262–264.
33. Serrao JM, Marks RL, Morley SJ, et al: Intrathecal midazolam for the treatment of chronic mechanical low-back pain: a controlled comparison with epidural steroid in a pilot study. Pain 1992; 48:5–12.
34. Thorén T, Holmström B, Rawal N, et al: Sequential combined spinal epidural block versus spinal block for cesarean section: effects on maternal hypotension and neurobehavioral function of the newborn. Anesth Analg 1994; 78:1087–1092.
35. Arkoosh VA, Sharkey SJ, Norris MC, et al: Subarachnoid labor analgesia: fentanyl and morphine versus sufentanil and morphine. Reg Anesth 1994; 19:243–246.

36. Caldwell LE, Rosen MA, Schnider SM: Subarachnoid morphine and fentanyl for labor analgesia. Reg Anesth 1994; 19:2–8.
37. Collis RE, Davies DWL, Aveling W: Randomised comparison of combined spinal-epidural and standard epidural analgesia in labour. Lancet 1995; 2:1413–1416.
38. Riley ET, Cohen SE, Macario A, et al: Spinal versus epidural anesthesia for cesarean section: a comparison of time efficiency, costs, charges, and complications. Anesth Analg 1995; 80:709–712.
39. Hood DD, Mallak KA, Eisenach JC, et al: Interaction between intrathecal neostigmine and epidural clonidine in human volunteers. Anesthesiology 1996; 85:315–325.
40. Roux M, Wattrisse G, Subtil D, et al: A comparison of early combined spinal epidural analgesia versus epidural analgesia on labor stage duration and outcome [abstract]. Anesthesiology 1996; 85(3A):A851.
41. Backus A, Scanlon J, Calmes S: Epidural bupivacaine compared to intrathecal sufentanil in early labor [abstract]. Anesthesiology 1996; 85(3A):A868.
42. Scott NB, James K, Murphy M, et al: Continuous thoracic epidural analgesia versus combined spinal/thoracic epidural analgesia on pain, pulmonary function and the metabolic response following colonic resection. Acta Anaesthesiol Scand 1996; 40:691–696.
43. Kartawiadi SL, Vercauteren MP, van Steenberge AL, et al: Spinal analgesia during labor with low-dose bupivacaine, sufentanil, and epinephrine—a comparison with epidural analgesia. Reg Anesth 1996; 21:191–196.
44. Suresh MS, Wali A, Panchal S, et al: Determination of dose response for intraspinal bupivacaine in laboring parturients using the combined spinal epidural technique [abstract]. Anesth Analg 1997; 84:S409.
45. Ferouz F, Norris MC, Arkoosh VA, et al: Baricity, needle direction, and intrathecal sufentanil labor analgesia. Anesthesiology 1997; 86:592–598.
46. James KS, McGrady E, Patrick A: Combined spinal-extradural anaesthesia for preterm and term Caesarean section: is there a difference in local anaesthetic requirements? Br J Anaesth 1997; 78:498–501.
47. Viscomi CM, Rathmell JP, Pace NL: Duration of intrathecal labor analgesia: early versus advanced labor. Anesth Analg 1997; 84:1108–1112.
48. Riley ET, Walker D, Hamilton CL, et al: Intrathecal sufentanil for labor analgesia does not cause a sympathectomy. Anesthesiology 1997; 87:874–878.
49. Peutrell J, Hughes D: Combined spinal and epidural anaesthesia for inguinal hernia repair in babies. Pediatr Anaesth 1994; 4:221–227.
50. Williams RK, McBride WJ, Abajian JC: Combined spinal and epidural anaesthesia for major abdominal surgery for infants. Can J Anaesth 1997; 44:511–514.
51. Wakamatsu M, Katoh H, Kondo U, et al: Combined spinal and epidural anesthesia for orthopaedic surgery in the elderly [in Japanese]. Masui 1991; 40:1766–1769.
52. Rawal N: European trends in the use of combined spinal epidural technique—a 17-nation survey [abstract]. Reg Anesth 1995; 20(2S):162.
53. Holmström B, Rawal N, Arner S: The use of central regional anesthesia techniques in Sweden—results of a nation-wide survey. Acta Anaesthesiol Scand 1997; 41:565–572.
54. Rawal N, Van Zundert A, Holmström B, et al: Combined spinal-epidural technique. Reg Anesth 1997; 22:406–423.
55. Blumgart CH, Ryall D, Dennison B, et al: Mechanism of extension of spinal anaesthesia by extradural injection of local anaesthetic. Br J Anaesth 1992; 69:457–460.
56. Stienstra R, Dahan A, Alhadi ZRB, et al: Mechanism of action of an epidural top-up in combined spinal epidural anesthesia. Anesth Analg 1996; 83:382–386.
57. Mardirosoff C, Dumont L, Lemedioni P, et al: Sensory block extension during combined spinal and epidural. Reg Anesth Pain Med 1998; 23:92–95.
58. Urmey WF, Stanton J: Combined spinal epidural vs epidural anesthesia for outpatient knee arthroscopy [abstract]. Reg Anesth 1997; 22:(2 suppl.):6.
59. Moir DD: Extradural analgesia for caesarean section. [editorial]. Br J Anaesth 1979; 51:1093.
60. Morgan BM, Aulakh JM, Barker JP, et al: Anaesthesia for caesarean section—a medical audit of junior anaesthetic staff practice. Br J Anaesth 1983; 55:885–889.
61. Datta S, Alper MH, Ostheimer GW, et al: Method of ephedrine administration and nausea and hypotension during spinal anesthesia for cesarean section. Anesthesiology 1982; 56:68–70.
62. Van Zundert A, Vaes L, Van der Aa P, et al: Motor blockade during epidural anesthesia. Anesth Analg 1986; 65:333–336.
63. Lewis M, Thomas P, Wilkes RG: Hypotension during epidural analgesia for caesarean section. Anaesthesia 1983; 38:250–253.
64. Lussos S, Datta S: Anesthesia for cesarean delivery. II. Epidural anesthesia: Intrathecal and epidural opioids; venous air embolism. Int J Obstet Anesth 1992; 1:208–211.
65. Kileff ME, James FM, Dewan DM, et al: Neonatal neurobehavioral responses after epidural anesthesia for caesarean section using lidocaine and bupivacaine. Anesth Analg 1984; 63:413–417.
66. Thorburn J, Moir DD: Bupivacaine toxicity in association with extra-dural analgesia for caesarean section. Br J Anaesth 1984; 56:551–553.
67. Carrie LES: Extradural, spinal or combined spinal block for obstetric surgical anaesthesia. Br J Anaesth 1990; 65:225–233.
68. Larsen JV: Obstetric analgesia anaesthesia. Clin Obstet Gynaecol 1982; 9:685–709.
69. Clark RB, Thompson DS, Thompson CH: Prevention of spinal hypotension associated with cesarean section. Anesthesiology 1976; 45:670–674.
70. Datta S, Alper MH: Anesthesia for cesarean section. Anesthesiology 1980; 53:142–160.
71. Lussos SA, Datta S: Anesthesia for cesarean delivery. I. General considerations and spinal anesthesia. Int J Obstet Anesth 1992; 1:79–91.
72. Robson SC, Boys RJ, Rodeck C, et al: Maternal and fetal haemodynamic effects of spinal and extradural anaesthesia for elective caesarean section. Br J Anaesth 1992; 68:54–59.
73. Santos A, Pedersen H: Current controversies in obstetric anesthesia. Anesth Analg 1994; 78:753–760.
74. Abboud T, Dror A, Mossad P: Mini-dose intrathecal morphine for relief of postcesarean section pain. Anesth Analg 1988; 67:370–374.
75. Clerckx K, van Aken H, van Hemelrijck J, et al: Combined spinal epidural anesthesia in cesarean section. Acta Anaesthesiol Belg 1991; 42:123–124.
76. Fan S-Z, Susetio L, Wang Y-P, et al: Low dose of intrathecal hyperbaric bupivacaine combined with epidural lidocaine for cesarean section—a balance block technique. Anesth Analg 1994; 78:474–477.
77. Vucevic M, Russell IF: Spinal anaesthesia for caesarean section: 0.125% plain bupivacaine 12 ml compared with 0.5% plain bupivacaine 3 ml. Br J Anaesth 1992; 68:590–595.
78. Randalls B, Broadway JW, Browne DA, et al: Comparison of four subarachnoid solutions in needle-through-needle technique for elective caesarean section. Br J Anaesth 1991; 66:314–318.
79. Davies SJ, Paech MJ, Welch H, et al: Maternal experience during epidural or combined spinal-epidural anesthesia for cesarean section: a prospective, randomized trial. Anesth Analg 1997; 85:607–613.
80. Vandermeersch E: Combined spinal-epidural anaesthesia. Baillieres Clin Anaesth 1993; 7:691–708.
81. Swami A, McHale S, Abbott P, et al: Low dose spinal anesthesia for cesarean section using combined spinal-epidural (CSE) technique [abstract]. Anesth Analg 1993; 76:S423.
82. Stacey RGW, Watt S, Kadim MY, et al: Single space combined spinal-extradural technique for analgesia in labour. Br J Anaesth 1993; 71:499–502.
83. Campbell DC, Camann WC, Datta S: The addition of bupivacaine to intrathecal sufentanil for labor analgesia. Anesth Analg 1995; 81:305–309.
84. Kang M, Orebaugh S, Ramanathan S: The analgesic effect of hyperbaric subarachnoid fentanyl in parturients [abstract]. Anesthesiology 1996; 85(3A):A862.

85. Palmer CM, Marquez RC, Nogami WM, et al: Epinephrine as an adjunct to intrathecal fentanyl/bupivacaine for labor analgesia [abstract]. Anesthesiology 1996; 85(3A):A866.
86. Campbell DC, Banner R, Crone L-A, et al: Addition of epinephrine to intrathecal bupivacaine and sufentanil for ambulatory labor analgesia. Anesthesiology 1997; 86:525–531.
87. Honet JE, Arkoosh VA, Norris MC, et al: Comparison among intrathecal fentanyl, meperidine and sufentanil for labor analgesia. Anesth Analg 1991; 75:734–739.
88. Camann WR, Denney RA, Holby ED, et al: A comparison of intrathecal, epidural, and intravenous sufentanil for labor analgesia. Anesthesiology 1992; 77:884–887.
89. Grieco WM, Norris MC, Leighton BL, et al: Intrathecal sufentanil labor analgesia: the effects of adding morphine or epinephrine. Anesth Analg 1993; 77:1149–1154.
90. Cohen SE, Cherry CM, Holbrook RH, et al: Intrathecal sufentanil for labor analgesia: sensory changes, side effects, and fetal heart rate changes. Anesth Analg 1993; 77:1155–1160.
91. Riley ET, Ratner EF, Cohen S: Intrathecal sufentanil for labor analgesia: do sensory changes predict better analgesia and greater hypotension? Anesth Analg 1997; 84:346–351.
92. Pan PH, Fragneto R, Moore C, et al: Effects of bupivacaine on intrathecal fentanyl for labor analgesia [abstract]. Anesthesiology 1996; 85(3A):A865.
93. Herman NL, Calicott R, Van Decar TK, et al: Determination of the dose-response relationship for intrathecal sufentanil in laboring patients. Anesth Analg 1997; 84:1256–1261.
94. Arkoosh V, Cooper M, Norris M, et al: Intrathecal sufentanil dose response in nulliparous patients. Anesthesiology 1998; 89:364–370.
95. Thorp JA, Hu DH, Albin RM, et al: The effect of intrapartum epidural analgesia on nulliparous labor: a randomized, controlled prospective trial. Am J Obstet Gynecol 1993; 169:851–858.
96. Nageotte M, Larson D, Rumney P, et al: Epidural analgesia compared with combined spinal-epidural analgesia during labor in nulliparous women. N Engl J Med 1998; 337:1715–1719.
97. Fernando R, Prior C: Posterior column sensory impairment during ambulatory extradural analgesia in labour. Br J Anaesth 1995; 74:349–350.
98. Plaat F, Alsaud S, Crowhurst JA, et al: Selective sensory blockade with low-dose combined spinal/epidural (CSE) allows safe ambulation in labour: a pilot study [letter]. Int J Obstet Anaesth 1996; 5:220.
99. Parry M, Bawa G, Poulton B, et al: Comparison of dorsal column functions in parturients receiving epidural and combined spinal epidural (CSE) for labour and elective caesarean section [letter]. Int J Obstet Anaesth 1996; 5:213.
100. Buggy D, Hughes N, Gardiner J: Posterior column sensory impairment during ambulatory extradural analgesia in labour. Br J Anaesth 1994; 73:540–542.
101. Bloom S, McIntire D, Kelly M, et al: Lack of effect of walking on labor and delivery. N Engl J Med 1998; 339:76–79.
102. Morgan BM: "Walking" epidurals in labour [editorial]. Anaesthesia 1995; 50:839–840.
103. Nikalls RWD, Dennison B: A modification of the combined spinal and epidural technique. Anaesthesia 1984; 39:935–936.
104. Hoffman VLH, Vercauteren MP, Buczkowski PW, et al: A new combined spinal-epidural apparatus: measurement of the distance to the epidural and the subarachnoid spaces. Anaesthesia 1997; 52:350–355.
105. Norris MC, Grieco WM, Borkowski M, et al: Complications of labor analgesia: epidural versus combined spinal epidural techniques. Anesth Analg 1994; 79:529–537.
106. Holmström B, Rawal N, Axelsson K, et al: Risk of catheter migration during combined spinal epidural block—percutaneous epiduroscopy study. Anesth Analg 1995; 80:747–753.
107. Phillip J, Brown W: Total spinal anesthesia late in the course of obstetric bupivacaine epidural block. Anesthesiology 1976; 44:340–341.
108. Robson JA, Brodsky JB: Latent dural puncture after lumbar epidural block. Anesth Analg 1977; 56:725–726.
109. Riegler R, Pernetzky A: Irremovable epidural catheter due to a sling and a knot: a rare complication of epidural anaesthesia in obstetrics [in German]. Reg Anaesth 1983; 6:19–21.
110. Reynolds F, Speedy H: The subdural space: the third place to go astray. Anaesthesia 1990; 45:120–123.
111. Joshi G, McCaroll S: Evaluation of combined spinal-epidural anesthesia using two different techniques. Reg Anesth 1994; 19:169–174.
112. Lyons G, MacDonald R, Mikl B: Combined epidural spinal anaesthesia for caesarean section: through the needle or in separate spaces? Anaesthesia 1992; 47:199–201.
113. Eldor J, Chaimsky G: Combined spinal-epidural needle (CSEN). Can J Anaesth 1988; 35:537–538.
114. Patel M, Swami A: Spinal anaesthesia for Caesarean section [letter]. Br J Anaesth 1992; 69:662.
115. Beck GN, Griffiths AG: Failed extradural anaesthesia for caesarean section: complication of subsequent spinal block. Anaesthesia 1992; 47:690–692.
116. Mets B, Broccoli E, Brown AR: Is spinal anesthesia after failed epidural anesthesia contraindicated for cesarean section? Anesth Analg 1993; 77:629–631.
117. Hodgkinson R: Total spinal block after epidural injection into an interspace adjacent to an inadvertent dural perforation. Anesthesiology 1981; 55:593–595.
118. Morgan B: Unexpectedly extensive conduction blocks in obstetric epidural analgesia. Anaesthesia 1990; 45:148–152.
119. Dawson P, Rosenfeld JV, Murphy MA, et al: Epidural abscess associated with postoperative epidural analgesia. Anaesth Intensive Care 1991; 19:569–572.
120. Harding SA, Collis RE, Morgan BM: Meningitis after combined spinal-extradural anaesthesia in obstetrics. Br J Anaesth 1994; 73:545–547.
121. Stallard N, Barry P: Another complication of the combined extradural-subarachnoid technique [letter]. Br J Anaesth 1995; 73:370–371.
122. Eldor J, Brodsky V: Danger of metallic particles in the spinal-epidural spaces using the needle-through-needle approach [letter]. Acta Anaesthesiol Scand 1991; 35:461.
123. Patel M: Combined spinal and extradural anesthesia [letter]. Anesth Analg 1992; 75:640–641.
124. Robbins PM, Fernando R, Lim GH: Accidental intrathecal insertion of an extradural catheter during combined spinal-extradural anaesthesia for Caesarean section. Br J Anaesth 1995; 75:355–357.
125. Crawford JS: Some maternal complications of epidural analgesia for labour. Anaesthesia 1985; 40:1219–1225.
126. Phillips DC, MacDonald R, Lyons G: Possible subarachnoid migration of an epidural catheter. Anaesthesia 1986; 41:653–654.
127. Ravindran R, Albrecht W, Mckay M: Apparent intravascular migration of epidural catheter. Anesth Analg 1979; 58:252–253.
128. Zebrowski ME, Gutsche BB: More on intravascular migration of epidural catheter [letter]. Anesth Analg 1979; 58:531.
129. Ready LB, Wild LM: Organization of an acute pain service: training and manpower. Anesth Clin North Am 1989; 7:229–239.
130. Van Zundert A, Vaes L, Soetens M, et al: Every dose given in epidural analgesia for vaginal delivery can be a test dose. Anesthesiology 1987; 67:436–440.
131. Morton CP, Armstrong PJ, McClure JH: Continuous subarachnoid infusion of local anaesthetic. Anaesthesia 1993; 48:333–336.
132. Hughes JA, Oldroyd GJ: A technique to avoid dural puncture by the epidural catheter [letter]. Anaesthesia 1991; 46:802.
133. Ferguson DJM: Dural puncture and epidural catheters [letter]. Anaesthesia 1992; 47:272.
134. Meiklejohn B: The effect of rotation of an epidural needle: an in vitro study. Anaesthesia 1987; 42:1180–1182.
135. Hollway TE, Tedford RJ: Observations on deliberate dural puncture with a Tuohy needle: depth measurements. Anaesthesia 1991; 46:722–724.
136. Carter LC, Popat MT, Wallace DH: Epidural needle rotation and inadvertent dural puncture with catheter. Anaesthesia 1992; 47:447–448.

137. Duffy BL: "Don't turn the needle!" Anaesth Intensive Care 1993; 21:328–330.
138. Kumar C: Combined subarachnoid and epidural block for cesarean section. Can J Anaesth 1987; 34:329–330.
139. Dennison B: Combined subarachnoid and epidural block for caesarean section. Can Anaesth Soc J 1987; 34:105–106.
140. Russell IF: Effect of posture during the induction of subarachnoid analgesia for caesarean section. Br J Anaesth 1987; 59:342–346.
141. Niemi L, Tuominen M, Pitkänen M, et al: Effect of late posture change on the level of spinal anaesthesia with plain bupivacaine. Br J Anaesth 1993; 71:807–809.
142. Zaric D, Axelsson K, Hallgren S, et al: Evaluation of epidural sensory blockade by thermostimulation, laser stimulation and recording of somatosensory evoked potentials. Reg Anesth 1996; 21:124–130.
143. Bernards CM, Kopacz DJ, Michel MZ: Effect of needle puncture on morphine and lidocaine flux through the spinal meninges of the monkey in vitro: implications for combined spinal-epidural anesthesia. Anesthesiology 1994; 80:853–858.
144. Suzuki N, Koganemaru M, Onizuka S, et al: Dural puncture with a 26 G spinal needle affects epidural anesthesia [abstract]. Reg Anesth 1995; 20(2S):118.
145. Holmström B, Rawal N, Beckman K-W: The dural hole does not cause any significant drug flux during combined spinal epidural block. *In* Van Zundert A (ed): The International Monitor. Proceedings of the XVth Annual European Society of Regional Anaesthesia Congress, Nice, France, September, 1996. London: Medicom Excel; 1990, 113.
146. Swenson JD, Wisniewski M, McJames S, et al: The effect of prior dural puncture on cisternal cerebrospinal fluid morphine concentrations in sheep after administration of lumbar epidural morphine. Anesth Analg 1996; 83:523–525.
147. Bromage P: Mechanism of action of extradural anaesthesia. Br J Anaesth 1975; 47:199–212.
148. Carrie LES: Epidural versus combined spinal-epidural block for caesarean section. Acta Anaesthesiol Scand 1988; 32:595–596.
149. Takiguchi T, Okano T, Egawa H, et al: The effect of epidural saline injection on analgesic level during combined spinal and epidural anesthesia assessed clinically and myelographically. Anesth Analg 1997; 85:1097–1100.
150. Sykes MK: Delayed spinal anaesthesia: A complication of epidural analgesia. Anaesthesia 1958; 13:78–83.
151. Leach A, Smith G: Subarachnoid spread of epidural local anesthetic following dural puncture. Anaesthesia 1988; 43:671–674.
152. Cruickshank RH, Hopkinson JM: Fluid flow through dural puncture sites: an in vitro comparison of needles point types. Anaesthesia 1989; 44:414–418.
153. Ready LB, Cuplin S, Haschke RH, et al: Spinal needle determinants of rate of transdural fluid leak. Anesth Analg 1989; 69:457–460.
154. Westbrook JL, Uncles DR, Sitzman BT, et al: Comparison of the force required for dural puncture with different spinal needles and subsequent leakage of cerebrospinal fluid. Anesth Analg 1994; 79:769–772.
155. Rawal N: Epidural and intrathecal opioids for postoperative pain management in Europe—a 17-nation questionnaire study of selected hospitals. Acta Anaesthesiol Scand 1996; 40:1119–1126.
156. Holmström B: Combined Spinal Epidural (CSE) Block: Clinical and Experimental Studies [Thesis]. *In* Acta Universitatis Upsaliensis: Comprehensive Summaries of Uppsala Dissertations from the Faculty of Medicine, No. 652. Uppsala, Sweden: University of Uppsala; 1996:1–48.
157. Sjöström S, Tamsen A, Persson P, et al: Pharmacokinetics of intrathecal morphine and meperidine in humans. Anesthesiology 1987; 67:889–895.
158. Yamaguchi H, Watanabe S, Harukuni I, et al: Effective doses of epidural morphine for relief of postcholecystectomy pain. Anesth Analg 1991; 72:80–83.
159. Cousins MJ, Veering BT: Epidural neural blockade. *In* Cousins MJ, Bridenbaugh P (eds): Neural Blockade in Clinical Anesthesia and Management of Pain, 3rd ed. Philadelphia: Lippincott-Raven; 1998:243–320.
160. Suzuki N, Koganemaru M, Onizuka S, et al: Dural puncture with a 26 gauge spinal needle affects spread of epidural anesthesia. Anesth Analg 1996; 82:1040–1042.
161. Felsby S, Juelsgaard P: Combined spinal and epidural anesthesia. Anesth Analg 1995; 80:821–826.
162. Barclay D, Renegar O, Nelson E: The influence of inferior vena cava compression on the level of spinal anesthesia. Am J Obstet Gynecol 1968; 101:792–800.
163. Tunstall M: Incremental spinal anaesthesia and caesarean section—relevance to the test dose for extradural analgesia [letter]. Br J Anaesth 1991; 67:227–228.
164. Russell IF: Spinal anaesthesia for caesarean section—the use of 0.5% bupivacaine. Br J Anaesth 1983; 55:309–313.
165. Ramsay M: Epidural injection does cause an increase in CSF pressure [letter]. Anesth Analg 1991; 73:668.
166. Carpenter RL, Hogan QH, Liu SS, et al: Lumbosacral cerebrospinal fluid volume is the primary determinant of sensory block extent and duration of spinal anesthesia. Anesthesiology 1998; 89:24–29.
167. Cascio M, Heath G: Meningitis following a combined spinal-epidural technique in a labouring term parturient. Can J Anaesth 1996; 43:399–402.
168. Bouhemad B, Dounas M, Mercier F, et al: Bacterial meningitis following combined spinal-epidural analgesia for labour. Anaesthesia 1998; 53:290–295.
169. Aldebert S, Sleth J: Meningite bacterieme apres anesthesie rachidienne et peridurale combinee en obstetrique. Ann Fr Anesth Reanim 1996; 15:687–688.
170. Lee J, Parry H: Bacterial meningitis following spinal anaesthesia for Caesarean section. Br J Anaesth 1991; 66:383–386.
171. Davis L, Hargreaves C, Robinson PN: Postpartum meningitis. Anaesthesia 1993; 48:788–789.
172. Berga S, Trierwieler M: Bacterial meningitis following epidural analgesia for vaginal delivery: a case report. Obstet Gynecol 1989; 74:437–439.
173. Donnelly T, Koper M, Mallaiah T: Meningitis following spinal anaesthesia—a coincidal infection. Int J Obstet Anesth 1998; 7:170–172.
174. Ready L, Helfer D: Bacterial meningitis in parturients after epidural anesthesia. Anesthesiology 1989; 71:988–990.
175. Bromage P: Postpartum meningitis. Anaesthesia 1994; 49:260.
176. Crowhurst J, Simmons S: Safety of epidural infusion mixtures using the Polybag. Anaesth Intensive Care 1994; 22:741–743.
177. Sosis MB, Braverman B, Ivankovich AD: Growth of *Candida albicans* and *Staphylococcus aureus* in fentanyl/bupivacaine mixtures for epidural administration [abstract]. *In* Proceedings of Society for Obstetric Anesthesia and Perinatology 25th Annual Meeting, 1993:92.
178. Crowhurst J, Simmons S: Patient-controlled analgesia in pregnancy. Int Anesth Clin 1994; 32:55.
179. Lee J, Atkinson R (eds): Sir Robert Macintosh's Lumbar Puncture and Spinal Analgesia: Intradural and Extradural. 4th ed. Edinburgh: Churchill Livingstone; 1978:129–131.
180. Burke D, Wildsmith JAW: Meningitis after spinal anaesthesia [editorial]. Br J Anaesth 1997; 78:635–636.
181. Frumin J: Spinal anesthesia using a 32-gauge needle. Anesthesiology 1969; 30:599–603.
182. Slattery PJ, Rosen M, Rees GAD: An aid to identification of the subarachnoid space with a twenty-five gauge needle [letter]. Anaesthesia 1980; 35:391.
183. Kho HG, van Egmond J: A double-needle technique for spinal anaesthesia to prevent postspinal headache. Eur J Anaesth 1990; 7:403–410.
184. Cesarini M, Torrielli R, Lahaye F, et al: Sprotte needle for intrathecal anaesthesia for caesarean section: incidence of postdural puncture headache. Anaesthesia 1990; 45:656–658.
185. Naulty JS, Hertwig L, Hunt CO, et al: Influence of local anesthetic solution on postdural puncture headache. Anesthesiology 1990; 72:450–454.
186. Brownridge P: Spinal anaesthesia in obstetrics [letter]. Br J Anaesth 1991; 67:663.
187. Westbrook JL, Donald F, Carrie LES: An evaluation of a combined spinal epidural needle set utilizing a 26-gauge, pencil point spinal needle for caesarean section. Anaesthesia 1992; 47:990–992.

188. Carrie LES: 29-Gauge spinal needles. Br J Anaesth 1991; 66:145–147.
189. Birnbach DJ, Stein DJ, Hartman JK, et al: Complications of combined spinal epidural (CSE) analgesia compared with lumbar epidural analgesia [abstract]. Anesthesiology 1996; 85(3A):A860.
190. Cox M, Lawton G, Gowrie-Mohan S, et al: Ambulatory extradural analgesia [letter]. Br J Anaesth 1995; 74:114.
191. Newman LM, Perez EC, Ivankovich D: In vivo evaluation of some spinal needles used for the combined spinal epidural [abstract]. Anesth Analg 1996; 82:S337.
192. Lambert DH: Continuous spinal anesthesia. *In* Van Zundert A (ed): Highlights in Regional Anesthesia and Pain Therapy. Third Joint European Society of Regional Anesthesia–American Society of Regional Anesthesia Congress, Brussels, 1992:339–348.
193. Boskovski N, Lewinski A: Epidural morphine for the prevention of headache following dural puncture [letter]. Anaesthesia 1982; 37:217–218.
194. Johnson MD, Hertwig L, Vehring PH, et al: Intrathecal fentanyl may reduce the incidence of spinal headache [abstract]. Anesthesiology 1989; 71:A911.
195. Abboud T, Zhu J, Reyes A, et al: Effect of subarachnoid morphine on the incidence of spinal headache. Reg Anesth 1992; 17:34–36.
196. Eldor J, Guedj P, Cotev S: Epidural morphine injections for the treatment of postspinal headache. Can J Anaesth 1990; 37:710–711.
197. Van Zundert A: Epidural anesthesia: test dose. *In* Van Zundert A, Ostheimer G (eds): Pain Relief and Anesthesia in Obstetrics. New York: Churchill Livingstone; 1996; 322–330.
198. Dogliotti AM: Segmented peridural spinal anesthesia. Am Surg 1933; 20:107–118.
199. Morgan BM: Is an epidural test dose necessary? Eur J Obstet Gynecol 1995; 59:559–560.
200. Recommended minimum standards for obstetric anaesthesia services. Obstetric Anaesthetists' Association (UK), 1995.
201. Crowhurst J: Fractured fine-gauge spinal needles. Anaesth Intensive Care 1997; 25:317–318.
202. Simsa J: Device to maintain the position of a 29-gauge spinal needle. Anaesthesia 1990; 45:593–594.
203. Tarkkila PJ, Heine H, Tervo RR: Comparison of Sprotte and Quincke needles with respect to postdural puncture headache and backache. Reg Anesth 1992; 17:283–287.
204. Lyons G: Epidural is an outmoded form of regional anaesthesia for elective caesarean section. Int J Obstet Anaesth 1995; 4:34–39.
205. Serpell MG, Gray WM: Flow dynamics through spinal needles. Anaesthesia 1997; 52:229–236.
206. Horlocker TT, Wedel DJ, Wilson PR: Effect of injection rate on sensory level and duration of hypobaric bupivacaine spinal anesthesia for hip arthroplasty. Anesth Analg 1994; 79:773–777.
207. Abouleish E, Mitchell M, Taylor G, et al: Comparative flow rates of saline in commonly used spinal needles including pencil-tip needles. Reg Anesth 1994; 19:34–42.
208. Patel M, Samsoon G, Swami A, et al: Flow characteristics of long spinal needles. Anaesthesia 1994; 49:223–225.
209. Wills R, Kopacz D: Flow characteristics of long spinal needles used for the combined spinal/epidural anesthesia (CSEA) [abstract]. Anesth Analg 1996; 82:S495.
210. Teh J: Breakage of Whitacre 27 gauge needle during performance of spinal anaesthesia for caesarean section [letter]. Anaesth Intensive Care 1997; 25:96.
211. Hoskin M: Spinal anaesthesia—the current trend towards narrow gauge atraumatic (pencil point) needles: case reports and review. Anaesth Intensive Care 1997; 26:96–106.
212. Kopacz DJ, Allen HW: Comparison of needle deviation during regional anesthetic techniques in a laboratory model. Anesth Analg 1995; 81:630–633.
213. Sitzman BT, Uncles DR: The effects of needle type, gauge, and tip bend on spinal needle deflection. Anesth Analg 1996; 82:297–301.
214. Katz J: Spinal and epidural anatomy. *In* Katz J (ed): Atlas of Regional Anaesthesia. Norwalk, CT: Appleton-Century-Crofts; 1985:168–169.
215. Husemeyer RP, White DC: Topography of the lumbar epidural space—a study in cadavers using injected polyester resin. Anaesthesia 1980; 35:7–11.
216. Urmey WF, Stanton J, Sharrock NE: Combined spinal/epidural anesthesia for outpatient surgery—in reply. Anesthesiology 1996; 84:481–482.
217. Eldor J, Guedj P, Gozal Y: Combined spinal-epidural anesthesia using the CSEN [letter]. Anesth Analg 1992; 74:169–170.
218. Herman N, Molin J, Knape KG: No additional metal particle formation using the needle-through-needle combined epidural/spinal technique. Acta Anaesthesiol Scand 1996; 40:227–231.
219. Rosenberg PH, Pitkänen MT, Hakala P, et al: Microscopic analysis of the tips of thin spinal needles after subarachnoid puncture. Reg Anesth 1996; 21:35–40.
220. Finucane BT: Spinal anesthesia for cesarean delivery. The dosage dilemma [editorial]. Reg Anesth 1995; 20:87–89.
221. Abouleish EI: Post-partum tubal ligation requires more bupivacaine for spinal anesthesia than does cesarean section. Anesth Analg 1986; 65:897–900.
222. De Simone CA, Leighton BL, Norris MC: Spinal anesthesia for cesarean delivery: a comparison of two doses of hyperbaric bupivacaine. Reg Anesth 1995; 20:90–94.
223. Norris MC: Obstetric anesthesia. *In* Norris MC (ed): Obstetric Anesthesia. Philadelphia: JB Lippincott; 1993:419–446.

12

Continuous Spinal Anesthesia Techniques for Labor and Delivery

❖ RONALD J. HURLEY, MD

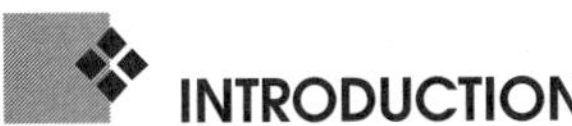

INTRODUCTION

After Bier's pioneering use of spinal anesthesia in 1898, many physicians, among them Henry Percy Dean, debated the relative merits of inhalation and regional methods of anesthesia. At the 75th Annual Meeting of the British Medical Society, in 1907, Dean[1] presented a paper concerning the deleterious effects of the commonly used agents of that era, ether and chloroform. Dean wrote:

> From the moment that the first portion of the vapor reaches the bronchial mucous membrane to the time that it passes out by the excreting organs, there is a summation of poisonous effects which contributes . . . largely to swell the death rate from all grave abdominal and other operations in which general anesthetics are employed . . . . In seeking an anesthetic that would avoid these dangers, it is obvious that we must endeavor to employ a drug that would not irritate in any serious way the mucous membranes of the bronchi and lungs. In the next place we should try and find an anesthetic that would act upon the peripheral part of the nervous system in such a way that stimuli would be prevented passing from the fields of operation upward to the vital centers—some drug that would paralyze all the afferent nerves passing from the region of operation.

In objecting to the "poisonous and treacherous character" of cocaine used by Bier, Dean proposed the use of stovaine, a chlorhydrate of one of the amino alcohols discovered by the French chemist Fourneau. Spinal headache, the bane of spinal anesthesia of all types, was described by Bier and again by Dean:[1] "In all probability the headache which is a constant after-effect of lumbar anesthesia is due to an increase in the cerebrospinal pressure induced by the inflammatory disturbance following the injection."

Dean had needles of three different lengths prepared for him and was, in fact, the first to describe continuous spinal anesthesia, stating:[1] "One can leave a needle in the canal during the operation, and at any moment some more drug can be injected without moving the patient" (Fig. 12–1).

Needle trauma and needle breakage plagued Dean's technique until Lemmon introduced the malleable needle with a split mattress during the Second World War (Fig. 12–2).[2] Lemmon and Paschal,[3] in their observations on the use of this continuous technique in their first 500 cases, described their attempts to eliminate the disadvantages of the single-dose spinal anesthetic, which were the toxic symptoms after intraspinal administration of a large dose of a toxic drug; failure of the drug to "take" or produce anesthesia to a desired level and degree; and cessation of drug action before conclusion of the operation. These limitations of the single-dose spinal are certainly familiar to today's practitioners. Lemmon's technique consisted of placing a 17- to 19-gauge malleable "German silver" needle in the subarachnoid space, bending the needle at the skin, and connecting the needle to a syringe of local anesthetic by a thick-walled rubber tubing. The patient was then placed on a special split mattress that permitted use of the supine position during surgery without interference with or dislodgement of the spinal needle. Hinebaugh and Lang[4] described the use of Lemmon's needle in 50 deliveries and achieved a

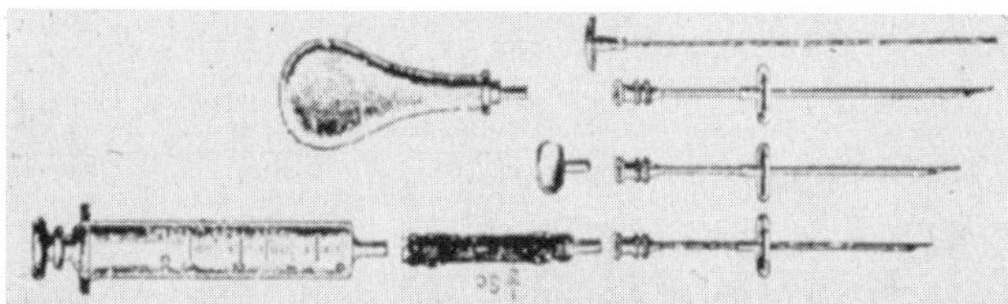

❖ **Figure 12-1** Dean's continuous spinal apparatus and the first description of a continuous spinal anesthetic.

spontaneous vaginal birth rate of 2%, with 98% requiring forceps. Thus the debate on the influence of regional anesthesia on the outcome of labor began! Interestingly, a major advantage of leaving the spinal needle in place was thought to be the ability to remove the local anesthetic should untoward events occur. These needle in situ techniques were obviously not suited for use in the active parturient, and useful continuous spinal analgesia and anesthesia in obstetrics awaited Tuohy's catheter technique in 1944.[5] However, Tuohy's 15-gauge needle and ureteral catheter resulted in a high percentage of post–dural puncture headaches (PDPHs) and thus the technique never gained great popularity. Bizzarri et al.[6] ushered in the modern era of continuous spinal anesthesia (CSA) in 1972 with a 21-gauge catheter. This was the smallest catheter that had been employed to date, and its use in 77 cesarean deliveries with procaine crystals utilized as the local anesthetic was reported.[7] The PDPH rate was 16% in this population, who are known to be at risk for this complication. In spite of the risk of headache, CSA with standard epidural equipment remained popular in some centers, especially in selected high-risk patients, such as the morbidly obese. Then in 1987, Hurley and Lambert[8] described their preliminary work with a 32-gauge microcatheter inserted through a 26-gauge Quincke-tipped spinal needle (Fig. 12–3). The technique rapidly gained acceptance in spite of difficulties with technical aspects such as difficulty threading the fine catheter, catheter breakage, and catheter kinking. Several manufacturers introduced 28-gauge tubing that fit through 22-gauge spinal needles. It looked as though CSA with a microcatheter would rival continuous epidural anesthesia for use in surgery and obstetrics. A special ramped 22-gauge Sprotte needle

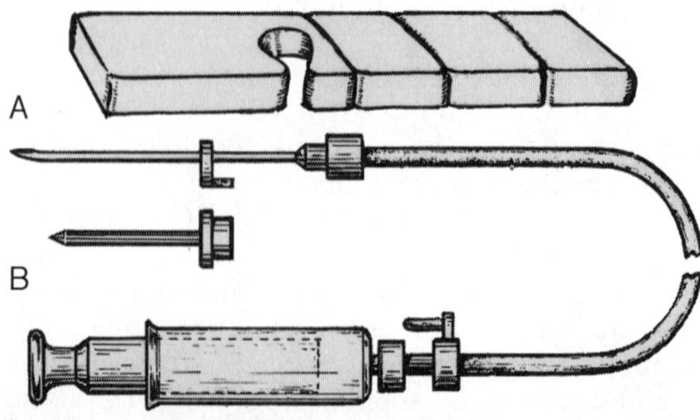

❖ **Figure 12-2** The Lemmon continuous spinal equipment.

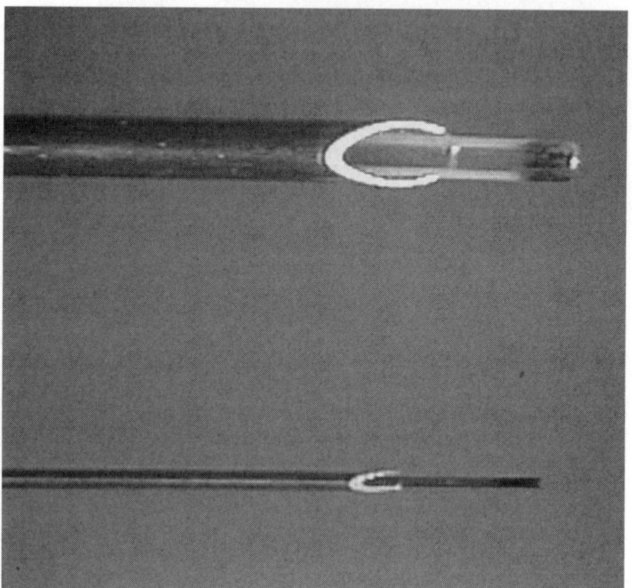

❖ **Figure 12-3** The 32-gauge spinal microcatheter exiting a 26-gauge Quincke needle contrasted with a conventional epidural catheter and needle combination.

that was compatible with the 28-gauge catheters offered the promise of anesthesia and analgesia with a low rate of PDPH (Fig. 12–4). A route was now available for the administration of subarachnoid opioids, and reports touted the advantages of these narcotics in labor analgesia and postoperative pain relief. Storm clouds appeared on the horizon, however. A report by Rigler et al.[9] documented four cases of cauda equina syndrome. Three of these cases involved the new microcatheters, and one a standard epidural catheter. Maldistribution of the local anesthetic was suspected, as excessive doses of 5% lidocaine and 1% tetracaine were required to achieve surgical levels. The United States Food and Drug Administration (FDA) withdrew approval of all microcatheters smaller than 24 gauge in the spring of 1992. Many countries followed the US ban; however, the microcatheters are still being used successfully in Europe.

ADVANTAGES OF CONTINUOUS SPINAL ANESTHESIA AND ANALGESIA

Continuous spinal anesthesia has many potential advantages over both single-dose spinal and continuous epidural techniques.

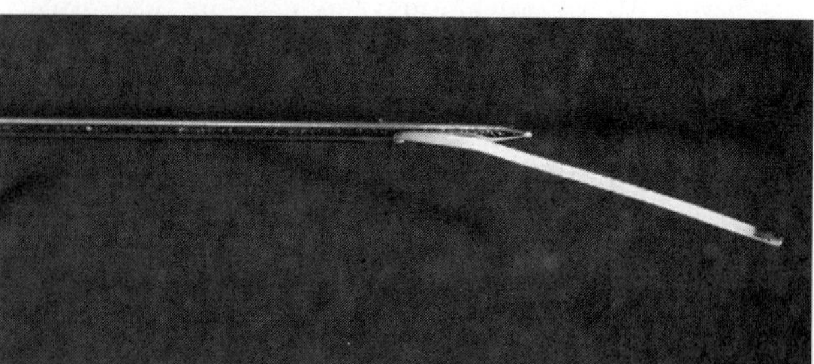

❖ **Figure 12-4** A 28-gauge spinal microcatheter exiting a ramped Sprotte spinal needle.

1. CSA requires 10% or less of the local anesthetic required for continuous epidural anesthesia, thus eliminating the possibility of systemic toxic reactions.
2. CSA may be instituted after patient positioning, thus minimizing the potential for cardiovascular instability.
3. The CSA catheter may be placed outside the operating room, thus facilitating the surgical schedule.
4. Careful titration of the developing anesthetic is possible, thus decreasing the likelihood of cardiovascular instability during induction.
5. Through the use of low doses of dilute, short-acting local anesthetic or narcotic, the recovery period is shortened.
6. The definitive end point (cerebrospinal fluid) of subarachnoid penetration enhances the likelihood of success.
7. The duration of the block can be prolonged indefinitely. Subarachnoid catheters have been used successfully for years in patients with chronic pain.
8. Microcatheters may minimize the incidence of PDPH, although large-scale studies proving this are lacking.
9. Continuous spinal catheters eliminate the need for vasoconstrictors. Phenylephrine was recently shown to increase the incidence of radicular irritation after tetracaine single-shot spinal anesthesia.[10]

Neurotoxicity

The microcatheter neurotoxicity issue has had one major benefit, albeit at the expense of continuous spinal techniques. The issue uncovered the relative toxicity of concentrated solutions of lidocaine. No sooner had the microcatheters been withdrawn in 1992 than reports of transient radicular irritation (TRI) appeared. It rapidly became clear that not all local anesthetics were created equal. Lambert et al.[11] were the first to show that 5% lidocaine appeared to be quite toxic to frog sciatic nerves in vitro. TRI was shown to be much more common with lidocaine spinal injections than with bupivacaine. In 1994, the FDA issued a letter concerning the 5% hyperbaric lidocaine solution, urging physicians to dilute the lidocaine with cerebrospinal fluid or saline before injection. These precautions were incorporated into the package insert by the drug manufacturers. Unfortunately, more recent data indicate that the 2.5 and 2.0% solutions do not reduce the incidence of TRI.[12] The irritation seems to be exacerbated by the lithotomy position[13] and minimized by the prone position.[14] The lithotomy position encourages pooling of local anesthetic around the most dorsal fibers and subjects these nerves to stretching, which may increase their vulnerability. Many anesthesiologists currently limit the concentration of subarachnoid lidocaine to 1.5% and epidural lidocaine to 2.0%.

Safety of Bupivacaine

Although TRI has been reported after subarachnoid bupivacaine,[15] the incidence appears to be low, and most clinicians believe it to be the safest subarachnoid drug (which is in contrast to its systemic reputation). Questions remain regarding whether TRI is a warning that the toxicity threshold is being approached, whether conduction blockade is really just reversible toxicity, and the safety of other local anesthetics. Data on the rarely used local anesthetics, such as prilocaine and mepivacaine, and on the opioids with local anesthetic action, such as meperidine and sameridine, are just starting to appear in the journals. The definitive answers are not yet in, but the next few years' research will probably give the anesthesia community a scale of the relative direct local toxicity potential of all the local anesthetics.

Maldistribution

Microcatheters and macrocatheters used for CSA shouldered the blame for the use of large quantities and high concentrations of local anesthetics (e.g., why was 5% lidocaine used in the subarachnoid space when 2% was adequate on the sheathed nerves of the epidural space?) that led to the horrific complications of the cauda equina syndrome. However, the catheters probably contributed. First, their small cross-sectional area limited flow (Fig. 12–5) and local anesthetic dripping slowly from the tip moved only short distances, presumably leading to maldistribution and occasionally toxicity. But the smallest catheters (32-gauge) were never implicated—although perhaps not as many were used because of high cost and handling difficulties—and the largest catheters (epidural) were found to be responsible more than once. More importantly, in vitro modeling showed that the caudally directed catheters led to a higher incidence of sacral pooling and maldistribution.[16]

Most authors recommended and anatomy dictated that spinal needles and therefore catheters be directed cephalad. Catheters are notoriously uncooperative, however, and a significant fraction of cephalad-directed catheters end up traveling in a caudad direction. In June of 1998, an important study by Biboulet et al.[17] appeared, concerning the causes and prediction of maldistribution during CSA. The authors employed 19-gauge catheters inserted 4 cm after the Tuohy bevel was turned cephalad. Fourteen percent ultimately had the tip pointed in the caudad direction, and this caudad orientation correlated highly with maldistribution. The previous in vitro studies had already suggested that this caudad pointing was a problem, but Biboulet showed that maldistribution could be predicted in the elderly patients studied. No maldistribution occurred if the upper sensory level was at the level of or cranial to L3, 10 minutes after 2.5 mg of isobaric bupivacaine (0.5 mL) or at the level of or cranial to L5 after 2.5 mg of hyperbaric bupivacaine (0.5 mL). The authors state, "The danger appears to lie in missing the diagnosis rather than in the occurrence of maldistribu-

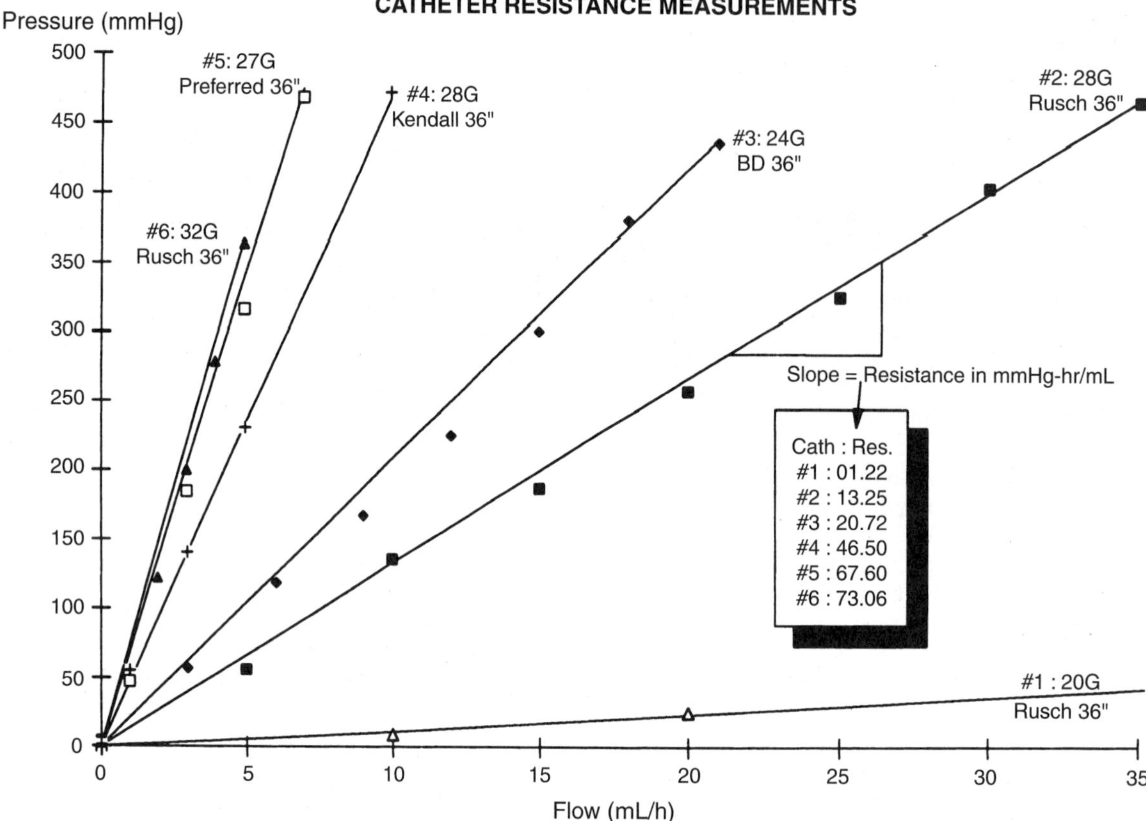

❖ **Figure 12–5** Flow-pressure characteristics of five spinal microcatheters and a conventional 20-gauge epidural catheter.

tion."[17] In their study, when maldistribution was diagnosed, changing the position of the patient or changing the baricity of a supplemental dose allowed an adequate level of sensory anesthesia for the surgery without necessitating administration of excessive amounts of local anesthetic. Although the study remains to be replicated in the younger obstetric patient, the news is encouraging. Why should we restrict the use of microcatheters when macrocatheters have also been implicated and the problem can be diagnosed and prevented with avoidance maneuvers?

PRACTICAL USE OF CONTINUOUS SPINAL ANESTHESIA CATHETERS IN OBSTETRICS

Until spinal microcatheters return to the American market, epidural catheters will continue to be used for CSA in special cases.

Management of the "Wet Tap" After Attempted Epidural Catheter Placement

Conventional management of the dural puncture during epidural placement usually involves withdrawing the epidural needle and inserting the catheter into the epidural space at another intervertebral space. This approach has limitations, however. If the placement was initially difficult, the next interspace may be no less so and another dural puncture raises the risk of PDPH to an extremely high likelihood and still no anesthesia or analgesia has been achieved. There is also the possibility that the catheter will arrive in the subarachnoid space from the second placement through the original hole in the dura, leading to unexpected high levels of block if not managed very carefully. The dural hole may also unpredictably facilitate the transfer of local anesthetic from the epidural to subarachnoid spaces, again leading to excessive sensory and motor block, hypotension, and potential fetal distress.

An alternative approach when the dura is unintentionally breached is to institute CSA without delay. At least then the catheter will be known to be subarachnoid and surprises will be minimized. We have gained considerable knowledge of subarachnoid dosing for labor via the combined spinal epidural technique. A conventional initial intervention would be to administer 2.5 mg of isobaric bupivacaine with 25 μg of fentanyl or 5 μg of sufentanil. This rapidly provides labor analgesia for 1 to 2 hours. Dextrose can be added to provide sacral spread if delivery is imminent. If labor is prolonged beyond the initial analgesic period, pain relief can be provided via a constant infusion pump infusing a standard epidural labor local anesthetic and opioid solution at 1 to 2 mL per hour. This mixture consists of 0.125% bupivacaine with 2 μg/mL of fentanyl at Brigham and Women's Hospital in Boston. Of course, if cesarean delivery becomes necessary, it is easy and rapid to administer local anesthetics such as hyperbaric 0.75% bupivacaine, which is adequate for surgery. One caveat: the catheter MUST be clearly labeled as a spinal catheter, and all health care providers that could potentially administer medications through the catheter must be warned. One potential ally is the patient, who is usually happy to remind practitioners that she has a spinal catheter. A well-functioning continuous infusion will decrease the likelihood that supplemental medications will be necessary, which is an advantage of this technique.

Use of the Continuous Spinal Catheter to Deliver Opioids

The use of subarachnoid opioids as a labor analgesic is appealing. The opioids produce dose-dependent analgesia without significant sympathetic or motor block, and this analgesia is reversible. Scott et al.[18] described the use of subarachnoid preservative-free morphine as a sole analgesic in 1980. However, the slow onset (up to 60 minutes) and the high incidence of side effects (pruritus and nausea) limited morphine's appeal. The lipid-soluble opioids fentanyl and sufentanil have a rapid onset and fewer side effects but may produce tachyphylaxis. Opioids have been used successfully for labor analgesia in patients who have a relative contraindication to sympathetic block. Examples include patients with severe pulmonary hypertension,[19] Wolff-Parkinson-White syndrome,[20] or a single ventricle.[21] In addition, meperidine has been used via the subarachnoid route to provide analgesia to a patient with allergy to conventional local anesthetics.[22]

The Morbidly Obese Parturient

As discussed in Chapter 37, the morbidly obese parturient represents a particular challenge to the obstetric anesthesiologist. These women are often at high risk for surgical delivery, have potentially difficult if not impossible airways, and often present with coexisting conditions such as diabetes and preeclampsia. The epidural space is often difficult to identify, and epidural catheters have a higher than normal risk of failure. CSA with conventional catheters is an attractive alternative. The positive end point of cerebrospinal fluid return increases the potential for a successful block; aspiration can usually (but not always) prove that the catheter is still properly located; and the rapid response characteristic of CSA prevents delays in deciding whether that catheter really works. PDPH is a problem, but a manageable one. A living patient with a headache that can be treated with an epidural blood patch is preferable to the nightmare of a failed intubation for general anesthesia in the morbidly obese parturient.

Special Cases

Special cases in obstetrics requiring CSA occasionally occur on the busy labor floor. Patients with spinal surgery in whom the epidural space has been obliterated may be candidates if the subarachnoid space can be reached. Patients with severe scoliosis may have more predictable analgesia with a CSA catheter than with conventional epidural block. Any patient with

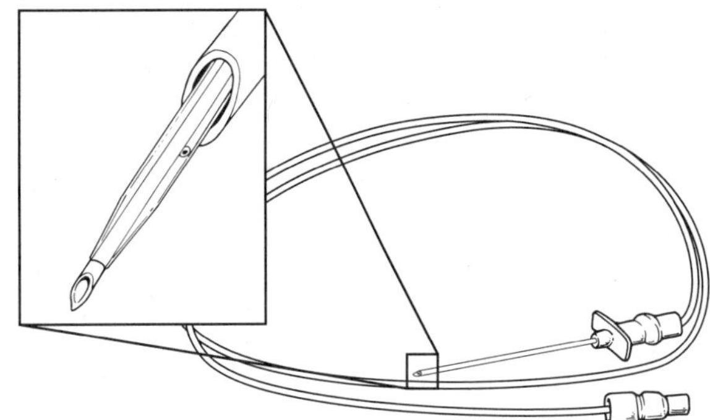

❖ **Figure 12-6** The Spinocath over-the-needle equipment that is currently being marketed outside the United States.

❖ SUMMARY

Key Points

- Continuous spinal anesthesia is not a new technique. The first description of this technique was published in 1907.
- The FDA withdrew approval of all microcatheters smaller than 24 gauge in 1992. Continuous spinal anesthesia via a macrocatheter technique (epidural needle and catheter into subarachnoid space) can still be used.
- Continuous spinal anesthesia has many potential advantages in a select group of high-risk parturients, especially the morbidly obese parturient with a difficult airway.
- Following an unintentional dural puncture during placement of an epidural ("wet tap"), the epidural catheter can be threaded subarachnoid and used for CSA for labor or cesarean section.

Key Reference

Biboulet P, Capdevila X, Aubas P, et al: Causes and prediction of maldistribution during continuous spinal anesthesia with isobaric or hyperbaric bupivacaine. Anesthesiology 1998; 88:1487–1494.

Case Stem

During placement of a labor epidural at the L3–L4 interspace in a morbidly obese parturient, free-flowing cerebrospinal fluid is noted in the 18-gauge Tuohy needle. Discuss your management of a spinal catheter for labor. Five hours later, the decision is made to proceed with a cesarean section. How would you manage the catheter for operative delivery?

severe systemic illnesses who is a candidate for regional anesthesia may benefit from the sure and stable analgesia or anesthesia that is a hallmark of CSA.

THE FUTURE

Interest in CSA with microcatheters was certainly dealt a devastating blow after the FDA withdrawal in the early 1990s, but, recently, interest in the technique seems to be reviving. The annual meeting of the Society for Obstetric Anesthesia and Perinatology in 1998 saw a presentation of preliminary data from a multicenter study evaluating microcatheters inserted through a ramped Sprotte needle used for labor analgesia employing bupivacaine and sufentanil. The data were encouraging, but any conclusions would be premature. Work with the catheters has continued apace in Europe, where the technique was never abandoned. New catheter prototypes have been proposed, such as a catheter (22-gauge Spinocath; Fig. 12–6) over the needle (27-gauge), which would provide rapid injection and presumably good mixing with a small dural hole. A recent small study claimed improved insertion, maintenance, and clinical effects of the 22-gauge Spinocath over a standard 28-gauge microcatheter.[23] The combined spinal epidural technique has seen an explosion of interest in spinal adjuvants such as clonidine and neostigmine. However, the subarachnoid space is only visited once with this technique. Perhaps the turn of the millennium will see the return of CSA with 21st century catheters that incorporate the knowledge gained in the last decade of the 20th century.

References

1. Dean HP: Discussion on the relative value of inhalation and injection methods of inducing anaesthesia. Br Med J 1907; 5:869–877.
2. Lemmon WT: A method for continuous spinal anesthesia. Ann Surg 1940; 111:141–144.
3. Lemmon WT, Paschal GW: Continuous spinal anesthesia: With observation on the first 500 cases. Penn Med J 1941; 44:975–981.
4. Hinebaugh MC, Lang WR: Continuous spinal anesthesia for labor and delivery. Ann Surg 1944; 120:143–151.
5. Tuohy EB: The use of continuous spinal anesthesia. JAMA 1945; 128:262–263.
6. Bizzarri D, Giuffrida JG, Brandoc L, et al: Continuous spinal anesthesia using a special needle and catheter. Anesth Analg 1964; 43:393–399.
7. Giuffrida JG, Bizzari DV, Masi R, et al: Continuous procaine spinal anesthesia for cesarean section. Anesth Analg 1972; 51:117–124.
8. Hurley RJ, Lambert DH: Continuous spinal anesthesia with a microcatheter technique: Preliminary experience. Anesth Analg 1990; 70:97–102.
9. Rigler ML, Drasner K, Krejcie TC, et al: Cauda equina syndrome after continuous spinal anesthesia. Anesth Analg 1991; 72:275–281.
10. Sakura S, Sumi M, Sakaguchi Y, et al: The addition of phenylephrine contributes to the development of transient neurologic symptoms after spinal anesthesia with 0.5% tetracaine. Anesthesiology 1997; 87:771–778.
11. Lambert LA, Lambert DH, Strichartz GR: Irreversible conduction block in isolated nerve by high concentrations of local anesthetics. Anesthesiology 1994; 80:1082–1093.
12. Pollock JE, Neal JM, Stephenson CA, et al: Prospective study of the incidence of transient radicular irritation in patients undergoing spinal anesthesia. Anesthesiology 1996; 84:1361–1367.
13. Hampl K, Schneider M, Ummenhofer W, et al: Transient neurologic symptoms after spinal anesthesia. Anesth Analg 1993; 81:1148–1153.
14. Morisaki H, Masuda J, Kaneko S, et al: Transient neurologic syndrome in one thousand forty-five patients after 3% lidocaine spinal anesthesia. Anesth Analg 1998; 86:1023–1026.
15. Tarkkila P, Huhtala J, Tuominen M, et al: Transient radicular irritation after bupivacaine spinal anesthesia. Regional Anesthesia 1996; 21:26–29.
16. Ross BK, Coda B, Heath CH: Local anesthetic distribution in a spinal model: A possible mechanism of neurologic injury after continuous spinal analgesia. Reg Anesth 1992; 17:69–77.
17. Biboulet P, Capdevila X, Aubas P, et al: Causes and prediction of maldistribution during continuous spinal anesthesia with isobaric or hyperbaric bupivacaine. Anesthesiology 1998; 88:1487–1494.
18. Scott PV, Bowen FE, Cartwright P, et al: Intrathecal morphine as sole analgesic during labor. Br Med J 1980; 281:351–353.
19. Abboud TK, Raya J, Noueihed R, et al: Intrathecal morphine for relief of labor pain in a parturient with severe pulmonary hypertension. Anesthesiology 1983; 59:477–479.
20. Brizgys RV, Shnider SM: Hyperbaric intrathecal morphine analgesia during labor in a patient with Wolff-Parkinson-White syndrome. Obstet Gynecol 1984; 64:44S–46S.
21. Copel JA, Harrison D, Whittemore R, et al: Intrathecal morphine analgesia for vaginal delivery in a woman with a single ventricle. J Reprod Med 1986; 31:274–276.
22. Johnson MD, Hurley RJ, Gilbertson LI, Datta S: Continuous microcatheter spinal anesthesia with subarachnoid meperidine for labor and delivery. Anesth Analg 1990; 70:658–661.
23. Muralidhar V, Kaul HL, Mallick P: Over-the-needle versus microcatheter-through-needle technique for continuous spinal anesthesia: A preliminary study. Regional Anesth Pain Med 1999; 24:417–421.

13

Patient-Controlled Epidural Analgesia

❖ MICHAEL PAECH, MBBS, DRCOG, FRCA, FANZCA, FFPWANZCA

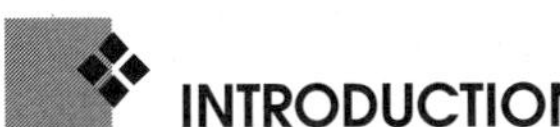

INTRODUCTION

The concept of patient-controlled analgesia (PCA) for acute pain management has been embraced with enthusiasm by clinicians and patients throughout the world in the last decade, and many would consider it one of the most important recent advances in pain management. Anesthesiologists are familiar with the principles pertaining to the safe and effective use of PCA, and with the documented benefits, in particular those related to patient satisfaction. It is interesting then to reflect on 10 years of personal experience with PCA using the epidural route of administration (PCEA), to review the literature and an abundance of clinical experience, particularly in obstetric analgesia, and to speculate on why obstetric PCEA appears to remain a relatively poorly utilized technique. On first appearances, PCEA would seem an ideal approach to obstetric epidural analgesia during labor, in which maternal perception of control is integral to high levels of satisfaction with childbirth. It is also eminently well-suited to postoperative analgesia, in which the efficacy of epidural opioids can be exploited in patients who already have an epidural catheter in place. Is PCEA an inappropriate method of PCA; is it a method that meets, or has failed to meet, expectations; is it unsafe; and if it is underutilized, why should this be and is the situation changing?

PATIENT-CONTROLLED EPIDURAL ANALGESIA FOR LABOR AND DELIVERY

Patient-controlled techniques have played a prominent role in obstetric analgesia for most of the 20th century, commencing with the self-administration of nitrous oxide. Intravenous patient-controlled analgesia (PCA) was given a trial in labor in the late 1960s,[1] and modern techniques gained impetus after the development of the Cardiff palliator by Evans and colleagues in the 1970s.[2] However, it was not until the 1980s that technologic advances leading to the development of improved PCA pumps heralded the widespread application of PCA for acute pain management. During this period, in many countries, the popularity of obstetric epidural analgesia was also increasing, and investigators from Vancouver were the first to report the obstetric use of patient-controlled epidural analgesia, or PCEA.[3]

The application of PCEA to labor pain management is conceptually appealing. The feeling of control, including control of panic and pain and involvement in decision making, is a complex perception that is central to maternal psychologic and emotional well-being and satisfaction. A common feature of women who are highly satisfied with their childbirth experience is a very positive perception of the control they experienced.[4] PCEA provides the psychologic benefits of self-administration and self-titration of solution to individually acceptable analgesic end points throughout labor and gives immediate access to more epidural solution. Midwifery, nursing, and anesthetic staff workload should be reduced, and lower rates of drug delivery may minimize side effects and risks. Perceived disadvantages of PCEA include the delayed feedback loop associated with the slow onset of epidural drugs and concerns about equipment function, safety, monitoring, and education.

There is now almost a decade of clinical experience with PCEA in labor, and more than 25 publications involving over 2750 parturients. The benefits and advantages of PCEA during labor have been reviewed.[5, 6]

Five years ago, Eisenach[7] considered PCEA a useful alternative, and "safe when small doses of dilute bupivacaine are administered with each bolus, reasonable hourly limits are prescribed, and periodic assessments by anesthesiologists are made." It is interesting to speculate on why PCEA during labor does not appear to have been embraced with widespread enthusiasm. Although PCEA is popular in many units, and clinical practice data are seldom reported, it appears that continuous infusion and intermittent bolus techniques predominate in most obstetric epidural services. Do the detractors of PCEA make valid points?[8] Has PCEA fulfilled its promise compared with alternative delivery techniques, and how is it best used? Are there problems associated with PCEA in labor or issues that have not been adequately addressed? Is PCEA safe in this setting?

Comparison with Continuous Infusion or Intermittent Staff-Administered Bolus Techniques in Labor

Pain Relief, Satisfaction, and Requirement for Supplementation

Most studies comparing PCEA with continuous infusion epidural analgesia (CIEA) have not demonstrated advantages with respect to either analgesic quality or satisfaction but found PCEA to be associated with either lower bupivacaine usage (by 25–50%) or a lower rate of supplementation and fewer staff management interventions.[3, 9–17] Outcome differences in randomized comparisons of PCEA and intermittent bolus epidural analgesia (IBEA) should be considered cautiously, because no study attempted to blind participants or observers and results may therefore have been influenced by investigator bias and confounding factors. Nevertheless, analgesia and satisfaction appear to be at least equivalent,[18–22] and one study reported higher satisfaction scores with PCEA.[3] Recently, a survey of 500 parturients using either PCEA or IBEA identified PCEA as independently associated with higher levels of satisfaction.[23] PCEA, which avoids potential delays in staff responding to requests and obtaining and administering further epidural drugs and also prevents the fluctuations in pain intensity associated with IBEA, provided more uniform pain relief.[22] Unilateral block and unblocked segments, as might be expected, probably do not differ in incidence with PCEA, CIEA, and IBEA (Figs. 13–1 and 13–2).[21]

Not all,[11, 12, 18] but most, clinical trials have found a reduced need for supplementation or intervention with PCEA compared with other techniques.[10, 14, 16, 21] No, or one, intervention was required in 89% and 87%, respectively, of parturients receiving PCEA or IBEA compared with 64% for CIEA.[21] Fewer supplements may indicate fewer episodes of unrelieved pain, and reduced workload has implications in situations in which anesthetic staff are required to provide all supplementation, or for more efficient utilization of midwifery time.

In contrast to the conditions pertaining during a controlled clinical trial, in which support and supervision are optimal, normal management practice in a busy delivery unit may alter the frequency of staff intervention or supplementation. A randomized series of midwifery-managed PCEA or IBEA reported an increased number of staff-administered extra boluses and greater total bupivacaine use with PCEA.[22] If the documented advantages of PCEA are to be realized, attention must be paid to personnel levels and education of staff with respect to the appropriate type and timing of supplementation and to management of the second stage of labor.

Rate of Bupivacaine Use, Motor Block, and the Effect of Patient-Controlled Epidural Analgesia on Delivery

Most studies show a 25% to 50% reduction in bupivacaine requirement with PCEA compared with alternatives,[3, 9–11, 15–17, 19] but some trials have not demonstrated any advantage.[14, 18, 22] Excellent pain relief is obtained with demand-only PCEA using only 3 to 8 mg/h of bupivacaine,[24] and the use of a concurrent background may or may not increase total drug usage.[15, 25, 26]

One of the prime aims of modern epidural analgesia in labor is the minimization of motor block, because retention of mobility (even if walking is neither desired nor permitted) is a feature important to most parturients[27] and avoidance of numb, heavy legs

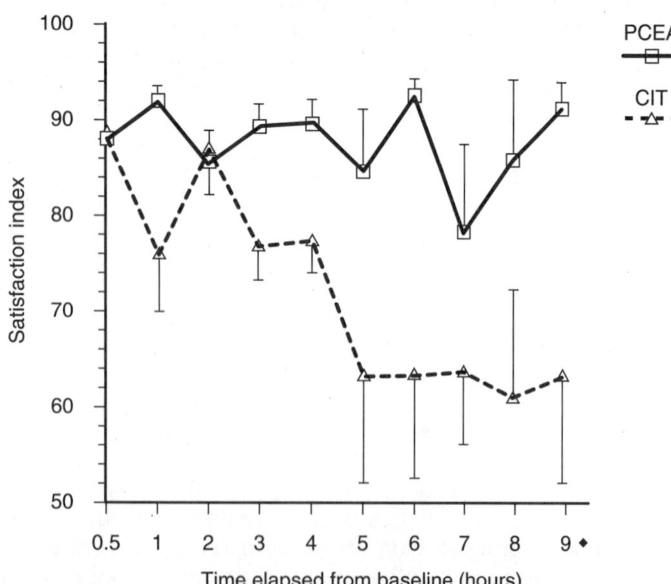

Figure 13–1 Patient satisfaction expressed as a Satisfaction Index. Patient-controlled epidural analgesia (PCEA) *(open squares)* versus conventional intermittent top-ups (CIT) *(open triangles)* (From Gambling DR, McMorland GH, Yu P, Laszlo C: Comparison of patient-controlled epidural analgesia and conventional intermittent "top-up" injections during labor. Anesth Analg 1990; 70:256–261.)

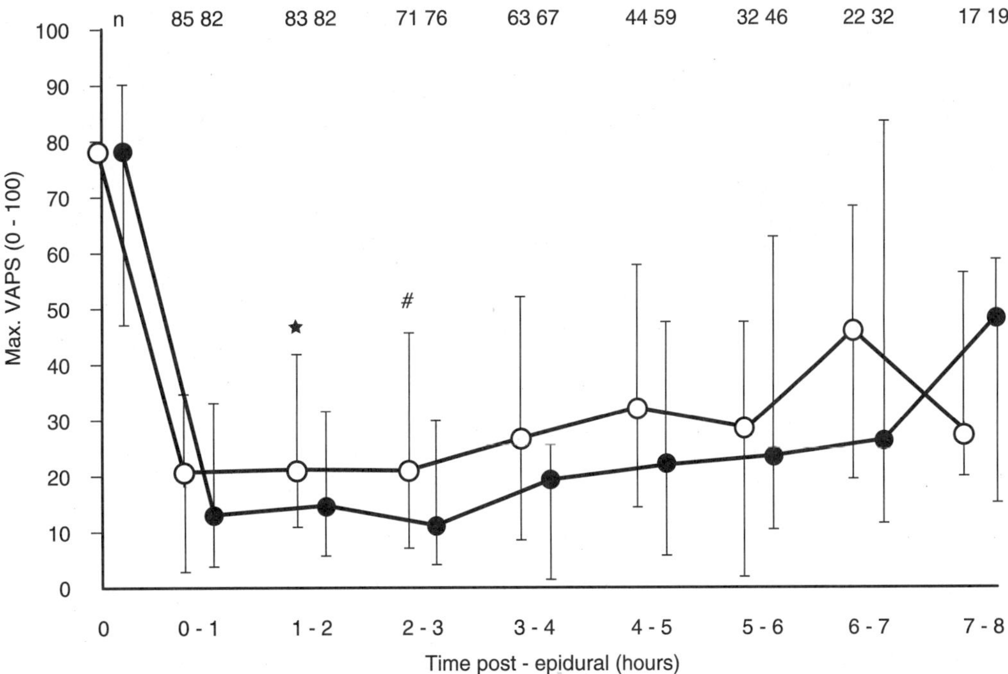

❖ **Figure 13–2** Maximum pain score (median and interquartile range) in the previous hour during labor. *Closed circles* represent patient-controlled epidural analgesia (PCEA) and *open circles* intermittent boluses. **P* < .05 second hour after epidural; #*P* < .02 third hour after epidural. (From Paech MJ, Pavy TJG, Sims C, et al: Clinical experience with patient-controlled and staff-administered intermittent bolus epidural analgesia in labour. Anaesth Intensive Care 1995; 23:459–463.)

is associated with greater maternal satisfaction.[28] A large randomized series comparing PCEA and IBEA (with bupivacaine 0.25%) and CIEA (with bupivacaine 0.125%) found that significantly more parturients using PCEA or IBEA had no leg muscle weakness.[21] PCEA solutions containing bupivacaine 0.0625% to 0.125% with opioid further reduce the risk of muscle weakness.[24] Full hip and knee flexion is retained during the first 3 to 4 hours of demand-only PCEA,[11, 15] and motor block is less than that associated with the infusion of similar solution.[17] With bupivacaine 0.0625%, fentanyl, and adrenaline, 80% of parturients using PCEA over a 6-hour period were able to temporarily demonstrate a sustained straight-leg raise,[24] although as the duration of labor increases, 20% to 30% develop profound leg weakness irrespective of the bupivacaine concentration.[9, 21, 24, 29] PCEA is nevertheless associated with good potential for ambulatory regional analgesia. If the analgesia is established with bupivacaine 0.125% with opioid or bupivacaine 0.25% and maintained with bupivacaine 0.0625% to 0.125%, about 80% of parturients can walk (Fig. 13–3).[22, 25, 29]

There is no convincing evidence that PCEA, by reducing local anesthetic requirement and minimizing motor block, reduces the duration of labor or improves spontaneous vaginal delivery rate. In small trials involving healthy nulliparous women[12] or those of mixed parity,[3, 9, 14, 16] the type of delivery was not influenced by epidural technique. Two small studies suggested a higher spontaneous vaginal delivery rate with PCEA than with CIEA,[13, 15] but a randomized series, stratified for parity, found that both the duration of the second stage and the incidence of instrumental delivery were higher with PCEA than IBEA.[22] Studies of both CIEA and combined spinal-epidural analgesia have also failed to identify an advantage with respect to labor and delivery outcome when techniques that minimize, and almost eliminate, motor block are used. This issue is unlikely to be resolved without very large, well-controlled trials, which are particularly difficult to perform (Table 13–1).

Drug Selection

Although no advantage was demonstrated when an initial bolus of bupivacaine 0.125% with opioid was

Table 13–1 ADVANTAGES OF PATIENT-CONTROLLED EPIDURAL ANALGESIA IN LABOR OVER ALTERNATIVES

Well-Documented Advantages
Reduced drug utilization
Reduced rates of intervention or supplementation
Potential Advantages
Greater maternal satisfaction
Reduced motor block
Lower risk of intravenous local anesthetic toxicity or total spinal block
No Significant Advantage, But No Disadvantage
Quality of analgesia
Maternal hypotensive episodes and high blocks
Effect on delivery outcome

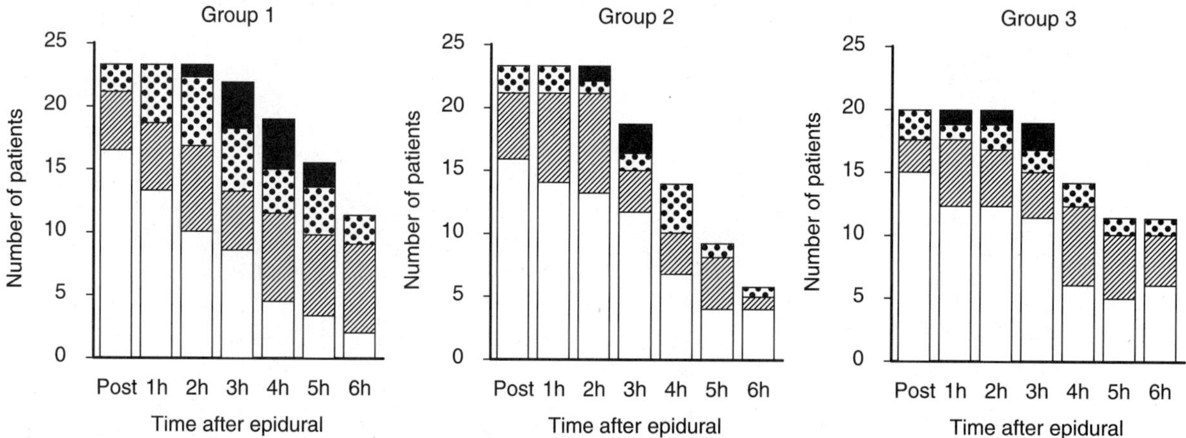

Figure 13–3 Distribution of motor block after epidural analgesia during labor. *Open bar* indicates no weakness, able to maintain straight leg raise; *hatched bar,* unable to maintain straight leg raise but full hip and knee flexion; *dotted bar,* able to flex ankle easily but weak hip and knee flexion; *solid bar,* no hip or knee flexion, ankle flexion present or absent. Group 1 represents patient-controlled epidural analgesia (PCEA) with 0.25% bupivacaine; group 2 represents PCEA with 0.125% bupivacaine and fentanyl 3 μg/mL; group 3 represents PCEA with 0.0625% bupivacaine and fentanyl 3 μg/mL and epinephrine 4 μg/mL. (From Paech MJ: Patient-controlled epidural analgesia during labour: Choice of solution. Int J Obstet Anesth 1993; 2:68.)

compared with bupivacaine 0.25% prior to CIEA, my practice before PCEA is to commence with bupivacaine 0.1% to 0.125% or ropivacaine 1 mg/mL, both with fentanyl 3 to 5 μg/mL (10–15 mL). Neither lignocaine nor chloroprocaine has been evaluated as a local anesthetic for PCEA because of the well-recognized disadvantages of each during labor.

The new local anesthetic ropivacaine offers potential advantages over bupivacaine with respect to reduced motor block intensity,[30] and early comparative studies with bupivacaine are now appearing in the literature. A 1.25 mg/mL concentration of both drugs (which represents a more potent dose of bupivacaine, the potency ratio of ropivacaine to bupivacaine in labor being about 0.6[31]) produces similar analgesia and motor block.[32] When fentanyl was combined to produce a dose-sparing effect with the same concentrations, reduction in motor block with ropivacaine was noted.[33] A study comparing equipotent concentrations, for example, bupivacaine 0.625% and ropivacaine 1 mg/mL (plus opioid), is awaited before it can be confirmed that ropivacaine offers a clinically important advantage for PCEA. The only PCEA study to include the α_2-adrenergic agonist clonidine found bupivacaine and fentanyl dose sparing, with fewer supplements and higher levels of satisfaction, without adverse side effects, suggesting that it may be a useful adjunct.[34]

Current data suggest that the most appropriate PCEA solutions are bupivacaine 0.0625% to 0.125% with fentanyl or sufentanil. Demand boluses of bupivacaine 8 mg (0.25% 4 mL), 5 mg (0.125% 4 mL), or 2.5 mg (0.0625% 4 mL), the latter two combined with fentanyl 3 μg/mL and the last also with epinephrine 1:400,000, produce equivalent pain relief, but the largest dose results in increased drug use and more profound motor block.[24] Compared with CIEA, both using 0.125% bupivacaine with fentanyl, PCEA is equally effective and lowers bupivacaine requirement by 40%.[16] The addition of epinephrine to PCEA solutions has been common[9, 15, 19, 20, 24] but should be avoided, because it has no benefit and significantly increases the density of motor block after 2 or 3 hours of PCEA.[9] Bupivacaine 0.0625% with opioid has been confirmed as effective and safe,[17] and I believe it can be recommended (Fig. 13–4).[35]

Choice of Regimen

The prescribed PCA variables should permit delivery of an adequate volume of solution, a further demand

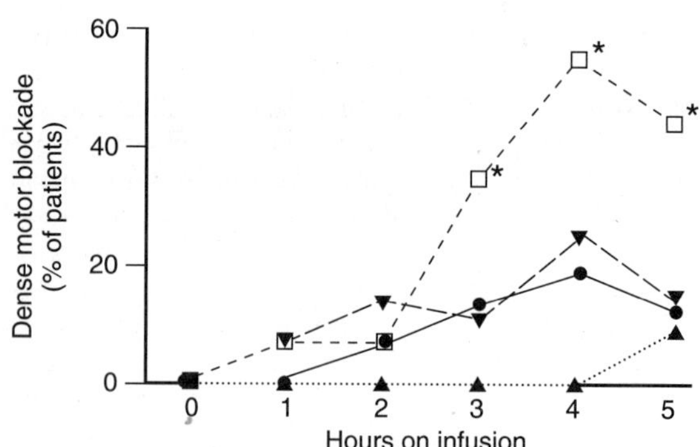

Figure 13–4 Percentage of patients with dense motor block (defined as unable to flex knees, able or unable to move feet) after epidural in labor. *Circles* represent continuous epidural infusion with 0.125% bupivacaine; *inverted triangles* represent patient-controlled epidural analgesia (PCEA) with 0.125% bupivacaine; *upright triangles* represent PCEA with 0.125% bupivacaine and fentanyl 1 μg/mL; *squares* represent PCEA with 0.125% bupivacaine and fentanyl 1 μg/mL and epinephrine 2.5 μg/mL. $P < .05$ for the last PCEA solution versus time zero. (From Lysak SZ, Eisenach JC, Dobson CE II: Anesthesiology 1990; 72:47.)

after 10 or more minutes, and safe maximum hourly drug doses. Untested ideas are to base the demand bolus volume on the response to the initial epidural bolus, or to allow more rapid initial access to demands rather than regular spacing over time. A study addressing the interrelation of demand bolus size and lockout time found little difference between a range of volume-lockout time combinations.[13] There was a trend, however, for larger demand bolus dose to be associated with higher sensory levels and more motor block. Most demand-only PCEA regimens prescribe 3 to 5 mL boluses with a 10 to 15 minute lockout interval.

The use of a background infusion is controversial, and clinical trials are contradictory.[15, 25, 26] All studies addressing the merit of a patient-assisted infusion approach versus a demand-only approach used 0.125% bupivacaine with opioid, and two found similar analgesia and satisfaction, but lower drug usage with the latter.[25, 36] Preliminary results from a study not yet reported in a peer-reviewed journal noted better analgesia with a background infusion (which is surprising).[26] In another study, the investigators found fewer anesthetist-administered supplements in the first stage of labor when an infusion at about a third of the maximum hourly demand dose was added, compared with demand-only or a lower infusion rate, and they concluded that such an infusion was appropriate.[15] Depending on the PCEA technique used, 10% to 50% of parturients require a supplement, although usually only one or two.[10, 14, 24, 25] Many studies indicate that excellent results are achieved without an infusion, and, unless patient benefits can be demonstrated, like others I will continue to favor a "bolus-only" technique (Fig. 13–5).[37–39]

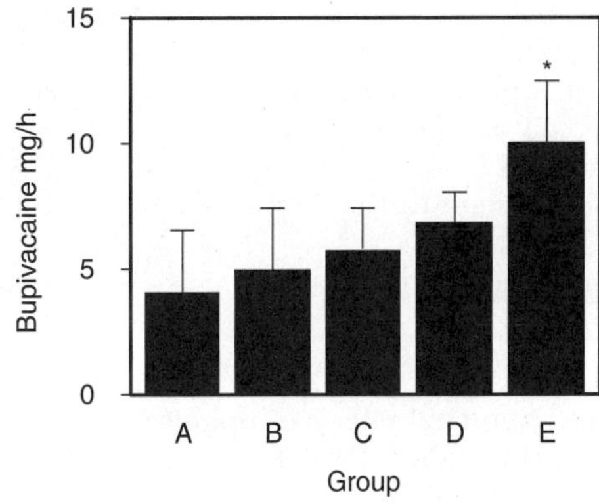

❖ **Figure 13–5** Bupivacaine consumption during labor (mean ± SD). All groups received 0.125% bupivacaine and fentanyl 2.5 μg/mL and epinephrine 2.5 μg/mL. Group A represents patient-controlled epidural analgesia (PCEA) 2 mL bolus/10 minute lockout; group B 3 mL/15 minute; group C 4 mL/20 minute; group D 6 mL/30 minute; and group E continuous epidural infusion at 8 mL/h. $P < .0001$ for group E versus all other groups. (From Gambling DR, Huber CJ, Berkowitz J, et al: Patient-controlled epidural analgesia in labor: Varying bolus dose and lockout interval. Can J Anaesth 1993; 40:211–217.)

Maternal Safety

Hypotension

Hypotension associated with epidural analgesia almost always follows bolus administration, especially if large doses are given. Risk is maximal during the initial sympathetic block, whereas during maintenance of analgesia, PCEA provides good hemodynamic stability comparable to that of CIEA.[10, 11, 18, 21] Hypotensive episodes from self-administered bupivacaine boluses during PCEA are rare if individual doses are limited to 2.5 to 6 mg.[11, 21, 22, 24, 25, 29, 40] Self-administration when standing, compared with lying in the lateral position, offers better blood pressure stability, possibly because of the avoidance of concealed aortocaval compression and a compensatory heart rate increase when upright.[40] It seems prudent to maintain recumbency for 20 to 30 minutes after establishing epidural analgesia, and to monitor blood pressure at least every 30 minutes, but more intensive monitoring during PCEA is unnecessary except after staff-administered additional larger boluses.

Catheter Misplacement and High Block

Although reservations continue to be expressed,[8] widespread clinical experience now attests to the safety of PCEA when appropriate variables and solutions are used in well-monitored delivery units. PCEA is associated with very low rates of local anesthetic use and reduces the number of extra boluses of concentrated solution, so should theoretically be safer than alternative techniques.[39, 41] At hourly bupivacaine dose rates of less than 10 mg and with 3 to 6 mg demand boluses, bupivacaine toxicity appears highly unlikely, even in the rare event of intravascular migration of the epidural catheter.[42] High subarachnoid block after accidental subarachnoid injection is also unlikely, because doses of about 5 mg of bupivacaine given intrathecally reliably produce sacral analgesia and cephalad dermatomal sensory change to T6-T10.[43]

About 20% of parturients titrate to a sensory level of T8, with extension above T7 in 5% to 10%.[3, 15, 17, 18] Similar[3, 9, 10, 18] or significantly higher levels[17] are noted with physician-controlled alternatives such as IBEA and CIEA. Frequent, ideally continuous, midwifery care, good maternal monitoring, assessment of the dermatomal distribution of sensory changes, and preparation for the occasional high block, which causes symptoms, are requirements irrespective of the method of drug delivery.

Respiratory Depression

Severe respiratory depression from intraspinal opioids in labor occurs rarely but should be anticipated. Pump mishaps during patient-controlled intravenous analgesia may have serious consequences, but there have been almost no recent reports, and no problems described during labor PCEA. The advent of simple, nonelectronic PCA devices should further reduce such events. Staff and parturient education is nevertheless important if unusual events are to be identified early and potentially dangerous practices such as PCA by proxy avoided.[44] Currently, no serious adverse events have been described during labor PCEA (Fig. 13–6).

Fetal and Neonatal Effects

Opioids

The fetal and neonatal effects of epidural fentanyl and sufentanil during labor have been well investigated, although not after PCEA. Fetal heart rate variability does not differ from control when a bolus of epidural fentanyl is administered, and boluses of epidural bupivacaine and fentanyl in labor do not affect neonatal sucking characteristics. PCEA studies have found that a solution containing fentanyl 1 to 3 μg/mL results in utilization rates of between 8 and 20 μg/h[9, 11, 13, 24] and a solution containing sufentanil 0.75 to 1 μg/mL results in rates of 5 to 15 μg/h.[19, 20, 26] Fentanyl 3 μg/mL maximizes bupivacaine dose sparing (mean minimum local anesthetic concentration, 0.03%), without increasing pruritus, when bolus doses are administered.[45] Extrapolating from studies using other techniques in labor, these epidural doses do not appear to have clinically important effects on the neonate. Fentanyl at rates of 20 μg/h for up to 15 hours does not produce neonatal respiratory or neurobehavioral effects,[46] although doses above 200 μg may have transient negative effects.[47]

Sufentanil up to 45 μg results in neurobehavioral scores similar to those of epidural bupivacaine alone.[48] Fentanyl and sufentanil have not been compared using a PCEA technique, but with CIEA, neonates exposed to mean doses of 137 μg fentanyl versus 24 μg sufentanil (a comparable potency ratio) have lower neurobehavioral scores at 24 hours after fentanyl.[49]

Local Anesthetics

Meta-analysis of clinical trials of ropivacaine versus bupivacaine for epidural analgesia in labor identified better neurobehavioral scores after ropivacaine, and analysis of fetal and neonatal adverse events after these local anesthetics for cesarean section indicates fewer events with ropivacaine.[30, 50] Although the reason is not understood, ropivacaine in adults has higher lipid solubility and a shorter half-life, and thus it is possible that bupivacaine persists in the neonatal tissues for a longer period.

Management of a Service

Patient-controlled epidural analgesia in labor is a safe technique that is associated with high levels of maternal satisfaction and perception of control. In my opinion, it should be an option provided by all maternity units that offer a regional analgesia service for labor and delivery. Nevertheless, although consumer response to labor PCEA is usually enthusiastic, and some units use it exclusively, I do not believe that it should be viewed as a panacea.

Some parturients prefer not to assume the responsibilities inherent in PCA, whether because of personality or situational factors, including extreme fatigue or the effects of systemic drugs. In addition, in some obstetric circumstances, especially regional analgesia commenced in late labor or when delivery appears imminent, the advantages of PCEA are largely negated.

Two important considerations when establishing a PCEA service are the acquisition of appropriate equipment and the education of both staff and parturients.

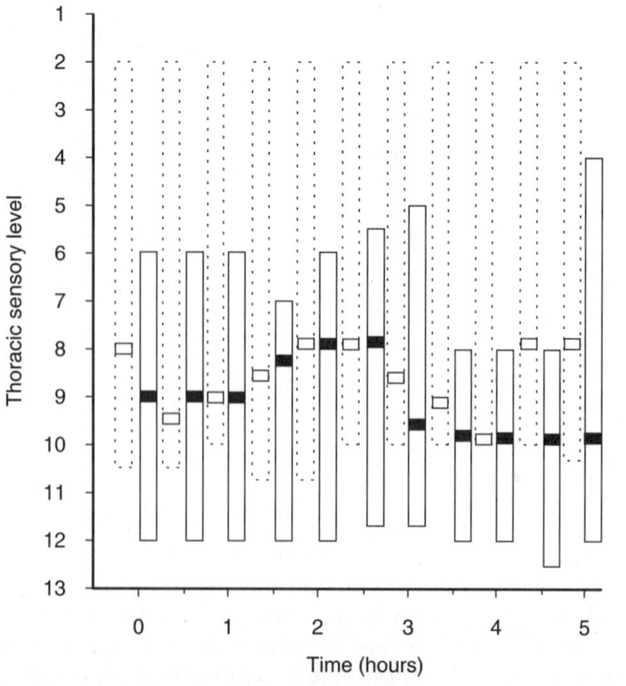

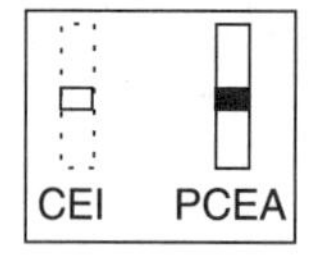

Figure 13–6 Cephalad extension of sensory block (median and range) with patient-controlled epidural analgesia (PCEA) (with 0.0625% bupivacaine and fentanyl 2 μg/mL) and continuous epidural infusion (CEI) (with 0.125% bupivacaine and fentanyl 2 μg/mL at 12 mL/h) during labor. The level with PCEA was significantly lower ($P < .03$) during both the first and second stages of labor. (From Ferrante FM, Barber MJ, Segal M, et al: 0.0625% bupivacaine with 0.0002% fentanyl via patient-controlled epidural analgesia for pain of labor and delivery. Clin J Pain 1995; 11:121–126.)

Anesthesia, midwifery, nursing, and technical staff should be aware of both the principles of PCA and the practicalities of managing PCEA, in particular monitoring policies, appropriate use of supplementary doses, and PCA pump function. It may be necessary to collaborate with obstetric medical and midwifery staff in reviewing attitudes and policies regarding mobility, management of the second stage of labor, and fetal monitoring. It is preferable to discuss PCEA and the appropriate use of PCA pumps in the antenatal period, by means of parenting classes, outpatient clinics, and written or visual resource materials. PCEA can nevertheless be implemented at any time, including in established labor, provided good pain relief and communication are established initially. It is worthwhile emphasizing how best to use the PCA pump, the place of supplementation and ambulation, and the relevance of notifying staff about unexpected sensations or events, including the gradual onset of dense motor block. If education or supervision is less than optimal, PCEA may fail to demonstrate its potential advantages over alternative approaches.[22]

POST-CESAREAN SECTION PATIENT-CONTROLLED EPIDURAL ANALGESIA

Although PCEA can be applied to any surgical procedure performed in a pregnant patient, either antenatally or postpartum, the predominant surgical operation in established pregnancy is cesarean section (CS) and the vast majority of clinical trials have investigated this setting. Despite the increasing popularity of spinal anesthesia, epidural anesthesia is recommended in cases in which operative delivery or procedures are required in parturients with effective epidural analgesia and remains widely used alone or as part of combined spinal-epidural anesthesia for elective CS.

Postoperative PCEA combines the effectiveness of epidural opioid analgesia with the flexibility and patient benefits of PCA, and from the maternal perspective appears ideal. Postpartum patients are usually healthy and well motivated and require opioid analgesia for the first 24 to 48 hours after CS. A technique that provides high-quality pain relief with few side effects, and does not restrict mobility, optimizes mother-infant bonding and the successful establishment of breast-feeding.

Although postoperative PCEA was described several years before obstetric use after CS, the first post-CS PCEA trials postdate those describing PCEA during labor.[51–53] Interest was generated, despite some problems being encountered, particularly when a retrospective study suggested that high-quality analgesia associated with PCEA might reduce the length of hospital stay.[54] In addition, a randomized study demonstrated improved maternal outcome (times to return of bowel function, resumption of solid diet, and shorter postoperative stay) compared with intravenous PCA (PCIA).[52] How then does PCEA compare with alternative approaches and what drugs and variables are most appropriate?

Clinical Efficacy

Comparison with Systemic Opioid Techniques

Patient-controlled epidural analgesia is a highly effective approach to postoperative analgesia that compares favorably with most alternatives, although some issues remain unresolved. As might be expected, PCEA clearly provides superior pain relief to intramuscular opioid and is preferred by both patients and nurses.[55] When compared with PCIA, the advantages of PCEA are partly dependent on the choice of drug or drug combination. Many studies show significantly reduced drug consumption with the epidural route (even with lipophilic opioids that do not always show dose sparing when administered epidurally rather than systemically). Examples are hydromorphone,[52] fentanyl,[56–58] and meperidine.[58, 59] Whether this translates into patient benefit, for example with respect to reduction of side effects, is the question. Sedation is usually less,[52, 57] but there is no evidence for a reduction in nausea, and PCEA with most opioids produces a higher incidence of pruritus.[52, 56, 57, 59] Better analgesia cannot be demonstrated with all opioids, but clinically significant improvement in analgesia both at rest and with coughing is seen with PCEA using fentanyl or meperidine (Figs. 13–7 and 13–8).[56–60]

Comparison with Other Spinal Opioid Techniques

Compared with a single bolus of epidural morphine, PCEA with either fentanyl or meperidine does not

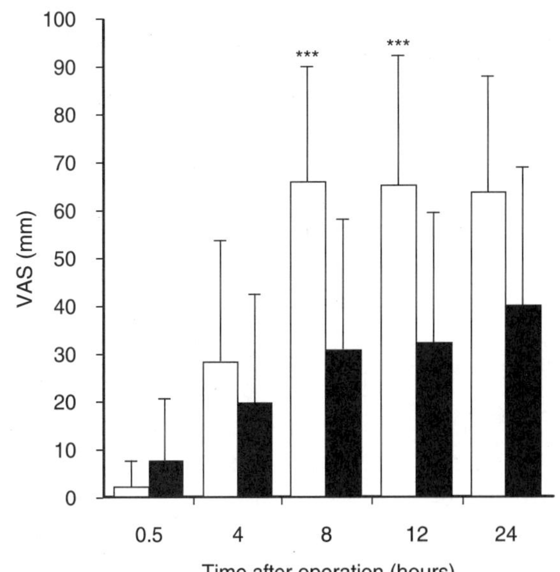

❖ **Figure 13–7** Pain scores (mean ± SD) with coughing after cesarean section. *Open bars* represent patient-controlled intravenous analgesia (PCIA) and *solid bars* patient-controlled epidural analgesia (PCEA), both with fentanyl 20 μg bolus and 10 minute lockout. $***P < .005$. (From Cooper DW, Ryall DM, Desira WR: Extradural fentanyl for postoperative analgesia: predominant spinal or systemic action? Br J Anaesth 1995; 74:184–187.)

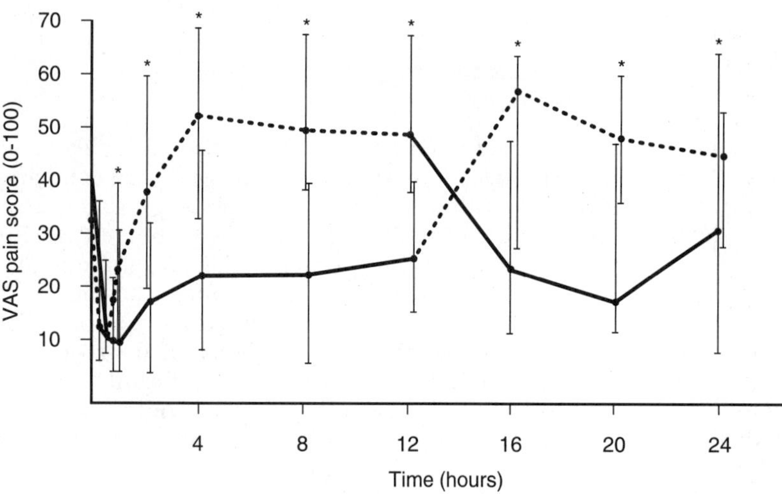

❖ **Figure 13–8** Pain scores with coughing (median and interquartile range) during post-cesarean patient-controlled epidural analgesia (PCEA) or patient-controlled intravenous analgesia (PCIA) with meperidine 20 mg bolus and 5 minute lockout. *Crosses* indicate PCEA for 12 hours, then PCIA for 12 hours; *circles*, PCIA for 12 hours, then PCEA for 12 hours. *$P < .05$. (From Paech MJ, Moore JS, Evans SF: Meperidine for patient-controlled analgesia after cesarean section: Intravenous versus epidural administration. Anesthesiology 1994; 80:1268–1276.)

improve initial analgesia but does reduce side effects and provide flexibility with respect to continued analgesia.[61, 62] Up to 10% of patients who have been distressed by epidural morphine-induced pruritus refuse it subsequently,[63] so for these patients and those with herpes simplex labialis, in whom intraspinal morphine risks reactivating lesions, meperidine PCEA appears a better option. There is considerable argument as to the relative merits of spinal anesthesia with subarachnoid morphine analgesia and epidural anesthesia or combined spinal-epidural analgesia (CSEA) with postoperative PCEA, and despite widespread use of these excellent techniques, no controlled comparison has been performed. In many units, adjunctive analgesia with nonsteroidal anti-inflammatory drugs is used to complement PCEA (Figs. 13–9 and 13–10).

Drug Selection

Opioids

Epidural drugs suitable for PCEA in this setting include local anesthetics (bupivacaine and ropivacaine), opioids (fentanyl, meperidine, and sufentanil), and α_2-adrenergic agonists (adrenaline, clonidine). Opioids of low lipid solubility, such as morphine, can be used for PCEA and compare very favorably with intermittent epidural morphine boluses,[64] but the onset of action is slow and the incidence of maternal side effects high compared with alternative opioids.[65] A highly lipophilic

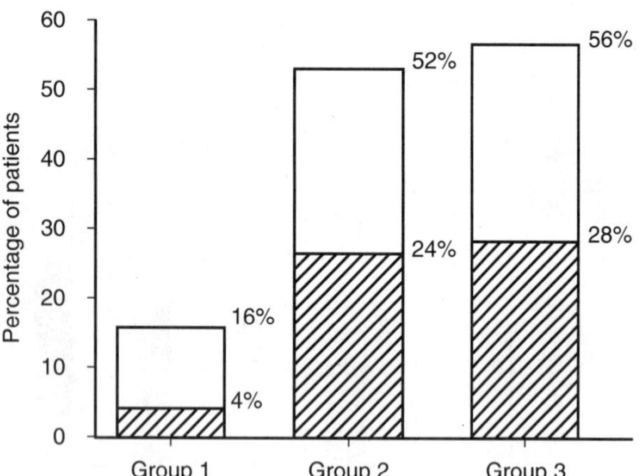

❖ **Figure 13–9** Percentage of patients with nausea (*cross-hatched bars* represent the percentage requiring treatment). Group 1 represents postcesarean patient-controlled epidural analgesia (PCEA) with meperidine; group 2 represents epidural morphine 3 mg bolus with placebo PCEA; group 3 represents epidural morphine 3 mg and epidural catheter removed. $P < .05$ group 1 versus groups 2 and 3. (From Roseag OP, Lindsay MP: Epidural opioid analgesia after caesarean section: A comparison of patient-controlled analgesia with meperidine and single bolus injection of morphine. Can J Anaesth 1994; 41:1063–1068.)

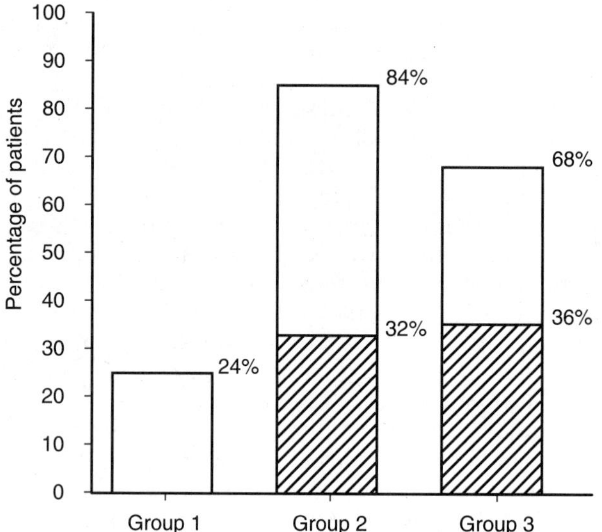

❖ **Figure 13–10** Percentage of patients with pruritus (*cross-hatched bars* represent the percentage requiring treatment). Group 1 represents postcesarean patient-controlled epidural analgesia (PCEA) with meperidine; group 2 represents epidural morphine 3 mg bolus with placebo PCEA; group 3 represents epidural morphine 3 mg and epidural catheter removed. $P < .001$ group 1 versus groups 2 and 3. (From Roseag OP, Lindsay MP: Epidural opioid analgesia after caesarean section: A comparison of patient-controlled analgesia with meperidine and single bolus injection of morphine. Can J Anaesth 1994; 41:1063–1068.)

opioid such as sufentanil is only marginally more effective than morphine PCIA,[66] causes more light-headedness, nausea, and pruritus than fentanyl,[60] and is expensive. Buprenorphine offers no advantages over fentanyl,[51] and the suitability of fentanyl has been challenged.[66] Opioids of intermediate solubility, such as hydromorphone, are effective but also result in pruritus in over two thirds of patients.[52, 53] Diamorphine, apart from very commonly causing mild pruritus, appears suitable but internationally has limited availability and minimal clinical evaluation.[67] The addition of nalbuphine modestly reduces the severity of adverse symptoms but is counterproductive, increasing pain scores.[68] Meperidine has been well investigated and has several attractive features.[58, 59, 65, 70, 71] Its onset of action is rapid (5–10 minutes) and a 20 mg epidural bolus produces similar pain relief to that of the same dose intravenously after 9 minutes.[72] Patient bolus doses of 20 mg during PCEA result in median pain scores during coughing of 20 or less and meperidine consumption of 15 to 17 mg/h.[59] The latter reflects a dose-sparing effect after epidural administration (compared with intravenous) of more than 50%[59, 73] and, for fentanyl, dose sparing of 10% to 30%.[57] The incidence and severity of nausea, dizziness, and pruritus after PCEA meperidine are very low.[59, 70, 71] Three studies comparing PCEA fentanyl with PCEA meperidine after CS have reached similar conclusions, favoring meperidine (Fig. 13–11).[65, 70, 71] Side effects, including pruritus (incidence, 7%)[65] and nausea (less than 10% requiring antiemetic treatment over 48 hours), are reduced,[65, 71] and two crossover studies confirm that meperidine is preferred to fentanyl by patients.[70, 71] Similar findings are reported when opioids are compared for PCEA after abdominal surgery (see Figs. 13–9 and 13–10).[74]

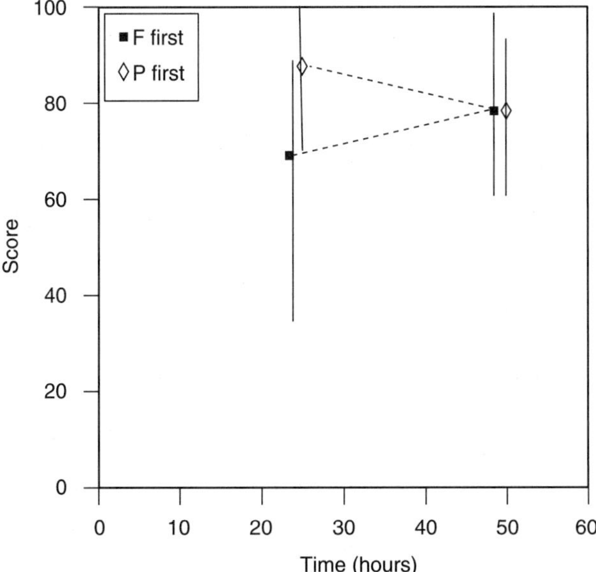

Figure 13–11 Satisfaction scores (median and interquartile range) during postcesarean patient-controlled epidural analgesia (PCEA). *Squares* (F) represent fentanyl for the first 24 hours and meperidine the second 24 hours, and *diamonds* (P) meperidine first and fentanyl second. *P* < .02 for meperidine versus fentanyl in the first 24 hours. (From Goh JL, Evans SF, Pavy TJG: Patient-controlled epidural analgesia following caesarean delivery: a comparison of pethidine and fentanyl. Anaesth Intensive Care 1996; 24:45–50.)

Local Anesthetics and Other Analgesics

There is convincing evidence that the addition of bupivacaine to epidural opioid improves neither analgesia nor satisfaction with post-CS PCEA (Fig. 13–12).[53, 75] Indeed, I believe local anesthetics should be avoided because of complications such as impairment of ambulation, unpleasant numbness, and reports of pressure sores on the heels or coccyx (within 24 hours).[53, 75, 76] A similar recommendation has been made for other surgical populations,[77] although large series without such events have now been reported.[78] Both epinephrine (up to 25 μg/h) and clonidine (up to 30 μg/h) have been used as adjuncts to PCEA opioid and confer a dose-sparing effect of about 15% with sufentanil but do not significantly improve analgesia or reduce sedation. Epinephrine also increases the incidence of pruritus.[51, 79–81]

Choice of Regimen

Although studies conflict, most anesthetists agree that there is usually no advantage in using a background infusion with PCIA and that the safety of the technique may be compromised if this is routine. The limited data available comparing PCEA demand-only with demand plus continuous infusion in the postoperative setting strongly support this opinion. A background infusion does not improve the quality of analgesia obtained with sufentanil, fentanyl, or meperidine, and drug consumption is increased.[53, 71, 80–82] The lockout time when lipophilic opioids are used for PCEA is calculated on the basis of onset of effect and a reasonable maximum hourly or four-hourly dose limit. In most cases 15 to 30 minutes is suitable, although no systematic evaluation has been performed. The optimum dilution volume for PCEA meperidine is about 5 mL, because a 2 mL volume has been shown to delay the onset of analgesia,[83] and in Asian patients (who may have lower dose requirements), the optimal staff-administered intermittent bolus dose is 25 mg.[72] Extensive clinical experience in Australia involves staff administered doses of 50 mg, and although dose-response data are not available for PCEA demand boluses, meperidine 20 mg (4 mL, 5 mg/mL, or 5 mL, 4 mg/mL) is effective and popular.[59, 71]

Maternal Respiratory Depression

Providing established guidelines for the safe use of epidural opioids on postoperative wards are followed,[84] epidural opioid techniques (including epidural morphine, which carries the highest risk of delayed respiratory depression) have an excellent safety record in the obstetric population. Youth, lack of respiratory disease or the sedative effects of general anesthetic or sedative drugs, and pregnancy-induced increases in respiratory

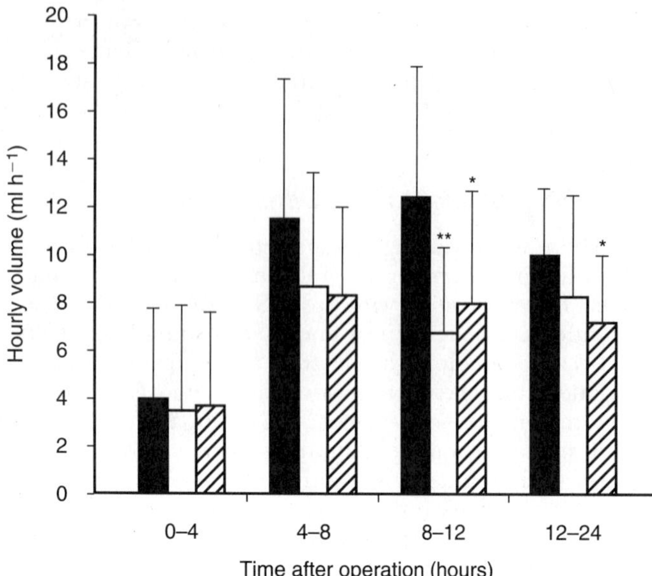

❖ **Figure 13–12** Hourly volumes of solution self-administered during postcesarean patient-controlled epidural analgesia (PCEA) (5 mL bolus and 10 minute lockout). *Solid bars* represent 0.1% bupivacaine; *open bars* represent fentanyl 4 μg/mL; and *hatched bars* represent 0.05% bupivacaine and fentanyl 2 μg/mL. *$P < .05$, **$P < .01$ compared with the solution 0.1% bupivacaine. (From Cooper DW, Ryall DM, McHardy FE, et al: Patient-controlled extradural analgesia with bupivacaine, fentanyl, or a mixture of both, after Caesarean section. Br J Anaesth 1996; 76:613.)

drive may protect pregnant women. Furthermore, PCEA minimizes opioid dose requirements, and there are no reported cases of severe respiratory depression in postpartum women receiving PCEA. There are sporadic case reports of severe depression after epidural fentanyl and sufentanil, and although there are no denominator data, the incidence must be exceptionally low. Whenever opioids are administered by any route, vigilance and preparation for such events must be exercised. Although poorly documented, the use of epidural meperidine (mainly by nurse-administered boluses, but also by PCEA) post-CS has an exceptional safety record involving hundreds of thousands of administrations since the early 1980s in Australia,[59] and a prospective audit of almost 4000 patients who received epidural meperidine after CS also supports its safety.[85] Severe respiratory depression from epidural meperidine is exceptionally unlikely provided a 50 mg bolus dose is not exceeded,[86] and in the rare event of intravenous misplacement of the epidural catheter,[42] PCA boluses up to 25 mg or rates of less than 20 mg/h are unlikely to cause clinical concern. Subarachnoid meperidine has been deliberately used in doses of 50 to 75 mg for spinal anesthesia and doses of 10 to 20 mg for labor analgesia.[87] It appears unlikely that 20 mg, injected into the subarachnoid space accidentally through an epidural catheter that has "migrated" intrathecally, would produce respiratory depression. We have seen two cases of repeated staff-administered subarachnoid boluses of meperidine 50 mg, in which catheter misplacement was eventually detected following patient description of profound lower limb weakness. Neither woman had any sign of sedation or change in respiratory parameters (M. Paech and colleagues, unpublished findings). When the patient is instructed about PCEA, a warning to report any unexpected side effects or events while using it will further improve safety.

Although there are no detailed audit data of postoperative obstetric PCEA, data from general surgical patient reviews indicate that the technique is very safe.[78, 88, 89] Under well-supervised conditions, a series of almost 1800 patients receiving PCEA with bupivacaine and sufentanil had no cases of severe sedation or respiratory depression,[89] and in another series respiratory depression occurred in 0.3% of patients (3 in 1030), only two of whom required naloxone.[78] When PCEA was compared with continuous epidural infusion, better results were obtained with PCEA, despite lower drug utilization and a similar incidence of side effects.[90] After major abdominal surgery, PCEA produced better analgesia and fewer side effects at similar cost to an epidural bolus technique.[91] In comparison with an epidural infusion with nurse-controlled supplements, or to PCEA with a background infusion, demand-bolus-only PCEA patients having abdominal surgery spend less time at low saturation and the severity of desaturation is less.[82]

Safety During Lactation

Although meperidine PCEA post-CS is ideal from a maternal perspective, the potential for effects on the breast-fed neonate due to transfer of meperidine and normeperidine into breast milk has not been investigated. Intravenous meperidine PCIA adversely affects neonatal neurobehavioral scores, including sucking reflexes and alertness, on the third day of life, compared with morphine PCIA, the effect of which is comparable to that in unmedicated control subjects.[92] Both meperidine and its major metabolite normeperidine accumulate in colostrum and breast milk and persist for at least 4 days. Even after doses of intravenous meperidine similar to those used with PCEA, infants are less alert than infants whose mothers received morphine, although bottle-fed infants had similar scores to neonates exposed to meperidine, so the clinical relevance is arguable.[93] The concurrent use of nonsteroidal anti-inflammatory drugs should produce further PCEA dose-sparing, and lower systemic plasma levels (and thus probably breast milk levels and infant exposure) result from equivalent doses epidurally compared with intravenously. Extensive clinical experience suggests that meperidine PCEA does not cause difficulties to breast-fed infants, but the impact of epidural opioids during lactation warrants further investigation.

Conclusion

Post-CS PCEA combines the benefits of PCA and the flexibility of catheterization with excellent pain relief that is superior to that achieved with systemic opioids, equivalent to that achieved with other epidural and, probably, subarachnoid analgesic techniques, and associated with fewer side effects. A demand-only regimen with the inexpensive and widely available opioid meperidine is better than alternative regimens. PCEA allows comfortable and safe maternal-infant interaction in the early postpartum period, allows patient independence, and reduces staff workload in drug preparation and management of side effects. Monitoring policies can be institution-specific and should be based on established guidelines for the postoperative use of epidural opioids on general wards.

Large prospective obstetric series would be helpful to confirm the clinical impression and results from general surgical populations that PCEA is very safe. Comparison with other intraspinal opioid techniques, for example subarachnoid morphine analgesia after single-shot spinal anesthesia, is needed. Further studies addressing cost-effectiveness and examining postoperative outcome, and the effect of epidural drugs during lactation and breast-feeding, would be of interest. In an era in which improvements continue to occur with respect to spinal analgesia and in which cost evaluation is important, these unresolved issues might continue to constrain the more widespread application of PCEA in this population.

PATIENT-CONTROLLED EPIDURAL ANALGESIA FOR MANAGEMENT OF OTHER ACUTE AND CHRONIC OBSTETRIC PAIN

Acute Pain

Severe acute pain in the antenatal period may occur owing to several pathologic conditions, including abdominal problems (pelvic cyst accidents, ischemic degeneration of uterine fibroids, appendicitis, or other pelvic or gastrointestinal tract conditions) and orthopedic problems (severe pelvic diastasis, local or radicular back pain of various types). PCEA may be a very effective approach to postoperative or short- to medium-term pain management and has the advantage of minimizing fetal drug exposure.

Chronic Pain

Epidural analgesia, including PCEA, has a small but important role in the palliative care of cancer patients with intractable pain.[94] Successful pain management is determined by factors such as careful patient selection, to confirm initial response to epidural opioid and adjuvant therapy; the reduction of technical catheter-related complications, especially dislodgment and infection; and reduction of the impact of tachyphylaxis to morphine by the judicious addition of adjuvant analgesics such as clonidine and possibly ketamine and other drugs. Most patients using PCEA will benefit from tunneling of their epidural catheter, implanted injection ports, and ambulatory-style PCA devices.[95]

Management of cancer pain in the pregnant woman is complex and carries the additional concern of drug effects on fetal development and well-being. Potential advantages of a PCEA technique include minimization of fetal opioid exposure and hemodynamic or respiratory effects, especially if the circulatory and respiratory systems are already compromised. An example is a case report describing the effective short-term use of sufentanil PCEA in a pregnant woman who was no longer responding to oral therapy and PCEA for severe pain from lumbosacral plexus compression secondary to a metastatic pelvic mass.[96]

PATIENT-CONTROLLED ANALGESIA PUMPS FOR EPIDURAL ADMINISTRATION

In the past, the lack of suitable pumps for PCEA and the disruption to nursing care and to patients were drawbacks that represented a major deterrent to the use of obstetric (and possibly nonobstetric) PCEA. Parturients were occasionally dissatisfied with PCEA because of the repeated sounding of the alarm in pumps designed for intravenous PCA,[25, 29] and it was noted that satisfaction with PCEA compared with epidural morphine may have been influenced by the pump, because 13% of patients felt the apparatus impeded their mobility.[62] The advent of purpose-designed PCA pumps for epidural use (which permit higher injection pressures and have the facility to provide a large reservoir of solution, but remain compact and lightweight) has been a major advance. Although such features are not essential, some provide the ability to program a variable bolus delivery rate, involving a maximum demand rate per hour or a dose limit in a specified period of time, and to eliminate the alarm because of air entrainment into the line.

When a PCEA service is implemented, either for labor or for postoperative analgesia, the acquisition cost of sophisticated electronic PCA pumps must be considered, but the cost-benefit ratio should be assessed against reduction in drug costs and nursing time, and with respect to patient satisfaction. In addition, several relatively inexpensive, user-friendly, disposable, nonelectronic PCA devices are now commercially available or under development,[97, 98] at least one of which is an acceptable alternative to electronic pumps.[99] Disposable devices have limitations such as lack of flexibility, data recording, alarm functioning, and security, but these are rarely an issue in the obstetric setting, and my experience over several years is very favorable. Further development and availability

❖ Summary

Key Points

- PCEA provides an increased maternal perception of self-control and may therefore improve patient satisfaction. Many studies, however, have shown that the analgesic quality of PCEA is similar to that of continuous epidural infusion.
- According to several studies, PCEA offers potential advantages as compared with continuous infusion or intermittent bolus. These benefits include a lower bupivacaine usage or a lower rate of supplementation and fewer staff management interventions.
- A variety of PCEA infusion regimens have been reported. Current data suggest that the most appropriate PCEA solutions are bupivacaine 0.0625% to 0.125% with opioid. New amide local anesthetics can be substituted for bupivacaine.

Key Reference

Paech MJ: Patient-controlled epidural analgesia in obstetrics. Int J Obstet Anesth 1996; 5:115–125.

Case Stem

A multiparous patient requests an epidural for labor, but she states that during her last delivery she was not satisfied with the epidural because the continuous infusion did not keep her comfortable enough, and that each time that she received a "top-off," she developed a motor block. Would you offer her a PCEA, and, if so, what local anesthetic solution and which settings would you advocate?

of appropriate devices may be crucial to the future of PCEA.

References

1. Scott JS: Obstetric analgesia. Am J Obstet Gynecol 1970; 106:959–978.
2. Evans JM, McCarthy JP, Rosen M, Hogg MIJ: Apparatus for patient-controlled administration of intravenous narcotics during labour. Lancet 1976; 1:17–18.
3. Gambling DR, Yu P, Cole C, et al: A comparative study of patient-controlled epidural analgesia (PCEA) and continuous infusion epidural analgesia (CIEA) during labour. Can J Anaesth 1988; 35:249–254.
4. Slade P, MacPherson SA, Hume A, Maresh M: Expectations, experiences, and satisfaction with labour. Br J Clin Psychol 1993; 32:469–483.
5. Gambling DR, White PF: Role of patient-controlled epidural analgesia in obstetrics. Eur J Obstet Gynecol Reprod Biol 1995; 59:S39–46.
6. Paech MJ: Patient-controlled epidural analgesia in obstetrics. Int J Obstet Anesth 1996; 5:115–125.
7. Eisenach JC: Patient-controlled epidural analgesia during labor, or whose finger do you want on the button? [editorial]. Int J Obstet Anesth 1993; 2:63–64.
8. Bogod D: Opposer: Epidural infusions in labour should be abandoned in favour of patient-controlled epidural analgesia. Int J Obstet Anesth 1996; 5:61–63.
9. Lysak SZ, Eisenach JC, Dobson CE II: Patient-controlled epidural analgesia during labor: A comparison of three solutions with a continuous infusion control. Anesthesiology 1990; 72:44–49.
10. Viscomi C, Eisenach JC: Patient-controlled epidural analgesia during labor. Obstet Gynecol 1991; 77:348–351.
11. Ferrante FM, Lu L, Jamison SB, Datta S: Patient-controlled epidural analgesia: Demand dosing. Anesth Analg 1991; 73:547–542.
12. Purdie J, Reid J, Thorburn J, Asbury AJ: Continuous extradural analgesia: Comparison of midwife top-ups, continuous infusions and patient controlled administration. Br J Anaesth 1992; 68:580–584.
13. Gambling DR, Huber CJ, Berkowitz J, et al: Patient-controlled epidural analgesia in labour: Varying bolus dose and lockout interval. Can J Anaesth 1993; 40:211–217.
14. Fontenot RJ, Price RL, Henry A, et al: Double-blind evaluation of patient-controlled epidural analgesia during labor. Int J Obstet Anesth 1993; 2:73–77.
15. Ferrante FM, Rosinia FA, Gordon C, Datta S: The role of continuous background infusions in patient-controlled epidural analgesia for labor and delivery. Anesth Analg 1994; 79:80–84.
16. Curry PD, Pacsoo C, Heap DG: Patient-controlled epidural analgesia in obstetric anaesthetic practice. Pain 1994; 57:125–128.
17. Ferrante FM, Barber MJ, Segal M, et al: 0.0625% bupivacaine with 0.0002% fentanyl via patient-controlled epidural analgesia for pain of labor and delivery. Clin J Pain 1995; 11:121–126.
18. Gambling DR, McMorland GH, Yu P, Lazlo C: Comparison of patient-controlled epidural analgesia and conventional intermittent "top-up" injections during labor. Anesth Analg 1990; 70:256–261.
19. Kumar AA, Vertommen JD, Van Aken H: Patient-controlled epidural analgesia during labor using 0.125% bupivacaine and sufentanil [abstract]. Anesth Analg 1993; 76:S198.
20. Baudot J, Vertommen JD, Van Aken H: Patient-controlled epidural analgesia vs. intermittent injections during labor using 0.125% bupivacaine and sufentanil [abstract]. Br J Anaesth 1993; 70S:A170.
21. Tan S, Reid J, Thorburn J: Epidural analgesia in labour: Complications of three techniques of insertion. Br J Anaesth 1994; 73:619–623.
22. Paech MJ, Pavy TJG, Sims C, et al: Clinical experience with patient-controlled and staff-administered intermittent bolus epidural analgesia in labour. Anaesth Intensive Care 1995; 23:459–463.
23. Dubost T, Coltat JC, Roulier JP, et al: Maternal satisfaction with patient-controlled extradural analgesia during labour: Results of a 6-month survey (500 questionnaires) [abstract]. Br J Anaesth 1996; 76(2S):A328.
24. Paech MJ: Patient-controlled epidural analgesia during labour: Choice of solution. Int J Obstet Anesth 1993; 2:65–72.
25. Paech MJ: Patient-controlled epidural analgesia in labour: Is a continuous infusion of benefit? Anaesth Intensive Care 1992; 20:15–20.
26. Davin C, Brichant JF, Falieres X, et al: Patient-controlled epidural analgesia during labor: Pure demand dosing or continuous infusion plus demand dosing? [abstract]. Anesthesiology 1994; 81:A1161.
27. Plummer JL, Brownridge P: Epidural analgesia in labour using intermittent doses determined by midwives. Int J Obstet Anesth 1998; 7:88–97.
28. Murphy JD, Henderson K, Bowden MI, et al: Bupivacaine versus bupivacaine plus fentanyl for epidural analgesia: Effect on maternal satisfaction. Br Med J 1991; 302:564–567.
29. Paech MJ: Epidural analgesia in labour: Constant infusion plus patient-controlled boluses. Anaesth Intensive Care 1991; 19:32–39.
30. Writer WD, Stienstra R, Eddleston JM, et al: Neonatal outcome and mode of delivery after epidural analgesia for labour with ropivacaine and bupivacaine: a prospective meta-analysis. Br J Anaesth 1998; 81:713–717.
31. Polley LS, Columb MO, Naughton NN, et al: Relative analgesic potencies of ropivacaine and bupivacaine for epidural

analgesia in labor: implications for therapeutic indexes. Anesthesiology 1999; 90:944–950.
32. Owen MD, D'Angelo R, Gerancher JC, et al: 0.125% ropivacaine is similar to 0.125% bupivacaine for labor analgesia utilizing patient-controlled epidural infusion. Anesth Analg 1998; 86:527–531.
33. Meister G, Owen M, D'Angelo R, Gaver R: Ropivacaine/fentanyl provided equivalent analgesia with less motor block than bupivacaine/fentanyl [abstract]. Anesthesiology 1998; SOAP '98 Supplement:A5.
34. Paech MJ, Pavy TJ, Orlikowski CE, Evans SF: Patient-controlled epidural analgesia in labor: the addition of clonidine to bupivacaine-fentanyl. Reg Anesth Pain Med 2000; 25:34–40.
35. Paech M: Patient-controlled epidural analgesia during labor [letter]. Clin J Pain 1996; 12:79.
36. Tong WN, Ng KF, Sze TS, Tsui SL: Patient controlled epidural analgesia (PCEA) in labour: a comparison of three dose regimens with continuous epidural infusion [abstract]. 11th World Congress of Anaesthesiologists Abstracts, Sydney, Australia, 1996:448; P796.
37. Paech MJ: Patient controlled epidural analgesia for labor [letter]. Anesth Analg 1995; 80:1064.
38. White PF, Gambling DR, Parker RK: Role of continuous background infusion with patient-controlled analgesia [letter]. Anesth Analg 1995; 80:646.
39. Gambling DR: Proposer: Epidural infusions in labour should be abandoned in favour of patient-controlled epidural analgesia. Int J Obstet Anesth 1996; 5:59–61.
40. Al-Mufti R, Morey R, Shennan A, Morgan B: Blood pressure and fetal heart rate changes with patient-controlled combined spinal epidural analgesia while ambulating in labour. Br J Obstet Gynaecol 1997; 104:554–558.
41. Eisenach JC: In reply: Patient-controlled epidural analgesia during labor may be hazardous [letter]. Anesthesiology 1990; 73:790.
42 Bush DJ, Kramer DP: Intravascular migration of an epidural catheter during postoperative patient-controlled epidural analgesia. Anesth Analg 1993; 76:1150–1151.
43. Fan S-Z, Susetio L, Wang Y-P, et al: Low dose of intrathecal hyperbaric bupivacaine combined with epidural lidocaine for cesarean section: A balance block technique. Anesth Analg 1994; 78:474–477.
44. Lam FY: Patient-controlled analgesia by proxy [letter]. Br J Anaesth 1993; 70:113.
45. Lyons G, Columb M, Hawthorne L, Dresner M: Extradural pain relief in labour: Bupivacaine sparing by extradural fentanyl is dose dependent. Br J Anaesth 1997; 78:493–497.
46. Cohen S, Amar D, Pantuck CB, et al: Epidural analgesia for labour and delivery: Fentanyl or sufentanil? Can J Anaesth 1996; 43:341–346.
47. Brix JL, Yoshii WY, Kotelko DM, et al: Effects of cumulative doses of epidural fentanyl in labor on the neuroadaptive capacity of the neonate [abstract]. Anesthesiology 1994; 81:A1165.
48. Mandell G, Adler L, Ramanathan S, Malley B: Maternal and neonatal effects of epidural sufentanil administration for labor analgesia [abstract]. Anesthesiology 1997; 87:A901.
49. Loftus JR, Hill H, Cohen SE: Placental transfer and neonatal effects of epidural sufentanil and fentanyl administered with bupivacaine during labor. Anesthesiology 1995; 83:300–308.
50. Larsson LE, Selander D, Waldenlind L: Neonatal adaptation after Caesarean section: A comparison between ropivacaine and bupivacaine [abstract]. Int Monitor Reg Anesth 1997; X:41.
51. Cohen S, Amar D, Pantuck C, et al: Epidural patient controlled analgesia after cesarean section: Buprenorphine-0.015% bupivacaine with epinephrine versus fentanyl-0.015% bupivacaine with and without epinephrine. Anesth Analg 1992; 74:226–230.
52. Parker RK, White PF: Epidural patient-controlled analgesia: An alternative to intravenous patient-controlled analgesia for pain relief after cesarean delivery. Anesth Analg 1992; 75:245–251.
53. Parker RK, Sawaki Y, White PF: Epidural patient-controlled analgesia: Influence of bupivacaine and hydromorphone basal infusion on pain control after Cesarean delivery. Anesth Analg 1992; 75:740–746.
54. Grass JA, Zuckerman RL, Tsao H, et al: Patient-controlled epidural analgesia results in shorter hospital stay after cesarean section [abstract]. Reg Anesth 1991; 16:S26.
55. Yarnell RW, Polis T, Reid GN, et al: Patient-controlled analgesia with epidural meperidine after elective cesarean section. Reg Anesth 1992; 17:329–333.
56. Cooper DW, Ryall DM, Desira WR: Extradural fentanyl for postoperative analgesia: Predominant spinal or systemic action? Br J Anaesth 1995; 74:184–187.
57. Fragneto R, Moore C, Long S, et al: Comparison of epidural and IV fentanyl PCA after cesarean delivery using epidural 2-chloroprocaine [abstract]. Anesthesiology 1997; 87:A881.
58. Ngan Kee WD, Lam KK, Chen PP, Gin T: Comparison of patient-controlled epidural analgesia with patient-controlled intravenous analgesia using meperidine and fentanyl. Anaesth Intensive Care 1997; 25:126–132.
59. Paech MJ, Moore JS, Evans SF: Meperidine for patient-controlled analgesia after cesarean section. Intravenous versus epidural administration. Anesthesiology 1994; 80:1268–1276.
60. Cohen S, Amar D, Pantuck C, et al: Postcesarean delivery epidural patient-controlled analgesia. Fentanyl or sufentanil? Anesthesiology 1993; 78:486–491.
61. Yu PYH, Gambling DR: A comparative study of patient-controlled epidural fentanyl and single dose epidural morphine for post-Caesarean analgesia. Can J Anaesth 1993; 40:416–420.
62. Roseag OP, Lindsay MP: Epidural opioid analgesia after Caesarean section: A comparison of patient-controlled analgesia with meperidine and single bolus injection of morphine. Can J Anaesth 1994; 41:1063–1068.
63. Harrison DM, Sinatra R, Morgese L, Chung JH: Epidural narcotic and patient-controlled analgesia for post-cesarean section pain relief. Anesthesiology 1988; 68:454–457.
64. Tan PH, Chia YY, Perng JS, et al: Intermittent bolus versus patient-controlled epidural morphine for postoperative analgesia. Acta Anaesthesiol Sinica 1997; 35:149–154.
65. Perez EC, Newman LM, Hopkins EM, Ivankovich AD: Post cesarean delivery patient-assisted analgesia: A comparison of three epidural infusions [abstract]. Anesthesiology 1995; 83:A972.
66. Grass JA, Zuckerman RL, Sakima NT, Harris AP: Patient-controlled analgesia after cesarean delivery. Epidural sufentanil versus intravenous morphine. Reg Anesth 1994; 19:90–97.
67. Chrubasik J, Martin E, Chrubasik S, Friedrich G: Is fentanyl appropriate for postoperative epidural PCA? [letter]. Anesth Analg 1993; 76:1162–1163.
68. Kunst G, Chrubasik S, Black AM, et al: Patient-controlled epidural diamorphine for post-operative pain: Verbal and visual analogue assessments of pain. Eur J Anaesthesiol 1996; 13:117–129.
69. Parker RK, Bottros L, Sawaki Y, White PF: Epidural PCA: Use of hydromorphone versus hydromorphone-nalbuphine after cesarean delivery [abstract]. Anesthesiology 1992; 77:A1014.
70. Goh JL, Evans SF, Pavy TJG: Patient-controlled epidural analgesia following Caesarean delivery: A comparison of pethidine and fentanyl. Anaesth Intensive Care 1996; 24:45–50.
71. Ngan Kee WD, Khaw KS, Ma ML: Patient-controlled epidural analgesia after Caesarean section using meperidine. Can J Anaesth 1997; 44:702–706.
72. Ngan Kee WD, Lam KK, Chen PP, Gin T: Epidural meperidine after cesarean section: A dose response study. Anesthesiology 1996; 85:289–294.
73. Kowbel M, Comfort VK, Lang SA, Yip RW: PCA meperidine analgesia study: PCA intravenous vs. PCA epidural. Anesth Analg 1995; 80:S249.
74. Smith AJ, Haynes TK, Roberts DE, Harmer M: A comparison of opioid solutions for patient-controlled epidural analgesia. Anaesthesia 1996; 51:1013–1017.
75. Cooper DW, Ryall DM, McHardy FE, et al: Patient-controlled extradural analgesia with bupivacaine, fentanyl, or a mixture of both, after Caesarean section. Br J Anaesth 1996; 76:611–615.
76. Smet IGG, Vercauteren MP, De Jongh RF, et al: Pressure sores as a complication of patient-controlled epidural analgesia after cesarean delivery. Reg Anesth 1996; 21:338–341.
77. Etches RC, Gammer T-L, Cornish R: Patient-controlled

epidural analgesia after thoracotomy: A comparison of meperidine with and without bupivacaine. Anesth Analg 1996; 83:81–86.

78. Liu SS, Allen HW, Olsson GL: Patient-controlled epidural analgesia with bupivacaine and fentanyl on hospital wards: Prospective experience with 1,030 surgical patients. Anesthesiology 1998; 88:688–695.
79. Vercauteren MP, Vandeput DM, Meert TF, Adrianesen HA: Patient-controlled epidural analgesia with sufentanil following Caesarean section: The effect of adrenaline and clonidine admixture. Anaesthesia 1994; 49:767–771.
80. Vercauteren MP, Saldien V, Bosschaerts P, Adrianesen HA: Potentiation of sufentanil by clonidine in PCEA with or without basal infusion. Eur J Anaesthesiol 1996; 13:571–576.
81. Vercauteren MP, Coppejans HC, ten Broecke PW, et al: Epidural sufentanil for postoperative patient-controlled analgesia (PCA) with or without background infusion: A double-blind comparison. Anaesth Analg 1995; 80:76–80.
82. Owen H, Kluger MT, Isley AH, et al: The effect of fentanyl administered epidurally by patient-controlled analgesia, continuous infusion, or a combined technique of oxyhaemoglobin saturation after abdominal surgery. Anaesthesia 1993; 48:20–25.
83. Ngan Kee WD, Lam KK, Chen PP, Gin T: Epidural meperidine after cesarean section: The effect of diluent volume. Anesth Analg 1997; 85:380–384.
84. Ready LB, Loper KA, Nessly M, Wild L: Postoperative epidural morphine is safe on surgical wards. Anesthesiology 1991; 75:452–456.
85. Paech MJ, Godkin R, Webster S: Complications of obstetric epidural analgesia and anaesthesia: A prospective analysis of 10 995 cases. Int J Obstet Anesth 1998; 7:5–11.
86. Etches RC, Sandler AN, Daley MD: Respiratory depression and spinal opioids. Can J Anaesth 1989; 36:165–185.
87. Ngan Kee WD: Intrathecal meperidine: Pharmacology and clinical applications. Anaesth Intensive Care 1998; 26:137–146.
88. Steude GM, Hasselbach N, Urbanski B: Complications associated with bupivacaine-fentanyl epidural infusion with PCEA for pain control in postoperative patients [abstract]. Anesth Analg 1995; 80:S473.
89. Brodner G, Pogatzki E, Wempe H, Van Aken H: Patient-controlled postoperative epidural analgesia: Prospective study of 1799 patients. Anaesthetist 1997; 46S:S165–171.
90. Lubenow TR, Tanck EN, Hopkins EM, et al: Comparison of patient-assisted epidural analgesia with continuous-infusion epidural analgesia for postoperative patients. Reg Anesth 1994; 19:206–211.
91. Rockemann MG, Seeling W, Duschek S, et al: Epidural bolus clonidine/morphine versus epidural patient-controlled bupivacaine/sufentanil: Quality of postoperative analgesia and cost-identification analysis. Anesth Analg 1997; 85:864–869.
92. Wittels B, Scott DT, Sinatra RS: Exogenous opioids in human breast milk and acute neonatal neurobehavior: A preliminary study. Anesthesiology 1990; 73:864–869.
93. Wittels B, Glosten B, Faure EAM, et al: Postcesarean analgesia with both epidural morphine and intravenous patient-controlled analgesia: Neurobehavioral outcomes among nursing neonates. Anesth Analg 1997; 85:600–606.
94. Chrubasik J, Chrubasik S, Martin E: Patient-controlled spinal opiate analgesia in terminal cancer. Has its time really arrived? Drugs 1992; 43:799–804.
95. Kwan JW: Use of infusion devices for epidural or intrathecal administration of opioids. Am J Hosp Pharm 1990; 47:S18–23.
96. McGrady EM, Malinow AM, Paly DA, Mokriski BK: Metastatic pain in the parturient: Treatment with patient-controlled epidural sufentanil. Acta Anaesthesiol Scand 1993; 37:594–596.
97. O'Keefe D, O'Herlihy C, Gross Y, Kelly JG: Patient-controlled analgesia using a miniature electrochemically driven infusion pump. Br J Anaesth 1994; 73:843–846.
98. Ngan Kee WD, Lam KK, Twyford CJ, Gin T: Evaluation of a disposable device for patient-controlled epidural analgesia after caesarean section. Anaesth Intensive Care 1996; 24:51–55.
99. Ngan Kee WD, Ma ML, Gin T: Patient-controlled epidural analgesia after caesarean section using a disposable device. Aust N Z J Obstet Gynaecol 1997; 37:304–307.

14

Nonpharmacologic Alternatives for Obstetric Analgesia

❖ JORGE RIQUELME, MD

❖ HECTOR J. LACASSIE, MD

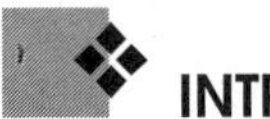

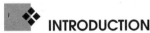

INTRODUCTION

"In sorrow you shall give birth to children" (Genesis 3:16).[1] This sentence condemned the human species to experience pain in labor, ranging from agony to ecstasy.[2] Mankind survived this punishment. Evidence of this is the permanence of humanity on the face of the earth.

The remedy has been the attenuation of pain, which is not easy even in our time. Considering today's approach to health care in which the triad of cost, benefit, and satisfaction of the patient is the primary concern, the pharmacologic attention to pain management should focus on factors significantly associated with high levels of satisfaction. This includes good analgesia as judged by parturients.[3]

Many therapeutic interventions have been tried and tested over the ages. What we currently know as "natural" childbirth is merely the systematization of ancient practices and beliefs, as well as scientific documentation and validation of the benefits of these interventions, in reducing labor pain.

Pain, as defined by the International Association for the Study of Pain is "an unpleasant sensory and emotional experience associated with actual or potential damage or described in terms of such damage."[4] This definition embraces various concepts, especially the subjectivity of the symptom, which is the basis of the nonpharmacologic options in the treatment of labor pain.

Pain and associated responses to noxious stimulation provoked by uterine contractions and other tissue-damaging factors during labor and vaginal delivery are the net effect of highly complex interactions of various neural systems, modulating influences, and psychologic and cultural factors. Through the interaction of the afferent systems and neocortical processes, the parturient receives perceptual and discriminant information that is analyzed and usually activates a series of motivational or cognitive processes. These, in turn, act on the motor system and initiate psychodynamic mechanisms of anxiety and apprehension that produce the complex physiologic, behavioral, and affective responses that characterize acute pain.[5]

A number of different methods of psychologic anesthesia have been used with varying degrees of success. These include psychologic training and support, and sensory stimulation.

PSYCHOLOGIC TRAINING AND SUPPORT

This heading is used to describe the many nonpharmacologic alternatives available today for the amelioration of pain in childbirth. They include childbirth education, hypnosis, and emotional support.

Childbirth Education

Childbirth education originated in Europe in the 1930s and in America in the 1950s as a method to alleviate labor pain. The premise is that labor and birth do not have to be painful if women are informed, relaxed, and well supported, and if they learn self-help measures to deal with this pain. *Natural childbirth,* the first of the nonpharmacologic alternatives for obstetric analgesia, was named by Dick-Read in England in 1933 and was based on the description of the fear-tension-pain vicious cycle. To combat this cycle he proposed education to dispel fear and taught muscular relaxation as well as specific and progressive breathing patterns. In the late 1940s natural childbirth was modified to meet American needs, and the introduction of the father as a "coach" was added.

Fernand Lamaze popularized *psychoprophylaxis* in 1958. It was based on Pavlov's conditioned reflex theory. It recognized the potentially painful stimulus of uterine contractions, but in the Lamaze method women were taught the development of new conditioned reflexes by which pain transmission or perception could be inhibited or blocked.

Both methods have in common (1) a series of lectures or discussions for imparting knowledge and attitudes; (2) training in voluntary muscle relaxation; (3) breathing techniques; (4) human support during labor; (5) the importance of a strong focus of attention; and (6) specific activities during labor contractions to block pain and achieve relaxation.[10]

Scientific Evidence. Numerous studies purporting to compare outcomes in prepared and unprepared women have appeared since the 1950s. If one considers only the best-designed trials which include well-controlled, cohort, and randomized studies, there is a clear tendency to the reduced use of analgesia among the trained patients,[6–8] even in high-risk patients such as low-income parturients.[9] It cannot be assumed, however, that a reduction in the use of pain medication is necessarily associated with reduced pain. No recent systematic trials have reported consistently low levels of pain among prepared women.

Hypnosis

Hypnosis is a temporarily altered state of consciousness in which the individual is in a state of increased suggestibility. Hypnosis has the following characteristics: (1) physical and mental relaxation; (2) increased focus of concentration; (3) an ability to modify perception; and (4) an ability to control normally uncontrollable physiologic responses. It has been used since the early 19th century on a limited scale, with a peak in the 1950s and 1960s. Its mechanism of action is not fully understood. A theoretic explanation, using the gate control theory (see Sensory Stimulation) might be that hypnosis works in at least three ways: (1) by not recognizing painful stimuli or by reinterpreting them as benign sensations, the brain centers are prevented from sending impulses that further "open" the gate to painful stimuli; (2) dampening the perception of pain by enhancing the descending inhibitory pathways from the brain to the dorsal horn; (3) dampening of the autonomic nervous system and the consequent release of stress hormones.

Hypnosis is used in two ways to control pain during labor: self-hypnosis or posthypnotic suggestion. In self-hypnosis the woman enters into a self-induced trance state during labor. Self-hypnosis techniques include visualization, relaxation, distraction, and glove anesthesia. In contrast to self-hypnosis, patients in posthypnotic suggestion are not encouraged to enter into a hypnotic trance but are asked to rely on posthypnotic suggestions of a previously taught sensation called "relaxed, fearless and happily expectant mother."

Scientific Evidence. Only a few randomized controlled trials have been conducted. Among retrospective trials there is a tendency to a reduced use of chemical analgesia and a lower perceived pain in women using hypnosis. In a prospective randomized trial, in patients who took childbirth classes and had self-hypnosis training, there was a reduction in analgesic use among good and moderately hypnotizable subjects. There was no statistical difference in maternal satisfaction with pain relief or duration of labor compared with controls.[10]

In a semi-prospective case-control study a significant reduction was found in analgesic requirements compared with controls as well as a reduction in the length of first-stage labor in both primiparae and multiparae, with a pain reduction in second-stage labor only in multiparae.[11]

Emotional Support

In the past, the labor took place in the woman's home where she was surrounded by female relatives or neighbors who assisted her in the process by advising, encouraging, and reassuring her as well as looking after her needs and giving emotional support during labor. This was so until the birth experience moved to hospitals, where the busy environment and current medical opinion were resistant to the emotional support offered by the hospital staff. It didn't take long to realize that the father was a very important part of the puzzle. So, in the 1960s the father was designated by childbirth educators as the "coach" and was trained for a dominant role. This was a hard task for most fathers and various studies have shown that only a few can fulfill their mate's needs; but they do exert an important role by providing companionship. Furthermore, health care givers have a high workload and cannot be centered on the needs of one parturient at a time. In fact, the mean supportive care provided by maternity nurses in a 4000 birth per year facility in Montreal, Canada, was only 6% of the entire time.[12]

Emotional support can be accomplished by any trained person. There are groups especially designed for this task called *doulas*. The term *doula* is the Greek word for slave or servant. Doulas provide emotional and physical support during pregnancy, labor, birth, and postpartum; give explanations of medical procedures; offer emotional support and advice during pregnancy; train mothers by exercise and physical suggestion to make pregnancy more comfortable; help with preparation of a birth plan; offer massage and other nonpharmacologic pain relief measures; give positioning suggestions during labor and birth; help support the partners so that they can love and encourage the laboring woman; aim to avoid unnecessary interventions; help with breast-feeding preparation and initiation; keep a written record of the birth; and offer many variations on the theme that varies from doula to doula. This is a service that has a monetary cost.

Scientific Evidence. A randomized controlled trial of labor support by doulas showed a reduction in cesarean section and instrumental delivery rates as well as a decrease in epidural analgesia use compared with controls. The authors suggest that it may be due to a calming and soothing effect of the doula on maternal anxiety-stress and also to reduced levels of stress hormones.[13]

SENSORY STIMULATION

As discussed in Chapter 1, labor pain is mediated by somatic fibers that enter the spinal cord via the T10 to L1 nerve roots for the first stage of labor and the S2 to S4 nerve roots in the second and third stages of labor. The pain message received by the brain is modified in numerous ways between the site of the stimulus and the cortex. The gate control theory of Wall and Melzack[14] postulates that the dorsal horn in the spinal cord is the site where impulses converge, some of which are excitatory to noxious impulse transmission and others inhibitory. Depending on the balance of impulses, the conscious perception will be of greater or lesser pain.

While small, thinly myelinated and unmyelinated afferent fibers (A-delta and C fibers, respectively) transmit pain impulses relatively slowly, the opposite is true for the large myelinated A-alpha and A-beta fibers that run adjacent to them, transmitting innocuous stimuli, such as touch and pressure. These fibers activate cells located in the substantia gelatinosa in the dorsal horn, inhibit transmission of noxious impulses, and decrease pain perception at the level of the spinal cord. The faster transmission over these fibers helps to "close" the gate to pain sensations. In addition, descending fibers from centers in the brain stem and cortex to the dorsal horn can modulate the excitability of the cells that transmit pain information.[14] This modulation permits us to define many interventions that have a scientific basis and in which we do not have to deal with the concept of placebo or a distracting maneuver.

A number of accessory stimuli that have been acknowledged as effective in controlling labor pain are

- maternal movement and position changes
- massage and touch
- superficial heat and cold
- hydrotherapy
- acupuncture and acupressure
- transcutaneous electrical nerve stimulation
- the needle effect
- intradermal sterile water blocks
- counterpressure and bilateral hip pressure
- music and audio analgesia

Maternal Movement and Position Changes

Among primitive women the position preferred during labor was either upright or semierect with some inclination.[15] If we analyze animal behavior, their labors are often achieved while in motion, probably as a way to cope with pain.

Today, women are confined to a bed with restriction of movement as a result of intravenous lines, tocodynamometers, and lack of physical space in labor wards. Most women prefer freedom of movement in or out of bed.[16] The intrinsic tendency of laboring women is to seek comfort, so that the preferred positions are sitting, standing, kneeling, leaning forward, and walking. The rationale for these maneuvers is to alter the relationship between gravity, uterine contractions, fetus, and the pelvis as well as to offer distraction and activation of joint receptors as stimuli to compete with pain for recognition at a supraspinal level.

Scientific Evidence. There are no randomized trials assessing this point. Only observational studies have been done to determine the parturients' attitude during labor. They were observed to adopt more than seven different positions, with more frequent variations observed in the late first and second stage than earlier in labor.[16]

Massage and Touch

There are two mechanisms by which massage and touch act to relieve pain:

1. By increasing neural activity in larger myelinated fibers (A-alpha and A-beta) after activating mechanoreceptors in the skin, thus stimulating the central nervous system with innocuous or pleasing stimuli and biasing cortical perceptions away from the awareness of pain. This is the scientific basis involved in the relief of pain in the injured child by the comforting touch of the mother.
2. By enhancing the descending inhibitory pathways from the limbic system in the midbrain (where the motivational-affective component of response to pain originates) as well as by means of a sensation of well-being generated by a soothing touch.

Scientific Evidence. Although this issue has not been studied systematically, there are some benefits reported when comparing a low versus a high degree of physical contact during alternating sets of three contractions during labor. There was an improvement in patients' coping ability and comfort along with drops in systolic blood pressure and pulse rate when the patients had a high degree of physical contact with the nurse.[17]

Superficial Heat and Cold. Labor pain may sometimes be reduced by the application of cold packs or hot compresses to the abdomen, groin, anus, or perineum. Temperature transmission is accomplished by A-delta fibers, just as is pain and touch. Higher brain centers discriminate between peripheral temperature and visceral pain in a counterstimulant fashion that causes stimuli to compete for recognition at the conscious level. There are other physiologic responses that indirectly act as pain relievers, such as reduction of muscle spasms or cramps, changes in circulation to an area, decreased inflammatory response, and relaxation of tiny muscles in the capillaries and hair follicles of the skin.

Scientific Evidence. The therapeutic use of temperature has not been subjected to randomized controlled trials as regards its efficacy. Case reports and personal communications have shown that there is partial relief from labor pain, so it must be considered only as an adjunct therapy.

Hydrotherapy

The benefits of hydrotherapy result from the combination of various mechanisms:

1. Warm water provides muscular relaxation.
2. Immersion buoyancy and hydrostatic pressure result in a feeling of weightlessness and a relief of pressure on the abdomen as well as relaxation of the sacroiliac joint.
3. Superficial thermal and tactile receptors are activated by immersion in water and more so if the water is sprayed (by a shower) or agitated as in the swirling of a whirlpool bath.

The dorsal column receives stimuli from throughout the periphery and the gate to pain is "closed," inhibiting transmission of pain impulses to the cortex.

Scientific Evidence. There are some reports that hydrotherapy provides no objective pain relief. However, it may have a temporal pain-stabilizing effect possibly mediated through the improved ability to relax in between contractions.[18] A recent report showed a reduction in operative delivery rates, a shorter second stage of labor, reduced analgesic requirements, and a lower incidence of perineal trauma in those using hydrotherapy.[19] Others have reported a longer time period from established labor to delivery as well as a higher proportion of women needing oxytocin administration when immersed in warm water.[20] Evidence so far is inconclusive, so further trials are needed.

Acupuncture and Acupressure

These techniques block sensory and emotional components of pain. Expressed in terms of the gate control theory (see earlier in chapter), the higher brain centers transmit strong inhibitory impulses to the dorsal horn, "closing" the gate to pain. A second proposed mechanism is enhanced liberation of endogenous endorphins after stimulation.

Acupuncture consists of the insertion of strategically placed needles of varying size and using different methods of insertion in more than 360 places along the 14 meridians in the body described in ancient oriental lore.[21] It is sometimes combined with electrical current, which augments the pain-relieving effect (electroacupuncture).

Acupressure is the application of pressure or deep massage to the traditional acupuncture points, with thumb, fingertip, fingernail, or palm of hand. Theoretically, it works in the same way as acupuncture by raising local endorphin levels in the treated area or by activating the central biasing mechanism in the brain to inhibit painful stimuli.

Scientific Evidence. There are a few controlled studies on acupuncture and acupressure. The results as to whether they reduce analgesic requirements are contradictory. Lyrenas and coworkers[22] found that pretreatment with acupuncture from the 38th week of gestation until delivery did not reduce the need for analgesics in labor. Furthermore, during labor, all women experienced successively rising pain irrespective of whether they had been treated with acupuncture prior to labor or delivered under local anesthesia. Despite this, 95% of the women stated that they would request acupuncture treatment prior to a future delivery. Abouleish and Depp[23] studied the efficacy of electroacupuncture in 12 parturients and on average it produced 66% analgesia in 7 patients for 139 minutes while patients were in active, progressive labor. No patient was completely free of pain. Patient satisfaction was 75%. This group stated that they would like to have acupuncture in future labors because no drugs were used, they were alert, and they experienced no aftereffects. The authors found acupuncture impractical, time-consuming, and restrictive to the patient, and that it interfered with electronic fetal monitoring.

Transcutaneous Electrical Nerve Stimulation

Transcutaneous electrical nerve stimulation (TENS) is a noninvasive method of pain relief and it has been used in labor to cope with uterine contractions. Two sets of electrodes are set in strategic points, one paravertebrally at the T10 to L1 vertebrae and the second set at the S2 to S4 vertebrae. A low-voltage electric current is transmitted which results in a "buzzing," tingling, or prickling sensation. The patient may vary the intensity, frequency, and patterns of stimulation, so that she can increase, decrease, or pulse the sensations as she wishes.

TENS is thought to work by bombarding large-diameter afferent fibers (A-alpha and A-beta) with innocuous electrical stimuli, thus "closing" the gate to pain and liberating endorphins after low-frequency and high-intensity transcutaneous stimulation.[11]

Scientific Evidence. TENS was reintroduced into medical practice in the early 1970s. Since that time, numerous studies, both controlled and uncontrolled, have suggested its utility for the treatment of pain. Others have found no difference compared with placebo.[24] In a recent systematic review of randomized controlled trials of TENS in pain during labor (which included 712 women), the evidence of reduced pain using TENS in labor was weak, although an analgesic-sparing effect was suggested.[25]

The Needle Effect and Intradermal Sterile Water Blocks

In the 1950s several independent investigators discovered that the insertion of a hypodermic needle through the skin without injecting an anesthetic or injecting only normal saline often produced a dramatic relief of myofascial pain. Later on, it was established that saline injected in a myofascial trigger point was more effective than the injection of mepivacaine for the relief of pain.[26]

Among laboring patients, one third have severe, continuous low back pain and an additional number of parturients feel the pain of contractions primarily in the back, possibly owing to a stretching of sacroiliac joints by the fetal presentation.[27]

The two hypotheses for the mechanism responsible for the needle effect are (1) stimulation of fast-conducting nerve fibers may inhibit the visceral pain of the contractions either at the level of the dorsal column of the spinal cord or the midbrain, as described in the gate control theory; and (2) a possible rise in β-endorphin levels is produced by the painful injection.

Scientific Evidence. In a prospective, double-blind, randomized trial in 272 Danish women in labor complaining of severe low back pain, it was demonstrated that four 0.1-mL intradermal papules in the low back area injected with sterile water resulted in a significantly higher degree of analgesia compared with normal saline, with no adverse effects and with high patient acceptability.[28]

Counterpressure and Bilateral Hip Pressure

This maneuver alleviates low back pain in parturients by applying a steady strong force to a spot on the low back during labor contractions. Bilateral hip pressure involves a steady pressure with both hands applied to the lateral aspects of the hips and directed toward the center. The steady pressure probably relieves strain against the sacroiliac ligaments caused by the fetal presentation.

Scientific Evidence. To date, there are no randomized controlled trials on the subject. Only empiric evidence and testimonials from users as to the benefits are available.[10]

Music and Audio Analgesia

The analgesic properties of music are explained using the gate control theory by which enhancement of descending inhibitory pathways occurs secondary to a variety of factors, for example, distraction, endorphin production,[29] relaxation, and reinforcement of other behaviors such as rhythmic breathing. Both music familiar to the patient as well as white noise (sound consisting of all frequencies), which dampens other incoming stimuli from the environment and from other parts of the body, have been used with varying success.

Scientific Evidence. Both music and white noise, alone or in combination, have been studied for their effectiveness in reducing childbirth pain. Obstetric applications were inspired by its success in controlling dental pain reported during the 1950s. Initial reports were nonrandomized and nonblinded. Their results were nonconclusive in terms of reduction of analgesic requirements, but there was a high degree of acceptability among patients.[30, 31] Other small randomized studies of childbirth pain showed that music or auditory stimulation has the capacity to reduce pain, at least in selected patients.

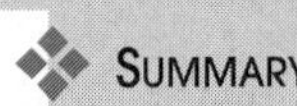

SUMMARY

Key Points

- A number of different psychologically based methods have been used with varying success. Even if they do not provide adequate analgesia, they may often be used as an adjunct to pharmacologic techniques.
- The success rate of nonpharmacologic methods is very poor for the second stage of labor, and other methods, (i.e., regional techniques) should be used.
- TENS, acupuncture, hypnosis, and biofeedback do not appear to decrease the pain associated with labor and delivery.
- Childbirth preparation is associated with increased maternal control and decreased anxiety. It does not, however, decrease the need for pharmacologic intervention.

Key Reference

Melzack R: The myth of painless childbirth. Pain 1984; 19:321–337.

Case Stem

A 24-year-old primiparous patient at 41 weeks' gestation is admitted for induction of labor. Although she is only 1 cm dilated, she is screaming in pain and is requesting pain relief. Her husband and her doula insist that she receive a nonpharmacologic technique. How would you handle this situation and what alternatives can be offered to this patient?

References

1. La Biblia: Ediciones Paulinas, LXXXIV edition. Verbo Divino (editors). Madrid: 1989.
2. Hughes S, DeVore J: Psychologic and alternative techniques for obstetric anesthesia. *In* Shnider S, Levinson G (eds): Anesthesia for Obstetrics, 3rd ed. Baltimore: Williams & Wilkins; 1993:103–111.
3. Geary M, Fanagan M, Boylan P: Maternal satisfaction with management in labour and preference for mode of delivery. J Perinat Med 1997; 25:433–439.
4. International Association for the Study of Pain (Subcommittee on Taxonomy): 1979 Pain Terms: a list with definitions and notes on usage. Pain 1979; 6:249–252.
5. Bonica JJ: Labour pain. *In* Melzak R, Wall PD (eds): Textbook of Pain, 3rd ed. New York: Churchill Livingstone; 1994:615–641.
6. Enkin M, Smith S, Dermer S: An adequately controlled study

of the effectiveness of PPM training. *In* Morris N (ed): Psychosomatic Medicine in Obstetrics and Gynecology. Basel: Karger; 1972.
7. Doering S, Entwisle D: Preparation during pregnancy and ability to cope with labor and delivery. Am J Orthopsychiatry 1975; 45:825–837.
8. Hetherington A: A controlled study of the effect of prepared childbirth classes on obstetric outcome. Birth 1990; 17:86–90.
9. Timm M: Prenatal education evaluation. Nurs Res 1979; 28:338–342.
10. Simkin P: Psychologic and other nonpharmacologic techniques. *In* Bonica JJ, McDonald J (eds): Principles and Practice of Obstetric Analgesia and Anesthesia, 2nd ed. Philadelphia: Williams & Wilkins; 1995;715–746.
11. Jenkins M, Pritchard M: Hypnosis: practical applications and theoretical considerations in normal labour. Br J Obstet Gynaecol 1993; 100:221–226.
12. Gagnon A, Waghorn K, Covell C: A randomized trial of one-to-one nurse support of women in labour. Birth 1997; 24:71–77.
13. Kennell J, Klaus M, McGrath S, et al: Continuous emotional support during labor in a US hospital. JAMA 1991; 265:2197–2201.
14. Melzak R, Wall PD: Pain mechanisms: a new theory. Science 1965; 150:971–979.
15. Engelmann G: Labor Among Primitive Peoples. St Louis: JH Chambers and Co; 1882.
16. Carlson J, Diehl J, Shachtelben-Murray M, et al: Maternal position during parturition in normal labor. Obstet Gynecol 1986; 68:443–447.
17. Saltenis I: Physical Touch and Nursing Support in Labor. Unpublished Master's Thesis, Yale University, 1962.
18. Cammu H, Clasen K, Van Wettere L, et al: 'To bathe or not to bathe' during the first stage of labor. Acta Obstet Gynecol Scand 1994; 73:468–472.
19. Aird I, Luckas M, Buckett W, et al: Effects of intrapartum hydrotherapy on labour-related parameters. Aust N Z J Obstet Gynaecol 1997; 37:137–142.
20. Eriksson M, Mattsson LA, Ladfors L: Early or late bath during the first stage of labour: a randomised study of 200 women. Midwifery 1997; 13:146–148.
21. Kao F: Acupuncture Therapeutics. New Haven; CT: Eastern Press; 1973.
22. Lyrenäs S, Lutsch H, Hetta J, et al: Acupuncture before delivery: effect on pain perception and the need for analgesics. Gynecol Obstet Invest 1990; 29:118–124.
23. Abouleish E, Depp R: Acupuncture in obstetrics. Anesth Analg 1975; 54:83–88.
24. van der Ploeg JM, Vervest HA, Liem AL, et al: Transcutaneous nerve stimulation (TENS) during the first stage of labour: a randomized clinical trial. Pain 1996; 68:75–78.
25. Carroll D, Tramèr M, McQuay H, et al: Transcutaneous electrical nerve stimulation in labour pain: a systematic review. Br J Obstet Gynaecol 1997; 104:169–175.
26. Frost F, Jessen B, Sigaard-Andersen J: A controlled, double-blind comparison of mepivacaine injection versus saline injection for myofascial pain. Lancet 1980; 1:499–501.
27. Melzack R, Schaffelberg D: Low back pain during labor. Am J Obstet Gynecol 1987; 156:901–905.
28. Trolle B, Moller M, Kronborg H, et al: The effect of sterile water blocks on low back labor pain. Am J Obstet Gynecol 1991; 164(5, pt 1):1277–1281.
29. Goldstein A: Thrills in response to music and other stimuli. Physiol Psychol 1980; 8:126–131.
30. Burt R, Korn G: Audio analgesia in obstetrics: "white sound." Am J Obstet Gynecol 1964; 88:361–366.
31. Moore W, Browne J, Hill I: Clinical trial of audio analgesia in childbirth. J Obstet Gynaecol Br Commonw 1965; 72:626–630.

15

Systemic Analgesia for Labor

❖ SHUSEE VISALYAPUTRA, MD

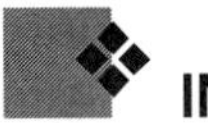

INTRODUCTION

Acute pain management (e.g., labor pain, postoperative pain) can be problematic. Postoperative pain is not necessarily improved by better patient education or communication, probably because of lack of innovative thinking and control, time pressure on the hospital staff, and, sometimes, a subservient attitude of the patient.[1] Analgesic requirements can be influenced by ethnic differences in pain perceptions, the attitudes of patients and health professionals toward pain management, and pharmacologic differences in the response to opioids. People of Asian ethnicity may receive less analgesia because they are more likely to experience, or are less tolerant of, the adverse effects of opioids.[2]

Labor pain, especially during the late first stage and second stage, is usually too strong to respond to systemic analgesics.[3] Although regional anesthesia can provide more pain relief during labor than systemic analgesics, major neuraxial blockade is only possible in the medical centers where anesthesiologists are available 24 hours a day. In many health centers, labor pain relief is still provided using systemic narcotics. A 1981 survey of obstetricians and anesthesiologists showed that only 16% of parturients received an anesthetic for labor other than parenteral medication.[4] A similar survey in 1992 showed that only 37% received analgesia.[5] It is, therefore, important that the physician be familiar with the pharmacology and application of systemic drugs and aware of their effects on the mother and the neonate.

HISTORY

Systemic analgesics for labor have been used since 1847, when Sir James Young Simpson gave ether for pain relief in a parturient with a deformed pelvis. Serturner, a German pharmacologist, isolated codeine and morphine from a crude extract of the poppy seed in 1803. Since then, about 25 alkaloids (such as morphine, codeine, papaverine, and thebaine) have been extracted from the juice of *Papaver somniferum*. The hypodermic needle was introduced by Wood and the hypodermic syringe by Pravaz (in 1853). The combination of opioids and scopolamine to make women amnesic and comfortable during labor ("twilight sleep") was not introduced for 50 years.[6]

In 1915, an antagonist of morphine was discovered and the safety of morphine was then established.[7] Endogenous opioids and opioid receptors were discovered in the mid-1970s, but it was not until 1979 that Wang et al.[8] reported success in the use of intrathecal morphine in patients suffering from cancer pain. The first report was followed by many others using epidural morphine for cancer pain,[9] for postoperative pain,[10] and for labor pain.[11]

Atropine is a product of the plant extract *atropa bella donna* that does not cross the blood-brain barrier. Scopolamine does get into the brain and can cause unconsciousness and hallucinations. Scopolamine, with opioid, was used for obstetrics between 1950 and 1960 to induce analgesia, sedation, and amnesia during labor and delivery.[12]

In 1864, barbiturate and several analogues were synthesized. In 1869, chloral hydrate was introduced and was followed by paraldehyde. In 1960, chlordiazepoxide (Librium) was the first benzodiazepine used as an anxiolytic agent, followed by diazepam, which then became one of the most popular drugs for sedation because of its oral availability and rapid onset. With a short duration of action and lack of venous irritability, midazolam, which was introduced later in 1978, has gained in popularity.

PLACENTAL TRANSFER OF DRUGS

All analgesics and anesthetics can cross the placenta.[13] Drugs injected into the bloodstream of the mother distribute to all internal organs, including the uterus. Eighty percent of uterine blood flow goes to the placenta while 20% goes to the myometrium.[14] Once in the fetal circulation, an aliquot of the drug will travel through the liver and is metabolized there. The remainder is shunted across the ductus venosus into the inferior vena cava. This portion will reach the right atrium, enter the right ventricle, and then go to the pulmonary artery, where 90% is shunted directly across the ductus arteriosus to the lower part of the body. Another 10% is shunted across the foramen ovale and via the right atrium, left atrium, left ventricle, and aorta to the upper part of the body, including the brain, where the drug effect occurs.

Most drugs, including analgesics, cross the placenta by the mechanism called "simple diffusion." Factors that affect diffusion across the placenta are described by the Fick principle.[15]

$$Q/T = \text{the rate of diffusion} = [K\,A\,(C_m - C_t)]/X$$

where

K = diffusion constant of the drug (molecular weight, spatial configuration, degree of ionization, lipid solubility and protein binding)

A = the available area of placenta (approximately 11 m^2)

C_m = the maternal blood concentration

C_t = the fetal blood concentration

X = the thickness of the membrane

The more lipid soluble the drug is, the more freely it can pass through the placental membrane. Once in the fetal system, lipid solubility enables the drug to be taken up by the fetal tissue rapidly. This will lower the blood concentration of the drug. Most drugs are in ionized and non-ionized form, and only the non-ionized form can cross the placenta. The degree of ionization is influenced by the pH of the blood. If the maternal pH is normal (7.4) but the fetal pH is low (7.0), the non-ionized part of the drug that crosses to the fetus becomes ionized and remains in the fetus, potentially causing enhanced effects of the drugs in that acidotic fetus (ion trapping).

OPIOIDS

Pharmacokinetics and Pharmacodynamics

Pharmacokinetics involves absorption, distribution and elimination of the drug. Pharmacodynamics involves the mechanism of action of the drug.

Factors that favor movement of the drug to the sites of action include lower protein binding, lower ionization, and high lipid solubility.

The diffusible fraction (i.e., the unbound, non-ionized portion) is free to leave the vasculature. The rate of movement from plasma to extracellular fluid is dependent on the lipid solubility. The ratio of diffusion potential (diffusion fraction and lipid solubility) of an opioid compared with morphine is known as the lipid diffusion index. The lipid diffusion index of morphine is 1, that of meperidine (pethidine) is 14, and that of fentanyl is 160.

Morphine has the lowest diffusion potential as compared with other common opioids. This results in some delay between intravenous morphine administration and the development of maximal brain concentration or the onset of maximal effects. Morphine is also slow to leave the plasma. Biotransformation and elimination decrease the plasma concentration, causing a further reduction in the rate of diffusion into the central nervous system (CNS). The low lipid solubility is responsible for a slow dynamic interaction between the plasma and the CNS. Diffusion back from CNS to the plasma is also slow.

Biotransformation occurs by enzymatic transformation (conjugation) with microsomal enzymes to produce glucuronide. Glucuronide compounds are excreted into the urine (renal system) and feces (gastrointestinal tract).

The minimal effective analgesic concentration is the minimal plasma level of an opioid that can control pain in a particular patient. Opioid concentration exhibits about a twofold intrasubject variation. Austin[16] found that the minimal effective analgesic concentration of meperidine was 460 ng/mL (range, 270–700) which was an eightfold variation among subjects. Morphine has a minimal effective analgesic concentration of about 16 ng/mL (range, 6–33).[17]

The mechanism of action of opioids is still unclear, owing to a multiplicity of opioid substances that may have more than one action.[18] Also, at different dosages, opioids can act as agonist and antagonist to the receptor. For example, naloxone is a μ agonist at low dose but an antagonist at high dose.[19]

Site of Action

There is still some controversy regarding the site of action of opioids in the CNS. Opioids induce analgesia by acting at the different levels of the central nervous system.[20] Herz and Teschemacher[21] suggested that morphine might activate the descending inhibitory system in the brain stem, which then inhibits transmission of noxious stimuli at the spinal cord level. At the spinal cord level, opioids inhibit substance P in the transmission of nociceptive impulses from the periphery to the CNS. At the level of basal ganglia, opioids activate a serotoninergic descending system that impairs peripheral impulses. At the limbic system, opioid (morphine) was found to reduce the maximal binding capacity with the muscarinic receptors, resulting in a diminution of pain and disappearance of dullness.[22] In the descending antinociceptive system, opioids act at the receptors in the anterior part of the periaqueductal area of the brain stem. If high cerebrospinal fluid (CSF) concentrations of opioids are obtained, activation of opioid receptors in the spinal cord is the major mechanism of analgesia.[23]

Opiate Receptors

An *opiate* is an alkaloid of opium plus semisynthetic derivatives. *Opioids* are synthetics and naturally occurring morphine-like compounds. A *receptor* is a macromolecule located on the cell membrane. Opioids have two different affinities at receptor sites: an affinity toward the binding site and an affinity toward the effector mechanism. An agonist has both affinity toward the binding site and affinity to activate the effector mechanism. An antagonist has only the receptor binding affinity (Table 15–1).[24]

The μ receptor is responsible for supraspinal analgesia, euphoria, respiratory depression, constipation, pruritus, urinary retention, nausea, vomiting, and physical dependence.[25] The δ receptor is responsible for analgesia and potentiation of morphine analgesia.[26] The κ receptor is responsible for spinal analgesia, miosis, and sedation.[27] The ϵ receptor's function is still unknown.[28] The σ receptor is responsible for dysphoria, hallucination, and stimulation of respiration and vasomotor centers. Sigma receptor agonists include ketamine and phencyclidine, which cannot be reversed by naloxone.[29]

Pharmacology

Opioids can control all types of pain in a dose-dependent fashion but are limited in their use by sedation and respiratory depression, which increase with the dose. If the plasma level needed for analgesic effects were distant from the plasma levels producing side effects, this would make for an ideal drug. In reality, the plasma levels producing side effects such as emesis, dizziness, or sedation are quite close to the level of minimal effective analgesic effect. A higher plasma concentration is required to produce respiratory depression. Although the plasma levels for minimal analgesic effect in individual patients are different, we still use "standard" doses for most patients. These standard doses might not reach the minimal effective dose in some patients. Different severities of pain require different minimal analgesic levels of opioid (e.g., severe pain will need a more potent opioid or a higher blood level of the same opioid).

Clinical Effects

The effects on the CNS include analgesia, euphoria, sedation, drowsiness, emesis, dizziness, hypoventilation, miosis, and pruritus.

Euphoria may occur in some patients and an unpleasant dysphoria in others. Dizziness, confusion, sedation, and drowsiness may follow opioid usage and can be ameliorated by a reduction in the dose or by the concomitant use of CNS stimulants such as amphetamine or caffeine or both.[30]

Chronic use of meperidine (pethidine) can produce multifocal myoclonic seizures because of the effects of the active metabolite normeperidine. Normeperidine can produce CNS hyperexcitability and lower the seizure threshold. This cannot be reversed by naloxone but can be suppressed by anticonvulsants.[31]

Esophageal Reflux. Morphine reduces reflux by increasing residual lower esophageal sphincter pressure during transient lower esophageal sphincter relaxation. Penagini and Bianchi[32] found that morphine reduces reflux in patients with reflux disease by decreasing the number of transient lower esophageal sphincter relaxations.

Gastric Emptying Time. One disadvantage of opioid analgesia is the effect of prolonged gastric emptying. When parenteral or epidural opioids are used, gastric emptying is prolonged.[33, 34] This may increase the risk of aspiration if a general anesthetic is administered after the opioid.

Constipation. Opioids can produce uncomfortable side effects such as constipation. This can be used to advantage in patients with diarrhea. Constipation can be a problem during analgesic therapy. Stool softeners and fluids should be given to patients who use opioids for prolonged periods.

Urinary Retention. Opioids can cause urinary retention by relaxing the detrusor muscle (by a local sacral spinal action when given intrathecally).[35]

Biliary Spasm. Radnay et al.[36] studied the effect of equianalgesic doses of fentanyl, morphine, meperi-

Table 15–1 **Characteristics of Opioid Receptors**

System	μ_1	μ_2	δ	κ	σ	ϵ
Central nervous	Analgesia, supraspinal sedation	Analgesia, spinal Euphoria Pruritus Miosis	Analgesia, spinal Pruritus	Sedation, dysphoria, hallucination, delirium, diuresis	Mydriasis	Unknown
Respiratory		Depression		Depression	Stimulation	
Cerebrovascular		Bradycardia			Tachycardia, hypertension, hallucination, delirium	
Gastrointestinal		Inhibits peristalsis Nausea, vomiting				
Urinary		Urinary retention				

dine, and pentazocine on common bile duct pressure and found that these opioids increased biliary pressure by up to 99%, 61%, 53%, and 15%, respectively.

Nausea and Vomiting. Ambulatory patients suffer more emesis because opioids potentiate vestibular stimulation.

Pruritus. The mechanism by which opioids cause pruritus is not well understood but is possibly central and μ receptor-mediated.[37] Pruritus can be reversed by nalbuphine, which is a κ agonist and μ antagonist. Naloxone and nalbuphine were studied in the prophylaxis of pruritus in post-cesarean section patients who received epidural morphine. Both naloxone and nalbuphine provided good relief of pruritus. However, there was evidence of shortening of the duration of analgesia in patients receiving naloxone and some reversal of analgesia in patients receiving nalbuphine.[38]

Tolerance. Tolerance or a decreased analgesic effect of opioids is faster when continuous intravenous (IV) infusion rather than patient-controlled analgesia (PCA) is used.[39] The earliest sign of tolerance is a patient's complaint that the duration or the degree of analgesic effect has decreased. Cross-tolerance can also occur but is usually incomplete. Switching to other opioids often results in adequate pain relief.

Physical Dependence. This is a neuroadaptive response to the pharmacologic effects of opioids. Opioids inhibit adenylate cyclase, which in turn is compensated for by increasing cAMP. Abrupt withdrawal of opioids may cause the development of abstinence syndrome, which consists of yawning, lacrimation, sneezing, agitation, tremor, insomnia, tachycardia, and other signs of hyperactivity of the sympathetic nervous system. Hagopian et al.[40] found that treatment with higher doses of methadone during pregnancy could improve gestational age but was associated with increased risk of more severe neonatal withdrawal symptoms.

Psychologic Dependence. Fear of addiction is one factor that leads to inadequate use of opioids in patients with severe pain. Psychologic dependence is a rare occurrence in medical use.[41]

Respiratory Depression. By acting through the μ receptor, opioids depress the responsiveness of the medullary respiratory center to carbon dioxide tension. Opioids depress both respiratory rate and tidal volume. Respiratory depression is usually preceded by sedation and followed by apnea. It can be treated with naloxone 0.1 to 0.4 mg IV. Caution is necessary, since, on rare occasion, naloxone can produce pulmonary edema.[42]

Circulation. Opioids, especially morphine, can cause peripheral vasodilatation by releasing histamine. The bradycardia is caused by stimulation of the vagus nerve at the level of the dorsal nucleus of the vagus in the medulla, which results in orthostatic hypotension. Patients treated with parenteral opioids should not ambulate, because hypotension may cause nausea, vomiting, vertigo, or loss of consciousness. In patients with hypotensive problems such as acute or chronic blood loss, the use of opioids for pain relief should be achieved using intravenous titration at small doses. Pregnant patients should be in the lateral position to prevent aortocaval compression. Even a therapeutic dose of opioid can cause bradycardia and a decrease in cardiac output, if given by rapid intravenous injection.

Effects on Labor

If systemic opioid is given in the latent phase of labor, it may slow cervical dilation and prolong labor, but when given during the active phase of labor, it should not have these effects and may even enhance labor by decreasing pain and catecholamine release.

Effects on the Neonate

Opioids can cause acidemia at birth. Other causes include breech presentation, administration of oxytocin, and cord entanglement.[43] Because of their lipid solubility and low molecular weight, all opioids can easily cross the placenta by diffusion and can cause neurobehavioral changes or neonatal respiratory depression because the blood-brain barrier is not well developed in the newborn. Use of parenteral opioids during labor often results in decreased beat-to-beat variability in the fetal heart rate (FHR), which does not reflect fetal oxygenation or acid-base status. Although there may be no obvious signs of neonatal depression, there may be a change in neurobehavioral scores for several days after parenteral administration of an opioid[44] (Fig. 15–1).

Opioids have more depressant effects in the neonate than in the adult. This is caused by a direct effect on the respiratory center of the fetus after opioids are given to the mother.[45] Epidural opioids (doses as high as morphine 3 mg, fentanyl 75 μg, sufentanil 50 μg, buprenorphine 0.2 mg, or oxymorphone 1 mg) given to the mother before delivery have no depressant effects on the neonate.[46] Depression is more prevalent in the premature baby and is potentiated by hypoxemia, hypercarbia, anesthetics, hypotension, prolonged labor, or trauma during delivery and can persist for a few days. More than one factor may be at play at the same time. Wittels et al.[47] found that nursing infants exposed to morphine were more alert and oriented than those exposed to meperidine. Another study confirmed the neonatal depressant effects of meperidine and suggested that the course of behavioral maturation during certain periods of infancy is influenced by meperidine administration at birth.[48]

Route of Application

Oral route. Oral morphine can be used for chronic pain at a dose of up to 120 mg daily with low risk of addiction.[49]

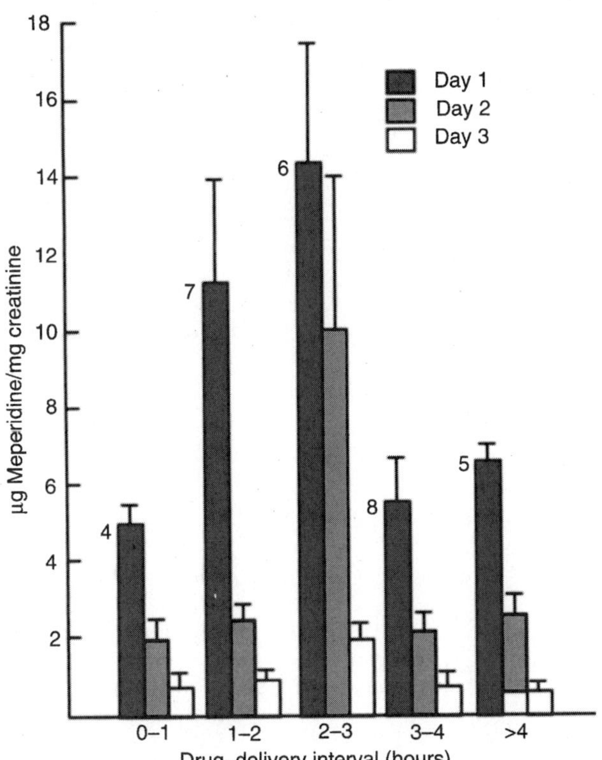

❖ **Figure 15–1** Following maternal administration of meperidine (50 mg IV) during labor, meperidine excretion was measured in the neonate's urine for the first 3 days. The relationship between the drug-delivery interval and the urinary excretion of meperidine by the neonate is shown. For each bar, the mean, standard error, and number of infants are given. Infants whose mothers received meperidine 1 to 2 and 2 to 3 hours prior to delivery excreted more meperidine. (From Kuhnert BR, Kuhnert PM, Tu ASL, et al: Meperidine and normeperidine levels following meperidine administration during labor. II. Fetus and neonate. Am J Obstet Gynecol 1979; 133:909.)

Intermittent Subcutaneous, Intramuscular, or Intravascular Injection. Owing to its ease of administration, intramuscular injection is still occasionally used for pain relief during labor. Many factors influence the plasma level after intramuscular injection (e.g., site of injection). Injection into the deltoid muscle, which is a better perfused muscle, will result in better absorption than injection into a less perfused muscle such as the gluteus muscle.

Following intramuscular injection, there are some variations in time to onset, duration, and intensity of pain relief. Intravascular injection has the advantage of rapid onset, albeit with a shorter duration of action.

Patient-Controlled Analgesia. PCA has been widely used for postoperative pain relief. It is claimed to have many beneficial effects (e.g., better pain relief with lower dosage, less maternal respiratory depression, less placental transfer, less requirement for antiemetics, and higher patient satisfaction). PCA in labor has its limitation in that it cannot "cover" the severe pain of the late first stage or the second stage of labor.[50] However, PCA is a reasonable alternative method for pain relief during labor in which neuraxial anesthesia is not available or is contraindicated. Although PCA may have an advantage in improved maternal satisfaction, the dose was not reduced and the analgesia was not improved when compared with intermittent injection in one study.[51] Ngan Kee et al.[52] compared patient-controlled epidural analgesia (PCEA) with patient-controlled intravenous analgesia (PCIA) using meperidine or fentanyl in patients after cesarean section and found that PCEA has advantages over PCIA. Wittels et al.[47] studied the neurobehavioral outcomes among neonates of nursing parturients after cesarean delivery. PCIA with meperidine was associated with more neonatal neurobehavioral depression than PCEA with morphine. They found that nursing infants exposed to morphine were more alert and oriented to animate human cues than those exposed to meperidine.[47]

Intraspinal Injection of Opioids. Traditionally, continuous epidural analgesia with local anesthetics has been used as the reference standard for providing analgesia during labor. Intrathecal opioids represent a safe and effective alternative that provides significant, rapid relief of pain during the first stage of labor. The drugs most often used for intrathecal administration include sufentanil, fentanyl, meperidine, and morphine. Use of intrathecal narcotics does not significantly affect the natural progression of labor, and no adverse fetal outcomes have been reported.[53] Intraspinal fentanyl 15–25 μg plus morphine 0.25 mg has a similar analgesic effect and duration of analgesia as intraspinal sufentanil 5–10 μg plus morphine 0.25 mg during labor.[54]

Combined Spinal-Epidural Injection of Opioids. Although intraspinal analgesia from opioids may not provide absolute pain relief during advanced labor,[55, 56] when used during the first stage of labor it will result in satisfactory pain relief. A combination of fentanyl or sufentanil with bupivacaine will provide excellent analgesia even in the second stage of labor. These drugs are discussed in detail in Chapters 7 and 11. The combination of opioids with low concentrations of local anesthetics can be used epidurally (e.g., 50 μg of fentanyl with 8 to 12 mL of 0.065 to 0.125% bupivacaine as an initial dose and followed by continuous infusion of 0.0625 to 0.125% bupivacaine with 1 to 2 μg/mL of fentanyl at 10 to 12 mL/hr). At these dilutions, the motor function is retained and can be used for the "walking epidural" technique.[57]

Opioids in Labor. Owing to their ease of use, in many parts of the world systemic opioids are still the most widely used medication for labor analgesia, even though they can provide only partial pain relief and cause maternal side effects such as nausea, vomiting, drowsiness, dysphoria, hypoventilation, delayed gastric emptying, and neonatal respiratory depression.

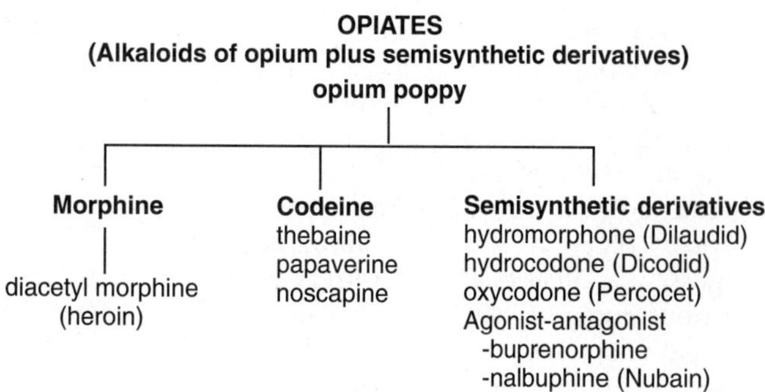

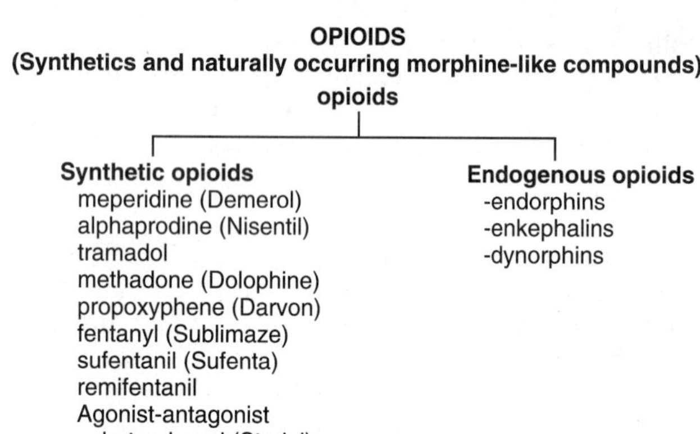

Figure 15–2 Narcotic analgesics.

AGONIST OPIOIDS (Fig. 15–2)

Morphine

In the past, morphine was used with scopolamine to provide "twilight sleep" during labor and delivery. It provided good pain relief but produced heavy sedation and neonatal depression. The onset was 3 to 5 minutes after IV administration and 20 to 40 minutes after intramuscular (IM) injection. Peak effect was 20 minutes after IV and 1 to 2 hours after IM injection. The effect lasted 1.5 to 2 hours after IV and 2.5 to 4 hours after IM injection (Table 15–2).[58]

Morphine is metabolized by the liver to the major metabolites morphine-3-glucuronide (M3G) and morphine-6-glucuronide (M6G). M6G has been shown to be relatively more selective for μ receptors than for δ and κ receptors, whereas M3G does not appear to compete for opioid receptors. M3G exhibits no analge-

Table 15–2 Opioid Analgesics Used for Labor Analgesia

Drugs	Dose (mg)	Peak (hr)	Duration (hr)	Precaution
Morphine	10 (IM)	1–2	2.5–4	Impaired ventilation
	2.5 (IV)	0.3	1.5–2	Asthma, liver failure, ↑ intracranial pressure
Meperidine, pethidine (Demerol)	50–75 (IM)	0.5–1	3–4	Accumulation of normeperidine can cause seizures; severe adverse reaction with monoamine oxidase inhibitors
	25–50 (IV)		2–3	
Fentanyl (Sublimaze)	50–100 μg (IM)		1–2	Cumulative effect of large dose
	25–50 μg (IV)		0.5–1	
Pentazocine (Talwin)	40–60 (IM)	0.5–1		May cause psychotomimetic effects
	20–40 (IV)			
Butorphanol (Stadol)	2 (IM)	0.5–1	4–6	Psychotomimetic effects, maternal sedation
	1 (IV)		3–4	
Nalbuphine (Nubain)	20 (IM)	0.5–1	4–6	Psychotomimetic effects
	10 (IV)		3–4	

sic effect after IV or intrathecal administration and may be responsible for the hyperalgesia/allodynia and myoclonus seen after high-dose morphine treatment.[59]

Although systemic use of morphine in labor is usually best avoided because of depressant effects on the newborn,[51] use via the epidural route (3 to 5 mg) or spinal route (0.2 to 0.4 mg) during the early phase of the first stage of labor produces satisfactory analgesia. In the later phase of labor, local anesthetics are usually necessary.[54] Because of the risk of respiratory depression, which may occur more than 12 hours following administration, neuraxial morphine is not commonly used to provide labor analgesia.

Effects on Labor. The depressant effect of morphine on human uterine activity has been studied.[60] In an animal study, Kowalski et al.[61] found that the decrease in uterine contractions after morphine is primarily due to an inhibition of oxytocin release. There was no evidence of a direct tocolytic effect of morphine on the uterus. Lindow et al.[62] found that maternal oxytocin secretion was inhibited by exogenous opiates (IV morphine, 5 mg) in the first stage of labor. An effect of opiate antagonism (naloxone) to oxytocin secretion was not demonstrated. These studies support the contention that morphine inhibits uterine contraction.

Effects on the Newborn. Surveys of drug use in pregnancy demonstrate that a significant proportion of human fetuses are exposed to prescription and nonprescription drugs antenatally or during labor.[63] Gerdin et al. reported the large plasma clearance, shorter elimination half-life, and higher M3G-to-morphine ratio in pregnant women compared with nonpregnant women. They observed no neonatal depression as judged by Apgar scores. Rapid elimination of morphine in the mother can decrease the period of intrauterine exposure of the fetus. The use of parenteral morphine for analgesia should be reconsidered and needs re-evaluation.[64]

Codeine

Although less commonly used during labor, codeine is, on a worldwide basis, the most commonly used opioid. Its advantages include high oral efficacy and low physical dependence. Tolerance can develop. The disadvantage is that it has an inferior analgesic effect. The antinociceptive and immunosuppressive effects of codeine and codeine 6-glucuronide were determined in rats after intracerebroventricular administration. Additionally, codeine 6-glucuronide showed significantly fewer immunosuppressive effects than codeine in vitro and may have clinical benefit in the treatment of pain in the immunocompromised patient.[65]

Tramadol

Tramadol is a synthetic analogue of codeine that binds to μ-opiate receptors and inhibits norepinephrine (noradrenalin) and serotonin (5HT) reuptake. It is rapidly and extensively absorbed after oral doses and is metabolized in the liver. Analgesia begins within 1 hour and starts to peak in 2 hours. In patients with moderate postoperative pain, IV or IM tramadol is roughly equal in efficacy to meperidine or morphine. For acute severe pain, tramadol is less effective than morphine. For labor pain, IM tramadol works as well as meperidine and is less likely to cause neonatal respiratory depression. Common adverse effects of tramadol include dizziness, nausea, dry mouth, and sedation.[66] The abuse potential seems to be low.[67]

MORPHINE DERIVATIVES (SEMISYNTHETIC)

Dihydromorphine, Hydromorphone (Dilaudid)

Hydromorphone 1.5 mg has an analgesic effect equipotent to 10 mg of morphine. It is easily absorbed by the gastrointestinal tract after oral or rectal administration and starts producing an analgesic effect within 30 minutes. It is associated with fewer side effects than morphine. A comparison of morphine and hydromorphone showed that both drugs provide adequate analgesia with no difference in side effect profile. Hydromorphone appears to result in improved mood and may be a suitable alternative to morphine.[68] Hydromorphone hydrochloride is approximately five times as potent as morphine sulfate on a milligram basis. After intravenous bolus doses of hydromorphone (10, 20, 40 μg/kg body weight), the onset of analgesia was rapid (within 5 minutes) and the maximal analgesic effect was seen between 10 and 20 minutes after the demonstrated peak plasma hydromorphone concentration.[69] Parker et al.[70] used the combination of hydromorphone (Dilaudid) 0.075 mg/mL and nalbuphine (Nubain) 0.04 mg/mL via PCEA with a 3 mL bolus dose, 2 mL on demand, and a 30-minute lockout interval. They found a lower incidence of nausea and urinary retention compared with hydromorphone alone, without an increased opioid analgesic requirement.[70]

Diacetyl Morphine (Heroin)

Heroin has faster onset but shorter duration of action than morphine. It is easily absorbed through nasal, oral, and gastrointestinal tissue and is rapidly metabolized by the liver enzymes to yield 6-monoacetyl morphine and morphine before entering the CNS. There is no advantage of heroin over morphine in equipotent doses.[71]

Oxycodone

Oxycodone is a semisynthetic codeine with equipotency to morphine. The pharmacokinetics of oxycodone have been determined after single-dose administration by the intravenous route (4.6–7.3 mg), oral route (tablets 9.1 mg and syrup 9.1 mg), and rectal route (30 mg).[72] Its use in a combination with aspirin (Percodan) or acetaminophen (Percocet) is effective for moderate postoperative pain.

SYNTHETIC COMPOUNDS RESEMBLING MORPHINE

Meperidine, Pethidine (Demerol)

Meperidine, a combined μ- and κ-receptor agonist, in 50-, 75-, and 100-mg dosages has equianalgesic effect to 6, 8, and 10 mg of morphine, but with shorter duration of action (2–3 hrs) and less depressant effect on respiration of the newborn.[73] Meperidine is a widely prescribed opioid analgesic used in a variety of clinical situations. The parent compound has CNS depressant effects. However, the sole active metabolite, normeperidine, is a CNS excitatory agent and has the ability to cause seizures. If the drug is used in large doses at frequent dosing intervals, seizures may occur.[31]

Small doses (15–25 mg) can control the shivering that is associated with labor and delivery, especially following epidural or spinal analgesia. The anti-shivering efficacy of meperidine results from a reduction in the shivering temperature rather than from thermoregulatory inhibition. This pattern of thermoregulatory impairment differs from those produced by alfentanil, clonidine, propofol, and the volatile anesthetics, all of which are comparable at reducing the vasoconstriction and increasing shivering thresholds.[74] Meperidine also slightly increases the threshold for sweating and reduces the thresholds for vasoconstriction. The special anti-shivering action of meperidine appears to result, at least in part, from its κ-receptor activity.[75]

Meperidine has been used to treat labor pain for more than 50 years. It is the most widely used parenteral opioid for labor analgesia. Recently, Olofson et al.[3] used intravenous morphine (up to 0.15 mg/kg body weight) or meperidine (up to 1.5 mg/kg body weight) for labor pain. They found that, even though very high pain scores were seen in each group as assessed by a visual analogue scale, the parturients were all significantly sedated and several fell asleep but were awakened by pain during contractions. They concluded that labor pain cannot be eliminated by systemically administered morphine or meperidine.

Onset of analgesia is within 5 minutes after IV administration and within 45 minutes after IM injection of meperidine. Its half-life is 2.5 to 3 hours in the mother but 18 to 23 hours in the neonate.[76, 77] It is metabolized in the liver to normeperidine, meperidic acid, and normeperidic acid. Normeperidine, which is the active metabolite and a potent respiratory depressant, crosses the placenta and has a half-life of 60 hours in the neonate.[78, 79] PCA meperidine produced better patient satisfaction than IV meperidine.[80] There were no differences in analgesia and maternal side effects compared with IV meperidine, and neonatal behavioral scores were comparable.[81]

Effects on the Mother. Rapid IV injection of meperidine can cause vasodilatation, tachycardia, and histamine release and can depress the myocardium and vasomotor center. Meperidine differs from other μ-agonists in that it produces a direct positive chronotropic effect. This probably results from the structural similarity of meperidine and atropine. It may also result from a central stimulatory effect of meperidine and normeperidine.[82] Meperidine is contraindicated in patients using monoamine oxidase inhibitors such as phenelzine (Nardil) and tranylcypromine (Parnate).

Two forms of the monoamine oxidase inhibitor–meperidine interaction exist. One is the excitatory form characterized by agitation, rigidity, hyperpyrexia, convulsions, hemodynamic instability, and coma. It is thought to be related to the blockade of neuronal uptake of serotonin by meperidine. The second or "depressive" type manifests as respiratory depression, hypotension, and coma and is due to the inhibition of microsomal enzymes by monoamine oxidase inhibitors, resulting in meperidine accumulation.[83]

Opioids are traditionally avoided during sphincter of Oddi manometry because of indirect evidence suggesting that these agents cause spasm of the sphincter of Oddi. The basal sphincter pressures of the biliary sphincter, pancreatic sphincter, and the combined sphincter group were not significantly altered by meperidine.[84]

Effect on Labor. It is still controversial whether meperidine depresses, has no effect on, or increases uterine contractility.[60, 85, 86] This is dependent, in part, on the time of the administration of meperidine. If given during the latent phase, it can delay contraction of the uterus; if given during active phase or in the hypertonic uterus, it has no effect or may even enhance the progress of labor. Epidural analgesia (0.125% bupivacaine with 2 μg/mL of fentanyl) produces better pain relief than PCIA meperidine (10 mg every 10 minutes) with the same cesarean section rate.[87] A previous study, however, suggested a two- to threefold increase in cesarean section rate when epidural analgesia was compared to parenteral meperidine.[88]

Effect on the Newborn. Meperidine readily crosses the placenta by passive diffusion. Like other opioids meperidine can decrease FHR variability. This occurs 25 minutes after IV injection and 40 minutes after IM injection.[89] Residual depressant effects, as demonstrated by decreased oxygen saturation, persist for several hours after delivery.[90] Nissen et al.[91] found that IM injection of meperidine 100 mg given under routine conditions may have unfavorable effects on infants' developing breast-feeding behavior if the drug-to-delivery interval is short (1.1–5.3 hours).

The optimal time for delivery after maternal administration of meperidine is within the first hour or more than 4 hours after a single IV dose. This is because maximal fetal uptake of normeperidine (an active metabolite) occurs 2 to 3 hours after maternal administration.[92] Normeperidine concentration increases as meperidine plasma level decreases. It is more slowly excreted than meperidine and may cause neurobehavioral changes for 3 to 5 days in the newborn. Meperidine, even in low doses (25–100 mg), can affect the performance as judged by the Brazelton Neonatal Behavioral Assessment Scale. The score is dependent on drug-to-delivery interval and levels of normeperidine. The greater the drug-to-delivery interval, the higher the fetal levels of normeperidine.[93]

Kuhnert and colleagues found that multiple doses of meperidine resulted in greater accumulation of both meperidine and normeperidine in fetal tissue.[94, 95] The amount of meperidine excreted into breast milk is small and does not warrant interruption of breast-feeding (the same applies to methohexital and diazepam).[96]

Alphaprodine (Nisentil)

Alphaprodine was initially popular in obstetrics because of its rapid onset (2–3 minutes after IV injection and 5–15 minutes after subcutaneous injection) and reasonable (60–90 minutes) duration of action. Although it provided good analgesia, its use in obstetrics was limited because it produced profound respiratory depression to both mother and neonate.[97] Alphaprodine in doses of 30, 40, or 50 mg has the equipotency of 6, 8, or 10 mg of morphine. Murakawa et al.[98] reported that IV alphaprodine 40 mg has an umbilical-to-maternal vein ratio of 0.52 and no adverse effects on the neonatal Apgar scores, neonatal acid-base status, or neurologic and adaptive capacity scores. There were also no differences between meperidine and alphaprodine on the length of labor.[99] One study, however, reported that alphaprodine decreased uterine contraction in 50% of patients receiving it.[100]

Effects on infants are similar to those seen with other opioids. Adams[101] found that newborns in the no-medication group had visual stimuli fixation for much longer periods than did infants in the alphaprodine group. This implied that babies of medicated and unmedicated mothers differ in the manner in which they respond to visual stimuli.[102] Alphaprodine is believed to affect the fetal cardioregulatory center in such a manner as to cause a sinusoidal FHR pattern, but it seems to cause no increase in perinatal morbidity or mortality when given in nontoxic doses.[103] The pattern may, however, alarm obstetricians and cause them to perform an emergency cesarean section for presumed fetal jeopardy. Matthews[104] found that even small doses of alphaprodine, when administered 1 to 3 hours prior to delivery, can delay effective feeding by several hours or, in some cases, days.[104]

Fentanyl (Sublimaze)

Fentanyl is a highly lipid soluble, highly protein bound, synthetic opioid with no active metabolites. It is 100 times as potent as morphine. It is a phenylpiperidine related, lipophilic agent of rapid onset and short duration of action. With larger doses, fentanyl does not behave as a short-acting drug. Craft et al.,[105] in an animal study, found that fentanyl in a dose less than 100 μg had no cardiovascular effects and did not alter uterine blood flow or maternal or fetal acid-base status. An intravenous dose of fentanyl 50 μg during early active labor was associated with temporary depressant effects on fetal biophysical parameters (decreased FHR and beat-to-beat variability and decreased body and breathing movement) without apparent harm being observed at delivery as assessed by Apgar score and umbilical artery pH.[106] Rayburn et al.[107] used fentanyl in the doses of 50 to 600 μg during labor and found that it provided transient analgesic effect and lasted about 30 minutes, with decreased FHR variability but no differences in Apgar scores, respiratory rate, or neurobehavioral scores of the newborn. They also compared the effects of giving fentanyl 50 to 100 μg hourly with meperidine 25 to 50 mg every 2 to 3 hours during labor and found that both drugs gave ineffective pain relief, although fentanyl caused fewer side effects and less neonatal depression.[108] Rayburn et al.[109] also compared PCA fentanyl (10 μg bolus, 10 μg continuous with 12-minute lockout) with intermittent injection (50-μg bolus, 50–199 μg hourly) for labor analgesia and found no differences in pain relief. Fentanyl was ineffective during late labor and had some maternal and neonatal side effects. Fentanyl PCA was used in a thrombocytopenic patient in high doses (1025 μg/12 hours) during labor with good analgesia except during the late second stage. It caused only minimal sedation, side effects, or neonatal depression (Apgars were 9 and 9 at 1 and 5 minutes).[110]

Sufentanil

Sufentanil, a lipophilic opioid, is sometimes administered parenterally to provide analgesia for labor and cesarean section, but it may cause neonatal depression. Sufentanil crosses the placenta by passive diffusion and accumulates in placental tissue, which in turn acts as a drug depot, slowing the initial transfer. Placental transfer is influenced by maternal plasma protein levels, but not by albumin. Fetal acidosis increases placental transfer. Owing to its low initial umbilical vein concentration, sufentanil may be the opioid of choice when delivery is to occur within 45 minutes.[111] Herman et al.[112] studied intrathecal sufentanil 2.5 to 15 μg in six groups of parturients using 2.5, 5, 7.5, 10, 12.5, and 15 μg and found that there was a trend toward increasing analgesic duration with increasing sufentanil dose. The maternal side effect profile did not differ among groups. FHR did not appreciably change for any group or individual studied. Assisted delivery and cesarean section rates were similar for all groups.[112] To prove that the analgesic effects of highly lipid-soluble opioids are not similar when these agents are administered either epidurally or intravenously in parturients, Camann et al.[113] studied this and found that sufentanil 10 μg intrathecally provides rapid and effective analgesia of 1 to 2 hours' duration during labor, whereas epidural and IV use of this dose of sufentanil did not provide evidence of satisfactory analgesia.[113]

Alfentanil

Alfentanil has more rapid analgesic onset and time to peak effect as well as the shortest distribution and elimination half-lives as compared with fentanyl and sufentanil. The volume of distribution and total body clearance of alfentanil are also smaller when compared with those of fentanyl and sufentanil.[114] Hill et al.[115] found that 266 μg/hr of alfentanil or 400 μg/hr of diamorphine added to 0.375% epidural bupivacaine could prolong duration of analgesia during labor, and that perineal analgesia was better as compared with the control group. When combined with low-dose bupivacaine (0.125%), epidurally administered alfentanil was not more effective than when it was administered IV for postoperative pain management. The spinal mechanism of action for alfentanil could, therefore, not be demonstrated.[116]

Remifentanil

Remifentanil is an esterase-metabolized opioid with a rapid clearance. Compared with alfentanil, the high clearance of remifentanil, combined with its small steady-state distribution volume, results in a rapid decline in body concentration after termination of an infusion. With the exception of remifentanil's nearly 20-times greater potency than alfentanil (30-times if alfentanil partioning between whole blood and plasma is considered), the drugs are pharmacodynamically similar.[117] Remifentanil, a new μ-opioid agonist with an extremely short duration of action, is metabolized by circulating and tissue esterase; therefore, its clearance should be relatively unaffected by changes in hepatic or renal function.[118] Its brevity of action ensures not only a rapid resolution of adverse effects but also a rapid offset of analgesic effect. Therefore, appropriate postoperative analgesia, when necessary, should be established before discontinuation of a remifentanil infusion.[119] Possible disadvantages of the drug include (1) the need to mix the lyophilized drug with a diluent, (2) the requirement of administration as a continuous infusion, (3) risk of rapid loss of analgesic and anesthetic effects if the infusion is interrupted accidentally, and (4) difficulty in judging the dose of another, longer-lasting opioid that will be required to control postoperative pain without producing excessive ventilatory depression.[120] A smooth transition must be made from remifentanil total IV anesthesia to either epidural analgesia or PCIA with morphine for postoperative analgesia by titration in the recovery room.

Methadone (Dolophine)

Methadone is a synthetic opioid with more potency but less dependence potential, less euphoria, and less sedation than morphine. Another advantage is its good absorption through the gastrointestinal tract and longer duration of action.[121] The usual dosage in cancer patients varies from 5 to 10 mg every 6 hours to 20 to 30 mg orally every 4 hours.

Propoxyphene (Darvon)

Propoxyphene 90 to 120 mg has the same analgesic effects as 60 mg of codeine. Its popularity is due to decreased dependence potential, but this is offset by its being a less effective analgesic and its being more expensive than codeine. Propoxyphene overdose can cause widening of the QRS complex on the electrocardiogram. If this uncommon complication occurs, it can be reversed by sodium bicarbonate.[122]

AGONIST-ANTAGONIST DERIVATIVES

Buprenorphine (Buprenex)

Buprenorphine, the semisynthetic of thebaine, is 20 to 30 times more potent than morphine. It has a good absorption through the oral mucosa, so the sublingual tablet is widely used and has an onset time of 45 to 60 minutes and a duration of approximately 8 hours.[123] Its common side effects include sedation and nausea.

Roy and Basu[124] used buprenorphine hydrochloride 6 μg/kg body weight sublingually during the first stage of labor and showed that the analgesic action started 30 minutes after administration of drug, increased gradually, and reached its peak level 3 hours after administration of the drug. There was no cardiorespiratory depression, no nausea or vomiting, and no change in FHR or Apgar scores of neonates. Mild withdrawal syndrome was reported on the second day of neonatal life in those who received buprenorphine through the milk of a heroin-addicted mother treated with buprenorphine 4 mg/day. Buprenorphine might be a good alternative to methadone in the treatment of pregnant heroin addicts to prevent marked withdrawal syndromes in newborns.[125]

Low doses of buprenorphine antagonized morphine analgesia, whereas high doses of buprenorphine administered with morphine elicited increasing analgesia in a dose-dependent manner. These findings suggest that buprenorphine produced analgesia through an interaction with κ_3 receptors and to a lesser extent with κ_1. It is also a partial μ-receptor agonist.[126]

Butorphanol (Stadol)

Butorphanol is similar to pentazocine. It is five times as potent as morphine and 40 times as potent as meperidine and has fewer side effects (such as nausea and vomiting) but produces excessive sedation. It is metabolized by the liver and is primarily excreted by the kidney. Some is eliminated by the biliary system.[127] Butorphanol in an equianalgesic low dose (such as 2 mg) produces the same degree of respiratory depression as morphine 10 mg or meperidine 70 mg, but butorphanol 4 mg produces less respiratory depression than morphine 20 mg or meperidine 140 mg.[128] Intravenous butorphanol 1 to 2 mg was compared with 40 to 80 mg of meperidine for labor analgesia in a double-blind study by Hodgkinson et al.[129] They found similar analgesic effects with fewer maternal side effects in the butorphanol group. Quilligan et al.[130] reported better analgesia in the butorphanol group with no difference in Apgar scores as compared with the meperidine group. A larger transnasal butophanol dose (2 mg) caused an impaired psychomotor performance for up to 2 hours, but a smaller dose (1 mg) had no psychomotor-impairing effects. These results suggest that patients should use caution when using the 1 mg dose of transnasal butorphanol and should curtail certain activities if they are administered the 2 mg dose of transnasal butorphanol for analgesia.

Wahab et al.[131] found that maternal acidemia and fetal acidosis were most marked with pentazocine, moderate with nalbuphine, and minimal with butorphanol. Butorphanol therapy during labor, however, is strongly associated with the appearance of a sinusoidal FHR pattern, which can be alarming. There were no short-term maternal or neonatal adverse sequelae. In the absence of other FHR signs suggestive of fetal distress, the presence of sinusoidal FHR pattern after butorphanol administration does not indicate fetal hypoxia.[132]

Epidural butorphanol 1 mg may be effective for the treatment of postepidural shivering.[133] Atkinson et al.[134] compared the use of 50 to 100 μg of fentanyl with 1 to 2 mg of butorphanol hourly during labor and found greater improvement in pain relief after the first dose of butorphanol than after fentanyl, with fewer patient requests for more medication or epidural analgesia.

Nalbuphine (Nubain)

Nalbuphine is a κ and σ agonist and a moderate μ antagonist. It is about 0.7 to 0.8 times as potent as morphine. In equipotent doses, it has the same degree of respiratory depression as morphine, but there seems to be no further depression after 30 mg of nalbuphine (ceiling effect). Side effects include euphoria, dysphoria, psychomimetic reaction, and also sedation. Nalbuphine tends to produce "irritability" at higher doses. At a dose of 10 to 20 mg, nalbuphine has an onset of action of 2 to 3 minutes after the IV injection and of about 15 minutes after IM injection with a duration of action of 3 to 6 hours. Wilson et al.[135] compared IM nalbuphine 20 mg with meperidine 100 mg and found no differences in analgesic effects. Nalbuphine caused less nausea and vomiting but a higher degree of sedation and dizziness. The mean maternal-to-umbilical drug ratio was higher with nalbuphine (0.78) as compared with meperidine (0.61), and the neonatal neurobehavioral scores were lower at 2 and 4 hours in the nalbuphine group. There were no demonstrable differences at 24 hours. Frank et al.[136] compared PCA nalbuphine (3 mg IV bolus with 10-minute lockout) and PCA meperidine (15 mg IV bolus with 10-minute lockout) and found that nalbuphine produced better analgesia with a similar pattern of maternal and neonatal side effects. Podlas and Breland[137] compared PCA nalbuphine (1 mg IV bolus with 6–10-minute lockout) with intermittent IV injection of 10 to 20 mg every 4 to 6 hours with similar results in analgesia and maternal and neonatal effects. More patients, however, preferred PCA over intermittent injection. Nalbuphine is more effective than diphenhydramine in relieving pruritus caused by intrathecal morphine, and the cost differences are small.[138]

Pentazocine (Talwin, Fortral)

Pentazocine is an agonist–weak antagonist opioid and at 30 to 60 mg is equipotent to morphine 10 mg. The peak analgesic level occurs 10 minutes after IV injection and 15 to 60 minutes after IM injection.[139] The ceiling effects occur at the doses of 40 to 60 mg. Neonatal respiratory depression from pentazocine 40 to 45 mg is similar to the depression from 100 mg of meperidine, but repeated doses of pentazocine do not increase neonatal respiratory depression, as is seen when repeated doses of meperidine are given.[140]

Pentazocine was introduced on the erroneous assumption that it has no dependence potential. It has the same side effects as other opioids, such as respiratory depression, somnolence, nausea, and unpleasant hallucinations. Psychomimetic effects such as dysphoria or the fear of impending death, which usually occurs after the larger doses of pentazocine, may also occur in some patients following a standard dose. These side effects have limited its use in obstetrics.[141] Discontinuation after prolonged use can cause an even worse abstinence syndrome than seen with other opioids.[142] The use of an agonist-antagonist following a pure agonist may induce reversal of the analgesic effects.

For labor pain, Refstad and Lindbaek[143] compared 45 mg of pentazocine with 100 mg of meperidine and found that labor pain relief was similar but that repeated injection of meperidine was associated with greater neonatal depression.

OPIOID ANTAGONISTS

Naloxone (Narcan)

Naloxone, the (*N*-allyl) derivative of oxymorphone, can be used to reverse respiratory depression and other side effects of neuraxial opioids such as pruritus, urinary retention, nausea, and vomiting without significantly decreasing analgesic effect.

Because of its rather short duration of action, it might not reverse the depression caused by the long-acting opioids for the whole duration, so that either repeated administration or IV infusion of 5 μg/kg/hr may be necessary.

Rapid IV injection may cause nausea and vomiting. Tachycardia, hypertension, and pulmonary edema were reported following the use of naloxone due to a sudden increase in sympathetic nervous system activity.[42, 144] A few patients (0.4–3%) suffered severe adverse effects (asystole, generalized convulsions, pulmonary edema, and violent behavior) within 10 minutes of naloxone administration. These serious complications are unacceptable and could, theoretically, be reduced by artificial respiration with a bag valve device (hyperventilation), as well as by administering naloxone slowly in small, incremental, and divided doses.[145]

It is not a good practice to give naloxone in the mother just before delivery to prevent respiratory depression in the newborn. This practice will reverse analgesia in the mother with uncertain or incomplete reversal of depressant effects in the neonate. Naloxone should be given directly to the newborn, if necessary. Naloxone may precipitate a withdrawal reaction in the newborn of the opioid-dependent mother.

The newly recommended dose (0.1 mg/kg) in newborns is higher than the previous one but may secure increased effectiveness.[146] If there is no response after repeated doses, the depression may not be due to opioid effect.[147]

Naltrexone is similar to naloxone in that it is a μ antagonist. Naltrexone is active when given orally, and its effect is sustained for 24 hours.

Cholecystokinin

Cholecystokinin is an octapeptide, secreted by the duodenum, that can increase the contractility of the gallbladder and relax the sphincter of Oddi. It can antagonize the analgesic effect of opioids; that is, it is an endogenous opioid antagonist. Cholecystokinin and its receptors are also widely distributed in the CNS and contribute to the regulation of anxiety, analgesia, and dopamine-mediated behavior.[148]

The cholecystokinin antagonist, proglumide, has been shown to have analgesic effects in animals.[149] Schafer et al.[150] found that cholecystokinin can inhibit peripheral opioid analgesia in inflamed tissue.

BARBITURATES

The use of barbiturates, such as secobarbital (Seconal), pentobarbital (Nembutal), amobarbital (Amytal), and cyclobarbital, as sedatives has diminished, especially since the benzodiazepine group has been introduced (Table 15–3). Since they have no analgesic effect (or may even cause hyperalgesia if given in the presence of pain), they should be used only in the very early phases of labor in parturients with mild pain to relieve anxiety.[151] Pregnant women who take barbiturates during the third trimester can give birth to addicted infants who undergo an extended withdrawal syndrome. In the presence of severe pain, administration of barbiturates may cause immense difficulty in management of the uncooperative patient. The most commonly used barbiturates for this purpose are pentobarbital (Nembutal) 100 to 200 mg orally or intramuscularly and secobarbital (Seconal) 100 mg orally or intramuscularly.

As their primary effect is sedation, barbiturates can provide good sleep in a patient in the very early phases of labor. Although small therapeutic doses of barbiturates cause minimal effects in mothers, the larger dose can depress respiration and cardiovascular parameters. Barbiturates in therapeutic doses can improve uterine activity in anxious patients but, in high doses, they can indirectly depress uterine activity. All barbiturates are lipid soluble and readily cross the placenta. Although barbiturates do not have significant neurobehavioral effects in the mature infant,[152] they may delay the rate of recovery from birth asphyxia.[153] The signs of overdosage of barbiturate in the newborn include somnolence, sluggish reflexes, flaccidity, bradycardia, and hypothermia.[154]

Benzodiazepines

Benzodiazepines activate supraspinal γ-aminobutyric acid-A receptors, resulting in antagonism of opioid analgesia. Gear et al.[155] found that the benzodiazepine antagonist flumazenil enhances morphine analgesia and decreases side effects as well as the requirement for analgesic medication. Drugs in this group, such as diazepam (Valium), lorazepam (Ativan), and midazolam (Versed) can be used as a sedative, anxiolytic, anticonvulsant, or muscle relaxant. They also produce amnesia.

Diazepam

Diazepam readily crosses the placenta, with an elimination half-life of 24 to 48 hours and a half-life of 51 to 120 hours for its main metabolite, *N*-desmethyldiazepam.[156] There is evidence from a previous study that first-trimester exposure to benzodiazepines (diazepam, chlordiazepoxide) in utero has resulted in the birth of some infants with facial clefts, cardiac malformations, and other multiple malformations.[157] In a further study involving first trimester use of benzodiazepines, the majority of infants were normal at birth and had normal postnatal development.[158]

Late third trimester use and exposure during labor seem to be associated with greater risks to the

Table 15–3 NONOPIOID SEDATIVES FOR LABOR ANALGESIA

CLASS OF DRUG	NAME	DOSE/ROUTE	ONSET (min)	DURATION
Anticholinergics	Scopolamine	0–0.6 IM/IV	15–60	90–120 min
Antihistamines	Hydroxyzine	50 mg IM	30	2–4 h
	Diphenhydramine	25–50 mg IV	1–15	1–3 h
Barbiturates	Pentobarbital	100–200 mg PO	15–60	1–4 h
		150–200 mg IM	10–25	15 min
	Secobarbital	100–200 mg PO	15–30	1–4 h
		100 mg IM/IV	2–10	15 min
Benzodiazepines	Diazepam	2–10 mg IV	5	1–2 h
	Lorazepam	1–2 mg IV	15–20	4–6 h
	Midazolam	1–5 mg IV	3–5	1–2 h
Dissociative Drugs	Ketamine	10–20 mg IV in doses up to 1 mg/kg	1	5–10 min
Phenothiazines	Promethazine	25 mg IV 50 mg IM	15–20	4 h

fetus and neonate. Some infants exposed at this time exhibit either the "floppy infant syndrome" or marked neonatal withdrawal symptoms. Symptoms vary from mild sedation, hypotonia, and reluctance to suck to apneic spells, cyanosis, and impaired metabolic responses to cold stress. This correlates well with the pharmacokinetics and placental transfer of the benzodiazepines and their disposition in the neonate. However, there seemed to be no significant increase in the incidence of neonatal jaundice and kernicterus in term infants, as previously reported.[158] Kanjilal et al.[159] studied 25 neonates of eclamptic mothers receiving diazepam and found that the effect of low-dose diazepam was minimal apart from a lowering of rectal temperature, which lasts for a period of 12 hours. High doses (>30 mg) of diazepam or prolonged duration of diazepam therapy in mothers caused significant depression of the newborn, and the effects lasted for a period of 36 to 48 hours. As the clinical condition of the newborn is not related to the diazepam concentration in cord blood, cord blood estimation is not helpful in the assessment of clinical effects of the drug in the newborn. The tissue storage of the drug in the newborn appears to be responsible for the clinical effects.[159] Smaller doses of diazepam (2.5–10 mg) did not alter the Apgar scores and could affect newborn muscle tone at 4 hours but not at 24 hours.[160]

Lorazepam (Ativan)

Lorazepam has a half-life of 12 hours, and its primary metabolite is an inactive glucoronide. Lorazepam 2 mg given before meperidine 100 mg provided better analgesia with no significant respiratory depression and no differences in neonatal behavioral scores, as compared with the group without lorazepam. Recall of labor was less in the lorazepam group.[161]

Midazolam (Versed)

Midazolam is a water-soluble drug that causes no pain on intramuscular or intravenous injection. It has a more rapid onset and shorter duration of action than diazepam.[162] When administered before cesarean section, it readily crosses the placenta, with an umbilical-to-maternal vein ratio of approximately 0.65 and a neonatal elimination half-life of 6.3 hours.[163]

Higher doses given for induction of general anesthesia produced higher incidences of respiratory depression, decreased muscle tone, and decreased body temperature in the newborn, as compared with the group using thiopental.[164] Since it is a potent amnesic that might reduce maternal recall of labor and delivery, its use should be avoided in mothers who want to appreciate and participate in their labor and delivery.[165]

Midazolam is metabolized by the cytochrome P450 enzyme system to several metabolites, including an active metabolite, α-hydroxymidazolam. Cytochrome P450 inhibitors such as cimetidine can profoundly reduce the metabolism of midazolam. Midazolam has a half-life of approximately 1 hour, but this half-life may be prolonged in patients with renal or hepatic dysfunction. Hiccups, cough, nausea, and vomiting are the most commonly reported adverse effects. Many of the adverse effects associated with midazolam can be reversed rapidly by the administration of flumazenil, a competitive benzodiazepine-receptor antagonist.[166] Midazolam neither potentiates nor decreases the analgesia produced by fentanyl.[167]

Scopolamine

Scopolamine, or hyoscine, has been used in the past in obstetrics together with other analgesic drugs to produce "twilight sleep," even though it also causes delirium, agitation, and excitement, which make the mother difficult to control. It can cross the maternal blood-brain barrier and placenta but usually does not cause neonatal depression. It increases the FHR but decreases the beat-to-beat variability without changes in Apgar scores.[168] Its use in the form of a transdermal patch 1.5 mg with oral promethazine 10 mg can reduce the incidence of postoperative nausea and vomiting following intrathecal morphine.[169]

PHENOTHIAZINE DERIVATIVES

Promethazine (Phenergan) and propiomazine (Largon) produce less hypotension than chlorpromazine (Thorazine) or promazine (Sparine) and prochlorperazine. Their α-adrenergic blocking effects may cause maternal hypotension, and consequently they are rarely used in obstetric practice.

Promethazine (Phenergan)

Promethazine is the most commonly used phenothiazine in obstetrics. Promethazine in a dose of 25 to 50 mg can be used together with meperidine to prevent emesis, but the potentiation of analgesic effects of opioids is still in doubt.[170] It is a mild respiratory stimulant and may counteract the respiratory depressant effects of meperidine. Promethazine minimally affects autonomic cardiovascular mechanisms and appears in the fetal blood within 1 to 2 minutes after IV injection in the mother and reaches equilibrium within 15 minutes.[171]

Propiomazine (Largon)

Propiomazine has short onset and duration as compared with promethazine. It has a mild respiratory depressant effect, which is additive to the respiratory depression of opioids. Ullery and Bair[172] found that propiomazine and promethazine can produce sedative effects in the mother and can cause an additive effect to meperidine analgesia.

Hydroxyzine (Atarax, Vistaril, Marax)

In a dose of 50 to 75 mg, hydroxyzine can be used to treat anxiety and also to prevent nausea and vomiting because of its antiemetic action. Owing to venous irritation and possible thrombophlebitis, its use via the intravenous route is not recommended. Intramuscular injection is also painful and may cause tissue necrosis.[173] Use of hydroxyzine or its metabolite, cetirizine, during pregnancy was not associated with increased teratogenic risk,[174] and the use of hydroxyzine in labor is not associated with neonatal respiratory depression.[175] It is suitable as a premedicant in the anxious mother scheduled to have elective cesarean section. It can also prevent pruritus caused by epidural or intrathecal opioids.[176] Since very high doses can cause malformations in pregnant rats, its use during early pregnancy is not recommended.[177]

Ketamine

Ketamine can produce dissociative anesthesia (functional electrical physiologic dissociation between the limbic system and the thalamocortical pathways)[178] characterized by catalepsy and nystagmus with intact corneal and light reflexes. As a phencyclidine derivative, the mechanism of action is possibly mediated by its interaction with phencyclidine receptors, which are found predominantly in the limbic and corticothalamic area.

Ketamine is an *N*-methyl D-aspartate (NMDA) receptor antagonist. These receptors are located on the postsynaptic membrane in the dorsal horn of the spinal cord.[179] There is now considerable evidence that NMDA antagonism is a central mechanism that contributes to the amnesic, analgesic, anesthetic, and psychotomimetic as well as neuroprotective actions of ketamine.[180] Antagonists of this receptor-channel complex have the potential to not totally abolish pain, but to prevent or block hyperalgesic states induced by tissue damage, inflammation, nerve damage, and ischemia. Aanonsen and Wilcox[181] reported that the intrathecal administration of excitatory amino acids in mice caused hyperalgesia to noxious stimuli, and ketamine could decrease this hyperalgesia response.[182]

In subanesthetic dosage, ketamine produces intense analgesia. Its main disadvantage is its potential for cardiovascular stimulation and emergence reactions. Ketamine in low dose (0.2–0.5 mg/kg) IV injection produces nondepressed neonates and has few effects on the mothers. Ketamine in a dose of 25 to 50 mg can be used to supplement incomplete neural blockade from epidural anesthesia for labor and delivery.

In a dose of 1 to 2 mg/kg, it can be used as the induction agent for cesarean section or for instrumental delivery. Its use in preeclamptic patients should be avoided because it stimulates the sympathetic nervous system and may exacerbate hypertension. It is beneficial as an induction agent in hypovolemic or asthmatic patients. It should be remembered that ketamine at a dose low enough to avoid dysphoric reactions (0.1 mg/kg bolus and 0.5 mg/kg/hr) did not have any bronchodilatory effect.[183] High doses of ketamine ($\geq$ 2 mg/kg) can cause psychotomimetic effects. Midazolam 2 to 4 mg IV can decrease the emergence reaction or hallucination associated with high-dose ketamine. Yang et al.[184] found that intrathecal ketamine enhances the analgesic effect of intrathecal morphine in patients with terminal cancer pain. Neonatal behavioral scores were better in the group using ketamine than in the group using thiopental.[185] Ketamine may be used in subanesthetic doses (0.5–1 mg/kg or 10 mg IV every 2–5 minutes up to 1 mg/kg in 30 minutes) during the late second stage of labor or just before delivery to supplement inadequate regional anesthesia or pudendal nerve block for instrumental vaginal delivery. Larger doses ($\geq$ 2 mg/kg) can increase uterine tone and may be associated with a low Apgar score or abnormally increased neonatal muscle tone.[186]

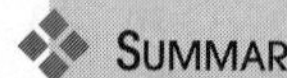

Summary

Key Points

- All parenterally administered opioids cross the placenta and can cause decreased beat-to-beat variability of the fetal heart rate tracing and can have a negative impact on neurobehavioral scores.
- Large doses of meperidine administered at short intervals can precipitate convulsions, owing to normeperidine, its active metabolite. Both meperidine and normeperidine easily cross the placenta and can cause neonatal respiratory and neurobehavioral depression.
- Agonist-antagonist drugs, including pentazocine, butorphanol, and nalbuphine, produce less respiratory depression than agonists. They do, however, have side effects, including sedation, dizziness, and psychotomimetic effects.

Key Reference

Reisine T, Pasternak G: Opioid analgesics and antagonists. In Hardman JG, Gilman AG, Limbird LE (eds.): Goodman and Gilman's The Pharmacological Basis of Therapeutics, 9th ed. New York: McGraw-Hill; 1996:521–554.

Case Stem

A primiparous patient in early labor is complaining of severe pain and requests labor analgesia. She has a platelet count of 48,000, and, on hearing the risks associated with the administration of neuraxial analgesia in the parturient with thrombocytopenia, she requests systemic opioids. How would you manage this patient's labor analgesia?

Metoclopramide

Although metoclopramide is usually used to treat nausea and vomiting and to decrease gastric emptying time before surgery, it was demonstrated to have an analgesic effect when used during labor.[187] It also reduced the requirement for nitrous oxide during labor when metoclopramide was used with meperidine as compared with meperidine alone.[188] It decreases the duration of labor and pain scores and reduces the need for morphine as compared with placebo in patients scheduled to have termination of pregnancy with prostaglandin.[189] However, Danzer et al.[190] found that metoclopramide decreased intraoperative nausea but did not supplement the analgesic effects in patients undergoing elective cesarean delivery.

NONSTEROIDAL ANTI-INFLAMMATORY DRUGS

Nonsteroidal anti-inflammatory drugs are prostaglandin synthetase inhibitors which can depress uterine contraction and cross the placenta to cause closure of the fetal ductus arteriosus. Walker et al.[191] used 10 mg IM ketorolac in labor and found that the cord blood level was 10 to 20% of the concentration in maternal blood. A dose of 10 mg of ketorolac produces higher pain scores than 50 to 100 mg meperidine. Both drugs were ineffective in producing effective pain relief in labor. Patients in the ketorolac group were less sedated and their neonates had higher 1-minute Apgar scores. There was no difference in the duration of labor.[192]

References

1. Boer C, Treebus AN, Zurmond WW, et al: Compliance in administration of prescribed analgesics. Anaesthesia 1997; 52:1177–1181.
2. Lee A, Gin T, Oh TE: Opioid requirements and responses in Asians. Anaesth Intensive Care 1997; 25:665–670.
3. Olofsson C, Ekblom A, Ekman Ordeberg G, et al: Lack of analgesic effect of systemically administered morphine or pethidine on labour pain. Br J Obstet Gynaecol 1996; 103:968–972.
4. Gibbs CP, Krischer J, Peckham BM, et al: Obstetric anesthesia: A national survey. Anesthesiology 1986; 65:298–306.
5. Hawkins JL, Gibbs CP, Orleans M, et al: Obstetric anesthesia workforce survey: 1992 versus 1981. Anesthesiology 1997; 87:135–143.
6. Safer DJ, Allen RP: The central effects of scopolamine in man. Biol Psychiatry 1971; 3:347–355.
7. Eckenhoff JE, Hoffman GL, Dripps RK: N-Allyl-normorphine: An antagonist to the opiates. Anesthesiology 1952; 13:242–251.
8. Wang JK, Nauss LA, Thomas JE: Pain relief by intrathecally applied morphine in man. Anesthesiology 1979; 50:149–151.
9. Cousins MJ, Mather LE, Blynn CJ, et al: Selective spinal analgesia. Lancet 1979; 1:1141–1142.
10. Bromage PR, Camporesi E, Chestnut D: Epidural narcotics for postoperative analgesia. Anesth Analg 1980; 59:473–480.
11. Scott PV, Bowen FE, Cartwright P, et al: Intrathecal morphine as sole analgesic during labour. Br Med J 1980; 281:351–355.
12. Eger EI II: Atropine, scopolamine and related compounds. Anesthesiology 1962; 23:365–383.
13. Dilts PV: Placental transfer. Clin Obstet Gynecol 1981; 24:555–559.
14. Makowski EL, Meschia G, Droegemueller W, et al: Distribution of uterine blood flow in the pregnant sheep. Am J Obstet Gynecol 1968; 101:409–412.
15. Moya F, Thorndike V: Passage of drugs across the placenta. Am J Obstet Gynecol 1962; 84:1778–1798.
16. Austin KL, Stapleton JV, Mather LE: Relationship of meperidine concentration and analgesic response. A preliminary report. Anesthesiology 1980; 53:460–466.
17. Dahlstrom B, Tamsen A, Paalzow L, et al: Patient-controlled analgesic therapy, part IV: pharmacokinetics and analgesic plasma concentration of morphine. Clin Pharmacokinet 1982; 7:266–279.
18. Kosterlitz HW: Opioid peptides and their receptors. The Wellcome Foundation Lecture, 1982. Proc R Soc Lond B Biol Sci 1985; 225:27–40.
19. Kosterlizt HW, Paterson SJ: Types of opioid receptors: Relation to antinociception. Philos Trans R Soc Lond B Biol Sci 1985; 308:291–297.
20. Duggan AW, North RA: Electrophysiology of opioids. Pharmacol Rev 1983; 35:219–281.
21. Herz A, Teschemacher H: Activities and sites of antinociceptive action of morphine-like analgesics and kinetics of distribution following intravenous, intracerebral and intraventricular application. Adv Drug Res 1971; 6:79–119.
22. Ma XF, Duan-Mu ZX, Yi QZ: Effects of morphine on muscarinic receptors in limbic system in acute adjuvant-induced arthritic rats. Acta Pharmacol Sinica 1993; 14:421–423.
23. Nordberg G: Pharmacokinetic aspects of spinal morphine analgesia. Acta Anaesthesiol Scand 1984; 28(Suppl 79):1–38.
24. Ling GSF, Spiegel K, Lockhart SH, et al: Separation of opioid analgesia from respiratory depression: Evidence for different receptor mechanisms. J Pharmacol Exp Ther 1985; 232:149–155.
25. Millan MJ. Kappa-opioid receptors and analgesia. Trends Pharmacol Sci 1990; 11:70–76.
26. Quirion R, Zajac JM, Morgat JL, et al: Autoradiographic distribution of mu and delta opiate receptors in rat brain using highly selective ligands. Life Sci 1983; 33(Suppl I):227–230.
27. Stein C: Peripheral mechanisms of opioid analgesia. Anesth Analg 1993; 76:182–191.
28. Pleuvry BJ: Opioid receptors and their relevance to anaesthesia. Br J Anaesth 1993; 71:119–126.
29. Deutsch SI, Weizman A, Goldman ME, et al: The sigma receptor: A novel site implicated in psychosis and antipsychotic drug efficacy. Clin Neuropharmacol 1988; 11:105–119.
30. Forrest WH, Brown BW Jr, Brown CR, et al: Dextroamphetamine with morphine for the treatment of postoperative pain. N Engl J Med 1977; 296:712–715.
31. Marinella MA: Meperidine-induced generalized seizures with normal renal function. South Med J 1997; 90:556–558.
32. Penagini R, Bianchi PA: Effect of morphine on gastroesophageal reflux and transient lower esophageal sphincter relaxation. Gastroenterology 1997; 113:409–414.
33. Wright PMC, Allen RW, Moore J, et al: Gastric emptying during lumbar extradural analgesia in labour: Effect of fentanyl supplementation. Br J Anaesth 1992; 68:248–251.
34. O'Sullivan GM, Sutton AJ, Thompson SA, et al: Noninvasive measurement of gastric emptying in obstetric patients. Anesth Analg 1987; 66:505–511.
35. Dray A: Epidural opiates and urinary retention: New models provide new insights. Anesthesiology 1988; 68:323–324.
36. Radnay PA, Brodman E, Mankikar D, et al: The effect of equianalgesic doses of fentanyl, morphine, meperidine, and pentazocine on common bile duct pressure. Anaesthetist 1980; 29:26–29.
37. Henderson SK, Cohen H: Nalbuphine augmentation of analgesia and reversal of side effects following epidural hydromorphine. Anesthesiology 1986; 65:216–218.
38. Kendrick WD, Woods AM, Daly MY, et al: Naloxone versus nalbuphine infusion for prophylaxis of epidural morphine-induced pruritus. Anesth Analg 1996; 82:641–647.
39. Hill HF, Chapman CR, Kornel JA, et al: Self-administration of morphine in bone marrow transplant patients reduces drug requirement. Pain 1990; 40:121–129.
40. Hagopian GS, Wolfe HM, Sokol RJ, et al: Neonatal outcome following methadone exposure in utero. J Matern Fetal Med 1996; 5:348–354.
41. Kanner RM, Foley KM: Patterns of narcotic drug use in a cancer pain clinic. Ann N Y Acad Sci 1981; 362:161–172.
42. Flacke JW, Flacke WE, Williams GD: Acute pulmonary edema

following naloxone reversal of high-dose morphine anesthesia. Anesthesiology 1977; 47:376–378.
43. Herbst A, Wolner Hanssen P, Ingemarsson I: Risk factors for acidemia at birth. Obstet Gynecol 1997; 90:125–130.
44. Hodgkinson R, Bhatt M, Wang CN: Double blind comparison of the neurobehavior of neonate following the administration of different doses of meperidine to the mother. Can Anaesth Soc J 1978; 25:405–411.
45. Bonica JJ: Effects of analgesia and anesthesia on the fetus and newborn. In Caldyro-Barcia R (ed.): Effects of Labor and Delivery on the Fetus and Newborn. New York: Pergamon Press, 1967.
46. Celleno D, Capogna G, Sebastiani M, et al: Epidural analgesia during and after cesarean delivery: Comparision of five opioids. Reg Anesth 1991; 16:79–83.
47. Wittels B, Glosten B, Faure EA, et al: Postcesarean analgesia with both epidural morphine and intravenous patient-controlled analgesia: Neurobehavioral outcomes among nursing neonates. Anesth Analg 1997; 85:600–606.
48. Golub MS: Labor analgesia and infant brain development. Pharmacol Biochem Behav 1996; 55:619–628.
49. Moulin DE, Iezzi A, Amireh R, et al: Randomized trial of oral morphine for chronic non-cancer pain. Lancet 1996; 347:143–147.
50. McIntosh DG, Rayburn WF: Patient-controlled analgesia in obstetrics and gynecology. Obstet Gynecol 1991; 78:1129–1135.
51. Benhamou D: The use of patient-controlled analgesia by the obstetrical patient Cah Anesthesiol 1993; 41:599–602.
52. Ngan Kee WD, Lam KK, Chen PP, et al: Comparison of patient-controlled epidural analgesia with patient-controlled intravenous analgesia using pethidine or fentanyl. Anaesth Intensive Care 1997; 25:126–132.
53. Stephens MB, Ford RE: Intrathecal narcotics for labor analgesia. Am Fam Physician 1997; 56:463–470.
54. Arkoosh VA, Sharkey SJ Jr, Norris MC, et al: Subarachnoid labor analgesia. Fentanyl and morphine versus sufentanil and morphine. Reg Anesth 1994; 19:243–246.
55. Husemeyer RP, O'Connor MC, Davenport HT: Failure of epidural morphine to relieve pain in labour. Anaesthesia 1980; 35:161–163.
56. Crawford JS: Experiences with epidural morphine in obstetrics. Anaesthesia 1981; 36:207–209.
57. Nageotte MP, Larson D, Ramney PJ, et al: Epidural analgesia compared with combined spinal epidural analgesia during labour in multiparous women. N Engl J Med 1997; 337:1715–1719.
58. Stoelting RK: Opioid agonists and antagonists. In Stoelting RK (ed): Pharmacology and Physiology in Anesthetic Practice, 2nd ed. Philadelphia: JB Lippincott, 1991: 70.
59. Christrup LL: Morphine metabolites. Acta Anaesthesiol Scand 1997; 41:116–122.
60. Patrie RH, Wu R, Miller FC: The effect of drug on uterine activity. Obstet Gynecol 1976; 48:431–435.
61. Kowalski WB, Parsons MT, Pak SC, et al: Morphine inhibits nocturnal oxytocin secretion and uterine contractions in the pregnant baboon. Biol Reprod 1998; 58:971–976.
62. Lindow SW, van der Spuy ZM, Hendricks MS, et al: The effect of morphine and naloxone administration on plasma oxytocin concentrations in the first stage of labour. Clin Endocrinol (Oxf) 1992; 37:349–353.
63. Rurak DW, Wright MR, Axelson JE: Drug disposition and effects in the fetus. J Dev Physiol 1991; 15:33–44.
64. Gerdin E, Salmonson T, Lindberg B, Rane A: Maternal kinetics of morphine during labor. J Perinat Med 1990; 18:479–487.
65. Srinivasan V, Wielbo D, Simpkins J, et al: Analgesic and immunomodulatory effects of codeine and codeine 6-glucuronide. Pharm Res 1996; 13:296–300.
66. Radbruch L, Grond S, Lehmann KA: A risk-benefit assessment of tramadol in the management of pain. Drug Safety 1996; 15:8–29.
67. Lewis KS; Han NH: Tramadol: A new centrally acting analgesic. Am J Health Syst Pharm 1997; 54:643–652.
68. Rapp SE, Egan KJ, Ross BK, et al: A multidimensional comparison of morphine and hydromorphone patient-controlled analgesia. Anesth Analg 1996; 82:1043–1048.
69. Coda B, Tanaka A, Jacobson RC, et al: Hydromorphone analgesia after intravenous bolus administration. Pain 1997; 71:41–48.
70. Parker RK, Holtmann B, White PF: Patient-controlled epidural analgesia: Interactions between nalbuphine and hydromorphone. Anesth Analg 1997; 84:757–763.
71. Kamendulis LM, Brzezinsbi MR, Pindel EV, et al: Metabolism of cocaine and heroin is catalyzed by the same human liver carboxylase. J Pharmacol Exp Ther 1996; 279:713–717.
72. Leow KP, Smith MT, Watt JA, et al: Comparative oxycodone pharmacokinetics after intravenous, oral, and rectal administration. Ther Drug Monit 1992; 14:479–484.
73. Way WL, Costey EC, Way EL: Respiratory sensitivity of the newborn infant to meperidine and morphine. Clin Pharmacol Ther 1965; 6:454.
74. Kurz A, Ikeda T, Sessler DI, et al: Meperidine decreases the shivering threshold twice as much as the vasoconstriction threshold. Anesthesiology 1997; 86:1046–1054.
75. Ikeda T, Kurz A, Sessler DI, et al: The effect of opioids on thermoregulatory responses in humans and the special antishivering action of meperidine. Ann N Y Acad Sci 1997; 813:792–798.
76. Kuhnert BR, Kuhnert PM, Tu AL, et al: Meperidine and normeperidine levels following meperidine administration during labor: I. Mother. Am J Obstet Gynecol 1979; 133:904–914.
77. Caldwell J, Notarianni LJ: Disposition of pethidine in childbirth [letter]. Br J Anaesth 1978; 50:307–308.
78. Clark RF, Wei EM, Anderson PO: Meperidine: Therapeutic use and toxicity. J Emerg Med 1995; 13:797–802.
79. Caldwell J, Wakile LA, Notarianni LJ, et al: Maternal and neonatal disposition of pethidine in childbirth—a study using quantitative gas chromotography-mass spectrometry. Life Sci 1978; 22:589–596.
80. Erskine WA, Dick A, Morrell DF, et al: Self-administered intravenous analgesia during labour: A comparison between pentazocine and pethidine. S Afr Med J 1985; 67:764–787.
81. Rayburn W, Leuschen MP, Earl R, et al: Intravenous meperidine during labor: A randomized comparison between nursing and patient-controlled administration. Obstet Gynecol 1989; 74:702–704.
82. Huang YF, Upton RN, Rutten RJ, et al: The hemodynamic effects of intravenous bolus doses of meperidine in conscious sheep. Anesth Analg 1994; 78:442–449.
83. Callingham BA: Drug interaction with reversible monoamine oxidase-A inhibitors. Clin Neuropharmacol 1993; 16:S42–50.
84. Sherman S, Gottlieb K, Uzer MF, et al: Effects of meperidine on the pancreatic and biliary sphincter. Gastrointest Endosc 1996; 44:239–242.
85. DeVoe SJ, DeVoe K Jr, Rigsby WC, et al: Effect of meperidine on uterine activity. Am J Obstet Gynecol 1969; 105:1004–1007.
86. Filler WW Jr, Hall WC, Filler NW: Analgesia in obstetrics. The effect of analgesia on uterine contractility and fetal heart rate. Am J Obstet Gynecol 1967; 98:832–846.
87. Sharma SK, Sidawi JE, Ramin SM, et al: Cesarean delivery: A randomized trial of epidural versus patient-controlled meperidine analgesia during labor. Anesthesiology 1997; 87:487–494.
88. Ramin SM, Gambling DR, Lucas MJ, et al: Randomized trial of epidural versus intravenous analgesia during labor. Obstet Gynecol 1995; 86:783–789.
89. Yeh SY, Forsythe A, Hon EH: Quantification of fetal heart beat to beat interval differences. Obstet Gynecol 1973; 41:363.
90. Taylar ES, von Fumetti HH, Essig LL, et al: The effects of demerol and trichlorethylene on arterial oxygen saturation in the newborn. Am J Obstet Gynecol 1955; 69:348–351.
91. Nissen E, Widström AM, Lilja G, et al: Effects of routinely given pethidine during labour on infants' developing breastfeeding behaviour. Effects of dose-delivery time interval and various concentrations of pethidine/norpethidine in cord plasma. Acta Paediatr 1997; 86:201–208.

92. Shnider S, Moya F: Effects of meperidine on the newborn infant. Am J Obstet Gynecol 1964; 89:1009–1015.
93. Kuhnert BR, Linn PL, Kennard MJ, et al: Effects of low doses of meperidine on neonatal behavior. Anesth Analg 1985; 64:335–342.
94. Kuhnert BR, Philipson EH, Kuhnert PM, Syracuse CD: Disposition of meperidine and normeperidine following multiple doses during labor: I. Mother. Am J Obstet Gynecol 1985; 151:406–409.
95. Kuhnert BR, Kuhnert PM, Philipson EH, et al: Disposition of meperidine and normeperidine following multiple doses during labor. II. Fetus and neonate. Am J Obstet Gynecol 1985; 151:410–415.
96. Borgatta L, Jenny RW, Gruss L, et al: Clinical significance of methohexital, meperidine, and diazepam in breast milk. J Clin Pharmacol 1997; 37:186–192.
97. Fuller JD, Crombleholme WR: Respiratory arrest and prolonged respiratory depression after one low subcutaneous dose of alphaprodine for obstetric analgesia: A case report. J Reprod Med 1987; 32:149–151.
98. Murakawa K, Abboud TK, Yanagi T: Neonatal responses to alphaprodine administered during labor. Anesth Analg 1986; 65:392–394.
99. Hingson RA, Hellman LM: Eight thousand parturients evaluate drugs, techniques, and doctors during labor and delivery. Am J Obstet Gynecol 1954; 68:262.
100. Ekelman SB, Reynolds SRM: Effect of the analgesic nisentil on uterine contractions: Considered by parity, stage of labor and status of membranes. Obstet Gynecol 1955; 6:644–651.
101. Adams RJ: Obstetrical medication and the human newborn: The influence of alphaprodine hydrochloride on visual behaviour. Dev Med Child Neurol 1989; 31:650–656.
102. Powell PO Jr, Savage JE: Nisentil in obstetrics. Obstet Gynecol 1953; 2:658–670.
103. Veren D, Bochm FH, Killam AP: The clinical significance of a sinusoidal fetal heart rate pattern associated with alphaprodine administration. J Reprod Med 1982; 27:411–414.
104. Matthews MK: The relationship between maternal labour analgesia and delay in the initiation of breastfeeding in healthy neonates in the early neonatal period. Midwifery 1989; 5:3–10.
105. Craft JB Jr, Coaldrake LA, Bolan JC, et al: Placental passage and uterine effects of fentanyl. Anesth Analg 1983; 62:894–898.
106. Smith CV, Rayburn WF, Allen KV, et al: Influence of intravenous fentanyl on fetal biophysical parameters during labor. J Matern Fetal Med 1996; 5:89–92.
107. Rayburn W, Rathke A, Leuschen P, et al: Fentanyl citrate analgesia during labor. Am J Obstet Gynecol 1989; 161:202–206.
108. Rayburn WF, Smith CV, Parriott JE, Woods RE: Randomized comparison of meperidine and fentanyl during labor. Obstet Gynecol 1989; 74:604–606.
109. Rayburn WF, Smith CV, Leuschen MP, et al: Comparison of patient controlled and nurse-administered analgesia using intravenous fentanyl during labor. Anesth Rev 1991; 18:31.
110. Rosaeg OP, Kitts JB, Koren G, et al: Maternal and fetal effects of intravenous patient-controlled fentanyl analgesia during labour in a thrombocytopenic parturient. Can J Anesth 1992; 39:277–281.
111. Krishna BR, Zakowski MI, Grant GJ: Sufentanil transfer in the human placenta during in vitro perfusion. Can J Anaesth 1997; 44:996–1001.
112. Herman NL, Calicott R, Van Decar TK, et al: Determination of the dose-response relationship for intrathecal sufentanil in laboring patients. Anesth Analg 1997; 84:1256–1261.
113. Camann WR, Denney RA, Holby ED, Datta S: A comparison of intrathecal, epidural, and intravenous sufentanil for labor analgesia. Anesthesiology 1992; 77:884–887.
114. Scholz J, Steinfath M, Schulz M: Clinical pharmacokinetics of alfentanil, fentanyl and sufentanil: An update. Clin Pharmacokin 1996; 31:275–292.
115. Hill DA, Mc Carthy G, Bali IM: Epidural infusion of alfentanil or diamorphine with bupivacaine in labour: A dose finding study. Anaesthesia 1995; 50:415–419.
116. van den Nieuwenhuyzen MC, Stienstra R, Burm AG, et al: Alfentanil as an adjuvant to epidural bupivacaine in the management of postoperative pain after laparotomies: Lack of evidence of spinal action. Anesth Analg 1998; 86:574–578.
117. Egan TD, Minto CF, Hermann DJ, et al: Remifentanil versus alfentanil: Comparative pharmacokinetics and pharmacodynamics in healthy adult male volunteers. Anesthesiology 1996; 84:821–833.
118. Dershwitz M, Hoke JF, Rosow CE, et al: Pharmacokinetics and pharmacodynamics of remifentanil in volunteer subjects with severe liver disease. Anesthesiology 1996; 84:812–820.
119. Minto CF, Schnider TW, Shafer SL: Pharmacokinetics and pharmacodynamics of remifentanil. II. Model application. Anesthesiology 1997; 86:24–33.
120. Michelsen LG, Hug CC Jr: The pharmacokinetics of remifentanil. J Clin Anesth 1996; 8:679–682.
121. Gourlay GK, Wilson RR, Glynn CJ: Methadone produces prolonged post-operative analgesia. Br Med J 1982; 284:630–631.
122. Stork CM, Redd JT, Fine K, Hoffman RS: Propoxyphene-induced wide QRS complex dysrhythmia responsive to sodium bicarbonate: A case report. J Toxicol Clin Toxicol 1995; 33:179–183.
123. Lewis JW, Rance MJ, Sanger DJ: The pharmacology and abuse potential of buprenorphine: A new antagonist analgesic. Adv Substance Abuse 1983; 3:103–154.
124. Roy S, Basu RK: Role of sublingual administration of tablet buprenorphine hydrochloride on relief of labour pain. J Indian Med Assoc 1992; 90:151–153.
125. Marquet P, Chevrel J, Lavignasse P, et al: Buprenorphine withdrawal syndrome in a newborn. Clin Pharmacol Ther 1997; 62:569–571.
126. Pick CG, Peter Y, Schreiber S, et al: Pharmacological characterization of buprenorphine, a mixed agonist-antagonist with kappa 3 analgesia. Brain Res 1997; 744:41–46.
127. Del Pizzo A: A double-blind study of the effects of butorphanol compared with morphine in balanced anesthesia. Can Anesth Soc J 1978; 25:392–397.
128. Kallos T, Caruso FS: Respiratory effects of butorphanol and pethidine. Anaesthesia 1979; 633–637.
129. Hodgkinson R, Huff RW, Hayashi RH: Double-blind comparison of maternal analgesia and neonatal neurobehavior following intravenous butorphanol and meperidine. J Int Med Res 1979; 7:224–230.
130. Quilligan EJ, Keegan KA, Donahue MJ: Double-blind comparison of intravenously injected butorphanol and meperidine in parturients. Int J Gynaecol Obstet 1980; 18:363–367.
131. Wahab SA, Askalani AH, Amar RA, et al: Effect of some recent analgesics on labor pain and maternal and fetal blood gases and pH. Int J Gynaecol Obstet 1988; 26:75–80.
132. Hatjis CG, Meis PJ: Sinusoidal fetal heart rate pattern associated with butorphanol administration. Obstet Gynecol 1986; 67:377–380.
133. Juneja M, Ackerman WE 3d, Heine MF, et al: Butorphanol for the relief of shivering associated with extradural anesthesia in parturients. J Clin Anesth 1992; 4:390–393.
134. Atkinson BD, Truitt LJ, Rayburn WF, et al: A double-blind comparison of intravenous butorphanol (Stadol) and fentanyl (Sublimaze) for analgesia during labor. Am J Obstet Gynecol 1994; 171:993–998.
135. Wilson CM, McClean E, Moore J, Dundee JW: A double-blind comparison of intramuscular pethidine and nalbuphine in labour. Anaesthesia 1986; 41:1207–1213.
136. Frank M, McAteer EJ, Cattermole R, et al: Nalbuphine for obstetric analgesia: A comparison of nalbuphine with pethidine for pain relief in labour when administered by patient-controlled analgesia. Anaesthesia 1987; 42:697–703.
137. Podlas J, Breland BD: Patient controlled analgesia with nalbuphine during labor. Obstet Gynecol 1987; 70:202–204.
138. Alhashemi JA, Gosby ET, Grodecki W, et al: Treatment of intrathecal morphine induced pruritus following caesarean section. Can J Anaesth 1997; 44:1060–1065.

139. Jaffe JH, Martin WR: Opioids with mixed actions: partial agonists. In Gilman AG, Rall TW, Nies AS, Taylor P (eds): The Pharmacological Basis of Therapeutics, 8th ed. New York: Pergamon Press, 1990:512.
140. Coalson DW, Glosten B: Alternatives to epidural analgesia. Semin Perinatol 1991; 15:375–385.
141. Jasinski DR, Martin WR, Hoeldtke RD: Effects of short and long-term administration of pentazocine in man. Clin Pharmacol Ther 1970; 11:385–403.
142. Stevens CW, Rothe KS: Supraspinal administration of opioids with selectivity for mu-, delta- and kappa-opioid receptors produces analgesia in amphibians. Eur J Pharmacol 1997; 331:15–21.
143. Refstad SO, Lindbaek E: Ventilatory depression of the newborn of women receiving pethidine or pentazocine. Br J Anaesth 1980; 52:265–271.
144. Vitalone V, Lopresti C: Acute pulmonary edema after intravenous naloxone. Minerva Anestesiol 1992; 58:225–227.
145. Osterwalder JJ: Naloxone—for intoxications with intravenous heroin and heroin mixtures—harmless or hazardous? A prospective clinical study [see comments]. J Toxicol Clin Toxicol 1996; 34:409–416.
146. Anonymous: Guidelines for cardiopulmonary resuscitation and emergency cardiac care. Emergency Cardiac Care Committee and Subcommittees, American Heart Association. Part VII. Neonatal resuscitation. JAMA 1992; 268:2276–2281.
147. Committee on Obstetrics: Maternal and Fetal Medicine: Naloxone Use in Newborns. Washington, DC: American College of Obstetricians and Gynecologists, 1989.
148. Wank SA: Cholecystokinin receptors. Am J Physiol 1995; 269:G628–646.
149. Price DD, von der Gruen A, et al: Potentiation of systemic morphine analgesia in humans by proglumide, a cholecystokinin antagonist. Anesth Analg 1985; 64:801–806.
150. Schafer M, Zhou L, Stein C: Cholecystokinin inhibits peripheral opioid analgesia in inflamed tissue. Neuroscience 1998; 82:603–611.
151. Coupey SM: Barbiturates. Pediatr Rev 1997; 18:260–264.
152. Moya F, Thorndike V: Effects of drugs used in labor on the fetus and newborn. Clin Pharmacol Ther 1963; 4:628.
153. Stechler G: Newborn attention as affected by medication during labor. Science 1964; 144:315–317.
154. Root B, Eichner E, Sunshine I: Blood secobarbital levels and their clinical correlation in mothers and newborn infants. Am J Obstet Gynecol 1961; 81:948–956.
155. Gear RW, Miaskowski C, Heller PH, et al: Benzodiazepine mediated antagonism of opioid analgesia. Pain 1997; 71:25–29.
156. Mandelli M, Tognoni G, Garatini S: Clinical pharmacokinetics of diazepam. Clin Pharmacokinet 1978; 3:72–91.
157. Shiono PH, Mills JL: Oral clefts and diazepam use during pregnancy. N Engl J Med 1984; 311:919–920.
158. Mc Elhatton PR: The effects of benzodiazepine use during pregnancy and lactation. Reprod Toxicol 1994; 8:461–475.
159. Kanjilal S, Pan NR, Chakraborty DP, et al: Cord blood diazepam: Clinical effects in neonates of eclamptic mothers. Indian J Pediatr 1993; 60:257–263.
160. Pan B, Lu Y, Wang D: Determination of diazepam concentration in maternal and fetal serum after intravenous administration during active phase of labor and its effects on neonates. Chung Hua Fu Chan Ko Tsa Chih 1995; 30:707–710.
161. McAuley DM, O'Neill MP, Moore J, et al: Lorazepam premedication for labour. Br J Obstet Gynecol 1982; 89:149–154.
162. Nordt SP, Clark RF: Midazolam: A review of therapeutic uses and toxicity. J Emerg Med 1997; 15:357–365.
163. Bach V, Carl P, Ravlo O, et al: A randomized comparison between midazolam and thiopental for elective cesarean section anesthesia. III. Placental transfer and elimination in neonates. Anesth Analg 1989; 68:238–242.
164. Ravlo O, Carl P, Crawford ME, et al: A randomized comparison between midazolam and thiopental for elective cesarean section anesthesia. II. Neonates. Anesth Analg 1989; 68:234–242.
165. Seidman SF, Marx GF: Midazolam in obstetric anesthesia. Anesthesiology 1987; 67:443–444.
166. Nordt SP, Clark RF: Midazolam: A review of therapeutic uses and toxicity. J Emerg Med 1997; 15:357–365.
167. Zacny JP, Coalson DW, Klafta JM, et al: Midazolam does not influence intravenous fentanyl-induced analgesia in healthy volunteers. Pharmacol Biochem Behav 1996; 55:275–280.
168. Aroomlooi J, Tobias M, Berg P: The effect of scopolamine and ancillary analgesics upon the fetal heart rate. J Reprod Med 1980; 25:323–326.
169. Tarkkila P, Töm K, Tuominen M, et al: Premedication with promethazine and transdermal scopolamine reduces the incidence of nausea and vomiting after intrathecal morphine. Acta Anaesthesiol Scand 1995; 39:983–986.
170. McQuitty FM: Relief of pain in labour: A controlled double-blind trial comparing pethidine and various phenothiazine derivatives. J Obstet Gynaecol Br Commonw 1967; 74:925–928.
171. Eisenstein JI, Rubin EJ, Arnold M, et al: Propiomazine hydrochloride in obstetrics. Am J Obstet Gynecol 1964; 88:606–611.
172. Ullery JC, Bair JR: Maternal-fetal effects of propiomazine-meperidine analgesia. Am J Obstet Gynecol 1962; 84:1051–1056.
173. Tokodi G Jr, Huber FC: Massive tissue necrosis after hydroxyzine injection. J Am Osteopath Assoc 1995; 95:609–612.
174. Einarson A, Bailey B, Jung G, et al: Prospective controlled study of hydroxyzine and cetirizine in pregnancy. Ann Allergy Asthma Immunol 1997; 78:183–186.
175. Zsigmond EK, Patterson RI: Double-blind evaluation of hydroxyzine hydrochloride in obstetric anesthesia. Anesth Analg 1967; 46:275–280.
176. Juneja MM, Ackerman WE, Bellinger K: Epidural morphine pruritus reduction with hydroxyzine in parturients. J Ky Med Assoc 1991; 89:319–321.
177. King CT, Howell J: Teratogenic effect of buclizine and hydroxzyzine in the rat and chlorcyclizine in the mouse. Am J Obstet Gynecol 1966; 95:109–111.
178. White PF, Way WL, Trevor AJ: Ketamine: Its pharmacology and therapeutic uses. Anesthesiology 1982; 56:119–136.
179. Detsch O, Kochs E: Effects of ketamine on CNS-function. Anaesthesist 1997; 46(Suppl 1):S20–29.
180. Kress HG: Mechanisms of action of ketamine. Anaesthesist 1997; 46(Suppl 1):S8–19.
181. Aanonsen LM, Wilcox GL: Nociceptive action of excitatory amino acids in the mouse: Effects of spinally administered opioids, phencyclidine and sigma agonists. J Pharmacol Exp Ther 1987; 243:9–19.
182. Sher GD, Mitchell D: *N*-Methyl-D-aspartate receptors mediate responses of rat dorsal horn neurones to hind limb ischemia. Brain Res 1990; 522:55–62.
183. Howton JC, Rose J, Duffy S, et al: Randomized, double-blind, placebo-controlled trial of intravenous ketamine in acute asthma. Ann Emerg Med 1996; 27:170–175.
184. Yang CY, Wong CS, Chang JY, et al: Intrathecal ketamine reduces morphine requirements in patients with terminal cancer pain. Can J Anaesth 1996; 43:379–383.
185. Hodgkinson K, Marx GF, Kim SS, et al: Neonatal neurobehavioral tests following vaginal delivery under ketamine, thiopental, and extradural anesthesia. Anesth Analg 1977; 56:548–553.
186. Akamatsu TJ, Bonica JJ, Rehmet R, et al: Experiences with the use of ketamine for parturition. I. Primary anesthesia for vaginal delivery. Anesth Analg 1974; 53:284–287.
187. Lisander B: Evaluation of the analgesic effect of metoclopramide after opioid free analgesia. Br J Anaesth 1993; 70:631–633.
188. Rosenblatt WH, Cioffi AM, Sinatra R, et al: Metoclopramide: An analgesic adjunct to patient-controlled analgesia. Anesth Analg 1991; 73:553–555.
189. Rosenblatt WH, Cioffi AM, Sinatra R, et al: Metoclopramide-enhanced analgesia for prostaglandin-induced termination of pregnancy. Anesth Analg 1992; 75:760–763.

190. Danzer BI, Birnbach DJ, Stein DJ, et al: Does metoclopramide supplement postoperative analgesia using patient-controlled analgesia with morphine in patients undergoing elective Cesarean delivery? Reg Anesth 1997; 22:424–427.
191. Walker JJ, Johnstone J, Lloyd J, et al: The transfer of ketorolac tromethamine from maternal to foetal blood. Eur J Clin Pharmacol 1988; 34:509–511.
192. Walker JJ, Johnston J, Fairlie FM, et al: A comparative study of intramuscular ketorolac and pethidine in labour pain. Eur J Obstet Gynecol Repod Biol 1992; 46:87–94.

16

Inhalation Agents for Labor

❖ Sun Sunatrio, MD

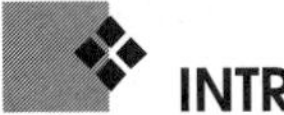

INTRODUCTION

The introduction and development of obstetric anesthesia by Sir James Y. Simpson was one of the most dramatic advances in medicine.[1] More than 150 years later, proper administration of obstetric analgesia to a suffering parturient remains one of the most humane practices in medicine. Improved labor and delivery practices and the development of superior local anesthetics and conduction techniques have caused a reduction in the number of inhalational anesthetics used for delivery.

Inhalation of subanesthetic doses of nitrous oxide, trichloroethylene, methoxyflurane, enflurane, and isoflurane can provide safe and effective analgesia during labor and delivery in patients for whom epidural analgesia is contraindicated or not available.

Inhalation anesthesia and analgesia for vaginal delivery might be needed for the following patients:

1. Patients who want to be asleep to avoid severe pain. In the present day, this is a rare indication. This patient's desire is usually due to lack of proper preparation for labor and delivery or the presence of obstetric complications.
2. Patients whose delivery process must be ended rapidly because of obstetric complications potentially lethal to the fetus, such as fetal "distress," premature separation of the placenta, or prolapse of the umbilical cord. These patients, however, tend to need anesthesia for emergent cesarean delivery.
3. Patients who are anesthetized for vaginal delivery for the sake of the physician. Patients who are hysterical at the time of delivery tend to unsettle some physicians. In extremely rare circumstances, some physicians request that patients be anesthetized for vaginal delivery.
4. In hospitals where facilities, equipment, or adequate knowledge does not exist to allow the safe administration of spinal, epidural, or combined spinal-epidural analgesia.

Even if pudendal nerve blocks are being used, the administration of analgesic concentrations of nitrous oxide, ethylene, trichloroethylene, or methoxyflurane after the patient is placed on the delivery table will make pudendal block placement more comfortable.

INHALATION ANALGESIA

Inhalation analgesia is the administration of subanesthetic concentrations of inhalation anesthetic agents (either alone or as a supplement to regional or local anesthesia) to relieve pain during the first and second stages of labor. This technique allows the mother to remain awake and cooperative and to maintain protective laryngeal reflexes, while enjoying good analgesia. The anesthetic agent may be administered via a mask or mouthpiece. This pain relief technique is not to be confused with inhalational anesthesia, which is intended to produce unconsciousness.

Although inhalation analgesia provides some pain relief, it is not comparable with that obtained by regional anesthesia. Many women elect not to have regional anesthesia because they fear needles and spinal headaches; are alarmed by the possibility, however remote, of neurologic damage; or believe that regional anesthesia would render them unable to participate in the delivery. In these cases, inhaled anesthetics may be used to provide pain relief during the first stage of labor or when a brief period of analgesia is needed during the second stage of labor.

An inhaled analgesic is usually administered from either a standard anesthetic machine or a flow-over vaporizer. Precision vaporizers attached to the anesthetic machine make the concomitant use of oxygen possible. They must be capable of delivering a reliable range of anesthetic vapor concentrations, without being significantly influenced by the patient's minute ventilation or peak flow or by variations in room temperature. These considerations are especially important because wide variations in ventilation occur during labor.

Inhaled analgesics are administered either intermittently (only during contractions) or continuously (during and between contractions). The dose should not be a fixed concentration of anesthetic but rather an amount regulated according to the patient's response. If the patient becomes confused, drowsy, excited or uncooperative, the inspired concentration should be lowered quickly. Continuous verbal contact should be kept with the patient. Not only does this provide constant reassurance and encouragement, but it also allows for monitoring of the depth of anesthesia. The major risk of inhalation analgesia is accidental anesthetic overdose which, in turn, can cause loss of protective reflexes, silent regurgitation, aspiration pneumonitis, obstruction, or asphyxia.

Inhaled analgesics may also be self-administered. The technique is the same as when intermittent analgesia is administered by an anesthetist. The patient should have an experienced attendant standing by to ensure proper use of the equipment and to monitor any change in the level of consciousness.

During the late second stage, when delivery is imminent, it is preferable to administer the inhalational agent continuously. Between contractions a lower concentration of the agent should be given, and the concentration should be increased as each contraction starts. This technique allows the analgesic concentration in the blood during each contraction to be achieved with less delay.

The addition of methoxyflurane or any other volatile agent to a mixture of nitrous oxide and oxygen may produce general anesthesia rather than the desired analgesia. This danger may be more pronounced if a plastic circuit rather than a rubber one is used. The latter absorbs larger amounts of methoxyflurane and, therefore, keeps the inspired concentration lower.

Some advantages of inhalational analgesics are as follows:

1. Satisfactory analgesia and amnesia can be achieved.
2. Laryngeal and cough reflexes are preserved at the lower concentrations.
3. The fetus is rarely influenced.
4. The contractility of the uterus is not significantly depressed.
5. Expulsive powers are not affected; the mother can often push better if pain is abolished.
6. Toxicity is eliminated by the use of low concentrations.
7. The use of inhalational analgesics combined with a pudendal block are sufficient for most low forceps deliveries.
8. They permit the use of higher oxygen concentrations which raise the maternal Pa_{O_2}.

There are limitations to the use of potent inhalational agents in the first and second stages of labor:

1. Insufficient analgesia for some parturients
2. Possible loss of protective airway reflexes and attendant pulmonary aspiration of gastric contents
3. Possibility of maternal amnesia
4. The need for a specialized vaporizer
5. Air pollution

Inhalation agents that may be used in obstetric analgesia and anesthesia are presented in Table 16–1, which shows the relationship between the chemical formulas and the concentration of agents that will produce analgesia and anesthesia. Although inhalational agents continue to be used in Third World countries, they have been replaced by neuraxial techniques in most developed countries.

Nitrous Oxide

For a long time, 50% nitrous oxide (N_2O) in air was a standard analgesic agent in spite of the obvious disadvantage of reducing the fraction of inspired oxygen concentration to 0.1. In some countries, the old opinion that the analgesic effect of nitrous oxide depended primarily on concomitant hypoxia proved difficult to change. In 1962 Cole and Nainby-Luxmore[2] still attracted attention to the lowered arterial oxygen saturation during the use of nitrous oxide and air. In the early 1960s, special machines such as the Lucy-Baldwin were designed to provide a 50:50 mixture of nitrous oxide and oxygen. Nevertheless, the major advance was the production of Entonox, a premixture of nitrous oxide and oxygen in the same cylinder.[3]

Entonox is a very stable mixture providing constant percentages of nitrous oxide and oxygen if the cylinder is not allowed to cool excessively. The critical temperature (i.e., the temperature above which no amount of increased pressure will produce liquefaction) of nitrous oxide is 36.5°C, that of oxygen is −118.8°C, and that of the mixture is −7°C. If the mixture is allowed to cool below −7°C, partial liquefaction occurs resulting in the proportions of gases released no longer being constant, even after the mixture is rewarmed. Initially, a relatively high concentration of oxygen is released but, with time, there is a gradual decrease in oxygen to below 21%. Agitation of the tank does not reconstitute the correct mixture.[4] The only effective method to reachieve the original mixture concentrations is to leave the tank horizontal for 24 hours at a temperature of above 5°C.[5]

A 60:40 mixture of nitrous oxide and oxygen delivered through a blender (e.g., Midogas, Ohmeda) provides favorable analgesia at the end of the first stage of labor and during the second stage. This mixture is especially useful during a pudendal block placement or as a preanesthetic for general anesthesia. For example, for a simple low forceps delivery, when the patient is placed on the delivery table, a 60:40 mixture of nitrous oxide and oxygen produces analgesia for painless pudendal block.

Satisfactory maternal analgesia, normal blood oxygen saturation, and normal infant blood chemistry can be maintained with a 60:40 mixture of nitrous oxide and oxygen for about 45 minutes to an hour before delivery. However, this mixture may cause some disorientation. If nitrous oxide is administered for longer

Table 16–1 Pharmacologic Comparison of Inhalation Analgesic and Anesthetic Agents Used in Obstetrics*

Agent	Chemical Formula	Inflammable Range (%)		Ignition Temp (°C)		% Concentration Inhaled for			Blood Concentration (mg%)	
		In Air	In Oxygen	In Air	In Oxygen	Analgesia	Anesthesia	Respiratory Arrest	Anesthesia	Respiratory Arrest
Nitrous oxide	N_2O	Supports combustion only		Supports combustion only		35–40	Not recommended			
Ethylene	$CH_2{=}CH_2$	3.05–28.6		490	485	20–35	Not recommended		140	
Cyclopropane	CH_2 / \ CH_2——CH_2	2.40–10.3		498	454	3-5	20–25	35–39	16–20	
Diethyl ether	$(C_2H_5)_2O$	1.85–36.5		304	182		3.5–4.5	6.7–8.0	90–130	140–180
Chloroform	$CHCl_3$	Oxidized by flame: $2\ CHCl_3 + O_2 \cdot$ $2\ COCl_2 + 2\ HCl$		Oxidized by flame: $2\ CHCl_3 + O_2 \cdot$ $2\ COCl_2 + 2\ HCl$			1.35–1.65	2.0	20–30	40–60
Trichloroethylene	$CCl_2 — CHCl$	Above 32°C, only: 15	10.3–64.5		419	0.28	0.55–0.70			
Fluroxene	$CF_3CH_2OCH{=}CH_2$	Dry 4.2 Sat. with H_2O 7.5–78	4.0–80			1.0-2.0	2.4–8.2	12.9	9.3	38.7
Halothane	$CF_3CHBrCl$	Nonflammable		Nonflammable			0.8–1.2	3.6–4.0		
Methoxyflurane	$C_2HFCl_2 — O — CH_3$	Flammable only at abnormally high vapor conc. (4%) and temp (75°C (167°F))				0.8	1.0–1.5		0.5–0.8	1.5–3.0

*Adapted from WHL Dornette for Ohio Chemical Company.

than 30 minutes, a 50:50 mixture of nitrous oxide and oxygen should be used, because analgesia can be achieved at this concentration without causing disorientation.

The administration of nitrous oxide and oxygen in 60:40 or 50:50 concentrations has no effect on hepatic, renal, cardiac, or pulmonary function. The mixture is nonexplosive and is reasonably inexpensive.

To achieve a near-maximal analgesic effect, intermittent inhalational analgesia with a nitrous oxide and oxygen mixture for 45 seconds is required. This was shown in practice by Minnitt in 1933 and has been calculated on theoretic grounds by Waud and Waud.[6]

It is therefore important to start the inhalation of the nitrous oxide and oxygen mixture about 45 seconds before pain is experienced to achieve satisfactory analgesia. In the first stage of labor the initial painless phase of the uterine contractions should indicate at which point inhalation should start so that analgesic concentration of nitrous oxide can rise. Needless to say, the inhalation should be continued during the painful phase of the contraction. Analgesia will not be satisfactory if inhalation is begun when pain is already present.

Inhalational analgesia may be helpful during procedures that may be associated with discomfort such as vaginal examination, placement of an epidural block, and delivery of the placenta. However, the use of nitrous oxide analgesia alone is not satisfactory for forceps delivery, perineal suture, and manual removal of the placenta, although it may be helpful during forceps or breech delivery if combined with a pudendal nerve block. Artificial rupture of the membranes causes pain in about 25% of mothers.[7] The inhalation of nitrous oxide is helpful to these women.

Unlike trichloroethylene and methoxyflurane, nitrous oxide does not accumulate in maternal and fetal tissues and, therefore, there is no restriction on the time over which it can be used in labor. Although at one time it was customary to restrict the administration of nitrous oxide to the second stage and the late part of the first stage of labor, it appears to be safe and, in some cases, even helpful to use nitrous oxide analgesia for the greater part of the labor process.

Nitrous oxide analgesia is at times imperfect. The explanation for this may lie with the agent and not the parturient or the technique of administration. Hence, the wider acceptability of more effective analgesic methods, such as epidural analgesia.

Ethylene

Ethylene (C_2H_4) provides satisfactory obstetric analgesia but it is not widely used because it is explosive and expensive and has a pungent smell that is not tolerated by many patients and obstetricians. The gas should never be used in a closed system because of its explosive hazard. Ethylene, like nitrous oxide, has essentially no deleterious effect on cardiopulmonary, renal, or hepatic function.[8] It may also be administered to the mother for long periods of time (45 minutes or more) without causing changes in maternal oxygen saturation or altering placental gaseous exchange or blood chemistry of infants at birth.[9] When ethylene is used for analgesia, it should be administered at a minimum of 2 L/min flow rate. When untrained personnel are charged with administering the analgesic, a responsible physician or anesthetist must stand by at frequent intervals to check the flow of gas being administered. The administration of higher concentrations, such as 60:40 ethylene and oxygen mixture, may result in greater patient irritability and in light anesthesia. It is best used for "terminal" analgesia (during the last 10–15 minutes of the second stage) or at the time of delivery. The expiratory valve should be left open. A transparent face mask should be used such that any vomiting can be observed. However, with this mixture of ethylene and oxygen, aspiration of vomitus is unlikely to occur because the pharyngeal reflexes are retained.

Nitrous oxide or ethylene and oxygen analgesia combined with a pudendal block is popular in smaller hospitals in some Third World countries where anesthetists are not available.

Trichloroethylene

Trichloroethylene (Trilene) has many practical uses in the management of obstetric pain. It is a very pleasant, effective, and relatively safe analgesic. Proper use of trichloroethylene is not associated with any harmful effects to the mother or infant.[10–12] It has no deleterious effect on the cardiovascular, pulmonary, hepatic, or renal systems.[12] In 1943, Freedman[13] reported its satisfactory use in over 2000 patients. Its apparent advantage over nitrous oxide was its higher potency. Seward[14] showed that a maximum concentration of trichloroethylene in air of 0.5% by volume was sufficient, and that 0.33% was adequate after a period of inhaling the 0.5% mixture.

The technique of using trichloroethylene to relieve the pain of a labor contraction is the same as that for nitrous oxide. It has been suggested that inhalation of the agent, in either of the available concentrations, must be continued for 3 to 4 minutes before a significant reduction in pain sensibility is obtained.[15] However, the kinetics of uptake and elimination of trichloroethylene are different from those of nitrous oxide, and the former is unlikely to be entirely excreted between contractions. The first few episodes of inhalation might not provide adequate analgesia, but later on the extent of pain relief is usually satisfactory. Therefore, when using trichloroethylene it might be a good practice to let the patient inhale the 0.5% mixture during the first few contractions. Once adequate analgesia has been attained, the weaker 0.33% mixture should be given. Use of the stronger mixture should be reserved for those patients whose pain is not relieved adequately.

The intermittent inhalation of trichloroethylene should not continue for longer than 6 hours. Many practitioners do not advocate the use of trichloroethylene for a period lasting more than 1 hour. Accumulation of the drug and its metabolites (which include trichloroacetic acid) in tissues of the mother and her fetus does occur. Prolonged intermittent inhalation of trichloroethylene may result in sleepiness and uncooperativeness of the mother, and drug-induced depression of the newborn. Therefore it is recommended that trichloroethylene, in contrast to nitrous oxide, should be reserved for use in the late phase of first-stage labor.

Although the interaction of trichloroethylene with soda lime (producing the toxic products phosgene and dichloroacetylene) has limited it use, the agent has been in considerable use for some time. It has one stunning advantage for use in the Third World; it is very inexpensive.

Trichloroethylene, given in the recommended manner, may be slightly more likely to produce satisfactory analgesia than is 50% nitrous oxide. The results of a comparison will, as is so often the case, depend on the eagerness of the observers. However, midwives usually report that parturients dislike the smell of trichloroethylene. This factor reduces its potential effectiveness.

During the second stage of labor, when contractions last, generally, for around 1 minute with a 2-minute interval (and are accompanied by a desire to bear down), the self-administration mode for an inhalational agent is significantly different from that relating to the first stage. In the second stage, the contraction is usually painful throughout and, therefore, it is necessary that the parturient start to inhale the analgesic agent 20 to 30 seconds prior to the beginning of a contraction to attain satisfactory analgesia. Fortunately, second-stage contractions happen at regular intervals, so that the parturient is able to anticipate the beginning of a contraction and can start her inhalation at the right time. Failure to follow this simple rule may result in extremely poor analgesia because (1) the beginning of the contraction is painful and (2) if a parturient bears down and holds her breath several times during each contraction, many of the remaining contractions are distressing. Each episode of bearing down lasts about 10 to 12 seconds, and between contractions the parturient hyperventilates. She could inhale from her face mask during these hyperventilation periods. During delivery of the fetal head, the parturient should be encouraged to hyperventilate, inhaling the analgesic agent throughout the contraction to produce a well-controlled delivery.

Chloroform

Chloroform is an extremely potent anesthetic that is pleasant to take and is associated with a smooth induction. It was used successfully for many thousands of deliveries over a span of 120 years.[16] Many women have been thankful that their general practitioner administered a few drops of chloroform at the time when their babies were pushed across the perineum. Chloroform provides simple and very pleasant analgesia for delivery if only a few drops are poured through a face mask that is held at least "one fist" away from the patient's face. Trichloroethylene and methoxyflurane are safer and more satisfactory anesthetics than chloroform even though chloroform, if given in low concentrations and intermittently during the terminal expulsion stages of labor, has been administered with relative safety by untrained personnel.

Chloroform used to be an ideal anesthetic to produce uterine relaxation for version and extraction of the breech; however, in using this agent to achieve relaxation, extreme skill is necessary. Since anesthetics are more familiar with current agents that are safer, chloroform is rarely, if ever, used anymore.

Halothane

Halothane is a highly potent anesthetic that must be administered from a special vaporizer and must not be used for a delivery in a greater concentration than 2%.[17–20] Halothane should be given with at least a 60:40 mixture of nitrous oxide and oxygen.

After moving the patient to the delivery table, inhalation of 60% nitrous oxide and 40% oxygen should be started and a transvaginal pudendal block should be performed. When a low forceps or spontaneous delivery is feasible, halothane can be added to the nitrous oxide mixture with the vaporizer set at 1%. If the patient tolerates the halothane satisfactorily, the vaporizer may be set at 1.5% as needed. Induction is usually rapid and within 3 minutes the baby can be delivered easily. As soon as the shoulders have been delivered, halothane is discontinued and the patient is continued on the 60:40 mixture of nitrous oxide and oxygen—without flushing the bag—until delivery is complete. The anesthetic bag is then compressed, nitrous oxide is discontinued, and the patient continues to inhale oxygen at 4 L/min. The repair of episiotomy may then be performed under pudendal block. This technique unfortunately exposes the mother to considerable risk of aspiration of gastric contents. As with any potent volatile anesthetic, the parturient may lose the ability to protect her airway and thus be at risk for aspiration.

Fluroxene

Fluroxene is trifluoroethylvinyl ether, with the physical and anesthetic characteristics as described in Table 16–1. It has great potential advantages for obstetrics.[21, 22] It is nonexplosive in the concentrations required for obstetrics and nonflammable when administered under the circle absorption technique. Fluroxene is a pleasant anesthetic agent capable of providing safe and efficient inhalation anesthesia with rapid induction and rapid recovery. During a 3-year period (1963–1965) at the University of North Carolina, junior and senior medical students (trained in an abbreviated course in anesthesia given by the Department of Anesthesiology) used fluroxene with nitrous oxide and oxygen almost exclusively for vaginal delivery with safety.[16] This experience suggests that the administration of fluroxene for obstetric anesthesia may be used by many Third World hospitals where there is a paucity of anesthetists and lack of proper obstetric anesthesia.

When the parturient is placed on the delivery table, she is given a 60:40 mixture of nitrous oxide and oxygen and a pudendal block is then performed. Fluroxene is, preferably, given through a special vaporizer with 2 L/min of nitrous oxide when delivery is feasible. Because it is not irritating, the concentration of fluroxene can be increased rapidly as tolerated to around 3%. This is maintained until the shoulders have been delivered, at which time the administration of fluroxene is stopped. Thereafter, a 60:40 mixture of nitrous oxide and oxygen is continued without flushing the bag. After complete delivery of the infant, the bag is flushed and the parturient is given 3 L/min of oxygen. The episiotomy is then repaired under pudendal block.

Methoxyflurane

Methoxyflurane was introduced into obstetric analgesia in 1962[23, 24] and soon proved to be a superior analgesic. An inhaled concentration of 0.35% in air provides significantly better analgesia than a concentration of 0.25%, while an inhaled concentration of 0.45% produces unacceptable drowsiness.[25] Major and her colleagues[26] had already shown a more positive response to methoxyflurane than trichloroethylene by patients, anesthetists, and midwives.

Unfortunately, nephrotoxicity following the use of methoxyflurane in surgical patients was first reported in 1966.[27] The biodegradation of methoxyflurane in the body produces both organic fluoride and oxalic acid, but it is the inorganic fluoride that is almost certainly responsible for the renal failure reported following the administration of methoxyflurane.[28] A dose of methoxyflurane that results in a serum inorganic fluoride level of over 50 μmol/L is required to cause this syndrome of vasopressin-resistant polyuria, hypernatremia, serum hyperosmolality, and increased serum urea nitrogen.[29]

Studies on inorganic fluoride levels in obstetric patients following the use of methoxyflurane, either for delivery alone or during labor as an intermittent inhalational analgesic in the late first stage and second stage, have been reported as remaining below the 50 μmol/L mark.[30] Methoxyflurane concentrations of up to 0.5% used during cesarean section produce similarly low levels of inorganic fluoride.[31]

Studies designed to compare the relative analgesic properties of methoxyflurane (0.35%), trichloroethylene (0.35% and 0.5%), and Entonox were not conclusive,[32, 33] and experience in other obstetric units has led to agreement that there is little to choose between the three agents in this respect. It seems that the two major determinants of acceptability and effectiveness are enthusiasm of the local midwifery staff, and the patients' personal reaction to the odor of the analgesic. However, two further points are worth noting. First, the report of a field trial conducted by Rosen and associates[33] referred to the observation that there was a tendency for methoxyflurane to induce restlessness in patients who had been given pethidine previously. Second, although the physical characteristics of methoxyflurane promote the supposition that prolonged intermittent inhalation would lead to an accumulation of the drug in maternal and fetal tissues, it appears that in clinical situations the laboring parturient regulates her intake of methoxyflurane, so that having, after the first few contractions, built up a baseline level of concentration, she inhales a smaller total mass of the agent during subsequent contractions.[34] Also, since trichloroethylene so nearly resembles methoxyflurane in its physical characteristics, a similar maternal feedback response is likely to occur. To date, no investigation of this has been reported.

Enflurane and Isoflurane

Isoflurane[35] and enflurane[36] have both been used as analgesics in obstetrics. Their effectiveness appears to be comparable to a 40:60 to 50:50 nitrous oxide and oxygen mixture. If a high concentration of oxygen is not indicated, they appear to have very little advantage over a 50:50 nitrous oxide and oxygen mixture. Furthermore, in equal MAC doses they appear to exert as much myometrial depression as does halothane.[37]

Abboud and coworkers[38] suggested that enflurane and nitrous oxide were equipotent, but McGuinness and Rosen[39] reported that a small series of volunteer parturients got better pain relief from 1% enflurane than from Entonox. Drowsiness, however, was more apparent with enflurane. These observations were rather surprising because enflurane is not particularly noted for its analgesic properties. It is also curious that the interest in enflurane should coincide with the near demise of two established effective inhalation agents: trichloroethylene and methoxyflurane. Enflurane has no deleterious effect on renal function and serum inorganic fluoride concentrations are not raised.[38]

In a small preliminary series by McLeod and colleagues[40] it was reported that 0.75% isoflurane produced superior analgesia compared with 50% nitrous oxide, but drowsiness, an unpleasant smell, and high cost were potential drawbacks.

GENERAL ANESTHESIA

The use of general anesthesia in the delivery room should be required only very rarely if ever. Administration by unskilled hands should be totally avoided and general anesthesia should never be used for the obstetrician's convenience. Even in locations where regional anesthesia is not available, general anesthesia is rarely required for vaginal delivery. Because of the major problems it poses, it has been abandoned by most practitioners. There are, however, times when it has its value, for example, in the parturient who refuses regional anesthesia or in whom regional anesthesia is contraindicated, or when analgesia by inhalation techniques does not provide sufficient pain relief. General anesthesia may also be required for the application of midcavity forceps or vacuum extractor in locations where epidural and spinal anesthesia are not available. Certain obstetric emergencies may also call for general anesthesia, such as relief of tetanic contraction, breech extraction, version, delivery of a second twin, manual exploration of the uterus, placenta previa, abruptio placentae, and the need for immediate

❖ SUMMARY

Key Points

- The use of inhalational analgesia for labor is no longer common in the U.S.; however, it is still used in other countries. In the U.K., Entonox (nitrous oxide and oxygen mixture) is still administered for labor analgesia, especially in hospitals where regional analgesia is not offered.
- When appropriately administered, 50% nitrous oxide provides pain relief to approximately half of parturients receiving it. Analgesia will not be adequate unless the mother is fully cooperative. To achieve an optimal analgesic effect, intermittent inhalational analgesia with nitrous oxide is required for approximately 45 seconds so that analgesic concentrations of nitrous oxide are present in the brain at the peak of contractions.
- Volatile halogenated agents are not routinely used for labor because of concerns regarding the loss of maternal airway reflexes and subsequent aspiration, uterine relaxation, and the pollution of the labor and delivery suite.

Key Reference

Irestadt L: Current status for nitrous oxide for obstetric pain relief. Acta Anaesthesiol Scand 1994; 38:771–772.

Case Stem

A multiparous patient at 36 weeks' gestation who delivered her last two children with Entonox analgesia at a hospital in the U.K. now requests that she be allowed to use nitrous oxide for her upcoming delivery. Your hospital does not have a policy for its use and has never offered it. How would you handle this situation?

cesarean section. In the presence of fetal distress, induction of general anesthesia can often be performed more rapidly than regional block, especially in the obese parturient.

The disadvantages of general anesthesia are the following:

1. The patient is exposed to the risk of pulmonary aspiration.
2. The placenta is no barrier to general anesthetics and the fetus is exposed to the danger of medullary depression.
3. The mother loses her ability to push.
4. Uterine contractility may be diminished, leading to postpartum hemorrhage.
5. The parturient is exposed to all the other complications of general anesthesia including arrhythmias, hypotension, and respiratory inadequacy.

The dangers of general anesthesia are the same whether it is used for forceps delivery or cesarean section. Certain general principles apply in both situations:

1. The airway must be protected.
2. The possibility of acid aspiration must be prevented.
3. Choice of agents and depth of anesthetic must be carefully gauged to minimize neonatal depression, and staff must be available to administer neonatal resuscitation.
4. Maternal hypotension must be avoided.

References

1. Simpson JY: Anesthesia, Or the Employment of Chloroform and Ether in Surgery, Midwifery, etc. Philadelphia: Lindsay and Blakiston; 1849.
2. Cole PV, Nainby-Luxmore RC: The hazards of gas and air in obstetrics. Anaesthesia 1962; 17:505.
3. Tunstall MF: Obstetric analgesia: the use of a fixed N_2O and O_2 mixture from one cylinder. Lancet 1961; 2:964.
4. Crawford JS, Ellis DB, Hill DW, Payne JP: Effects of cooling on the safety of premixed gases. BMJ 1967; 15:138–142.
5. Bracken A, Broughton GB, Hill DW: Safety precautions to be observed with cooled premixed gases. BMJ 1968; 3:715–716.
6. Waud BE, Waud DR: Calculated kinetics of distribution of nitrous oxide and methoxyflurane during intermittent administration in obstetrics. Anesthesiology 1970; 32:306–316.
7. Caseby N: Epidural analgesia for the surgical induction of labour. Br J Anaesth 1974; 46:747–751.
8. Adrini J: The Pharmacology of Anesthetic Drugs. Springfield, IL: Charles C Thomas; 1950.
9. Flowers CE: Effects of analgesia and anesthesia on the fetus. Clin Obstet Gynecol 1960; 3:890.
10. Fabian LW, Stephen CR, Bourgeois-Gavardin M: Place of trichloroethylene in obstetrical and anesthetic practice. South Med J 1956; 49:808.
11. Morgan HS, Cole F: Trichloroethylene in obstetrics. Obstet Gynecol 1955; 6:416.
12. Flowers CE: Trilene: an adjunct to obstetrical analgesia and anesthesia. Am J Obstet Gynecol 1953; 65:1027.
13. Freedman A: Trichloroethylene-air analgesia in childbirth: an investigation with a suitable inhaler. Lancet 1943; 2:696.
14. Seward EH: Self-administered analgesia during labour with special reference to trichloroethylene. Lancet 1949; 2:781.
15. Dundee JW, Moore J: Alterations in response to somatic pain associated with anaesthesia. IV. Effect of sub-anaesthetic concentration of inhalational agents. Br J Anaesth 1960; 32:453.
16. Flowers CE Jr: Inhalation analgesia and anesthesia and intravenous anesthesia for delivery. *In* Flowers CE Jr: Obstetric Analgesia and Anesthesia. New York: Harper & Row; 1967:136–162.
17. Sheridan CA, Rabson JG: Fluothane in obstetrical anaesthesia. Can Anaesth Soc J 1959; 6:365.
18. Albert C, Anderson G, Wallace W, et al: Fluothane for obstetrical anaesthesia. J Obstet Gynaecol Br Emp 1959; 13:282.
19. Stoelting VK: Fluothane in obstetric anesthesia. Anesth Analg Curr Res 1964; 43:243.
20. Cutter JA, King BD: Use of halothane (Fluothane) in obstetric anesthesia. N Y Med J 1960; 60:503.
21. Cavallaro RJ, Dornetti WHL: Fluoromar anesthesia in obstetrics. Obstet Gynecol 1961; 17:447.
22. Martin EM, Bosnak JN: Trifluoroethylvinyl ether (Fluoroxene, Fluoromar) in obstetrics. Can Anaesth Soc J 1962; 9:419.
23. Boisvert M, Hudon F: Clinical evaluation of methoxyflurane in obstetrical anaesthesia: a report on 500 cases. Can Anaesth Soc J 1962; 9:325.
24. Romagnoli A, Korman D: Methoxyflurane in obstetrical anaesthesia and analgesia. Can Anaesth Soc J 1962; 9:414.
25. Major V, Rosen M, Mushin WW: Concentration of

methoxyflurane for obstetric analgesia by self-administered intermittent inhalation. BMJ 1967; 4:767.
26. Major V, Rosen M, Mushin WW: Methoxyflurane as an obstetric analgesic: a comparison with trichloroethylene. BMJ 1966; 2:1554.
27. Crandell WB, Papper SG, MacDonald A: Nephrotoxicity associated with methoxyflurane anesthesia. Anesthesiology 1966; 27:591.
28. Mazze RI, Toudell JR, Cousins MJ: Methoxyflurane metabolism and renal dysfunction: clinical correlation in man. Anesthesiology 1971; 35:247–252.
29. Cousins MJ, Mazze RI: Methoxyflurane nephrotoxicity: a study of dose-response in man. JAMA 1973; 225:1611–1616.
30. Palahniuk RJ, Cumming M: Plasma fluoride levels following obstetric use of methoxyflurane. Can Anaesth Soc J 1975; 22:291–297.
31. Young SR, Stoelting RK, Bond VK, Peterson C: Methoxyflurane biotransformation and renal function following methoxyflurane administration for vaginal delivery or cesarean section. Anesth Analg 1976; 55:415–419.
32. Jones PL, Rosen M, Mushin WW, et al: Methoxyflurane and nitrous oxide as obstetric analgesics. II. A comparison by self-administered intermittent inhalation. BMJ 1969; 3:259–262.
33. Rosen M, Mushin WW, Jones PL, et al: Field trial of methoxyflurane, nitrous oxide and trichloroethylene as obstetric analgesics. BMJ 1969; 3:263–267.
34. Latto IP, Rosen M, Molloy MJ: Absence of accumulation of methoxyflurane during intermittent self-administration for pain relief in labour. Br J Anaesth 1972; 44:391–400.
35. Hicks JS, Shnider SM, Cohen H: Isoflurane (Forane) analgesia in obstetrics [abstracts of scientific papers]. Presented at the Annual Meeting of the American Society of Anesthesiologists, Chicago, IL, Oct 1975:99–100.
36. Ball GF, Marcias-Loza MD, Cohen H: Enflurane analgesia in obstetrics [abstracts of scientific papers]. Presented at the Society for Obstetric Anesthesia and Perinatology, Orlando, FL, 1976.
37. Munson ES, Embro WJ: Enflurane, isoflurane and halothane and isolated human uterine muscle. Anesthesiology 1977; 46:11–14.
38. Abboud TK, Shnider SM, Wright RH: Enflurane analgesia in obstetrics. Anesth Analg Curr Res 1981; 60:133–137.
39. McGuinness C, Rosen M: Enflurane as an analgesic in labour. Anaesthesia 1984; 39:24–26.
40. McLeod DD, Ramayya GP, Tunstall ME: Self-administered isoflurane in labour: a comparative study with Entonox. Anaesthesia 1985; 40:424–426.

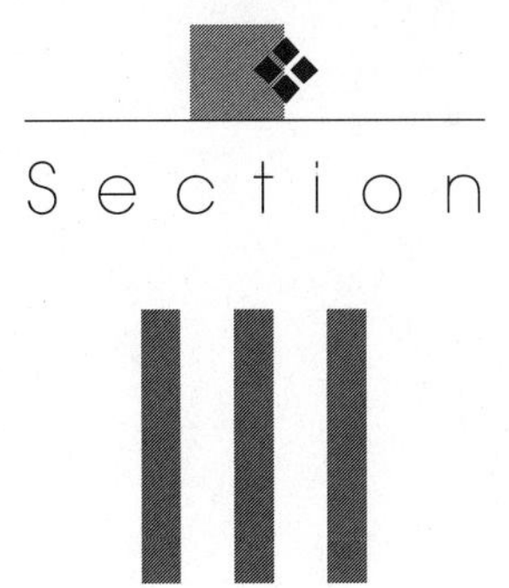

Operative Anesthesia

17

General Anesthesia for Cesarean Section

❖ Marewenteiti Ali Biribo, DSM(Fiji), DA(UP&FSM), FPBA

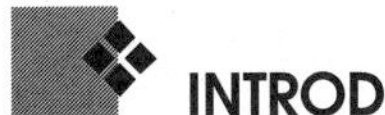

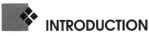

INTRODUCTION

Although regional anesthesia is the preferred method for cesarean section in the healthy woman, general anesthesia is still necessary in selected cases. In the United States, approximately 15% of cesarean sections are performed under general anesthesia, although that number is decreasing.[1] The frequency of use of general anesthesia is dependent on many factors, including the percentage of parturients who receive epidural analgesia, the percentage of high-risk parturients, and the skills of the particular anesthesiologist.

INDICATIONS AND CONSIDERATIONS FOR GENERAL ANESTHESIA

General anesthesia is not routinely used for elective cesarean section but is still necessary for certain obstetric and maternal conditions. Table 17–1 reviews indications for the use of general anesthesia.

The choice of anesthetic technique and the method of delivery must be appropriate to the clinical situation. The indications for general anesthesia vary greatly between individual hospitals. In Fiji, the indications for general anesthesia are most often dystocia and fetal "distress." When time is the limiting factor, general anesthesia is sometimes necessary because it offers speed of induction, reliability, controllability, reproducibility, and avoidance of sympathectomy-induced hypotension. Patient refusal should not be a major factor in choice of anesthetic technique if the anesthesiologist presents the patient with all the necessary information to make an informed decision. A recent survey suggested that many women who are given general anesthesia are not given a choice. In emergency situations, allowing the patient a choice may not be realistic.[2] The problems associated with general anesthesia principally involve failed intubation and aspiration. As discussed in Chapter 2, the physiologic changes of pregnancy may increase the incidence of failed intubation and its associated maternal morbidity and mortality.

The physiologic changes affecting the gastrointestinal system and the accompanying anatomic changes include decreased gastric and intestinal motility, relaxation of lower esophageal sphincter tone, increased intra-abdominal pressure, and increased gastric acid secretion. Since general anesthesia is often necessary for obstetric emergencies, many patients will not be fasting. With the pathophysiologic changes described, parturients should also be considered to be at risk for aspiration. The often emergent nature of the obstetric situation requiring general anesthesia may present numerous dilemmas but should never compromise an anesthesiologist's preoperative evaluation.

Table 17–1 INDICATIONS FOR GENERAL ANESTHESIA

Contraindications to regional anesthesia
Massive hemorrhage
Hemodynamic instability
Maternal coagulopathy
Sepsis
Fetal "distress"
Patient refusal
Failed block

Preparation for General Anesthesia

Airway Evaluation

Physical factors, including weight gain, enlarged breasts, and the other physiologic changes of pregnancy, can complicate endotracheal intubation. Associated anatomic changes of the oropharynx and tracheobronchial tree may make intubation even more difficult. Certain disease states, such as preeclampsia, may also predispose to difficult intubation.[3] Preanesthetic evaluation must always start with a complete evaluation of the mother's airway. To decrease the risks associated with general anesthesia, it is vital to identify patients with problematic airways early, so that regional anesthesia with a catheter can be utilized early, thus precluding the use of general anesthesia. It has been reported that airway evaluation can usually identify the patient with a difficult airway and was not performed in up to 10% of cases in which mortality occurred.[4] Rocke et al.[5] evaluated the risk factors associated with difficult intubation in obstetric patients and suggested that the largest risks were associated with a Mallampati IV airway classification and mandibular recession. Active labor can also change the Mallampati views after an initial airway evaluation has occurred.[6, 7] Airway evaluation is discussed in greater detail in Chapters 32 and 37.

Aspiration Prophylaxis

Pharmacologic agents are available to decrease the risk of acid aspiration associated with induction of general anesthesia. Although no agent or combination of agents can guarantee that a parturient will not aspirate or develop pneumonitis following a failed intubation, there are several agents that can dramatically decrease these risks. Antacids are the mainstay of treatment because animal evidence suggests that the acidity of the pulmonary aspirate is the most important factor.[8] Administration of 30 mL of 0.3 M sodium citrate increases the pH of intragastric contents, and because it is nonparticulate it does not increase the risk of pneumonitis.[9, 10] The simultaneous administration of an H_2-blocking agent such as ranitidine will maintain prolonged intragastric alkalinization.[11] This effect is not immediate, however, and becomes significant only after 2 hours. Metoclopramide is often administered before induction of general anesthesia to further decrease the risk of aspiration. Given intravenously, it produces an increase in lower esophageal sphincter tone and a reduction in residual gastric volume.[12]

Experienced Personnel

The anesthesiologist's experience is an important factor in anesthetic-related maternal mortality.[4] A recent study reviewed a 17-year experience in a teaching hospital and reported that most cases of failed intubation occurred when patients were cared for by less experienced anesthesiologists.[13] Proper application of cricoid pressure (Sellick's maneuver[14]) by a skilled assistant facilitates tracheal intubation and reduces gastric aspiration.

Backup Plans and Failed-Airway Algorithm

Anesthesiologists must be aware that failed intubations do occur and must be able to react immediately in such an event. Appropriate planning is essential and includes the use of alternative methods in the patient with a known or suspected difficult airway. These include awake intubation, fiberoptic intubation, and surgical airway. Should failed intubation occur, the anesthesiologist should know an algorithm for airway management. Management of the failed intubation is discussed in detail in Chapter 32.

Preoxygenation (Denitrogenation)

The induction of general anesthesia is associated with varying degrees of apnea.[15] Filling the lungs with 100% oxygen will delay the onset of hypoxemia following induction of anesthesia. A well-applied, tight-fitting mask is required for denitrogenation with 100% oxygen for 3 minutes or four maximal breaths.[16] Table 17–2 illustrates the changes that occur following preoxygenation. Parturients drop their Pa_{O_2} by about 80 mm Hg per minute when under anesthesia.[15] Marx and Mateo[17] confirmed that maximal fetal oxygenation occurs at Pa_{O_2} of approximately 300 mm Hg including normal blood gases.

Fetal Considerations

Current evidence suggests that normal blood gases as well as acid-base status are similar whether the fetus is delivered by regional or general anesthesia, in babies weighing more than 2500 g.[18] In a study of emergency cesarean section deliveries due to fetal "distress," the neonatal blood gas and acid-base values were similar in the regional and general anesthesia groups.[19] Ong et al.[20] showed that Apgar scores of babies born by cesarean section either electively or emergently under general anesthesia have a higher percentage of neurobehavioral depression. Abboud et al.[21] found that general anesthesia reduces neurobehavioral scores in the first 24 hours. Briefly, the following steps must be carried out to ensure optimal fetal outcome:

1. Acute maternal denitrogenation
2. Adoption of the lateral uterine displacement position to prevent aortocaval compression
3. Preinduction fluid loading to avoid maternal hypotension
4. Prevention of maternal hypocarbia

UTERINE INCISION TO DELIVERY TIME

Crawford et al.,[22] in 1973, reported the significance of prompt delivery of the fetus within a certain time following uterine incision. This observation was confirmed by Datta et al.[23] in 1981, when they demonstrated that neonates delivered after 3 minutes following uterine incision had lower Apgar scores and acidotic blood gases. Factors such as maternal catecholamine release in relation to uterine incision, vasoconstrictor prostaglandin release from fetus and perhaps

Table 17–2 PULMONARY CHANGES THAT OCCUR AFTER PREOXYGENATION

		3 Minutes	Four Deep Breaths
Baseline	Pa_{O_2}	101	103
	Pc_{O_2}	31	32
Post-denitrogenation	Pa_{O_2}	376	408
	Pc_{O_2}	32	31
Post-intubation	Pa_{O_2}	264	313
	Pa_{CO_2}	40	40

from placental separation, including contraction of the myometrial muscles, probably result in uterine artery spasm and consequent fetal compromise.

CONDUCT OF GENERAL ANESTHESIA

Basic Preparation

- Check the anesthesia machine, including back-up cylinders, for oxygen and nitrous oxide and vaporizers.
- Check monitors, including capnography.
- Draw up clearly labeled induction and emergency drugs, including vasopressors.
- Prepare fluid warmers.
- Have a difficult-intubation cart available.
- Recheck the laryngoscopes.
- Load all endotracheal tubes with stylets, check balloons to make sure that there are no leaks.
- Set out assorted face masks and oropharyngeal airways.
- Check suction.
- Have a skilled assistant ready.
- Check for intravenous line function.

Positioning

- Lay patient in the supine position with a wedge under the right hip.
- Table must be able to allow Trendelenburg positioning.

Monitors

- Connect electrocardiographic electrodes, blood pressure cuff, pulse oximeter probe.
- Connect capnograph.
- Check that Foley contents can be seen.

Denitrogenation

As previously discussed, the patient must breathe 100% O_2. The basis for this is to wash out nitrogen from the lungs and to raise both the maternal and fetal Po_2 by increasing oxygen saturation. Ninety-eight percent nitrogen can be washed out within 80 seconds in a parturient.[24] In urgent situations, the parturient should be instructed to take four deep breaths while keeping the face mask firmly in position.

Induction

Rapid sequence induction is the standard technique, starting with sodium thiopental 3 to 5 mg/kg body weight intravenously. Ketamine hydrochloride 1 to 1.5 mg IV, or propofol 1 to 2.5 mg/kg IV may also be used to induce general anesthesia. Thiopental is the most frequently used induction agent for cesarean section in the United States. Thiopental appears in the fetal blood within 45 seconds of maternal administration, with fetal drug concentrations peaking at less than 3 minutes.[25] Rapid redistribution and nonuniform intervillous blood flow are responsible for the wide variability in ratios of umbilical venous and maternal venous blood thiopental concentrations.[26] Ketamine is generally selected for cases in which there is significant maternal hemorrhage or in parturients with asthma. Apgar scores are similar in neonates delivered after induction of anesthesia with ketamine 1 mg/kg or thiopental (3 mg/kg).[27] Ketamine in doses of greater than 2 mg/kg is associated with neonatal depression.[28] Etomidate, though not routinely used for induction of general anesthesia for cesarean section, has been used and may have a place in the management of the parturient who could not handle cardiorespiratory perturbations.[29] Propofol is an intravenous agent that provides a rapid induction and rapid awakening. It is a lipophilic agent with a low molecular weight that rapidly crosses the placenta. Propofol has been used to induce general anesthesia for cesarean section[30] but is associated with a greater potential for hypotension than thiopental.[31] There is controversy regarding whether propofol produces neurobehavioral changes.[32] Propofol does not appear to have any significant advantage over thiopental for induction of general anesthesia in the healthy parturient and it is also much more expensive than thiopental.

Succinylcholine 1 to 1.5 mg/kg is used for neuromuscular blockade to facilitate intubation. Succinylcholine is rapidly metabolized by plasma pseudocholinesterase. Although the levels of plasma pseudocholinesterase are decreased in pregnancy, recovery from an intubating dose of succinylcholine is unchanged in the pregnant patient, perhaps in part due to the parturient's increased volume of distribution.[33] Cricoid pressure is applied until successful cannulation of the trachea, inflation of the cuff, and confirmation of correct positioning are achieved. Breath sounds must be appreciated bilaterally before the cricoid pressure is released, to rule out endobronchial intubation. If intubation fails, cricoid pressure must be maintained until either the patient is awakened or the trachea is intubated by an alternative means. The use of prefasciculating doses of nondepolarizing agents before administration of succinylcholine is not standard practice, in part because pregnancy decreases the incidence of fasciculations[34] and also because pretreatment has not been found to decrease the incidence of myalgias. Rapacuronium, a newly introduced nondepolarizing muscle relaxant with fast onset, may prove to be an alternative to succinylcholine in the parturient undergoing general anesthesia.

Maintenance

Inhalational agents can be administered to maintain general anesthesia during the cesarean section. Nitrous oxide should be limited to 50% until delivery. The volatile agent should be discontinued following delivery to prevent postpartum hemorrhage due to the uterine relaxant effect of volatile agents. Oxytocin (20–30 U/L IV fluid) should be administered following delivery. After delivery, an intravenous opioid should be administered and the nitrous oxide increased to 70%. Muscle relaxation can be provided by continuous infusion of succinylcholine or nondepolarizing neuromuscular blockade.

Benzodiazepines are also advisable following delivery to ensure amnesia. The obstetric anesthesiologist should be aware of the potential for maternal awareness during general anesthesia. This problem is particularly prevalent during the period between induction and delivery of the infant, when the 50% nitrous oxide is the only amnestic agent being used and is associated with high awareness rates.[35] The use of a volatile agent, such as 0.5 MAC of isoflurane, will decrease the risk of intraoperative awareness to less than 1%.[36] Recent studies have reported the safe use of sevoflurane and desflurane for maintenance of general anesthesia for cesarean section, but they have not been found to offer advantages as compared with isoflurane.[37, 38]

❖ SUMMARY

Key Points

- Regional anesthesia techniques are usually utilized for cesarean section; however, general anesthesia continues to be essential in certain scenarios, such as dire fetal "distress," maternal hemorrhage and hypovolemia, and coagulopathy.
- When administering general anesthesia to a parturient, the anesthesiologist should attempt to minimize the risks of failed intubation and aspiration. This includes an adequate preoperative assessment, denitrogenation, and rapid sequence induction with cricoid pressure.
- Although thiopental readily crosses the placenta, peak barbiturate concentrations in the fetal brain are generally below the threshold for depression. This is explained by many factors, including the preferential uptake of thiopental by the fetal liver, the rapid redistribution of the drug back into maternal tissues, and the higher relative water content of the fetal brain.
- Ketamine, in doses of less than 1.5 mg/kg, is the induction agent of choice for the asthmatic or hypotensive parturient.

Key Reference

Hawkins JL, et al.: Anesthesia-related deaths during obstetric delivery in the United States, 1979–1990. Anesthesiology 1997; 86:277–284.

Case Stem

A patient is to undergo an emergency cesarean section for acute hemorrhage secondary to abruptio placentae. Her estimated blood loss is 2000 mL, and her blood pressure is 70/40. The fetal heart rate is 70. Discuss your proposed anesthetic management for this cesarean section.

Reversal

The stomach must be emptied via an orogastric tube. The succinylcholine infusion should be discontinued or the nondepolarizing neuromuscular blockade reversed (e.g., with neostigmine and glycopyrrolate). When ventilatory exchange is appropriate and the patient is awake, extubation can be accomplished. If, however, the patient is considered unstable, the endotracheal tube should remain in place. Intermittent intramuscular opioids still can play a significant role in pain relief, especially in the underdeveloped countries, but its efficacy is inferior when compared with the current alternatives of epidural opioids or intravenous patient-controlled analgesia.[39–41]

Postoperative Pain Relief

The subject of postoperative pain relief is covered in Chapter 24. It is important to realize that following a general anesthetic the patient will need active management of analgesia, unlike with regional anesthesia, in which the block continues to provide pain relief in the early recovery period.

CONSIDERATIONS FOR GENERAL ANESTHESIA

As in any other situation, certain fundamental steps must be executed to prevent delays and to facilitate delivery of a fetus in the presence of maternal disease or ongoing fetal emergencies, including fetal distress, prolapsed cord, or sudden intrauterine death. Maternal conditions include obstructed labor, hemorrhage, preeclampsia, asthma, and sepsis. Irrespective of whether the delivery is elective or urgent, delays must be minimized. Communication between anesthesiologists, obstetricians, and labor nurses is essential to ensure optimal care for these patients.

References

1. Hawkins JL, Gibbs C, Orleans M, et al: Obstetric Anesthesia Workforce Survey. Anesthesiology 1997; 87:135–143.
2. Ngan Kee WD, Hung VYS, Roach VJ, Law TK: A survey of factors influencing patients' choices of anaesthesia for caesarean section. Aust N Z J Obstet Gynaecol 1997; 37:300–303.
3. Dupont X, Hamza J, Julien P, et al: Is pregnancy-induced hypertension a risk factor for difficult intubation? [Abstract.] Anesthesiology 1990; 73:A985.
4. Morgan M: Anaesthetic contribution to maternal mortality. Br J Anaesth 1987; 59:842–855.
5. Rocke DA, Murray WB, Rout CC, Gouws E: Relative risk analysis of factors associated with difficult intubation in obstetric anesthesia. Anesthesiology 1992; 77:67–73.
6. Mallampati SR, Gatt SP, Gugino LD, et al: A clinical sign to predict difficult tracheal intubation: A prospective study. Can Anaesth Soc J 1985; 32:429–434.
7. Farcon EL, Kim MH, Marx GF: Changing Mallampati score during labour. Can J Anaesth 1994; 41:50–51.
8. James CF, Modell JH, Gibbs CP, et al: Pulmonary aspiration: Effects of volume and pH in the rat. Anesth Analg 1984; 63:665–668.
9. Gibbs CP, Spohr L, Schmidt D: The effectiveness of sodium citrate as an antacid. Anesthesiology 1982; 57:44–46.

10. O'Sullivan GM, Bullingham RE: Non-invasive assessment by radiotelemetry of antacid effect during labor. Anesth Analg 1985; 64:95–100.
11. Thompson EM, Loughran PG, McAuley DM, et al: Combined treatment with ranitidine and saline antacids prior to obstetric anaesthesia. Anaesthesia 1984; 39:1086–1090.
12. Bylsma-Howell M, Riggs KW, McMorland GH, et al: Placental transport of metoclopramide: Assessment of maternal and neonatal effects. Can Anaesth Soc J 1983; 30:487–492.
13. Hawthorne L, Wilson R, Lyons G, et al: Failed intubation revisited: 17-year experience in a teaching maternity unit. Br J Anaesth 1996; 76:680–684.
14. Sellick BA: Cricoid pressure to control regurgitation of stomach contents during induction of anaesthesia. Lancet 1961; 2:404–406.
15. Archer GW, Marx GF: Arterial oxygen tension during apnea in parturient women. Br J Anaesth 1974; 46:358–360.
16. Russell GN, Smith CL, Snowdon SL, et al: Preoxygenation and the parturient patient. Anaesthesia 1987; 42:346–351.
17. Marx GF, Mateo CV: Effects of different oxygen concentrations during general anaesthesia for elective caesarean section. Can Anaesth Soc J 1971; 18:587–593.
18. Evans CM, Murphy F, Gray OP, et al: Epidural versus general anaesthesia for elective Caesarean section. Anaesthesia 1989; 44:778–782.
19. Marx GF, Luykx WM, Cohen S: Fetal-neonatal status following caesarean section for fetal distress. Br J Anaesth 1984; 56:1009–1013.
20. Ong BY, Cohen MM, Palahniuk RJ: Anaesthesia for Caesarean section—effects on neonates. Anesth Analg 1989; 68:270–275.
21. Abboud TK, Nagappala S, Muratawa K, et al: Comparison of the effects of general and regional anaesthesia for caesarean section on neurologic and adaptive capacity scores. Anesth Analg 1985; 64:996–1000.
22. Crawford JS, Burton M, Davies P: Anaesthesia for section: Further refinements of a technique. Br J Anaesth 1973; 45:726–732.
23. Datta S, Ostheimer GW, Weiss JB, et al: Neonatal effect of prolonged anesthetic induction for cesarean section. Obstet Gynecol 1981; 58:331–335.
24. Byrne F, Oduro-Dominah A, Kipling R: The effect of pregnancy on pulmonary nitrogen wash-out: a short study of preoxygenation. Anaesthesia 1987; 42:148–150.
25. McKechnie FB, Converse J: Placental transmission of thiopental. Am J Obstet Gynecol 1955; 71:639–644.
26. Datta S, Alper MA: Anesthesia for cesarean section. Anesthesiology 1980; 53:142–160.
27. Peltz B, Sinclair DM: Induction agents for caesarean section: A comparison of thiopentone and ketamine. Anaesthesia 1973; 28:37–42.
28. Chantigian RC, Ostheimer GW: Effects of maternally administered drugs in the fetus and newborn. *In* Freidman E (ed): Advances in Perinatal Medicine, Vol 5. New York: Plenum; 1986:181.
29. Downing JW, Buley RJR, Brock-Utne JG, Houlton PC: Etomidate for induction of anesthesia at cesarean section: Comparison with thiopentone. Br J Anaesth 1979; 51:135–140.
30. Valtonen M, Kanto J, Rosenberg P: Comparison of propofol and thiopentone for induction of anaesthesia for elective Caesarean section. Anaesthesia 1989; 44:758–762.
31. Capogna G, Celleno D, Sebastiani M, et al: Propofol and thiopentone for cesarean section: maternal effects and neonatal outcome. Int J Obstet Anesth 1991; 1:19.
32. Celleno D, Capogna G, Tomassetti M, et al: Neurobehavioural effects of propofol on the neonate following elective caesarean section. Br J Anaesth 1989; 62:649–654.
33. Leighton BL, Cheek TG, Gross JB, et al: Succinylcholine pharmacodynamics in peripartum patients. Anesthesiology 1986; 64:202–205.
34. Cook WP, Schultetus RR, Caton D: A comparison of d-tubocurarine pretreatment and no pretreatment in obstetric patients. Anesth Analg 1987; 66:756–760.
35. Crawford JS: Awareness during operative obstetrics under general anesthesia. Br J Anaesth 1971; 43:179–182.
36. Tunstall ME: The reduction of amnesic wakefulness during caesarean section. Anaesthesia 1979; 34:316–319.
37. Gambling DR, Sharma SK, White PF, et al: Use of sevoflurane during elective cesarean birth: A comparison with isoflurane and spinal anesthesia. Anesth Analg 1995; 81:90.
38. Abboud TK, Zhu M, Peres E, et al: Desflurane: A new volatile anesthetic for cesarean section: maternal and neonatal effects. Acta Anaesthesiol Scand 1995; 39:723–726.
39. Eisenbach JC, Grice SC, Dewan DM: Patient-controlled analgesia following caesarean section: a comparison with epidural and intramuscular narcotics. Anesthesiology 1988; 68:444–448.
40. Harrison DM, Sinatra R, Morgese L, Chung JH: Epidural narcotic and patient-controlled analgesia for post-caesarean pain relief. Anesthesiology 1988; 68:454–457.
41. Cade L, Ashley J: Towards optimal analgesia after caesarean section: comparison of epidural and intravenous patient-controlled opioid analgesia. Anaesth Intensive Care 1993; 21:416–419.

18

Regional Anesthesia for Cesarean Section

❖ CHRISTOPHER C. ROUT, FRCA

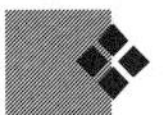

INTRODUCTION

Recent decades have seen the development of regional anesthesia as the method of choice for cesarean delivery. In terms of safety, indirect evidence from mortality reports suggests that regional anesthesia is safer than general anesthesia for the mother, and direct evidence from studies comparing the two techniques has demonstrated advantages for the neonate associated with well-conducted regional anesthesia. However, there are times when regional techniques are contraindicated. Disturbing aspects of increased use of regional anesthesia are the decreased exposure of trainees to general anesthesia for obstetrics and the increased proportion of general anesthetics being administered to patients with severe comorbidity.[1] It is important that obstetric anesthesia be developed worldwide as a specialty with adequate expert supervision and training, lest these factors cause increased mortality with general anesthesia to be a self-fulfilling prophecy.

Choice between epidural and spinal anesthesia is mostly dictated by circumstances. There is very little difference between the two techniques regarding maternal and neonatal outcome, but spinal anesthesia tends to give better operative analgesia and because it is a simpler technique, with lower drug dosage, there are fewer things that can go wrong. Epidural anesthesia, however, is increasingly being used in patients with epidural catheters presited for labor analgesia. No anesthetic method is without limitations and hazards, and the techniques and drugs that anesthesiologists use are continually being modified in an attempt to surmount the challenges posed. As our knowledge and understanding of central neuronal transmission of pain has increased, so has the array of agents being injected into the epidural space and the subarachnoid space. Often, for every problem solved a new one is created, for example, the use of neuraxial opiates and their association with pruritus.

Spinal and epidural anesthesia each have advantages and disadvantages. Combined spinal-epidural (CSE) techniques have been developed in the hope of combining the advantages of both techniques, without the disadvantages of either. Whether this can be achieved remains to be seen. Currently problems associated with each component of the CSE technique are still featured in published reports, and the combined technique presents more new challenges. Combined spinal-epidural anesthesia has gained wide acceptance by both patients and practitioners in a relatively short time since its introduction into obstetric practice. It is a welcome addition to the range of techniques available to the obstetric anesthetist and increases the flexibility of regional anesthesia.

GENERAL VERSUS REGIONAL ANESTHESIA

The Mother

Epidemiologic considerations have played a major role in the trend from general to regional anesthesia for cesarean section. The series of triennial *Confidential Enquiries into Maternal Deaths in the United Kingdom*[2, 3] has documented an overall reduction in anesthesia-related mortality despite increasing numbers of deliveries and an increasing cesarean section rate. These reports have been dominated by mortality associated with general anesthesia, in particular, pulmonary aspiration of gastric contents and difficulties with tracheal intubation. This has led to a perception that anesthetic risk is greater with general than regional anesthesia. However, it has been argued[4] that the continuing downward trend in anesthetic mortality in the United Kingdom has been associated with increasing cesarean section rates and a relatively static number of general anesthetics. Thus, there may be factors responsible for improved obstetric anesthesia safety other than the use of regional anesthesia, and in the United Kingdom at any rate, general anesthesia has also been associated with an improved safety record. There is very little, if any, direct evidence that regional anesthesia is inherently safer than general anesthesia for cesarean section.

The best evidence for increased safety of regional anesthesia comes from the United States. The American Society of Anesthesiologists' Closed Claims Study demonstrated that maternal death claims were largely due to complications of general anesthesia.[5] More significantly, in the first national review of anesthesia-related maternal deaths, Hawkins and colleagues[6] clearly demonstrated an increase in the case-fatality risk ratio of general to regional anesthesia between the periods 1979 to 1984 and 1985 to 1990. This was partly due to reduced risk associated with regional anesthesia. At the same time, the mortality rate associated with general anesthesia increased, despite reduced use of the technique.[6]

With the current trend favoring the use of regional anesthesia in obstetrics, the use of general anesthesia may be increasingly confined to patients with associated disease. In a series of over 500 consecutive cases of general anesthesia for cesarean section, Tsen and coworkers[8] documented a constant proportion of general anesthetics used between 1990 and 1995, set against a gradually reducing obstetric workload. During the period studied, however, the indications for general anesthesia for cesarean section relating to maternal disease increased from 17.2% to 35%.

The reduced use of general anesthesia in obstetrics has implications for both trainees and occasional practitioners, in whom the required level of expertise may be insufficiently developed or maintained. A clear difference in practice is seen between the United States and the United Kingdom. In 1992 general anesthesia was used in approximately 12% to 22% of cesarean deliveries in the United States[7] and approximately 44% in the United Kingdom[4] (the latter including 29% of elective cases). Overall maternal mortality associated with elective cesarean section is not much different from that associated with vaginal delivery (90 per million compared with 60 per million[2]), whereas emergency cesarean section has consistently emerged as a risk factor. Morbidity is also much higher following emergency (24.2%) compared with elective (4.7%) cesarean delivery, with an 11-fold difference in the incidence of major complications.[9] Another transatlantic difference in practice is the continuing provision of obstetric anesthesia care in the United States by nonanesthesiologists practicing without the supervision of an anesthesiologist. In 1992 approximately 25% of anesthetics for cesarean section were provided by independent nurse anesthetists not medically directed by an anesthesiologist.[7] In contrast, the United Kingdom has seen an increasing involvement of experienced anesthesiologists in obstetric anesthesia[10] and has eliminated the provision of obstetric anesthesia care by anyone other than anesthesiologists trained or in training. Despite this, lack of experience is still cited as a factor in anesthesia-related mortality. Nevertheless, the Confidential Enquiry for the triennium 1994 to 1996[3] reported only one death directly attributable to anesthesia (associated with a regional technique), a truly remarkable achievement.

Thus, there is epidemiologic evidence of an association between increased use of regional techniques and decreasing maternal mortality, and an overall increased risk ratio of mortality for general anesthesia compared with regional anesthesia. Despite this epidemiologic evidence, it is not possible to apply these general data directly to an individual patient. Given a normal healthy woman requiring elective cesarean section under the care of an experienced anesthesiologist, there is probably little difference between general and regional anesthesia in terms of mortality risk. Nevertheless, collective experience suggests that the unpredictable complications of general anesthesia are more likely to result in an adverse outcome compared with those occurring during regional anesthesia.

Regional anesthesia does offer several clear advantages. The most frequently cited causes of maternal mortality are pulmonary aspiration of gastric contents and difficulty with or failure of tracheal intubation. Both these complications can be avoided by the use of regional anesthesia. Aspiration is still possible during regional anesthesia but requires the combination of gastric regurgitation with obtunded laryngeal reflexes owing to sedation or to profound hypotension or hypoxia (either of which must be treated promptly and may require tracheal intubation and ventilation). All patients requiring cesarean delivery should therefore receive preoperative nonparticulate antacid prophylaxis. The argument that unexpectedly high motor block may demand immediate intubation in patients with potentially difficult airways receiving regional anesthesia is not sufficient reason to avoid regional blockade in these patients. However, facilities for management of difficult or failed intubation should always be available, even when regional anesthesia is being used.

Although uncomplicated surgical delivery does not usually cause sufficient blood loss to require transfusion, epidural anesthesia is associated with significantly less bleeding than general anesthesia.[11] An additional hazard of general anesthesia is the rare but devastating problem of intraoperative awareness. Although the incidence has decreased following the reintroduction of volatile agents as part of the technique, it remains a danger with the light anesthesia used for cesarean delivery.

In Western society regional anesthesia has become the method of maternal choice for cesarean delivery. In maintaining consciousness, the mother remains part of the delivery process. The presence of the child's father, routinely allowed during regional but not general anesthesia, provides emotional support at a time when the mother is feeling most vulnerable. In addition to the psychologic advantage, early maternal-child contact may enhance bonding, increase self-confidence, and improve success and subsequent infant care and breast-feeding.[12, 13]

In non-Western societies, however, cultural and religious influences may create a reluctance to be awake during an embarrassing or proscribed public display, and the presence of the father during childbirth may be unthinkable. With increasing migration and pluralism in Western society, these influences may create a conflict with current anesthetic practice and standards of care. In situations in which the mother insists on general anesthesia, her wishes should be respected and she should not be made to feel that she is increasing the risk to her child, which only increases internal conflict and anxiety.

Fetal and Neonatal Considerations

The baby can be affected directly by transplacental drug transfer or indirectly by alteration of fetal-placental perfusion, or both. The risk of direct effects from placental transfer are greatest with general anesthesia, because maternal drug exposure is greater, but it might also occur with epidural anesthesia, particularly when a preexisting labor epidural catheter is "topped up" for cesarean delivery. Although the direct effects of general anesthesia are short-lived following delivery, they may become significant, particularly in the premature or low birthweight baby. Early neonatal sedation can adversely affect onset of respiration, thermoregulation, and feeding. Indirect effects, on the other hand, have the potential for more permanent harm, for example, intrauterine fetal asphyxia due to prolonged hypotension or maternal hypoxia.

Studies of the effects of general or regional anesthesia on the baby have used various means of assessment including cardiotocography, uteroplacental blood flow, fetal arterial flow velocity waveforms, acid-base status at delivery, Apgar scores, and neurobehavioral scoring systems. Ultimately, the most important outcome variables are perinatal morbidity and mortality and long-term assessment of child development. However, the large numbers required for prospective studies are prohibitive, and few studies exist. Also it is impossible to control for the various environmental factors influencing child development, and it is unlikely that mode of anesthesia for cesarean section could be isolated as an independent risk factor.

Cardiotocographic studies have occasionally demonstrated direct effects of epidurally administered local anesthetic agents on fetal heart rate variability, but most studies have been performed in laboring patients and are subject to various interpretations. Although it is true that changes in fetal heart rate and heart rate variability can occur following the administration of anesthesia, they are usually short-lived.[14–18] The most common abnormalities seen are loss of variability and occasional decelerations, but increased beat-to-beat variability[14] and fetal tachycardia[15] have also been observed. Changes in fetal heart rate patterns owing to direct placental transfer are probably unimportant and certainly negligible compared with the changes that can transpire secondary to maternal physiologic derangement as can occur during untreated hypotension or aortocaval compression. Severe or prolonged hypotension commonly causes fetal bradycardia. Maternal systolic blood pressures below 70 mm Hg[19] or below 80 mm Hg for 4 minutes or more may cause fetal bradycardia. Transient or less severe hypotension is unlikely to result in fetal heart rate changes.

Studies of uteroplacental blood flow generally have shown either no adverse effects or even an improvement in perfusion during regional anesthesia, provided that hypotension does not occur. Placental intervillous blood flow is largely dependent on maternal arterial pressure and cardiac output. Radioisotope studies have demonstrated no significant decrease in intervillous blood flow associated with subarachnoid blockade for elective cesarean section[20] accompanied by liberal intravenous ephedrine and volume preloading. Epidural anesthesia may be associated with a reduction in placental blood flow, directly related to changes in mean arterial pressure, which is preventable by prophylactic ephedrine.[21] Intravenous colloid volume preloading may also prevent a decrease in placental blood flow associated with epidural anesthesia for cesarean section, again by preventing hypotension.[22] In the presence of pregnancy-induced hypertension, epidural anesthesia can improve maternal hemodynamics[23] and actually increase intervillous blood flow.[24]

Hypotension associated with either epidural[25] or spinal[26] anesthesia may decrease maternal cardiac output leading to reduced uterine blood flow. Fetal aortic or umbilical blood flow may be unaffected by epidural anesthesia[27] or may increase.[28] Umbilical and placental vascular resistance may decrease slightly.[29] No significant changes in fetal blood flow occur if blood pressure is maintained under spinal anesthesia.[30]

In summary, indices of uteroplacental and fetal blood flow are either unchanged or slightly improved by regional anesthesia, provided that maternal blood pressure and cardiac output are maintained.

General anesthesia, on the other hand, is associated with a maternal adrenergic response[31] that may lead to uteroplacental vasoconstriction and decreased placental blood flow. These changes may impair fetal oxygenation and worsen preexisting fetal compromise. Jouppila and associates[32] demonstrated reduced placental blood flow following general anesthesia induction with thiopental, 4 mg/kg, for elective cesarean section. Measurement of intervillous blood flow was made before intubation, which is a major stimulus to adrenergic response; thus their observation was probably a direct pharmacologic effect of thiopental. Adverse effects of adrenergic stimulation on uterine blood flow have been demonstrated in animal models.[33–35]

Ideally, the best combination is low maternal catecholamine concentrations with preserved fetal and neonatal adrenergic responses, which assist in the transition from intrauterine to extrauterine life.[36] While general anesthetics tend to suppress the fetal adrenergic stress response,[37] neonatal catecholamine concentrations are higher following cesarean delivery under epidural compared with general anesthesia.[38]

Blood gas and acid-base status at delivery, obtained from a double-clamped segment of umbilical cord, tend to reflect the indirect effects of anesthetic techniques on the fetus rather than direct pharmacologic effects. Thus, provided that conditions which may lead to intrauterine fetal asphyxia (aortocaval compression, maternal hypoxia or hyperventilation, hypotension, adrenergic stress response) are avoided, there should be no difference in umbilical blood gas status between general and regional anesthesia. This is generally the case with both elective and emergency cesarean sections.[39–46] In the case of emergency cesarean delivery for presumptive acute "fetal distress," umbilical arterial pH at delivery is usually higher than that obtained from a predelivery scalp sample, irrespective of method of anesthesia.[46] Presumably this is due to lower maternal catecholamine concentrations during anesthesia compared with those during labor.[47] Any deleterious effects of anesthesia technique might be expected to emerge in relation to duration of exposure. With general anesthesia, an association between induction-to-delivery interval and neonatal acidosis has been observed.[48] Neonatal acidosis may occur despite the use of high inspired oxygen concentration.[49] The acidosis may be due to adrenergic stress with light anesthesia or to more prolonged exposure to nitrous oxide,[50] although one would expect any vasoconstrictor effect of the latter agent to be offset by concomitant use of an inhalational agent. Umbilical acid-base status is unaffected by induction-to-delivery time under regional anesthesia, provided that hypotension is avoided or promptly treated.[48] The interval between uterine incision (when reflex uterine contraction may decrease placental blood flow) and delivery has a greater effect on acid-base status. Uterine incision-to-delivery times greater than 3 minutes are associated with decreased umbilical blood pH irrespective of anesthetic method,[48] although regional anesthesia may be somewhat protective.[51, 52] Relative intrauterine asphyxia during the uterine incision-to-delivery interval is reflected by an association between higher umbilical arterial concentrations of catecholamines, lower umbilical arterial blood pH, and prolonged uterine incision-to-delivery times.[53]

Clinical neonatal outcome assessed by Apgar scores is useful to determine the need for and the response to active resuscitation. With modern anesthetic techniques, however, Apgar scores may not be sensitive enough to detect differences between general and regional anesthesia. Several studies have shown no difference,[39–41, 54, 55] and those studies that have demonstrated a difference have shown a transient effect of general anesthesia affecting scores only at 1 minute postdelivery.[42, 46, 56] Apgar scores depressed at 5 minutes may well reflect preexisting fetal asphyxia rather than anesthetic effect. No study has ever demonstrated lower Apgar scores following regional anesthesia compared with general anesthesia. Most studies have examined elective cesarean section in uncomplicated cases, and results cannot necessarily be extrapolated to an emergency delivery with preexisting fetal compromise. Hypotension during regional anesthesia must be immediately treated, however, since it may cause fetal acidosis and poor Apgar scores.[57] In a nonrandomized prospective study of emergency cesarean section in cases with preexisting evidence of fetal distress, Marx and colleagues[46] demonstrated significantly higher 1-minute Apgar scores in infants delivered under regional blockade compared with general anesthesia. These authors concluded that, considering time requirements for urgent delivery, subarachnoid blockade was the most suitable and was safe in the presence of fetal distress.

Neonatal neurobehavioral testing can detect more subtle changes in clinical status than Apgar scores following delivery. General anesthesia can reduce neurobehavioral scores for up to 2 days following delivery in comparison with regional anesthesia.[54, 58] Following general anesthesia, neonates have reduced adaptive capacity, lower tone, and depressed primal reflexes at 15 minutes and at 2 hours but by 24 hours there is no significant difference compared with babies of mothers delivered under regional anesthesia.[54] Using modern general anesthetic techniques and agents, no differences in neonatal outcome may be detectable between general and regional anesthesia.[59]

There have been no prospective randomized studies of perinatal mortality comparing general with regional anesthesia for cesarean section. Retrospective studies are clouded by preexisting maternal or neonatal conditions that might have dictated the choice of anesthesia, and their results should be interpreted with caution. In a study of outcome in 3940 cesarean deliveries, it was reported that the neonatal mortality rate associated with general anesthesia was twice that associated with regional anesthesia. Overall rates were so low, however, that this did not achieve statistical significance.[56]

SPINAL VERSUS EPIDURAL ANESTHESIA

Choice between spinal and epidural anesthesia may be dictated by circumstances (urgency and whether there is a presited epidural catheter) or maternal comorbidity (e.g., valvular heart disease). The main differences between spinal and epidural anesthesia are rate of onset, quality of neural blockade, and dosage, all of which have an impact on side effects. These differences are due to the site of action of the local anesthetic at the spinal nerve roots. Epidurally administered drug must penetrate the dura and reach an effective concentration in the nerve roots. The epidural "space" contains fat and vessels, both of which absorb drug and may impede its spread within the epidural space. Thus epidural anesthesia requires high drug doses, has a delayed onset of action, and is prone to patchy or incomplete blockade. In addition, radiographic studies have demonstrated folds of dura in the midline of the epidural space which, although usually incomplete, may impede spread of local anesthetic and result in unilateral blocks or segmental failure of neural blockade.[60, 61] By comparison, subarachnoid anesthesia is administered directly into the cerebrospinal fluid and gains rapid access to the exposed nerve roots. The factors affecting spread of solution also affect response to changes in drug concentration and dosage. Epidural anesthesia requires high concentration of local anesthetic, and high volumes help the spread of solution to the nerve roots (both important factors when considering toxicity). Spinal anesthesia is more dependent on the dose administered, and increasing the volume (decreasing concentration) does not affect the extent of blockade.

There have been surprisingly few studies directly comparing spinal with epidural anesthesia. Helbo-Hansen[62] demonstrated no better intraoperative analgesia with spinal 0.5% plain bupivacaine, 13 mg, compared with epidural 1.5% bupivacaine (median dose 155 mg). Alahuhta[63] also demonstrated no difference in patient visual analogue scores for visceral pain between spinal and epidural anesthesia. Both these studies, however, are contrary to the clinical experience of obstetric anesthesiologists and the indirect evidence of supplementary analgesic requirements reported in studies of epidural or spinal anesthesia. For example, Riley and coworkers[64] observed reduced requirement for supplementary sedation with spinal anesthesia compared with epidural anesthesia for cesarean section. Russell[65] compared 10 mg to 17.5 mg of hyperbaric subarachnoid bupivacaine with epidural anesthesia using 0.5% bupivacaine or 2% lidocaine with epinephrine for cesarean section. Significantly more patients were pain-free with spinal anesthesia (87%) than with epidural anesthesia (67%). Keohane[66] reported less discomfort at elective cesarean section in women receiving spinal anesthesia than in those receiving epidural anesthesia. Of those women who had experienced both techniques for cesarean delivery, 80% preferred the spinal anesthetic.

PREOPERATIVE PREPARATION

Because there is a risk of a sudden requirement for securing the airway or administering general anesthesia in the event of a major complication, much of the preoperative preparation of the patient is the same as for general anesthesia. The patient should have had an appropriate period of fasting and should receive antacid prophylaxis. Anesthesia should be performed in an environment that permits administration of general anesthesia with all necessary equipment, drugs, and trained assistance immediately available.

Preoperative evaluation of the patient should include a history and examination looking specifically for contraindications to regional anesthesia and potential hazards to general anesthesia and airway management. Inquiry should be made into previous obstetric and anesthetic experiences that may affect the patient's attitude to anesthesia and surgery. Evidence of comorbidity that might affect the outcome or performance of regional anesthesia should be sought. Specifically, the back should be examined for infection and spinal deformity. While neurologic disease and back pain need not contraindicate regional anesthesia, existing symptoms and signs must be documented preoperatively. The anesthesiologist must have a clear understanding of the obstetric indications for cesarean delivery and how these may affect conduct of the planned anesthetic technique.

Preoperative laboratory investigations are generally unnecessary before initiating neuraxial analgesia in the healthy parturient. If the patient requires a cesarean section, blood group type and screening for antibodies and hemoglobin concentration must be available, and therefore these tests are usually ordered on admission. Any other investigations should be dictated by comorbidity.

Before commencing regional anesthesia, a functional intravenous line should be secured, equipment checked, and intravenous drugs that might be required drawn into syringes. These should include an intravenous induction agent, succinylcholine, atropine, and a vasopressor (usually ephedrine, 50 mg diluted to 5 mg/mL). A full aseptic technique should be used including sterile gloves and mask, antiseptic skin preparation, and sterile drapes to the patient's back. Some anesthesiologists perform a surgical scrub and wear a gown. Although infection is rare following regional anesthesia, it will only remain so if steps are always taken to avoid it.

In the absence of preoperative dehydration or hypovolemia, administration of large volumes of intravenous fluids is unnecessary before regional anesthesia. Generally, intravenous fluid is allowed to run freely during preparation and insertion of the regional anesthetics and is continued during onset of neural blockade. Solutions containing large amounts of dextrose should be avoided, as they may contribute to fetal acidosis and neonatal hypoglycemia.[67, 68] Maternal hypoglycemia can occur following prolonged fasting before elective cesarean section, and it has been suggested that the use of a 1% dextrose solution might be of benefit without risk to the neonate,[69] but even with such a dilute solution it is possible to give more than 10 g of glucose over a short period before delivery. Ringer's lactate is the solution most often used. Concerns regarding hyperchloremic acidosis following the use of 0.9% sodium chloride are unwarranted in the amounts used preoperatively.[70]

Preoperative preparation can be severely constrained in emergency cases. Equipment should be regularly checked and maintained in any operating room used for emergency obstetrics, and emergency drugs can be predrawn, labeled, and stored. Obstetric anesthesiologists should be regarded as part of the labor and delivery team and be made aware of all admissions to labor and delivery suites, and they should also be notified whenever scalp pH determinations are to be performed. Emergency cesarean section is always a possibility in any labor, and much time can be gained by proactive awareness of potentially problematic labors.

CONTRAINDICATIONS TO REGIONAL ANESTHESIA

Absolute Contraindications

Maternal refusal is a clear contraindication to regional anesthesia. Some patients may initially refuse the procedure through fear or ignorance, in which case gentle persuasion by reassurance and explanation can often change their view. Others will never be persuaded, and it is important that the mother's anxiety is not heightened by unwarranted emphasis on the dangers of general anesthesia.

Sepsis over the site of the injection is another obvious contraindication. It is not clear how close a septic focus on the skin has to be to the site of insertion to pose a threat. In the case of multiple, purulent inflamed spots that are thought to be due to bacterial infection, it may be unwise to perform regional anesthesia at all. Isolated lesions distant from the lumbar region apparently pose no threat.

Coagulopathy and hypovolemia, while absolute contraindications, are relative terms. Many patients with severe pregnancy-induced hypertension have low platelet counts and have varying degrees of intravascular hypovolemia, yet may greatly benefit from regional anesthesia. Both can be corrected, if time is available. The potential for bleeding presented by placenta previa or obstructed labor in the second stage need not contraindicate regional block, but the possibility of major hemorrhage should be anticipated. Severe antepartum hemorrhage with uncorrected hypovolemia and continued bleeding is an absolute contraindication to regional anesthesia. Similarly, overt bleeding, either spontaneously from gums or skin puncture sites, is also a contraindication, as is established disseminated intravascular coagulation (DIC) with abnormal coagulation indices, or a patient on full anticoagulant therapy.

Relative Contraindications

Patients with neurologic disease or chronic back pain who receive regional anesthesia may subsequently ascribe worsening of symptoms to the regional procedure. Despite the lack of evidence that regional anesthesia exacerbates chronic low back pain, some anesthesiologists are reluctant to undertake regional procedures in these patients. Obviously, full documentation is essential. Intracranial tumors causing raised intracranial pressure pose an increased risk of cerebellar herniation following dural puncture. Unless there is a pressing reason to avoid general anesthesia because of pathology elsewhere, neuraxial anesthesia is probably best avoided. Benign intracranial hypertension and surgically corrected hydrocephalus are not contraindications.

Severe infection, such as pneumonia or pyelonephritis, may be associated with bacteremia which theoretically may increase the risk of epidural or meningeal infection following regional anesthesia. The most common infection seen in the parturient is chorioamnionitis, which may be associated with bacteremia yet also may not be diagnosed until after delivery. Thus regional anesthesia is commonly used unwittingly in the presence of sepsis, usually with no untoward effects.[71] Some judgment is required in those patients with a known infection but no systemic manifestations of sepsis, those responding to treatment, or those who had a catheter placed before becoming symptomatic. In those situations it is accepted practice to proceed with regional anesthesia. However, if patients are having rigors, have high fevers and have not received antibiotics, or are showing signs of septic shock general anesthesia should be used.

Fetal heart rate abnormalities do not necessarily preclude the use of regional techniques. While profound bradycardia or decelerations in association with abruption necessitate anesthesia by the fastest possible route, there is usually sufficient time with less severe conditions to supplement an existing epidural or administer spinal anesthesia. Neonatal condition at delivery is better following regional anesthesia in these circumstances.[46]

Many cardiac lesions do well with regional anesthesia. Conditions that will not withstand significant reductions in systemic vascular resistance, such as moderate to severe aortic stenosis, primary pulmonary hypertension, and cyanotic lesions, are best operated on under general anesthesia. In a recent change in practice, pregnant patients with mitral stenosis requiring cesarean section are now delivered under epidural anesthesia, unless they are anticoagulated.

EPIDURAL ANESTHESIA

Choice of Local Anesthetic Agent

The ideal local anesthetic agent for epidural use should combine rapid onset of sensory blockade with a duration of action that permits completion of surgery but without prolonged postoperative motor blockade. Systemic absorption should not be associated with plasma levels likely to cause toxicity in the mother or affect the clinical condition of the neonate. Unfortunately, all agents fall short of this ideal in one way or another. Because of the large doses required for epidural anesthesia, prilocaine is unsuitable owing to associated methemoglobinemia[72] and mepivacaine is also unsuitable owing to prolonged fetal metabolism causing significant effects in the neonate.[73] The regularly used agents are bupivacaine, lidocaine, and 2-chloroprocaine. It remains to be seen whether ropivacaine[4] or levobupivacaine will have a significant influence on obstetric anesthesia practice.

Bupivacaine. Bupivacaine has the greatest potency of agents in current use and a 0.5% solution provides adequate surgical anesthesia in many, but not all, cases. It does not cause prolonged troublesome motor blockade postoperatively, and its duration of action in a dose up to 2 mg/kg is 2 to 3 hours. The main problems with epidural bupivacaine are its slow onset of action and increased risk of cardiotoxicity. Time to onset of action for bupivacaine depends on how this is defined and how the drug is administered. Defining onset time as a sensory level (loss of pinprick sensation) to the T6 nerve root, Thompson and colleagues[74] recorded a mean onset time of 40 minutes following rapid injection (20 mL of 0.5% bupivacaine over 20 seconds following a 3-mL test dose) through a 16-gauge catheter. This time to onset of surgical anesthesia is somewhat longer than one would expect in clinical practice and may relate to dosage and timing of increments. Using the same definition Abboud and colleagues[75] recorded an onset time of 23 minutes using a similar initial dose, with further increments up to a mean of 27 mL. At the opposite extreme, McMorland and coworkers[76] recorded a mean onset time (from test dose to the L1 sensory level) detected by loss of temperature sensation to ice of 6.4 minutes using a fractionated technique following pH adjustment. In routine practice, however, it is unusual to be able to commence surgery in less than 20 minutes following the test dose using a fractionated technique with unmodified 0.5% bupivacaine. Although onset times may be reduced when presited catheters have been used for labor, the delay associated with bupivacaine makes it unsuitable for use in urgent cesarean section.

The toxicity issue with bupivacaine primarily concerns its effect on the heart. In general, depression of myocardial contractility by local anesthetic agents is a function of potency,[77, 78] and the relative effects of bupivacaine to lidocaine on myocardial depression is about 4:1, which is what one would expect from their relative potency. The problem with bupivacaine is that it has a greater effect on conduction tissue than lidocaine[77, 79] and is more likely to cause arrhythmias. Also, because of its physical characteristics, bupivacaine has a greater affinity for the sodium channels in the myocardial cells than lidocaine[80] and requires more prolonged resuscitative efforts before its effects can be reversed.[81] The latter effect is further exaggerated by hypoxia and acidosis occurring during convulsions associated with neurotoxicity or during cardiorespiratory resuscitation.[82] It should be emphasized at this point that correct acceptable anesthetic practice in obstetrics precludes the rapid injection of large volumes of bupivacaine into the epidural space.

2-Chloroprocaine. As an ester-linked agent, 2-chloroprocaine is the least likely agent to directly affect the fetus and neonate. It is rapidly metabolized by plasma esterases and in the absence of pseudocholinesterase deficiency,[83, 84] maternal or neonatal toxicity is highly unlikely following systemic absorption. It has the fastest onset of action, surgical anesthesia (test dose to at least the T6 sensory level) developing rapidly.[75] Problems with 2-chloroprocaine lie with its low potency and short duration of action (about 45 minutes), and its propensity to interact with other agents. James and colleagues[85] compared 3% 2-chloroprocaine with 0.5% bupivacaine in 30 women presenting for elective cesarean section and found it an acceptable alternative, although maternal hypotension occurred more frequently in patients receiving 2-chloroprocaine. As seen in clinical practice, they also reported that surgical anesthesia was achieved much faster with 2-chloroprocaine than with bupivacaine. Writer and Dewan[86] have demonstrated acceptable analgesia in 41 of 44 parturients receiving a minimum dose of 25 mL of 3% 2-chloroprocaine.

Since further top-ups of 2-chloroprocaine can be given through the epidural catheter (and toxicity is not an issue with this agent), the short duration of action is not necessarily a problem. However, when analgesia extending into the postoperative period is required, 2-chloroprocaine can interfere with the action of epidurally administered bupivacaine,[87–89] clonidine,[90] and opiates[91–94] and may increase dose requirements of postoperative patient-controlled opiate analgesia.[94] Interactions with opiates may be due to 2-chloroprocaine acting as an antagonist at opiate μ and κ receptors.[95]

Reports of neurologic symptoms[96] and back pain[97, 98] following epidural 2-chloroprocaine have been ascribed to the preservatives used in earlier preparations but are not seen in obstetric patients. Now that a preservative-free solution is available, this should no longer be a problem.

Lidocaine. Epidural lidocaine temporarily fell into disfavor in obstetric anesthesia following reports of neonatal effects with its use in labor,[73] which were not seen with bupivacaine.[99] Later studies[17, 100] could not reproduce these questionable findings and while bupivacaine remains the most widely used drug for epidural analgesia in labor, lidocaine has regained its popularity and is very commonly used to provide epidural anesthesia for cesarean section. Onset of action of a 2% solution is closer to 2-chloroprocaine than bupivacaine and duration of action is approximately 1 hour. In a comparison of 0.5% bupivacaine, 3% 2-chloroprocaine, and 2% lidocaine, the protocol had to be modified, because 2% lidocaine was associated with discomfort unless epinephrine was added.[75] For this reason and more importantly to increase safety, lidocaine is most commonly used in combination with epinephrine 5 μg/mL, which provides a quality of analgesia equal to[101] or slightly better than[102] 0.5% bupivacaine. Lidocaine has a tendency to produce a greater degree of motor blockade than bupivacaine and a difference can be detected in respiratory performance.[103] Although this might have implications for patients with extensive preexisting respiratory compromise, it is of no clinical significance in the healthy parturient.

Ropivacaine. Ropivacaine is produced as a stereoisomerically pure S-enantiomer rather than a racemic mixture. It has similar properties to bupivacaine in terms of onset and duration of sensory blockade but it is reported to have less motor blockade[104, 105] and to be less cardiotoxic.[106–108] Unfortunately the clinical picture is not yet clear. Studies of epidural drug concentrations at the top of the dose-response curve for analgesia may mask subtle differences in potency.[109] Studies comparing ropivacaine with bupivacaine at cesarean section have used 0.5% concentrations of each agent. Studies of lower concentrations for analgesia in labor[110] suggest that the two drugs are not equipotent and that ropivacaine is the less potent of the two agents. This has been confirmed using sequential dose adjustment to determine the median effective dose (ED_{50}) for epidural analgesia (minimum local analgesic concentration [MLAC]) for the two agents.[111] It would appear that ropivacaine is approximately one third less potent than bupivacaine. Viewed in this light, the equipotent equivalent of 0.5% bupivacaine would be 0.75% ropivacaine. Studies in a nonobstetric population suggest that motor blockade is comparable between the two agents at these concentrations.[112] Nevertheless, studies have demonstrated that 0.5% ropivacaine can be effective for cesarean section. Comparative cardiotoxicity of the two agents needs to be reexamined in light of the difference in potency. How much of the difference in toxicity is due to the chemical differences between the two agents and how much is due to the stereospecificity of the ropivacaine preparation? Studies of bupivacaine have demonstrated the D-enantiomer to be the most cardiotoxic with a twofold difference in median lethal dose (LD_{50}) values in small mammals.[109] Similar differences have been found comparing lethal doses of ropivacaine with bupivacaine in sheep, with fatalities occurring with bupivacaine at half the dose of ropivacaine. When adjustment is made for the difference in potency between the two agents, the difference in toxicity may not be as great.

Decreasing the Onset Time of Epidural Anesthesia

Sodium Bicarbonate. Local anesthetics are all weak bases and they are commercially prepared in an acidic solution in order to maintain their water solubility in the ionized form. Ionized compounds, however, do not cross lipid membranes as readily as their un-ionized counterparts. The addition of small quantities (0.1–2.0 mEq to 20 mL of solution) of bicarbonate immediately prior to epidural injection increases the pH of the solution, and thereby increases the proportion of un-ionized local anesthetic and decreases the time to onset of action.[113] Alkalinization significantly reduces the onset time of 2-chloroprocaine[114] and lidocaine.[115] Bupivacaine tends to precipitate when alkalinized, so less bicarbonate should be added to bupivacaine. Addition of sodium bicarbonate can significantly reduce the onset time of bupivacaine,[76] although not all studies have demonstrated a significant effect.[116, 117] Decreasing the onset time of epidural anesthesia may reproduce the effects of spinal anesthesia on maternal blood pressure, and hypotension may occur more frequently.[118] Therefore, any method used to reduce onset time should be monitored with more frequent measurements of maternal blood pressure.

Carbonated Solutions. Carbon dioxide rapidly diffuses across all membranes, increasing intracellular hydrogen ion concentration. This has at least two effects which may explain the more rapid onset of action of carbonated local anesthetics. First, the decreased intracellular pH increases the ionization of the local anesthetic, thus "trapping" it intracellularly, increasing both the concentration gradient for un-ionized drug and the availability of local anesthetic in its active form at the intracellular sodium channel. Second, either carbon dioxide itself or hydrogen ions can cause a conformational change in the sodium channel which increases its affinity for blockade by the local anesthetic. Bicarbonate may also work in this way and may have its principal effect indirectly on intracellular carbon dioxide, rather than through its effects on drug ionization.[119, 120] Carbonization of lidocaine reduces latency by about 33%,[121] but seems to have little effect on bupivacaine.[122]

Epinephrine. Commercially prepared solutions of local anesthetics with epinephrine have a lower pH than plain solutions. Thus their use may be associated with a delayed onset of action. However, addition of epinephrine to the local anesthetic immediately before epidural injection has been shown to decrease the latency of lidocaine[123] but not bupivacaine.[124, 125]

Epidural Opioids. The lipid-soluble opioids fentanyl and sufentanil have a rapid onset of action when administered epidurally. While they are usually administered with the intention of improving the quality of intraoperative analgesia, they have been noted to shorten the onset of epidural anesthesia with bupivacaine.[126, 127]

Techniques of Injection and Patient Position. Although it is difficult to imagine, intravascular or subarachnoid position of an epidural needle has been missed. Therefore, bolus injection of large volumes of local anesthetic through the needle should always be avoided in the pregnant patient. Large-volume boluses are also dangerous when given through an epidural catheter, which may have penetrated a vessel or the dura during insertion or relocated thereafter. Epidural catheter injection should be routinely performed via intermittent injection of 3- to 5-mL boluses following a test dose. Subsequent doses can be given with increasing confidence in the absence of indications of intravascular or subdural injection. It seems pointless to administer the solution in increments through the needle[124] and then insert and tape the catheter, when the time could best be used by skin preparation and draping for surgery. In any case, epidural administration in a situation of urgency is invariably associated with a presited catheter used for labor analgesia. Without a preexisting epidural catheter, urgency indicates spinal anesthesia. Although patient position during injection may cause different patterns of onset of blockade, studies have revealed no consistent advantage in terms of block latency.[128, 129]

Enhancing the Quality of Epidural Blockade

The limited efficacy of epidural anesthesia is due, in part, to varying patient requirements. Choice of local anesthetic agent might make a difference, but this is often determined more by requirements for onset time and duration of effect. Increased concentration of local anesthetic improves the quality of block. For some time 0.75% bupivacaine was popular as an agent for epidural cesarean sections, particularly in North America; its advantage was that it gave a denser block than 0.5% bupivacaine. Unfortunately, because of the requirement for volume as well as concentration of local anesthetic solution injected epidurally, large doses were administered. Following a number of deaths associated with epidural anesthesia with 0.75% bupivacaine[130, 131] in the United States, the Food and Drug Administration banned its use in obstetric anesthesia. Although fewer deaths associated with bupivacaine toxicity have been reported in the United Kingdom, the majority were associated with 0.75% bupivacaine,[132, 133] and as in the United States, the preparation was withdrawn from obstetric anesthesia. It is probable that most of the deaths associated with 0.75% bupivacaine were due to inadvertent intravenous injection rather than to toxicity from absorption. In a study comparing 0.5% with 0.75% solution for cesarean section, almost half of those patients receiving the 0.75% solution received more than the recommended maximum dose; nevertheless, plasma bupivacaine concentrations were within acceptable limits in both groups.[134] However, in the deaths reported in the United Kingdom, toxicity was regarded as being due to systemic absorption from the epidural space.

A number of agents have been added to local anesthetic drugs in an attempt to enhance the quality of blockade.

Epinephrine. The majority of local anesthetics are weak vasodilators in the concentration used for epidural anesthesia.[135] This can lead to their more rapid uptake from the epidural space, resulting in higher plasma concentration and thus leaving less drug available within the epidural space. It is therefore logical that the addition of epinephrine might not only prolong the duration of blockade but also enhance its quality. As previously mentioned, addition of epinephrine is more effective with lidocaine than with bupivacaine. Dose requirements, however, are reduced with bupivacaine,[124] and plasma bupivacaine concentration is reduced[124, 125] when epinephrine is added. Although Abboud and coworkers[54] did not observe a significant reduction in plasma bupivacaine concentration when adding epinephrine to the local anesthetic, efficacy seemed to be enhanced. The effect of epinephrine on epidural lidocaine is significant, producing enhanced blockade of more rapid onset, with significantly lower plasma concentration.[136] An epinephrine concentration of 5 μg/mL is the most commonly used, but half this concentration may be equally effective in enhancing the quality of blockade.[137]

Some anesthesiologists have been concerned that the use of epidural or spinal epinephrine may lead to neurologic sequelae. This concern is unwarranted. While direct application of epinephrine to rat sciatic nerve may cause ischemic neural damage,[138] no case of spinal cord damage has ever been caused by the use of epinephrine in obstetric regional anesthesia. In fact, epidural doses as high as 1 mg have been used with no subsequent neurologic damage.[139] Systemic absorption of epinephrine (or inadvertent intravenous injection) may cause uterine arterial vasoconstriction and reduced placental blood flow. Although this has been demonstrated in animal models,[140–143] human placental blood flow measured using radioactive xenon was unchanged following epidural administration of epinephrine.[144] Use of epinephrine-containing solutions in labor has been found to have no effect on uterine activity, fetal heart rate and variability, or the incidence of abnormal fetal heart rate patterns. In addition, neonatal outcome is unaffected by epidural local anesthetic containing epinephrine.[54] Systemic absorption of epinephrine might possibly have an adverse effect in patients with uteroplacental insufficiency[145] and severe preeclampsia.[146] On balance, the advantages of adding epinephrine to lidocaine for epidural cesarean section clearly outweigh any potential hazards.

Clonidine. Epinephrine itself has an analgesic action via α_2-adrenergic receptors in the spinal cord,[139, 147] and this may contribute to analgesic enhancement of epidural local anesthetics. Clonidine has also been used as an additive to both spinal and epidural anesthetics, although there have been few reports of its use in obstetric anesthesia. Its main effect is to prolong analgesia into the postoperative period but it has also been used to enhance labor analgesia by intrathecal opiates.[148] Problems encountered include sedation, bradycardia, and hypotension, which can lead to impaired airway control and hypoxemia.[149] Prolonged motor blockade following bupivacaine can also be a problem.

Opioids. Opioids are commonly added to an epidural anesthetic to improve intraoperative analgesia and to extend analgesia into the postoperative period. Fentanyl[126, 127, 150, 151] and sufentanil[152] can both improve the quality of epidural anesthesia without neonatal impairment, although high doses of sufentanil (80 μg) may cause some depression of neurobehavioral scores.[152] A direct comparison of epidural fentanyl with sufentanil added to 2% lidocaine with epinephrine demonstrated a rapid onset with both agents but suggested that fentanyl was more effective in the doses used.[153]

Morphine is more suited to providing prolonged postoperative analgesia but may also improve intraoperative analgesia.[154, 155] Since it is more water soluble than the other agents, morphine can cause delayed respiratory depression. No more than 4 mg should be administered epidurally, because doses greater than this are not more effective but increase the incidence of untoward effects. All epidural opiates may cause nausea and pruritus, but these side effects may be prolonged with morphine. Urinary retention can also occur. Pethidine (meperidine) has both opiate and local anesthetic properties and has been used epidurally, improving quality of analgesia and having a duration of effect between that of fentanyl and morphine.[156, 157]

PRACTICAL ISSUES

Patient Comfort. Patients are frequently afraid of pain during epidural catheter placement. It is important that the patient understands the stages involved in the procedure and that she is warned what to expect before every skin contact. Although the patient may have a preferred position, if there are any factors that are going to make insertion more difficult in one position or the other, then ultimately she will be more comfortable in the position preferred by the anesthesiologist. The presence of the father during placement of an epidural catheter can be a comfort, but he must understand that he is there to comfort the patient, not to be a spectator.

If the patient experiences pain during the procedure, always apologize, withdraw the needle, inject more local anesthetic if necessary, and make another pass in a slightly different direction. Never ignore complaints of pain, particularly if radicular in nature, as pain during insertion may be associated with subsequent neurologic symptoms and back pain. Never continue injecting a local anesthetic if the patient complains of radicular pain.

Identifying the Interspace. This can be difficult in an obese patient. Always try to maintain maximum flexion of the back to reduce the lumbar lordosis. In the sitting position, the patient must not use her arms for weight bearing and her shoulders should be relaxed. The most important landmarks to identify are midline and the posterior iliac crests, which are at the level of the upper border of the L4 vertebra. There is often more fat over the L4 to L5 interspace, so that the L3 to L4 or L2 to L3 spaces may be more easily identifiable. Avoid applying excessive pressure when palpating the spine, because it may cause pain.

Location of the Epidural Space. Although a number of methods have been described to identify the epidural space, the most commonly used technique is loss of tissue resistance. Both air and saline have their advocates. Using saline, the needle should be advanced under continuous pressure on the plunger (not the barrel) of the syringe. Tissue resistance to injection permits both needle and syringe to move until the epidural "space" is encountered, at which point resistance to injection disappears. Theoretically, the ejection of saline from the needle displaces the dura away from the tip of the needle and decreases the risk of dural puncture. Also, since air injected into the epidural space may collect around nerve roots and subsequently interfere with local anesthetic distribution, missed segments or "patchy" blocks are less likely.

Irrespective of which method of insertion is used, key elements are first to ensure that the tip of the needle is in the interspinous ligament before starting to test for resistance, and second, to use the nondominant hand to apply counterpressure to the needle hub (or wings) in order to control entry speed and direction.

If the needle entry point is directly between two vertebrae, there need be only slight cephalad angulation of the needle during entry. Unlike the thoracic spine, lower lumbar spinous processes project almost at right angles to the spine. If in the midline, the epidural needle should not be angled in a caudad direction.

Catheter Insertion. Inserting the catheter too far increases the risk of the catheter emerging laterally from the epidural space, which may result in a unilateral block. Beilin and associates recommend 5 cm as the optimal insertion length for multiorifice catheters.[158] If the patient straightens her back before the catheter is secured, the risk of catheter movement is decreased.[159]

Testing the Catheter. The fallibility of tests of catheter position is no reason for their abandonment. Routine performance of tests is a worthwhile discipline that focuses attention on prevention of life-threatening complications of epidural anesthesia. It requires little effort to inspect the catheter for the presence of blood. Unusually excessive backflow of clear fluid following a loss of tissue resistance by the saline technique can be tested for glucose and protein using a reagent strip, although both are fallible, particularly if tested following local anesthetic injection.[160] Cerebrospinal fluid only tests weakly positive for protein and glucose, and pH may be a more reliable indicator.[161] Looking for passive backflow should be followed by gentle aspiration before injecting any test drug. A number of methods have been used for epidural catheter testing. Epinephrine, 15 μg, is the most commonly used but does not always cause tachycardia.[162] Also spontaneous tachycardia owing to pain in labor can cause a false-positive response.[163] Isoproterenol, 5 μg, more consistently produces tachycardia and although not regularly used, it may be safer for use in preeclampsia than epinephrine because it is a pure β-adrenergic agent.[164, 165] A more specific indicator of intravenous catheter placement is injection of 1 to 2 mL of air in conjunction with precordial Doppler monitoring for 15 seconds.[166, 167] If an inadvertent dural puncture is recognized following the needle or catheter insertion, many anesthesiologists thread the catheter intrathecally rather than resiting it at another interspace. Replacing the catheter is time-consuming, uncomfortable for the patient, does not guarantee that another dural puncture will be avoided, and introduces the additional problem of increased drug transfer across the dura. If the catheter is to remain subarachnoid, it is important that everyone involved with patient care knows exactly where the catheter is sited. Postdural puncture headache is not inevitable and if it occurs, it can be managed by a postpartum epidural blood patch.

The appearance of blood in the epidural catheter is a more common problem, occurring in up to 15% of cases. If frank blood appears and is flowing through the catheter, the catheter should be replaced at another interspace. If there is no flowing of blood, the catheter may be flushed with saline and withdrawn slightly. If blood does not reappear either passively or after gentle aspiration, a test dose should be administered, watching closely for signs of intravenous injection. If blood reappears or a test dose is positive, withdraw the catheter and resite at another interspace.

Many obstetric anesthesiologists routinely use lidocaine, 3 mL, with epinephrine, 5 μg/mL, as a test dose, except in cases (such as severe preeclampsia) when intravenous injection of epinephrine might compromise placental blood flow. Regardless of test dose used, remember that every epidural injection is a test dose if injection does not exceed 3- to 5-mL increments.

Considerations During Surgery. All patients must have uterine displacement maintained at approximately 20 to 30 degrees via a wedge or a rolled blanket under the right buttock and hip. Oxygen supplementation by face mask improves placental oxygen delivery and umbilical venous saturation. Onset and level of the block should be tested and further epidural incremental injections administered via the catheter, as necessary to achieve a block at the T4 interspace. Unilateral blocks are uncommon but can occur, so that dermatomal levels should be assessed bilaterally. Resiting a catheter or converting to spinal anesthesia may be necessary if the block does not develop. This is best done before the patient is fully prepped and draped, so sensory blockade should be present bilaterally before allowing skin preparation to proceed. Most anesthesiologists attempt to achieve a T4 level, since peritoneal manipulation requires a minimum block height at the T5 dermatomal level.[168]

Pain occurring during the procedure occasionally occurs with an adequate upper sensory level. It is due either to a "patchy" block or missed segment or to inadequate density of the block. When this occurs, it usually manifests after delivery at the time that the surgeon exteriorizes the uterus and is often accompanied by nausea. Management depends on the severity of the pain. Intravenous fentanyl in doses up to 100 μg often provides successful pain relief. Although some anesthesiologists administer nitrous oxide, some patients lose airway control when receiving 50% nitrous oxide in oxygen. If intravenous fentanyl plus small doses of ketamine is insufficient to control the pain, the induction of general anesthesia may be necessary. Nausea and vomiting with shivering are recognized problems associated with regional anesthesia. Shivering is thought to be due to thermal redistribution from the body core to the periphery associated with the sympathetic block and inevitable with regional anesthesia. Its incidence can be reduced, but not entirely eliminated, by the use of warm intravenous fluids and epidural solutions and the use of epidural fentanyl or sufentanil.[169–172]

Nausea and vomiting can often be the first signs of hypotension following regional blockade or can accompany visceral pain sensation. Having excluded these as the cause, metoclopramide (10 mg) or droperidol (0.625–1.0 mg) can be effective treatment. A high incidence of this complication probably justifies the prophylactic use of antiemetics. Metoclopramide, droperidol, and ondansetron have all been used with varying degrees of success.[173, 174]

Postanesthesia Care. Postoperatively, the patient should be accompanied by the anesthesiologist to a recovery area and handed over to appropriately trained staff. It is important that recovery staff are aware of any preexisting morbidity or anesthetic or surgical problems occurring during the procedure. In the absence of complications or comorbidity, the patient who has not received intravenous medications may not require oxygen therapy following regional anesthesia and can be discharged to the ward when signs of recovery of sensory (two-block regression) and motor function are observed. The epidural catheter can be left in situ for postoperative pain management if adequate ward staffing levels are met and protocols for management are in place. Catheter removal can rarely cause problems; however, the patient may have to adopt either flexed or hyperextended positions to assist removal.[175, 176]

SPINAL ANESTHESIA

Choice of Local Anesthetic Agent

As with epidural anesthesia, choice of agent for spinal anesthesia is limited in practice to three or four agents. Because of its short duration of action and previously documented problems with preservative, 2-chloroprocaine is not used by the intrathecal route. Because spinal drugs are administered directly into the cerebrospinal fluid, onset of action is rapid with all agents. Issues affecting choice relate to duration of action and efficacy and agent-specific adverse effects.

Bupivacaine. Bupivacaine approaches the ideal for subarachnoid blockade for cesarean section. It is a potent agent and if an adequate block height is achieved, the agent alone provides satisfactory anesthesia in the majority of parturients. Duration and extent of blockade are dose related, although the latter can be modified by baricity and patient positioning. Dose requirements may vary between patient populations. In Durban, South Africa, 7.5 mg of bupivacaine can be sufficient to provide anesthesia for cesarean section,[177] whereas in Europe and North America doses of 12 to 15 mg are used. Doses above 15 mg significantly increase the risk of high motor block and are not recommended. Bupivacaine is produced in concentrations of 0.5%, 0.75%, and 1%, although availability of these products varies worldwide. Because of the low dose used for spinal anesthesia, systemic toxicity is not an issue. Regarding transient neurologic symptoms, spinal bupivacaine appears to be the least likely of the three most commonly used agents to cause problems[178] or transient neurologic deficits. Although the extent of neuronal blockade is largely unaffected by concentration,[179–181] density of sensory blockade may be better with the 0.75% than the 0.5% solution. However, there seems little point in increasing the concentration to 1%. Runza and colleagues[182] compared hyperbaric

0.75% with 1% bupivacaine and found no difference in onset times or quality of block; however, postoperative backache was more commonly reported after the 1% solution (24% vs. 1%). These investigators also noted a significantly shorter time to first request for postoperative analgesia with the 1% solution (3 hours vs. 4.3 hours).

Lidocaine. Lidocaine has also been a popular choice for cesarean sections under spinal anesthesia, particularly in developing countries where the newer agents are not always available. It is invariably used as the hyperbaric solution. Doses of 80 mg can provide acceptable conditions for cesarean section lasting up to 70 minutes, but this is stretching the limit of lidocaine's duration of action and patients may have significant pain at the end of surgery or during transfer to the recovery room.[183] Some investigators have found lidocaine to be less predictable when used in doses of 65 to 75 mg, with sensory levels reaching as high as the C2 dermatome in some patients and only the L1 level in others.[184]

Recently, subarachnoid lidocaine has fallen out of favor because of reports of cauda equina syndrome, radicular pain, and transient neurologic symptoms following its use.[185, 186] Initially this was believed to be a problem mainly confined to the 5% solution, particularly with the use of intraspinal catheters. However, symptoms have been observed following spinal anesthesia with concentrations as low as 0.5%.[187]

Logistic regression analysis of 1863 patients receiving spinal anesthesia has demonstrated an increased risk of developing transient neurologic symptoms following lidocaine compared with bupivacaine (relative risk, 5.1) and tetracaine (relative risk, 3.2).[188] Data such as these are worrisome, but their clinical significance is not clear. If the symptoms are due to the lidocaine itself, one might expect a dose-response relationship of incidence to concentration, which was not seen in Pollock's study.[187] However, something is happening with lidocaine that does not seem to happen as frequently with either tetracaine or bupivacaine. Subarachnoid lidocaine has served well over the years and apart from cases using 5% lidocaine in conjunction with spinal microcatheters, there have been no reports of permanent neurologic damage because of lidocaine. If bupivacaine is available, it is clearly the superior agent for cesarean section under spinal anesthesia.

Tetracaine. Tetracaine (7–10 mg) is a long-acting agent with a duration of action similar to bupivacaine, but it tends to be associated with more prolonged motor blockade and a sensory block that is not as dense.[189, 190] Addition of a vasoconstrictor can improve the efficacy of low-dose tetracaine in nonobstetric cases,[191] but it also may increase the incidence of transient neurologic symptoms,[192] which is normally between that of lidocaine and bupivacaine.

Other Agents. Procaine has been used for spinal anesthesia in obstetrics either on its own or in combination with tetracaine. Unfortunately, its duration of action is shorter than lidocaine and it is best used for procedures of short duration. In combination with tetracaine, it produces a block of better quality than tetracaine alone and of longer duration, but the prolonged motor block conferred by tetracaine is often excessive.[189] Ropivacaine, available currently only as a plain solution, has been used spinally in nonobstetric cases.[193] Decreased potency may make the 0.75% solution a more appropriate choice. From the pharmacology, one would expect effects between those of bupivacaine and mepivacaine. As systemic toxicity is not an issue with subarachnoid block, there does not appear to be any particular advantage over bupivacaine. Preservative-free pethidine (meperidine) may be a useful alternative in developing countries where local anesthetics may be in short supply. Although having a short duration of action, meperidine has been used successfully as the sole intrathecal agent for cesarean section,[194] and postpartum tubal ligation.[195] Side effects include hypotension, nausea, and pruritus, as one would expect from a combination of local anesthetic and opiate action.

Patient Position and Baricity

Subarachnoid injection can be performed with the patient in the sitting or lateral position using either plain or hyperbaric solutions. Each method has its advocates and it remains a matter of personal choice. From the patient's point of view, those with a higher body mass tend to prefer the sitting position. Most importantly, the anesthesiologist should be aware that patient position and movement following injection can affect the performance of spinal blockade and that hyperbaric and plain solutions behave differently.

Although one might expect a plain solution to stay in a fairly coherent bolus following slow injection into the subarachnoid space and therefore produce a more predictable block, this is not the case. Russell[196] studied the effects of increasing dosage of plain bupivacaine administered in the lateral position to patients for elective cesarean section. He turned one group of patients into the supine wedged position immediately following injection of 10 to 15 mg of bupivacaine. A second group received 15 to 17.5 mg of bupivacaine then waited 15 minutes before turning, and a third group received 15 to 17.5 mg then waited 15 minutes, when an additional 2.5- to 5-mg dose was administered and then the patients were turned. The final block height was similar for all three groups and the process of turning the patient appeared to be the most important factor in developing the block. During the process of turning, increases in epidural venous flow caused by transient vena caval compression or increased abdominal pressure create a surge of cerebrospinal fluid that carries the local anesthetic in a cephalad direction. This contributes to the unpredictability of block height following spinal anesthesia with plain solutions. In fact, plain bupivacaine is slightly hypobaric, and maintaining the patient in the lateral position for any length of time may actually cause more extensive block on the nondependent side.

The effect of patient position on spread of hyperbaric solutions is as predicted, with the drug following the effect of gravity. In the supine position the normal thoracic curvature of the spine prevents excessively high blockade by impeding cephalad spread of the agent. It is important to remember that this effect is lost once the patient is in the lateral position. Indeed, because many pregnant women are wider at the hips than the shoulders, the effect of gravity in the lateral position often encourages cephalad spread. This can be prevented by placing pillows under the patient's head and shoulders in the lateral position.[197]

Comparisons of plain/hypobaric with hyperbaric solutions have failed to produce consistent results, perhaps owing to the use of additional agents and dose. Because of the effects of gravity on hyperbaric solutions, one would expect any differences in distribution of block to show up more with smaller doses. Also, because of the effects of the gravid uterus on the distribution of plain solutions, the drugs may behave differently between pregnant and nonpregnant patients. Height of block is dose dependent. Both Vucevic and Russell[181] and Van Zundert and colleagues[179] have demonstrated that the same height of block is achieved with increased volumes of plain solutions diluted with 0.9% saline, provided that the dose remains the same. With hyperbaric solutions the effect of gravity dominates the effect of dose on distribution of block. Increasing the dose of hyperbaric bupivacaine from 7.5 to 10 mg to 10 to 12.5 mg produces similar heights of sensory block[198] but improves the density of analgesia within the blocked segments. The same factors may explain why patient variables such as height and spinal column length may influence the dose requirement per segment of block for plain solutions[199, 200] but not for hyperbaric solutions.[201–203] There is a limit to this phenomenon, however, and it is important to reduce the dose of hyperbaric bupivacaine by 40% in achondroplastic dwarves.[204]

Extending the Duration of Action of Spinal Analgesia

Despite the excellent quality of analgesia provided by spinal anesthesia, both epinephrine and opiates are often added to the local anesthetic. Although this is often done to increase the duration of the block, improved quality of intraoperative anesthesia may also be seen. Fentanyl in doses as low as 6.25 μg can improve intraoperative analgesia and prolong the duration of analgesia to greater than 100 minutes.[205] The addition of 15 μg of fentanyl to intrathecal hyperbaric 0.5% bupivacaine (2.5 mL) significantly improves the quality of surgical anesthesia without affecting the incidence of maternal side effects, although onset of hypotension may be earlier with fentanyl.[206] Higher doses have been used, but are associated with an increase in the incidence of side effects without improving the quality of surgical anesthesia.[205] Higher doses, however, may prolong the duration of action[207] at the cost of increased sedation and pruritus. Following the administration of doses as high as 0.75 μg/kg, a decrease in respiratory rate was observed as early as 4 minutes following injection, but clinically significant maternal respiratory depression was not seen.[207] This is reassuring to anesthesiologists who might be concerned about neuraxial opiate-induced respiratory depression. Intrathecal fentanyl also decreases the need to administer epidural anesthesia in combined spinal-epidural techniques.[208] An interesting phenomenon of acute tolerance to subsequently administered morphine may occur with the intrathecal use of fentanyl. Cooper and colleagues[208] observed increased patient-controlled postoperative morphine requirements in patients receiving 25 μg of intrathecal fentanyl with 10 mg of 0.5% hyperbaric bupivacaine, compared with spinal bupivacaine alone for cesarean section. Patients were all given 10 mL of epidural bupivacaine (45 mg) with fentanyl (50 mg) following surgery. There was no difference in patient-controlled morphine requirements between the two groups for the first 6 hours, but thereafter increased morphine usage was seen in those patients who had received intrathecal fentanyl.

Although most studies have examined the effect of intrathecal fentanyl when added to bupivacaine, similar effects are seen when fentanyl is added to lidocaine[209, 210] and tetracaine.[211] One would expect the effects of intrathecal sufentanil to be similar to those of fentanyl. Courtney and associates[212] demonstrated improved intraoperative analgesia and prolonged duration of effective analgesia in patients receiving 10, 15, or 20 μg of subarachnoid sufentanil added to 10.5 mg of hyperbaric bupivacaine compared with saline controls. No respiratory depression was seen but pruritus was problematic. A comparison of sufentanil, 10 μg, with fentanyl, 15 μg, added to 7.5 mg of bupivacaine gave similarly satisfactory intraoperative analgesia (better than bupivacaine alone) with a longer duration of action in the sufentanil group. The incidence of pruritus and number of episodes of desaturation were, however, higher with sufentanil. The longer action of sufentanil versus fentanyl has also been observed in other studies.[213, 214]

Unlike fentanyl,[215] intrathecal sufentanil has a greater tendency to cause hypotension.[216] Also, there have been several reports of significant respiratory depression following intrathecal sufentanil administration.[217–220] The longer duration and increased incidence of side effects compared with fentanyl may be related to dosage issues. The maximum effect with sufentanil is seen between 10 and 15 μg[221] and about 25 μg for fentanyl[222]; however, lower doses of both agents are often used. With epidural analgesia, both agents have a similar duration of action if equianalgesic doses are used.[223]

Although intrathecal morphine can improve the quality of intraoperative analgesia,[224] its onset of action is slower than the more lipid-soluble agents. Its main advantage is its long duration of action. Abouleish[225] studied intrathecal morphine, 0.2 mg, added to spinal hyperbaric bupivacaine for cesarean section and observed prolonged postoperative analgesia. Larger doses have been used and there appears to be a correlation between dose and duration of effect[226]; with larger doses, however, pruritus becomes a problem. A dose-response study[227] confirmed the value of intrathecal morphine in reducing postoperative patient-controlled analgesia requirements, but demonstrated no advantage in increasing the dose beyond 75 μg. Pruritus and the need for its treatment increased as intrathecal morphine dose increased. Addition of epinephrine to the spinal mixture improves intraoperative analgesia[228] and reduces systemic morphine uptake.[229] Intrathecal diamorphine (heroin) has also been used successfully to prolong analgesia into the postoperative period. The use of 200 μg of intrathecal diamorphine gives similarly effective postoperative analgesia as the same dose of morphine, with less pruritus.[230] Doses above 250 μg usually confer no added advantage.[231] Because of its lipophilicity diamorphine should have a more rapid onset of action and be less susceptible to cephalad spread. As with other intrathecal opioids, intraoperative analgesia is improved with its use.[231]

Unpredictability

The biggest drawback of spinal anesthesia is the inherent unpredictability of a "single shot" technique. There are many factors that influence extension of neuronal blockade, and it is difficult to know exactly how they are going to interact in a given patient. This can cause failure of the spinal anesthetic to achieve either sufficient height or duration of block or, at the other extreme, a dangerously high block associated with profound hypotension, respiratory paralysis, and loss of consciousness.

Failed Spinal. Intraoperative failure of spinal anesthesia represents a hazard because the only practical way of dealing with it is conversion to general anesthesia, with all its attendant risks. Rarely, complete failure to establish a block may be due to injection of the local anesthetic outside of the subarachnoid space. If this occurs, it is often appropriate to repeat the spinal. However, sufficient time must be allowed for a delayed onset of block, which sometimes may not appear for up to 10 minutes following injection. Unlike epidural anesthesia, density of blockade is seldom a problem with spinal anesthesia (with the exception of tetracaine), and failure is usually associated with inability to locate the subarachnoid space or administration of an insufficient dose. Hyperbaric solutions have an advantage, because in the event of an inadequate level of block, the patient may be placed in the Trendelenburg position, which displaces the agent cephalad and increases the block height.

High Block/Total Spinal. In addition to the intended spinal anesthesia, this potentially life-threatening complication can also occur during epidural anesthesia if inadvertent spinal injection occurs owing to unrecognized penetration of the dura by the epidural needle or catheter. An unexpectedly high block can also result from a subdural, extra-arachnoid injection.[232] A review of serious complications of spinal and epidural blockade in obstetrics documented an incidence of approximately 1 in 500 epidural blocks and 1 in 3000 spinal procedures.[233] Paech and coworkers[234] reported eight high blocks occurring in 10,995 epidural procedures (incidence 1 in 1400), with two of these patients requiring intubation. The onset can be sudden and the outcome catastrophic unless immediately treated. Motor weakness, hypotension, apnea, and loss of consciousness can quickly lead to hypoxia, bradycardia, and cardiac arrest without intubation and blood pressure support. Other cases can present more insidiously as a progressive onset of higher and higher levels of blockade. As the level reaches the cervical dermatomes, the patient usually complains of shortness of breath. As the level continues to rise, her complaints become a whisper, and as the diaphragm is affected, the patient is unable to phonate. Hypotension is common but not invariable. Initial stages may be difficult to distinguish from an excessively anxious patient unable to take a deep breath owing to abdominal pressure in the supine position; however, there is no other cause than high block for the parturient who, following a neuraxial block, complains of shortness of breath, is unable to grasp your fingers in her hand, and is unable to speak.

Management. Treatment must be immediate. If apnea and desaturation have occurred, commence hand ventilation with 100% oxygen through the anesthetic gas delivery system with an assistant applying cricoid pressure, open the intravenous line to run freely, and administer a vasoconstrictor. If the patient is conscious, administer a reduced dose of an intravenous induction agent immediately followed by succinylcholine and tracheal intubation; thereafter, proceed with general anesthesia. No further neuromuscular blockade is required and depending on the local anesthetic used, the patient often starts breathing again before completion of surgery. Rarely, unconsciousness and apnea can also be caused by profound hypotension with resultant brain stem hypoperfusion. In these cases the patient may recover promptly following ephedrine. If in any doubt, however, proceed with securing the airway.

Oxygen saturation is not a useful early monitor in these cases. If profound desaturation occurs, it means action should have been taken 1 to 2 minutes previously.[235]

Spinal Anesthesia Following Epidural Blockade

Occasionally a patient presents for cesarean section with a unilateral or patchy epidural block that has been used for labor. If a one-shot spinal anesthetic is administered, a sensory block above the C8 dermatome may occur.[236] A high sensory level alone is not a problem, but when it is associated with high motor block and apnea,[237] the spinal level poses an immediate threat to life. Whether or not spinal anesthesia is relatively contraindicated following a failed epidural block is a subject for debate.[237–239] Part of the problem is that without knowing the exact mechanism that produces high blocks, it is difficult to prevent this occurrence.

There are several possible mechanisms for these high spinal blocks following failed epidural blocks. Expansion of the epidural space may compress the spinal canal, encouraging cephalad spread of intrathecal drugs. Rapid transfer of local anesthetic from the epidural space across the dural hole may occur. Alternatively, although the epidural block is inadequate, sufficient local anesthetic may be present in the nerve roots to decrease the dose requirement of subsequent spinal anesthesia. While a recently administered large-volume epidural supplement might cause volume and pressure changes sufficient to compress the spinal canal, several of the reported cases[237] have followed continuous epidural infusions. The epidural space is a very leaky structure,[240] and it is difficult to envisage a persistent large-volume effect in these cases. Also, if the process were mechanically mediated, one would expect high blocks to be less likely with hyperbaric solutions, any dural compression impeding cephalad spread of the agent. Yet high blocks have also been reported with hyperbaric agents. Any transfer of drug from the epidural space through the dural puncture would require a very large amount of epidural pressure, which is unlikely in young patients.[241] The high blocks reported by Gupta and coworkers[237] had an onset time of 1 to 2 minutes, suggesting an immediate effect of the subarachnoid injection itself, which favors the pharmacologic theory.

If a pharmacologic etiology is indeed the cause of this problem, then the dose of spinal anesthetic should be reduced; but by how much? Without knowing the degree of receptor occupancy produced by the previously administered epidural agent, it is impossible to gauge any modified spinal dose. Alternatively, a method of limitation of cephalad spread of hyperbaric agent by altering patient position to restrict the level of block to the T4 dermatome might be used.[242]

In the case of a nonemergent cesarian section in a patient with a "patchy" epidural block, several anesthetic options other than a one-shot spinal block exist. The epidural catheter can be resited or a combined spinal-epidural anesthetic can be prepared, using a markedly decreased spinal dose (≤7.5 mg)[243] and using the epidural catheter to supplement the block, if necessary. If the case is more emergent, a spinal macrocatheter can be inserted (via an epidural needle) and a spinal dose given in small incremental boluses. Of course, the entire situation can usually be avoided if inadequately functioning labor epidural blocks are detected early and the catheter resited.

COMBINED SPINAL-EPIDURAL ANESTHESIA

The combined spinal-epidural (CSE) technique has gained popularity rapidly following its introduction to obstetric practice in 1984.[244] Although it is most often described in relation to labor analgesia, CSE is also used for cesarean section. The advantage of this technique when used for cesarean section is that it provides the rapid onset of surgical anesthesia afforded by one-shot spinal anesthesia as well as the flexibility of an epidural catheter, which allows extension of an inadequate height of block and may be used to provide prolongation during surgery of unexpectedly longer duration or for postoperative analgesia. Given the ability to supplement the block, the CSE technique permits the use of smaller doses of subarachnoid local anesthetic, which may reduce the incidence of hypotension and the risk of inadvertent high motor blockade.

The CSE technique is technically more demanding than either spinal or epidural anesthesia alone and the equipment is more costly. There is no consensus as to the best method of achieving both epidural and subarachnoid penetration. The most popular method appears to be the single interspace approach using either a standard epidural needle with a long spinal needle, or a specially modified epidural needle that either has two barrels or a hole on the tip curvature which permits passage of the spinal needle. There is a theoretic risk of the epidural catheter passing through the hole created in the dura by the spinal needle if both emerge from the tip of the epidural needle at the same angle. Studies have demonstrated that it is possible to pass an epidural catheter through holes created by spinal needles larger than 25 gauge,[245, 246] but it seems almost impossible to push a 16- or 18-gauge catheter through the hole created by a 25-gauge needle, although this might occur following multiple punctures.[246] The risk of unrecognized dural perforation by the epidural needle is probably of greater concern.[247] This risk, however, is not unique to combined spinal-epidural anesthesia and can occur with any epidural technique.

Deviation of the epidural needle away from the midline may prevent subarachnoid penetration by the spinal needle. Other problems include inadequate length of spinal needle, and "tenting" but no penetration of the dura by pencil-point needles.[247] Thus, technical difficulties may cause failure of the needle-through-needle single interspace technique, leading some to prefer a sequential double interspace technique. Lyons and coworkers[248] documented a 16% failure of the spinal element of a combined technique using a needle-through-needle method, compared with 4% of sequential placements. Failure rates in clinical practice are, however, generally much lower than 16%.[245, 249, 250] Failure rates may decrease with increasing familiarity with the technique and equipment. Lyons' group reported a prior failure rate of 25% during evaluation of a 30-gauge spinal needle as part of the CSE technique.

Others advocate a needle-beside-needle single interspace technique. This can be done using a standard pencil-point needle to identify the subarachnoid space then passing an epidural needle parallel to it.[251] This technique, however, might result in damage to the spinal needle by subsequent passage of the epidural needle. Alternatively, the epidural needle can be inserted first, a spinal introducer placed next to it, the epidural catheter inserted and the needle withdrawn, and the spinal needle then introduced through the introducer.[252] The risk of possible catheter damage by the spinal needle is probably reduced by placing the needle in a different direction than that taken by the epidural catheter.

Whether or not complications are reduced depends largely on what is injected and how much. The incidence of puncture headaches is similar to conventional spinal anesthesia; nausea and vomiting are associated with hypotension; and as with other techniques, pruritus will occur if opiates are used. The incidence of hypotension depends on the rapidity of onset and height of block, which in turn depends on subarachnoid local anesthetic dose, baricity, and patient position during injection. Studies using a dose of subarachnoid bupivacaine similar to conventional spinal anesthesia have demonstrated similar incidence of hypotension. In Turner and Reifenberg's study,[252] "hypotension was almost universal, requiring treatment in 83%" using 12.5 mg of 0.5% hyperbaric bupivacaine.

Randalls and colleagues,[249] using hyperbaric bupivacaine, 12.5 mg, with or without epinephrine or fentanyl, observed hypotension in 24% of subjects, despite intravenous fluid preloading and prophylactic ephedrine infusion. Others have found a greater requirement for ephedrine when using the combined technique as compared with epidural anesthesia alone—the result of denser blocks of more rapid onset.[253] When the onset of action is delayed (e.g., using a hyperbaric solution in the sitting position), the incidence of hypotension and nausea can be reduced, but more patients may require epidural supplementation.[254] Deliberate reduction of the intrathecal dose with the intention of early epidural supplementation may decrease the incidence and severity of side effects. Vercauteren[255] used a dose of bupivacaine, 6.6 mg, with sufentanil, 3.3 μg, and recorded an overall incidence of hypotension of 13%, but noted that the incidence of hypotension was less using a hyperbaric solution (6%) compared with plain bupivacaine (21%).

Initiating epidural anesthesia with a preexisting spinal block presents its own problems.[256] Injecting large volumes epidurally can displace free drug within the CSF, thus extending the height of the subarachnoid block. This may be advantageous in the intraoperative setting where CSE is used, in that the subarachnoid block can be extended rapidly, but it also introduces an element of unpredictability. The effects vary depending on timing of epidural injection in relation to spinal injection. Myelographic studies demonstrate significant compression of the subarachnoid space by epidural injection 10 mL of saline.[257] This effect can be seen up to 20 minutes following spinal injection,[258] but can be modified by keeping patients in the sitting position for 5 minutes following injection with a hyperbaric solution[259] in nonobstetric patients. Once two-segment regression has been observed, there appears to be no significant volume effect,[260] so it is a phenomenon relevant largely to supplementation of a spinal block at the start of surgery, rather than to epidural injections administered at the end of the procedure or for postoperative pain relief.

Commencing epidural anesthesia via a catheter in a patient with an existing subarachnoid block also may strain interpretation of epidural test doses. Rapid onset of segmental blockade following a small-volume epidural local anesthetic injection cannot be used as an indicator of subarachnoid placement. However, the use of small fractionated epidural doses following aspiration through the catheter should obviate the need to test the subarachnoid position. Testing for intravascular catheter placement using the combined technique by use of epinephrine- or isoprenaline-containing solutions is still a worthwhile exercise. The presence of preexisting tachycardia owing to pain is not a problem because of the existing block, but heart rate responses to intravenous ephedrine can also create difficulties in interpretation. The need to treat hypotension with ephedrine is more likely with higher blocks; in which case activation of the epidural component may be unnecessary.

Concern has been expressed that it is possible for epidurally administered agents to pass into the subarachnoid space through the dural puncture site following the CSE technique. This dural flux may have resulted in severe respiratory depression[261] and cardiorespiratory arrest following cesarean section[262] during which epidural diamorphine was administered to patients who had previously received CSE. Animal studies have demonstrated that it is possible for epidural drugs

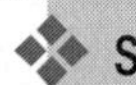

Summary

Key Points

- Most cesarean sections are performed with the patient under regional anesthesia, which is safer than general anesthesia for this surgery. Since the advent of "atraumatic" spinal needles, most elective cesarean sections have been performed with the patient under spinal anesthesia.
- Catheter techniques (e.g., epidural) allow the anesthesiologist more control, because the level of block can be titrated slowly.
- Hypotension is common following initiation of spinal anesthesia and is often heralded by nausea and vomiting. Ephedrine, intravenous fluids, and an increase in left uterine displacement should be used to treat hypotension.
- A T4 dermatome level is optimal for cesarean section.

Key Reference

Hawkins JL, Koonin LM, Palmer SK, Gibbs CP: Anesthesia-related deaths during obstetric delivery in the United States, 1979–1990. Anesthesiology 1997; 86:277–284.

Case Stem

A patient with an indwelling epidural catheter is brought to the operating room for a cesarean section due to arrest of dilatation. Twenty-five minutes following the administration of 20 mL of 0.5% bupivacaine, the patient has a "patchy" block at the T10 dermatome. How would you manage this patient?

administered adjacent to a dural puncture to cross into the subarachnoid space.[263] This risk may be reduced by using the smallest possible spinal needle. Radiographically demonstrated spread of contrast medium from the epidural to subarachnoid space has been reported following use of the CSE technique in gynecologic patients,[264] but a subsequent study failed to document spread in 15 patients. Assuming adequate postoperative care, the provision of costly postoperative monitoring facilities in the hope of preventing these exceedingly rare adverse events following what is generally held to be a safe technique is unwarranted. Effective opiate analgesia by any route can cause respiratory depression and it is therefore important that everyone involved in the postoperative care of these patients is aware of the method of analgesia used. In addition, anesthesiologists must ensure the development and observance of nursing protocols that mandate frequent patient observation.

References

1. Hawkins JL, Gibbs CP: General anesthesia for cesarean section: are we really prepared? Int J Obstet Anesth 1998; 7:145–146.
2. Report on Confidential Enquiries into Maternal Deaths in the United Kingdom, 1985–1987. London: Her Majesty's Stationer's Office; 1987.
3. Report on Confidential Enquiries into Maternal Deaths in the United Kingdom, 1994–1996. London: Her Majesty's Stationer's Office; 1996.
4. Brown GW, Russell IF: A survey of anaesthesia for caesarean section. Int J Obstet Anesth 1995; 4:214–218.
5. Chadwick HS, Posner K, Caplan RA, et al: A comparison of obstetric and nonobstetric anesthesia malpractice claims. Anesthesiology 1991; 74:242–249.
6. Hawkins JL, Koonin LM, Palmer SK, Gibbs CP: Anesthesia-related deaths during obstetric delivery in the United States, 1979–1990. Anesthesiology 1997; 86:277–284.
7. Hawkins JL, Gibbs CP, Orleans M, et al: Obstetric anesthesia work force survey, 1981 versus 1992. Anesthesiology 1997; 87:135–143.
8. Tsen LC, Pitner R, Camann WR: General anesthesia for cesarean section at a tertiary care hospital, 1990–1995: indications and implications. Int J Obstet Anesth 1998; 7:147–152.
9. Nielsen TF, Hökegård K-H: Postoperative cesarean section morbidity: A prospective study. Am J Obstet Gynecol 1983; 146:911–916.
10. Thomas TA: Maternal mortality. *In* Russell IF, Lyons G (eds): Clinical Problems in Obstetric Anaesthesia. London: Chapman & Hall; 1997:1–9.
11. Moir DD: Anaesthesia for caesarean section. Br J Anaesth 1970; 42:136–142.
12. Morgan BM, Aulakh JM, Barker JP, et al: Anaesthetic morbidity following caesarean section under epidural or general anaesthesia. Lancet 1984; 1:328–330.
13. Lie B, Juul J: Effect of epidural vs general anaesthesia on breast feeding. Acta Obstet Gynecol Scand 1988; 67:207–209.
14. Lavin JP, Samuels SV, Miodovnik M, et al: The effects of bupivacaine and chloroprocaine as local anesthetics for epidural anesthesia on fetal heart rate monitoring parameters. Am J Obstet Gynecol 1981; 141:717–722.
15. Lavin JP: The effects of epidural anesthesia on electronic fetal heart rate monitoring. Clin Perinatol 1982; 9:55–62.
16. Rickford WJK, Reynolds F: Epidural analgesia in labour and maternal posture. Anaesthesia 1983; 38:1169–1174.
17. Abboud TK, Afrasiabi A, Sarkis F, et al: Continuous infusion epidural analgesia in parturients receiving bupivacaine, chloroprocaine or lidocaine—maternal, fetal and neonatal effects. Anesth Analg 1984; 63:421–428.
18. Nel JT: Clinical effects of epidural block during labour: a prospective study. S Afr Med J 1985; 63:371–374.
19. Ebner H, Barcohana J, Bartoshuk AK: Influence of postspinal hypotension on the fetal electrocardiogram. Am J Obstet Gynecol 1960; 80:569–572.
20. Jouppila P, Jouppila R, Barinoff T, Koivula A: Placental blood flow during caesarean section performed under subarachnoid blockade. Br J Anaesth 1984; 56:1379–1382.
21. Hollmén AI, Jouppila R, Albright GA, et al: Intervillous blood flow during caesarean section with prophylactic ephedrine and epidural anaesthesia. Acta Anaesthesiol Scand 1984; 28:396–400.
22. Huovinen K, Lehtovirta P, Forss M, et al: Changes in placental intervillous blood flow measured by the ^{133}Xenon method during lumbar epidural block for elective caesarean section. Acta Anaesthesiol Scand 1979; 23:529–533.
23. Newsome LR, Bramwell RS, Curling PE: Severe preeclampsia: hemodynamic effects of lumbar epidural anesthesia. Anesth Analg 1986; 65:31–36.
24. Jouppila P, Jouppila R, Hollmén A, Koivula A: Lumbar epidural analgesia to improve intervillous blood flow during labor in severe preeclampsia. Obstet Gynecol 1982; 59:158–161.
25. Robson S, Hunter S, Boys R, et al: Changes in cardiac output during epidural anaesthesia for caesarean section. Anaesthesia 1989; 44:475–479.
26. Robson SC, Boys RJ, Rodeck C, Morgan B: Maternal and fetal haemodynamic effects of spinal and extradural anaesthesia for elective caesarean section. Br J Anaesth 1992; 68:54–59.
27. Lindblad A, Marsál K, Vernersson E, Renck H: Fetal circulation during epidural analgesia for caesarean section. BMJ 1984; 288:1329–1330.
28. Lindblad A, Bernow J, Marsál K: Obstetric analgesia and fetal aortic blood flow during labour. Br J Obstet Gynaecol 1987; 94:306–311.
29. Giles WB, Lah FX, Trudinger BJ: The effect of epidural anaesthesia for caesarean section on maternal uterine and fetal umbilical artery blood flow velocity waveforms. Br J Obstet Gynaecol 1987; 94:55–59.
30. Lindblad A, Bernow J, Marsál K: Fetal blood flow during intrathecal anaesthesia for elective caesarean section. Br J Anaesth 1988; 61:376–381.
31. Loughran PG, Moore J, Dundee JW: Maternal stress response associated with caesarean delivery under general and epidural anaesthesia. Br J Obstet Gynaecol 1986; 93:943–949.
32. Jouppila P, Kuikka J, Jouppila R, Hollmén A: Effect of induction of general anesthesia for cesarean section on intervillous blood flow. Acta Obstet Gynecol Scand 1979; 58:249–253.
33. Greiss FC: The uterine vascular bed: effect of adrenergic drug stimulation. Obstet Gynecol 1963; 21:295–299.
34. Greiss FC, Pick JR: The uterine vascular bed: adrenergic receptors. Obstet Gynecol 1964; 23:209–213.
35. Greiss FC, Gobble FL: Effect of sympathetic nerve stimulation on the uterine vascular bed. Am J Obstet Gynecol 1967; 97:962–967.
36. Irestedt L: How does anaesthesia influence fetal and neonatal stress? Abstracts of the European Society of Regional Anaesthesia, Oulu, Finland, 1989; 27.
37. Barrier G, Sureau C: Effects of anaesthetic and analgesic drugs on labour, fetus and neonate. Clin Obstet Gynaecol 1982; 9:351–367.
38. Hagnevik K, Irestedt L, Lundek B, Skolderfors E: Cardiac function and sympathoadrenal activity in the newborn after caesarean section under spinal and epidural anaesthesia. Acta Anaesthesiol Scand 1988; 32:234–238.
39. Fox GS, Smith JB, Namba Y, Johnson RC: Anesthesia for cesarean section: further studies. Am J Obstet Gynecol 1979; 133:15–19.
40. James FM, Crawford JS, Hopkinson R, et al: A comparison of general anesthesia and lumbar epidural analgesia for elective cesarean section. Anesth Analg 1977; 56:228–235.
41. Downing JW, Houlton PC, Barclay A: Extradural analgesia for caesarean section: a comparison with general anaesthesia. Br J Anaesth 1979; 51:367–374.

42. Crawford JS, Davies P: Status of neonates delivered by elective caesarean section. Br J Anaesth 1982; 54:1015–1022.
43. Milsom I, Forssman L, Biber B, et al: Maternal haemodynamic changes during caesarean section: a comparison of epidural and general anaesthesia. Acta Anaesthesiol Scand 1985; 29:161–167.
44. Evans CM, Murphy JF, Gray OP, Rosen M: Epidural versus general anaesthesia for elective caesarean section: effect on Apgar score and acid-base status of the newborn. Anaesthesia 1989; 44:778–782.
45. Datta S, Brown WU: Acid-base status in diabetic mothers and their infants following general or spinal anesthesia for cesarean section. Anesthesiology 1977; 47:272–276.
46. Marx GF, Luykx WM, Cohen S: Fetal-neonatal status following caesarean section for fetal distress. Br J Anaesth 1984; 56:1009–1013.
47. Irestedt L, Lagercrantz M, Mjemdahl P, et al: Fetal and maternal plasma catecholamine levels at elective cesarean section under general or epidural anesthesia versus vaginal delivery. Am J Obstet Gynecol 1982; 142:1004–1010.
48. Datta S, Ostheimer GW, Weiss JB, et al: Neonatal effect of prolonged anesthetic induction for cesarean section. Obstet Gynecol 1981; 58:331–335.
49. Robertson A, Fothergill RJ, Hall RA, et al: Effects of anesthesia with a high oxygen concentration on the acid-base state of babies delivered at elective cesarean section. S Afr Med J 1974; 48:2309–2313.
50. Marx GF, Joshi CW, Orkin LR: Placental transmission of nitrous oxide. Anesthesiology 1970; 32:429–432.
51. Dick W, Traub E, Kraus H, et al: General anaesthesia versus epidural anaesthesia for primary caesarean section—a preliminary study. Eur J Anaesthesiol 1992; 9:15–21.
52. Kamat SK, Shah MV, Chaudary LS, et al: Effect of induction–delivery and uterine incision–delivery on Apgar scoring of the newborn. J Postgrad Med 1991; 37:125–127.
53. Bader AM, Datta SS, Arthur GR, et al: Maternal and fetal catecholamines and uterine incision-to-delivery interval during elective cesarean. Obstet Gynecol 1990; 75:600–603.
54. Abboud TK, Sheik-ol-Eslam A, Yanagi T, et al: Safety and efficacy of epinephrine added to bupivacaine for lumbar epidural analgesia in obstetrics. Anesth Analg 1985; 64:585–591.
55. Hollmén AI, Jouppila R, Koivisto M, et al: Neurological activity of infants following anesthesia for cesarean section. Anesthesiology 1978; 48:350–356.
56. Ong BY, Cohen MM, Palahniuk RJ: Anesthesia for cesarean section—effects on neonates. Anesth Analg 1989; 68:270–275.
57. Wollman SB, Marx GF: Acute hydration for prevention of hypotension of spinal anesthesia in parturients. Anesthesiology 1968; 29:374–380.
58. Hodgkinson R, Bhatt M, Kim SS, et al: Neonatal neurobehavioral tests following cesarean section under general and spinal anesthesia. Am J Obstet Gynecol 1978; 132:670–674.
59. Gambling DR, Sharma SK, White PF, et al: Use of sevoflurane during elective cesarean birth: a comparison with isoflurane and spinal anesthesia. Anesth Analg 1995; 81:90–95.
60. Luyendijk W, Van Voorthuisen AE: Contrast examination of the spinal epidural space. Acta Radiol 1966; 5:1051–1066.
61. Luyendijk W: The plica mediana dorsalis of the dura mater and its relation to lumbar peridurography (canalography). Neuroradiology 1976; 11:147–149.
62. Helbo-Hansen S, Bang U, Garcia RS, et al: Subarachnoid versus epidural bupivacaine 0.5% for caesarean section. Acta Anaesthesiol Scand 1988; 32:473–476.
63. Alahuhta S, Kangas-Saarela T, Hollmén AI, Edström HH: Visceral pain during caesarean section under spinal and epidural anaesthesia with bupivacaine. Acta Anaesthesiol Scand 1990; 34:95–98.
64. Riley ET, Cohen SE, Macario A, et al: Spinal versus epidural anesthesia for cesarean section: a comparison of time efficiency, costs, charges, and complications. Anesth Analg 1995; 80:709–712.
65. Russell IF: Levels of anaesthesia and intraoperative pain at caesarean section under regional block. Int J Obstet Anesth 1995; 4:71–77.
66. Keohane M: Patient comfort: spinal versus epidural anesthesia for cesarean section. Anesth Analg 1996; 82:219.
67. Kenepp NB, Kumar S, Shelley WC, Gabbe SG: Fetal and neonatal hazards of maternal hydration with 5% dextrose before caesarean section. Lancet 1982; 1:1150–1152.
68. Philipson EH, Kalham SC, Riha MM, Pimental R: Effects of maternal glucose infusion on fetal acid-base status in human pregnancy. Am J Obstet Gynecol 1987; 157:866–873.
69. Peng ATC, Shamsi HH, Blancato LS, et al: Euglycemic hydration with dextrose 1% in lactated Ringer's solution during epidural anesthesia for cesarean section. Reg Anesth 1987; 12:184–188.
70. Norris MC, Leighton BL, DeSimone CA, et al: Influence of the choice of crystalloid solution on neonatal acid-base status at cesarean section [abstract]. Anesthesiology 1987; 67:A458.
71. Bader AM, Gilbertson L, Kirz L, Datta S: Regional anesthesia in women with chorioamnionitis. Reg Anesth 1992; 17:84–86.
72. Arens JF, Carrera AE: Methemoglobin levels following peridural anesthesia with prilocaine for vaginal deliveries. Anesth Analg 1970; 49:219–222.
73. Scanlon JW, Brown WU, Weiss JB, Alper MH: Neurobehavioral responses of newborn infants after maternal epidural anesthesia. Anesthesiology 1974; 40:121–126.
74. Thompson EM, Wilson CM, Moore J, et al: Plasma bupivacaine levels associated with extradural anaesthesia for caesarean section. Anaesthesia 1985; 40:427–432.
75. Abboud TK, Kim KC, Noueihed R, et al: Epidural bupivacaine, chloroprocaine, or lidocaine for cesarean section—maternal and neonatal effects. Anesth Analg 1983; 62:914–919.
76. McMorland GH, Douglas MJ, Kim JHK, et al: The effect of pH adjustment of bupivacaine on onset and duration of epidural anaesthesia for caesarean section. Can J Anaesth 1988; 35:457–461.
77. Nath S, Haggmark S, Johansson G, Reiz S: Differential depressant and electrophysiologic cardiotoxicity of local anesthetics: an experimental study with special reference to lidocaine and bupivacaine. Anesth Analg 1986; 65:1263–1270.
78. Buffington CW: The magnitude and duration of direct myocardial depression following intracoronary local anesthetics: a comparison of lidocaine and bupivacaine. Anesthesiology 1989; 70:280–287.
79. Moller RA, Covino BG: Cardiac electrophysiologic effects of lidocaine and bupivacaine. Anesth Analg 1988; 67:107–114.
80. Clarkson CW, Hondeghem LM: Mechanism for bupivacaine depression of cardiac conduction: fast block of sodium channels during the action potential with slow recovery from block during diastole. Anesthesiology 1985; 62:396–405.
81. Albright GA: Cardiac arrest following regional anesthesia with etidocaine or bupivacaine. Anesthesiology 1979; 51:285–287.
82. Rosen MA, Thigpen JW, Shnider SM, et al: Bupivacaine-induced cardiotoxicity in hypoxic and acidotic sheep. Anesth Analg 1985; 64:1089–1096.
83. Smith AR: Grand mal seizures after 2-chloroprocaine epidural anesthesia in a patient with plasma cholinesterase deficiency. Anesth Analg 1987; 66:677–678.
84. Kuhnert BR, Philipson EH, Pimental R, Kuhnert PM: A prolonged chloroprocaine epidural block in a postpartum patient with abnormal pseudocholinesterase. Anesthesiology 1982; 56:477–478.
85. James FM, Dewan DM, Floyd HM, et al: Chloroprocaine vs. bupivacaine for lumbar epidural analgesia for elective cesarean section. Anesthesiology 1980; 52:488–491.
86. Writer WDR, Dewan DM: Three per cent 2-chloroprocaine for caesarean section: appraisal of a standardized dose technique. Can Anaesth Soc J 1984; 31:559–564.
87. Cohen SE, Thurlow A: Comparison of a chloroprocaine–bupivacaine mixture with chloroprocaine and bupivacaine used individually for obstetric epidural analgesia. Anesthesiology 1979; 51:288–292.
88. Corke BC, Carlson CG, Dettbarn W-D: The influence of 2-chloroprocaine on the subsequent analgesic potency of bupivacaine. Anesthesiology 1984; 60:25–27.
89. Grice SC, Eisenach JC, Dewan DM: Labor analgesia with epidural bupivacaine plus fentanyl: enhancement with

epinephrine and inhibition with 2-chloroprocaine. Anesthesiology 1990; 72:623–628.
90. Huntoon M, Eisenach JC, Boese P: Epidural clonidine after cesarean section: appropriate dose and effect of prior local anesthetic. Anesthesiology 1992; 76:187–193.
91. Camann WR, Hartigan PM, Gilbertson LI, et al: Chloroprocaine antagonism of epidural opioid analgesia: a receptor-specific phenomenon? Anesthesiology 1990; 73:860–863.
92. Eisenach JC, Schlairet TJ, Dobson CE, Hood DH: Effect of prior anesthetic solution on epidural morphine analgesia. Anesth Analg 1991; 73:119–123.
93. Camann WR, Hurley RH, Gilbertson LI, et al: Epidural nalbuphine for analgesia following caesarean delivery: dose-response and effect of local anaesthetic choice. Can J Anaesth 1991; 38:728–732.
94. Karambelkar DJ, Ramanathan S: 2-Chloroprocaine antagonism of epidural morphine analgesia. Acta Anaesthesiol Scand 1997; 41:774–778.
95. Coda B, Bausch S, Haas M, Chavkin C: The hypothesis that antagonism of fentanyl analgesia by 2-chloroprocaine is mediated by direct action on opioid receptors. Reg Anesth 1997; 22:43–52.
96. Ravindran RS, Bond VK, Tasch MD, et al: Prolonged neural blockade following regional analgesia with 2-chloroprocaine. Anesth Analg 1980; 59:447–451.
97. Stevens RA, Chester WL, Arthuso JD, et al: Back pain after epidural anesthesia with chloroprocaine in volunteers: preliminary report. Reg Anesth 1991; 16:199–203.
98. Allen RW, Fee JPH, Moore J: A preliminary assessment of epidural chloroprocaine for day procedures. Anaesthesia 1993; 48:773–775.
99. Scanlon JW, Ostheimer GW, Lurie AO, et al: Neurobehavioral responses and drug concentrations in newborns after maternal epidural analgesia with bupivacaine. Anesthesiology 1976; 45:400–406.
100. Abboud TK, Sarkis F, Abilikan A, et al: Lack of adverse neonatal neurobehavioral effects of lidocaine. Anesth Analg 1983; 63:421–428.
101. Norton AC, Davies AG, Spicer RJ: Lignocaine 2% with adrenaline for epidural caesarean section: a comparison with 0.5% bupivacaine. Anaesthesia 1988; 43:844–849.
102. Reid JA, Thorburn J: Extradural bupivacaine or lignocaine anaesthesia for elective caesarean section: the role of maternal posture. Br J Anaesth 1988; 61:149–153.
103. Yun E, Topulos GP, Body SC, et al: Pulmonary function changes during epidural anesthesia for cesarean delivery. Anesth Analg 1996; 82:750–753.
104. Datta S, Camann W, Bader A, Vanderburgh L: Clinical effects and maternal and fetal plasma concentrations of epidural ropivacaine versus bupivacaine for cesarean section. Anesthesiology 1995; 82:1346–1352.
105. Griffin RP, Reynolds F: Extradural anaesthesia for caesarean section: a double-blind comparison of 0.5% ropivacaine with 0.5% bupivacaine. Br J Anaesth 1995; 74:512–516.
106. Reiz S, Häggmark S, Johansson G, Nath S: Cardiotoxicity of ropivacaine—a new amide local anaesthetic agent. Acta Anaesthesiol Scand 1989; 33:93–98.
107. Feldman HS, Arthur GR, Covino BG: Comparative systemic toxicity of convulsant and supraconvulsant doses of intravenous ropivacaine, bupivacaine, and lidocaine in the conscious dog. Anesth Analg 1989; 69:794–801.
108. Santos AC, Arthur GR, Pedersen H, et al: Systemic toxicity of ropivacaine during ovine pregnancy. Anesthesiology 1991; 75:137–141.
109. Reynolds F: Does the left hand know what the right hand is doing? An appraisal of single enantiomer local anaesthetics. Int J Obstet Anesth 1997; 6:257–269.
110. Zaric D, Nydahl P-A, Philipson L, et al: The effect of continuous lumbar epidural infusion of ropivacaine (0.1%, 0.2%, and 0.3%) and 0.25% bupivacaine on sensory and motor block in volunteers: A double-blind study. Reg Anesth 1996; 21:14–25.
111. Capogna G, Celleno D, Fusco P, et al: Relative potencies of bupivacaine and ropivacaine for analgesia in labour. Br J Anaesth 1999; 82:371–373.
112. Wolff AP, Hasselström L, Kerkkamp HE, Gielen MJ: Extradural ropivacaine and bupivacaine in hip surgery. Br J Anaesth 1995; 74:458–460.
113. Bromage PR: Epidural Analgesia. Philadelphia: WB Saunders; 1978:78–85.
114. Stevens RA, Chester WL, Schubert A, et al: pH adjustment of 2-chloroprocaine quickens the onset of epidural anaesthesia. Can J Anaesth 1989; 36:515–518.
115. DiFazio CA, Carron H, Grosslight RR, et al: Comparison of pH-adjusted lidocaine solutions for epidural anesthesia. Anesth Analg 1986; 65:760–764.
116. Benhamou D, Labaille T, Bonhomme L, Perrachon N: Alkalinization of epidural 0.5% bupivacaine for cesarean section. Reg Anesth 1980; 14:240–243.
117. Stevens RA, Chester WL, Grueter JA, et al: The effect of pH adjustment of 0.5% bupivacaine on the latency of epidural anesthesia. Reg Anesth 1989; 14:236–239.
118. Parnass SM, Curran MJA, Becker GL: Incidence of hypotension associated with epidural anesthesia using alkalinized and nonalkalinized lidocaine for cesarean section. Anesth Analg 1987; 66:1148–1150.
119. Ackerman WE, Denson DD, Juneja MM, et al: Alkalinization of chloroprocaine for epidural anesthesia: effects of pCO_2 at constant pH. Reg Anesth 1990; 15:89–93.
120. Wong K, Strichartz GR, Raymond SA: On the mechanisms of potentiation of local anesthetics by bicarbonate buffer: drug structure-activity studies on isolated peripheral nerve. Anesth Analg 1993; 76:131–143.
121. Bromage PR, Burfoot MF, Crowell DE, Truant AP: Quality of epidural blockade. III: Carbonated local anesthetic solutions. Br J Anaesth 1967; 39:197–209.
122. Brown DT, Morison DH, Covino BG, Scott DB: Comparison of carbonated bupivacaine and bupivacaine hydrochloride for extradural anaesthesia. Br J Anaesth 1980; 52:419–422.
123. Eisenach JC, Grice SC, Dewan DM: Epinephrine enhances analgesia produced by bupivacaine during labor. Anesth Analg 1987; 66:447–451.
124. Laishley RS, Morgan BM: A single dose epidural technique for caesarean section: a comparison between 0.5% bupivacaine plain and 0.5% bupivacaine with adrenaline. Anaesthesia 1988; 43:100–103.
125. Wilson CM, Moore J, Ghaly RG, et al: Plasma concentrations of bupivacaine during extradural anaesthesia for caesarean section. Anaesthesia 1988; 43:12–15.
126. Noble DW, Morrison LM, Brockway MS, McClure JH: Adrenaline, fentanyl or adrenaline and fentanyl as adjuncts to bupivacaine for extradural anaesthesia in elective caesarean section. Br J Anaesth 1991; 66:645–650.
127. Preston PG, Rosen MA, Hughes SC, et al: Epidural anesthesia with fentanyl and lidocaine for cesarean section: maternal effects and neonatal outcome. Anesthesiology 1988; 68:38–43.
128. Reid J, Thornburn J: Bupivacaine and lignocaine for epidural caesarean section and the role of maternal posture. Br J Anaesth 1988; 61:149–153.
129. Norris MC, Dewan DM: Effect of gravity on the spread of extradural anaesthesia for caesarean section. Br J Anaesth 1987; 59:338–341.
130. Albright GA: Cardiac arrest following regional anesthesia with etidocaine or bupivacaine [editorial]. Anesthesiology 1979; 51:285–287.
131. Writer WDR, Davies JM, Strunin L: Trial by media: the bupivacaine story. Can Anaesth Soc J 1984; 31:1–4.
132. Thorburn J, Moir DD: Bupivacaine toxicity in association with extradural analysis for caesarean section. Br J Anaesth 1984; 56:551–552.
133. Crawford JS, Davies P, Lewis M: Some aspects of epidural block provided for elective caesarean section. Anaesthesia 1986; 41:1039–1046.
134. Dutton DA, Moir DD, Howe HB, et al: Choice of local anaesthetic drug for extradural caesarean section: comparison of 0.5% and 0.75% bupivacaine and 1.5% etidocaine. Br J Anaesth 1984; 56:1361–1368.
135. Blair MR: Cardiovascular pharmacology of local anaesthetics. Br J Anaesth 1975; 47:247–252.
136. Burm AGL, van Kleef JW, Gladines MPRR, et al: Epidural

anesthesia with lidocaine and bupivacaine: effects of epinephrine on the plasma concentration profiles. Anesth Analg 1986; 65:1281–1284.
137. Brose WG, Cohen SE: Epidural lidocaine for cesarean section: effect of varying epinephrine concentration. Anesthesiology 1988; 69:936–940.
138. Partridge BL: The effects of local anesthetics and epinephrine on rat sciatic nerve flow. Anesthesiology 1991; 75:243–250.
139. Priddle MD, Andros GJ: Primary spinal anesthetic effects of epinephrine. Anesth Analg 1950; 29:156–162.
140. Rosenfeld CR, Barton MD, Meschia G: Effects of epinephrine on distribution of blood flow in the pregnant ewe. Am J Obstet Gynecol 1976; 124:156–163.
141. Wallis KL, Shnider SM, Hicks JS, Spivey HT: Epidural anesthesia in the normotensive pregnant ewe: effects on uterine blood flow and fetal acid-base status. Anesthesiology 1976; 44:481–487.
142. Chestnut DH, Weiner CP, Herrig JE, Wang J: Effect of intravenous epinephrine upon uterine blood flow velocity in the pregnant guinea pig [abstract]. Anesthesiology 1985; 63:A453.
143. Hood DD, Dewan DM, James FM: Maternal and fetal effects of epinephrine in gravid ewes. Anesthesiology 1986; 64:610–613.
144. Albright GA, Jouppila R, Hollmén AI, et al: Epinephrine does not alter human intervillous blood flow during epidural anesthesia. Anesthesiology 1981; 54:131–135.
145. Marx GF, David-Elstein ID, Schuss M, et al: Effects of epidural block with lignocaine and lignocaine-adrenaline on umbilical artery velocity wave ratios. Br J Obstet Gynaecol 1990; 97:517–520.
146. Hadzic A, Vloka J, Patel N, Birnbach D: Hypertensive crises after a successful placement of an epidural anesthetic in a hypertensive parturient. Reg Anesth 1995; 20:156–158.
147. Eisenach J, Detweiler D, Hood D: Hemodynamic and analgesic actions of epidurally administered clonidine. Anesthesiology 1993; 78:277–287.
148. Mercier FJ, Boulay G, Ben Ayed M, Benhamou D: Analgesie rachidienne et peridurale combinee pour le travail: prolongation par l'adjonction d'une minidose de clonidine au sufentanil. Etude preliminaire. Ann Fr Anesth Reanim 1996; 15:263–265.
149. Narchi P, Benhamou D, Hamza J, Bouaziz H: Ventilatory effects of epidural clonidine during the first 3 hours after caesarean section. Acta Anaesthesiol Scand 1992; 36:791–795.
150. Gaffeld MP, Bansal P, Lawton C, et al: Surgical analgesia for cesarean delivery with epidural bupivacaine and fentanyl. Anesthesiology 1986; 65:331–334.
151. Paech MJ, Speirs HM: A double-blind comparison of epidural bupivacaine and bupivacaine-fentanyl for caesarean section. Anaesth Intensive Care 1990; 18:22–30.
152. Capogna G, Celleno D, Tomassetti M: Maternal analgesia and neonatal effects of epidural sufentanil for cesarean section. Reg Anesth 1989; 14:282–287.
153. Madej TH, Strunin L: Comparison of epidural fentanyl with sufentanil. Anaesthesia 1987; 42:1156–1161.
154. Celleno D, Capogna G, Sebastian M: Epidural analgesia during and after cesarean delivery: comparison of five opioids. Reg Anesth 1991; 16:79–83.
155. Palmer CM, Petty JV, Nohami WM, et al: What is the optimal dose of epidural morphine for post-cesarean analgesia [abstract]? Anesthesiology 1996; 85:A909.
156. Glynn CJ, Mather LE, Cousins MJ, et al: Peridural meperidine in humans. Anesthesiology 1981; 55:520–526.
157. Nyan Kee WD, Lam KK, Chen PP, Gin T: Epidural meperidine after cesarean section: a dose response study. Anesthesiology 1996; 85:289–294.
158. Beilin Y, Bernstein HH, Zucker-Pinchoff B: The optimal distance that a multiorifice epidural catheter should be threaded into the epidural space. Anesth Analg 1995; 81:301–304.
159. Hamilton CL, Riley ET, Cohen SE: Changes in the position of epidural catheters associated with patient movement. Anesthesiology 1997; 86:778–784.
160. Reisner LS: Epidural test solution or spinal fluid? Anesthesiology 1976; 44:451.
161. Rosenberg H: pH in differentiating CSF from local anesthesia in peridural anesthesia. Anesthesiology 1976; 45:579.
162. Leighton BL: Intraoperative anesthetic complications. *In* Norris MC (ed): Obstetric Anesthesia, 2nd ed. Philadelphia: Lippincott Williams & Wilkins; 1999:593–618.
163. Leighton BL, Norris MC, Sosis M, et al: Limitations of epinephrine as a marker of intravascular injection in laboring women. Anesthesiology 1987; 66:688–691.
164. Leighton BL, DeSimone CA, Norris MC, Chayen B: Isoproterenol is an effective marker for intravenous injection in laboring women. Anesthesiology 1989; 71:206–209.
165. Marcus MAR, Vertommen JD, Van Aken H, et al: Hemodynamic effects of intravenous isoproterenol versus saline in the parturient. Anesth Analg 1997; 84:1113–1116.
166. Leighton BL, Norris MC, DeSimone CA, et al: The air test is a clinically useful indicator of intravenously placed epidural catheters. Anesthesiology 1990; 73:610–613.
167. Leighton BL, Gross JB: Air: an effective marker of intravenously located catheters. Anesthesiology 1989; 71:848–851.
168. Russell IF: Levels of anaesthesia and intraoperative pain at caesarean section under regional block. Int J Obstet Anesth 1995; 4:71–77.
169. Workhoven MN: Intravenous fluid temperature, shivering and the parturient. Anesth Analg 1986; 65:496–498.
170. Johnson MD, Sevarino FB, Lena MJ: Cessation of shivering and hypothermia associated with epidural sufentanil. Anesth Analg 1989; 68:70–71.
171. Sessler DI, Poute J: Shivering during epidural anesthesia. Anesthesiology 1990; 72:816–821.
172. Capogna G, Celleno D: IV clonidine for post-extradural shivering in parturients: a preliminary study. Br J Anaesth 1993; 71:294–295.
173. Chestnut DH, Vandewalker GE, Owne CL, et al: Administration of metoclopramide for prevention of nausea and vomiting during epidural anesthesia for elective cesarean section. Anesthesiology 1987; 66:563–566.
174. Pan PH, Moore CH: Intraoperative antiemetic efficacy of prophylactic ondansetron versus droperidol for cesarean section patients under epidural anesthesia. Anesth Analg 1996; 83:982–986.
175. Boey SK, Carrie LES: Withdrawal forces during removal of lumbar extradural catheters. Br J Anaesth 1994; 73:833–835.
176. Balance JHW: Difficulty in removal of an epidural catheter. Anaesthesia 1981; 36:71–72.
177. Rout CC, Rocke DA, Levin J, et al: A reevaluation of the role of crystalloid preload in the prevention of hypotension associated with spinal anesthesia for elective cesarean section. Anesthesiology 1993; 79:262–269.
178. Freedman JM, Li DK, Drasner K, et al: Transient neurologic symptoms after spinal anesthesia: an epidemiologic study of 1863 patients. Anesthesiology 1998; 89:633–641.
179. Van Zundert AA, DeWolf AM, Vaes L: High-volume spinal anesthesia with bupivacaine 0.125% for cesarean section. Anesthesiology 1988; 69:998–1003.
180. Russell IF: Spinal anesthesia for cesarean delivery with dilute solutions of plain bupivacaine: the relationship between infused volume and spread. Reg Anesth 1991; 16:130–136.
181. Vucevic M, Russell IF: Spinal anaesthesia for caesarean section: 0.125% plain bupivacaine 12 ml compared with 0.5% plain bupivacaine 3 ml. Br J Anaesth 1992; 68:590–595.
182. Runza M, Albani A, Tagliabue M, Haiek M, et al: Spinal anesthesia using 3 ml hyperbaric 0.65% versus hyperbaric 1% bupivacaine for cesarean section. Anesth Analg 1998; 87:1099–1103.
183. Palmer CM, Voulgaropoulos D, Alves D: Subarachnoid fentanyl augments lidocaine spinal anesthesia for cesarean delivery. Reg Anesth 1995; 20:389–394.
184. Bembridge M, MacDonald R, Lyons G: Spinal anaesthesia with hyperbaric lignocaine for elective caesarean section. Anaesthesia 1986; 41:906–909.
185. Schneider M, Ettlin T, Kaufmann M, et al: Transient neurologic toxicity after hyperbaric subarachnoid anesthesia with 5% lidocaine. Anesth Analg 1993; 76:1154–1157.
186. Hampl KF, Schneider MC, Pargger H, et al: A similar

incidence of transient neurologic symptoms after anesthesia with 2% and 5% lidocaine. Anesth Analg 1996; 83:1051–1054.
187. Pollock JE, Liu SS, Neal JM, Stephenson CA: Dilution of spinal lidocaine does not alter the incidence of transient neurological symptoms. Anesthesiology 1999; 90:445–450.
188. Freedman JM, Li DK, Drasner K, et al: Transient neurologic symptoms after spinal anesthesia: an epidemiologic study of 1,863 patients. Anesthesiology 1998; 89:633–641.
189. Chantigian RC, Datta S, Burger GA, et al: Anesthesia for cesarean delivery utilizing spinal anesthesia: tetracaine versus tetracaine and procaine. Reg Anesth 1984; 9:195–200.
190. Michie AR, Freeman RM, Dutton DA, Howie HB: Subarachnoid anaesthesia for elective caesarean section: a comparison of two hyperbaric solutions. Anaesthesia 1988; 43:96–99.
191. Carpenter RL, Smith HS, Brindenbaugh LD: Epinephrine increases the effectiveness of tetracaine spinal anesthesia. Anesthesiology 1989; 71:33–36.
192. Sakura S, Sumi M, Sakaguchi Y, et al: The addition of phenylephrine contributes to the development of transient neurologic symptoms after spinal anesthesia with 0.5% tetracaine. Anesthesiology 1997; 87:771–778.
193. Wahedi W, Nolte H, Klein P: Ropivacaine for spinal anesthesia: a dose-finding study. Anesthetist 1996; 45:737–744.
194. Nguyen Thi TV, Orliaguet G, Ngu TH, Bonnet F: Spinal anesthesia with meperidine as the sole agent for cesarean delivery. Reg Anesth 1994; 19:386–389.
195. Norris MC, Honet JE, Leighton BL, Arkoosh VA: A comparison of meperidine and lidocaine for spinal anesthesia for postpartum tubal ligation. Reg Anesth 1996; 21:84–88.
196. Russell IF: Spinal anaesthesia for caesarean section: the use of 0.5% bupivacaine. Br J Anaesth 1983; 55:309–314.
197. Carrie LES: Combined spinal-epidural anesthesia for cesarean section. Tech Reg Anesth Pain Manage 1997; 1:118–123.
198. Pedersen H, Santos AC, Steinberg ES, et al: Incidence of visceral pain during cesarean section: the effect of varying doses of spinal bupivacaine. Anesth Analg 1989; 69:46–49.
199. Pitkänen MT: Body mass and spread of spinal anesthesia with bupivacaine. Anesth Analg 1987; 66:127–131.
200. Schnider TW, Minto CF, Bruckert H, Mandema JW: Population pharmacodynamic modeling and covariate detection for central neural blockade. Anesthesiology 1996; 85:502–512.
201. Norris MC: Patient variables and the subarachnoid spread of hyperbaric bupivacaine in the term parturient. Anesthesiology 1990; 72:478–482.
202. Norris MC: Height, weight and the spread of spinal anesthesia for cesarean section. Anesth Analg 1988; 67:555–558.
203. Hartwell BL, Aglio LS, Hauch MA, Datta S: Vertebral column length and spread of hyperbaric subarachnoid bupivacaine in the term parturient. Reg Anesth 1991; 16:17–19.
204. Ravenscroft A, Govender T, Rout C: Spinal anaesthesia for emergency caesarean section in an achondroplastic dwarf. Anaesthesia 1998; 53:1236–1237.
205. Hunt CO, Naulty JS, Bader AM, et al: Perioperative analgesia with subarachnoid fentanyl-bupivacaine for cesarean delivery. Anesthesiology 1989; 71:535–540.
206. Shende D, Cooper GM, Dowden MI: The influence of intrathecal fentanyl on the characteristics of subarachnoid block for caesarean section. Anaesthesia 1998; 53:706–710.
207. Belzarena SD: Clinical effects of intrathecally administered fentanyl in patients undergoing cesarean section. Anesth Analg 1992; 74:653–657.
208. Cooper DW, Lindsay SL, Ryall DM, et al: Does intrathecal fentanyl produce acute cross-tolerance to i.v. morphine? Br J Anaesth 1997; 78:311–313.
209. Liu S, Chiu AA, Carpenter RL, et al: Fentanyl prolongs lidocaine spinal anesthesia without prolonging recovery. Anesth Analg 1995; 80:730–734.
210. Connelly NR, Dunn SM, Ingold V, Villa EA: The use of fentanyl added to morphine-lidocaine-epinephrine spinal solution in patients undergoing cesarean section. Anesth Analg 1994; 78:918–920.
211. Pan MH, Wei TT, Shieh BS: Comparative analgesic enhancement of alfentanil, fentanyl and sufentanil to spinal tetracaine anesthesia for cesarean delivery. Acta Anaesthesiol Sin 1994; 32:171–176.
212. Courtney MA, Bader AM, Hartwell B, et al: Perioperative analgesia with subarachnoid sufentanil administration. Reg Anesth 1992; 17:274–278.
213. Dahlgren G, Hultstrand C, Jakobsson J, et al: Intrathecal sufentanil, fentanyl, or placebo added to bupivacaine for cesarean section. Anesth Analg 1997; 85:1288–1293.
214. Ngiam SK, Chong JL: The addition of intrathecal sufentanil and fentanyl to bupivacaine for caesarean section. Singapore Med J 1998; 39:290–294.
215. Grant GJ, Susser L, Cascio M, et al: Hemodynamic effects of intrathecal fentanyl in non-laboring term parturients. J Clin Anesth 1996; 8:99–103.
216. Lin BC, Lin PC, Lai YY, et al: The maternal and fetal effects of the addition of sufentanil to 0.5% spinal bupivacaine for cesarean delivery. Acta Anaesthesiol Sin 1998; 36:143–148.
217. Hays RL, Palmer CM: Respiratory depression after intrathecal sufentanil during labor. Anesthesiology 1994; 81:511–512.
218. Baker MN, Sarna MC: Respiratory arrest after second dose of intrathecal sufentanil. Anesthesiology 1995; 83:231–232.
219. Ferouz F, Norris MC, Leighton BL: Risk of respiratory arrest after intrathecal sufentanil. Anesth Analg 1997; 85:1088–1090.
220. Greenhalgh CA: Respiratory arrest in a parturient following intrathecal injection of sufentanil and bupivacaine. Anaesthesia 1996; 51:173–175.
221. Herman NL, Calicott R, Van Decar TK, et al: Determination of the dose-response relationship for intrathecal sufentanil in laboring patients. Anesth Analg 1997; 84:1256–1261.
222. Palmer CM, Cork RC, Hays R, et al: The dose-response relation of intrathecal fentanyl for labor analgesia. Anesthesiology 1998; 88:355–361.
223. Grass JA, Sakima NT, Schmidt R, et al: A randomised double-blind, dose-response comparison of epidural fentanyl versus sufentanil analgesia after cesarean section. Anesth Analg 1997; 85:365–371.
224. Abouleish E, Rawal N, Fallon K, Hernandez D: Combined intrathecal morphine and bupivacaine for cesarean section. Anesth Analg 1988; 67:370–374.
225. Abouleish E, Rawal N, Fallon K, Hernandez D: Combined intrathecal morphine and bupivacaine for cesarean section. Anesth Analg 1988; 67:370–374.
226. Chadwick HS, Ready LB: Intrathecal and epidural morphine sulfate for post-cesarean analgesia—a clinical comparison. Anesthesiology 1988; 68:925–929.
227. Palmer CM, Emerson S, Volgaropoulos D, Alves D: Dose-response relationship of intrathecal morphine for post-cesarean analgesia. Anesthesiology 1999; 90:437–444.
228. Abouleish E, Rawal N, Tobon-Randall B, et al: A clinical and laboratory study to compare the addition of 0.2 mg of morphine, 0.2 mg of epinephrine, or their combination to hyperbaric bupivacaine for spinal anesthesia in cesarean section. Anesth Analg 1993; 77:457–462.
229. Zakowski MI, Ramanathan S, Sharnick S, Turndorf H: Uptake and distribution of bupivacaine and morphine after intrathecal administration in parturients: effects of epinephrine. Anesth Analg 1992; 74:664–669.
230. Husaini SW, Russell IF: Intrathecal diamorphine compared with morphine for postoperative analgesia after caesarean section under spinal anaesthesia. Br J Anaesth 1998; 81:135–139.
231. Kelly MC, Carabine UA, Mirakhur RK: Intrathecal diamorphine for analgesia after caesarean section. Anaesthesia 1998; 53:231–237.
232. Collier CB: Accidental subdural block: four more cases and a radiographic review. Anaesth Intensive Care 1992; 20:215–232.
233. Scott DB, Tunstall ME: Serious complications associated with epidural/spinal blockade in obstetrics: a two-year prospective study. Int J Obstet Anesth 1995; 4:133–139.
234. Paech MJ, Godkin R, Webster S: Complications of obstetric epidural analgesia and anaesthesia. Int J Obstet Anesth 1998; 7:5–11.
235. Baraka AS, Hanna MT, Jabbour SI, et al: Preoxygenation of pregnant and non-pregnant women in the head-up versus supine position. Anesth Analg 1992; 75:757–759.

236. Furst SR, Reisner LS: Risk of high spinal anesthesia following failed epidural block for cesarean delivery. J Clin Anesth 1995; 7:71–74.
237. Gupta A, Enhund G, Bengtsson M, Sjöberg F: Spinal anaesthesia for caesarean section following epidural analgesia in labour: a relative contraindication. Int J Obstet Anesth 1994; 3:153–156.
238. Mets B, Broccoli E, Brocou AR: Is spinal anesthesia after failed epidural anesthesia contraindicated for cesarean section? Anesth Analg 1993; 77:629–631.
239. Vickers R, Wilkey A: Spinal anaesthesia for caesarean section. Br J Anaesth 1996; 77:301–302.
240. Bromage PR: Epidural Analgesia. Philadelphia: WB Saunders; 1978:31.
241. Bromage PR: Epidural Analgesia. Philadelphia: WB Saunders; 1978:173.
242. Stoneham M, Souter A: Spinal anaesthesia for caesarean section in women with incomplete epidural analgesia. Br J Anaesth 1996; 77:476.
243. Norris MC: Spinal anesthesia for cesarean delivery. *In* Norris MC (ed): Obstetric Anesthesia. Philadelphia: Lippincott Williams & Wilkins; 1999:415–439.
244. Carrie LES, O'Sullivan GM: Subarachnoid bupivacaine 0.5% for caesarean section. Eur J Anaesth 1984; 1:275–283.
245. Rawal N, Schollin J, Wesstrom G: Epidural versus combined spinal epidural block for caesarean section. Acta Anaesthesiol Scand 1998; 32:61–66.
246. Holmström B, Rawal N, Axelsson K, Nydahl P-A: Risk of catheter migration during combined spinal epidural block: percutaneous epiduroscopy study. Anesth Analg 1995; 80:747–753.
247. Rawal N: Problems with combined spinal-epidural anaesthesia. *In* Russell IF, Lyons G (eds): Clinical Problems in Obstetric Anaesthesia. London: Chapman & Hall; 1997:213–220.
248. Lyons G, MacDonald R, Mikl B: Combined epidural spinal anaesthesia for caesarean section: through the needle or in separate spaces? Anaesthesia 1992; 47:199–201.
249. Randalls B, Broadway JW, Browne DA, Morgan BM: Comparison of four subarachnoid solutions in needle-through-needle technique for elective caesarean section. Br J Anaesth 1991; 66:314–318.
250. Carrie LES: Extradural spinal or combined spinal block for obstetric surgical anaesthesia. Br J Anaesth 1990; 65:225–233.
251. Cook TM: Combined spinal epidural anaesthesia: a new technique. Int J Obstet Anesth 1999; 8:3–6.
252. Turner MA, Reifenberg NA: Combined spinal epidural anaesthesia: the single space double-barrel technique. Int J Obstet Anesth 1995; 4:158–160.
253. Davies SJ, Paech MJ, Welch H, et al: Maternal experience during epidural or combined spinal-epidural anesthesia for cesarean section: a prospective, randomized trial. Anesth Analg 1997; 85:607–613.
254. Patel M, Samsoon G, Swami A, Morgan B: Posture and the spread of hyperbaric bupivacaine in parturients using the combined spinal epidural technique. Can J Anaesth 1993; 40:943–946.
255. Vercauteren MP, Coppejans HC, Hoffmann VL, et al: Small-dose hyperbaric versus plain bupivacaine during spinal anesthesia for cesarean section. Anesth Analg 1998; 86:989–993.
256. Stienstra R, Dahan A, Alhadi BZ, et al: Mechanism of action of an epidural top-up in combined spinal epidural anesthesia. Anesth Analg 1996; 83:382–386.
257. Takiguchi T, Okano T, Egawa H, et al: The effect of spinal saline injection on analgesic level during combined spinal and epidural anesthesia assessed clinically and myelographically. Anesth Analg 1997; 85:1097–1100.
258. Kase S, Kobayashi T, Takiguchi T, Kitajima T: The effect of epidural saline injection on analgesic level during combined spinal and epidural anesthesia. Masui 1998; 47:1080–1084.
259. Mardirosoff C, Dumont L, Lemedioni P, et al: Sensory block extension during combined spinal and epidural. Reg Anesth Pain Med 1998; 23:92–95.
260. Trautman WJ III, Liu SS, Kopacz DJ: Comparison of lidocaine and saline for epidural top-up during combined spinal-epidural anesthesia in volunteers. Anesth Analg 1997; 84:575–577.
261. Corke CF, Wheatley RG: Respiratory depression complicating epidural diamorphine: two case reports of administration after dural puncture. Anaesthesia 1985; 40:1203–1205.
262. Myint Y, Bailey PW, Milne BR: Cardiorespiratory arrest following combined spinal epidural anaesthesia for caesarean section. Anaesthesia 1993; 48:684–686.
263. Swenson JD, Wisniewski M, McJames S, et al: The effect of prior dural puncture on cisternal cerebrospinal fluid morphine concentrations in sheep after administration of lumbar epidural morphine. Anesth Analg 1996; 83:523–525.
264. Collier CB: Cardiorespiratory arrest following combined spinal epidural anaesthesia. Anaesthesia 1994; 49:259.

19

Anesthesia for Presumed Fetal Jeopardy

❖ MICHAEL A. FRÖLICH, MD, DEAA

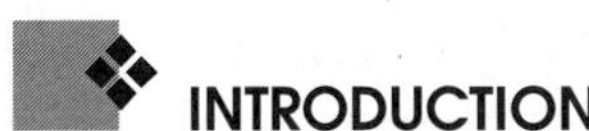

INTRODUCTION

The management of the stressed fetus is one of the most challenging tasks for both the obstetrician and the anesthesiologist. There is an extensive list of obstetric emergencies that demand prompt intervention. The consequences of unrecognized or poorly managed perinatal emergencies can be devastating, ranging from neurologic impairment to intrauterine fetal death. Perinatal asphyxia at term remains a significant cause of infant death and developmental impairment. In recent years, a variety of epidemiologic studies have shown that most cases of hypoxic-ischemic encephalopathy observed in children are not related to intrapartum asphyxia.[1–10] Nevertheless, if one excludes premature infants, approximately 12% to 23% of cerebral palsy can be related to intrapartum asphyxia.[11] A large body of experimental, clinical, and brain imaging data shows that brain injury occurs intrapartum in a significant number of infants.[12, 13] Even a relatively small percentage of cases of cerebral palsy caused by intrapartum events, 2 to 3 cases per 1000 children born in the United States, translates into a large absolute number considering that approximately 4 million live births take place every year.

One important element in the care of the compromised fetus is the well-coordinated teamwork of anesthesiologist, obstetrician, and neonatologist. The collaboration of the involved specialists is often hindered by the indifferent understanding of the medical terms used to describe fetal status and the urgency of the necessary intervention. Fetal jeopardy, fetal asphyxia, and stat or emergent cesarean section are terms that may be used to describe a variety of clinical situations and are not indicative of a single clinical entity.

To administer the best possible care to both mother and newborn, the anesthesiologist must have a clear understanding of certain obstetric emergencies and the possible management modalities, and at the same time there must be a uniform agreement on the terms used to describe the fetus at risk. The anesthesiologist's expertise is called for in particular if the obstetric intervention necessitates an operative mode of delivery.

This chapter reviews the terminology used to describe the status of the compromised fetus as well as the different terms used to indicate the urgency of an operative mode of delivery. The pathophysiologic effects following fetal hypoxia and anoxia as well as the role of different intrapartum fetal surveillance modalities are discussed. Recommendations for anesthetic management follow an overview of emergent obstetric treatment modalities.

TERMINOLOGY

The term *fetal distress* is widely used as an indication for an emergent cesarean section, or as justification for operative delivery. It is often prefaced by the term acute or chronic. Some authors have equated fetal distress with "late decelerations" or "severe variable decelerations," or "tachycardia with total loss of short-term variability" of the fetal heart rate.[14, 15] Physicians frequently use the terms "fetal distress" interchangeably with "asphyxia of the newborn"; some view asphyxia as the cause of fetal distress. It appears that the confusion of the definition compounds the difficulty in making an accurate diagnosis and initiating appropriate treatment. According to some authors and to the American College of Obstetricians and Gynecologists, the poor definition of the term *fetal distress* as well as varied interpretations of it is felt to be a "disservice to obstetrics."[16]

Parer and Livingston[17] attempted to define "fetal distress" by reviewing the fetal physiologic adaptations that occur with decreased oxygenation to protect the brain, heart, and adrenals. The definition they have developed is logical: fetal distress is progressive fetal asphyxia that, if not corrected or circumvented, results in decompensation of physiologic responses (primarily redistribution of blood flow to preserve oxygenation of vital organs) and causes permanent central nervous system and other organ damage or death. The difficulty lies in the use of this definition clinically. Clinicians rely on indirect parameters such as fetal heart rate to evaluate fetal status, because the underlying pathophysiologic events unfortunately cannot be measured clinically.

Most physicians recognize that fetal distress is related to asphyxia. The word *asphyxia* has a Greek derivation, indicating a "stopping of the pulse." It is defined in *Dorland's Illustrated Medical Dictionary* as "pathological changes caused by lack of oxygen in respired air, resulting in hypoxia and hypercapnia."[18] *Webster's Medical Dictionary* defines asphyxia as "a lack of oxygen or excess of carbon dioxide in the body that is usually caused by interruption of breathing and that causes unconsciousness."[19]

In this chapter the terms *asphyxia* and *fetal distress (nonreassuring status)* are used to describe "a condition resulting from compromised fetal gas exchange." The term *fetal anoxia* is used to describe "a condition resulting from complete cessation of fetal gas exchange." Most clinical scenarios fall into the category of "fetal distress" (nonreassuring status) or asphyxia. There are, however, certain circumstances in which fetal anoxia has to be suspected, and the understanding that fetal gas exchange has stopped completely must govern therapeutic interventions. Figure 19–1 describes the categories of intrapartum asphyxia.

Cerebral palsy can be defined as a nonprogressive disorder of the central nervous system (CNS) that has been present since birth and that includes some impairment of motor function and posture. Sometimes the term *cerebral palsy* is equated with hypoxic-ischemic encephalopathy. Since peripartum asphyxia accounts for only the minority of cases of cerebral palsy, this simplification of terminology is misleading. A multivariate analysis of risk revealed that the leading factors associated with cerebral palsy are (1) maternal mental retardation, (2) birthweight less than 2001 g, and (3) fetal malformation. Other factors involved are (4) breech presentation, (5) severe proteinuria in the second half of pregnancy, and (6) third trimester bleeding.

Several intrapartum emergencies may necessitate delivery by emergent cesarean section. To ensure proper coordination of perioperative care, all involved health professionals must have a clear understanding of the desired time to delivery. In general, *elective* or *nonemergent* cesarean sections can be distinguished from *unplanned or emergency* cesarean sections.

Harris[20] divides emergency cesarean sections into three categories: stable, urgent, and "stat" (immediate surgery). According to his classifications stable emergency cesarean sections are performed in patients with stable maternal and fetal physiology but who need surgery before destabilization occurs (e.g., chronic placental insufficiency with nonreactive nonstress test or in a footling breech but with no signs of labor). Urgent cesarean sections refer to situations in which maternal and/or fetal physiology is unstable (e.g., variable decelerations with prompt recovery), whereas the term stat cesarean section is used for situations with immediate life-threatening conditions for mother and/or fetus (e.g., cord prolapse with fetal bradycardia). This classification is practical and helps the anesthesiologist to appreciate the urgency of certain obstetric entities. Unfortunately, there is significant overlap between the three categories.

The clinical diagnosis per se is often not precise and the desired time frame to delivery is subject to the obstetrician's judgment of the individual clinical presentation. In most cases the key to adequate patient management is the prompt communication between obstetrician and anesthesiologist. The desired time frame from diagnosis to delivery in cases with presumed fetal anoxia is strictly "as soon as possible." Only a well-planned emergency protocol with a clear understanding of the sequence of events of all involved specialties will guarantee optimal patient management in this type of scenario. Conditions in which the fetus appears to be at risk but stable for the time being are labeled as "compromised fetal state" (compromised fetus). In the latter category, a complete cessation of gas exchange is not suspected (see Table 19–1).

PATHOPHYSIOLOGY OF FETAL ASPHYXIA

Fetal asphyxia is the condition resulting from failure to maintain gas exchange. Arterial carbon dioxide partial

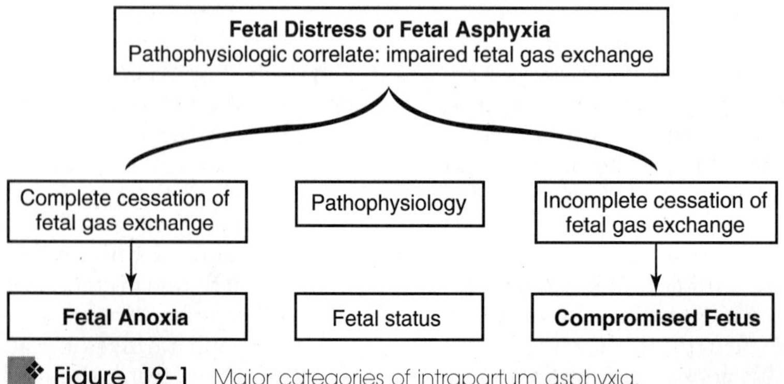

Figure 19–1 Major categories of intrapartum asphyxia.

pressure ($Paco_2$) rises, and arterial oxygen partial pressure (Pao_2) and pH fall. Despite the low Pao_2, tissues continue to consume oxygen. In the presence of very low Pao_2, anaerobic metabolism results, producing metabolic acidosis. These are partly buffered by bicarbonate in the blood.[21]

A particularly vulnerable time for the infant is the perinatal period. During normal labor, transient hypoxemia occurs with uterine contractions, but the healthy fetus tolerates this well. There are five basic causes of asphyxia in the peripartum period:

1. Inadequate perfusion of the maternal side of the placenta (e.g., severe hypotension)
2. Failure of gas exchange across the placenta (e.g., placental abruption)
3. Interruption of umbilical blood flow (e.g., cord compression)
4. The effect of transient, intermittent hypoxia of normal labor in the compromised fetus (e.g., the anemic or growth-retarded fetus)
5. Failure to inflate the lungs and complete the change in ventilation and lung perfusion that must occur at birth (e.g., airway obstruction, excessive fluids in the lungs, or weak respiratory effort)

The umbilical cord blood pH, partial pressure of oxygen (Po_2), partial pressure of carbon dioxide (Pco_2), and the calculated base excess are standard measures of fetal asphyxia.[22, 23] With fetal acidosis, the pH can vary over a wide range. The gradient in blood gas tension between umbilical artery and vein may be an indication of placental perfusion at the time of birth. The slower the flow of fetal blood through the placenta, the more complete the equilibration of gas tensions between fetal and maternal blood. For example, an arterial Pao_2 of 25 mm Hg with a venous Pao_2 of 32 mm Hg suggests good placental flow. An arterial Pao_2 of 12 mm Hg with a venous Pao_2 of 45 mm Hg suggests suboptimal flow. Metabolic acidosis suggests asphyxia, although some increased lactic acid in the blood may be due to reduced uptake of lactate by the asphyxiated liver rather than the result of increased lactate production from anaerobic metabolism.[24] If asphyxia occurred just before birth, there may be lactic acid in the tissues that has not yet reached the central circulation. This is detectable only by blood gas measurements a few minutes after birth. If the fetus was asphyxiated an hour before delivery and recovered, that event is not reflected in the umbilical cord blood gases at birth. Other indicators of asphyxia include plasma hypoxanthine, which increases because of lack of aerobic metabolism, and plasma erythropoietin, which increases in response to fetal hypoxia.[25, 26]

The speed and extent of fetal asphyxia are highly variable. Fetal anoxia (severe asphyxia) can be lethal in less than 10 minutes. Repeated episodes of brief, mild asphyxia may reverse spontaneously but produce a cumulative effect of progressive asphyxia. Figure 19–2 schematically represents the sequence of events that accompany asphyxia.[27]

Cardiac output is maintained early in asphyxia, but its distribution changes radically. Selective regional vasoconstriction reduces blood flow to less vital organs and tissues such as gut, kidneys, muscle, and skin.[28] Blood flow to the brain and myocardium increases, thereby maintaining adequate oxygen delivery despite reduced oxygen content of the arterial blood. Other organs and tissues must depend on increased oxygen extraction to maintain oxygen consumption.[29, 30] Pulmonary blood flow is also decreased and oxygen consumption reduced further. Although vigorous respiratory efforts may be noticeable initially, as asphyxia becomes more severe, the respiratory center is depressed. Fetal respiratory efforts decrease and pulmonary perfusion is reduced even more.

At the advanced stage of asphyxia, oxygen delivery to the brain and heart decreases and the myocardium consumes glycogen reserves. Evolving lactic acidosis and progressively lower Po_2 and pH lead to myocardial dysfunction and decreased blood flow to vital organs.[31, 32]

Tachycardia is an early response to hypoxia and is usually followed by hypertension and reflex bradycardia. This initial adaptation of the systemic circulation is mediated by several reflexes.[33] Catecholamines, which are produced in the fetal adrenal medulla, maintain myocardial function in the presence of asphyxia, thereby increasing survival.[34, 35] Arginine vasopressin helps maintain the hypertension, bradycardia, and redistribution of systemic flow,[36] whereas increased hepatic glycogenolysis helps maintain plasma glucose concentration.

Early in asphyxia, central venous (i.e., right atrial) pressure may rise slightly, owing to pulmonary hypertension and constriction of systemic capacitance vessels. When the myocardium finally fails, central venous pressure increases significantly and aortic pressure decreases, with further reduction in the fetal heart rate ensuing. Generally, myocardial failure does not occur until both pH and Pao_2 are extremely low, approximately 6.9 and 20 mm Hg, respectively.

DIAGNOSIS OF INTRAPARTUM ASPHYXIA

The hallmarks of intrapartum asphyxia have traditionally been the occurrence of fetal bradycardia and the passage of meconium in utero. The alterations in fetal heart rate that occur with disturbances in fetal well-being have been defined in great detail in the past several decades with refinement of electronic fetal monitoring, as well as with the use of fetal blood sampling to assess acid-base status.

Meconium Passage in Utero. In most cases, the finding of meconium-stained amniotic fluid is not of serious importance, since it is not necessarily indicative of intrauterine asphyxia. Although the presence of meconium-stained amniotic fluid during labor is a potentially ominous sign, controversy exists over its relative impact on fetal status.[37–50] Data indicate that timing

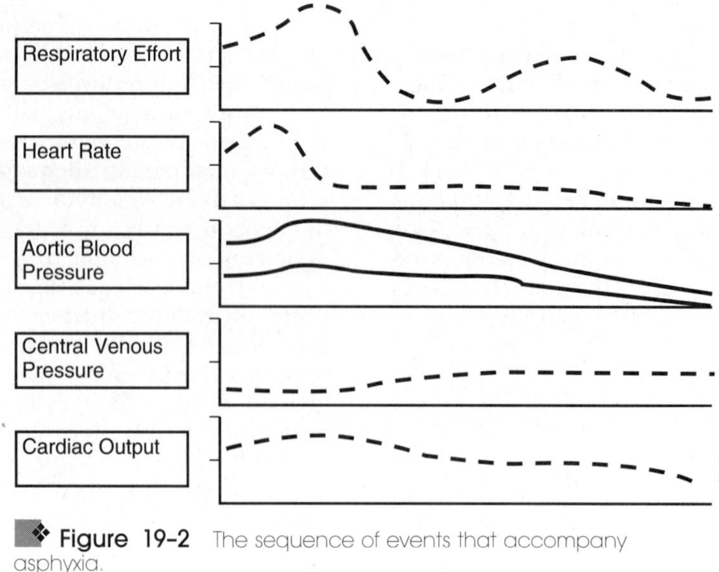

Figure 19–2 The sequence of events that accompany asphyxia.

and quantity of meconium passage are critical variables in attempting to assess the significance of this occurrence for fetal well-being. Presumably, these two aspects of meconium passage correlate with the duration and severity of the intrauterine insult.[51]

Fetal Heart Rate Alterations. The necessity and relative merits of electronic heart rate monitoring have been the subject of disagreement.[52–63] Nevertheless, whether intermittent or continuous, use of such monitoring during labor is a standard part of obstetric practice in most Western countries (Table 19–1). The basis for the controversy concerning the value of electronic monitoring of fetal heart rate is (1) abnormalities are detected in a large number of infants who are normal at birth and on follow-up and (2) the increase in operative deliveries provoked by the finding of such abnormalities has little or no impact on adverse neurologic outcome, particularly cerebral palsy. It should be noted that only in the so-called Dublin trial of nearly 13,000 women, a study generally acknowledged to be among the best designed of all trials, was the use of electronic fetal heart rate monitoring followed by a decrease in the incidence of neonatal seizures. In this study the presence of certain heart rate patterns was an important predictor of abnormal neonatal neurologic examinations.[64, 65]

Assessment of fetal heart rate begins with the fact that normal rate ± 2 standard deviations is 120 to 160 beats/min.[49] In general, when a consistent heart rate is found above or below these values, a second method of fetal assessment is recommended, usually fetal acid-base determination. The loss of beat-to-beat variability coupled with variable or late decelerations significantly increases the likelihood of significant fetal hypoxia. Indeed, there is ample documentation of the association between decreased fetal heart rate variability and decelerations with fetal acidosis, intrauterine fetal death, and low Apgar scores.[17, 66]

Fetal Acid-Base Status. Alterations in fetal acid-base measurements, particularly when combined with fetal heart rate assessment, are effective predictors of the condition of the infant at birth.[67, 68] According to Low,[69] fetal blood gas values indicative of significant fetal metabolic acidosis occur at a fetal pH of less than 7.15 and a buffer base of less than 34 mmol/L. There is an association between complications and severe metabolic acidosis, but not with respiratory acidosis.[69] Current observations demonstrate the predictive value of intrapartum monitoring of fetal acid-base status.[70, 71]

Moreover, fetal blood gas sampling provides major insight into the importance of both severity and critical threshold of duration of the hypoxic insult. The latter observations are supported by experimental data obtained in fetal monkeys, which suggest that several hours of compromised (incomplete interruption of) fetal gas exchange result in neurologic deficits.[72] The relationship between severity of fetal acidosis and neo-

Table 19–1 Fetal Heart Rate Patterns: Causes and Clinical Interpretation

Fetal Heart Rate Pattern	Cause	Clinical Interpretation
Loss of beat-to-beat variability	Multiple	Variable
Early decelerations	Head compression	Benign
Variable decelerations	Umbilical cord compression	Variable
Late decelerations with loss of beat-to-beat variability	Uteroplacental insufficiency	Ominous

Table 19–2 RELATIONSHIP BETWEEN FETAL BLOOD pH AND NEONATAL NEUROLOGIC AND SYSTEMIC MANIFESTATIONS

	UMBILICAL ARTERY pH			
CLINICAL DYSFUNCTION	6.61–6.70	6.71–6.79	6.80–6.89	6.90–6.99
Hypoxic-ischemic encephalopathy	80%	60%	33%	12%
Renal dysfunction	60%	53%	26%	16%
Cardiac dysfunction	60%	60%	30%	18%
Pulmonary dysfunction	80%	47%	30%	12%
None	20%	40%	48%	75%

From Goodwin TM, Belai I, Hernandez P, et al: Asphyxial complications in the term newborn with severe umbilical acidemia. Am J Obstet Gynecol 1992; 167:1506–1512.

natal symptoms has been demonstrated by Goodwin and coworkers[71] (Table 19–2).

Transcutaneous Monitoring of Fetal pH, PO_2, and PCO_2. The continuous transcutaneous measurement of pH,[73] PO_2,[74] and PCO_2[75] is possible in the fetus. The technique may be of particular value for demonstrating the temporal course of the infant's condition and thus can be very useful in making judgments for interventions. However, there are still a few technical problems regarding the use of these electrodes. Hence, further design changes are necessary to allow for broader clinical application.

Fetal Electroencephalography. Fetal electroencephalography (EEG) is the most direct means of assessing the status of the central nervous system in utero.[76] Prolonged voltage suppression and persistent sharp waves have been shown to be associated with neurologic abnormalities in the neonatal period and at 1 year of age.[77, 78] When data related to fetal heart rate, Apgar scores, and neonatal neurologic examination were considered in addition to the fetal EEG findings, accuracy of prediction increased to 80%. Because of methodologic difficulties, however, use of fetal EEG has not reached wide clinical acceptance, despite attempts to develop electrodes more easily used in clinical obstetrics.[79]

Doppler Measurements of Blood Flow. The measurement of blood flow velocities in umbilical and fetal cerebral arteries is a relatively new and valuable tool in antepartum surveillance. In the peripartum period there is particular interest in the determination of blood flow velocity during labor in the fetal anterior and middle cerebral arteries, insonated either through the anterior fontanel by transvaginal Doppler ultrasound or via the transabdominal approach with duplex Doppler.[80, 81] Doppler ultrasound is currently used as an investigational tool to assess the intracerebral blood flow distribution in asphyxia.[82]

Near-Infrared Spectroscopy. By applying a near-infrared light source and a photon counting device to the cranium of the newborn and appropriate selection of light wavelengths, information concerning intracranial concentration of oxygenated and deoxygenated hemoglobin can be obtained. With such data, information concerning cerebral hemoglobin oxygen saturation, cerebral oxygen delivery, and cerebral blood volume can be determined.[83, 84] Initial studies show that with normal labor contractions, a decrease in cerebral content of both oxygenated and deoxygenated hemoglobin, and thereby total hemoglobin, occurs. Clearly this technique holds great promise for the intrapartum monitoring of the fetus, because unlike fetal heart rate monitoring and fetal acid-base measurement, information about intracranial physiology is obtained directly.

Fetal Pulse Oximetry. The development of a pulse oximeter that can be used to monitor fetal oxygen saturation during labor is most promising.[85, 86] Carbonne and colleagues[87] have showed that the predictive value of intrapartum fetal pulse oximetry could be favorably compared with that of fetal blood gas analysis. Randomized controlled management trials are presently being performed to assess the potential clinical use of this new tool.

SELECTED PERIPARTUM FETAL EMERGENCIES

The list of potential sudden and unexpected fetal or obstetric occurrences demanding prompt action is extensive. There are, nevertheless, only a few emergency situations in which fetal anoxia is expected (Table 19–3). Some of these situations necessitate a stat cesarean section. Since there is usually limited time available to discuss the necessary therapeutic steps in these types of situations, the anesthesiologist needs to have a clear understanding of the pathophysiology as well as diagnostic procedures and management options.

Table 19–3 SITUATIONS SUGGESTIVE OF FETAL ANOXIA

Cord prolapse with complete cord occlusion
Shoulder dystocia with fetal bradycardia
Extensive uterine rupture with maternal hypovolemic shock
Unresolved tetanic uterine contraction

Anesthesia can then be conducted in an efficient and safe fashion.

The obstetric diagnosis is obvious in most of these cases. Occasionally, only indirect evidence (e.g., prolonged fetal bradycardia) for fetal anoxia is available and an emergency cesarean section needs to be performed with only a presumptive diagnosis. Animal studies evaluating the pathophysiology of fetal asphyxia have shown that irreversible brain damage occurs approximately 10 minutes after the onset of fetal anoxia without immediate intervention.[88] It is also well known that signs of fetal anoxia become obvious a few minutes after the onset of the actual anoxic event. This implies that the clinical time frame from diagnosis of the fetal emergency situation to desired delivery is even shorter. It is for this reason that anesthesia for the emergency cesarean section must be conducted in the shortest possible time frame without sacrificing safety.

Shoulder Dystocia

Shoulder dystocia, or impacted shoulder, is an infrequently encountered obstetric emergency. It occurs in 0.15% to 2.0% of all deliveries.[89, 90] Nevertheless, it is one of the primary causes of birth trauma and is associated with significant perinatal and maternal morbidity. This complication is typically unexpected and difficult to predict.

Shoulder dystocia is best defined as the arrest of spontaneous delivery owing to impaction of the anterior shoulder against the symphysis pubis.[91] The greatest risk factor for shoulder dystocia is the presence of fetal macrosomia, with the incidence of shoulder dystocia increasing as birthweight increases. In 1960 Schwarz[92] found the incidence of shoulder dystocia to be 0.15% for infants weighing greater than 2500 g and 1.7% for infants weighing greater than 4000 g. The frequency increases acutely as weights increase from 4100 g (3% incidence) to 4500 g (8% incidence).[93] Sacks[94] reported an incidence of 10% when newborn weight exceeded 4500 g. The risk factors for shoulder dystocia can be separated into antepartum and intrapartum clinical factors (Table 19–4). The influence of these risk factors on the incidence of shoulder dystocia is cumulative.

The perinatal mortality associated with shoulder dystocia varies from 19 to 289 per 1000 deliveries.[95, 96] The most acute consequence of shoulder dystocia is fetal asphyxia, which is directly related to the delay in completing delivery. It has been suggested that the umbilical artery pH declines at a rate of 0.04 pH units/min.[97] Therefore, delivery must be completed within several minutes to avoid fetal acidemia and possible consequent neurologic impairment or death.

Table 19–4 RISK FACTORS FOR SHOULDER DYSTOCIA

ANTEPARTUM	INTRAPARTUM
Cephalopelvic dysproportion	Prolonged second stage of labor
Maternal obesity[98]	Oxytocin use[99]
Diabetes[100]	Midpelvic delivery
Post-term pregnancy	
Advanced maternal age	

When shoulder dystocia occurs, a number of possible maneuvers can be carried out in an attempt to complete delivery. Suprapubic pressure (not fundal pressure) should be used initially.[101] This maneuver directs the anterior shoulder underneath the symphysis pubis. Fundal pressure should be avoided because this may further impact the anterior shoulder against the symphysis pubis. The Roberts maneuver requires two assistants who each grasp one leg of the parturient and sharply flex the maternal thigh against the abdomen. This position serves to straighten the sacrum relative to the lumbar vertebrae and causes cephalic rotation of the pelvis to occur, which helps to free the impacted shoulder. The Wood's screw maneuver entails rotation of the posterior shoulder 180 degrees in a corkscrew fashion, clockwise or counterclockwise, so that the impacted anterior shoulder can be released. The Zavanelli maneuver may be resorted to when feasibility of a vaginal delivery is excluded. This maneuver involves cephalic replacement with subsequent delivery by cesarean section.[102]

Anesthetic Considerations. If adequate regional anesthesia is not present at the time, induction of general anesthesia should be performed to carry out the more invasive procedures, particularly the Zavanelli maneuver. Adequate relaxation of the pelvic floor must be provided to relieve the dystocia. This can occasionally be accomplished with a repeated bolus dose using a previously placed epidural[103] or spinal macrocatheter. For clinical as well as technical reasons, single-shot spinal anesthesia may not be practical. In the patient with several risk factors for shoulder dystocia (e.g., obesity, diabetes mellitus, and advanced maternal age), the prophylactic placement of a spinal macrocatheter (i.e., diameter >24 gauge) should be considered. This technique should be given serious consideration if there are any concerns with respect to airway management. If the Zavanelli maneuver is selected, tocolysis must be provided to allow for cephalic replacement. This can be achieved with an intravenous or subcutaneous terbutaline bolus (250 μg) or, alternatively, with intravenous nitroglycerin (100–200 μg[104]) or as amyl nitrite inhalational.[106]

Uterine Rupture

The incidence of uterine rupture with the modern transverse uterine incision ranges from 0.02% to 0.08%.[105, 106] This obstetric catastrophe may occur in primagravidae and multigravidae.[107] The key to a favorable outcome is early recognition, prompt exploratory laparotomy, and appropriate blood product replacement therapy. Plauche and colleagues[108] defined uterine rupture as complete separation of the wall of the pregnant uterus with or without expulsion of the fetus. Asymptomatic uterine scar dehiscence is not included in this definition.

Table 19–5 CLINICAL CONDITIONS WITH POSSIBLE ASSOCIATION WITH UTERINE RUPTURE

Prior cesarean section
Oxytocin
Parity ≥4
Abruptio placentae
Midforceps delivery
Breech version/extraction

There are a number of conditions that may be associated with uterine rupture (Table 19–5). There is some controversy over the significance of a previous cesarean section. Of patients with a uterine rupture, the average incidence of those who had a prior cesarean section ranges from 21% to 79%.[109] However, data in these patients with one[110] or multiple[111] previous cesareans fail to demonstrate an increased risk of uterine rupture. Oxytocin administration has been theoretically linked to the risk of uterine rupture. The risk of uterine rupture in patients with or without a uterine scar has been linked rather to the duration of labor than to the use of oxytocin.[112]

Although there is no clinical evidence, it has been suggested that epidural anesthesia may be a potential source for uterine rupture. There is also the theoretic possibility of delaying the diagnosis owing to a masking of the pain associated with uterine rupture, but Rodriguez[113] and Rowbottom[114] and their colleagues found no such masking of pain. Epidural analgesia is a practical option in the patient with previous uterine scar undergoing trial of labor as well as vaginal birth after cesarean section (VBAC). The incidence of epidural analgesic use in patients with uterine rupture is small, in the range of 6% to 21%,[115] and no causal relationship between epidural analgesia and uterine rupture has ever been demonstrated.

In a contemporary perspective, Rodriguez and coworkers[113] observed that the most consistent clinical feature of uterine rupture was the sudden appearance of a nonreassuring fetal heart tracing during labor (81%) (Table 19–6). The most common fetal heart rate pattern associated with uterine rupture was the sudden appearance of variable decelerations during labor in an unexpected situation. Traditionally, severe abdominal pain that is unrelated to contractions has been a sine qua non of uterine rupture. However, these investigators were able to identify abdominal pain in only 18% of patients with uterine rupture.[113]

Uterine rupture is associated with significant maternal and fetal morbidity and mortality. Perinatal mortality rate associated with uterine rupture patients ranges from 8% to 56%.[109, 115, 116] Maternal morbidity is associated with gravid hysterectomy and a high rate of blood loss, with increased utilization of blood transfusion.

Table 19–6 SYMPTOMS OF UTERINE RUPTURE

Fetal distress
Abdominal pain
Vaginal bleeding
Uterine hyperstimulation
Recession of presenting part
Altered uterine contour

Anesthetic Considerations. Uterine rupture is a sudden, unexpected event. In the majority of cases uterine rupture is associated with fetal compromise or anoxia. This is an indication for immediate cesarean section. If operative delivery is delayed, the effect of the disruption of the placental blood flow is compounded by the developing maternal hypovolemia. Because of the high incidence of maternal hemorrhage, general anesthesia is often chosen since the vasodilation associated with a neuraxial block might add to the instability associated with evolving maternal hypovolemia. Adequate intravenous access is crucial as well as the provision of adequate blood products and volume expanders. Puncture of the subclavian or internal jugular vein may be necessary if other sites of venous access are not feasible because of hypovolemia or peripheral vasoconstriction. The possibility of hypothermia should be considered, and appropriate preventive measures should be taken as soon as possible.

Umbilical Cord Prolapse

Umbilical cord prolapse is another condition that can cause fetal asphyxia. Several techniques have been described in an attempt to reduce the pressure of the presenting part on the umbilical cord with each contraction. Katz and coworkers[117] have described the successful use of retrograde bladder filling with 500 to 600 mL of saline in combination with intravenous ritodrine. The bladder filling may reduce the pressure on the umbilical cord by displacement and elevation of the presenting part. Manual reduction alone[118] or manual head elevation and subsequent cesarean section[119] have also been described.

Whether the umbilical cord compression is partial or complete is difficult to predict and depends on the stage of the presenting part. If umbilical cord prolapse is associated with refractory fetal bradycardia, fetal anoxia must be suspected and a cesarean section performed immediately.

ANESTHETIC CONSIDERATIONS IN THE COMPROMISED FETUS

Anesthesia for Presumed Fetal Anoxia/ "Code" Cesarean Section

When formulating an anesthetic plan, one must distinguish elective cesarean from emergent cesarean section. The desired time frame from diagnosis to delivery has been subject to discussion for many years. In 1969 the German Society for Perinatal Medicine proposed a 10-minute time frame from diagnosis to delivery.[120] The American College of Obstetricians and Gynecologists published similar guidelines in 1982,[121] in which they proposed a 15-minute time frame. These guidelines, however, were revised in 1988,[122] at which time the 15-minute recommendation was extended to 30 minutes. The latest recommendation of the German Society for Gynecology and Obstetrics demands a 20-minute time frame for the decision-to-delivery time.[123]

The 20- or 30-minute time frame is reported to be adequate for the majority of emergency cesarean sections.[124] Nevertheless, Korhonen and Kariniemi[125] have reported evidence for an increased risk of fetal loss if the "alarm to surgery" interval exceeds 20 minutes. From early studies on the pathophysiology of fetal asphyxia, there is evidence that permanent fetal central nervous system damage may begin after approximately 10 minutes of fetal anoxia.[74] Fortunately, most cases of fetal asphyxia are not the result of absolute fetal anoxia (complete cessation of fetal gas exchange). In most instances, partial fetal gas exchange continues and the time frame until permanent central nervous system damage ensues is longer. In cases of fetal asphyxia in which total fetal anoxia is suspected, delivery should be attempted as soon as possible, but optimally within 10 minutes. Since this can happen any time, the anesthesiologist must always be prepared.

A "stat" cesarean section is initiated once the obstetrician in charge establishes the diagnosis of "fetal jeopardy." In Germany, a "code C-section" is performed for the most extreme cases, in which fetal asphyxia is present and every second counts. The code is engaged (by telephone or by pressing a designated button) and the anesthesiologist and the neonatologist receive a code cesarean section page by means of an automated paging algorithm. The patient's verbal consent is obtained and nonparticulate antacid is administered. As preparations proceed, the anesthesiologist evaluates the airway and obtains the basic medical information if the patient has not been evaluated yet. Usual preparations such as the application of support hose or shaving are not performed. The patient is not transported to the nearby surgical suite, in order to prevent any time delay or interruption of fetal monitoring. Every delivery room is set up with an oxygen outlet and wall suction. The anesthesia machine and all anesthesia supply—including equipment for alternative airway management—is transported to the delivery room. Time taken to complete surgical disinfection is reduced by use of a quick alcohol disinfection of the surgeons' hands and single disinfection of the patient's abdomen with povidone-iodine (Betadine); povidone-iodine solution is also poured over the surgical area. Anesthesia in these critical situations often consists of general anesthesia with rapid-sequence induction. The decision regarding whether to perform the surgery in the delivery room or the operating room in this scenario partly depends on the room layout and size as well as the accessibility of equipment and varies from one institution to another. Although the use of a "code" cesarean section ("stat" c-section performed in a delivery room) is now accepted practice in a few European countries,[128] it is not commonly accepted practice in the United States, where almost all patients are transported to the operating room.

It is difficult to demonstrate that the incidence of hypoxic-ischemic encephalopathy can be reduced by institution of a "code" cesarean section drill. Perinatal statistics suggest that perinatal mortality has not been subject to major changes in the last 30 years despite a larger percentage of cerebral palsy as a result of prematurity.[126] This suggests that the care of term infants must have improved. This may, at least in part, be attributable to improved perinatal care. If one considers the pathophysiology of peripartum fetal anoxia and the limited time from onset of fetal anoxia to the beginning of permanent fetal brain damage (i.e., 10 minutes),[74] the benefit of a well-organized cesarean section drill in selected fetal emergencies is obvious.

There is some discussion over the routine administration of antibiotics in cesarean sections. The benefit of the routine administration of antibiotics in the emergency cesarean section situation, nevertheless, is well accepted.[127] The administration of multiple antibiotic doses or the use of antibiotic combination does not appear to offer an advantage over the single-dose regimen.

Comparison of General Anesthesia Versus Regional Anesthesia

Clinical studies on the effect of intravenous and inhalational anesthetics on the asphyxiated fetus suffer from the imprecise definition and nonuniform interpretation of the terms "fetal distress" and "asphyxia." Several studies have attempted to compare general anesthesia with regional techniques.[128–131] Review of those data suggests that infants of mothers who received regional anesthesia fared at least as well or better than those infants whose mothers received general anesthesia. However, many of these studies were retrospective and nonrandomized and may have had a selection bias.

Regional Anesthesia in the Compromised Fetus

The choice of anesthetic technique for emergency cesarean sections is determined by the fetal and maternal condition as well as the anesthesiologist's preference and experience with certain techniques. Certain maternal conditions favor a regional anesthetic technique. (e.g., airway abnormalities). Some anesthesiologists prefer a regional technique even in the severely asphyxiated fetus. When deciding which anesthetic technique to use, the anesthesiologist should attempt to differentiate "suspected fetal anoxia" (the absolute cessation of fetal gas exchange) from the "compromised fetus" (diminished but persisting gas exchange). This can only be achieved if clear communication between the anesthesiologist and obstetrician occurs.

Regional techniques are appropriate anesthetic choices in most situations with a compromised but not anoxic fetus and in situations in which general anesthesia appears to be contraindicated. Spinal anesthesia has the advantage of a rapid and predictable onset. Compared with epidural anesthesia, spinal anesthesia has the advantage of providing a faster and more dense sensory block. Disadvantages of spinal anesthesia include the limited duration of action and the faster onset of sympathectomy, often associated with hypotension.[132] In recent years spinal anesthesia has become popular for elective as well as emergency cesarean section. This development can be attributed to the improved design of spinal needles, which has resulted in a dramatically reduced incidence of postdural puncture headache.

Several of the measures necessary for the preparation of a patient undergoing an emergency cesarean section under general anesthesia are also applicable for regional anesthetic techniques. Aspiration prophylaxis can successfully be accomplished with Bicitra (30 mL PO) alone or in combination with metoclopramide (10 mg IV).[133]

Many anesthesiologists prefer the patient to be in the sitting position for the insertion of a spinal or epidural needle. The sitting position has the advantage of better conceptualization of anatomic landmarks. Technical disadvantages of the sitting position include the necessity to have one person dedicated to stabilizing the patient and the higher likelihood of monitor dislocation with movement of the patient from the sitting into the supine position. In addition, certain obstetric conditions (e.g., prolapsed umbilical cord) may contraindicate the use of a sitting position. It is therefore advisable to be familiar with both sitting and lateral positions for the placement of a spinal or epidural anesthetic.

In the case of an emergency cesarean section under spinal anesthesia, time can be saved in the presence of a helpful hand who applies patient monitors and draws up the local anesthetic solution at the same time as the patient's back is prepped and draped (Fig. 19–3). Some anesthesiologists feel that there is no time disadvantage associated with the use of spinal anesthesia for emergency cesarean sections as long as the spinal anesthetic can be rapidly placed and help is readily available. It is also advisable to choose a needle that is technically easy to use (stiff design, possibly larger gauge) in the emergency setting. It has recently been shown that the time to appearance of fluid at the needle hub of a spinal needle is shorter if the stylet is withdrawn slowly, owing to a "suction effect" of the spinal needle stylet.[134] One must also consider the possibility of continuous spinal anesthesia in such a situation by using an epidural needle and catheter (macrocatheter), especially in morbidly obese patients. If spinal anesthesia is used, prevention of maternal hypotension becomes extremely important. Aggressive treatment with vasopressors, ephedrine, or, if necessary, small doses of phenylephrine may be used.

Epidural Anesthesia for Emergency Cesarean Section

Frequently, patients who present for nonelective cesarean section may have an indwelling epidural catheter that was previously placed for the relief of labor pain. Depending on the acuity and the severity of the compromised fetal gas exchange, maternal hemodynamics, and the level and density of the preexisting epidural blockade, there is usually adequate time to supplement the epidural blockade to provide surgical anesthesia. The use of bicarbonate with the local anesthetic, whether lidocaine or chloroprocaine, speeds up the onset. The epidural catheter can also be used for postoperative pain relief.[135]

Drawbacks of a rapid epidural anesthetic are similar to those associated with a single-shot spinal anesthetic. Both incidence and severity of hypotension appear to be comparable.[136, 137] The time from dosage to the onset of hypotension varies and is primarily determined by the dosing mode (fractioned vs. single bolus dosing). Prophylaxis of hypotension is best accomplished with intravenous ephedrine as an infu-

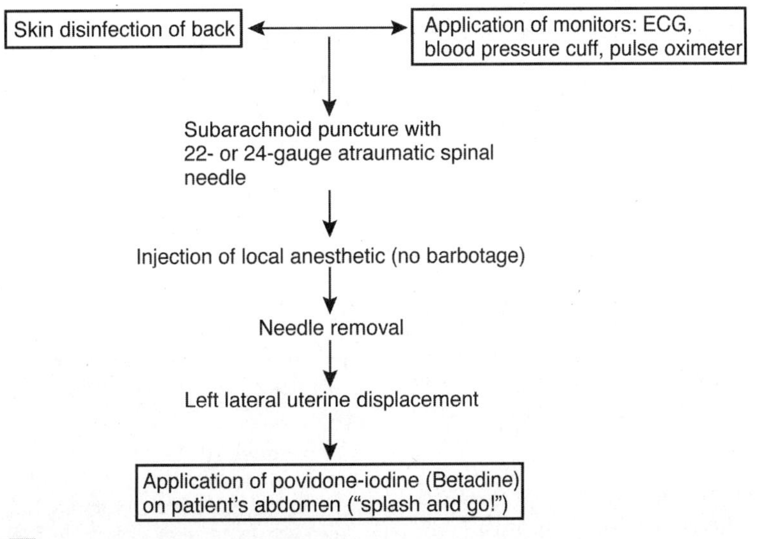

Figure 19–3 Emergency cesarean section under spinal anesthesia.

sion[138] or bolus doses concurrent with crystalloid or colloid fluid expansion.[139] The use of prophylactic intramuscular or epidural ephedrine, although not popular, has been described.[140] Most obstetric anesthesiologists, however, prefer the use of intravenous vasopressors over the intramuscular or subcutaneous routes.

Nausea is observed during spinal anesthesia and is associated with the degree of maternal hypotension. Adequate surgical anesthesia as well as a stable hemodynamic condition lowers the incidence of nausea and vomiting. Additionally, metoclopramide (10 mg IV) or droperidol (0.625 to 1.25 mg IV) can be administered to further lower the incidence of nausea and vomiting. The relatively frequent shivering (observed in approximately 80% of patients[141]) can be effectively treated with warming of the intravenous fluids and the epidural injectate[142] and the administration of 25 to 50 mg of meperidine (pethidine) after clamping of the umbilical cord. Epidural fentanyl may have a prophylactic effect as well.[143]

Two percent lidocaine with or without epinephrine can be given via the existing epidural catheter that has been used for labor analgesia. Although there is some controversy, there is the potential risk of fetal ion trapping of the local anesthetic in the presence of severe fetal acidosis (see Chapter 6). In the acidotic fetus, 3% 2-chloroprocaine may be preferable since it is almost completely hydrolyzed by maternal plasma esterases before it reaches the fetal circulation. Unfortunately, chloroprocaine is not approved in many European countries. A possible alternative is the use of 0.75% ropivacaine.[144]

One of the most popular and effective techniques to achieve a fast onset of block is the use of pH-adjusted local anesthetic. The addition of sodium bicarbonate to the injectate increases the uncharged, nonionized, lipid-soluble form of the local anesthetic and thus speeds up its onset (Table 19–7).

If the epidural catheter has been used successfully during labor and tested to exclude subarachnoid or intravascular placement of the catheter, an adequate amount of local anesthetic in divided doses given over a short time period can be used to achieve the fastest possible onset of block for an emergency cesarean section.[145] There is, nevertheless, the theoretic possibility of epidural catheter migration from the epidural space into the intravascular or subarachnoid space. Thus, some authorities recommend repeated test dosing of the epidural catheter before bolus dosing.

Local Anesthetics and Fetal Acidosis

The balance of ionized and nonionized forms of a local anesthetic is shifted toward the ionized, poorly lipid-soluble form in the acidotic environment. This has led many investigators to believe that local anesthetics (in particular, lidocaine) may accumulate in the acidotic environment.[146] However, several authors doubt the clinical importance of ion trapping.[147, 148] This subject is covered in greater detail in Chapter 6.

Table 19–7 pH Adjustment of Local Anesthetics

1 mL sodium bicarbonate 8.4% +
10 mL 2% lidocaine
10 mL 2% mepivacaine
10 mL 3% 2-chloroprocaine
Only 0.1 mL 8.4% sodium bicarbonate to 10 mL 0.5% bupivacaine

General Treatment Measures in Fetal Distress (Nonreassuring Fetal Status)

The majority of cases of presumed fetal jeopardy (nonreassuring fetal status) are diagnosed based on a suspicious fetal heart tracing. The concerning fetal heart trace can be a temporary event and an emergent cesarean section is not always warranted, since other therapeutic measures may successfully resuscitate the fetus in utero (Table 19–8). A first step in the general treatment of presumed fetal jeopardy is the discontinuation of oxytocin, if used. The position of the parturient should be changed to maximize left uterine displacement, oxygen given by means of a face mask, and rate of intravenous fluid infusion maximized.

Some obstetricians attempt to stimulate the fetus displaying a suspicious tracing with a vibro-acoustic transducer or direct stimulation if possible. Fetal reactivity would argue against fetal acidosis. If the suspicious fetal heart tracing is associated with uterine hyperactivity, intravenous tocolysis is indicated (e.g., 250 μg of intravenous terbutaline).[149] The absence of fetal reactivity following treatment is further evidence of fetal asphyxia, usually necessitating an emergent cesarean section.

Often, a fetal scalp pH is obtained when fetal well-being is being evaluated. A fetal scalp pH below 7.20 is usually indicative of compromised fetal gas exchange and necessitates an emergency cesarean section. A fetal scalp pH between 7.20 and 7.25 is equivocal and should be repeated after 10 to 15 minutes. Also important is the fetal base excess (a fetal base excess of 8.0 mmol/L is concerning), since metabolic acidosis is usually indicative of a longer duration of diminished fetal gas exchange.

Since presumed fetal jeopardy can potentially result in an emergency cesarean section, resuscitation of a depressed neonate is always a possibility. Hence, the help of a neonatologist or pediatrician should be called for whenever scalp pH is performed.

Table 19–8 In Utero Resuscitation

Maternal oxygen via face mask (6 L/min)
Intravenous (IV) fluid bolus
Discontinue oxytocin, consider IV terbutaline
Change maternal position, consider knee-chest
Treat hypotension if indicated

❖ SUMMARY

Key Points

- The term *fetal distress* is imprecise and has a low positive predictive value.
- In utero fetal resuscitation should be implemented when fetal jeopardy is diagnosed. Resuscitation includes the administration of intravenous fluids, the discontinuation of oxytocin, the normalization of blood pressure, and the administration of supplemental oxygen. In addition, the administration of a tocolytic agent and the initiation of amnioinfusion have been suggested.
- Communication between the obstetrician and the anesthesiologist is imperative so that the optimal anesthetic can be selected for these cases. Emergency cesarean section, by itself, does not preclude the use of regional anesthesia. If complete anoxia is suspected, cesarean section should be initiated as rapidly as possible.
- The fetal heart rate tracing should be monitored during the initiation of anesthesia for urgent cesarean section.

Key Reference

American College of Obstetricians and Gynecologists, Committee on Obstetric Practice: Inappropriate Use of the Terms Fetal Distress and Birth Asphyxia. ACOG Committee Opinion No. 197. Washington, DC; 1998.

Case Stem

A 28-year-old G2P1 in active labor is found to have a prolapsed cord with a fetal heart rate of 60 beats/min. Discuss the obstetric and anesthetic management of this patient.

References

1. Hagberg B, Hagberg G, Zetterstrom R: Decreasing perinatal mortality—increase in cerebral palsy morbidity. Acta Paediatr Scand 1989; 78:664–670.
2. Hagberg B, Hagberg G, Olow I, et al: The changing panorama of cerebral palsy in Sweden. V. The birth period 1979–82. Acta Paediatr Scand 1989; 78:283–290.
3. Hagberg B, Hagberg G: The changing panorama of infantile hydrocephalus and cerebral palsy over forty years—a Swedish survey. Brain Dev 1989; 11:368–373.
4. Hagberg B, Hagberg G, Olow I: The changing panorama of cerebral palsy in Sweden: prevalence and origin during the birth year period 1983–1986. Acta Paediatr Scand 1993; 82:387–393.
5. Riikonen R, Raumavirta S, Sinivouri E, et al: Changing pattern of cerebral palsy in the southwest region of Finland. Acta Paediatr Scand 1989; 78:581–587.
6. Nelson KB, Ellenberg JH: Antecedents of cerebral palsy: multivariate analysis of risk. N Engl J Med 1986; 315:81–86.
7. Blair E, Stanley FJ: Intrapartum asphyxia: a rare cause of cerebral palsy. J Pediatr 1988; 112:515–519.
8. Grant A, O'Brien N, Joy MT, et al: Cerebral palsy among children born during the Dublin randomised trial of intrapartum monitoring. Lancet 1989; 2:1233–1236.
9. MacDonald D, Grant A, Sheridan-Pereira M, et al: The Dublin randomized controlled trial of intrapartum fetal heart rate monitoring. Am J Obstet Gynecol 1985; 152:524–539.
10. Kuban KC, Leviton A: The epidemiology of cerebral palsy. N Engl J Med 1994; 330:188–195.
11. Truwit CL, Barkowich AJ, Koch TK, et al: Cerebral palsy: MR findings in 40 patients. Am J Neuroradiol 1992; 13:67–78.
12. Volpe JJ: Value of MR in defining the neuropathology of cerebral palsy in vivo. AJNR Am J Neuroradiol 1992; 13:79–83.
13. Hope PL, Moorcraft J: Cerebral palsy in infants born during trial of intrapartum monitoring. Lancet 1990; 335:238.
14. Haverkamp AD, Orleans M, Langendoerfer S, et al: A controlled trial of the differential effects of intrapartum fetal monitoring. Am J Obstet Gynecol 1979; 134:399–408.
15. Haeslein HC, Niswander KR: Fetal distress in term pregnancies. Am J Obstet Gynecol 1980; 137:245–253.
16. Steer P: Has the expression "fetal distress" outlived its usefulness? Br J Obstet Gynaecol 1982; 89:690–693.
17. Parer JT, Livingston EG: What is fetal distress? Am J Obstet Gynecol 1990; 162:1421–1425.
18. Dorland's Illustrated Medical Dictionary, 28th ed. Philadelphia: WB Saunders; 1994.
19. Webster's Medical Dictionary, 2nd ed. Springfield, MA: Merriam-Webster, Inc, 1993.
20. Harris AP: Emergency cesarean section. *In* Rogers MC (ed): Current Practice in Anesthesiology. Toronto: BC Decker; 1990: 361–367.
21. Torrance S, Wittnich C: The effect of varying arterial oxygen tension on neonatal acid-base balance. Pediatr Res 1992; 31:112–116.
22. James LS, Weisbrot IM, Prince CE, et al: The acid-base status of human infants in relation to birth asphyxia and onset of respiration. J Pediatr 1958; 52:379–394.
23. Yeomans ER, Hauth JC, Gilstrap LC, et al: Umbilical cord pH, pCO_2, and bicarbonate following uncomplicated term vaginal deliveries. Am J Obstet Gynecol 1985; 151:798–800.
24. Rudolph CD, Roman C, Rudolph AM: Effect of acute umbilical cord compression on hepatic carbohydrate metabolism in the fetal lamb. Pediatr Res 1989; 25:228–233.
25. Ruth V, Fyhrquist F, Clemons G, et al: Cord plasma vasopressin, erythropoietin and hypoxanthine as indices of asphyxia at birth. Pediatr Res 1988; 24:490–494.
26. Fahnenstich H, Dame C, Alléra A, Kowalewski S: Biochemical monitoring of fetal distress with serum-immunoreactive erythropoietin. J Perinat Med 1996; 24:1, 85–91.
27. Dawes G: Fetal and Neonatal Physiology. Chicago: Year Book Medical Publishers; 1968.
28. Cohn HE, Sacks FJ, Heymann MA, et al: Cardiovascular responses to hypokalemia and acidemia in fetal lambs. Am J Obstet Gynecol 1974; 120:817–824.
29. Fisher DJ: Increased regional myocardial blood flows and oxygen deliveries during hypoxemia in lambs. Pediatr Res 1984; 18:602–606.
30. Boyle DW, Host K, Zerbe GO, et al: Fetal hind limb oxygen consumption and blood flow during graded hypoxia. Pediatr Res 1990; 28:94–100.
31. Fisher DJ: Acidemia reduces cardiac output and left ventricular contractility in conscious lambs. J Dev Physiol 1986; 8:23–31.
32. Downing SE, Talner NS, Gardner TH: Influences of hypoxemia and acidemia on left ventricular function. Am J Physiol 1966; 210:1327–1334.
33. Itskovitz J, LaGamma EF, Bristow J, et al: Cardiovascular responses to hypoxemia in sinoaortic-denervated fetal sheep. Pediatr Res 1991; 30:381–385.
34. Fisher DJ: β-Adrenergic influence on increased myocardial oxygen consumption during hypoxemia in awake newborn lambs. Pediatr Res 1989; 25:585–590.
35. Slotkin TA, Seidler FJ: Adrenomedullary catecholamine release in the fetus and newborn: secretory mechanisms and their role in stress and survival. J Dev Physiol 1988; 10:1–16.
36. Perez R, Espinoza M, Riquemez R, et al: Arginine vasopressin mediates cardiovascular responses to hypoxemia in fetal sheep. Am J Physiol 1989; 256:R1011–1018.
37. Hobel CJ: Intrapartum clinical assessment of fetal distress. Am J Obstet Gynecol 1971; 110:336–342.

38. Spellacy WN, Buhi WC, Birk SA, et al: Human placental lactogen levels and intrapartum fetal distress: meconium-stained amniotic fluid, fetal heart rate patterns, and Apgar scores. Am J Obstet Gynecol 1972; 114:803–808.
39. Low JA, Pancham SR, Piercy WN, et al: Intrapartum fetal asphyxia: clinical characteristics, diagnosis, and significance in relation to pattern of development. Am J Obstet Gynecol 1977; 129:857–872.
40. Saldana LR, Schulman H, Yang WH: Electronic fetal monitoring during labor. Obstet Gynecol 1976; 47:706–710.
41. Fujikura T, Klionsky B: The significance of meconium staining. Am J Obstet Gynecol 1975; 121:45–50.
42. Gregory GA, Gooding CA, Phibbs RH, et al: Meconium aspiration in infants—a prospective study. J Pediatr 1974; 85:848–852.
43. Wood C, Pincerton J: Foetal distress. Br J Obstet Gynaecol 1961; 68:427–437.
44. Miller FC, Sacks DA, Yeh SY, et al: Significance of meconium during labor. Am J Obstet Gynecol 1975; 122:573–580.
45. Abramovici H, Brandes JH, Fuchs K, et al: Meconium staining during delivery: a sign of compensated fetal distress. Am J Obstet Gynecol 1974; 118:251–255.
46. Meis PJ, Hall M 3rd, Marshall JR, et al: Meconium passage: a new classification for risk assessment during labor. Am J Obstet Gynecol 1978; 131:509–513.
47. Krebs HB, Petres RE, Dunn LJ, et al: Intrapartum fetal heart rate monitoring. III. Association of meconium with abnormal fetal heart rate patterns. Am J Obstet Gynecol 1980; 137:936–943.
48. Meis PJ, Hobel CJ, Ureda JR: Late meconium passage in labor—a sign of fetal distress? Obstet Gynecol 1982; 59:332–335.
49. Schifrin BS: The diagnosis and treatment of fetal distress. *In* Hill A, Volpe JJ (eds): Fetal Neurology. New York: Raven Press; 1989: 743–789.
50. Nathan L, Leveno KJ, Carmody TJ, et al: Meconium—a 1990s perspective on an old obstetric hazard. Obstet Gynecol 1994; 83:329–332.
51. Spinillo A, Fazzi E, Capuzzo E, et al: Meconium-stained amniotic fluid and risk for cerebral palsy in preterm infants. Obstet Gynecol 1997; 90:519–523.
52. Haverkamp AD, Orleans M, Langendoerfer S, et al: A controlled trial of the differential effects of intrapartum fetal monitoring. Am J Obstet Gynecol 1979; 134:399–412.
53. Zuspan FP, Quilligan EJ, Iams JD, et al: NICHD Consensus Development Task Force report: predictors of intrapartum fetal distress—the role of electronic fetal monitoring. J Pediatr 1979; 95:1026–1030.
54. Thacker SB: The efficacy of intrapartum electronic fetal monitoring. Am J Obstet Gynecol 1987; 156:24–30.
55. Jenkins HM: Thirty years of intrapartum fetal heart rate electronic monitoring: discussion paper. J R Soc Med 1989; 82:210–214.
56. Steer PJ, Eigbe F, Lissauer TJ, et al: Interrelationships among abnormal cardiotocograms in labor, meconium staining of the amniotic fluid, arterial cord blood pH, and Apgar scores. Obstet Gynecol 1989; 74:715–721.
57. Colditz PB, Henderson-Smart DJ: Electronic fetal heart rate monitoring during labour: does it prevent perinatal asphyxia and cerebral palsy? Med J Aust 1990; 153:88–90.
58. Shy KK, Luthy DA, Bennett FC, et al: Effects of electronic fetal heart-rate monitoring, as compared with periodic auscultation, on neurologic development of premature infants. N Engl J Med 1990; 322:588–593.
59. Freeman R: Intrapartum fetal monitoring—a disappointing story. N Engl J Med 1990; 322:624–626.
60. Anthony MY, Levene MI: An assessment of the benefits of intrapartum fetal monitoring. Dev Med Child Neurol 1990; 32:547–553.
61. Morrison JC, Chez BF, Davis ID: Intrapartum fetal heart rate assessment—monitoring by auscultation or electronic means. Am J Obstet Gynecol 1993; 168:63–66.
62. Vintzileos AM, Antsaklis A, Varvarigos I, et al: A randomized trial of intrapartum electronic fetal heart rate monitoring versus intermittent auscultation. Obstet Gynecol 1993; 81:899–907.
63. de Haan HH, Gunn AJ, Gluckman PD: Fetal heart rate changes do not reflect cardiovascular deterioration during brief repeated umbilical cord occlusions in near-term fetal lambs. Am J Obstet Gynecol 1997; 176:8–17.
64. MacDonald D, Grant A, Sheridan-Pereira M, et al: The Dublin randomized controlled trial of intrapartum fetal heart rate monitoring. Am J Obstet Gynecol 1985; 152:524–539.
65. Ellison PH, Foster M, Sheridan-Pereira M, et al: Electronic fetal heart monitoring, auscultation, and neonatal outcome. Am J Obstet Gynecol 1991; 164:1281–1289.
66. Martin C Jr: Physiology and clinical use of fetal heart rate variability. Clin Perinatol 1982; 9:339–352.
67. Low JA: Fetal acid-base status and outcome. *In* Hill A, Volpe JJ (eds): Fetal Neurology. New York: Raven Press; 1989: 195–214.
68. Low JA, Muir DW, Pater EA, et al: The association of intrapartum asphyxia in the mature fetus with newborn behavior. Am J Obstet Gynecol 1990; 163:1131–1135.
69. Low JA, Panagiotopoulos C, Derrick EJ: Newborn complications after intrapartum asphyxia with metabolic acidosis in the term fetus. Am J Obstet Gynecol 1994; 170:1081–1087.
70. Tejani N, Verma UL: Correlation of Apgar scores and umbilical artery acid-base status to mortality and morbidity in the low birth weight neonate. Obstet Gynecol 1989; 73:597–600.
71. Goodwin TM, Belai I, Hernandez P, et al: Asphyxial complications in the term newborn with severe umbilical acidemia. Am J Obstet Gynecol 1992; 167:1506–1512.
72. Brann AW Jr, Myers RE: Central nervous system findings in the newborn monkey following severe in utero partial asphyxia. Neurology 1975; 25:327–338.
73. Small ML, Beall M, Platt LD, et al: Continuous tissue pH monitoring in the term fetus. Am J Obstet Gynecol 1989; 161:323–329.
74. Weber T, Secher NJ: Continuous measurement of transcutaneous fetal oxygen tension during labour. Br J Obstet Gynaecol 1979; 86:954–958.
75. Hansen PK, Thompson SG, Secher NJ, et al: Transcutaneous carbon dioxide measurement in the fetus during labor. Am J Obstet Gynecol 1984; 150:47–51.
76. Rosen MG, Scibetta JJ, Hochberg CJ: Human fetal electroencephalogram. 3. Pattern changes in presence of fetal heart rate alterations after use of maternal medications. Obstet Gynecol 1970; 36:132–140.
77. Chik L, Sokol R, Rosen MG: Computer interpreted fetal encephalogram: sharp wave detection and classification of infants for one year neurologic outcome. Encephalogr Clin Neurophysiol 1977; 42:745–753.
78. Chik L, Sokol RJ, Rosen MG, et al: Computer interpreted fetal monitoring data: discriminant analysis of perinatal data as a model for prediction of neurologic status at one year of age. J Pediatr 1977; 90:985–989.
79. Weller C, Dyson RJ, McFadyen IR, et al: Fetal electroencephalography using a new, flexible electrode. Am J Obstet Gynecol 1981; 88:983–986.
80. Mirro R, Gonzalez A: Perinatal anterior cerebral artery blood flow during normal active labour and in labour with variable decelerations. Br J Obstet Gynaecol 1987; 156:1227–1231.
81. Yagel S, Anteby E, Lavy Y, et al: Fetal middle cerebral artery blood flow during normal active labour and in labour with variable decelerations. Br J Obstet Gynaecol 1992; 99:483–485.
82. Owen P, Harrold AJ, Farrell T: Fetal size and growth velocity in the prediction of intrapartum caesarean section for fetal distress. Br J Obstet Gynaecol 1997; 104:445–459.
83. Peebles DM, Edwards AD, Wyatt JS, et al: Changes in human fetal cerebral hemoglobin concentration and oxygen during labor measured by near-infrared spectroscopy. Am J Obstet Gynecol 1992; 166:1369–1373.
84. Peebles DM, Spencer JAD, Edwards AD, et al: Relation between frequency of uterine contractions and human fetal cerebral oxygen saturation studied during labour by near infrared spectroscopy. Br J Obstet Gynaecol 1994; 101:44–48.
85. Johnson N, Johnson VA: Continuous fetal monitoring with a pulse oximeter: a case of cord compression. Am J Obstet Gynecol 1989; 161:1295–1296.

86. McNamara H, Chung DC, Lilford R, et al: Do fetal pulse oximetry readings at delivery correlate with cord oxygenation and acidaemia? Br J Obstet Gynaecol 1992; 99:735–738.
87. Carbonne B, Langer B, Goffinet F, et al: Multicenter study on the clinical value of fetal pulse oximetry. II. Compared predictive values of pulse oximetry and fetal blood analysis. The French Study Group on Fetal Pulse Oximetry. Am J Obstet Gynecol 1997; 177:593–598.
88. Brann AW Jr, Myers RE: Central nervous system findings in the newborn monkey following severe in utero partial asphyxia. Neurology 1975; 25:327–338.
89. Acker DB, Sachs BP, Friedman EA: Risk factors for shoulder dystocia in the average weight infant. Obstet Gynecol 1986; 67:614–618.
90. Schwarz BC, Dixon DM: Shoulder dystocia. Obstet Gynecol 1958; 11:468–471.
91. Beneditti TJ, Gabbe SG: Shoulder dystocia: Complication of fetal macrosomia and prolonged second stage of labor with midpelvic delivery. Obstet Gynecol 1978; 52:526–529.
92. Schwarz DP: Shoulder girdle dystocia in vertex delivery: clinical study and review. Obstet Gynecol 1960; 15:194–206.
93. Golditch IM, Kirkman K: The large fetus: management and outcome. Obstet Gynecol 1978; 52:26–30.
94. Sacks RA: The large infant: a study of maternal, obstetric, fetal, and newborn characteristics: including a long-term pediatric follow-up. Am J Obstet Gynecol 1969; 104:195.
95. Seigworth GR: Shoulder dystocia: review of 5 years experience. Obstet Gynecol 1966; 28:764–777.
96. McCall JO: Shoulder dystocia: review of 5 years experience. Obstet Gynecol 1962; 83:1486–1490.
97. Wood C, Ng KH, Houndslow D, Benning H: Time: an important variable in normal delivery. Br J Obstet Gynaecol 1973; 80:295–300.
98. Johnson SR, Kolberg BH, Varner MW: Maternal obesity and pregnancy. Surg Gynecol Obstet 1987; 164:431.
99. Cunningham FG, MacDonald PC, Gant NF: Williams Obstetrics, 18th ed. Norwalk, CT: Appleton & Lange; 1989.
100. Nathanson JN: The excessively large fetus as an obstetric problem. Am J Obstet Gynecol 1950; 60:54.
101. Resnick R: Management of shoulder girdle dystocia. Clin Obstet Gynecol 1980; 23:559–564.
102. Sandberg EC: The Zavanelli maneuver: a potentially revolutionary method for resolution of shoulder dystocia.
103. Hepner DL, Gaiser RR, Cheek TG, Gutsche BB: The Zavanelli maneuver does not preclude regional anesthesia (case report). Anesth Analg 1997; 84:1145–1146.
104. Bayhi DA, Sherwood CDA, Campbell CE: Intravenous nitroglycerine for uterine inversion. J Clin Anesth 1992; 4:487–488.
105. Rodriguez MH, Masaki DI, Phelan JP, Diaz FG: Uterine rupture: are intrauterine pressure catheters useful in the diagnosis? Am J Obstet Gynecol 1989; 161:666–669.
106. Eden RD, Parker RT, Gall SA: Rupture of the pregnant uterus: a 53-year review. Obstet Gynecol 1986; 68:671–674.
107. Dainer MJ: Spontaneous uterine rupture. J Reprod Med 1981; 26:35–37.
108. Plauche WC, von Almen W, Müller R: Catastrophic uterine rupture. Obstet Gynecol 1984; 64:792–797.
109. Spaulding LB, Gallup DG: Current concepts for management of rupture of the gravid uterus. Obstet Gynecol 1979; 54:437–441.
110. Phelan JP, Clark SL, Diaz F, et al: Vaginal birth after cesarean. Am J Obstet Gynecol 1987; 157:1510–1515.
111. Phelan JP, Clark SL, Diaz F, et al: Vaginal birth after multiple prior cesareans. *In* Phelan JP, Clark SL (eds): Cesarean Delivery. New York: Elsevier; 1988:491.
112. Lynch JC, Pardy JP: Uterine rupture and scar dehiscence: a five-year survey. Anaesth Intensive Care 1996; 24:699–704.
113. Rodriguez MH, Masaki DI, Phelan JP, Diaz FG: Uterine rupture: are intrauterine pressure catheters useful in the diagnosis? Am J Obstet Gynecol 1989; 161:666–669.
114. Rowbottom SJ, Critchley LA, Gin T: Uterine rupture and epidural analgesia during trial of labour. Anaesthesia 1997; 52:486–488.
115. Golan A, Sandbank O, Rubin A: Rupture of the pregnant uterus. Obstet Gynecol 1980; 56:549–554.
116. Suner S, Jagminas L, Peipert JF, Linakis J: Fatal spontaneous rupture of a gravid uterus: case report and literature review of uterine rupture. J Emerg Med 1996; 14:181–185.
117. Katz Z, Shoham Z, Lancet M, et al: Management of labor with umbilical cord prolapse: a 5-year study. Obstet Gynecol 1988; 72:278–281.
118. Bartrett JM: Funic reduction for the management of umbilical cord prolapse: a 5-year study. Obstet Gynecol 1988; 31:1023–1026.
119. Duval C, Lemoine JP, Ba S, Demory JE: Prolapse of the umbilical cord: 79 cases. Rev Fr Gynecol Obstet 1987; 82:163–167.
120. Empfehlungen der Deutschen Gesellschaft für Perinatale Medizin (1969): Erfassung und Betreuung von Risikofällen während der Schwangerschaft, Geburt und Neugeborenenperiode. Perinatal Medizin 1989; 1(suppl 1):56–62.
121. American College of Obstetricians and Gynecologists: Committee on Professional Standards. *In* Standards for Obstetric-Gynecologic Services, 5th ed. Washington, DC: ACOG; 1982.
122. American College of Obstetricians and Gynecologists: Committee on Professional Standards. *In* Standards for Obstetric-Gynecologic Services, 7th ed. Washington, DC: ACOG; 1989.
123. Stellungnahme der Deutschen Gesellschaft für Gynaekologie und Geburtshilfe. Mindestanforderungen an prozessuale, strukturelle und organisatorische Voraussetzungen für geburtshilfliche Abteilungen. Der Frauenarzt 1995; 36:27.
124. Chauhan SP, Roach H, Naef RW 2nd, et al: Cesarean section for suspected fetal distress: does the decision-incision time make a difference? J Reprod Med 1997; 42:347–352.
125. Korhonen J, Kariniemi V: Emergency cesarean section: the effect of delay on umbilical arterial gas balance and Apgar scores. Acta Obstet Gynecol Scand 1994; 73:782–786.
126. Ulsenheimer K, Schlüter U, Böker MH, Bayer M: Rechtliche Probleme in Geburtshilfe und Gynäkologie. Stuttgart: Enke; 1990.
127. Roex AJ, Puyenbroek JI, MacLaren DM, et al: A randomized clinical trial of antibiotic prophylaxis in cesarean section: maternal morbidity, risk factor and bacteriological changes. Eur J Obstet Gynecol Reprod Biol 1986; 22:117–124.
128. Hoffmen WE, Pellegrino D, Werner C, et al: Ketamine decreases plasma catecholamines and improves outcome from incomplete cerebral ischemia in rats. Anesthesiology 1992; 76:755–762.
129. Gale R, Zalkinder-Luboshitz I, Slater PE: Increased neonatal risk from the use of general anesthesia in emergency cesarean section: a retrospective analysis of 374 cases. J Reprod Med 1982; 27:715–719.
130. Marx GF, Luykx WM, Cohen S: Fetal-neonatal status following caesarean section for fetal distress. Br J Anaesth 1984; 56:1009–1013.
131. Eisenach JC: Fetal stress/distress. Probl Anesth 1989; 3:19–31.
132. Keohane M: Patient comfort: spinal versus epidural anesthesia for cesarean section [letter; comment]. Anesth Analg 1996; 82:219.
133. Manchikanti L, Grow JB, Colliver JA, et al: Bicitra (sodium citrate) and metoclopramide in outpatient anesthesia for prophylaxis against aspiration pneumonitis. Anesthesiology 1985; 63:378–384.
134. Personal communication: Herr Otto, Product Manager Regional Anesthesia. Melsungen, Germany: B. Braun Melsungen AG (011-5661-71-0 [tel.]).
135. Hirose M, Hara Y, Hosokawa T, Tanaka Y: The effect of postoperative analgesia with continuous epidural bupivacaine after cesarean section on the amount of breast feeding and infant weight gain. Anesth Analg 1996; 82:1166–1169.
136. Lussos A: Anästhesie bei Sectio caesarea. *In* Ullstein DS (ed): Anästhesie in der Geburtshilfe. St. Louis: Mosby; 1997.
137. Huang JS, I YY, Tung CC, Chou P: Comparison between the effects of epidural and spinal anesthesia for selective cesarean section. Chung Hua I Hsueh Tsa Chih (Taipei) 1993; 51:40–47.
138. Brizgys RV, Dailey PA, Shnider SM, et al: Incidence and

neonatal effects of maternal hypotension during epidural anesthesia for cesarean section. Anesthesiology 1987; 67:782.
139. Fong J, Gurewitsch ED, Press RA, et al: Prevention of maternal hypotension by epidural administration of ephedrine sulfate during lumbar epidural anesthesia for cesarean section. Am J Obstet Gynecol 1996; 175:985–990.
140. Fong J, Gurewitsch ED, Press RA, et al: Prevention of maternal hypotension by epidural administration of ephedrine sulfate during lumbar epidural anesthesia for ceasarean section. Am J Obstet Gynecol 1996; 175:985–990.
141. Casey WF, Smith CE, Katz JM, et al: Intravenous meperidine for control of shivering during caesarean section under epidural anaesthesia. Can J Anaesth 1988; 35:128–133.
142. Sessler DI, Ponte J: Shivering during epidural anesthesia. Anesthesiology 72:816–821.
143. Liu WH, Luxton MC: The effect of prophylactic fentanyl on shivering in elective caesarean section under epidural analgesia. Anaesthesia 1991; 46:344–348.
144. Morton CP, Bloomfield S, Magnusson A, et al: Ropivacaine 0.75% for extradural anaesthesia in elective caesarean section: an open clinical and pharmacokinetic study in mother and neonate. Br J Anaesth 1997; 79:3–8.
145. Karinen J, Mäkäräinen L, Alahuhta S, et al: Single bolus compared with a fractionated dose injection technique of bupivacaine for extradural Caesarean section: effect on uteroplacental and fetal haemodynamic state. Br J Anaesth 1996; 77:140–144.
146. Morishima HO, Pedersen H, Santos AC, et al: Adverse effects of maternally administered lidocaine on the asphyxiated preterm fetal lamb. Anesthesiology 1989; 71:110–115.
147. Morishima HO, Santos AC, Pedersen H, et al: Effect of lidocaine on the asphyxial responses in the mature fetal lamb. Anesthesiology 1987; 66:502–507.
148. Friesen C, Cumming M, Biehl D: The effect of lidocaine on regional blood flows and cardiac output in the nonstressed and the stressed foetal lamb. Can Anaesth Soc J 1986; 33:130–137.
149. Esteban-Altirriba J, Cabero L, Calaf F: Correction of fetal homeostatic disturbances. *In* Aladjem S, Brown AK, Sureau C (eds): Clinical Perinatology. St. Louis: Mosby–Year Book; 1980: 100–115.

20

Anesthesia for Postpartum Surgery

❖ REMI BOURLIER, MD

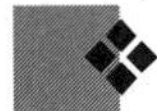 INTRODUCTION

This chapter examines the anesthetic implications of surgery in the postpartum patient. In this chapter, *postpartum* is defined as beginning immediately after the third stage of labor. When it ends, however, is somewhat controversial.[1] For the purpose of this chapter, we shall consider that "postpartum" includes the entire period of time during which the physiologic modifications of pregnancy are still present (puerperium) and lasting until the body returns to a nonpregnant state. This return to nonpregnant status generally takes 6 to 8 weeks.[2, 3]

Pregnancy is responsible for numerous physiologic changes, many of which may have an impact on anesthetic management. Although most anesthetic literature supports the assumption that pregnancy and the postpartum period are associated with delayed gastric emptying, not everyone agrees.[4, 5] There is no controversy, however, when it comes to airway management. It is universally recommended that these patients be treated as status "full stomach," regardless of the time of their last meal. If it becomes necessary, intubation should be rapid sequence. The physiologic changes of pregnancy do not disappear instantly following delivery and the return to a prepregnancy state can take months, depending on the degree of physiologic modifications.[3] Thus, a discussion of anesthesia for postpartum surgery can be summarized in a single key question: When is the new mother no longer pregnant as regards all physiologic systems?

Since the physiologic modifications of pregnancy continue following delivery, the anesthesiologist should consider postpartum patients as if they were still pregnant. In addition, many nonessential or nonemergency surgical procedures can be delayed to decrease anesthetic risk. Unfortunately, in the current era of managed care and cost containment, delays in elective postpartum surgery are often deemed inappropriate. This chapter considers the various surgical procedures that are performed on the postpartum patient, analyzes the risks and benefits associated with anesthetizing these patients, and finally reviews several anesthetic options that can be safely used.

PHYSIOLOGIC CHANGES IN THE POSTPARTUM PERIOD

Pregnancy and the postpartum period are associated with changes to all major organ systems, which are fully discussed in Chapter 2. Because of their importance to the anesthesiologist, this chapter concentrates on the postpartum patient with regard to airway, gastrointestinal tract, hemodynamics, and the pharmacology of commonly used drugs.

Airway

During the immediate postpartum period, elevated levels of estrogens and progesterone induce a capillary engorgement of the mucosa, especially of the upper airway.[6] Furthermore, airway changes such as decreased visualization on laryngoscopy and increased incidence of difficult intubations occur not only during labor but also in the postpartum period.[7] Disengorgement of airway mucosa should commence following the normalization of hormonal levels, which typically begins on the first postpartum day.[3, 8]

Thus, expecting the anatomically unanticipated difficult intubation remains of importance in the immediate postpartum period. In fact, the airway abnormalities shortly after delivery may even be greater than before labor, owing in part to airway changes produced by pushing.[7] As in other patients, a careful preoperative airway assessment is mandatory before performance of any anesthetic, either regional or general.

Gastrointestinal Physiology

Regurgitation and subsequent aspiration of gastric contents remains an important cause of morbidity and mortality related to anesthesia[9] and therefore should be of major concern to anesthesiologists caring for patients who are to undergo surgery in the postpartum period. The risk of aspiration and of developing aspiration pneumonitis following aspiration are discussed subsequently.

To assess the risk of aspiration in the postpartum patient, one must first examine the anatomy, gastric motility, secretions, and volume. Unfortunately, a review of this subject illustrates controversial and discordant results.[10] A recent study that evaluated gastric ultrasound examinations of women following delivery reported the presence of solid food particles and a delay in gastric emptying.[11] This, however, is not the only opinion. Using an epigastric impedance technique to compare gastric emptying times in women in their third trimester of pregnancy with women in the first hour post partum and in nonpregnant control subjects, O'Sullivan and coworkers[12] concluded that the rate of gastric emptying in postpartum women is delayed only if opioids have been administered during labor. This was also confirmed by Nimmo.[13] To add even more confusion, it has been reported that applied potential tomography measurements in 10 healthy patients during and following labor showed no difference in gastric emptying.[14]

Because there appears to be no clear way to assess the individual patient's risk of aspiration in the postpartum period, it is difficult to define the optimum timing and anesthetic management that allows an anesthesiologist to assure a postpartum patient that there is no risk of this potentially devastating complication.

Nevertheless, the concept of barrier pressure is a useful tool to help solve this troubling question. Barrier pressure is defined as the difference between intragastric pressure and the tone of the lower esophageal high-pressure zone.[10] Any factors that contribute to a decrease in barrier pressure (i.e., increased intragastric pressure or decreased tone of the lower esophageal sphincter) enhance the risk of aspiration. Integrity of barrier pressure, and thus a decreased aspiration risk, can be approximated by the presence of pyrosis, which is a clinical symptom of gastroesophageal reflux. Fifty percent to 80% of pregnant women have pyrosis.[15, 16] In these patients, a reduction of barrier pressure is more likely due to a decreased tone of the lower esophageal sphincter than to an increase in intragastric pressure.[16] However, since gastroesophageal reflux is often silent, using its presence to predict the proportion of women at risk for regurgitation and aspiration can clearly underestimate the problem.

Prevention of Pneumonitis. Gastric volume and pH have been specifically studied in an attempt to define the risk of aspiration pneumonitis. A critical combination of a gastric pH of less than 2.5 and gastric volume greater than 25 mL have been historically accepted as the criteria for risk of pneumonitis following aspiration.[17] Further studies emphasize not only the role of pH[18, 19] but the fact that critical volume is itself often dependent on the pH. Thus, the lower the pH, the smaller the volume necessary to produce pneumonitis.[18]

In a 1992 study, Lam and associates[20] demonstrated that between 1 and 5 days following delivery, 150 mL of water administered orally may be given safely 2 to 3 hours preoperatively. Intragastric volume and acidity were not increased, and the findings in postpartum patients were similar to those found in nonpregnant patients. Another study that also evaluated the effect of preoperative oral fluids on gastric volume and pH in postpartum patients demonstrated that ingestion of 150 mL of plain water approximately 2½ hours before the scheduled time of postpartum tubal ligation did not increase the risk of aspiration syndrome.[21] However, a recent study examining the stomach contents of women following delivery using ultrasound imaging has demonstrated the presence of solid food particles and a delay of gastric emptying in the postpartum period.[11]

James and colleagues[19] have studied postpartum patients up to 45 hours after delivery, and have reported that these patients did not have a statistically significant increase in the risk of aspiration pneumonitis when compared with a group of women undergoing elective gynecologic or orthopedic procedures. This said, it must be reiterated that the fact that there was no statistically significant difference between pregnant, postpartum, and nonpregnant patients in 1 or 2 studies does not mean that the pregnant and postpartum patient are not at risk for aspiration pneumonitis.

The Impact of Labor and Analgesia on Gastrointestinal Physiology. It has been suggested that labor produces a delay of gastric emptying[17] and increases gastric volume[17, 18] and that these effects may linger into the postpartum period. The impact of labor epidural analgesia on gastrointestinal physiology remains unclear. Parenteral opioids may change gastric motility times. Opioids decrease the barrier pressure by acting on the lower esophageal sphincter tone, and thus put the laboring woman at greater risk for aspiration.[22] It has also been suggested that epidural opioids may delay gastric emptying,[23] but a recent study has suggested that any negative effect would occur only at a cumulative dose of greater than 100 μg.[24] Nevertheless, Zimmermann and coworkers[25] did not find differences in gastric emptying when evaluating laboring parturients receiving either bupivacaine or bupivacaine plus fentanyl. Intrathecal opioids have also been incriminated as potentially delaying gastric emptying during labor, but the clinical significance of this finding is unclear.

The risk of anesthesia-induced aspiration and pneumonitis in the postpartum period is uncertain. Evidence that supports both increased or unchanged risk exists, and there is no compelling evidence that a postpartum patient's risk is decreased by delaying surgery, since no time interval has been shown to guarantee a risk-free anesthetic. However, since there is clinical evidence that aspiration does sometimes occur in these patients, there is no reason to withhold nonparticulate antacid prophylaxis in all postpartum patients undergoing any form of anesthesia. In addition, all efforts to decrease the risk of failed intubation and aspiration should be made.

Hemodynamic Changes in the Postpartum Period

As discussed in Chapter 2, cardiac output at term is dramatically increased as compared with prepregnancy values; this is due to an increase in both stroke volume and heart rate.[26, 27] Cardiac output in the second stage of labor is additionally increased over prelabor values.[28, 29] This increase in cardiac output peaks in the immediate postpartum period, mainly owing to increased stroke volume, and then decreases toward baseline values[30] approximately 1 hour following delivery. Noninvasive ultrasonic Doppler cardiac output has been used to evaluate hemodynamic changes in women undergoing cesarean section under epidural or general anesthesia.[31] This study demonstrated a similar pattern of increase in cardiac output with the two anesthesia techniques (36.7% and 28% at 15 minutes and 26.3% and 17.2% at 30 minutes postdelivery, respectively) and a return by 60 minutes to preoperative levels, which persisted for up to 24 hours after delivery. Thus, hemodynamic ramifications of anesthesia do not appear to be risk factors for the stable postpartum patient undergoing surgery under either regional or general anesthesia.

Blood loss at the time of vaginal delivery averages 450 mL, with 25% to 30% of the blood volume expansion owing to pregnancy.[32, 33] Loss of another third of the expanded blood volume occurs during the first 24 hours postpartum,[32, 34] which is followed by little change in blood volume for the next 3 to 6 days.[32–34] Subsequently, plasma volume continues to fall while red blood cell volume remains constant, which results in hemoconcentration, as reflected by the increasing hematocrit.[35] Blood volume returns to normal by 6 to 9 weeks postpartum.[35] During cesarean delivery, blood loss is approximately 900 mL.[32, 33] Therefore, except in cases of exaggerated blood loss, the postpartum period should be considered as a hypervolemic state compared with predelivery conditions.

Drug Metabolism

There is a decrease in the plasma cholinesterase activity of approximately 20% in the first trimester of pregnancy and this reduction is maintained until delivery.[36] Two to 4 days after delivery, there is a further 33% reduction in activity. It is not until the sixth postpartum week that there is a return to prepregnancy levels.[36] The cause of these changes cannot be explained by hemodilution alone as exemplified by the further postpartum diminution in activity when there is actually a reduction in blood volume. Regardless of these laboratory findings, clinical experience suggests that this cholinesterase "deficiency" should not cause prolongation of drug effect. Because an enzyme activity of less than 30% does not lead to succinylcholine sensitivity,[36] no healthy pregnant woman who is homozygous would be expected to experience prolonged apnea following an appropriate dose of succinylcholine. That said, patients who are 1 to 2 days postpartum may in fact exhibit a slightly prolonged recovery from succinylcholine compared with term pregnant and nonpregnant controls receiving the same dose of relaxant, and they may require a significantly reduced dose compared with nonpregnant controls for 80% depression of control muscle fiber twitch height.[37, 38] A modest prolongation of succinylcholine effect, however, even if it does occasionally occur, is usually undetected and generally clinically insignificant.

Mivacurium, a recently introduced short-acting nondepolarizing neuromuscular blocking agent, has been shown to be metabolized by plasma pseudocholinesterase at a rate between 70% and 88% of that of succinylcholine.[36] A recent study described a slightly prolonged neuromuscular block after the administration of mivacurium for a tubal ligation in postpartum patients.[39] However, although the prolongation of neuromuscular block was statistically significant, this finding is of questionable clinical significance. The median duration for recovery of 25% of the first twitch was increased by approximately 3 minutes.

Remifentanil, a new μ-agonist opioid, produces intense analgesia of rapid onset and very short duration. For these reasons, it may be considered for very short postpartum surgical procedures. Remifentanil is susceptible to rapid hydrolysis by nonspecific cholinesterases[36] and therefore should not be prolonged because of plasma cholinesterase deficiency.

A prolongation of action of vecuronium has been reported in patients undergoing postpartum tubal ligation,[40, 41] suggesting a potential for enhanced sensitivity to nondepolarizing muscle relaxants during the puerperium. This was subsequently confirmed by a study that compared vecuronium and atracurium in postpartum and nonpregnant patients.[42] Although the duration of action of atracurium in the two groups was not different, the clinical duration of vecuronium was significantly prolonged in the postpartum group (49 ± 10 vs. 32 ± 6 minutes). These authors concluded that pregnancy-induced changes in liver blood flow might interfere with the hepatic clearance of vecuronium and thereby cause the slight prolongation of neuromuscular blockade.

An extended duration of action of rocuronium has also been demonstrated. A study comparing nonpregnant and postpartum patients receiving a single bolus of 600 μg/kg[43] reported that the time to 25% twitch recovery was significantly longer in postpartum patients (31.1 ± 3.6 minutes) compared with the nonpregnant group (24.9 ± 4.0 minutes). Once again, this prolongation would be of clinical importance only in very short operative procedures.

Minimum alveolar concentration (MAC) during pregnancy is reduced by 20% to 40%. Possible explanations for this include the sedative effect of progesterone,[44] the increased central nervous system serotoninergic activity,[45] and the activation of the endorphin system[46] during pregnancy and the postpartum period. The MAC of isoflurane has been compared in three groups of patients undergoing bilateral tubal ligation: an early postpartum group (1–12 hours), a late postpartum group (12–25 hours), and a control group (>6 weeks postpartum).[47] The MAC in the early postpartum group was significantly less (0.75 ± 0.17) than in late postpartum (0.95 ± 0.2) or control groups (1.04 ± 0.12). However, there was no difference between late postpartum and control groups. Furthermore, there was no correlation between plasma progesterone or β-endorphin levels and MAC. Another study confirmed this decrease in the MAC of isoflurane in postpartum patients, but reported a delay of more than 72 hours for return to normal values.[48]

Volatile agents are also known to produce uterine vasodilatation, which may precipitate postpartum hemorrhage secondary to uterine atony in the early postpartum period. This is especially true in the grand multiparous patient for early postpartum tubal ligation, who is at greater risk for development of uterine atony. Both halothane and enflurane have been found to impair spontaneous uterine activity and to decrease the response to oxytocin in the early postpartum period.[49]

SURGERY PERFORMED DURING THE POSTPARTUM

Numerous operative procedures are performed in the postpartum period. These include elective surgeries (e.g., postpartum tubal ligation) and emergency procedures (e.g., cesarean hysterectomy, repair of perineal lacerations, repair of uterine inversion). Because the postpartum patient for emergency surgical intervention is often suffering from a life-threatening condition and may be profoundly hypovolemic, general anesthesia is most often used. This is not the case, however, with elective postpartum procedures, which are often performed under regional anesthesia techniques. The most common elective postpartum surgery, postpartum tubal ligation, is discussed in detail.

The following guidelines have been recommended for postpartum tubal ligation.[50] Although these guidelines are primarily geared to obstetricians, anesthesiologists should also be cognizant of these recommendations:

- The patient must be at least 21 years of age and mentally competent when consent is obtained.
- Informed consent for tubal ligation may not be obtained while the patient is in labor or during childbirth.
- Informed consent may not be obtained while the patient is undergoing an abortion or under the influence of alcohol or other substances.
- A total of 30 days must pass between the date the consent is signed and the day that the procedure is to be performed. Exceptions to this rule can be made for preterm delivery or emergency abdominal surgery.
- Consent is valid for only 180 days.

In some countries, laws forbid the use of sterilization surgery as a first-line birth control method.[51] In France, for example, tubal ligation can only be performed with a strong medical indication (e.g., a coexisting disease in which pregnancy would be life-threatening and any other contraceptive method contraindicated) or in some very specific economic and social settings.[52]

A more thorough explanation of the common surgical methods for postpartum tubal ligation may be helpful to the anesthesiologist:

- Irving procedure: the medial cut end of the fallopian tube is buried in the myometrium posteriorly and the distal cut end is buried in the mesosalpinx. This technique is least likely to fail but requires more extensive exposure and increases the risk of hemorrhage.
- Pomeroy procedure: the simplest of the procedures; a loop of oviduct is ligated, and the knuckle of tube above the ligature is excised.
- Parkland procedure: a midsegment of tube is separated from the mesosalpinx at an avascular site; the separated tubal segment is ligated proximally and distally and then excised.

ANESTHESIA FOR POSTPARTUM TUBAL LIGATION

Although some of the factors that predispose the pregnant patient to aspiration (such as increased intragastric pressure and decreased emptying caused by anatomic obstruction) are rapidly alleviated after delivery, the use of opioids in labor may dramatically increase the risk of aspiration. In order to decrease this risk, aspiration prophylaxis should be used in all postpartum patients receiving anesthesia. In addition, any patient requiring general anesthesia in the early postpartum period must be considered "full stomach" status and should therefore be intubated using a rapid-sequence induction with the Sellick maneuver.[19]

As in the pregnant patient, the airway examination in the postpartum patient is of paramount importance when considering the choice of anesthetic, so that general anesthesia can be avoided, if possible, in patients who are considered to be at high risk for failed intubation. Because of the risks of failed intubation, aspiration, and postpartum hemorrhage, many anesthesiologists prefer to use regional anesthesia for postpartum surgery, whenever possible.

Regional Anesthesia

Most elective procedures performed in the immediate postpartum period are of short duration and amenable to the use of epidural, spinal, or combined spinal-epidural techniques. If epidural analgesia was used in labor, the epidural catheter can be converted for operative use. Most often, 2% lidocaine or 3% 2-chloroprocaine are chosen owing to their short duration of action. If an epidural catheter is not in situ, spinal anesthesia offers the advantage of fast onset, density of block, and short duration of block. Epidural anesthesia is more time-consuming (its placement may require more time than the tubal ligation itself); epidurals require the use of a large volume of local anesthetic with greater potential toxicity; and epidural anesthesia is often more expensive to perform than a spinal block.[53] There are thus numerous reasons to favor the use of spinal anesthesia for postpartum tubal ligation, especially since the risk of postdural puncture can be greatly decreased by use of small-gauge pencil-point needles.[54–56]

Regardless of whether epidural or spinal anesthesia is chosen, a dermatone level of T4 is optimum to block the visceral pain that occurs during exposure and manipulation of the fallopian tubes.

Segmental local anesthetic dose requirements are known to be reduced during pregnancy, but the doses necessary to produce appropriate anesthetic levels return to those of nonpregnant women shortly after delivery, as demonstrated by the elevated segmental dose requirements within 8 to 24 hours postpartum,[57] the reduced spread of a fixed dose of bupivacaine in patients 2 to 51 hours postpartum,[58] and the significant increase in the postpartum dose requirement to achieve a certain level of anesthesia in individuals studied at term and again at 36 to 48 hours postpartum.[59]

In addition to local anesthetics, preservative-free intrathecal meperidine may be used to provide spinal anesthesia in the postpartum patient. A dose of 60 mg was recently compared with intrathecal lidocaine (70 mg) in patients undergoing postpartum tubal ligation.[60] Intraoperative anesthesia was equal and although the meperidine group patients experienced more pruritus, postoperative analgesia was much better in this group. Patient satisfaction was the same in both groups.

If an indwelling labor epidural catheter is to be used to provide anesthesia for postpartum tubal ligation, the possibility of failure of reactivation must be considered. Viscomi and Rathmell[53] performed a cost-comparison study that compared labor epidural catheter reactivation with spinal anesthesia for delayed postpartum tubal ligation. Adequate anesthesia for tubal ligation was achieved in only 78% of women after reinjection of their epidural catheter. Operating room and anesthesia times were highest when epidural catheter reactivation was unsuccessful, intermediate when epidural catheter reactivation was successful, and lowest with initial spinal anesthesia. Spinal anesthesia for postpartum tubal ligation was associated with lower anesthesia professional fees and operating room charges compared with attempted reactivation of epidural catheters placed during labor. Similar findings were also reported by Vincent and Reid,[61] who reported a 74% success rate for indwelling catheters when used for postpartum tubal ligation. Timing, however, appears to be a major factor in the success or failure of an indwelling epidural catheter. When evaluating the delay between delivery and surgery, reactivation was successful in 95% of patients when the catheter was reinjected within 4 hours after delivery, but success declined to only 67% for catheter reinjection after 4 hours postpartum. The increased failure in epidural catheters that have been dormant for many hours has also been reported by other authors.[62, 63] Some anesthesiologists, therefore, remove the epidural catheter and perform spinal anesthesia for postpartum tubal ligation if there will be a several-hour delay between delivery and the surgical procedure.

Appropriate sedative drugs may be given to supplement a regional anesthetic, if needed. Since most women, however, want to remember their first several hours of contact with their newborn, the anesthesiologist should minimize the use of benzodiazepines, owing to their amnesic effects.

Local Anesthesia

Cruishank and colleagues[64] reported on the use of intraperitoneal lidocaine to achieve anesthesia for tubal ligation. The effectiveness of this technique is demonstrated by the fact that most of their patients slept through the operative procedure. Merger and associates[52] have reviewed 732 laparoscopic postpartum tubal ligations done under local anesthesia (2nd to 6th day postdelivery), with good success rates.

ANESTHESIA AND BREAST-FEEDING

Breast milk is considered to be the optimal method of infant feeding. Therefore, many women who undergo postpartum surgery still want to breast-feed their newborn postoperatively. Most drugs given to the mother are secreted in breast milk, and thus the anesthesiologist should be aware of the implications of the drugs they administer in regard to breast-feeding. Many factors influence the excretion of drugs into breast milk, including lipid solubility, ionization, concentration in the plasma, degree of protein binding, and molecular weight.

The amount of drug ingested by the infant typically is small and, for most drugs, is insufficient to exert any clinical effects.[65, 66] Most pain relievers used for intraoperative and postoperative analgesia, including acetaminophen, codeine, meperidine, and morphine, do not appear to cause significant breast milk levels or neonatal depression when administered in therapeutic doses.[65, 66] Fentanyl, for example, has been extensively studied and cannot be found in breast milk when total doses of up to 400 μg were maternally administered during labor.[67]

Not all narcotics, however, are equivalent. For example, a comparison of neonatal neurobehavioral scores in infants of nursing mothers receiving either morphine or meperidine via intravenous patient-controlled analgesia following cesarean section has shown that the babies of mothers receiving morphine were significantly more alert, oriented, and had higher scores than the infants whose mothers received meperidine.[68] This advantage of morphine as compared with meperidine was similarly reported by Wittels and colleagues.[69] These authors demonstrated that mothers who had received meperidine intravenous patient-controlled analgesia following cesarean section had persistently elevated concentrations of normeperidine in breast milk for up to 96 hours. Although it has been suggested that maternally administered opioids may cause neonatal apnea or cyanosis,[70] most women who undergo cesarean section or postpartum surgery receive opioid medications and despite opioid levels in breast milk, have no neonatal sequelae. That said, if a newborn exhibits signs of apnea, bradycardia, or cyanosis, and if the mother has been receiving opioids, breast-feeding should be temporarily discontinued.

The American Academy of Pediatrics has classified the drugs that can be found in breast milk following maternal administration[71] into drugs that are compatible with breast-feeding, those that require temporary discontinuation of breast-feeding, and those that contraindicate breast-feeding. Of the commonly used analgesics, the American Academy of Pediatrics has listed butorphanol, codeine, and morphine as being compatible with breast-feeding. Although the evidence of newborn risk is inconclusive, it has been suggested that the following drugs be avoided, when possible, for the patient who will breast-feed:

Diazepam: prolonged presence of active metabolites in newborns.[72]

Atropine: anticholinergic effects in newborns.[73]

Antihistamines: decreased lactation.[73]

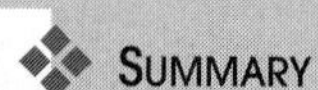

Summary

Key Points

- Postpartum sterilization is convenient for the patient and the surgeon and is cost-effective. It is, however, a totally elective procedure and therefore should never proceed unless the patient is stable and manpower is available.
- Postpartum procedures should be canceled or delayed in the patient with medical or obstetric complications.
- Epidural analgesia for labor can be used for these procedures, but the longer the delay, the greater the chance that the catheter will fail.
- If the procedure is delayed or if the patient has not received labor epidural anesthesia, spinal anesthesia is the favored technique.

Key References

American College of Obstetricians and Gynecologists Committee on Obstetrics, Maternal and Fetal Medicine: postpartum tubal sterilization. Committee Opinion 105. Washington, DC; 1992.

Goodman EJ, Dumas SD: The rate of successful reactivation of labor epidural catheters for postpartum tubal ligation surgery. Reg Anesth Pain Med 1998; 23:258–261.

Case Stem

A patient with an indwelling epidural catheter is brought to the operating room for a cesarean section, because of arrest of dilatation. Twenty-five minutes following the administration of 20 mL of 0.5% bupivacaine, the patient has a "patchy" T10 block. How would you manage this patient?

Regional anesthesia is also suitable for pain relief after surgery in the postpartum.[74, 75] Postoperative analgesia with continuous epidural bupivacaine for several days was recently shown to improve breast-feeding and the gain of infant weight after cesarean section.[74]

References

1. Frisoli G: Physiology and pathology of the puerperium. *In* Iffy L, Kaminetzky HA (eds): Principles and Practice of Obstetrics and Perinatology. New York: John Wiley & Sons; 1981:1657.
2. The puerperium. *In* Cunningham FG, MacDonald PC, Gant NF, et al (eds): Williams Obstetrics, 20th ed. Stamford, CT: Appleton & Lange; 1997:533–546.
3. Horovitz J, Hocke C, Roux D, et al: Suites de couches normales et pathologiques. *In* Papiernick E, Cabrol D, Pons JC (eds): Obstétrique. Paris: Flammarion; 1995:1455–1464.
4. Macfie AG, Magides AD, Richmond MN, et al: Gastric emptying in pregnancy. Br J Anaesth 1991; 67:54–57.
5. Gin T, Cho AMW, Lew JKL, et al: Gastric emptying in the postpartum period. Anaesth Intensive Care 1991; 19:521–524.
6. Leontic EA: Respiratory disease in pregnancy. Med Clin North Am 1977; 61:111–128.
7. Farcon EL, Kim MH, Marx GF: Changing Mallampati score during labour. Can J Anaesth 1994; 41:50–51.
8. Llauro JL, Runnebaum B, Zander J: Progesterone in human peripheral blood before, during and after labor. Am J Obstet Gynecol 1968; 101:867–873.
9. Hawkins JL, Koonin LM, Palmer SK, et al: Anesthesia-related deaths during obstetric delivery in the United States, 1979–1990. Anesthesiology 1997; 86:277–284.
10. Conklin KA: Maternal physiologic considerations during pregnancy and delivery. *In* Van Zundert A, Ostheimer G (eds): Pain Relief and Anesthesia in Obstetrics. New York: Churchill Livingstone; 1996:61–87.
11. Jarayam A, Bowen MP, Deshpande S, et al: Ultrasound examination of the stomach contents of women in the postpartum period. Anesth Analg 1997; 84:522–526.
12. O'Sullivan GM, Sutton AJ, Thompson SA, et al: Noninvasive measurement of gastric emptying in obstetric patients. Anesth Analg 1987; 66:505–511.
13. Nimmo WS: Gastric emptying and anesthesia. Can J Anaesth 1989; 36:S45–S47.
14. Sandhar BK, Elliott RH, Windram I, et al: Peripartum changes in gastric emptying. Anaesthesia 1992; 47:196–198.
15. Bassey OO: Pregnancy heartburn in Nigerians and Caucasians with theories about aetiology based on manometric recordings from the oesophagus and stomach. Br J Obstet Gynaecol 1977; 84:439–443.
16. Nagler R, Spiro HM: Heartburn in late pregnancy: manometric studies of esophageal motor function. J Clin Invest 1961; 40:954–970.
17. Roberts RB, Shirley MA: Reducing the risk of acid aspiration during cesarean section. Anesth Analg 1974; 53:859–868.
18. Taylor G, Pryse-Davies J: The prophylactic use of antacids in the prevention of the acid-pulmonary-aspiration syndrome (Mendelson's syndrome). Lancet 1966; 1:288–291.
19. James CF, Gibbs CP, Banner T: Postpartum perioperative risk of aspiration pneumonia. Anesthesiology 1984; 61:756–759.
20. Lam KK, So HY, Gin T: Gastric pH and volume after oral fluids in the postpartum patient. Can J Anaesth 1993; 40:218–221.
21. Somwanshi M, Tripathi A, Singh B, et al: Effect of preoperative oral fluids on gastric volume and pH in postpartum patients. Middle East J Anesthesiol 1995; 13:197–203.
22. Hey VMF, Ostick DG, Mazumder JK, et al: Pethidine, metoclopramide and the gastro-oesophageal sphincter: a study in healthy volunteers. Anaesthesia 1981; 36:173–176.
23. Wright PMC, Allen RW, Moore J, et al: Gastric emptying during lumbar extradural analgesia in labor: effect of fentanyl supplementation. Br J Anaesth 1992; 68:248–251.
24. Porter JS, Bonello E, Reynolds F: The influence of epidural

administration of fentanyl infusion on gastric emptying in labor. Anaesthesia 1997; 52:1151–1156.
25. Zimmermann DL, Breen TW, Fick G: Adding fentanyl 0.0002% to epidural bupivacaine 0.125% does not delay gastric emptying in laboring parturients. Anesth Analg 1996; 82:612–616.
26. Robson SC, Hunter S, Boys RJ, et al; Serial study of factors influencing changes in cardiac output during human pregnancy. Am J Physiol 1989; 256:H1060–H1065.
27. Robson SC, Hunter S, Moore M, et al: Haemodynamic changes during the puerperium: a Doppler and M-mode echocardiographic study. Br J Obstet Gynaecol 1987; 94:1028–1039.
28. Hansen JM, Ueland K: The influence of caudal analgesia on cardiovascular dynamics during normal labor and delivery. Acta Anaesthesiol Scand 1966; 23(suppl):449–452.
29. Kjeldsen J: Hemodynamic investigations during labor and delivery. Acta Obstet Gynecol Scand 1979; 89(suppl):1–252.
30. Ueland K, Hansen JM: Maternal cardiovascular dynamics. III. Labor and delivery under local and caudal analgesia. Am J Obstet Gynecol 1969; 103:8–18.
31. James CF, Banner T, Caton D: Cardiac output in women undergoing cesarean section with epidural or general anesthesia. Am J Obstet Gynecol 1989; 160:1178–1184.
32. Ueland K: Maternal cardiovascular dynamics. VII. Intrapartum blood volume changes. Am J Obstet Gynecol 1976; 126:671–677.
33. Pritchard JA, Baldwin RM, Dickey JC, et al: Blood volume changes in pregnancy and the puerperium. II. Red blood cell loss and changes in apparent blood volume during and following vaginal delivery, cesarean section, and cesarean section plus total hysterectomy. Am J Obstet Gynecol 1962; 84:1271–1282.
34. McLennan CE, Lowenstein JM: Blood volume changes immediately after delivery. Stanford Med Bull 1959; 17:152–156.
35. Lund CJ, Donovan JC: Blood volume during pregnancy: significance of plasma and red cell volumes. Am J Obstet Gynecol 1967; 98:393–403.
36. Davis L, Britten JJ, Morgan M: Cholinesterase: its significance in anaesthetic practice. Anaesthesia 1997; 52:244–260.
37. Leighton BL, Cheek TG, Gross JB, et al: Succinylcholine pharmacodynamics in peripartum patients. Anesthesiology 1986; 64:202–205.
38. Ganga CC, Heyduk JV, Marx GF, et al: A comparison of the response to suxamethonium in postpartum and gynaecological patients. Anaesthesia 1982; 37:903–906.
39. Gin T, Derrick JL, Chan MT, et al: Postpartum patients have slightly prolonged neuromuscular block after mivacurium. Anesth Analg 1998; 86:82–85.
40. Camp CE, Tessem J, Adenwala J, et al: Vecuronium and prolonged neuromuscular blockade in postpartum patients. Anesthesiology 1987; 67:1006–1008.
41. Hawkins JL, Adenwala J, Camp C, et al: The effect of H2-receptor antagonist premedication on the duration of vecuronium-induced neuromuscular blockade in postpartum patients. Anesthesiology 1989; 71:175–177.
42. Khuenl-Brady KS, Koller J, Mair P, et al: Comparison of vecuronium- and atracurium-induced neuromuscular blockade in postpartum and nonpregnant patients. Anesth Analg 1991; 72:110–113.
43. Puhringer FK, Sparr HJ, Mitterschiffthaler G, et al: Extended duration of action of rocuronium in postpartum patients. Anesth Analg 1997; 84:352–354.
44. Merryman W, Boiman R, Barnes L, et al: Progesterone "anesthesia" in human subjects. J Clin Endocrinol Metab 1954; 14:1567–1569.
45. Spielman FJ, Mueller RA, Corke BC: Cerebrospinal concentration of 5-hydroxyindoleacetic acid in pregnancy. Anesthesiology 1985; 62:193–195.
46. Genazzani AR, Facchinetti F, Parrini D: Beta-lipotrophin and beta-endorphin plasma levels during pregnancy. Clin Endocrinol 1981; 14:409–418.
47. Zhou HH, Norman P, De Lima LG, et al: The minimum alveolar concentration of isoflurane in patients undergoing bilateral tubal ligation in the postpartum period. Anesthesiology 1995; 82:1364–1368.
48. Chan MT, Gin T: Postpartum changes in the minimum alveolar concentration of isoflurane. Anesthesiology 1995; 82:1360–1363.
49. Marx GF, Kim YI, Lin CC, et al: Postpartum uterine pressures under halothane or enflurane anesthesia. Obstet Gynecol 1978; 51:695–698.
50. Medicaid. Sterilizations, hysterectomies and abortions. Consent form, Form No. 91860 MED-178 (revised February 6, 1979).
51. Code Civil (France), chapitre II: Du respect du corps humain, L. no. 94-653 du 29 juillet 1994, Art 16-3.
52. Merger C, Perdu M, Marchand F: Tubular sterilization in the immediate postpartum period using local anesthesia and laparoscopy. J Gynecol Obstet Biol Reprod 1995; 24:77–80.
53. Viscomi CM, Rathmell JP: Labor epidural catheter reactivation or spinal anesthesia for delayed postpartum tubal ligation: a cost comparison. J Clin Anesth 1995; 7:380–383.
54. Tarkkila P, Huhtala J, Salminen U: Difficulties in spinal needle use: insertion characteristics and failure rates associated with 25-, 27- and 29-gauge Quincke-type spinal needles. Anaesthesia 1994; 49:723–725.
55. Ross BK, Chadwick HS, Mancuso JJ, et al: Sprotte needle for obstetric anesthesia: decreased incidence of post–dural puncture headache. Reg Anesth 1992; 17:29–33.
56. Buettner J, Wresch KP, Klose R: Postdural puncture headache: comparison of 25-gauge Whitacre and Quincke needles. Reg Anesth 1993; 18:166–169.
57. Abouleish EI: Postpartum tubal ligation requires more bupivacaine for spinal anesthesia than does cesarean section. Anesth Analg 1986; 65:897–900.
58. DeSimone CA, Norris MC, Leighton BL, et al: Spinal anesthesia for cesarean section and postpartum tubal ligation [abstract]. Anesthesiology 1989; 71:A837.
59. Assali NS, Prystowsky H: Studies on autonomic blockade. I. Comparison between the effects of tetraethylammonium chloride (TEAC) and high selective spinal anesthesia on blood pressure of normal and toxemic pregnancy. J Clin Invest 1950; 29:1354–1366.
60. Norris MC, Honet JE, Leighton BL, et al: A comparison of meperidine and lidocaine for spinal anesthesia for postpartum tubal ligation. Reg Anesth 1996; 21:81–83.
61. Vincent RD Jr, Reid RW: Epidural anesthesia for postpartum tubal ligation using epidural catheters placed during labor. J Clin Anesth 1993; 5:289–291.
62. Kopacz DJ: Postpartum tubal ligation: timing and choice of regional anesthetic technique [abstract]. Reg Anesth 1990; 15:75S.
63. Ghost AK, Tipton RH: Early postpartum tubal ligation under epidural analgesia. Br J Obstet Gynaecol 1976; 83:731–732.
64. Cruishank DP, Laube DW, DeBacker LJ: Intraperitoneal lidocaine anesthesia for postpartum tubal ligation. Obstet Gynecol 1973; 42:127–130.
65. Findlay JWA, De Angelis RL, Kearney MF, et al: Analgesic drugs in breast milk and plasma. Clin Pharmacol Ther 1981; 29:625–633.
66. Borgatta L, Jenny RW, Gruss L, et al: Clinical significance of methohexital, meperidine, and diazepam in breast milk. J Clin Pharmacol 1997; 37:186–192.
67. Leuschen MP, Wolf LJ, Rayburn WF: Fentanyl excretion in breast milk. Clin Pharm 1990; 9:336–337.
68. Wittels B, Glosten B, Faure EAM, et al: Postcesarean analgesia with both epidural morphine and intravenous patient-controlled analgesia: neurobehavioral outcomes among nursing neonates. Anesth Analg 1997; 85:600–606.
69. Wittels B, Scott DT, Sinatra RS: Exogenous opioids in human breast milk and acute neonatal neurobehavior: a preliminary study. Anesthesiology 1990; 73:864–869.
70. Naumberg EG, Meny RG: Breast milk opioids and neonatal apnea. Am J Dis Child 1988; 142:11–12.
71. American Academy of Pediatrics: Transfer of drugs and other chemicals into human milk. Pediatrics 1989; 84:924–936.
72. Cole AP, Hailey DM: Diazepam and active metabolite in breast

milk and their transfer to the neonate. Arch Dis Child 1975; 50:741–742.
73. O'Brien TE: Excretion of drugs in human milk. Am J Hosp Pharm 1974; 31:844–854.
74. Hirose M, Hara Y, Hosokawa T, et al: The effect of postoperative analgesia with continuous epidural bupivacaine after cesarean section on the amount of breast feeding and infant weight gain. Anesth Analg 1996; 82:1166–1169.
75. Lie B, Jual J: Effects of epidural vs. general anesthesia on breast feeding. Acta Obstet Gynecol Scand 1988; 67:207–209.

21

Anesthesia for Nonobstetric Surgery in the Pregnant Patient

❖ FLORIAN R. NUEVO, MD

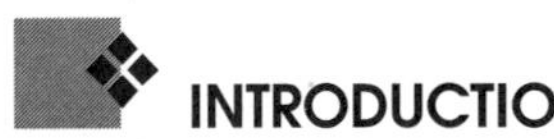

INTRODUCTION

One of the most challenging tasks that an anesthesiologist may face in clinical practice is the perioperative care of a pregnant patient for a nonobstetric surgical procedure. About 0.5% to 2.0% of all pregnant women undergo nonobstetric surgery during pregnancy.[1, 2] The difficulty arises when the surgical intervention must be carried out either during fetal organogenesis or when fetal viability may be compromised.

The primary condition that requires immediate surgical intervention can itself directly harm the mother and indirectly affect the fetus. Such clinical situations are frequently urgent, making it difficult to adequately prepare the pregnant woman emotionally, psychologically, or physically. The pregnant patient wishes to be assured of the well-being of her fetus, while also being concerned for her own health.

GOALS IN ANESTHETIC MANAGEMENT

There are two main goals in the perioperative care of these patients: maternal safety and fetal safety. Success in the perioperative care of the pregnant patient for nonobstetric surgery rests on the cooperation of obstetrician, surgeon, and anesthesiologist. The medical team members must communicate with each other and formulate the best plan for the patient. The team must also be able to prepare the patient and her family emotionally and to clearly explain the risks, benefits, and possible complications.

Fetal safety demands that spontaneous abortion or preterm labor be prevented. Surgical procedures in the abdominal or pelvic cavity may stimulate uterine activity and lead to uterine irritability and the untimely delivery or loss of the fetus.

The anesthesiologist must choose anesthetic agents free of any teratogenic effects. Episodes of intrauterine asphyxiation must be avoided by ensuring continuous intrauterine perfusion. The anesthetic technique employed must balance safety for both mother and fetus. Intensive perioperative monitoring must be directed at both mother and fetus.

Aside from these considerations, the anesthesiologist must pay attention to the duration of the planned surgical procedure, anticipating the most probable consequences of surgical and anesthetic interventions on maternal and fetal well-being.

The pregnant woman must be protected from psychologic harm and physical discomfort. Pain relief is necessary but must be done without causing fetal depression. It is quite a challenge to achieve optimum analgesic requirements during the perioperative period without exposing the fetus to risks of neurologic and respiratory depression.

Furthermore, the pregnant woman and her entire family must understand very well that nobody can fully assure that some adverse effects of surgery and teratogenicity will not occur. This underscores the importance of psychologic assistance that must be extended to the pregnant patient, her husband, and immediate family members.

The goals in the anesthetic management of the pregnant patient for nonobstetric surgery are

1. Maternal safety

- Aggressive preoperative preparation and evaluation

- Optimum anesthetic management
- Adequate analgesia during and after surgery
- Full perioperative emotional support

2. Fetal safety

- Prevention of preterm labor to avoid fetal loss
- Avoidance of teratogenic drugs
- Optimum uteroplacental perfusion to prevent fetal asphyxiation and hypoxemia

COMMON CAUSES OF NONOBSTETRIC SURGERY

The common indications for nonobstetric surgery among pregnant women can be generally grouped into two categories:

1. Procedures directly related to pregnancy

- Cerclage procedure
- Emergency pelvic laparotomy to repair twisted ovarian pedicle

2. Procedures incidental to pregnancy

- Surgery for maternal trauma
- Acute abdomen
- Correction of a neurologic problem
- Correction of a decompensating cardiac lesion

Surgery for Incompetent Cervix. The Shirodkar suture procedure and McDonald procedure are two frequently used interventions in the management of the incompetent cervix. Usually these are performed during the first and second trimesters of pregnancy. Both procedures are often associated with spontaneous abortion because the direct manipulations on the uterus can precipitate premature uterine contractions.

Ovarian Pathology. Torsion of the ovarian pedicle or presence of an enlarging ovarian cyst or tubo-ovarian abscess, with possible secondary rupture or hemorrhage, are also common indications for abdominal or pelvic explorations during pregnancy. Since these structures lie very close to the gravid uterus, gentle surgical manipulation is essential and all measures to prevent increases in uterine tone must be taken. Surgical intervention for these pathologic conditions cannot be delayed if either fetal well-being or maternal safety is endangered.

Maternal Trauma. In 1992, Fildes and colleagues[3] reported that maternal trauma secondary to vehicular accidents, suicide, and homicide has become the leading cause of maternal death. Most women today continue to work and travel throughout pregnancy, hence exposing themselves to risk. Fatigue and instability of gait make the pregnant female more prone to falls. The causes of severe trauma in pregnancy[4, 5] are given in Table 21–1. Of the homicides, 52% are due to gunshot wounds and 19% are due to stab wounds.[6]

In a review of blunt maternal trauma of 103 cases by Rothenberger and associates,[7] 20% were classified as major, consisting of skull fracture, cerebral contusion, intracerebral hemorrhage, spinal column fracture, chest injury necessitating thoracotomy, abdominal visceral and genitourinary injury, and pelvic fracture; 17% were minor and included head, chest, abdominal, and genitourinary injuries with deep lacerations, long bone fractures, and facial fractures; 63% were labeled insignificant, mostly consisting of soft tissue injuries, superficial lacerations, and fractures of the bones of the hands and the face. This study reaffirms that the best chance of fetal survival lies in securing maternal survival.

Table 21–1 Causes of Severe Trauma in Pregnancy

	Incidence (%)
Motor vehicular accidents	64
Falls	19
Penetrating wounds	10
Blunt trauma	6
Burns	1

Data from Lavery JP, State McCormack M: Management of moderate to severe trauma in pregnancy. Obstet Gynecol Clin North Am 1995; 22:69–72; and Rozycki G: Trauma during pregnancy: predicting pregnancy outcome. Arch Gynecol Obstet 1993; 253:S15–S18.

A major complication of blunt maternal abdominal trauma is placental abruption, which can occur in 38% of major cases.[8] Two percent to 4% of abruptions are associated with minor or insignificant injuries. The patient must be observed closely for abdominal and/or pelvic tenderness, uterine contractions, and vaginal bleeding. Signs and symptoms pertinent to abruption manifest within 48 hours. Abruption may present with frequent uterine contractions or profuse vaginal bleeding. However, the degree of vaginal bleeding may not correlate well with the degree of placental abruption. Serial hemoglobin determination and evaluation of the coagulation profile and ultrasound of the uterus are necessary to establish an early diagnosis.

The order of organ involvement in penetrating thoracoabdominal injuries, in decreasing order of frequency, is small bowel, liver, colon, and stomach. The uterus is almost always involved, particularly during the third trimester. Hence, fetal injury occurs in 59% to 89% of penetrating thoracoabdominal injury with fetal mortality rates of 41% to 71%.[9] Fetal mortality is higher if injury is sustained before 37 weeks' gestation. Fetal death can be a consequence of severe maternal hemorrhage, placental abruption, or direct injury to the fetus. Maternal mortality is about 7% to 9% for gunshot wounds to the uterus. Table 21–2 shows the indications for emergency cesarean section in a traumatized pregnant woman.[10]

The overall effect of trauma on pregnancy depends on (1) the gestational age of the fetus, (2) the type and severity of the injury, and (3) the extent of disruption of normal uterine and fetal physiology. Pelvic and abdominal ultrasonography should be done immediately to assess fetal viability. Survival of the fetus depends on adequate uterine perfusion and delivery

Table 21–2 INDICATIONS FOR EMERGENCY CESAREAN SECTION

Stable mother with a viable fetus in distress
Traumatic uterine rupture
Gravid uterus interfering with intra-abdominal surgical repairs in the mother
Severely injured mother but fetus is viable

From Hawkins J: Anesthesia for the pregnant patient undergoing nonobstetric surgery. ASA Refresher Course Lectures 1996; 235:1–7.

of oxygen. Every attempt must be made to stabilize the mother prior to surgery, as this greatly influences fetal outcome.

Acute Abdomen. Appendicitis occurs in 1 out of 2000 pregnancies,[11] while cholecystitis has been reported to have an incidence of 1 to 6 out of every 10,000 pregnancies.[12] These are the most common etiologies of acute abdomen in the pregnant patient. Both manifest as abdominal pain. Symptoms include nausea, vomiting, constipation, and abdominal distention, all of which are common to both normal pregnancy and most abdominal pathology. Abdominal tenderness may be difficult to distinguish from uterine contraction pains. Because of the enlarging gravid uterus, standard anatomic landmarks are hard to identify and have an altered position. Perforation of the appendix usually occurs owing to delayed or failed clinical diagnosis.

Abdominal pain during pregnancy can be due to a medical condition or may be gynecologic in origin. Other nongynecologic surgical problems associated with an acute abdomen are acute pancreatitis, intestinal obstruction, vascular accidents, peptic ulcer, visceral injury, or hemorrhage secondary to trauma.

Neurologic Surgery. Unless an intracranial aneurysm or arteriovenous malformation is a constant threat to the pregnant patient, neurologic repair procedures may be delayed until such time as the fetus is viable. Head trauma resulting in subdural hemorrhage or intracerebral bleeding warrants emergency evacuation of the hematoma.

The pregnant patient is at increased risk for any thromboembolic event because of the increase in clotting factors VII, VIII, and X, and high fibrinogen level and low fibrinolytic activity. It is not surprising that stroke or cerebrovascular accidents secondary to thromboembolism are relatively common but are best managed medically.

Cardiac and Related Surgery. During pregnancy, there is a physiologic increase in blood volume and cardiac output. These reach a peak at 28 to 30 weeks' gestation. Any gravida with coexisting heart disease has an increased risk of cardiac decompensation. Cardiac decompensation requires urgent intervention in those with valvular lesions, especially with mitral valve involvement. If the gravid cardiac patient fails to respond to aggressive medical management, surgical intervention can sometimes optimize maternal cardiac function.

A large left atrial tumor or mass (e.g., left atrial myxoma) can present for emergency correction in a pregnant woman. These tumors may severely affect cardiac output because they can occlude the valvular orifice. These masses are often friable and can send emboli to the brain which clinically manifest as stroke. The excision of left atrial myxoma necessitates open heart surgery under cardiopulmonary bypass. Often, the pregnancy is allowed to progress a little farther before surgery is undertaken. If the mass is large and pedunculated and has a high probability of constantly obstructing or even getting impacted in the valvular orifice, surgical intervention must be seriously considered. Cardiopulmonary bypass must be maintained at high flow rates, at normothermia, and with the shortest ischemic time posssible.[13, 14]

Fetal monitoring is very important during the operative procedure to enable early recognition and appropriate management of any adverse effects in the fetus. Fetal bradycardia is the most common response observed and this can be improved by increasing the flow rates through the oxygenator.

ISSUES AND CONCERNS

Gestational age is the key factor in management of pregnant patients for nonobstetric surgery. The obstetrician, surgeon, and anesthesiologist must discuss and plan the perioperative care of these patients. Should the plan also involve delivery of the fetus, a neonatologist and/or pediatrician must be consulted and included in the management team. One needs to be realistic about the capability of the neonatal intensive care unit to handle these delicate newborns. If the unit does not have the qualified staff, the necessary system in operation, or the equipment to take care of sick preterm babies at birth, delaying the delivery of the fetus must be considered.

Obstetric Viewpoint

The main focus of the obstetrician is fetal safety, regardless of gestational age, especially if surgery is imminent. The goal of the obstetrician is to preserve the pregnancy until term. Management is directed at the prevention of fetal loss, by preventing premature uterine contractions, spontaneous delivery, and premature birth, or by enhancing placental implantation and promoting the progress of the pregnancy until fetal viability is achieved. Pharmacologic agents and hormonal therapy to prevent uterine contractions can be used to prevent premature labor (Table 21–3). Tocolytic agents are usually administered before 32 weeks' gestation; they provide tocolysis for 48 hours.

β-Sympathomimetic drugs, such as terbutaline and ritodrine, are effective in inhibiting labor for 24 to 48 hours but have been shown to be ineffective for longer durations.[15] These drugs cause tachycardia, hypotension, and cardiac arrhythmia, particularly in anesthetized patients. Pulmonary edema, cerebral

Table 21-3 DRUGS THAT INHIBIT UTERINE CONTRACTIONS

β-Sympathomimetic agents
Terbutaline
Ritodrine
Calcium channel blockers
Nifedipine
Nimodipine
Magnesium sulfate
Prostaglandin synthesis inhibitors
Indomethacin
Oxytocin antagonists
Atosiban
Nitroglycerin
17-Alpha hydroxyprogesterone

Adapted with modifications from Douglas MJ: New drugs, old drugs and the obstetric anaesthetist. Can J Anaesth 1995; 42(5):R3–R8.

vasospasm, and ketoacidemia are other side effects associated with β-sympathomimetic therapy.

If magnesium sulfate is used to prevent premature uterine contractions, it should be remembered that this drug interacts with neuromuscular blockers and may also exert some central nervous system depression. The neonate can also manifest some alteration in neuromuscular function. The side effects of muscle weakness, decreased deep tendon reflexes, respiratory depression, and cardiac depression are dose related.[16]

Atosiban is an oxytocin inhibitor that competitively acts at the oxytocin receptors in the myometrial junction. It inhibits the second messenger release of free intracellular calcium which mediates uterine contraction.[16] In a clinical study by Goodwin and colleagues,[17] atosiban decreased the frequency of uterine contraction by 70.8% and stopped contractions in 61 of 62 subjects.

Nitroglycerin, a nitric oxide donor, is a potent smooth muscle relaxant. Lately, this drug has been used to relax the uterus to facilitate removal of retained placenta, perform uterine inversion, and allow delivery of a premature fetus or second twin.[18] The application of a nitroglycerin patch in inhibiting preterm labor was reported by Lees and coworkers[19] but further clinical trials are still needed.

Progesterone enhances placental implantation and has an effect on uterine contractility. During open heart surgery under cardiopulmonary bypass, there can be dilutional reduction in plasma levels of progesterone. Hydroxyprogesterone caproate, given intramuscularly preoperatively, can compensate for these induced hormone deficits. It renders the uterus quiescent and helps prevent spontaneous abortion. The fetus must be closely monitored by Doppler or electronic fetal heart rate monitoring for confirmation of fetal well-being because a quiescent uterus can "tolerate" a dead fetus in utero without trying to expel it. The possibility of teratogenic effects from hydroxyprogesterone in early pregnancy are still the subject of research.

If gestational age is compatible with life, the obstetrician may consider the delivery of a premature fetus, especially if this would make surgery easier or render medical therapy of the mother more effective. The obstetrician must work closely with a neonatologist if delivery of the fetus is being contemplated and, as mentioned earlier, the capabilities of the neonatal intensive care unit must be considered in prognosticating neonatal outcome.

Surgical Viewpoint

Timing of surgery is vital to the perinatal outcome of mother and fetus. The surgeon may wish to delay surgery to maximize fetal viability. In the interim, the surgeon strives to minimize the danger to mother and fetus. A detailed history and physical examination are imperative if the surgeon is to arrive at a more accurate clinical evaluation and diagnosis. The latter is essential in surgical decision making, especially with regard to the timing of surgery.

In maternal trauma or in emergency situations (e.g., acute surgical abdomen, cardiac-decompensated pregnant patient) in which immediate surgical intervention would improve maternal survival, the primary aim of the surgeon is the speed and safety with which surgery can be done. Prolonged surgery means longer exposure time to the anesthetic agents and more surgical manipulation, thus increasing the risks for the fetus.

The surgeon may also have to change the approach to the site of operation or the type of surgical procedure to be performed. Surgery in the abdomen or pelvic cavity brings the surgeon in close contact with the gravid uterus. Surgical handling of the viscera and other organs must be done with utmost gentleness. During the early weeks of gestation (i.e., at 15 weeks or less), the size of the uterus may not be a hindrance to exposing the surgical pathology but these patients are prone to spontaneous abortion.

In the second trimester and more so during the third trimester, the uterus is much bigger and heavier and may interfere with the surgical technique. This enlarging gravid uterus renders anatomic and surface landmarks unreliable. The inflamed appendix may be pushed higher up into the right upper quadrant of the abdomen and present as "cholecystitis." There is increased risk for premature uterine contractions in abdominal and pelvic cavity explorations during this time.

Abdominal laparoscopic procedures in the pregnant woman can present additional risks to the fetus. Abdominal laparoscopy in the pregnant woman requires general anesthesia and carbon dioxide is insufflated into the peritoneal cavity. Carbon dioxide insufflation can decrease uteroplacental perfusion and cause fetal acidemia. Pneumoperitoneum pressures should be minimized to around 8 to 12 mm Hg. Above this range, uterine blood flow may be severely compromised because of the increased intra-abdominal pressure. The placement of trocars and other instruments may injure the gravid uterus.[20, 21]

For cardiac surgery also, the surgeon must choose between closed or open heart surgery under cardiopulmonary bypass. If cardiopulmonary bypass is to be used, it is recommended that normothermia and high flow rates be maintained in order not to compromise the fetus. Cardiopulmonary bypass can dilute plasma progesterone levels. The posture of the pregnant patient on the operating table must also be considered. In the supine position the gravid uterus can reduce venous return to the maternal heart and cause hypotension owing to aortocaval compression. A wedge should be placed under the right hip to displace the gravid uterus to the left and relieve the pressure on major blood vessels.

Anesthesia Viewpoint

The anesthesiologist must grasp the implications of the physiologic changes of pregnancy for the conduct of anesthesia and must recognize the direct effects of anesthetic drugs on the fetus. These include teratogenicity, adverse effects on fetal physiology and well-being, and direct effects on uterine muscle tone, uterine blood flow, and uteroplacental perfusion. Many direct effects on the mother (e.g., maternal hypotension, acid-base imbalance, hypoxemia, hypercarbia, hypocarbia, pain, and anxiety) can indirectly affect the fetus.

Anesthetic Implications of the Physiologic Changes in Pregnancy

Respiratory System. The physiologic changes that occur involve the lung volumes, ventilation, and oxygen consumption in the mother. Table 21–4 shows the various parameter changes in respiratory function during pregnancy.[22] Arterial oxygen tension is higher, while carbon dioxide tension (about 30–32 mm Hg) is lower, in the pregnant state. This is compensated for by renal excretion of bicarbonate. The increased oxygen consumption reaches about 40% to 60% and can be explained by the growing fetus and increasing basal metabolic rate in the pregnant woman. The oxygen hemoglobin dissociation curve is shifted to the right, allowing increased oxygen unloading to the fetus.

Table 21–4 PHYSIOLOGIC CHANGES IN THE RESPIRATORY SYSTEM DURING PREGNANCY

	THROUGHOUT PREGNANCY
Expiratory reserve volume	25% decrease
Residual volume	15% decrease
Functional residual capacity	20% decrease
Total lung capacity	5% decrease
Inspiratory capacity	15% increase
Vital capacity	No change
Closing capacity	No change
	AT TERM
Alveolar ventilation	60% increase
Minute volume	50% increase
Tidal volume	40% increase
Respiratory rate	10% increase

Adapted from Cohen S: The physiology of pregnancy and the anesthetic meaning for the anesthesiologist. ASA Refresher Course Lectures 1996; 136:1–7.

The pregnant woman may present difficulty in airway management because of the increased body weight; short neck; enlarged breasts; and fragile, edematous endothelial lining of the nasopharyngeal tract, which can easily be traumatized or injured.

CLINICAL IMPLICATIONS. The pregnant patient is more prone to hypoxia and hypercarbia even during short periods of apnea because of decreased functional residual capacity and increased oxygen consumption. Supine posture further aggravates the decrease in functional residual capacity in relation to the closing capacity. It is imperative that oxygen saturation be monitored using pulse oximetry. Oxygen should be administered during surgery. Normocarbia should be aimed for during controlled ventilation under general anesthesia because very low levels of carbon dioxide can compromise uteroplacental perfusion owing to uterine artery vasoconstriction and decreased umbilical blood flow.

Inhalational induction is more rapid because of the small functional residual capacity and hyperventilation seen in pregnant women. Postoperative pain can lead to rapid, shallow respiration which can further decrease carbon dioxide levels.

Cardiovascular System. Generally, there is an observed increase in plasma volume (45%) and erythrocyte volume (20%) over prepregnancy levels. The plasma volume increase is greater than erythrocyte count, so that there is dilutional anemia. Clotting procoagulants, platelets, and fibrinogen are increased, while there is a progressive decrease in fibrinolytic activity during pregnancy. Cardiac output increases as early as the first trimester and progressively rises to about 30% to 50% in the third trimester. This is associated with a 15% increase in heart rate. Systemic vascular resistance and pulmonary vascular resistance are decreased.

CLINICAL IMPLICATIONS. The increased blood volume and red cell mass occur in anticipation of blood loss during delivery. During nonobstetric surgery, perioperative blood loss is more manageable but there is an increased predisposition to thromboembolic problems, which can be aggravated by confinement. In the second to third trimester, the enlarging gravid uterus can also alter maternal hemodynamics because of the pressure exerted by the gravid uterus on the vena cava and aorta while in the supine position. Unless the pregnant patient has hypertension or is preeclamptic, there is no significant increase in systemic arterial pressure because vascular resistance gets progressively lower as the pregnancy proceeds.

Gastrointestinal System. Most changes occur in the third trimester when the enlarging uterus causes increased intragastric pressure. There is also decreased lower esophageal sphincter tone, and gastric acid contents of the stomach are increased in volume compared with nonpregnant females. Delayed emptying time may be more relevant at term pregnancy or when the patient is anxious and in labor.

Clinical Implications. All pregnant females must be protected from the risk of regurgitation and aspiration during surgery. The increased acidity of the gastric contents makes the use of histamine type 2 (H_2) blockers indicated in the preoperative preparation of these patients for surgery.

Renal System. There is an increase in renal blood flow and glomerular filtration rate secondary to the cardiac output increase during pregnancy. The ureters and renal pelvis may be dilated owing to mechanical obstruction by the gravid uterus. Glucosuria and orthostatic proteinuria are also common.

Clinical Implications. Levels of blood urea nitrogen, creatinine, and uric acid are slightly lower in the pregnant woman compared with the nonpregnant female. In evaluating preeclamptic patients or those suspected of a renal complication perioperatively, a normal or slightly elevated plasma level may signify considerable renal insufficiency.

Central Nervous System. Progesterone is known to have a central nervous depressant effect. Central and peripheral sensitivity of the nerves occur (probably) secondary to the prolonged high levels of progesterone during gestation. Late in pregnancy, there is a decrease in the epidural space capacity because of the reflected increases in venous pressure secondary to the enlarging gravid uterus in the abdominal cavity and engorgement of the venous plexus.

Clinical Implications. There is a decrease in the dose-response relationship to inhalational agents as the pregnancy progresses. A central neural blockade (spinal or epidural) can be achieved with reduced doses of local anesthetics. Contributing to this decreased response is the observation that there is an increased proportion of free drug in the pregnant woman owing to lessened protein binding from diminished albumin levels. For example, bupivacaine, a local anesthetic agent, is highly protein bound and has increased myocardial toxicity in pregnancy.

Plasma cholinesterase levels have been noted to be low in pregnancy compared with the nonpregnant state. Muscle relaxant activity should be monitored, when agents such as succinylcholine and mivacurium are used. The duration of action of neuromuscular blockers is prolonged even further when magnesium sulfate is administered to pregnant patients.

Effects of Anesthetic Agents on the Fetus

Are anesthetic agents teratogenic? Animal and human studies have been done to investigate the direct effects of anesthesia on the fetus, especially during the first trimester. Several factors must be considered: (1) dose of the teratogen; (2) timing of exposure to the drug or the stage of development of the embryo when exposed to the teratogen; (3) applicability of animal teratogen experiments to human beings; and (4) genetic susceptibility or individual differences in susceptibility to malformations or congenital anomalies. Among different species, susceptibility and/or resistance may differ, making correlation between animal data and humans difficult.[23] Table 21–5 gives the incidence and etiology of congenital anomalies.[24]

There is still much to learn regarding which agent or physical insult can cause a morphologic, behavioral, or biochemical defect at a particular stage of gestation that is detectable either at birth or later in life. Results of multiple studies and surveys show no conclusive evidence of an increase in the incidence of congenital abnormalities in offspring of gravidae who have undergone surgery early in pregnancy.[25–29]

Inhalational Agents

Nitrous oxide has been widely used as an inhaled analgesic agent to supplement general inhalational anesthesia. Nitrous oxide inhibits maternal and fetal methionine synthetase activity. Inhibition of methionine synthetase decreases the production of endogenous folinic acid (vitamin B_{12}), which is necessary for the conversion of uridine to thymidine. This may result in impaired DNA synthesis and inhibition of cell division.[30]

Nitrous oxide has been known to be a consistent animal teratogen, specifically among rodents. In animal experiments, chronic exposure to nitrous oxide has been associated with spontaneous abortions. In humans, however, there have been conflicting results. Nitrous oxide may cause a slight increase in spontaneous abortions in chronically exposed pregnant health workers. Most studies suggest that it is the underlying illness or disease process that poses the greater risk of loss of the fetus and that the cause of the increase is not directly related to nitrous oxide exposure.[31, 32]

Halothane was found to cause fetal death, congenital anomalies, and growth retardation among mice but not in rat or rabbits exposed to the same agent.[33–35]

Table 21–5 INCIDENCE AND ETIOLOGY OF CONGENITAL ABNORMALITIES

Etiology	Incidence (%)
Genetic transmission	20
Chromosomal aberration	3–5
Environment (e.g., infection)	2–3
Maternal metabolic imbalance	1–2
Drugs or toxins	2–3
Radiation	<1
Unknown	65–70

Modified from Goldberg JD, Golbus MS: The value of case reports in human teratology. Am J Obstet Gynecol 1986; 154:479–482.

Instead, behavioral changes were observed among adult rats born to female rats anesthetized with halothane during pregnancy. Mazze and colleagues[36] also have demonstrated that halothane, when used in combination with nitrous oxide, prevented the latter's teratogenic effect on the rat by increasing uterine blood flow. The administration of folinic acid does not protect the pregnant woman from the adverse effects of nitrous oxide.[36]

Enflurane was associated with limb and abdominal wall defects in rabbits and with cleft palate, skeletal anomalies, and growth retardation in the offspring of mice who were exposed to this agent during pregnancy.[37] Other studies were unable to demonstrate the same effects.[35]

Isoflurane was associated with cleft palate, skeletal anomalies, and fetal growth retardation in a study by Mazze.[38] Interestingly, when given with nitrous oxide, isoflurane protected the rats from the teratogenic effects of nitrous oxide by decreasing the uterine muscular tone and preserving uterine blood flow.[35]

Intravenous Drugs

Benzodiazepines. An association between cleft palate and intake of diazepam during pregnancy has been reported by Safra and Oakley and by the Finnish Registry of Congenital Malformations.[39, 40] However, this was not observed in two separate studies conducted by Hartz[41] and Rosenberg.[42] While there is no conclusive evidence, it is best to avoid benzodiazepines (e.g., diazepam and chlordiazepoxide) and phenothiazines (e.g., chlorpromazine) during the period of organogenesis.

Narcotics. Early reported adverse effects in association with the use of morphine, meperidine, and methadone in animals may be secondary to excessively high doses that cause maternal cardiorespiratory depression, resulting in intrauterine fetal asphyxia.[43] More recent rodent experiments using fentanyl, sufentanil, and alfentanil delivered at a constant dose by infusion did not cause any maternal toxicity or teratogenic or adverse reproductive effects.[44, 45]

Muscle Relaxants. Because of their high molecular weight, neuromuscular blockers cannot cross the uteroplacental barrier. At very large doses, however, they can be detected in the fetal circulation. No adverse effects on fetal development or neonatal outcome have been reported.[46]

Local Anesthetics. Local anesthetic agents can cross the placental barrier. Dose-related effects on neurobehavioral consequences in the neonate have been reported.[47] So far, no teratogenic effects have been directly associated with the use of lidocaine, tetracaine, or bupivacaine in early pregnancy.[48]

Table 21-6 RECOMMENDED GUIDELINES IN THE MANAGEMENT OF THE PREGNANT PATIENT FOR NONOBSTETRIC SURGERY

Timing of surgery	• As much as possible, delay the proposed operative procedure into the second or third trimester. The fetus is most vulnerable with regard to teratogenic effects until the 12th week of pregnancy. • The risk of spontaneous abortion remains high even in the second trimester.
Choice of drugs	• Use anesthetic agents with a known history of fetal safety. Understandably, this is a must during the first trimester, but must also be observed beyond the stage of organogenesis. • Use drugs and techniques that preserve uteroplacental perfusion and prevent uterine irritability or premature contractions.
Promote fetal well-being	• Keep all maternal physiologic functions at an optimum. • Ensure good uteroplacental perfusion by (a) Maintaining normal maternal systemic arterial blood pressure. (b) Promoting maternal normocarbia and normal acid-base balance. (c) Preventing uterine irritability and hypertonicity. (d) Using drugs to achieve the desired therapeutic end points while avoiding fetal toxicity and depression. • Perform intensive fetal monitoring especially during surgery and in the immediate postoperative period.
Promote maternal well-being	• Provide optimal emotional and psychologic support, particularly during the preoperative preparation of the patient. • Allay anxiety and promote a stress-free environment perioperatively. • Perform intensive monitoring during surgery. • Ensure optimal postoperative pain control. • Encourage multidisciplinary care of the pregnant patient, particularly if medical problems are present. Involve the relevant specialty service to ensure that the nonobstetric problems of the mother are well managed.

Effects of Anesthetics on Fetal Physiology and Well-Being

Fetal bradycardia secondary to administration of large doses of narcotics may be observed but this can be reversed by intravenous atropine. Large doses of narcotics can also produce neonatal respiratory depression and changes in neonatal neurobehavioral status because these agents cross the placental barrier. Neurologic depression of the neonate by intravenous diazepam, given about 30 minutes prior to birth, has been reported.[49]

The depressant effects on the fetus should be transient; they disappear as the drugs are metabolized further and are excreted from the maternal system. Placental transfer and fetal depression secondary to spinal narcotics can be minimized by using very low doses. Lidocaine for epidural anesthesia has been shown to cause transient neurobehavioral effects on the neonate.[50] In a study by Scanlon and coworkers,[51] neonates using epidural bupivacaine showed no difference from the nonepidural-group neonates, suggesting that bupivacaine does not affect neonatal neurobehavior. Lidocaine crosses the placental barrier more than bupivacaine. Since these are transient neurobehavioral changes observed in neonates, it is possible that fetal well-being is not compromised so long as uterine perfusion is well maintained while the pregnant woman is under anesthesia.

The concentration of free drug in the fetus is determined by fetal circulation, plasma binding, metabolism by the fetal/neonatal liver, and renal excretion of the drug and its metabolites. Local anesthetics with increased lipid solubility pose a risk for fetal toxicity, especially at large doses.

Likewise, the drug effects of opioids and inhalational agents on the fetus should not be detrimental if the mother is well oxygenated and normal acid-base balance is maintained. Fetal well-being is directly tied to uteroplacental blood flow.

Effects of Anesthetics on the Uterus

Generally, inhalational agents affect the uterus in a dose-related manner. With increasing concentrations of inhalational agents, there is peripheral vasodilatation which can cause decreases in maternal systemic arterial pressure. This leads to decreased uterine blood flow, fetal asphyxiation, and fetal bradycardia. High concentrations of inhalational agents cause relaxation of the uterine musculature and prevent uterine hypertonicity.

There is no autoregulation in the uteroplacental circulation. The uterine vasculature is at its most dilated state during pregnancy, so that uterine blood flow is proportional to systemic maternal mean arterial pressure. Uterine vascular resistance is a major determinant of uteroplacental blood flow. Uterine vascular resistance is inversely related to uterine blood flow. Uterine blood flow is linearly related to the difference between uterine artery pressure and uterine venous pressure. Vena caval compression increases uterine venous pressure and indirectly decreases uterine artery pressure.

Exogenous vasopressors, endogenous catecholamines, and uterine contractions can increase uterine vascular resistance and reduce uterine blood flow. Among the vasopressors, drugs that exhibit a pure α-mimetic effect vasoconstrict the uterine arteries. Ephedrine acts on both α-adrenergic and β-adrenergic receptors, making it a drug of choice to treat maternal hypotension without causing vasoconstriction of the uterine vessels. Uterine tone (state of uterine musculature) also influences uterine vascular resistance.

Ketamine given in doses of 1.0 mg/kg or lower has been shown not to affect uteroplacental perfusion. Above this dose, it can trigger a tetanic uterine contraction that interrupts uteroplacental circulation and leads to fetal asphyxiation.

Neither depolarizing nor nondepolarizing muscle relaxants paralyze the uterine muscles. Accidental intravascular injection of local anesthetics or deposition of the drug close to the uterine arteries as in paracervical block, particularly when combined with epinephrine, can cause vasospasm of the uterine arteries and uterine hypertonicity.[52]

Effects of Anesthetics on the Mother

Central neural blockade or general anesthesia can cause significant maternal hypotension in the perioperative period. Maternal hypotension from any cause must be aggressively corrected so as not to compromise fetal well-being. Correction of hypovolemia by administration of crystalloids or colloids, followed by exogenous vasopressors, if necessary, must be undertaken immediately. Mechanical compression of the aorta and vena cava in the supine position must also be remedied expeditiously by displacing the gravid uterus laterally. This becomes a concern starting at 24 to 26 weeks' gestation, but not in the first trimester when uterine size has minimal potential for producing hypotension.

Maternal hyperventilation during general anesthesia or that caused by perioperative anxiety or pain leads to respiratory alkalemia. However, low arterial carbon dioxide tension causes uterine vasoconstriction. Respiratory alkalemia causes a leftward shift of the oxyhemoglobin dissociation curve making oxygen less available to the fetus.

In like manner, maternal hypoventilation secondary to the effect of large doses of opioid administered to control postoperative pain can lead to hypercarbia. This promotes maternal catecholamine release and causes a direct uteroplacental vasoconstriction. It is therefore best to maintain normocarbia to preserve good uteroplacental perfusion and to choose analgesic drugs free of sedative effects.

Throughout the perioperative period, the pregnant patient undergoing nonobstetric surgery must have optimum arterial oxygen tension to avoid fetal asphyxia. Pregnant patients are prone to hypoxemia because of the physiologic respiratory changes that occur during gestation, particularly the decreased functional residual capacity, increased oxygen demand, and increased basal metabolic rate.

ANESTHESIA PLAN AND MANAGEMENT

The choice of anesthetic for pregnant patients scheduled for nonobstetric surgery is determined by the following factors: (1) the surgical indication; (2) the proposed operative procedure; (3) the age of gestation; and (4) maternal condition. Neither general nor regional anesthesia is strongly associated with increased risk to pregnant patients. The issue of teratogenicity has been extensively studied by several authors and researchers, and only a select few anesthetic agents are likely to cause adverse effects.

If the proposed surgical procedure and the maternal condition allow, regional anesthesia is preferable because of the minimal drug exposure of the fetus, especially with spinal subarachnoid block. Central neural blockade (spinal, epidural, or combined spinal-epidural anesthesia) may be administered for lower abdominal surgery (e.g., appendectomy, excision of twisted ovarian cyst, open reduction for lower limb fracture).

General anesthesia using inhalational anesthetics, however, makes pregnant patients less anxious and more comfortable. This is recommended for upper abdominal surgery, such as cholecystectomy, or in laparoscopic procedures.

It should be emphasized that the anesthetic plan must be individualized and planned according to the best options to safeguard both mother and fetus. Adverse perioperative outcome may correlate more with the risk of the surgical procedure than with anesthesia technique.

Nevertheless, multiple factors in the perioperative period influence the outcome of pregnancy. Nutrition, environmental factors, and psychologic factors can in one way or another affect the outcome of pregnancy.

CONCLUSION

Aggressive preservation of maternal health can ensure improved fetal outcome at the time of birth. The objective of total quality care in pregnant patients for nonobstetric surgery is the promotion of both maternal and fetal safety during the preoperative evaluation and preparation phase and during the conduct of surgery and anesthesia. Such vigilance and care must be extended throughout the postoperative period.

The incidence of premature labor and fetal loss increases with increasing severity of underlying surgical disease and occurrence of perioperative complications.[53] It is important to prevent perioperative maternal hypoxemia and hypotension, as these increase risk to the fetus.

Success in outcome of pregnancy is influenced by four major factors: (1) timing of surgery; (2) choice of drugs; (3) promotion of fetal health; and (4) promotion of maternal well-being.

❖ SUMMARY

Key Points

- The anesthetic is not the only risk factor for adverse perinatal outcome following surgery during pregnancy; poor outcome may be due to maternal disease and the surgery itself.
- The incidence of premature labor and fetal loss increases with increasing severity of the underlying surgical disease and the occurrence of perioperative complications.
- Teratogenicity of anesthetic agents has been extensively studied, and no currently used anesthetic agents have been found to be teratogenic in humans. Some agents, however, have been found to be teratogenic in animals.

Key Reference

Duncan PG, Pope WEB, Cohen MM, Greer N: Fetal risks of anesthesia and surgery during pregnancy. Anesthesiology 1986; 64:790–794.

Case Stem

A 40-year-old G1P0 is admitted at 23 weeks' gestation with the diagnosis of acute appendicitis and is scheduled for emergency surgery. Discuss your proposed anesthetic management and its implications for mother and fetus.

References

1. Shnider SM, Webster GM: Maternal and fetal hazards of surgery during pregnancy. Am J Obstet Gynecol 1965; 192:891–900.
2. Brodsky JB, Cohen EN, Brown BW, et al: Surgery during pregnancy and fetal outcome. Am J Obstet Gynecol 1980; 138:1165–1167.
3. Fildes J, Reed L, Lones N, et al: Trauma: the leading cause of maternal death. J Trauma 1992; 32:643–645.
4. Lavery JP, State McCormack M: Management of moderate to severe trauma in pregnancy. Obstet Gynecol Clin North Am 1995; 22:69–72.
5. Rozycki G: Trauma during pregnancy: predicting pregnancy outcome. Arch Gynecol Obstet 1993; 253:S15–S18.
6. Dannenburg AL, Carter DM, Lawson HN, et al: Homicide and other injuries as causes of death in New York City. Am J Obstet Gynecol 1995; 172:1557–1559.
7. Rothenberger D, Quattlebaum F, Perry J, et al: Blunt maternal trauma: a review of 103 cases. J Trauma 1978; 18:173–179.
8. Dahmus M, Sibai BM: Blunt abdominal trauma: are there any predictive factors for abruptio placentae or maternal-fetal distress? Am J Obstet Gynecol 1993; 169:1054–1057.
9. Kuhlman RS, Cruikshank DP: Maternal trauma during pregnancy. Clin Obstet Gynecol 1994; 37:274.
10. Hawkins J: Anesthesia for the pregnant patient undergoing non-obstetric surgery. ASA Refresher Course Lectures 1996; 235:1–7.
11. Condon RE, Telford GE: Appendicitis. *In* Sabiston DC Jr (ed): Textbook of Surgery, 14th ed. Philadelphia: WB Saunders; 1991:884–898.
12. Hill MN, Johnson CE, Lee RA: Cholecystectomy in pregnancy. Obstet Gynecol 1975; 46:291–295.
13. Conroy JM, Bailey MK: Anesthesia for open heart surgery in the pregnant patient. South Med J 1989; 82:492–495.
14. Salerno TA, Houck JP, Barrozo CAM, et al: Retrograde continuous warm cardioplegia: a new concept in myocardial protection. Ann Thorac Surg 1991; 51:245–249.
15. Higby K, Xenakis EMJ, Paerstein CJ: Do tocolytic agents stop preterm labor? A critical and comprehensive review of efficacy and safety. Am J Obstet Gynecol 1993; 168:1247–1259.

16. Douglas MJ: New drugs, old drugs and the obstetric anaesthetist. Can J Anaesth 1995; 42(5):R3–R8.
17. Goodwin TM, Paul R, Silver H, et al: The effect of oxytocin antagonist atosiban on preterm uterine activity in human. Am J Obstet Gynecol 1994; 170:474–478.
18. Douglas MJ, Ward ME: Current pharmacology and the obstetric anesthesiologist. Int Anesthesiol Clin 1994; 32:1–10.
19. Lees C, Campbell S, Jauniaux E, et al: Arrest of preterm labour and prolongation of gestation with glyceryl trinitrate, a nitric oxide donor. Lancet 1994; 343:1325–1326.
20. Arvidsson D, Gerdin E: Laparoscopic cholecystectomy during pregnancy. Surg Laparosc Endosc 1991; 1:193–194.
21. Pucci RO, Seed RW: Case report of laparoscopic cholecystectomy in the third trimester of pregnancy. Am J Obstet Gynecol 1990; 165:401–402.
22. Cohen S: The physiology of pregnancy and the anesthetic meaning for the anesthesiologist. ASA Refresher Course Lectures 1996; 136:1–7.
23. Manilow A: Anesthetic management of the pregnant surgical patient. IARS Refresher Course Lectures 1998; 61–65.
24. Goldberg JD, Golbus MS: The value of case reports in human teratology. Am J Obstet Gynecol 1986; 154:479–482.
25. Brodsky JB: Anesthesia and the pregnant surgical patient. Reg Anesth 1984; 9(3):119–123.
26. Smith BE: Fetal prognosis after anesthesia during gestation. Anesth Analg 1963; 42:521–536.
27. Schnider SM, Webster GM: Maternal and fetal hazards of surgery during pregnancy. Am J Obstet Gynecol 1965; 192:891–900.
28. Konieczko KM, Chapek JC, Nunn JF: Fetotoxic potential of general anaesthesia in relation to pregnancy. Br J Anaesth 1987; 59:449–454.
29. Mazze RI, Kallen B: Reproductive outcome after anesthesia and operation during pregnancy: a registry study of 5,405 cases. Am J Obstet Gynecol 1989; 161:1178–1185.
30. Nunn JF: Clinical aspect of the interaction between nitrous oxide and vitamin B_{12}. Br J Anaesth 1987; 59:3–13.
31. Crawford JS, Lewis M: Nitrous oxide in early human pregnancy. Anaesthesia 1986; 41:900–905.
32. Duncan PG, Pope WEB, Cohen MM, Greer N: Fetal risks of anesthesia and surgery during pregnancy. Anesthesiology 1986; 64:790–794.
33. Wharton RS, Mazze RI, Baden JM, et al: Fertility, reproduction and postnatal survival in mice chronically exposed to halothane. Anesthesiology 1978; 48:167–174.
34. Kennedy GL, Smith SH, Keplinger ML, Calandra JC: Reproductive and teratologic studies with halothane. Toxicol Appl Pharmacol 1976; 35:467–474.
35. Mazze RI, Fujinaga M, Rice SA, et al: Reproductive and teratogenic effects of nitrous oxide, halothane, isoflurane and enflurane in Sprague-Dawley rats. Anesthesiology 1986; 64:339–344.
36. Mazze RI, Fujinaga M, Baden JM: Halothane prevents nitrous oxide teratogenicity in Sprague-Dawley rats: folinic acid does not. Teratology 1988; 38:121–127.
37. Wharton RS, Mazze RI, Wilson AI: Reproduction and fetal development in mice chronically exposed to enflurane. Anesthesiology 1981; 54:505–510.
38. Mazze RI, Wilson AI, Rice SA: Fetal development in mice exposed to isoflurane. Teratology 1985; 32:339–345.
39. Safra MJ, Oakley GP: Association between cleft lip with or without cleft palate and prenatal exposure to diazepam. Lancet 1975; 2:478–480.
40. Saxen I, Saxen L: Association between maternal intake of diazepam and oral clefts. Lancet 1975; 2:498–501.
41. Hartz SC, Heinomen OP, Shapiro S, et al: Antenatal exposure to meprobamate and chlordiazepoxide in relation to malformations, mental development and childhood mortality. N Engl J Med 1975; 292:726–728.
42. Rosenberg L, Mitchell AA, Parsells JL, et al: Lack of relation of oral clefts to diazepam use during pregnancy. N Engl J Med 1983; 309:1282–1285.
43. Geber WF, Schramm LC: Congenital malformations of the central nervous system produced by narcotic analgesics in the hamster. Am J Obstet Gynecol 1975; 123:705–713.
44. Fujinaga M, Stevenson JM, Mazze RI: Reproductive and teratogenic effects of fentanyl in Sprague-Dawley rats. Teratology 1986; 34:54–57.
45. Fujinaga M, Mazze RI, Jackson EC, Baden JM: Reproductive and teratogenic effects of sufentanil and alfentanil in Sprague-Dawley rats. Anesth Analg 1988; 67:166–169.
46. Fujinaga M, Baden JM, Mazze RI: Developmental toxicity of nondepolarizing muscle relaxants in cultured rat embryos [abstract]. Anesthesiology 1991; 75:A850.
47. Brown WU, Bell GC, Lurie AO, et al: Newborn blood levels of lidocaine and mepivacaine in the first post natal day following maternal epidural anesthesia. Anesthesiology 1975; 42:698–701.
48. Friedman JM: Teratogen update: anesthetic agents. Teratology 1988; 37:69–77.
49. Rolbin SH, Wright RG, Shnider SM, et al: Diazepam during cesarean section—effects on neonatal Apgar scores, acid-base status, neurobehavioral assessment, maternal and fetal plasma norepinephrine levels. *In* Abstracts of Scientific Papers, Annual Meeting of the American Society of Anesthesiologists, New Orleans, October, 1997; 449.
50. Scanlon JW, Brown WU, Weiss JB, Alper MH: Neurobehavioral responses of newborn infants after maternal epidural anesthesia. Anesthesiology 1974; 40:121–128.
51. Scanlon JW, Ostheimer GW, Lurie AO, et al: Neurobehavioral responses and drug concentration in newborns after maternal epidural anesthesia with bupivacaine. Anesthesiology 1976; 45:400–405.
52. Greiss F, Still JG, Anderson S: Effects of local anesthetics on the uterine vasculatures and myometrium. Am J Obstet Gynecol 1976; 124:889–899.
53. Kammerer WS: Non-obstetric surgery during pregnancy. Med Clin North Am 1979; 63:1157–1164.

22

Anesthesia for Fetal Surgery

❖ FRANK G. ZAVISCA, MD, PHD
❖ JONATHAN H. SKERMAN, BDSc, MScD, DSc
❖ MARK D. JOHNSON, MD

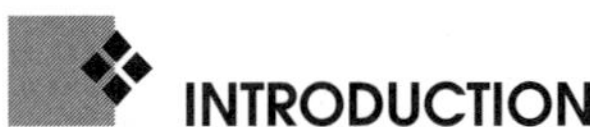

INTRODUCTION

Currently, the fetus is increasingly being treated as a patient in its own right. Advances in technology have made many medical and surgical procedures available earlier in gestation.[1–6] The first practical procedure for the treatment of erythroblastosis fetalis was intraperitoneal blood transfusion in 1963.[7, 8] In 1966, hysterotomy was used for intrauterine exchange transfusion, but maternal morbidity was unacceptable.[9] In 1984, fetoscopy was used for fetal transfusion.[10] Since 1986, ultrasound-guided umbilical venous transfusion has been used successfully.[11] Noninvasive procedures, such as administering steroids to hasten fetal lung maturation, are routine. Less invasive procedures, such as fetal blood sampling, are frequently done. Better methods and improved technology have permitted earlier diagnosis of a number of fetal disorders. A limited number of fetuses have abnormalities that progress to serious or nonviable conditions in utero, thus the rationale for in utero treatment.[12, 13] At present, intrauterine surgery is experimental and is performed at only a few centers, such as the University of California at San Francisco (UCSF).[1–4] However, this field of medicine is expanding, and more in utero surgery will undoubtedly be carried out at other major centers.

Although most anesthesiologists will not participate in fetal surgery, many will see patients who have had or who may be candidates for some of the procedures to be discussed. Therefore, we will review new developments and related issues that may be of interest to many anesthesiologists.

Diagnostic Methods

Noninvasive Methods. Noninvasive diagnostic methods to diagnose fetal disorders, for example, ultrasound, computed tomography (CT), and magnetic resonance imaging (MRI) have continued to improve.[1, 2, 5] In particular, high-resolution ultrasonography has dramatically improved and is an integral component of all fetal procedures.

Invasive Methods. Invasive diagnostic methods include fetoscopy, amniocentesis, and chorionic villous sampling for biochemical and cytogenetic diagnosis, and fetal viscocentesis for urine analysis, as well as fetal blood sampling.[1, 2, 5] For patients with a family history of inherited malformations, more specific diagnostic testing may be performed. However, malformations are often discovered during maternal ultrasound testing when done for obstetric indications.

THERAPEUTIC OPTIONS FOR FETAL MALFORMATIONS

The definition of what is treatable depends on our current state of knowledge and experience, which is constantly changing.[1, 2, 5]

Abnormalities That May Be Treated Medically

Drugs, cells, genes, and hormones may all be injected into the fetus. Abnormalities treated by these methods include deficiencies in surfactant, anemia caused by erythroblastosis fetalis, metabolic diseases, and cardiac arrhythmias. Diagnostic blood and skin sampling, as well as liver and muscle biopsies may be done using these methods. These may be performed percutaneously or endoscopically under ultrasonic guidance.[1, 2, 5] Several diseases treatable by hematopoietic stem cell transplantation (e.g., immunodeficiencies, hemoglobinopathies, storage diseases) may be treatable in utero, because before 15 weeks' gestation the fetus will not reject transplanted cells.[2]

Abnormalities Correctable by Fetal Surgery

For malformations interfering with organ development before the lungs mature, and which produce a poor outcome if not treated, surgical intrauterine correction may be appropriate.[1, 2, 5, 14] Anatomic malformations that may be corrected in the fetus include those resulting from failure of closure and obstruction of vital structures. These include hydronephrosis, diaphragmatic hernia, gastroschisis, cystic pulmonary adenoma, hydrocephalus, neural tube defects (spina bifida), cardiac defects, sacrococcygeal teratoma, acardiac and anencephalic twins, and skeletal defects. In recent years, endoscopic procedures have been intensively studied in an effort to be able to treat many of these fetal abnormalities less invasively.[15–19]

Such invasive therapy is justified, however, only when the results will be better than therapy after birth. Surgery is reasonable if

1. The lesion and its severity are diagnosed accurately.
2. The natural history of the lesion, and its pathophysiology, are well known.
3. Associated severe and uncorrectable anomalies are excluded.
4. Maternal risk is low.
5. The families are extensively counseled concerning the risks to the mother and the experimental nature of many of the treatments.
6. Fetal surgery is more successful than surgery performed after preterm or term delivery.
7. The required personnel and facilities are readily available (obstetrics, anesthesia, pediatrics, surgery, and others).

The following conditions may be correctable in the fetus.

Hydronephrosis. Fetal urinary obstruction results in oligohydramnios, pulmonary hypoplasia, and frequently, fatal renal damage. This can be corrected by decompression before birth.[1, 2, 5] Diagnostic criteria for intervention include fetal urine electrolytes, β_2-microglobulin levels, the ultrasound appearance of the kidneys, and the presence of oligohydramnios. Procedures include bladder decompression by open fetal vesicotomy, a catheter shunt placed percutaneously, and fetoscopic vesicotomy or placement of a wire mesh stent (all done under ultrasonic guidance). Use of fetoscopic techniques should allow treatment of these abnormalities less invasively.[20] It is unclear, however, whether these interventions improve renal development.[1, 2, 5]

Cystic Adenomatoid Malformations of the Lung and Fetal Hydrops. Most congenital lung cysts are benign, but large cysts can produce pulmonary hypoplasia and compression of the heart.[2, 21, 22] Heart failure and hydrops result from obstruction of cardiac venous return and central venous hypertension. If hydrops develops before 26 weeks' gestation, ultrasonic-guided thoracentesis, placement of a thoracoamniotic shunt, or open fetal pulmonary lobectomy may be done. Correction of these malformations in the fetus have produced good results.[2, 23] Other causes of fetal hydrops, such as pulmonary sequestration and pleural effusions, may also be corrected surgically in the fetus.[24–27]

Diaphragmatic Hernia. Despite heroic surgical interventions after birth, the mortality of infants born with congenital diaphragmatic hernia remains high.[2, 5] Pulmonary hypoplasia is usually reversible, but weeks or months are required, and the newborn often succumbs. Hypoplasia of the heart may also occur.[28] In utero correction may reverse these cardiac abnormalities[29]; however, repair in utero is difficult, especially when the left lobe of the liver is incarcerated in the chest. Reduction of the liver, reconstruction of the diaphragm, and enlargement of the abdomen to accept the returned viscera are done. Reduction of the liver often compromises umbilical blood flow. Fetuses with late herniation tend to do better, and may be treated after birth. However, those with early herniation, severe mediastinal shift and a dilated intrathoracic stomach with resulting gastric dilation and polyhydramnios have a poor prognosis. Despite heroic efforts, there were no survivors in fetuses in which liver herniation had occurred. Because results of open repair of fetuses without the liver in the chest are no better than those in untreated patients, this method has largely been abandoned.[6, 30, 31]

Studies in fetal lambs have shown that controlled occlusion of the trachea inhibits the normal egress of lung fluid, allowing development of the hypoplastic lungs that then push the viscera back into the abdomen.[32–35] However, overexpansion of the lungs may lead to compression of the fetal heart, resulting in hydrops.[36] In humans, open and endoscopic application of clips to the fetal trachea, followed by definitive correction postnatally, has been used to correct diaphragmatic hernia.[37, 38]

Sacrococcygeal Teratoma. Sacrococcygeal teratoma is usually benign, and is treated postnatally. However, larger lesions diagnosed prenatally by ultrasound and associated with elevated α-fetoprotein levels may produce rapid death. High-output cardiac failure and hydrops result from the large blood flow through the tumor.[2] Open resection in the fetus has been successful in several patients.[26]

Twin-Twin Transfusion Syndrome. In some twin pregnancies, high-output cardiac failure and hydrops may develop. Abnormal chorionic vessels in the placenta connect the circulation of the two fetuses.[2] This may occur with normal twins and acardiac-anencephalic twins. Serial amniocentesis of the polyhydramniotic sac may be successful. Also, occlusion of the umbilical circulation of one twin may be done percutaneously or endoscopically,[39] or by removing the abnormal twin by hysterotomy. Fetoscopic vessel ablation has also been reported.[40, 41]

Heart Block. Fetal heart block may occur in association with maternal collagen-vascular disease, and is treated with β-blockers or steroids. If hydrops develops from low-output heart failure, a pacemaker may be placed percutaneously or by open techniques.[2] Cryosurgical ablation of the fetal atrioventricular node has been performed in fetal lambs.[42]

AQUEDUCTAL STENOSIS. Obstruction of the flow of cerebrospinal fluid dilates the ventricles and damages the developing brain. Percutaneous placement of vesicoamniotic shunts have not improved outcome, and therefore this procedure is no longer done.[2] Hopefully, continuing development of newer techniques and selection criteria may improve shunting techniques in the future.

CONGENITAL CARDIAC DEFECTS. Pericardial effusion caused by a ventricular diverticulum[43] or pericardial teratoma may be treated by pericardiocentesis.[44, 45] Structural cardiac defects, such as pulmonary and aortic stenosis, may alter cardiac development.[2] In utero correction may alter cardiac development.[46] Experimental fetal cardiac surgery with improved techniques for cardiopulmonary bypass has produced better results.[47, 48] A significant problem during bypass has been greatly increased placental vascular resistance which can lead to decreased placental flow, acidosis, and death of the fetus. Indomethacin and high-dose steroids attenuate this increase and improve fetal survival, suggesting that prostaglandin imbalance may be responsible for this intense placental vasoconstriction.[49, 50] The use of total spinal anesthesia to block the stress response has also improved fetal survival following bypass.[51] Blockade of endothelin receptors also improves results, suggesting alteration of endothelial regulatory mechanisms.[52]

ABNORMALITIES OF THE AIRWAY. A fetus with intrinsic or extrinsic airway obstruction because of tumors often has overdistention of the lungs owing to retained fluid.[2] Fetal tracheostomy may prevent development of fetal hydrops. At term, the fetus may remain on placental support following delivery by cesarean section until the airway is secured.[37, 53–56] This may be done for fetuses with a congenital obstruction, or for those who had the trachea plugged to treat a congenital diaphragmatic hernia.

MYELOMENINGOCELE. Myelomeningocele may be diagnosed early in gestation by α-fetoprotein and by ultrasound, and may potentially be prevented by vitamin supplementation.[2] Studies in fetal lambs indicate that exposure of the spinal cord to the intrauterine environment causes neurologic damage, and that neurologic impairment may be prevented by in utero correction using a latissimus dorsi flap.[57–59] The possibility of using these same methods to treat patients has been studied intensively.[60–62] Recently, three human fetuses underwent open repair of a meningomyelocele, with survival of all three.[63] More recently, after a maternal laparotomy, maternal skin was placed over the fetal defect endoscopically in four patients.[64] In the two surviving fetuses, neurologic dysfunction was mild.

CLEFT LIP AND PALATE. Because fetal wounds heal without scarring, interest in correcting defects such as cleft lip and palate has increased.[2] Scarring, midfacial growth restriction, and nasal deformities may therefore be reduced. The reasons for this reduced scarring are under intensive study.[65–69] In sheep, fetal skin has been harvested and cultured to produce grafts that may be used to cover large defects after birth.[70]

Premature Delivery for Correction

Certain malformations may be corrected in the premature neonate after induction and early delivery.[71] These include obstructive hydrocephalus and hydronephrosis, amniotic band malformations, gastroschisis and omphalocele, intestinal volvulus, hydrops fetalis, intrauterine growth retardation, and arrhythmias causing cardiac failure. Close follow-up of the parturient is needed to determine the optimal timing of delivery, to balance the risk-benefit relationship between correction of the defect and the risks of prematurity.

Abnormalities Requiring Cesarean Section

Malformations that might interfere with delivery could require cesarean section. Such conditions include conjoined twins, and developmental disorders such as gastroschisis, omphalocele, hydrocephalus, sacrococcygeal teratoma, cystic hygroma, or meningomyelocele. In addition, airway abnormalities may require delivery by cesarean section.[37, 55, 56]

Abnormalities Optimally Corrected Following Delivery

For malformations best corrected after delivery at term, early diagnosis allows time for following the patient and referral to a center where such specialized procedures may be performed. These include intestinal atresia, meconium ileus, small and intact cysts, omphalocele, meningomyelocele, spina bifida, unilateral hydronephrosis, craniofacial and chest wall deformities, cystic hygroma, and small sacrococcygeal teratoma.

Untreatable Abnormalities

For severe abnormalities that are usually fatal and/or untreatable, counseling the parturient about alternatives, including termination of pregnancy, is appropriate. Patients with a family history of these malformations are likely to present early in gestation for diagnostic procedures. The definition of "untreatable" changes with advancing techniques. These abnormalities include severe deformities of the central nervous system (e.g., anencephaly, porencephaly, encephalocele, and severe hydrocephalus), chromosomal abnormalities (trisomy syndromes), metabolic and hematologic abnormalities, and lethal anatomic defects (including severe osteogenesis imperfecta).

ETHICAL CONSIDERATION

Because invasive fetal therapy and surgery is a new field that is rapidly developing and expanding, many unanswered ethical questions remain. These include the following:

1. *Allocation of resources:* Fetal surgery demands and consumes enormous resources from an already strained medical system. The questions of efficacy of diagnostic testing, cost-effectiveness, and long-term results for treating specific conditions will become more important as techniques are developed and improved. What is treatable and what is not will continually change with our evolution of knowledge and technology.
2. *Fetal rights and needs:* Today, the fetus is considered a patient.[72] Therefore, we may be obligated to provide lifesaving services just as we do to a child or adult. However, exactly when the fetus becomes a person (patient) is not defined in a consistent manner. For example, the same fetus that qualifies for surgery may also be aborted.
3. *Maternal rights and needs:* Intrauterine treatment of the fetus can place the mother at risk. Therefore, the mother must agree to the additional risk involved in the treatment of her fetus.
4. *Legal issues:* The legal responsibility of the mother to submit herself to additional risk for the benefit of the fetus is not well defined. The liability of the provider is not well defined at present, because many of these treatments have been experimental. A conflict may exist between liability and the ethical beliefs of the providers and the patient(s).

ANESTHETIC CONSIDERATIONS

These considerations closely follow the recommendations for nonobstetric surgery during pregnancy (for both mother and fetus),[73] considering the physiologic changes of pregnancy.[74]

Basic considerations include

1. Maternal safety. The mother is the primary patient.
2. Avoidance of teratogenic drugs, as for other surgery during pregnancy.
3. Avoidance of intrauterine fetal asphyxia.

In addition, there are special considerations for the specific procedure planned, and special considerations for the treatment of the fetus.

Special Considerations for Fetal Surgery

Fetal Safety. The fetus must be monitored and anesthetized, and premature labor must be prevented. Knowledge of fetal circulation, and how anesthesia affects it, is important. Factors that decrease uterine blood flow and therefore may lead to fetal acidosis must be considered.

Fetal Circulation. Study of the cardiovascular system in the human fetus is limited.[3, 4, 6] In the fetus, myocardial contractility is probably maximally stimulated, with limited capacity to increase.[75, 76] Recent information suggests that ventricular preload and therefore stroke volume may be limited by mechanical constraints in the fetus.[77] These constraints may be relieved at birth when the lungs are aerated. Therefore, fetal cardiac output is generally dependent on heart rate.[78] In fetal lambs, augmentation of preload by volume loading has only a small effect on cardiac output.[79] Therefore, the fetus depends on a high venous return.[80] β-Blockade may reduce the ability of the fetal heart rate to increase during stress, such as hypoxemia.[81]

Because heart rate is so important in determining cardiac output, baroreceptor and chemoreceptor functions are important. The aortic and carotid chemoreceptors are functional in fetal lambs.[82–87] Baroreflex sensitivity increases from midgestation to term.[76, 88–91] However, most studies have been short term and in anesthetized preparations.

Because the fetus has limited ability to increase cardiac output following stress, blood flow to more vital organs is preserved while less vital organs may be deprived.[92] Cerebral blood flow (CBF) in the fetal lamb is twice that in the adult, however, allowing some reserve.[93, 94] Factors that regulate CBF include cerebral metabolic rate, Pa_{CO_2}, Pa_{O_2}, blood pressure, and autoregulation.[89, 95–97] Autoregulation of CBF occurs in normoxic fetal lambs, but may be incomplete following hypoxia.[98]

Effects of Anesthesia on the Fetal Circulation. Observation of the cardiovascular effects of anesthetics in the preterm human fetus is limited. Therefore, much of our present-day knowledge concerning this issue has been derived from animal studies. Oxygenation by the uteroplacental unit determines the well-being of the fetus.[73, 99]

In fetal lambs, placental transfer of volatile halogenated agents is rapid, and the minimum alveolar concentration (MAC) is lower than that in the mother for both halothane[100] and isoflurane.[101] Both halothane[102] and isoflurane[103] levels remain lower in the fetus. Amnesia probably occurs, but the evidence is indirect.

In a very early sheep study, halothane at 1 MAC and isoflurane in the mother caused only a mild decrease in fetal blood pressure, with no change in other important parameters. However, at 2 MAC, large decreases occurred with severe cardiovascular depression and acidosis.[104] Other studies[102, 105–107] using short administrations of halothane at 2 MAC showed a decrease in fetal blood pressure and systemic vascular resistance, but no change in other important parameters. In yet another study,[103] isoflurane at 2 MAC was used for a longer time, but no decrease of fetal blood pressure occurred; however, a decrease in fetal cardiac output and acidosis resulted. These studies suggest that light anesthesia (1 MAC) is safe for the fetus. However, these studies were done in animals that were not stressed by in utero surgery or hypoxia.

Umbilical occlusion in animals produces characteristic fetal bradycardia and hypertension, resulting in decreased cardiac output and increased CBF.[108–112] These effects are thought to be mediated by the autonomic nervous system. In another study,[107] maternal halothane produced a decline of blood pressure to the same level as an unanesthetized asphyxiated fetus; the heart rate increased, and cardiac outputs, CBF, and oxygenation did not decline. In yet another study,[113] maternal halothane administration aggravated fetal acidosis and hypoxia, decreasing fetal blood pressure and CBF. During more prolonged administration of potent anesthetics, fetal CO and placental blood flow decreases, and placental vascular resistance increases disproportionately to fetal systemic vascular resistance. This shunting of blood away from the placental circulation leads to fetal acidosis.[114] The sensitivity of the fetal lamb heart to low doses of halothane[115] may account for some of these changes. A shorter duration of anesthesia (>60 minutes) and a moderate inspired concentration of volatile agents (1–1.5 MAC) are well tolerated by the fetus.

In fetal sheep, cervical subarachnoid tetracaine, 2 mg/kg, blocked the stress response to surgery, and produced higher cardiac outputs, as well as higher brain, body, and placental blood flow than in those given intramuscular ketamine, 25 mg/kg.[6, 51, 116] Also in fetal sheep, maternal propofol infusion (150–450 μg/kg/min) produced no adverse effects.[117] Decreased heart rate variability suggested the presence of fetal anesthesia.

Because only a small number of surgical procedures have been done on human fetuses, a controlled comparison of anesthetic techniques is unlikely. Neither have controlled acid-base studies following various anesthetic techniques been done in the human fetus.

Fetal Pain and Response to Surgical Stimulation. In the fetus, anesthetic goals are the same as for the mother. These include analgesia, amnesia, immobility, and physiologic homeostasis. Evidence of pain in the human fetus undergoing surgery is indirect. In premature human neonates undergoing surgery under light anesthesia, stress hormones are markedly elevated.[8, 118–123] However, these responses are attenuated with adequate anesthesia.[118, 124, 125] Spinal anesthesia of the fetus also attenuates the stress response.[6, 51, 116] Surgical stimulation of the unanesthetized fetus activates the stress response[126] and increases motor activity.[72] During late gestation, the fetus responds to a variety of environmental stimuli,[127] consistent with the development of pain perception.[128] The fetus responds to less invasive procedures, such as fetal hepatic vein puncture for transfusion, with elevations of stress hormones[129] and redistribution of blood flow to vital organs as is observed following hypoxemia.[130] Some believe that intrauterine stress may even lead to prolonged behavioral consequences.[131, 132] Despite the indirect nature of much of the evidence, today anesthesiologists proceed as if the fetus can feel pain and react adversely to it.

Maternal Considerations and the Effects on the Fetus. Uterine incision can stimulate uterine tone, and hence affect the placental circulation. Increased uterine activity, fetal manipulation, direct compression of vessels, anesthetics, maternal hypotension, hyperventilation, hypocarbia, and hypercarbia can also alter uterine and umbilical blood flow.[6, 99, 133] Although the mother is no longer the primary patient,[72] factors affecting the management of any surgery during pregnancy become important.[134] Aortocaval compression can become clinically important as early as the 10th week of gestation. Hypercoagulability and venous stasis may be associated with an increased risk of thrombophlebitis. Decreased functional residual capacity, increased oxygen consumption, and decreased buffering capacity all lead to reduced cardiopulmonary reserve. Pregnant patients are more sensitive to the effects of general anesthetic agents.

The Fetus as a Patient. The fetus tolerates surgery well and heals rapidly, with little or no scarring.

Special Fetal Monitoring Techniques. Invasive methods used in experimental preparations, such as flow probes and indwelling catheters, have limited application in human fetal surgery. Electronic fetal heart rate (FHR) monitoring is used to diagnose fetal asphyxia, hypoxia, and distress, and to monitor the response to corrective measures.[135] Currently, FHR monitoring, pulse oximetry, ultrasonography, and blood gases are monitored in human fetuses undergoing surgery.[3, 4, 6] Direct monitoring with modified atrial pacing wires using special signal processing is used. Implanted radiotelemetry devices can be used to continuously monitor the fetal electrocardiogram (ECG), temperature, uterine pressure during surgery, postoperative recovery, and for the remainder of gestation.[3, 136]

Pulse oximetry is done with a modified device wrapped around the hand or foot, using special signal processing.[3] In sheep, pulse oximetry is an excellent index of fetal well-being.[137] Intermittent ultrasonography is used to monitor FHR and umbilical blood flow, as well as fetal cardiac contractility and volume.[3] Capillary or umbilical venous samples can be obtained for blood gas, electrolyte, and glucose determinations. For prolonged procedures, a surgical cutdown of the internal jugular vein is used for fluid, drug, and blood administration.

Less invasive methods of monitoring with potential promise include detailed waveform analysis of the fetal electroencephalogram, fetal ECG, continuous monitoring of blood gases, cerebral oxygenation, tissue pH, and blood flow. The placental vessels may also be catheterized for blood pressure monitoring and sampling.[3, 4]

PREVENTION OF PRETERM LABOR

The incision and surgical stimulation increase contractions of the thick muscular wall of the uterus. Premature labor is an important cause of fetal loss after surgery,[1, 2, 5] and appears to be directly related to the degree of manipulation and invasion of the uterus. Strong contractions can reduce uteroplacental blood flow, displace intrauterine needles, and may even induce placental separation.

Ideally, prevention of contractions is preferred to treating them. Tocolytic agents have included preoperative indomethacin,[138, 139] intraoperative isoflurane,[54, 139, 140] intraoperative and postoperative magnesium sulfate,[139] and postoperative β-adrenergic and indomethacin therapy.[3, 141] Halogenated anesthetic agents can also reduce uterine tone, facilitating surgical exposure, but they also cause increased surgical bleeding when used in higher concentrations.[133] Recent work indicates that nitric oxide donors produce tocolysis in primates.[142] This is consistent with the uterine relaxation in patients produced by nitroglycerin.[143, 144]

Tocolysis is not usually needed for cordocentesis or intrauterine transfusion. β-Agonists may be used for prophylaxis of uterine irritability during more invasive procedures, such as percutaneous shunt catheter placement. The increased use of less invasive endoscopic procedures should greatly decrease the need for tocolysis.

ANESTHESIA TECHNIQUES

For surgery during pregnancy, local and regional anesthesia are intrinsically appealing because they limit fetal drug exposure, avoid major hemodynamic perturbations, reduce the risk of maternal aspiration, and facilitate postoperative analgesia.[140, 145] However, regional anesthesia in the mother cannot block maternal anxiety and the associated stress response, nor does it provide fetal anesthesia or block the fetal response to surgery-induced stress. Furthermore, it does not provide uterine relaxation.

Preparation. Less invasive procedures may be done in a clinic setting. However, surgical and anesthetic backup must be available for treating unusual but predictable complications. These include fetal distress from occlusion of vessels during attempted cannulation, and maternal bleeding. In addition to the usual preoperative evaluation, special considerations apply. These patients are usually very anxious and must be counseled about special invasive monitors, epidural catheters for postoperative pain control, and preoperative tocolytics when needed.

Patients must have adequate cardiopulmonary reserve to tolerate blood loss, which is frequently significant, and tocolytic therapy, which may be intense and prolonged. Some fetal anomalies may produce polyhydramnios, which increases the risk of maternal vomiting and aspiration.

Other important factors include the nature of the fetal lesion and the procedure planned, the need for and availability of blood for the mother or fetus, the location of the placenta, the planned site of incision, and the patient's obstetric condition (uterine activity, cervical dilatation, obstetric complications). For transfusion of the fetus, O-negative, cytomegalovirus-negative, irradiated blood is used.

Gestational age may determine which interventions, such as an emergency cesarean section, will be done for sudden fetal complications. More invasive procedures are carefully planned, usually by a multidisciplinary fetal therapy committee in specialized centers. For all procedures, the patient should fast overnight, receive an oral antacid, and be monitored at least for the requirements of conscious sedation, if needed. For the occasional very anxious patient, small doses of anxiolytics such as midazolam may be given preoperatively.

General Considerations. Normally, avoidance of aortocaval compression and maintenance of adequate maternal blood pressure and cardiac output by using adequate volume expansion and ephedrine will maintain fetal perfusion.[134]

Supplemental oxygen should be administered. There is no evidence that maternal hyperoxia produces in utero retrolental fibroplasia or premature closure of the ductus arteriosus. Maternal $Pa{CO_2}$ should be kept in the normal range. Maternal hypocapnia produced by overventilation may decrease venous return and decrease uterine blood flow. Maternal respiratory or metabolic alkalosis also produces direct umbilical vasoconstriction, reducing flow. Maternal alkalosis shifts the maternal oxyhemoglobin curve to the left, causing decreased release of oxygen at the placenta. Maternal hypercapnia may produce fetal acidosis and myocardial depression if it is severe.

Maternal stress and drugs that increase uterine tone (ketamine >1 mg/kg, toxic doses of local anesthetics, and neostigmine) should be avoided. Uterine vasoconstriction from endogenous or exogenous sympathomimetics increases uterine vascular resistance and decreases uterine blood flow. Drugs that have possible teratogenic potential should be avoided.

Monitoring

Mother. Standard noninvasive monitors are used (pulse oximetry, noninvasive blood pressure, ECG, end-tidal carbon dioxide, temperature) for all cases. For more invasive procedures, an arterial line and central venous pressure monitors, a Foley catheter, and a large-bore intravenous infusion may be needed for rapid treatment of fluid shifts and blood loss. Postoperatively, maternal pressures and uterine activity are monitored. External, internal, or telemetric fetal heart rate monitoring are continued, along with intermittent ultrasound examinations.

Fetus. For less invasive procedures, ultrasonic monitoring is used. Of importance is fetal heart rate, fetal positioning, instrumentation, and fetal movement. For more invasive procedures, special monitors, as discussed previously, are used.

Local Anesthesia. For percutaneous procedures, such as fetal blood sampling or intrauterine transfusions, local anesthetic infiltration of the maternal abdominal wall is sufficient. Intravenous fentanyl (25 μg) or midazolam (0.5 mg) may be needed, and are safe. Supplemental oxygen is administered.[3, 4]

For placement of vesicoamniotic catheter shunts,

larger needles or catheters and multiple attempts at placement may be needed. The fetus may be sedated via placental transfer of the drugs administered to the mother. If multiple attempts are needed, spinal, epidural, or general anesthesia may be indicated.

Fetal movement may render these procedures difficult or impossible. Displacement of a needle or catheter may lead to bleeding, trauma, or compromised umbilical circulation.[146, 147] Neuromuscular blockade of the fetus may be achieved by direct intramuscular or intravascular injection. Direct fetal intramuscular injection of d-tubocurarine (3 mg/kg) has been used.[148] Pancuronium (0.05–0.1 mg/kg) may be used.[149–154] With pancuronium, the fetus maintains a higher heart rate and blood pressure.[155] Vecuronium bromide (0.1 mg/kg) has similarly been injected into the umbilical vein.[156]

If assistance by the anesthesiologist is needed, the usual monitors (pulse oximetry, blood pressure, ECG) are placed, and supplemental oxygen is given. Left uterine displacement is maintained. Short-acting agents (such as propofol, midazolam, and fentanyl) are used.[145] Finally, local anesthesia given to the mother does not produce analgesia or amnesia in the fetus.

Regional Anesthesia. Some have advocated the use of regional or local anesthesia for fetal surgery.[145] The reduced risk of aspiration and the avoidance of major hemodynamic alterations are appealing. However, fetal movement may occur, but this can be controlled with the use of relaxants. Fetal anesthesia does not occur, and surgical stimulation may result in a fetal stress response. Finally, uterine relaxation does not occur, hindering surgery. The use of spinal anesthesia in the fetus may attenuate the stress response,[51, 116] but is not a practical method. The long-term effects of fetal pain and stress are unknown,[131] but the safety of general anesthesia has made regional anesthesia less popular in recent years.

General Anesthesia. For more invasive procedures, such as fetoscopy and/or hysterotomy, general anesthesia offers a number of advantages over regional anesthesia. Safe preparation, the use of antacids, an awareness of airway problems in pregnancy, and greater experience have made general anesthesia in the parturient a safe alternative to regional anesthesia, especially in the elective setting. For the fetus, general anesthesia offers immobility, anesthesia, and maintenance of normal maternal-fetal perfusion. For the mother, it offers muscle relaxation and uterine relaxation, as well as analgesia and amnesia.

A technique using a halogenated agent (usually isoflurane) to provide maternal and fetal anesthesia as well as uterine relaxation has been used by the San Francisco group for fetal surgery requiring hysterotomy, following initial studies in primates.[3, 4, 157] Left uterine displacement is used, and a rapid-sequence induction with succinylcholine or rocuronium is done. Anesthesia is maintained with low-dose isoflurane (1 MAC) and a 50% oxygen/nitrous oxide mixture. Opioids are given as needed.

For the fetus, anesthesia is provided with fentanyl, 25 to 50 μg, and paralysis is provided with pancuronium or rocuronium, 0.3 mg given intramuscularly. Tocolysis is maintained with nitroglycerin up to 20 μg/kg/min, which produces less severe cardiovascular effects than high-dose isoflurane.[158] Additional tocolysis may be obtained with terbutaline (0.35 mg) or magnesium sulfate (4 g/30 min followed by 1–2 g/h). Mean arterial pressure is maintained near 65 mm Hg.[138]

Alternatively, higher-dose isoflurane is used, with supplemental opioids to decrease the required concentration of isoflurane. Tocolysis is maintained with isoflurane and magnesium as needed.

Extubation is done using lidocaine or opioids to minimize straining. Postoperatively, premature labor is the most important complication.[2] Various tocolytics are used, including some nitrous oxide donors.[138] These patients are at risk for development of pulmonary edema, owing to the large volumes of fluid needed to maintain hemodynamic stability, and possible causative roles for decreased low oncotic pressure and increased pulmonary capillary permeability.[159, 160]

In recent years, more procedures are being performed using fetoscopy, which greatly reduces the risk of postoperative complications. In monkeys, postoperative uterine activity is absent 24 hours after fetoscopy.[161] In sheep, endoscopic procedures did not reduce uteroplacental oxygen delivery as much as did hysterotomy,[162] likely because of less manipulation of vessels. Anesthetic goals for fetoscopic procedures are the same as those for open surgery, with some additional considerations for the surgical methods. Carbon dioxide is used to displace amniotic fluid to allow visualization of the operative field.[15] In fetal lambs, hypercarbia and acidosis may result, which may be reversed by hyperventilation.[163, 164] Extreme insufflation pressure can lead to decreased placental flow and fetal hypoxia. Helium, water,[17] glycine,[165] and Hartmann's solution[166] have been used in sheep to avoid the acidosis following the use of carbon dioxide. Because there is less disturbance of the uterus, less tocolysis is needed, and a volatile anesthetic alone may be sufficient. Indeed, subsequent vaginal deliveries may be possible, in contrast to open hysterotomy, where an upper uterine incision mandates subsequent cesarean delivery. The operative team must always be prepared to convert to open hysterotomy if needed.

Occasionally, a fetus with a known obstruction of the upper airway must be delivered. This is referred to as OOPS (operation on placental support) or EXIT (ex utero intrapartum treatment).[37, 53–56] Anesthetic considerations are similar to those for other fetal conditions requiring hysterotomy. Once the airway is established, the fetus is delivered and care of the mother is routine. Because of prolonged uterine manipulation, uterine atony and postpartum bleeding may occur.

RESULTS AND COMPLICATIONS

Maternal Outcome. Significant risks to the mother occur following fetal surgery. The cost, as compared with treating a usually fatal defect in the fetus, must be determined, and is a highly individual matter.

Early complications of fetal surgery in primates include uterine rupture, wound infection and dehiscence, and decreased future fertility owing to exposure of the endometrial cavity to metal staples used for closure.[167] Improved techniques resulted in very few complications in human patients.[168]

At the UCSF Fetal Treatment Center, 6 of 50 patients required blood transfusion.[2] Almost all patients develop preterm labor, with pulmonary edema frequently occurring following intense, prolonged tocolysis.[159] Patients receiving nitroglycerin for tocolysis after fetal surgery demonstrated more prolonged and more severe pulmonary edema than the general obstetric population.[160] These authors hypothesized that high-dose intravenous nitroglycerin could act as a nitric oxide donor forming peroxynitrite, which has been implicated in immune complex–mediated lung injury and pulmonary edema, and may also damage the alveolar cells and inhibit surfactant function.

When high-output cardiac failure in the fetus and fetal hydrops result from a sacrococcygeal teratoma, the mother may also have high-output cardiac failure and findings consistent with preeclampsia.[168–170] This syndrome may persist after fetal hydrops is corrected, and may result from persistent placental hypertrophy. Termination of pregnancy may be required.[170]

The upper-segment incision used for open fetal surgery can place the patient at risk for scar dehiscence during subsequent pregnancies.[2] Future fertility is not altered.[2]

Fetal Outcome. Results vary with the lesion treated.[1, 2, 5] Open correction of congenital diaphragmatic hernia has not produced satisfactory results,[31] and the use of temporary tracheal occlusion appears more promising.[38] Fetal correction of congenital cystic adenomatoid malformation of the lung has produced good results in all nine patients treated.[2] Treatment of obstructive uropathy has also produced satisfactory results in some patients.[2]

Umbilical cord hematoma may form following intravascular transfusion, compromising fetal circulation.[171] Following chorioamniotic membrane separations, amniotic bands may form and strangulate the umbilical cord. This may occur spontaneously, or following fetal surgery.[172]

Of 33 infants born after open fetal surgery, seven treated for congenital diaphragmatic hernia had periventricular hemorrhage, intraventricular hemorrhage, and periventricular leukomalacia.[173] These authors believed that changes in fetal cerebral hemodynamics owing to maternal hypoxia or tocolytic drugs might account for some of these neurologic lesions.

FUTURE DIRECTIONS

Improved use of older methods or development of newer diagnostic methods should improve the precision of fetal diagnosis, allowing more precise planning of therapy. For example, MRI of congenital diaphragmatic hernia clearly defines liver herniation, which greatly alters prognosis.[174] Transesophageal echocardiography allows more precise diagnosis of structure and hemodynamics noninvasively.[175]

Improved technology will allow therapy unheard of just a few years ago. For example, a new device allows single-port tracheoscopic surgery, less invasive than earlier methods.[176] Chronic catheterization of the umbilical vein will make multiple cannulations now required for some diseases obsolete.[177]

Improvements in devices and techniques (such as fetoscopy) will allow less invasive treatments of many diseases with minimal maternal morbidity, and treatment thought impossible only a few years ago.

For more invasive therapy, such as correction of congenital cardiac defects, improved technology may allow correction before permanent damage is done following abnormal cardiac development. For complex defects such as craniofacial defects, improved anesthetic and surgical techniques may allow prolonged surgery with minimal cerebral edema and mortality.[178]

New animal models allow study from a different perspective because of anatomic differences, such as the Yucatan miniature swine.[179] Increasingly sophisticated techniques have allowed study of fetal surgery in smaller animals, such as rabbits.[180, 181]

Improved technology may also allow the use of genetic engineering to treat metabolic defects, with more precise placement of genes into the fetus.

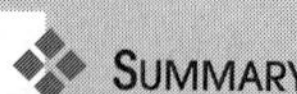

Summary

Key Points

- Some serious or potentially fatal developmental disorders may now be treated in utero, reducing or eliminating progression of the disorder.
- Anesthesia for fetal surgery must consider two patients—the mother and fetus. Maternal and fetal safety, optimal operating conditions, and prevention of premature labor must be considered.
- Improved technology, including fetoscopy, has allowed less invasive fetal surgery, resulting in a reduction in complications.
- The cost of fetal surgery must be balanced against the human tragedy and the financial burden of death and long-term disability.

Key Reference

Harrison MR: Fetal surgery. Am J Obstet Gynecol 1996; 174:1255–1264.

Case Stem

A fetal diagnosis of diaphragmatic hernia has been made by ultrasound in a 41-year-old primiparous patient. Discuss the obstetric and anesthetic implications of this finding and the possible role of in utero surgical repair.

References

1. Albanese CT, Harrison MR: Surgical treatment for fetal disease: the state of the art (review). Ann N Y Acad Sci 1998; 847:74.
2. Harrison MR: Fetal surgery. Am J Obstet Gynecol 1996; 174:1255.
3. Rosen MA: Anesthesia for fetal surgery. *In* Chestnut D (ed): Obstetric Anesthesia. Philadelphia: WB Saunders; 1994:110.
4. Rosen MA: Anesthesia for fetal procedures and surgery. *In* Shnider SM, Levinson G (eds): Anesthesia for Obstetrics, 3rd ed. Baltimore: Williams & Wilkins; 1993:281.
5. Manning FA: The future of intrauterine fetal surgery: a critical appraisal. *In* Harman CR (ed): Invasive Fetal Testing and Management. Oxford, England: Blackwell Scientific Publications; 1995:440.
6. Fogel ST, Langer JC: Anesthesia for fetal surgery. *In* Norris M (ed): Obstetric Anesthesia, 2nd ed. Baltimore: Lippincott Williams & Wilkins; 1998:187–210.
7. Liley AW: Intrauterine transfusion of the foetus in haemolytic disease. BMJ 1963; 2:1107.
8. Anand KJS: Hormonal and metabolic function of neonates undergoing surgery. Curr Opin Cardiol 1986; 1:681.
9. Adamsons K: Fetal surgery. New Engl J Med 1966; 275:204.
10. Rodeck CH, Nicolaides KH, Warsof SL: The management of severe rhesus isoimmunization by fetoscopic intravascular transfusion. Am J Obstet Gynecol 1984; 150:769.
11. Nicolaides K, Soothill PW, Rodeck C, et al: Rh disease: intravascular fetal blood transfusion by cordocentesis. Fetal Ther 1986; 1:185.
12. Harrison MR, Filly RA, Globus MS, et al: Fetal treatment 1982. New Engl J Med 1982; 307:1651.
13. Harrison MR: Fetal surgery for congenital hydronephrosis. N Engl J Med 1982; 306:591.
14. Pearson JF: Fetal surgery [editorial]. Arch Dis Child 1983; 58:324.
15. Estes JM, MacGillivray TE, Hedrick MH, et al: Fetoscopic surgery for the treatment of congenital anomalies. J Pediatr Surg 1992; 27:950.
16. Crombleholme TM, Dirkes K, Whitney TM, et al: Amniotic band syndrome in fetal lambs: fetoscopic release and morphometric outcome. J Pediatr Surg 1995; 30:974.
17. Pelletier GJ, Srinathan SK, Langer JC: Effects of intraamniotic helium, carbon dioxide, and water on fetal lambs. J Pediatr Surg 1995; 30:1155.
18. Skarsgard ED, Bealer JF, Meuli M, et al: Fetal endoscopic ('Fetendo') surgery: the relationship between insufflating pressure and the fetoplacental circulation. J Pediatr Surg 1995; 30:1165.
19. Skarsgard ED, Meuli M, VanderWall KJ, et al: Fetal endoscopic tracheal occlusion (Fetendo-PLUG) for congenital diaphragmatic hernia. J Pediatr Surg 1996; 31:1335.
20. Deprest JA, Luks FI, Peers KH, et al: Intrauterine endoscopic creation of urinary tract obstruction in the fetal lamb: a model for fetal surgery. Am J Obstet Gynecol 1995; 172:1442.
21. Cha I, Adzick NS, Harrison MR, et al: Fetal congenital cystic adenomatoid malformation of the lung: a clinicopathologic study of eleven cases. Am J Surg Pathol 1997; 21:537.
22. Rice HE, Estes JM, Hedrick MH, et al: Congenital cystic adenomatoid malformations: a sheep model of fetal hydrops. J Pediatr Surg 1994; 29:692.
23. Adzick NS, Harrison MR, Crombleholme TM, et al: Fetal lung lesions: management and outcome. Am J Obstet Gynecol 1998; 179:884.
24. Ahmad FK, Sherman SJ, Hagglund KH, et al: Isolated fetal pleural effusion: the role of sonographic surveillance and in utero therapy. Fetal Diagn Ther 1996; 11:383.
25. Becmeur F, Horta-Geraud P, Donato L, et al: Pulmonary sequestrations: prenatal ultrasound diagnosis, treatment, and outcome. J Pediatr Surg 1998; 33:492.
26. Bullard KM, Harrison MR: Before the horse is out of the barn—fetal surgery for hydrops. Semin Perinatol 1995; 29:462.
27. Petrikovsky B, Gross BR, Bialer M: Single-needle insertion technique for thoracocentesis for bilateral pleural effusion. Fetal Diagn Ther 1996; 11:26.
28. Allan LD, Irish M, Glick PL: The fetal heart in diaphragmatic hernia. Clin Perinatol 1996; 23:795.
29. Karamanoukian HL, O'Toole SJ, Rossman JR, et al: Fetal surgical interventions and the development of the heart in congenital diaphragmatic hernia. J Surg Res 1996; 65:5.
30. Langer JC: Congenital diaphragmatic hernia [review]. Chest Surg Clin North Am 1998; 8:295.
31. Harrison MR, Adzick NS, Bullard KM, et al: Correction of congenital diaphragmatic hernia in utero. VII: A prospective trial. J Pediatr Surg 1997; 32:1637.
32. Bealer JF, Skarsgard ED, Hedrick MH, et al: The PLUG odyssey: adventures in experimental fetal tracheal occlusion. J Pediatr Surg 1995; 30:361.
33. DiFiore JW, Wilson JM: Lung development [review]. Semin Pediatr Surg 1994; 3:221.
34. Luks FL, Gilchrist BF, Jackson BT, et al: Endoscopic tracheal obstruction with expanding device in a fetal lamb model: preliminary considerations. Fetal Diagn Ther 1996; 11:67.
35. Wilson JW, DiFiore JW, Peters CA: Experimental fetal tracheal ligation prevents the pulmonary hyperplasia associated with fetal nephrectomy: possible applications to congenital diaphragmatic hernia. J Pediatr Surg 1993; 28:1433.
36. Graf JL, Gibbs DL, Adzick NS, et al: Fetal hydrops after in utero tracheal occlusion. J Pediatr Surg 1997; 32:214.
37. Mychaliska GB, Bealer JF, Graf JL, et al: Operating on placental support: the ex-utero intrapartum treatment procedure. J Pediatr Surg 1997; 32:227.
38. VanderWall KJ, Skarsgard ED, Filly RA, et al: Fetendo-clip: a fetal tracheal clip procedure in a human fetus. J Pediatr Surg 1997; 32:970.
39. Quintero RA, Reich H, Puder KS, et al: Brief report: umbilical-cord ligation of an acardiac twin by fetoscopy at 19 weeks of gestation. N Engl J Med 1994; 330:469.
40. Ville Y, Hyett J, Kecher K, et al: Preliminary experience with endoscopic laser surgery for severe twin-twin transfusion syndrome. New Engl J Med 1995; 332:224.
41. De Lia JE, Cruikshank DP, Keye WR: Fetoscopic laser occlusion of choriopagus in severe twin transfusion syndrome. Obstet Gynecol 1990; 75:1046.
42. Assad RS, Aiello VD, Jatene MB, et al: Cryosurgical ablation of fetal atrioventricular node: new model to treat malignant tachyarrhythmias. Ann Thorac Surg 1995; 60:S629–S632.
43. Johnson JA, Ryan G, Toi A, et al: Prenatal diagnosis of a fetal ventricular diverticulum associated with pericardial effusion: successful outcome following pericardiocentesis. Prenat Diagn 1996; 16:954.
44. Bruch SW, Adzick NS, Reiss R, et al: Prenatal therapy for pericardial teratomas. J Pediatr Surg 1997; 32:1113.
45. Sklansky M, Greenberg M, Lucas V, et al: Intrapericardial teratoma in a twin fetus: diagnosis and management. Obstet Gynecol 1997; 89:807.
46. Saiki Y, Konig A, Waddell J, et al: Hemodynamic alteration by fetal surgery accelerates myocyte proliferation in fetal guinea pig hearts. Surgery 1997; 122:412.
47. Turley K, Vlahakes GJ, Harrison MR, et al: Intrauterine cardiothoracic surgery: the fetal lamb model. Ann Thorac Surg 1982; 34:422.
48. Reddy VM, Liddicoat JR, Klein JR, et al: Long-term outcome after fetal cardiac bypass: fetal survival to full term and organ abnormalities. J Thorac Cardiovasc Surg 1996; 111:536.
49. Sabik JF, Heinemann MK, Assad RS, et al: High dose steroids prevent placental dysfunction after fetal cardiac bypass. J Thorac Cardiovasc Surg 1994; 107:116.
50. Sabik JF, Assad RS, Hanley FL: Prostaglandin synthesis inhibition prevents dysfunction after fetal cardiac bypass. J Thorac Cardiovasc Surg 1992; 103:733.
51. Fenton KN, Zinn HE, Heinemann MK, et al: Long-term survivors of fetal cardiac bypass in lambs. J Thorac Cardiovasc Surg 1994; 107:1423.
52. Reddy VM, McEhinney DB, Rajasinghe HA, et al: Role of endothelium in placental dysfunction after cardiac bypass. J Thorac Cardiovasc Surg 1999; 117:345.
53. Langer JC, Tabb T, Thompson P, et al: Management of prenatally diagnosed tracheal obstruction: access to the airway in utero prior to delivery. Fetal Diagn Ther 1992;7:12.

54. Norris MC, Joseph J, Leighton BL: Anesthesia for perinatal surgery. Am J Perinatol 1989; 6:39.
55. Gaiser RR, Cheek TG, Kurth CD: Anesthetic management of cesarean delivery complicated by ex utero intrapartum treatment of the fetus. Anesth Analg 1997; 84:1150.
56. Skarsgard ED, Chitkara U, Krane EJ, et al: The OOPS procedure (operation on placental support): in utero airway management of the fetus with prenatally diagnosed tracheal obstruction. J Pediatr Surg 1996; 31:826.
57. Meuli M, Meuli-Simmen C, Yingling CD, et al: Creation of a myelomeningocele in utero: a model of functioning damage from spinal cord exposure in fetal sheep. J Pediatr Surg 1995; 30:1028.
58. Meuli M, Meuli-Simmen C, Hutchins GM, et al: In utero surgery rescues neurological function at birth in sheep with spina bifida. Nature Med 1995; 1:342.
59. Meuli-Simmen C, Meuli M, Hutchins GM, et al: Fetal reconstructive surgery: experimental use of the latissimus dorsi flap to correct myelomeningocele in utero. Plast Reconstr Surg 1995; 96:1007.
60. Hutchins GM, Meuli M, Meuli-Simmen C, et al: Acquired spinal cord injury in human fetuses with myelomeningocele. Pediatr Pathol Lab Med 1996; 16:701.
61. Meuli-Simmen C, Meuli M, Adzick NS, et al: Latissimus dorsi flap procedures to cover myelomeningocele in utero: a feasibility study in human fetuses. J Pediatr Surg 1997; 32:1154.
62. Meuli M, Meuli-Simmen C, Hutchins GM, et al: The spinal cord lesion in human fetuses with myelomeningocele: implications for fetal surgery. J Pediatr Surg 1997; 32:448.
63. Tulipan N, Bruner JP: Myelomeningocele repair in utero: report of three cases. Pediatr Neurosurg 1998; 28:177.
64. Bruner JP, Richards WO, Tulipan NB, et al: Endoscopic coverage of fetal myelomeningocele in utero. Am J Obstet Gynecol 1999; 180:143.
65. Estes JM, Whitby DJ, Lorenz HP, et al: Endoscopic creation and repair of fetal cleft lip. Plast Reconstr Surg 1992; 90:747.
66. Estes JM, Whitby DJ, Lorenz HP, et al: Mechanisms of wound healing in the embryo and fetus. Plast Reconstr Surg 1992; 90:743.
67. Estes JM, Adzick NS, Harrison MR, et al: Hyaluronate metabolism undergoes an ontogenic transition during fetal development: implications for scar-free wound healing. J Pediatr Surg 1993; 28:1227.
68. Martin P: Mechanisms of wound healing in the embryo and fetus. Curr Top Dev Biol 1996; 32:175.
69. Sullivan KM, Lorenz HP, Meuli M, et al: A model of scarless human fetal wound repair is deficient in transforming growth factor beta. J Pediatr Surg 1995; 30:198.
70. Fauza DO, Fishman SJ, Mehegan K, et al: Videofetoscopically assisted fetal tissue engineering: skin replacement. J Pediatr Surg 1998; 33:357.
71. Harrison MR: Selection for treatment: which defects are correctable. *In* Harrison MR, Globus MS, Filly RA (eds): The Unborn Patient: Prenatal Diagnosis and Treatment, 2nd ed. Philadelphia: WB Saunders; 1991; 159.
72. Liley AW: The foetus as a personality. Aust N Z J Psychiatry 1972; 6:99.
73. Parer JT: Uteroplacental circulation and respiratory gas exchange. *In* Shnider SM, Levinson G (eds): Anesthesia for Obstetics, 3rd ed. Baltimore: Williams & Wilkins; 1993:19.
74. Cheek TG, Gutsche BB: Maternal physiologic alterations during pregnancy. *In* Shnider SM, Levinson G (eds): Anesthesia for Obstetics, 3rd ed. Baltimore: Williams & Wilkins; 1993:3.
75. Friedman WF: The intrinsic physiologic properties of the developing heart. Prog Cardiovasc Dis 1972; 15:87.
76. Gilbert RD: Effects of afterload and baroreceptors on cardiac function in fetal sheep. J Devel Physiol 1982; 4:299.
77. Grant DA: Ventricular constraint in the fetus and newborn. Can J Cardiol 1999; 15:95.
78. Rudolph AM, Heymann MA: Cardiac output in the fetal lamb: the effects of spontaneous and induced changes of heart rate on right and left ventricular output. Am J Obstet Gynecol 1976; 124:183.
79. Gilbert RD: Control of fetal cardiac output during changes in blood volume. Am J Physiol 1980; 238:H80.
80. Gilbert RD: Determinants of venous return in the fetal lamb. Gynecol Invest 1977; 8:233.
81. Cohn HE, Piasecki GJ, Jackson BT: The effect of beta-adrenergic stimulation on fetal cardiovascular function during hypoxemia. Am J Obstet Gynecol 1982; 144:810.
82. Blanco CE, Dawes GS, Hanson MA, et al: The response to hypoxia of arterial chemoreceptors in fetal sheep and new-born lambs. J Physiol 1984; 351:25.
83. Dawes GS, Duncan SLB, Lewis BV, et al: Hypoxaemia and aortic chemoreceptor function in foetal lambs. J Physiol 1969; 201:105.
84. Dawes GS, Duncan SLB, Lewis BV, et al: Cyanide stimulation of the systemic arterial chemoreceptors in foetal lambs. J Physiol 1969; 201:117.
85. Dawes GS, Lewis BV, Milligan JE, et al: Vasomotor responses in the hind limbs of foetal and newborn lambs to asphyxia and aortic chemoreceptor stimulation. J Physiol 1968; 195:55.
86. Goodwin JW, Milligan JE, Thomas B, et al: The effect of aortic chemoreceptor stimulation on cardiac output and umbilical blood flow in the fetal lamb. Am J Obstet Gynecol 1973; 116:48.
87. Itskovitz J, Rudolph AM: Denervation of arterial chemoreceptors and baroreceptors in fetal lambs in utero. Am J Physiol 1982; 242:H916.
88. Dawes GS, Johnston BM, Walker DW: Relationship of arterial pressure and heart rate in fetal, new-born and adult sheep. J Physiol 1980; 310:405.
89. Gilbert RD, Pearce WJ, Ashwal S, et al: Effects of hypoxia on contractility of isolated fetal lamb cerebral arteries. J Devel Physiol 1990; 13:122.
90. Itskovitz J, LaGamma EF, Rudolph AM: Baroreflex control of the circulation in chronically instrumented fetal lambs. Circ Res 1983; 52:589.
91. Shinebourne EA, Vapaavouri EK, Williams RL, et al: Development of baroreflex activity in unanesthetized fetal and neonatal lambs. Circ Res 1972; 31:710.
92. Cohn HE, Piasecki GJ, Jackson BT: The effect of fetal heart rate on cardiovascular function during hypoxemia. Am J Obstet Gynecol 1980; 138:1190.
93. Jones MD, Rosenberg AA, Simmons MA, et al: Oxygen delivery to the brain before and after birth. Science 1982; 216:324.
94. Makowski EL, Schneider JM, Tsoulos NG, et al: Cerebral blood flow, oxygen consumption and glucose utilization of fetal lambs in utero. Am J Obstet Gynecol 1972; 114:292.
95. Rosenberg A, Jones MD, Traystman RJ, et al: Response of cerebral blood flow to changes in P_{CO_2} in fetal, newborn and adult sheep. Am J Physiol 1982; 242:H862.
96. Jones MDJ, Sheldon RE, Battaglia FC, et al: Fetal cerebral oxygen consumption at different levels of oxygenation. J Appl Physiol 1977; 43:1080.
97. Tweed WA, Cote J, Wade JG, et al: Preservation of fetal brain blood flow relative to other organs during hypovolemic hypotension. Pediatr Res 1982; 16:137.
98. Tweed WA, Cote J, Pash M, et al: Arterial oxygenation determines autoregulation of cerebral blood flow in the fetal lamb. Pediatr Res 1983; 17:246.
99. Shnider SM, Levinson G, Cosmi EV: Obstetric anesthesia and uterine blood flow. *In* Shnider SM, Levinson G (eds): Anesthesia for Obstetrics, 3rd ed. Baltimore: Williams & Wilkins; 1993:29.
100. Gregory GA, Wade JG, Biehl DR, et al: Fetal anesthetic requirement (MAC) for halothane. Anesth Analg 1983; 62:9.
101. Bachman CR, Biehl DR, Sitar D, et al: Isoflurane potency and cardiovascular effects during short exposures in the fetal lamb. Can Anaesth Soc J 1986; 33:41.
102. Biehl DR, Cote J, Wade JG, et al: Uptake of halothane by the foetal lamb in utero. Can Anaesth Soc J 1983; 30:24.
103. Biehl DR, Yarnell R, Wade JG, et al: The uptake of isoflurane by the foetal lamb in utero: effect on regional blood flow. Can Anaesth Soc J 1983; 30:581.
104. Palahniuk RJ, Shnider SM: Maternal and fetal cardiovascular and acid-base changes during halothane and isoflurane anesthesia in the pregnant ewe. Anesthesiology 1974; 41:462.

105. Biehl DR, Tweed WA, Cote J, et al: Effect of halothane on cardiac output and regional flow in the fetal lamb in utero. Anesth Analg 1983; 62:489.
106. Cheek DBC: Effect of halothane on regional cerebral blood flow and cerebral metabolic oxygen consumption in the fetal lamb in utero. Anesthesiology 1987; 67:361.
107. Yarnell R, Biehl DR, Tweed WA, et al: The effect of halothane anesthesia on the asphyxiated foetal lamb in utero. Can Anaesth Soc J 1983; 30:474.
108. Cohn HE, Sachs EJ, Heymann MA, et al: Cardiovascular responses to hypoxemia and acidemia in fetal lambs. Am J Obstet Gynecol 1974; 120:817.
109. Peeters LLH, Sheldon RE, Jones MD, et al: Blood flow to fetal organs as a function of arterial oxygen content. Am J Obstet Gynecol 1979; 35:637.
110. Reuss ML, Parer JT, Harris JL, et al: Hemodynamic effects of alpha-adrenergic blockade during hypoxia in fetal sheep. Am J Obstet Gynecol 1982; 142:410.
111. Court DJ, Parer JT, Block BSB: Effects of beta-adrenergic blockade on blood flow distribution during hypoxemia in fetal sheep. J Dev Physiol 1984; 6:349.
112. Johnson GN, Palahniuk RJ, Tweed WA, et al: Regional cerebral blood flow changes during severe fetal asphyxia produced by slow partial umbilical cord compression. Am J Obstet Gynecol 1979; 135:48.
113. Palahniuk RJ, Doig GA, Johnson GN, et al: Maternal halothane anesthesia reduces cerebral blood flow in the acidotic sheep fetus. Anesth Analg 1980; 59:35.
114. Sabik JF, Assad RS, Hanley FL: Halothane as an anesthetic for fetal surgery. J Pediatr Surg 1993; 28:542.
115. Davis DA, Speziali G, Wagerle CL, et al: Effects of halothane on the immature lamb heart. Ann Thoracic Surg 1995; 59:695.
116. Fenton KN, Heinemann MK, Hickey PR, et al: The stress response during fetal surgery is blocked by total spinal anesthesia. Surg Forum 1992; 43:631.
117. Alon E, Ball RH, Gillie MH, et al: Effects of propofol and thiopental on maternal and fetal cardiovascular and acid-base variables in the pregnant ewe. Anesthesiology 1993; 78:562.
118. Anand KJ: Clinical importance of pain and stress in the neonate. Biol Neonate 1998; 73:1.
119. Milne EMG, Elliott MJ, Pearson DT, et al: The effect on intermediary metabolism of open-heart surgery with deep hypothermia and circulatory arrest in infants of less than 10 kilograms body weight. Perfusion 1986; 1:29.
120. Anand KJS, Brown MJ, Bloom SR, et al: Studies on the hormonal regulation of fuel metabolism in the human newborn infant undergoing anesthesia and surgery. Horm Res 1985; 22:115.
121. Obra H, Sugiyama D, Maekawa N: Plasma cortisol levels in paediatric anaesthesia. Can Anaesth Soc J 1984; 31:24.
122. Srinvasan G, Jain R, Pildes RS, et al: Glucose homeostasis during anesthesia and surgery in infants. J Pediatr Surg 1986; 20:41.
123. Anand KJS, Broenk MJ, Causon RC, et al: Can the human neonate mount an endocrine and metabolic response to surgery? J Pediatr Surg 1985; 20:41.
124. Anand KJS, Sippell WG, Aynslwy-Green A: Randomized trial of fentanyl anaesthesia in preterm neonates undergoing surgery: effects on the stress response. Lancet 1987; 1:243.
125. Anand KJ, Hickey PR: Halothane-morphine compared with high-dose sufentanil for anesthesia and postoperative analgesia in neonatal cardiac surgery [comment]. New Engl J Med 1992; 326:1.
126. Rose JC, MacDonald AA, Heymann MA, et al: Developmental aspects of the pituitary-adrenal axis response to hemorrhagic stress in lamb fetuses in utero. J Clin Invest 1978; 61:424.
127. Smyth CN: Exploratory methods for testing the integrity of the foetus and neonate. J Obstet Gynaecol Br Commonw 1965; 72:920.
128. Anand KJS, Hickey PR: Pain and its effects in the human neonate and fetus. New Engl J Med 1987; 317:1321.
129. Giannakoulopoulos X, Speulveda W, Kourtis P: Fetal plasma cortisol and beta-endorphin response to intrauterine needling. Lancet 1994; 334:77.
130. Teixeira J, Fogliani R: Fetal haemodynamic stress response to invasive procedures [letter]. Lancet 1996; 347:624.
131. Glover V, Fisk N: We don't know; better to err on the safe side from midgestation. BMJ 1996; 313:796.
132. Meany M, Bhatnagar S, Diorio J, et al: Molecular basis for the development of individual differences in the hypothalamic-pituitary-adrenal response. Cell Mol Neurobiol 1993; 13:321.
133. Miller AC, DeVore JS, Eisler EA: Effects of anesthesia on uterine activity and labor. *In* Shnider SM, Levinson G (eds): Anesthesia for Obstetrics, 3rd ed. Baltimore: Williams & Wilkins; 1993:53–69.
134. Levinson G, Shnider SM: Anesthesia for surgery during pregnancy. *In* Shnider SM, Levinson G (eds): Anesthesia for Obstetrics, 3rd ed. Baltimore; Williams & Wilkins; 1993:259.
135. Parer J: Diagnosis and management of fetal asphyxia. *In* Shnider SM, Levinson G (eds): Anesthesia for Obstetrics, 3rd ed. Baltimore: Williams & Wilkins; 1993:657–670.
136. Jennings RW, Adzick NS, Longaker MT: Radiotelemetric fetal monitoring during and after open fetal operation. Surg Gynecol Obstet 1993; 176:59.
137. Luks FI, Johnson BD, Papadakis K, et al: Predictive value of monitoring parameters in fetal surgery. J Pediatr Surg 1998; 33:1297.
138. Cauldwell CB, Rosen MA, Harrison MR: The use of nitroglycerin for uterine relaxation during fetal surgery [abstract]. Anesthesiology 1995; 83:A929.
139. Gaiser RR, Cheek TG, Kurth CD, et al: Perioperative management of the parturient presenting for fetal surgery [abstract]. Soc Obstet Anesth Perinatol 1997:60.
140. Johnson MD, Birnbach DJ, Burchman C, et al: Fetal surgery and general anesthesia: a case report and review. J Clin Anesth 1989; 5:363.
141. Chestnut DH, Dailey PA: Anesthesia for preterm labor and delivery. *In* Shnider SM, Levinson G (eds): Anesthesia for Obstetics, 3rd ed. Baltimore: Williams & Wilkins; 1993:337.
142. Jennings RW, MacGillivray TE, Harrison MR: Nitric oxide inhibits preterm labor in the Rhesus monkey. J Maternal-Fetal Med 1993; 2:170–175.
143. Altabef KM, Spencer JT, Zinberg S: Intravenous nitroglycerin for uterine relaxation of an inverted uterus. Am J Obstet Gynecol 1992: 166:1237–1238.
144. Peng ATC, Gorman RS, Shulman SM, et al: Intravenous nitroglycerin for uterine relaxation in the postpartum patient with retained placenta. Anesthesiology 1989; 71:171.
145. Spielman FJ, Seeds JW, Corke BC: Anaesthesia for fetal surgery. Anaesthesia 1984; 39:756.
146. Reece EA, Copel JA, Scioscia AL, et al: Diagnostic fetal umbilical blood sampling in the management of isoimmunization. Am J Obstet Gynecol 1988; 159:1057.
147. Sacher RA, Falchuk SC: Percutaneous umbilical blood sampling. Crit Rev Clin Lab Sci 1990; 28:19.
148. DeCrespigny LC, Robinson HP, Ross AW, et al: Curarization of fetus for intrauterine procedures. Lancet 1985; 1:1164.
149. Moise KJ, Carpenter RJ, Deter RL, et al: The use of fetal neuromuscular blockade during intrauterine transfusions. Am J Obstet Gynecol 1987; 157:874.
150. Moise KJ, Deter RL, Kirshon B, et al: Intravenous pancuronium bromide for fetal neuromuscular blockade during intrauterine transfusion for red-cell alloimmunization. Obstet Gynecol 1989; 74:905.
151. Copel JA, Grannum PA, Harrison D, et al: The use of intravenous pancuronium bromide to produce fetal paralysis during intravascular transfusion. Am J Obstet Gynecol 1988; 158:170.
152. Byers JW, Aubrey RH, Feinstein SJ, et al: Intravascular neuromuscular blockade for fetal transfusion [letter]. Am J Obstet Gynecol 1988; 158:677.
153. Seeds JW, Corke BC, Spielman FJ: Prevention of fetal movement during invasive procedures with pancuronium bromide. Am J Obstet Gynecol 1986; 155:818.
154. Pielet BW, Socol ML, MacGregor SN, et al: Fetal heart rate changes after fetal intravascular treatment with pancuronium bromide. Am J Obstet Gynecol 1988; 159:640.
155. Chestnut DH, Weiner CP, Thompson CS, et al: Intravenous administration of d-tubocurarine and pancuronium in fetal lambs. Am J Obstet Gynecol 1989; 160:510.

156. Leveque C, Murat I, Toubas F, et al: Fetal neuromuscular blockade with vecuronium bromide: studies during intravascular intrauterine transfusion in isoimmunized pregnancies. Anesthesiology 1992; 76:642.
157. Harrison MR, Anderson J, Rosen MA, et al: Fetal surgery in the primate: anesthetic, surgical and tocolytic management to maximize fetal-neonatal survival. J Pediatr Surg 1982; 17:115.
158. de Rosaryo M, Nahrwold ML, Hill AB, et al: Plasma levels and cardiovascular effect of nitroglycerin in pregnant sheep. Can Anaesth Soc J 1980; 27:560.
159. DiFrederico EM, Harrison M, Matthay MA: Pulmonary edema in a woman following fetal surgery. Chest 1996; 109:1114.
160. DiFrederico EM, Burlingame JM, Kilpatrick SJ, et al: Pulmonary edema in obstetric patients is rapidly resolved except in the presence of infection or of nitroglycerin tocolysis after open fetal therapy. Am J Obstet Gynecol 1998; 179:925.
161. van der Wildt B, Luks FI, Steegers EAP, et al: Absence of electrical uterine activity after endoscopic access for fetal surgery in the rhesus monkey. Eur J Obstet Gynecol Reprod Biol 1995; 58:213.
162. Luks FI, Peers HHE, Deprest JA, et al: The effect of open and endoscopic fetal surgery on uteroplacental oxygen delivery in the sheep. J Pediatr Surg 1996; 31:310.
163. Saiki Y, Litwin DE, Bigras JL, et al: Reducing the deleterious effects of intrauterine CO_2 during fetoscopic surgery. J Surg Res 1997; 69:51.
164. Hunter JG, Swanstrom L, Thornburg K: Carbon dioxide pneumoperitoneum induces fetal acidosis in a pregnant ewe model. Surg Endosc 1995; 9:277.
165. Ford WD, Cool JC, Byard R, et al: Glycine as a potential window for minimal access fetal surgery. Fetal Diagn Ther 1997; 12:145.
166. Evrad VA, Verbeke K, Peers KH, et al: Amnioinfusion with Hartmann's solution: a safe distension medium for endoscopic fetal surgery in the ovine model. Fetal Diagn Ther 1997; 12:188.
167. Adzick NS, Harrison MR, Glick PL, et al: Fetal surgery in the primate. III. Maternal outcome after fetal surgery. J Pediatr Surg 1986; 21:477.
168. Longaker MT, Globus MS, Filly RA, et al: Maternal outcome after open fetal surgery: a review of the first 17 human cases. JAMA 1991; 265:737.
169. van Selm M, Kanhai HH, Gravenhorst JB: Maternal hydrops syndrome: a review. Obst Gynecol Surv 1991; 46:785.
170. Bock B, Riess R, Wunsch PH, et al: Prenatal diagnosis of a sacrococcygeal teratoma with hydrops fetalis and placental hypertrophy: consequences for the further course of pregnancy [in German]. Geburtshilfe Frauenheilkd 1990; 50:647.
171. Moise KJJ, Carpenter RJ, Huhta JC, et al: Umbilical cord hematoma secondary to in utero intravascular transfusion for RH isoimmunization. Fetal Ther 1987; 2:65.
172. Graf JL, Bealer JF, Gibbs DL, et al: Chorionic membrane separation: a potentially lethal finding. Fetal Diagn Ther 1997; 12:81.
173. Bealer JF, Raisanen J, Skarsgard ED, et al: The incidence and spectrum of neurological injury after open fetal surgery. J Pediatr Surg 1995; 30:1150.
174. Hubbard AM, Adzick NS, Crombleholme TM, et al: Left-sided congenital diaphragmatic hernia: value of prenatal MR imaging in preparation for fetal surgery. Radiology 1997; 203:636.
175. Kohl T, Stelnicki EJ, VanderWall KJ, et al: Transesophageal echocardiography in fetal sheep: a monitoring tool for open and fetoscopic cardiac procedures. Surg Endosc 1996; 10:820.
176. Papadakis K, Luks FI, Deprest JA, et al: Single-port tracheoscopic surgery in the fetal lamb. J Pediatr Surg 1998; 33:918.
177. Lemery DJ, Santolaya-Forgas J, Wilson LJ, et al: A non-human primate model for the in utero chronic catheterization of the umbilical vein: a preliminary report. Fetal Diagn Ther 1995; 10:326.
178. Sims CD, Butler PE, Casanova R, et al: Prolonged general anesthesia for experimental craniofacial surgery in fetal swine. J Invest Surg 1997; 10:53.
179. Swindle MM, Wiestt DB, Smith AC, et al: Fetal surgical protocols in Yucatan miniature swine. Lab Animal Sci 1996; 46:90.
180. Butler PE, Sims CD, Randolph MA, et al: Prolonged survival in fetal rabbit surgery. J Invest Surg 1998; 11:57.
181. Nelson JM, Krummel TM, Haynes JH, et al: Operative techniques in the fetal rabbit. J Invest Surg 1990; 3:393.

23

Anesthesia for Assisted Reproductive Technologies

❖ LAWRENCE C. TSEN, MD

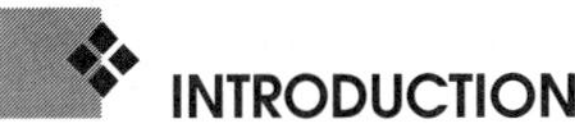

INTRODUCTION

The birth of the first in vitro fertilized baby in 1978[1] validated extracorporeal embryo fertilization and the scientific techniques known as assisted reproductive technologies (ART). As experience and refinements within the science occurred, live birth rates increased; in 1995, a survey of North American clinics reported more than 59,000 initiated cycles with 11,631 deliveries resulting.[2] Although the 1995 results are impressive, recent reported delivery rates per treatment cycle by the Society for Assisted Reproductive Technology (SART) in the United States and the Human Fertilisation and Embryology Authority (HFEA) in the United Kingdom were 19% and 15%, respectively.[3,4] The application of ART to increasingly broad etiologies of infertility may be responsible for these limited results; however, subtle differences in hormonal manipulation, techniques, and laboratory methods are known to affect results.[5] As such, anesthesiologists should be vigilant to the potential impact of anesthetic agents on the success of ART. This chapter reviews the techniques that ART comprises, and reviews the known relationship to and anesthetic management for these procedures.

ASSISTED REPRODUCTIVE TECHNOLOGIES

Although the umbrella of ART covers many techniques, the basic pattern remains essentially the same, and includes hormonal stimulation, oocyte retrieval, in vitro fertilization, and transfer to the fallopian or uterine cavities.

Hormonal Stimulation. The goal of hormonal manipulation is to produce a number of oocytes for retrieval. Although various regimens have been used, since the late 1980s most programs accomplish this by ovarian downregulation to prevent a single large follicle, followed by hyperstimulation to produce a number of follicles and oocytes. Downregulation of the ovary is accomplished via the pituitary with the administration of a gonadotropin-releasing hormone (GnRH) agonist, with leuprolide acetate (Lupron) being the most commonly used in the United States.[6] When given during the midluteal phase of the menstrual cycle, ovarian downregulation is achieved in approximately 10 to 14 days, and is confirmed by ultrasonographic visualization of quiescent ovaries and a low serum estrogen (E_2) level. This ovarian resting phase attempts to minimize the development of a single dominant follicle or the onset of premature ovulation.[7] Once downregulation is achieved, ovarian hyperstimulation with human menopausal gonadotropin (hMG) is initiated and followed by ultrasonographic confirmation of follicular growth and a progressive increase in serum E_2 levels. The GnRH agonist is continued to prevent a premature luteinizing hormone surge. When the follicles reach maturity, ovulation is induced by human chorionic gonadotropin (hCG), and oocyte recovery is performed.

Oocyte Retrieval. Historically performed by laparoscopy,[8] oocyte retrieval, through refinements in ultrasound technologies, has progressed from transabdominal to transvaginal aspirations. Thirty-four to 36 hours after hCG is given, retrieval is performed, allowing for

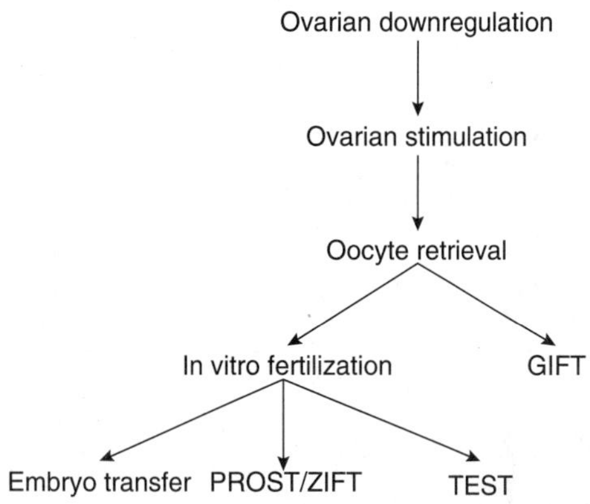

Figure 23–1 Assisted reproductive technology pathway. GIFT, gamete intrafallopian transfer; PROST, pronuclear stage tubal transfer; TEST, tubal embryo stage transfer; ZIFT, zygote intrafallopian transfer.

Procedures Following In Vitro Fertilization

ET (embryo transfer): The placement of fertilized oocytes into the female reproductive system.

PROST (pronuclear stage tubal transfer): The placement of fertilized oocytes at the pronuclei stage (usually 16–24 hr after insemination) into the female reproductive system.

ZIFT (zygote intrafallopian transfer): The placement of fertilized oocytes at the zygote stage (usually 24–26 hr after insemination) into the female reproductive system.

TEST (tubal embryo stage transfer): The placement of fertilzed oocytes at the 2- to 8-cell stage (usually 48 hr after insemination) into the female reproductive system.

the maximal number of oocytes; waiting longer could allow ovulation to reduce the number. Using a transvaginal ultrasound probe and needle, follicles are identified, punctured, and their contents suctioned into prewarmed tubes. The fluid is examined under a microscope, and the oocyte placed in a culture medium. Complications following transvaginal follicle aspiration are low,[9] mainly confined to infection and abscess formation, although hemoperitoneum and iliac hematomas have been reported.[10] Following oocyte retrieval, two major pathways are available: in vitro fertilization (IVF) or gamete intrafallopian transfer (GIFT) (Fig. 23–1).

In Vitro Fertilization. Although the term *in vitro fertilization* (IVF) is often used in reference to all ARTs, technically it applies only to the fertilization of an oocyte with a spermatozoon in a culture medium. Insemination occurs within the first 8 hours following retrieval, based on the maturity of the oocyte.[11] On occasion, oocyte or sperm micromanipulation (see box) is required to allow fertilization to occur, and the first child conceived in this way was born in 1992.[12] Following confirmation of fertilization by direct visualization of two pronuclei and two polar bodies in the perivitelline space, embryos are selected for intrauterine or intrafallopian placement, called a *transfer.* A number of transfer options are available (Fig. 23–1), including embryo transfer (ET), PROST/ZIFT, or TEST (see definitions in box). The advantage of IVF is the confirmation of fertilization prior to the subsequent procedures. By contrast, a GIFT procedure places the oocyte and sperm in the fallopian tubes, and thus direct confirmation of fertilization is not made.

Oocyte and Sperm Micromanipulation

PZD (partial zona dissection): Opening a window in the zona pellucida to allow ingress of sperm

SUZI (subzonal insemination): Injection of the sperm into the perivitelline space

ICSI (intracytoplasmic sperm injection): injection of sperm directly into the cytoplasm of the egg

Embryo Transfer. The term *embryo transfer* technically refers to the placement of embryos into the female reproductive system. The least complex technique occurs transcervically via a semirigid tube placed into the uterine cavity or the fallopian tubes.[13] As the placement of each additional embryo increases the chance of both pregnancy and multiple gestation, individual programs and even countries have placed limits on the number of embryos transferred at one time; in the United Kingdom, the maximum allowed by law is three embryos.[14] Transfers usually occur after 48 to 72 hours of incubation, when embryos have undergone at least one mitotic division. Embryos not used may be cryopreserved until a later date.

PROST, ZIFT, TEST. These procedures alter both the timing and the mechanism of the transfer, with most being performed via laparoscopic technique with placement into the distal portion of the fallopian tube. A pronuclear stage tubal transfer (PROST) occurs 16 to 20 hours after insemination, when the sperm head and ovum form visible pronuclei.[15] A zygote intrafallopian transfer (ZIFT) occurs after the pronuclei nuclear membranes have dissolved and the male and female chromosomes have intermingled. Tubal embryo transfer (TET), also called tubal embryo stage transfer (TEST) occurs after 48 hours of incubation when the embryo is at the 2- to 8-cell stage. With each of these procedures, fertilization is confirmed prior to transfer.

GIFT. Gamete intrafallopian transfer is unique in that oocytes and sperm are placed directly into the ampullary region of the fallopian tube; thus, fertilization occurs in vivo and cannot be confirmed visually. GIFT cycles include ovarian hyperstimulation procedures, retrieval by transvaginal or laparoscopic techniques, and laparoscopic oocyte and sperm placement.

EFFECTS OF ANESTHESIA ON ASSISTED REPRODUCTIVE TECHNOLOGIES

It is unclear what impact anesthesia has on embryogenesis. Although a few agents are believed to be devoid of mutagenic and/or teratogenic effects,[16] the relative overall safety and the lack of rigid cause and effect studies has led to the use of multiple anesthetic agents and techniques for ARTs. Robust causal relationships are difficult to establish due to the myriad of subtle and complex etiologies of infertility and responses to ART stimulation, retrieval, fertilization, and transfer procedures. Potential anesthetic interactions may include a direct or indirect effect of the anesthetic state or agents on gamete and embryo development.

Caution must be applied in evaluating the existing literature owing to differences in ART procedures, drug exposure, and study techniques. General anesthesia, for example, has been suggested to significantly alter the cleavage rate of harvested oocytes when compared with epidural anesthesia.[17] The general and epidural anesthetic agents, however, were used for laparoscopic and transvaginal retrievals, respectively, and the difference in the oocyte retrieval method could have partially accounted for the observed results. Moreover, the impact of carbon dioxide pneumoperitoneum for laparoscopy is not trivial, with decreases in both follicular fluid pH (to below 7.0)[18] and oocyte fertilization rates being noted.[19] In terms of drug exposure, ART protocols themselves can accentuate the pharmacologic effects of medications. Serial measurements of the serum proteins albumin and α_1-acid glycoprotein responsible for drug binding have been shown to significantly decrease with the hormonal manipulation of ART, thus allowing for greater concentrations of free drug.[20]

Broad statements on specific anesthetic drugs must be interpreted carefully. Different drug administration methods, doses, combinations, and timing of exposure may potentially alter results. A local anesthetic, for instance, yields dissimilar pharmacokinetic profiles when given paracervically, intrathecally, or epidurally. Moreover, although data exist on anesthesia's impact on animal and human fetal development, extrapolating these results to embryonic development is difficult. In that regard, anesthesia may have different effects on an oocyte versus an embryo, and thus the same anesthetic for a GIFT versus a TEST procedure, in which exposure occurs prior to and after fertilization, respectively, may yield different information. Interestingly, a few studies make strong conclusions on anesthesia but neglect to identify the actual agents used.[21]

The impact of anesthetic agents needs to be continually revisited. The applicability of interspecies data and assay methods, such as the two-cell mouse embryo model, to prediction of human reproductive toxicity has been challenged,[22, 23] although primarily on low sensitivity, and not specificity. Moreover, strict attention should be applied to whether the experiments were conducted on intact subjects, unfertilized oocytes, or fertilized embryos. With these considerations in mind, the available literature on this topic can be evaluated.

Local Anesthetics

The absolute dose of local anesthetics administered must be taken in context, since other determinants of systemic and ultimately follicular fluid concentrations, including the physiochemical and vasoactive properties, the presence of additives, and the site of injection, may play more important roles. In general, and independent of the agent used, absorption from different sites follows a particular order: paracervical, caudal, epidural, then spinal.[24] In addition, it has been demonstrated that significantly higher free fractions of the local anesthetic bupivacaine[20] exist when comparing concentrations prior to and after stimulation because of a decrease in serum binding proteins. Yet even with a knowledge of follicular concentrations, animal and human studies evaluating the potential toxicity of local anesthetics on embryogenesis have yielded conflicting results.

Animal Studies. The effect of local anesthetics appears related to the agent and the timing of exposure. Mouse oocytes incubated for 30 minutes in lidocaine or 2-chloroprocaine at concentrations of 1.0 and 0.1 μg/mL, respectively, exhibited abnormal fertilization and embryo development. Bupivacaine, by contrast, affected oocytes only at the highest studied concentration of 100 μg/mL.[25] Hamster oocytes exposed to procaine (3×10^{-3} M) or tetracaine (7.5×10^{-5} M) were noted to have impaired cortical granule release, thereby inhibiting the zona reaction.[26] Normally, when the first sperm passes through the zona pellucida, the zona reaction renders this layer impermeable to other sperm; alterations to this reaction can allow more than one sperm to enter the oocyte, creating abnormal chromosomal numbers (polyploidy). Clinically, this may have little significance because it is unknown how these levels correspond to those obtained during anesthesia, and more importantly, the impairment of cortical granules is reversed by washing the eggs. Moreover, all embryos are usually screened prior to uterine transfer.

By contrast, in vivo rat studies demonstrated that chronic administration of lidocaine (100–250 mg/kg/day) prior to mating and throughout pregnancy did not affect measures of reproduction, including implantation, rates of resorption, or teratogenic formation.[27] Moreover, two-cell mouse embryos noted no adverse affects when incubated for 4 hours with lidocaine in concentrations of 1 to 100 μg/mL.[28]

Human Studies. Local anesthetics appear to have minimal impact on ART outcome. Women undergoing paracervical blocks for embryo transfer, despite obtaining follicular fluid lidocaine concentrations of 1.1 μg/mL, demonstrated differences in fertilization, cleavage, or pregnancy rates when compared with women without blocks.[29] When compared with general anesthesia under halothane, patients undergoing epidural anesthesia with bupivacaine or lidocaine for GIFT procedures had significantly higher cleavage rates (47% vs. 37%).[17]

Barbiturates, Benzodiazepines, Opioids, and Propofol

Animal Studies. Two-cell mouse embryos cultured in midazolam, up to and including a concentration of 12.5 μg/mL, underwent normal development.[30] In vivo, midazolam in doses up to 500 times (35 mg/kg) greater than the dose administered when human ova were harvested (0.07–0.08 mg/kg), given via intraperitoneal injection in female mice prior to coitus, did not affect the fertilization or early development of the oocytes. Of interest, midazolam appeared to accelerate embryo development rather than inhibit it, which may raise the possibility that midazolam increases DNA replication or translation.[30]

Sea urchin eggs, when incubated in the presence of fentanyl, 3.3 nmol (equivalent to giving 344 μg to a 60-kg woman), as well as 7 and 14 times this amount, demonstrated no effects on fertilization or early development.[31] By contrast, earlier work with morphine in the same model, when fertilized in doses that would correspond to approximately 50 mg of morphine, had approximately 30% of the eggs exhibit polyspermy.[32] Following fertilization, two-cell mouse embryos, when incubated for 30 minutes in either fentanyl (1.5 ng/mL) or meperidine (250 ng/mL), underwent normal embryo development.[33]

Propofol, evaluated in clinically relevant concentrations, was noted to only minimally decrease hamster sperm motility,[34] a quality control method for water and culture media used in ART.

Human Studies. When given for laparoscopic egg retrieval as an induction dose of 5 mg/kg, thiopental and thiamylal were measurable in the follicular fluid as early as 11 minutes, and continued to increase up to 50 minutes despite decreasing plasma levels.[35] The effect of these medications on fertilization or embryo development was not reported. When an induction dose of thiopental (5.4 mg/kg) was compared with propofol (2.7 mg/kg) for GIFT procedures, no differences in clinical pregnancy rates were noted.[36]

Midazolam[37] and fentanyl,[38] given as premedication for general anesthesia for oocyte retrieval, when detected, were in extremely minimal follicular fluid concentrations.

Propofol, when given as an induction bolus of 2.5 mg/kg as part of a general anesthetic for oocyte retrieval, demonstrated no correlation between serum and follicular fluid concentrations, and no effect on the oocyte cleavage rates.[39] When compared to sedation with midazolam and fentanyl, the addition of propofol in doses of 1.87 to 8 mg/kg, did not have a negative impact on cumulative embryo scores, probability of clinical pregnancy, or implantation rate.[40] However, when a propofol/nitrous oxide technique was compared with an isoflurane/nitrous oxide technique for laparoscopic PROST procedures, the clinical and ongoing pregnancy rates were higher in the isoflurane group (54% vs. 30%).[41]

Nitrous Oxide

Noted to inhibit methionine synthetase activity and DNA synthesis in animal[42] and human[43] tissues, nitrous oxide was speculated to affect fertilization, and the cleavage of human oocytes may be affected.

Animal Studies. Mammalian HeLa cells, when exposed to hyperbaric nitrous oxide, demonstrated altered chromosomal alignment during mitosis.[44] When 30 minutes of nitrous oxide was administered 4 hours prior to expected cell cleavage, two-cell mouse embryos underwent slower development to the four-cell stage.[45] However, when two-cell mouse embryos were followed to the later blastocyst stage, no effect of nitrous oxide exposure was noted.[33]

Human Studies. In vivo, when an isoflurane/oxygen mixture was compared with and without nitrous oxide for laparoscopic oocyte retrieval, no differences in fertilization or pregnancy rates were noted.[46] Moreover, during PROST procedures, which transfer one-cell embryos into the fallopian tubes, the use of nitrous oxide,[41] although not directly studied, did not appear to be detrimental to reproductive success.

Volatile Inhalational Agents

Animal and human studies suggest that halogenated anesthetic agents depress DNA synthesis, and may have negative reproductive effects.

Animal Studies. Halogenated agents appear to affect cell division by disrupting the spindle-forming apparatus, thus creating multipolar spindles, unequal divisions, and chromosome lagging. Halothane and enflurane were noted to prevent cytoplasmic cleavage[47] and disrupt mitotic spindle microtubules,[48] respectively, thereby increasing the number of abnormal mitotic figures. Halothane, but not enflurane or methoxyflurane, inhibited cell development in sea urchin eggs.[49] Two-cell mouse embryos, when exposed for 30 minutes to 0.75% isoflurane/nitrous oxide/oxygen, had a reduction in development to the blastocyst stage in comparison to nitrous oxide/oxygen.[33] In an interesting study, when the sera from humans undergoing oocyte retrieval via laparoscopy with nitrous oxide/oxygen with 1% to 1.5% isoflurane were compared with the sera from patients undergoing spinal or intravenous sedation, a decrease in two-cell mouse embryo development was noted.[50] In vivo, however, when female hamsters were anesthetized with halothane and immediately mated, the cell cycle was prolonged, but the number of lethal mutations or implantations was not affected.[51]

Human Studies. Human studies seem to indicate that halogenated agents have some effect, and agent-specific differences exist. In human lymphoid cell lines, although halothane, enflurane, and methoxyflurane all increased mitotic abnormalities, when exposure was limited to the first 24 hours of a 48-hour time frame, only halothane increased the number of abnormal mitoses.[52] In addition, although a retrospective analysis comparing general anesthesia with halothane/nitrous oxide versus regional anesthesia via lidocaine epidural or paracervical techniques noted no differences in the embryo yield or quality, lower clinical pregnancy and delivery rates occurred in the general anesthesia group.[53] When general anesthesia was provided by fentanyl with nitrous oxide/oxygen, isoflurane/oxygen, or a combination, a negative influence of isoflurane was noted on cell cleavage, with immature oocytes being more susceptible.[54] When the first and last oocytes collected by laparoscopy under general anesthesia via 50:50 nitrous oxide/oxygen with 1.0% enflurane or 1.0% isoflurane, fertilization rates of the eggs collected later were decreased[19]; unclear, however, is the impact of carbon dioxide pneumoperitoneum.

Halothane, when compared with isoflurane in IVF, has been noted to significantly lower the pregnancy[55] and birth rates.[56] These data suggest that halogenated agents may affect IVF outcome differently, and caution is therefore advised in using new anesthetics (e.g., sevoflurane, desflurane). However, the applicability of this data to later stages of development may be limited, as the routine use of isoflurane for PROST with one-cell embryos has yielded high pregnancy rates.[57]

Although a number of factors including surgery[58] may affect its serum concentration,[59] prolactin has been hypothesized as a mechanism by which anesthesia may impact ARTs. By affecting both follicular development[60] and corpus luteum production of progesterone,[61] high prolactin levels may be potentially detrimental to oocyte production and embryo uterine receptivity. In this regard, halogenated agents may offer an advantage. When 0.5% to 1% halothane in nitrous oxide/oxygen was compared with "neuroleptanaesthesia" consisting of droperidol, 0.1 mg/kg, with fentanyl, 4 μg/kg, for transvaginal retrieval, higher plasma prolactin levels and lower plasma progesterone levels were noted in the latter group; owing to the small sample size, however, little can be concluded on the overall impact on pregnancy.[62] In addition, although a dramatic rise in plasma prolactin levels occurred with enflurane in nitrous oxide/oxygen, no changes were noted for the first 4 to 10 minutes after induction, no changes in follicular fluid prolactin levels were found, and no observed effects on the incidence of fertilization and early embryonic development in vitro were noted, although the incidence of pregnancy was highest in the group of patients with the lowest preanesthesia plasma prolactin levels.[63]

Antiemetic Drugs

The previous discussion on prolactin levels may have implications beyond anesthetic agents. The antiemetic drugs droperidol and metoclopramide have been known to affect prolactin levels. Metoclopramide has been noted to induce hyperprolactinemia, which has subsequently impaired ovarian follicle maturation and corpus luteum function in women.[64] The effect of other antiemetics on prolactin levels and reproductive success is unknown at this time. However, the likelihood of emesis increases with ART stimulation owing to the changes in plasma estradiol levels; patients undergoing IVF with estrogen levels that increased less than 10-fold and more than 10-fold, experienced 26% and 39% incidence of emesis, respectively.[65] Therefore with each case the risk of potentially impairing pregnancy outcome should be weighed against the benefit of potentially reducing nausea and emesis. Moreover, this risk-benefit ratio should be considered when aspiration prophylaxis is given to morbidly obese individuals.

ANESTHETIC MANAGEMENT FOR ASSISTED REPRODUCTIVE TECHNOLOGIES

In general, most patients undergoing ART procedures are young and otherwise healthy. In terms of preoperative studies, unless their history mandates otherwise, at the Brigham and Women's Hospital, we do not require preoperative laboratory studies, electrocardiograms, or chest radiographs. Preoperatively, all patients must remain nothing per os (NPO) status from the midnight prior to the day of retrieval. For patients with risk factors for aspiration (e.g., obesity, history of reflux), a nonparticulate antacid is given prior to the procedure.

On occasion, a patient may not adhere to strict NPO policies and consideration is given to delaying or cancelling the case. However, these decisions should not be taken without careful analysis of the potential risks and benefits. In terms of risks, the window for maximal oocyte retrieval (usually 36 hours following hCG) may be missed, leading to spontaneous ovulation and loss of oocytes. Moreover, should aspiration of follicles not be performed, an increased incidence of ovarian hyperstimulation syndrome,[66] with its potential for tension ascites, thromboembolic phenomena, renal and hepatic dysfunction, and adult respiratory distress syndrome[67] may be observed. Finally, a complete or even partial loss of a stimulation cycle may invalidate the considerable effort and expense leading to the retrieval or transfer procedure. In terms of benefits, the reduction in aspiration risk produced by delay or cancellation of the procedure is difficult to quantify. A review of the most recently approved practice guidelines of the American Society of Anesthesiologists demonstrates a relaxation of the standards for same-day admission or ambulatory procedures in healthy patients,[68] now allowing a 2-hour fast for clear liquids in unlimited amounts. In addition, the overall importance of gastric fluid volume has been questioned.[69] Although the use of regional anesthesia does not obviate the risk of aspiration, it can potentially reduce the risk; as such, it may represent a suitable alternative to delay or cancellation.

As with other-day surgery cases, the ideal anesthetic results in effective anesthesia with minimal postoperative nausea, sedation, pain, and psychomotor impairment.

Ultrasound-Guided Transabdominal Oocyte Retrieval. Although oocyte retrieval is more commonly performed transvaginally, the transabdominal approach is occasionally used. Although usually conducted under general anesthesia, local infiltration and epidural techniques have been used. When infiltration with 1% lidocaine, general anesthesia with ketamine and midazolam (1 mg/kg IV and 0.15 mg/kg IV, respectively), and epidural anesthesia with 10 to 15 mL of 0.25% bupivacaine were directly compared, local anesthesia was tolerated poorly, resulting in impaired recovery rates and frequent conversion to general anesthesia, although no differences in fertilization rates were noted.[70]

Ultrasound-Guided Transvaginal Oocyte Retrieval. With the shift of oocyte retrieval to transvaginal techniques, the anesthetic options have expanded to include paracervical, spinal, epidural, and general anesthetic techniques. Although the absence of anesthesia[71] and paracervical blocks has been reported, both of these techniques are often abandoned because of patient discomfort.[53] When asked to evaluate the experience of transvaginal follicle aspiration under a paracervical block with pethidine, 75 mg intramuscular premedication, 43% of patients reported pain, and 28% required additional sedation. Interestingly, the pain may not be overtly obvious; in 23% of the cases in which the patient reported pain, the physician performing the oocyte retrieval was not aware that the patient was experiencing discomfort.[72] The discomfort stems from the paracervical anesthetic covering only the vaginal, and not ovarian, wall.

Although sedation techniques have widespread acceptance,[73] the doses required may involve a loss of consciousness, allow the patient to move at critical times, and result in prolonged recovery room stays.[72] Moreover, one report noted that the number of unplanned hospital admissions was higher after the use of conscious sedation than general anesthesia; the overall rate of complications, however, was very low (0.16%), and most of the admissions were for intra-abdominal bleeding.[74]

Epidural[17] and spinal anesthesia have been used successfully. When compared with sedation techniques with propofol and mask-assisted ventilation with nitrous oxide, epidural anesthesia with bupivacaine provided fewer complications, especially the absence of nausea and emesis.[75] Spinal anesthesia may be preferable to epidural anesthesia owing to the lower systemic and hence follicular levels of anesthesia, a more rapid turnover, and a more reliable anesthetic.[76] At the Brigham and Women's Hospital, spinal anesthesia with lidocaine (45 mg) and fentanyl (10 μg) is the preferred method for oocyte retrieval owing to its excellent anesthesia, minimal exposure of oocytes to agents, and short recovery profile. The use of hyperbaric 1.5% lidocaine (45 mg) provides significantly shorter recovery time than an equivalent dose of 5% lidocaine.[77] Moreover, the addition of fentanyl (10 μg) to lidocaine improves postoperative analgesia for the first 24 hours, with no change in time for urination, ambulation, and discharge when compared with lidocaine alone.[78] The benefit of reducing the dose of local anesthetic by increasing the amount of narcotic is being studied at the present time with good success.

General anesthesia can be used, and it is our practice to use total intravenous anesthesia with propofol (titrated) and fentanyl (50–100 μg), with midazolam (1–2 mg) as an optional premedicant. Most patients are managed with spontaneous ventilation via high-flow oxygen mask and the use of carbon dioxide analysis. On rare occasion, or in individuals with a higher risk of aspiration, an endotracheal tube is placed. In individuals undergoing laparoscopic or ultrasound-guided oocyte harvesting, inhalational anesthesia with enflurane and 70% nitrous oxide produced significantly higher incidence of nausea and vomiting and unplanned admissions when compared with propofol with alfentanil with air/oxygen.[79]

Embryo Transfer. This procedure is relatively painless and usually done without analgesia or anesthesia. However, on occasion, intravenous sedation or general anesthesia is needed.

PROST, ZIFT, TEST, GIFT. These procedures, usually performed by laparoscopy, can be done under local, regional, or general anesthesia. General anesthesia is often employed to provide optimal immobile operating conditions for placement of embryos in the fallopian tubes. At my institution, endotracheal intubation follows an induction with intravenous propofol and succinylcholine, followed by maintenance with oxygen/isoflurane and either a short-acting nondepolarizing muscle relaxant (e.g., atracurium/vecuronium) or a succinylcholine drip. Patients undergoing PROST procedures with a propofol/nitrous oxide technique had lower postoperative sedation, visual analogue scale score, and emesis when compared with an isoflurane/nitrous oxide technique.[80]

Future Technologies. Ultrasound and fiberoptic methods of fallopian tube cannulation have been demonstrated.[81, 82] These alterations could make laparoscopic intervention unnecessary, and offer potential changes in the types of anesthesia provided.

Postanesthesia Care. Postoperatively, especially following a laparoscopy, patients may report abdominal pain (including uterine cramping) and shoulder pain. It is our practice to use small doses of intravenous fentanyl, 25 to 50 μg, to allay this discomfort. As changes in the prostaglandin milieu can affect embryo implantation, nonsteroidal anti-inflammatory drugs are avoided in these patients.[83] Nausea and emesis can also occur, although as discussed previously, we usually try to limit exposure to droperidol and metoclopramide. In the event that these symptoms do not abate, we use these medications in standard dosages. Patients must be hemodynamically stable, and be able to take and retain oral liquids, ambulate, and void prior to discharge. At my institution, every patient undergoing anesthesia for ART receives a follow-up call at 24 hours postprocedure to assess for questions or complications.

CONCLUSION

Advances in assisted reproductive therapies and technologies continue to underscore the importance of subtle differences in outcome. As such, attention and

❖ SUMMARY

Key Points

- Causal relationships between anesthesia and the effects on embryogenesis are difficult to establish owing to the myriad of subtle and complex etiologies of infertility and the responses to assisted reproductive technology (ART) stimulation, retrieval, fertilization, and transfer procedures.
- Animal and human studies exist for many anesthetic agents. Overall, anesthetic agents are relatively safe for these procedures and local, general, epidural, and spinal anesthesia all have been used. However, steps can be taken to reduce exposure to individual agents.
- Antiemetic drugs should be administered, with attention to the risk-benefit ratios, as some of these medications may have a deleterious impact on follicle maturation.

Key Reference

Ditkoff ECX, Plumb J, Selick A, Sauer MV: Anesthesia practices in the United States common to in vitro fertilization (IVF) centers. J Assist Reprod Genet 1997; 14:145–147.

Case Stem

A 38-year-old nulliparous woman 63 inches in height and weighing 90 kg, with no medical history other than infertility, is admitted to the assisted reproductive technology suite for transvaginal oocyte retrieval. The patient asks you about the anesthetic options and their potential impact on her ART procedure. What will you tell her?

vigilance should be given to each step to accurately assess and identify their etiologies, mechanisms, and implications. Anesthesiologists should not be disinterested in the impact of these technologies on anesthetic practice, nor in the potential impact of anesthetics on reproductive outcomes. Instead, with anesthesiologists' active participation in the enhancement of the care and anesthetics that are provided, improved outcomes for this particular patient group, as well as other patient populations undergoing physiologic or iatrogenic hormonal manipulation, may be realized.

References

1. Steptoe PC, Edwards RG: Birth after the reimplantation of a human embryo. Lancet 1978; 2:366.
2. Society for Assisted Reproductive Technology, The American Society for Reproductive Medicine: Assisted reproductive technology in the United States and Canada: 1995 results generated from The American Society for Reproductive Medicine/Society for Assisted Reproductive Technology Registry. Fertil Steril 1998; 69:389–398.
3. Assisted reproductive technology in the United States and Canada: 1994 results generated from the American Society for Reproductive Medicine/Society for Assisted Reproductive Technology Registry. Fertil Steril 1995; 66:697–705.
4. Sixth annual report. London: Human Fertilisation and Embryology Authority; 1997.
5. Yovich JL, Edirisinghe WR, Yovich JM: Methods of water purification for the preparation of culture media in an IVF-ET programme. Hum Reprod 1988; 3:245–248.
6. Meldrum DR, Wisot A, Hamilton F, et al: Routine pituitary suppression with leuprolide before ovarian stimulation for oocyte retrieval. Fertil Steril 1989; 51:455–459.
7. deZiegler D, Cedars MI, Randle D, et al: Suppression of the ovary using a gonadotropin-releasing hormone agonist prior to stimulation for oocyte retrieval. Fertil Steril 1987; 48:807–810.
8. Edwards RG, Steptoe PC, Purdy JM: Establishing full-term human pregnancies using cleaving embryos grown in vitro. Br J Obstet Gynaecol 1980; 87:737–756.
9. Evers JL, Larsen JF, Gnanny GG, Sieck UV: Complications and problems in transvaginal sector scan–guided follicle aspiration. Fertil Steril 1988; 49:278–282.
10. Bennet SJ, Waterstone JJ, Cheng WC, Parsons J: Complications of transvaginal ultrasound-directed follicle aspirations: a review of 2670 consecutive procedures. J Assist Reprod Genet 1993; 10:72–77.
11. Hammitt DG, Syrop CH, Hahn SJ, et al: Comparison of concurrent pregnancy rates for in vitro fertilization-embryo transfer, pronuclear stage embryo transfer, and gamete intrafallopian transfer. Hum Reprod 1990; 5:947–954.
12. Palermo G, Joris H, Devroey P, Van Steirteghem AC: Pregnancies after intracytoplasmic injection of single spermatozoon into an oocyte. Lancet 1992; 340:17–18.
13. Jansen RP, Anderson JC, Sutherland PD: Nonoperative embryo transfer to the fallopian tube. N Engl J Med 1988; 319:288–291.
14. Van Steirteghem A: Outcome of assisted reproductive technology. N Engl J Med 1998; 338:194–195.
15. Devroey P, Staessen C, Camus M, et al: Zygote intrafallopian transfer as a successful treatment for unexplained infertility. Fertil Steril 1989; 52:246–249.
16. Eger IE: Isoflurane: a review. Anesthesiology 1981; 55:559–576.
17. Lefebvre G, Vauthier D, Seebacher J, et al: In vitro fertilization: a comparative study of cleavage rates under epidural and general anesthesia—interest for gamete intrafallopian transfer. J In Vitro Fertil Embryo Transfer 1988; 5:305–306.
18. Degueldre M, Puissant F, Camus M, et al: Effects of carbon dioxide insufflation at laparoscopy on the gas phase in oocyte recovery fluids [abstract]. J In Vitro Fertil Embryo Transfer 1984: 1:106.
19. Boyers SP, Lavy G, Russell JB, DeCherney AH: A paired analysis of in vitro fertilization and cleavage rates of first- versus last-recovered preovulatory human oocytes exposed to varying intervals of 100% CO_2 pneumoperitoneum and general anesthesia. Fertil Steril 1987; 48:969–974.
20. Tsen LC, Arthur GR, Datta S, et al: Estrogen induced changes in protein binding of bupivacaine during in-vitro fertilization. Anesthesiology 1997; 87:879–883.
21. Lewin A, Margalioth EJ, Rabinowitz R, Schenker JG: Comparative study of ultrasonically guided percutaneous aspiration with local anesthesia and laparoscopic aspiration of follicles in an in vitro fertilization program. Am J Obstet Gynecol 1985; 151:621–624.
22. Rinehart JS, Bavister BD, Gerrity M: Quality control in the in vitro fertilization laboratory: comparison of bioassay systems for water quality. J In Vitro Fertil Embryo Transfer 1988; 5:335–342.
23. Davidson A, Vermesh M, Lobo RA, Paulson RJ: Mouse embryo culture as quality control for human in vitro fertilization: the one-cell versus the two-cell model. Fertil Steril 1988; 49:516–521.
24. Tucker GT, Mather LE: Properties, absorption, and disposition of local anesthetic agents. *In* Cousins MJ, Bridenbaugh PO (eds): Neural Blockade in Clinical Anesthesia and Management of Pain, 2nd ed. Philadelphia: JB Lippincott; 1988:47–110.
25. Schnell VL, Sacco AG, Savoy-Moore RT, et al: Effects of oocyte exposure to local anesthetics on in vitro fertilization and embryo development in the mouse. Reprod Toxicol 1992; 6:323–327.

26. Ahuja KK: In vitro inhibition of the block to polyspermy of hamster eggs by tertiary amine local anesthetics. J Reprod Fertil 1982; 65:15–22.
27. Fujinaga M, Mazze RI: Reproductive and teratogenic effects of lidocaine in Sprague-Dawley rats. Anesthesiology 1986; 65:626–632.
28. McFarland CW, Witt BR, Wheeler CA, Thorneycroft IH: Effects of short term exposure to lidocaine on mouse embryo development in vitro [abstract]. Abstract book, 45th Meeting of the American Fertility Society, 1989; 146:212.
29. Wikland M, Evers H, Jakobsson AH, et al: The concentration of lidocaine in follicular fluid when used for paracervical block in a human IVF-ET programme. Hum Reprod 1990; 5:920–923.
30. Swanson RF, Leavitt MG: Fertilization and mouse embryo development in the presence of midazolam. Anesth Analg 1992; 75:549–554.
31. Bruce DL, Hinkley R, Norman PF: Fentanyl does not inhibit fertilization or early development of sea urchin eggs. Anesth Analg 1985; 64:498–500.
32. Cardasis C, Schuel H: The sea urchin egg as a model system to study effects of narcotics on secretion. *In* Ford DH, Clouet DH (eds): Tissue Responses to Addictive Drugs. New York: Spectrum; 1976:631–640.
33. Chetkowski RJ, Nass TE. Isoflurane inhibits early mouse embryo development in vitro. Fertil Steril 1988; 49:171–173.
34. Vincent RD, Hammitt DG, Baker MT, et al: Evaluation of the potential embryo toxicity of propofol using an in vitro fertilization quality control test (hamster sperm motility assay) [abstract]. Abstract book, Annual Meeting of the Society of Obstetric Anesthesiology and Perinatology; 1992:58.
35. Endler GC, Stout M, Magyar DM, et al: Follicular fluid concentrations of thiopental and thiamylal during laparoscopy for oocyte retrieval. Fertil Steril 1987; 48:828.
36. Pierce ET, Smalky M, Alper MM, et al: Comparison of pregnancy rates following gamete intrafallopian transfer (GIFT) under general anesthesia with thiopental sodium or propofol. J Clin Anesth 1992; 4:394–398.
37. Chopineau J, Bazin JE, Terrisse MP, et al: Assay for midazolam in liquor folliculi during in vitro fertilization under anesthesia. Clin Pharm 1993; 12:770–773.
38. Schoeffler PF, Levron JC, Jany L, et al: Follicular concentration of fentanyl during laparoscopy for oocyte retrieval—correlation with in vitro fertilization results [abstract]. Anesthesiology 1988; 69:A573.
39. Palot M, Haarika G, Pigeon F, et al: Propofol in general anesthesia for IVF (by vaginal and transurethral route)—follicular fluid concentration and cleavage rate [abstract]. Anesthesiology 1988; 69:A573.
40. Rosenblatt MA, Bradford CN, Bodian CA, Grunfeld L: The effect of a propofol-based sedation technique on cumulative embryo scores, clinical pregnancy rates, and implantation rates in patients undergoing embryo transfers with donor oocytes. J Clin Anesth 1997; 9:614–617.
41. Vincent RD, Syrop CH, Van Voorhis BJ, et al: An evaluation of the effect of anesthetic technique on reproductive success after laparoscopic pronuclear stage transfer. Anesthesiology 1995; 82:352–358.
42. Baden JM, Serra M, Mazze RI: Inhibition of fetal methionine synthetase by nitrous oxide. Br J Anaesth 1984; 56:523–526.
43. Koblin DD, Waskell L, Watson JE, et al: Nitrous oxide inactivates methionine synthetase in human liver. Anesth Analg 1982; 61:75–78.
44. Rao PN: Mitotic synchrony in mammalian cells treated with nitrous oxide at high pressure. Science 1968; 160:774–776.
45. Warren JR, Shaw B, Steinkampf MP: Effects of nitrous oxide on preimplantation mouse embryo cleavage and development. Biol Reprod 1990; 43:158–161.
46. Rosen MA, Rozien MF, Eger EI, et al: The effect of nitrous oxide on in vitro fertilization success rate. Anesthesiology 1987; 67:42–44.
47. Sturrock JE, Nunn JF: Mitosis in mammalian cells during exposure to anesthetics. Anesthesiology 1975; 43:21–33.
48. Kusyk CJ, Hsu TC: Mitotic anomalies induced by three inhalation halogenated anesthetics. Environ Res 1976; 12:366–370.
49. Hinkley RE, Wright BD: Comparative effects of halothane, enflurane, and methoxyflurane on the incidence of abnormal development using sea urchin gametes as an in vitro model system. Anesth Analg 1985; 64:1005–1009.
50. Matt DW, Steingold KA, Dastvan CM, et al: Effects of sera from patients given various anesthetics on preimplantation mouse embryo development in vitro. J In Vitro Fertil Embryo Transfer 1991; 8:191–197.
51. Basler A, Rohrborn G: Lack of mutogenic effects of halothane in mammals in vivo. Anesthesiology 1981; 55:143–147.
52. Kusyk CJ, Hsu TC: Mitotic anomalies induced by three inhalation halogenated anesthetics. Environ Res 1976; 2:366–370.
53. Gonen O, Shulman A, Ghetler Y, et al: The impact of different types of anesthesia on in vitro fertilization-embryo transfer treatment outcome. J Assist Reprod Genet 1995; 12:678–682.
54. Hayes MF, Sacco AG, Savoy-Moore RT, et al: Effect of general anesthesia on fertilization and cleavage of human oocytes in vitro. Fertil Steril 1987; 48:975–981.
55. Fishel S, Webster J, Faratian B, Jackson P: General anesthesia for intrauterine placement of human conceptuses after in vitro fertilization. J In Vitro Fertil Embryo Transfer 1987; 4:260–264.
56. Critchlow BM, Ibrahim Z, Pollard BJ: General anesthesia for gamete intrafallopian transfer. Eur J Anaesthesiol 1991; 8:381–384.
57. Vincent RD, Syrop CH, Van Voorhis BJ, et al. An evaluation of the effect of anesthetic technique on reproductive success after laparoscopic pronuclear stage transfer. Anesthesiology 1995; 82:352–358.
58. Soules MR, Sutton GP, Hammond CB, Haney AF: Endocrine changes at operation under general anesthesia: reproductive hormone fluctuations in young women. Fertil Steril 1980; 33:364–371.
59. Kreitmann O, Nixon WE, Hodgen GD: Induced corpus luteum dysfunction after aspiration of preovulatory follicle in monkeys. Fertil Steril 1981; 35(suppl):236.
60. McNeilly AS, Glaisir A, Jonassen J, Howie P: Evidence for direct inhibition of ovarian function by prolactin. J Reprod Fertil 1982; 65:559–569.
61. Demura R, Ono M, Demura H, et al: Prolactin directly inhibits basal as well as gonadotrophin-stimulated secretion of progesterone in 17β-oestradiol in the human ovary. J Clin Endocrinol Metab 1982; 54:1246–1250.
62. Naito Y, Tamai S, Fukata J, et al: Comparison of endocrinological stress responses associated with transvaginal ultrasound-guided oocyte pick-up under halothane anaesthesia and neuroleptanaesthesia. Can J Anaesth 1989; 36:633–636.
63. Forman R, Fishel B, Edwards RG, Walters E: The influence of transient hyperprolactinemia on in vitro fertilization in humans. J Clin Endocrinol Metab 1985; 60:517–522.
64. Kauppila A, Leiononen P, Vihko R, Ylostalo P: Metoclopramide-induced hyperprolactinaemia impairs ovarian follicle maturation and corpus luteum function in women. J Clin Endocrinol Metab 1982; 54:955–960.
65. Coburn R, Lane J, Harrison K, Hennessey J: Postoperative vomiting factors in IVF patients. Aust N Z J Obstet Gynaecol 1993; 33:57–60.
66. Rabinowitz R, Simon A, Lewin A, et al: Manipulating the follicular phase in IVF cycles: a comparison of two HMG stimulation protocols. Gynecol Endocrinol 1989; 3:117–123.
67. Schenker JG: Prevention and treatment of ovarian hyperstimulation. Hum Reprod 1993; 8:653–659.
68. Practice guidelines for preoperative fasting and the use of pharmacologic agents to reduce the risk of pulmonary aspiration: application to healthy patients undergoing elective procedures: a report by the American Society of Anesthesiologists Task Force on Preoperative Fasting. Anesthesiology 1999; 90:896–905.
69. Schreiner MS: Gastric fluid volume: is it really a risk factor for pulmonary aspiration? Anesth Analg 1998; 87:754–756.
70. Sterzik K, Jonatha W, Keckstein G, et al: Ultrasonically guided follicle aspiration for oocyte retrieval in an in vitro fertilization program: further simplification. Int J Gynaecol Obstet 1987; 24:309–314.
71. Feichtinger W: Current technique of oocyte retrieval. Curr Opin Obstet Gynecol 1992; 4:697–701.

72. Hammarberg K, Wikland M, Nilsson L, Enk L: Patient's experience of transvaginal follicle aspiration under local anesthesia. Ann N Y Acad Sci 1988; 541:135–137.
73. Ditkoff ECX, Plumb J, Selick A, Sauer MV: Anesthesia practices in the United States common to in vitro fertilization (IVF) centers. J Assist Reprod Genet 1997; 14:145–147.
74. Oskowitz SP, Berger MJ, Mullen L, et al: Safety of a freestanding surgical unit for the assisted reproductive technologies. Fertil Steril 1995; 63:874–879.
75. Botta G, D'Angelo A, D'ari GD, et al: Epidural anesthesia in an in vitro fertilization and embryo transfer program. J Assist Reprod Genet 1995; 12:187–190.
76. Endler GC, Magyar DM, Hayes MF, Moghiosi KS: Use of spinal anesthesia in laparoscopy for IVF. Fertil Steril 1985; 43:809–810.
77. Manica V, Bader AM, Fragneto G, et al: Anesthesia for in vitro fertilization: a comparison of 1.5% and 5% spinal lidocaine for ultrasonically guided oocyte retrieval. Anesth Analg 1993; 77:453–456.
78. Martin R, Tsen LC, Tzeng G, et al: Anesthesia for in vitro fertilization: the addition of fentanyl to 1.5% lidocaine. Anesth Analg 1999; 88:523–526.
79. Raftery S, Sherry E: Total intravenous anaesthesia with propofol and alfentanil protects against postoperative nausea and vomiting. Can J Anaesth 1992; 39:37–41.
80. Vincent RD, Syrop CH, Van Voorhis BJ, et al: An evaluation of the effect of anesthetic technique on reproductive success after laparoscopic pronuclear stage transfer. Anesthesiology 1995; 82:352–358.
81. Yovich JL, Draper RR, Turner SR, Cummins JM: Transcervical tubal embryo-stage transfer (TC-TEST). J In Vitro Fertil Embryo Transfer 1990; 7:137–140.
82. Pearlstone AC, Surrey ES, Kerin JF: The linear everting catheter: a nonhysteroscopic, transvaginal technique for access and microendoscopy of the fallopian tube. Fertil Steril 1992; 58:854–857.
83. Von der Weiden RM, Helmerhorst FM, Keirse MJ: Influence of prostaglandins and platelet activating factor on implantation. Hum Reprod 1991; 6:436–442.

24

Postcesarean Analgesia: Patient-Controlled Analgesia and Neuraxial Techniques

❖ Raymond S. Sinatra, MD, PhD
❖ Chakib M. Ayoub, MD
❖ Ferne B. Sevarino, MD

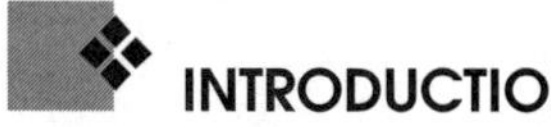

INTRODUCTION

In 1973, Marks and Sachar[1] published the classic report on the undermedication of pain in hospitalized patients. They found that more than 70% of patients experienced inadequate pain control as suboptimal doses of opioids were ordered, and less than one fourth of that amount was actually administered.

Undermedication and poorly controlled pain are important considerations in mothers recovering from cesarean section, as they interfere with ambulation, breast-feeding, and early maternal-infant bonding after cesarean delivery. These activities are further hampered by the sedation and other side effects associated with as needed intramuscular administration of analgesics. Nursing mothers are especially concerned about neonatal exposure to analgesics, and some women avoid medications, especially opioid analgesics, that may accumulate in breast milk.[2]

Most cesarean deliveries in the United States are performed with regional anesthesia,[3, 4] and the administration of epidural and intrathecal opioids (i.e., intraspinal or neuraxial administration) has become a common means of augmenting intraoperative anesthesia and optimizing postoperative analgesia.[3–5] More than 90% of obstetric anesthesiologists administer intraspinal opioids in this setting.[5] Postoperative pain control may be achieved by neuraxial opioids alone, intravenous patient-controlled analgesia (IV-PCA), or a multimodal approach employing both techniques. The following review outlines the application and benefits of IV-PCA as well as spinal/epidural opioid analgesia in this patient population.

INTRAVENOUS PATIENT-CONTROLLED ANALGESIA

Theory

Interpatient variability in postoperative pain perception and requirements for opioid analgesics are implied every time orders are written for pain medication to be given "as needed." Medication administered on an as needed, or *pro re nata* (PRN), basis requires multiple interventional steps, which are both time-consuming for the nursing staff and delay analgesic delivery to the patient. These steps include (1) nursing evaluation of patient status, (2) obtaining access to opioid analgesics, (3) preparation of medication and intramuscular (or subcutaneous) injection, and (4) delayed absorption and distribution to central nervous system receptors (Fig. 24–1). These variabilities can be minimized by employing IV-PCA.[6, 7]

The concept of PCA was introduced in 1965 when Sechzer[6] envisaged a demand system by which the patient could directly control the dosage of analgesic agent via a simple feedback loop. He hypothesized that patients would respond to their pain by pressing an analgesic "activation button" until a personal level of pain relief was attained.[6, 8] The frequency of button pushing provides an important measure of pain intensity and the cumulative dose administered correlates with the adequacy of pain relief.[6, 8] PCA devices consist of an infusion pump (which connects to the patient's indwelling intravenous catheter), a microprocessor (which contains programmable infusion parameters), and an activating button switch on an extension cord (by which the patient can initiate an incremental dose).[9] Potential overdosage is prevented by programming limits to the incremental opioid bolus dose and to the amount of opioid infusible over a specified time (1 hour or 4 hour dosage limit).[9, 10] More sophisticated systems allow a continuous infusion to be programmed in addition to the patient-activated bolus doses.[9] PCA systems operate under three basic assumptions.[9, 10] The first is that opioid-related side effects occur at higher brain concentrations of the drug than those needed to produce analgesia; the second is that pain intensity and analgesic requirements are rarely constant; and the third is that the entire spectrum of pain relief lies within a narrow plasma concentration range subject to individual variation. This has been described as the minimum effective analgesic concentration (MEAC),[7, 9, 11] above which there is a diminished return in analgesic effectiveness but an increased incidence of side effects. PCA therapy eliminates delays related to communication, patient evaluation, and drug preparation, allows rapid absorption and distribution of opioid (by intravenous delivery), and may be programmed to allow frequent self-administration (that is, every 6 minutes) of relatively small analgesic doses. In theory, plasma opioid concentrations show less variability over time, thus maintaining effective analgesia while avoiding periodic episodes of excessive sedation (Fig. 24–2).[7–10, 12]

The size of the incremental bolus and the duration of the lockout interval (in minutes) appear to influence the patient's perception of PCA effectiveness and may determine the success or failure of such therapy.[10, 11, 13] If the size of the incremental bolus is too small, a large proportion of patients will experience inadequate analgesia; however, too large a demand bolus may produce an unacceptable incidence of side effects. Optimal incremental bolus size may be defined as the minimum dose capable of consistently providing appreciable analgesia without causing either subjective or objective side effects.[10, 13] A prolonged lockout interval may also diminish analgesic effectiveness, as it is opioid-specific and is dependent on analgesic onset and duration of effect. PCA safety and efficacy can be improved by limiting incremental bolus size while minimizing the lockout interval.[9, 10]

The key to successful PCA therapy is the administration of an opioid "loading dose," which provides a baseline plasma concentration of analgesic, which is subsequently maintained within a narrow therapeutic range by patient-initiated boluses. The loading dose is administered in the postanesthesia care unit (PACU) upon recovery from general anesthesia or during regression of spinal or epidural blockade. Although intermittent activation of the PCA device maintains a consistent level of analgesia over time, plasma opioid levels decline during periods of sleep, and patients may awaken because of waning analgesia. These problems can be avoided by programming the PCA pump

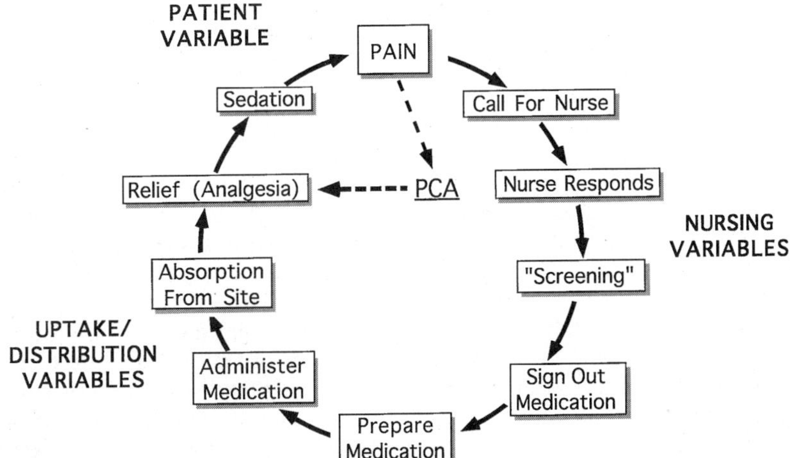

❖ **Figure 24–1** The postoperative pain cycle associated with intramuscular PRN doses of opioid analgesics. Patient-controlled delivery avoids nursing and absorption variables, thereby eliminating the cycle. PCA, patient-controlled analgesia. (Modified from Sinatra RS: Acute pain management and acute pain services. *In* Cousins MJ, Bridenbaugh PO (eds). Neural Blockade in Clinical Anesthesia and Management of Pain. Philadelphia: Lippincott-Raven Publishers; 1998:796.)

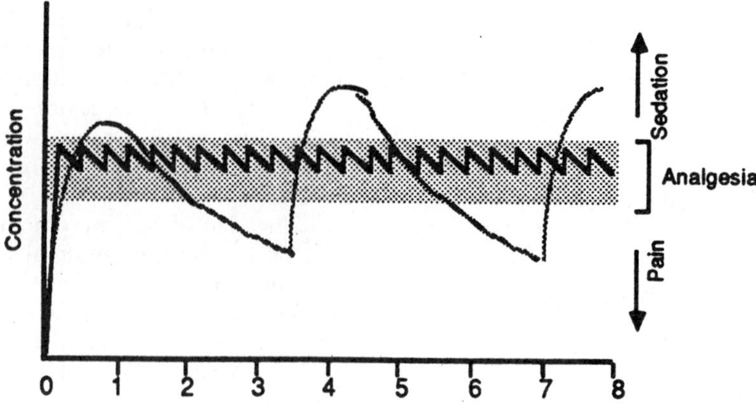

❖ **Figure 24–2** Theoretical plasma concentrations achieved with PRN IM bolus (large amplitude wave) and intravenous patient-controlled analgesia (IV-PCA) (small sawtooth wave form). Patients utilizing IV-PCA are more likely to remain in the analgesic "window" on plasma concentrations associated with the optional analgesia stipled region. (From Parker AJ, Sinatra RS, Glass PSA: Patient-controlled analgesia systems. *In* Sinatra RS, Hord AH, Ginsberg B, Preble LM (eds): Acute Pain: Mechanisms and Management. St. Louis, Mosby–Year Book, 1992: 205–224.)

to infuse opioid continuously, in addition to delivering bolus doses in response to patient activation.[9, 10, 14]

Agents and Methods of Delivery

In randomized studies comparing intramuscular, epidural, and PCA administration of morphine after cesarean delivery,[15–17] patients in the intramuscular group reported the poorest analgesia and lowest satisfaction. In contrast, patients receiving epidural morphine achieved the best pain relief but also had the highest incidence of pruritus. Even though sedation was more common with PCA, overall patient satisfaction was greatest in the PCA group. This type of outcome analysis demonstrates that the *degree of analgesia* achieved, though a primary objective of each therapeutic modality, is less important to patients than *overall satisfaction,* which may be diminished greatly by opioid-related side effects.

A wide variety of opioids may be administered by IV-PCA at equipotent dosages to provide equivalent analgesic responses; however, differences in opioid-specific pharmacokinetics, pharmacodynamics, and complications may result in varying degrees of effectiveness and overall satisfaction (Table 24–1). Depending on individual patient risk factors, patient preferences, and efficacy of supplemental medications to prevent or treat complications, each opioid has unique benefits and risks. An investigation of IV-PCA with morphine, meperidine, or oxymorphone after cesarean delivery showed that all patient groups had similar opioid requirements and achieved equivalent pain relief at rest.[18] PCA oxymorphone promoted the most rapid onset of analgesia, whereas patients receiving PCA morphine reported the lowest pain scores beyond 8 hours postoperatively. Meperidine was associated with the most pain during movement. Morphine was associated with the most sedation, and oxymorphone resulted in the greatest degree of nausea and emesis.[18]

Morbidly obese parturients using PCA meperidine may experience less than optimal pain control and be reluctant to ambulate. Remaining in bed could increase their risk of deep vein thrombosis and pulmonary embolus. Patients with renal insufficiency may accumulate normeperidine, a renally cleared metabolite of meperidine, and risk developing neuromuscular tremors or seizures.[19] PCA morphine-related sedation may adversely affect maternal-infant bonding. Conversely, after a prolonged course of labor followed by cesarean delivery, parturients may benefit from the sedating properties of PCA morphine postoperatively. Prophylaxis against nausea and emesis might be necessary for patients receiving PCA oxymorphone.[19]

Clinical comparison of PCA alone versus PCA plus a continuous basal infusion has been made in patients following cesarean delivery who received either morphine or oxymorphone (Fig. 24–3).[20] Among patients receiving oxymorphone, the addition of a basal infusion to PCA decreased pain scores at rest and with movement, further increased the incidence of nausea and emesis, but was not associated with excessive sedation or respiratory depression and did not influence patient satisfaction. For patients receiving morphine, the addition of a basal infusion decreased pain scores with movement but had no effect on satisfaction scores.[20] These results recapitulate the theme that although analgesia may be enhanced by adding a basal infusion of opioid, patient satisfaction varies independently. Rarely will postcesarean patients require PCA plus basal infusion; some, however, including those recovering from cesarean hysterectomy, might benefit from the improved pain control such therapy offers. In those instances, close attention must be given to assessing respiratory status and providing adequate treatment of side effects. It is evident that many factors contribute to the development of a logical plan for maintaining analgesia by PCA after cesarean delivery. In patients who receive neuraxial opioids, PCA may be

Table 24-1 **Dosing Guidelines for Intravenous Patient-Controlled Analgesia**

Opioid	Concentration	Loading Dose	Incremental Bolus Dose	Lockout Interval	Basal Infusion (Rate)	Comments
Morphine	1 mg/mL	3–10 mg	0.5–1.5 mg	6–8 min	0.5–1.5 mg/h	Slow onset to peak effect, sedation and pruritus common
Meperidine	10 mg/mL	25–50 mg	5–15 mg	6–8 min	Not recommended	Useful for visceral pain following tubal ligation, limit dose to 600 mg/24 h
Hydromorphone	0.2 mg/mL	0.5–1 mg	0.1–0.3 mg	6–8 min	0.1–0.3 mg/h	Rapid onset, fewer side effects than morphine
Oxymorphone	0.1 mg/mL	0.5–1 mg	0.1–0.2 mg	6–8 min	0.1 mg/h	Rapid onset, less sedating than morphine, increased risk of nausea and vomiting with higher doses
Fentanyl	20 µg/mL	30–100 µg	10–20 µg	5–6 min	10–20 µg/h	Rapid onset, short duration of effect, requires basal infusion

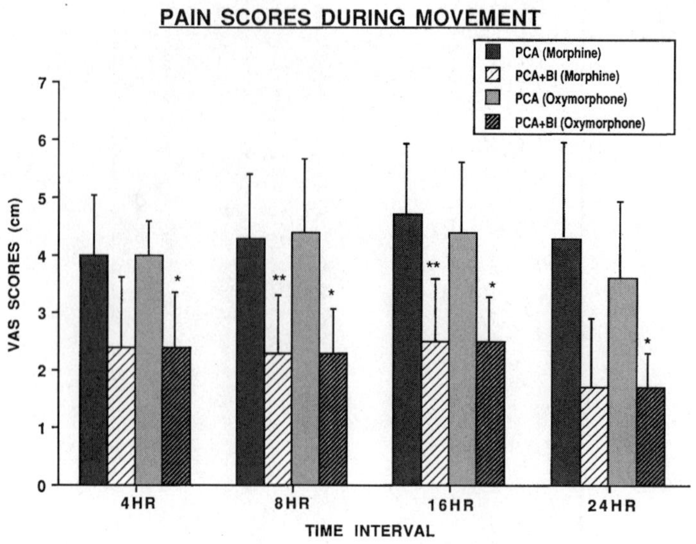

Figure 24–3 Visual analogue pain scores following deep cough or ambulation in patients recovering from cesarean section and treated with intravenous patient-controlled analgesia (IV-PCA) morphine or oxymorphone, with or without basal infusion (BI). (From Sinatra RS, Lodge K, Sibert K, et al: A comparison of morphine, meperidine, and oxymorphone as utilized in patient controlled analgesia following cesarean delivery. Anesthesiology 1989; 70:585–590.)

initiated as the spinal analgesic effect wanes, with less risk of a transitional hiatus of inadequate analgesia (refer to section on neuraxial opioids).[21] Neuraxial opioids with long durations (24 hours) may be employed to minimize or eliminate IV-PCA opioid use and to facilitate transition to oral therapy (Fig. 24–4).[22] The duration of analgesia averages only 2 to 12 hours after epidural fentanyl, meperidine, or hydromorphone bolus,[8, 10] thus necessitating early initiation of IV-PCA therapy.

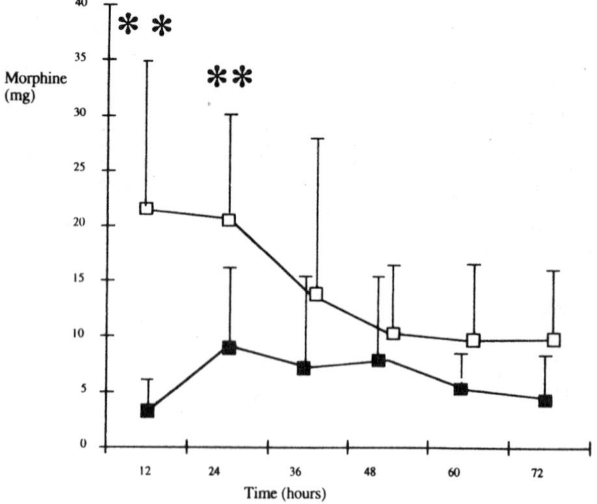

Figure 24–4 Intravenous patient-controlled analgesia morphine requirement per 12-hour period (mean ± SD). *White box*, control group; *black box*, group given 5 mg epidural morphine prior to surgery. $P < .01$ between groups. (From Negre I, Gueneron JP, Jamali SJ, et al: Preoperative analgesia with epidural morphine. Anesth Analg 1994; 79:298–302.)

Most parturients after cesarean delivery utilize PCA to achieve adequate but not complete analgesia.[20, 21] Limiting self-administered doses tends to reduce the incidence and severity of opioid-related side effects, thus enhancing patient satisfaction. On occasion, however, a postcesarean patient may complain of moderate to severe pain despite a loading dose and appropriate use of PCA. Parturients with chronic pain requiring opioid analgesics, as well as individuals abusing drugs (specifically opioids or cocaine), may present in this manner. Among patients with a remote history of drug abuse, inadequate postoperative analgesia may also occur, especially if a daily methadone maintenance dose is omitted on or before the day of surgery. Management of such patients should include (1) maintaining a daily methadone dose (oral or parenteral) throughout their hospitalization, (2) allowing normal utilization of PCA opioids after cesarean delivery, (3) avoiding the use of opioid antagonists or mixed agonist-antagonists,[23] and (4) anticipating increased opioid dose requirements to prevent acute withdrawal and to maintain adequate postoperative analgesia.

Adjunctive Agents

The two most common reasons why patients become dissatisfied and "fail" PCA therapy are inadequate analgesia and excessive nausea or emesis.[10, 13, 24] Several adjunctive agents and combination therapies have been evaluated to minimize total opioid dosage while maintaining excellent analgesia. Such reductions in opioid self-administration represent the key to minimizing dose-dependent side effects.

Ketorolac, a potent nonsteroidal anti-inflammatory drug, provides useful potentiation of PCA morphine analgesia. Fifteen milligrams administered intravenously every 6 hours reduces PCA morphine requirements by 40% to 50% and usually eliminates the need for basal opioid infusions (R. Sinatra and F. Sevarino, unpublished observations, 1992–1998). Doses of ketorolac reduced PCA morphine consumption and dose-dependent side effects in patients recovering from cesarean delivery and gynecologic surgery.[25, 26] Of note, Food and Drug Administration (FDA) restrictions contraindicate ketorolac in nursing mothers.

Visceral (spasmodic) pain and associated nausea may be reduced by the addition of metoclopramide or hydroxyzine to PCA therapy (R. Sinatra and F. Sevarino, unpublished observations, 1992–1998).[24] Metoclopramide appears to reduce peristalsis and spasm associated with tubal manipulation[25] and may decrease cramping uterine pain following hysterectomy. Promethazine and metoclopramide also reduced the incidence of nausea and emesis associated with PCA opioids in patients recovering from abdominal hysterectomy.

Neonatal Considerations

Maternal use of PCA after cesarean delivery carries the potential risk for neonatal central nervous system (CNS) depression secondary to opioid distribution and secretion in breast milk.

Given the same requirement for postcesarean analgesia and sufficient time to achieve equilibrium between maternal plasma and breast milk, accumulation of drug molecules in breast milk will be in proportion to the equivalent potency of the opioid being administered.[2, 21] Neonatal gastrointestinal absorption of ingested opioids will be greater with more lipid-soluble opioids and opioid metabolites. Finally, if neonates cannot adequately detoxify or excrete certain opioids (notably those that require renal excretion), neonatal CNS depression is more likely to occur.

Detection of subtle CNS depression among nursing neonates requires one or more neurobehavioral examinations performed by trained and certified personnel. Furthermore, to determine why this depression occurs requires quantitation of opioid concentrations in relevant tissue compartments. One study utilized both these approaches to assess the incidence, severity, and cause of neonatal depression among infants of nursing parturients who used PCA meperidine or PCA morphine after cesarean delivery.[2] Neonates in the morphine group were significantly more alert and significantly more responsive to human orientation cues than neonates in the meperidine group on their third day of life. Decrements in alertness and human orientation, seen with meperidine, not only reflect opioid-related neonatal depression but may also inhibit normal maternal-infant bonding interactions.

Because PCA with meperidine results in accumulation in breast milk of normeperidine and thus neonatal neurobehavioral depression, PCA with morphine or hydromorphone may be a better choice for postcesarean analgesia lasting longer than 24 hours in the parturient who nurses her infant. Especially with a low birthweight infant (<2500 g) who is already prone to seizures,[21] neonatal ingestion and accumulation of normeperidine would only exacerbate that risk. It is important to remember that, among infants of nursing parturients who receive PCA with morphine after cesarean delivery, neonatal neurobehavior is no different from that observed in normal infants with no drug exposure after vaginal delivery.[2, 21]

NEURAXIAL ANALGESIA: SPINAL AND EPIDURAL TECHNIQUES

Neuraxial Opioid Analgesia Theory

Using a variety of animal models, researchers[11, 16, 17] reported that neuraxially (intrathecally, epidurally) administered opioids produced naloxone-reversible analgesia of prolonged duration and that two or more distinct opioid receptor systems were likely involved in the modulation of pain at the spinal level.[27–30] In 1979, Wang and associates[31] published the first report of intraspinal opioid administration in humans. Subsequently, thousands of published documents have confirmed the analgesic efficacy of epidurally and intrathecally administered opioids.[32]

The epidural route of administration is complicated by several anatomic and physiologic factors, including (1) drug penetration of the dura and pia mater, (2) absorption by epidural fat, and (3) the consequences of vascular uptake and redistribution of drug to supraspinal sites (Fig. 24–5).[32, 33] A small portion of the epidural dose crosses the dura to enter the cerebrospinal fluid (CSF) and penetrates spinal tissue in amounts proportional to the agent's lipid solubility. By activating spinal opioid receptors, nociceptive input is blunted at the first synapse in the CNS. The remainder of the epidural dose is absorbed by the vasculature, producing plasma levels comparable to those achieved with intramuscular injections and providing some degree of supraspinal analgesia.[32–35]

Intrathecal administration allows injection of the drug directly into the CSF. This represents a more efficient method of delivering opioid to spinal cord opioid receptors. A bolus dose of intrathecal morphine 0.5 mg results in a CSF concentration greater than 10,000 ng/mL, with barely detectable plasma concentrations.[34]

Epidural and intrathecal opioids often produce analgesia of greater intensity than similar doses administered parenterally. A second advantage of intraspinal opioids is the selectivity of analgesia, which occurs in the absence of motor or sympathetic blockade. Unlike local anesthetic blockade, intraspinal opioid analgesia facilitates patient ambulation while minimizing the risk of hypotension.[35] The physiochemistry and pharmacodynamics of neuraxial opioids are presented in Table 24–2.

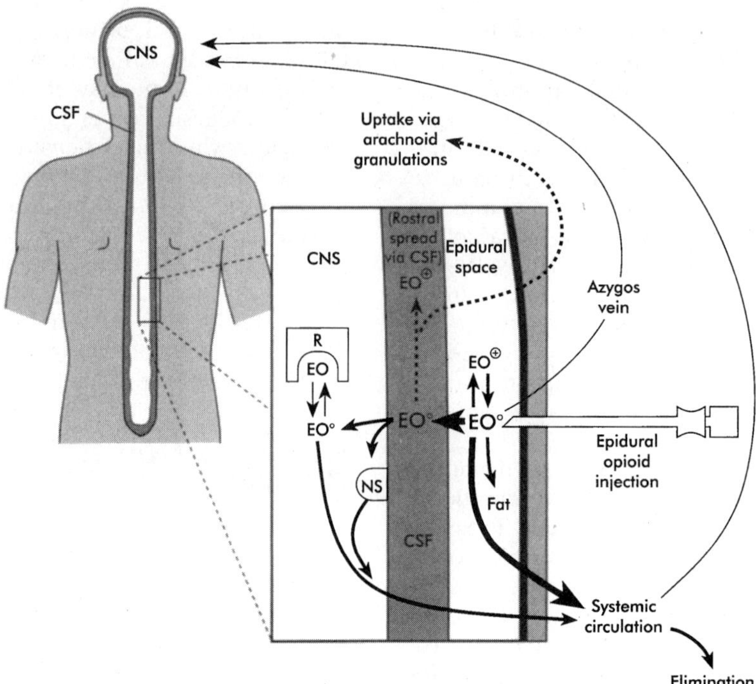

Figure 24–5 Factors that influence dural penetration, cerebrospinal fluid (CSF) sequestration, and vascular clearance of epidurally administered opioids. The major portion of epidurally administered opioids (EO) is absorbed by epidural and spinal blood vessels or dissolved into epidural fat. Molecules taken up by the epidural plexus and azygos system may recirculate to supraspinal centers and mediate central opioid effects. A smaller percentage of uncharged molecules (EO°) traverse the dura and enter the CSF. Lipophilic opioids rapidly exit the CSF and penetrate into spinal tissue. As with intrathecal dosing, the majority of these molecules are either trapped within lipid membranes (nonspecific binding sites, NS) or are rapidly removed by the spinal vasculature. A small fraction of molecules bind to and activate opioid receptors (R). Hydrophilic opioids penetrate pia-arachnoid membranes and spinal tissue slowly. A larger proportion of these molecules remain sequestered in CSF and are slowly transported rostrally. This CSF depot permits gradual spinal uptake, greater dermatomal spread, and a prolonged duration of activity. CNS, central nervous system. (From Sinatra RS: Pharmacokinetics and pharmacodynamics of spinal opioids. *In* Sinatra RS, Hord AH, Ginsberg B, Preble LM (eds): Acute Pain: Mechanisms and Management. St Louis, Mosby, 1992.)

Epidural Opioids

Morphine

After epidural administration, plasma morphine concentrations are similar to those observed after intramuscular injection; however, peak analgesic effect is delayed until 60 to 90 minutes following administration.[32, 36, 37] This latency results from morphine's low lipid solubility, which retards penetration into spinal tissue.[32, 33] Epidural morphine provides a prolonged duration of analgesia, which typically persists long after plasma concentrations have declined to subtherapeutic levels (Fig. 24–6). This finding reflects the fact that significant amounts of morphine become sequestered in CSF, which functions as an aqueous drug depot.[32, 33]

After cesarean delivery, 5 mg of epidural morphine provides reliable analgesia for up to 24 hours.[36, 37] Smaller doses of epidural morphine (3 to 4 mg) provide more than 12 hours of analgesia. Leicht et al[38] prospectively studied 1000 patients who received 5 mg of epidural morphine for postcesarean analgesia. Fuller and colleagues[39] reviewed the records of 4880 women who received 2 to 5 mg of epidural morphine at the conclusion of cesarean section. In both studies, the mean duration of analgesia was 23 hours, but the duration varied widely among patients.

The choice of local anesthetic used for epidural anesthesia may affect the subsequent efficacy of epidural morphine.[40, 41] Kotelko and colleagues[40] evaluated the epidural administration of 5 mg of morphine for postcesarean analgesia in 276 women. A high proportion of patients who received 2-chloroprocaine as the primary local anesthetic experienced unexpectedly poor postoperative analgesia, usually lasting less than 3 hours.

Patients treated with single bolus doses (5 mg) of epidural morphine experienced more effective postcesarean analgesia but with a higher incidence of adverse events than similar women who self-administered intravenous morphine or received intramuscular morphine

Table 24-2 **Spinal Opioid Physiochemistry and Pharmacodynamics**

Opioid	Molecular Weight	Lipid Solubility*	Parenteral Potency	pKa	Mu-Receptor Affinity	Dissociation Kinetics	Potency Gain (Epidural vs. IV or SC)	Onset of Analgesia	Duration of Analgesia
Morphine	285	1.4	1	7.9	Moderate	Slow	10	Delayed	Prolonged
Meperidine	247	39	0.1	8.5	Moderate	Moderate	2–3	Rapid	Intermediate
Methadone	309	116	2	9.3	High	Slow	2	Rapid	Intermediate
Hydromorphone	285	1.9	8	—	High	Slow	4	Rapid	Intermediate
Alfentanil	417	129	25	6.5	High	Very rapid	1	Very rapid	Short
Fentanyl	336	816	80	8.4	High	Rapid	1	Very rapid	Short
Sufentanil	386	1727	800	8.0	Very high	Moderate	1	Very rapid	Short

IV, intravenous; SC, subcutaneous.
*Octanol-water partition coefficient (at pH of 7.4)

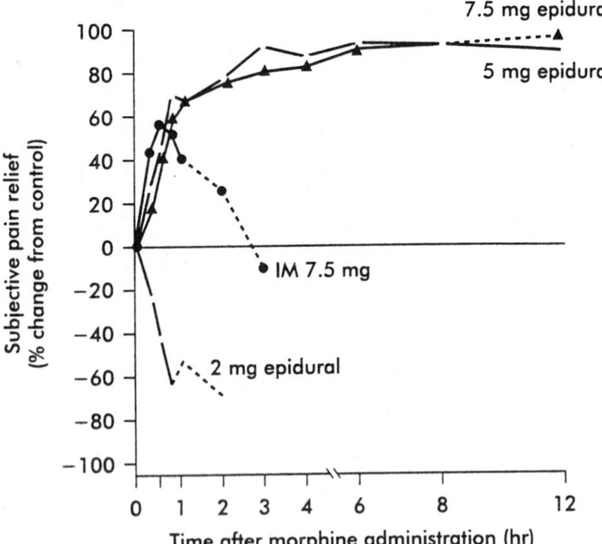

❖ **Figure 24-6** Percent changes in pain relief for patients recovering from cesarean section and treated with intramuscular (7.5 mg) or epidural (2 mg, 5 mg, or 7.5 mg) morphine. (From Rosen MA, Hughes SC, Shnider SM, et al: Epidural morphine for the relief of postoperative pain after cesarean delivery. Anesth Analg 1983; 62:666–672.)

(Fig. 24–7).[15, 16] Low-dose, continuous epidural infusions of morphine avoid initial peak and subsequent trough of CSF concentrations and provide more consistent analgesia with a reduced incidence of unpleasant side effects.[42, 43] In one study, patients who received an epidural morphine bolus of 2.6 mg and an infusion of 0.1 mg/h experienced more effective analgesia and a lower incidence of pruritus than patients who received a single 5-mg bolus.[35] The authors suggested that epidural morphine infusions are most cost effective in settings in which epidural analgesia is maintained for more than 24 hours and in which nurses do not have the option to reinject epidural opioids without physician supervision.

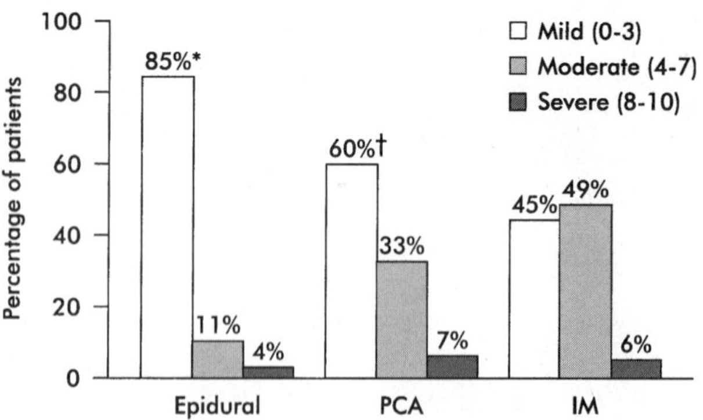

❖ **Figure 24-7** The percentage of patients recovering from cesarean section and treated with either epidural, patient-controlled, or intramuscular morphine and reporting mild, moderate, or severe discomfort over the 24-hour study period. $^*P < .05$ denotes epidural versus PCA and IM. $^\dagger P =$ NS denotes patient-controlled versus intramuscular. (From Harrison DM, Sinatra RS, Morgese L, et al: Epidural narcotic and PCA for post-cesarean section pain relief. Anesthesiology 1988; 68:454–457.)

Fentanyl

Fentanyl is more lipid-soluble than morphine, and it rapidly penetrates the dura and spinal tissues to bind and activate opioid receptors.[44–46] Naulty and coworkers[44] reported that in patients recovering from cesarean section performed with epidural bupivacaine (0.75%) anesthesia, an epidural fentanyl bolus (50–100 μg) provided 4 to 5 hours of postoperative analgesia and significantly reduced 24-hour analgesic requirements. Sevarino and colleagues[46] observed an analgesic duration of only 90 minutes and no reduction in 24-hour opioid requirements in patients who received 100 μg of epidural fentanyl during epidural lidocaine anesthesia (Fig. 24–8). This discrepancy in duration of analgesia was attributed to the potentiating effect of 0.75% bupivacaine (used in Naulty's study), which is no longer used or approved for use in obstetric patients. After resolution of motor blockade, residual quantities of bupivacaine can potentiate spinal opioid analgesia.

Fentanyl's rapid onset and short duration make it ideally suited for continuous epidural infusion. With this technique, the level of analgesia can be titrated to the pain stimulus, and the opioid effects can be terminated rapidly if problems occur. Youngstrom and associates[47, 48] evaluated the continuous epidural infusion of fentanyl 4 μg/mL and epinephrine 1.6 μg/mL for postcesarean analgesia. Patients who received a continuous epidural infusion at a rate of 15 mL/h

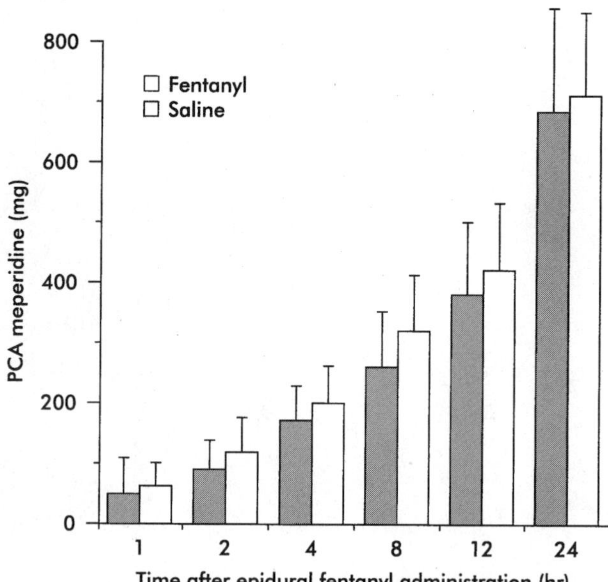

❖ **Figure 24-8** Patient-controlled meperidine requirements in patients recovering from cesarean delivery and administered either epidural fentanyl or saline during anesthesia with lidocaine 2% plus epinephrine. (From Sevarino FB, McFarlane C, Sinatra RS, et al: Epidural fentanyl does not influence intravenous PCA requirements in the post-caesarean patient. Can J Anaesth 1991; 38:450–453.)

obtained excellent pain relief and required fewer self-administered doses of intravenous opioid for supplementation of analgesia.

Epidural fentanyl administration results in significant systemic absorption of drug, and some have questioned the neuraxial specificity of epidural fentanyl analgesia.[49, 50] The high dose requirements (40 to 80 μg/h or 1000–2000 μg/day) underscore the relative inefficiency and potential toxicity of epidurally administered fentanyl and other lipophilic opioids.[51] Nonetheless, continuous epidural fentanyl infusions are widely used because they provide a uniform level of effective analgesia, with fewer adverse effects than those associated with epidural morphine.

Sufentanil

Sufentanil is a lipid-soluble opioid that has a parenteral potency 5 to 10 times greater than fentanyl. Epidural sufentanil provides effective pain relief that is rapid in onset, although dose requirements are high (Table 24–3).[52, 53] Among patients recovering from cesarean section, the analgesic potency of epidural sufentanil appears to be only 2 to 2.5 times greater than that of fentanyl.[53] The duration of analgesia is relatively brief. An epidural bolus of 25 μg sufentanil produces less than 2 hours of complete analgesia, whereas 50 μg provides only 3 to 4 hours of pain relief.[52, 53]

This duration of analgesia may be safely extended by adding epinephrine,[54] utilizing a large diluent volume,[55] or employing a continuous epidural infusion.[56–58] Sufentanil's rapid onset and short duration of action are highly desirable characteristics for use in this setting, as the anesthesiologist can titrate the level of analgesia and minimize the side effects and risk of respiratory depression associated with large bolus doses. Cheng and coworkers[57] reported that continuous epidural infusion of sufentanil (0.3 μg/kg/h) provided rapid and sustained analgesia with few side effects in patients recovering from intra-abdominal surgery.

Other Epidural Opioids

Less commonly administered epidural opioids include meperidine,[59] hydromorphone,[60, 61] diamorphine,[62] methadone,[63] buprenorphine,[51] and butorphanol.[64]

Meperidine is commonly used as a parenteral analgesic in patients recovering from cesarean section. Unlike other opioids, epidurally administered meperidine has local anesthetic qualities. Two clinical trials compared the safety and efficacy of epidural meperidine 50 mg and intramuscular meperidine 100 mg.[60, 65] Both studies noted that either route of administration provided 2.5 to 3 hours of analgesia, although the onset was faster in the epidural group. Patients preferred the epidural route of administration. Paech[59] evaluated the quality of analgesia and side effects produced by a single epidural bolus of meperidine 50 mg or fentanyl 100 μg in 50 women recovering from cesarean section. All patients experienced highly effective pain relief with few side effects. The onset was slightly faster with fentanyl, and the duration of analgesia was longer with meperidine.

Hydromorphone is a hydroxylated derivative of morphine. Available in preservative-free solution, it provides effective epidural analgesia in patients recovering from cesarean section.[60, 66, 67] Chestnut and colleagues[66] evaluated the epidural administration of hydromorphone 1 mg administered during wound closure in patients who had received epidural lidocaine or bupivacaine anesthesia. The mean time to first request for supplemental analgesia was 13 hours, and 92% of patients reported good or excellent pain relief. Henderson and coworkers[67] observed that the median duration of postcesarean analgesia provided by epidural hydromorphone 1 mg was 19.3 hours. In both studies, approximately 50% of patients reported mild-to-moderate itching, but not all required treatment.

Diamorphine is a lipid-soluble derivative of morphine that is available for use as an intravenous and epidural analgesic in the United Kingdom.[62] It provides rapid and effective epidural analgesia, but systemic absorption is high, and the duration of activity is limited to 6 to 8 hours.[68] Semple and associates[69] evaluated the effects of epinephrine on vascular uptake and analgesic duration of epidural diamorphine 5 mg in patients recovering from cesarean section. Plasma levels of the principal metabolite (morphine) were lower, whereas the duration of analgesia was longer in patients who received diamorphine plus epinephrine (12.5 hours) than in those who received diamorphine alone (9.9 hours). Unfortunately, these patients also

Table 24–3 ONSET AND DURATION OF ANALGESIA WITH EPIDURAL MORPHINE AND SUFENTANIL

	MORPHINE SULFATE 5 μg	SUFENTANIL 30 μg	SUFENTANIL 45 μg	SUFENTANIL 60 μg
Onset of 50% pain relief (min)	52*	15	15	15
Onset of 90% pain relief (min)	90*	30	30	15
Description of analgesia, first dose (h)	26*	3.9	4.5	5.6

Median values, *$P < .05$ compared to each sufentanil group.

From Rosen MA, Dailey PA, Hughes SC, et al: Epidural sufentanil for postoperative analgesia after cesarean section. Anesthesiology 1988; 68:448–452.

experienced a higher incidence of annoying side effects.

The mixed agonist-antagonist opioids such as butorphanol offer two theoretical advantages when administered epidurally: (1) the ability to selectively activate kappa-opioid receptors, which modulate visceral nociception,[29] and (2) a "ceiling effect," which minimizes severe respiratory depression. Early studies demonstrated that epidural butorphanol (2–4 mg) provided up to 8 hours of postcesarean analgesia without significant pruritus, but with significant dose-dependent increases in sedation.[70, 71] Subsequent studies have questioned the efficacy of epidural butorphanol. Camann and associates[72] noted that in patients recovering from cesarean section, epidural butorphanol 2 mg offered few if any advantages over a similar dose given intravenously.

Epidural Opioid Combinations

One method used to hasten the onset of epidural analgesia while providing a prolonged duration of effect is to combine fentanyl with small doses of morphine.[73, 74] Naulty and Ross[73] compared the epidural injection of 5 mg of morphine versus 50 μg of fentanyl plus 0, 1, 2, or 3 mg of morphine. All patients who received fentanyl had a rapid onset of analgesia. Among patients who received 50 μg of fentanyl and 3 mg of morphine, the duration of analgesia and the total 24-hour supplemental opioid dose were similar to those provided by 5 mg of morphine alone. The addition of sufentanil to morphine may also hasten the onset and prolong the duration of epidural analgesia.[75, 76] Naulty and coworkers[75] reported that the combination of sufentanil 20 μg and morphine 2.5 mg provided a very rapid onset and a prolonged duration of analgesia, with a low incidence of side effects. Dottrens and colleagues[76] randomized patients to receive a single epidural dose of either morphine (4 mg), sufentanil (50 μg), or morphine (2 mg) with sufentanil (25 μg). The morphine-sufentanil combination provided a more rapid onset of pain relief than did morphine alone. Dosing guidelines for single dose and continuous opioid infusions are presented in Table 24–4.

Patient-Controlled Epidural Analgesia

Self-administration techniques permit the patient to titrate analgesic agents in proportion to the intensity of post-surgical discomfort. This reduces patient anxiety while increasing patient control. Thus it seems reasonable to expect that epidural opioid analgesia might be combined with a self-administration dosing regimen to provide the psychologic benefits of PCA and the superior analgesia associated with intraspinal opioids. Table 24–5 lists the potential advantages of patient-controlled epidural analgesia (PCEA).[77, 78]

Chrubasik and coworkers[78] noted that the dose of self-administered morphine required to provide effective PCEA was significantly less than amounts used with either continuous epidural opioid or IV-PCA techniques. Walmsley[79] reported that PCEA morphine provided high clinical efficacy and safety in over 4000 patients recovering from a variety of surgical procedures at the University of Kentucky Medical Center. Walmsley described the following protocol: An epidural bolus injection of 2 to 3 mg of preservative-free morphine is followed by a continuous epidural infusion of morphine at 0.4 mg/h. Patients are allowed to self-administer 0.2 mg of morphine every 10 to 15 minutes, with a maximum hourly dose of 1.2 mg.

Disadvantages of using morphine for PCEA include its prolonged latency and the risk of delayed respiratory depression. For this reason, more lipophilic opioids (e.g., meperidine,[80] fentanyl,[68] hydromorphone,[81, 82] sufentanil[83, 84]) have been evaluated for PCEA use.

Yarnell and associates[80] noted that PCEA meperidine provided better postcesarean analgesia than intra-

Table 24-4 DOSING GUIDELINES FOR EPIDURAL OPIOID ANALGESIA*

Opioid	Intermittent Bolus Technique*	Continuous Infusion Technique*	Adjunctive Therapy
Morphine	Administer 2-3 mg bolus in 10 mL preservative-free saline every 8-24 h as clinically indicated	2-4 mg bolus followed by infusion (50 μg/mL) at 6-12 mL/h	IV ketorolac 15-30 mg q6h† Epidural bupivacaine 0.1-0.03%
Hydromorphone	0.5-1 mg bolus every 5-10 h	0.5-1.5 mg bolus followed by infusion (10 μg/mL) at 6-12 mL/h	IV ketorolac 15-30 mg q6h† Epidural bupivacaine 0.1-0.03%
Meperidine	50-75 mg bolus every 3-5 h	Not recommended	IV ketorolac 15-30 mg q6h†
Fentanyl	50-100 μg bolus every 2-3 h (not recommended)	50-100 μg bolus followed by infusion (5 μg/mL) at 8-15 mL/h	IV ketorolac 15-30 mg q6h† Epidural bupivacaine 0.05-0.1% or less
Sufentanil	20-30 μg bolus every 2-3 h (not recommended)	20-30 μg bolus followed by infusion (1-2 μg/mL) at 8-15 mL/h	IV ketorolac 15-30 mg q6h† Epidural bupivacaine 0.05-0.1% or less

*Dependent on physical status, height, extent of surgical dissection, and so on.
†Administration should be restricted to non-nursing mothers.

Table 24-5 POTENTIAL ADVANTAGES OF PCEA

Versus Epidural Opioid Boluses or Infusions
Patient control and autonomy
Increased patient satisfaction
Decreased anxiety
Reduced opioid requirement
Versus Intravenous Patient-Controlled Analgesia
Increased efficacy of analgesia
Increased patient satisfaction
Reduced opioid requirement
Decreased sedation
Shorter hospitalization (?)

muscular injections of the drug. Further, patients who received PCEA meperidine ambulated sooner and cared for their infants earlier. The incidence of maternal side effects was similar in the two groups. However, one patient in the PCEA group developed respiratory depression 25 minutes after receiving 75 mg of epidural meperidine in the operating room.

Boudreault and colleagues[68] noted that patients who received PCEA fentanyl required less drug than patients who received a continuous epidural infusion of fentanyl. The two groups of patients had similar analgesia. Because side effects and complications appear to be dose dependent, a decrease in dose associated with PCEA may improve safety. Cohen and associates[85] evaluated the effect of varying diluent volumes on the quality of analgesia, total dose requirement, and side-effect profile of PCEA fentanyl-bupivacaine. A higher infusion rate (15 mL/h) of a more dilute solution (bupivacaine 0.01% with fentanyl 2 μg/mL) provided effective postcesarean analgesia and was associated with the lowest incidence of adverse effects.

Parker and White[81] noted that patients who self-administered epidural hydromorphone required four to five times less drug than patients who received IV-PCA hydromorphone after cesarean section (see Fig. 24–9). The authors speculated that the dose sparing in the PCEA group was responsible in part for significant reductions in adverse effects, a more rapid return of bowel function, and a shortened hospital stay in that group. In a second study,[82] these investigators attempted to further increase the efficacy of PCEA hydromorphone by adding 0.08% bupivacaine or by using a basal infusion of hydromorphone in patients recovering from cesarean section. These adjuvant therapies did not improve pain scores, decrease PCA demands, or reduce 24-hour dose requirements but were associated with significant lower extremity sensory deficits (e.g., numbness) as well as a fivefold increase in nausea and vomiting. In a third study,[84] PCEA hydromorphone alone or with varying concentrations of nalbuphine was evaluated in 64 patients recovering from cesarean delivery. The addition of nalbuphine to the epidural infusate resulted in lower nausea scores and decreased urinary retention. Nalbuphine did not decrease the incidence of pruritus but was associated with a partial reversal of analgesia.

In an evaluation of 441 patients recovering from cesarean section, Grass and associates[87] noted that patients using PCEA sufentanil experienced superior analgesia and had a shorter duration of hospitalization (4.3 days versus 5.0 days) when compared with similar women who received intramuscular opioids. In a follow-up study, these authors noted that PCEA sufentanil resulted in a more rapid onset of peak analgesia and better analgesia with movement than did IV-PCA morphine.[88] The authors suggested that the superior analgesia associated with movement and the decreased level of sedation provided by PCEA sufentanil resulted in improved maternal-infant bonding. They also noted that earlier ambulation and hospital discharge should reduce overall hospital costs. It was unclear whether the improved outcome resulted from the opioid, the method of administration, or both.

In summary, PCEA appears to enhance the quality of analgesia (with perhaps a decreased total dose of opioid) when compared with IV-PCA. Further, PCEA provides greater patient satisfaction than either a single bolus dose or a continuous epidural infusion of opioid. Table 24–6 shows common PCEA dosing regimens for different opioids.

Intrathecal Opioids

Morphine

Given the increased safety and popularity of spinal anesthesia for cesarean section, intrathecal morphine has become an attractive option for postcesarean analgesia.[89–93] The duration of action and the side-effect profile are similar to those of epidural morphine. As one should expect, the dose requirements are much smaller (0.1–0.4 mg). This low dose requirement reflects the potency gain associated with subarachnoid deposition of drug and is advantageous in parturients who are concerned about the accumulation of opioids in breast milk.

Intrathecal morphine administration results in a

Table 24-6 EPIDURAL PATIENT-CONTROLLED ANALGESIA (PCA) DOSING GUIDELINES

OPIOID	CONCENTRATION (μg/mL)	LOADING DOSE	EPI-PCA DOSE (mL)	LOCKOUT (min)	CONTINUOUS RATE	4-H LIMIT (mL)
Morphine	50	1-3 mg	2-4	10-15	6-12 mL/h	40-70
Hydromorphone	10	500-1000 μg	2-4	6-10	6-12 mL/h	40-70
Fentanyl	5	75-100 μg	2-4	6	6-15 mL/h	40-70
Sufentanil	2	25-30 μg	2-4	6	0.1 μg/kg/h	40-70

faster onset of analgesia than does epidural morphine, but this technique still requires 45 to 60 minutes to achieve a peak effect. The duration of analgesia averages 18 to 24 hours.[89–91] Abboud and associates[90] observed prolonged postcesarean analgesia in patients who received either 0.1 or 0.25 mg of intrathecal morphine with hyperbaric bupivacaine for cesarean section. The mean durations of analgesia were 18.6 and 27.7 hours, respectively. Abouleish and colleagues[93] added either morphine 0.2 mg or saline-placebo to the solution of hyperbaric bupivacaine during administration of spinal anesthesia for cesarean section. The mean duration of analgesia was almost 27 hours in the morphine group, versus only 3 hours in the saline-placebo group. Pulse oximetry revealed no evidence of hypoxemia or respiratory depression in the two groups.

Fentanyl

Hunt and coworkers[94] examined intrathecal fentanyl dose response during and after cesarean section. Doses ranging from 6.25 to 50 μg of intrathecal fentanyl were administered with the hyperbaric bupivacaine. The time to first request for additional pain relief ranged from 3 to 4 hours in patients who received intrathecal fentanyl compared with approximately 1 hour for those who did not receive fentanyl. Administration of doses of fentanyl greater than 6.25 μg did not prolong the duration of analgesia. In contrast, we have observed that 12.5 to 25 μg of intrathecal fentanyl provides negligible postcesarean pain relief and that analgesia often wanes before or soon after the patient is discharged from the PACU. The primary advantage of intrathecal fentanyl is that it improves the quality of anesthesia during cesarean section.[95]

Sufentanil

Courtney et al.[96] examined intrathecal sufentanil dose response during and after cesarean section. Doses of 0, 10, 15, or 20 μg of intrathecal sufentanil were administered with hyperbaric bupivacaine. All three doses of sufentanil resulted in a mean duration of analgesia of approximately 3 hours. More than 90% of patients reported pruritus, but only one patient required treatment. Intrathecal sufentanil did not affect neonatal condition as assessed by umbilical cord blood gas and pH measurements and Apgar and neurobehavioral scores.

Meperidine

Unlike other opioids, meperidine has local anesthetic qualities. Some anesthesiologists have administered intrathecal meperidine (1 mg/kg) as the sole anesthetic agent for various surgical procedures. Intrathecal administration of a small dose of preservative-free meperidine reduces the intensity of pain associated with regression of spinal anesthesia and facilitates the transition to IV-PCA.[97] Intrathecal meperidine provides effective postoperative analgesia of intermediate duration (4–5 hours) (R. Sinatra and F. Sevarino, unpublished observations, 1992–1998). Feldman and coworkers[97] evaluated intrathecal meperidine dose response. They added either 10 or 20 mg of meperidine or saline-placebo to 12 mg of hyperbaric bupivacaine during administration of spinal anesthesia for cesarean section. Patients treated with either dose of meperidine reported lower pain scores and higher satisfaction with analgesia during the first 4 hours of recovery than the women who had received intrathecal saline-placebo.

Intrathecal Opioid Combinations

Intrathecal administration of both morphine and a lipophilic opioid offers some advantages. Because of morphine's delayed onset, patients recovering from spinal lidocaine anesthesia often report breakthrough pain in the PACU. Naulty[98] noted that the addition of both fentanyl 5 μg and morphine 0.1 mg to hyperbaric bupivacaine provided better intraoperative analgesia than bupivacaine alone and provided postcesarean analgesia with fewer side effects than morphine 0.2 mg without fentanyl.[98]

The rapid onset and intermediate duration of intrathecal meperidine also compensates for the prolonged latency of intrathecal morphine and provides a smooth transition during regression of spinal anesthesia. Chung et al.[99] evaluated the combination of meperidine 10 mg plus morphine 0.15 mg for postcesarean pain relief in 60 patients. They reported that this combination augmented intraoperative anesthesia and provided 8 to 12 hours of postcesarean analgesia with minimal side effects. Tables 24–3 and 24–4 include the doses of epidural and intrathecal opioids that have been advocated for postcesarean analgesia.

SIDE EFFECTS OF EPIDURAL AND INTRATHECAL OPIOIDS

Intraspinal opioid administration may result in annoying (and occasionally serious) side effects and complications, including pruritus, nausea and vomiting, urinary retention, somnolence, and respiratory depression.[101]

Pruritus

Pruritus occurs more often in obstetric patients than in any other patient group. The incidence ranges from 40% to 100% of parturients treated with epidural and intrathecal morphine, hydromorphone, or methadone.[101–105] Pruritus occurs somewhat less often after epidural or intrathecal administration of the lipid-soluble opioids. Mild pruritus, usually involving the face or chest, probably occurs even more frequently; however, patients may not mention it unless directly questioned. Occasionally, the intensity of itching is so annoying that it interferes with sleep and breast-feeding. In our experience, severe pruritus is the most frequent cause of patient dissatisfaction after administration of epidural and intrathecal opioids (R. Sinatra and F. Sevarino, unpublished observations, 1992–1999).

The etiology of pruritus is unclear, but its occurrence does not reflect an acute or excessive release of histamine.[103, 104] Indeed, pruritus is most severe 3 to 6 hours after intraspinal morphine administration. At this time, plasma concentrations of opioid and histamine are clinically insignificant. Further, pruritus often occurs after intraspinal administration of other opioids (e.g., fentanyl, sufentanil) that do not cause histamine release. Changes in spinal efferent outflow may indirectly release small amounts of histamine in tissues adjacent to peripheral nerve endings.[103, 104]

Mild facial pruritus may be relieved with cold compresses, whereas pruritus of moderate severity may respond to one or more doses of diphenhydramine 25 mg. Moderate-to-severe pruritus may be treated successfully with small intravenous doses of naloxone 0.04–0.08 mg), which typically relieves symptoms without reversing the analgesia (Table 24–7). Alternatively, some anesthesiologists prefer intravenous nalbuphine[106] (5–10 mg) or naltrexone[107] for treatment of pruritus.

Borgeat and colleagues[108, 109] reported that propofol relieved the pruritus caused by epidural and intrathecal morphine. Subhypnotic doses of intravenous propofol 10 mg provided rapid relief of mild-to-moderate pruritus; the relief lasted more than 60 minutes. The authors proposed that the anti-pruritus activity of propofol does not depend on specific antagonism of opioid receptors; rather, it may result from nonselective depression of neural transmission in the spinal cord.

Nausea and Vomiting

Although nausea and vomiting are common complaints in patients recovering from cesarean delivery, the incidence of symptoms is increased in patients treated with epidural and intrathecal opioids. In general, patients treated with morphine experience the highest incidence of nausea and vomiting,[32] whereas patients who receive a continuous fentanyl-epinephrine infusion are affected less often. Nausea may result from either rostral spread of the drug in the CSF to the brain stem or vascular uptake and delivery to the vomiting center and chemoreceptor trigger zone.[32, 101]

A variety of agents have been evaluated for prevention or treatment of intraspinal opioid-induced emesis, including intravenous metoclopramide 10 mg, low doses of droperidol (0.625–1.25 mg), or ondansetron 2 to 4 mg. In our experience, metoclopramide is an effective and inexpensive choice for prophylaxis for nausea and vomiting. It provides effective antiemesis, does not increase maternal sedation, and has no untoward effects on the neonate (R. Sinatra and F. Sevarino, unpublished observations, 1992–1999). In the presence of intractable nausea, intravenous boluses of naloxone, followed by a continuous infusion of 50 to 100 μg/kg/h, may be useful. Ondansetron may also be helpful in cases of intractable nausea. Small doses (2–4 mg) may effectively reduce the incidence and severity of intraspinal opioid-induced nausea. A major disadvantage of ondansetron is its cost.

Urinary Retention

Urinary retention is a common complication of intraspinal opioid administration in nonpregnant patients. However, this is an infrequent complication in patients who are recovering from cesarean delivery. This probably reflects the common practice of maintaining an indwelling urinary catheter for the first 24 hours after surgery. Evron and associates[110] reported that patients who received epidural morphine 4 mg had greater difficulty in micturition and an increased incidence of urinary retention than patients who received an equivalent dose of epidural methadone for postcesarean analgesia. Urinary retention may result from inhibition of sacral parasympathetic outflow, which results in relaxation of the bladder detrusor muscle and an inability to relax the sphincter.[111, 112] This effect may be relieved with a large intravenous dose (0.8 mg) of naloxone; unfortunately, reversal of analgesia may occur. Urocholine and apomorphine may also provide relief.[111, 112] Ambulation and intermittent bladder catheterization are more practical forms of treatment in this patient population.

Table 24–7 INFLUENCE OF NALOXONE INFUSION ON PAIN RELIEF AND ADVERSE EFFECTS OF EPIDURAL MORPHINE (4 mg)

	NALOXONE INFUSION 10 μg/kg⁻¹/h⁻¹	NALOXONE INFUSION 5 μg/kg⁻¹/h⁻¹	SALINE INFUSION
Duration of analgesia (h)	13.7*	17.8	18.5
Urinary retention (%)	33	53	67
Severe pruritus (%)	0	7	7
Nausea/vomiting (%)	7	13	20
Pulmonary complications (%)	7	7	20

*Significant difference.

From Rawal N, Schott U, Dahlstrom B, et al: Influence of naloxone infusion on analgesia and respiratory depression following epidural morphine. Anesthesiology 1986; 64:194–201.

Respiratory Depression

Respiratory depression is the most feared complication of epidural and intrathecal opioid administration.[32, 101, 113] Mild respiratory depression noted at 30 to 90 minutes results from systemic absorption of morphine from the epidural space. Delayed respiratory depression, which results from rostral spread of morphine in the CSF, may occur 6 to 10 hours later (Fig. 24–10).[32, 101, 102] After reaching the fourth ventricle, the drug rapidly equilibrates with intracranial CSF and interacts with the medullary respiratory centers to reduce the ventilatory response to carbon dioxide.[32, 101] Patients recovering from cesarean section are young and usually healthy, and they rarely present with significant pulmonary disease or other risk factors that might increase the likelihood of respiratory depression. Pregnant women also have an increased concentration of progesterone, which is a respiratory stimulant.[114] Nonetheless, Leicht and coworkers[38] reported four cases of respiratory depression (defined as a respiratory rate of less than 10 breaths per minute) among 1000 patients who received 5 mg of epidural morphine for postcesarean analgesia.

Single epidural or intrathecal doses of a lipophilic opioid are not associated with delayed respiratory depression.[32] However, early-onset respiratory depression, usually occurring within 30 minutes of administration, has been reported.[115, 116] Early-onset respiratory depression results from vascular uptake of the lipophilic opioid by the epidural or subarachnoid venous plexus and rapid transport via the systemic circulation to brain stem respiratory centers.[116, 117] Early-onset respiratory depression usually is of lesser significance than delayed-onset respiratory compromise; it is more likely to occur in a high-visibility, controlled setting (e.g., operating room, PACU, intensive care unit) where an anesthesiologist is present or immediately available.

There is no universal acceptance of the appropriate method of respiratory monitoring for patients treated with epidural or intrathecal morphine or a continuous epidural opioid infusion. Although various noninvasive monitors have been advocated, including pulse oximetry and end-tidal P_{CO_2} monitoring, none has become universally accepted. Vigilant nursing observation and hourly assessment of respiratory effort, respiratory rate, and unusual somnolence is probably the best form of monitoring in obstetric patients.[86] In our experience, the respiratory depression does not develop suddenly; rather, the rate of respiratory depression is slow and progressive, and it is usually preceded by increasing maternal somnolence. With appropriate nursing staff education and standardized orders (see Fig. 24–11), hospitals can provide safe care for the large majority of women who receive a modest dose of epidural (3–4 mg) or intrathecal (0.2–0.3 mg) morphine or a continuous epidural infusion of fentanyl. An anesthesia care provider should be readily available to manage complications that may arise.

SUPPLEMENTAL ANALGESIA

A significant number of patients treated with a single dose of intrathecal or epidural morphine will request

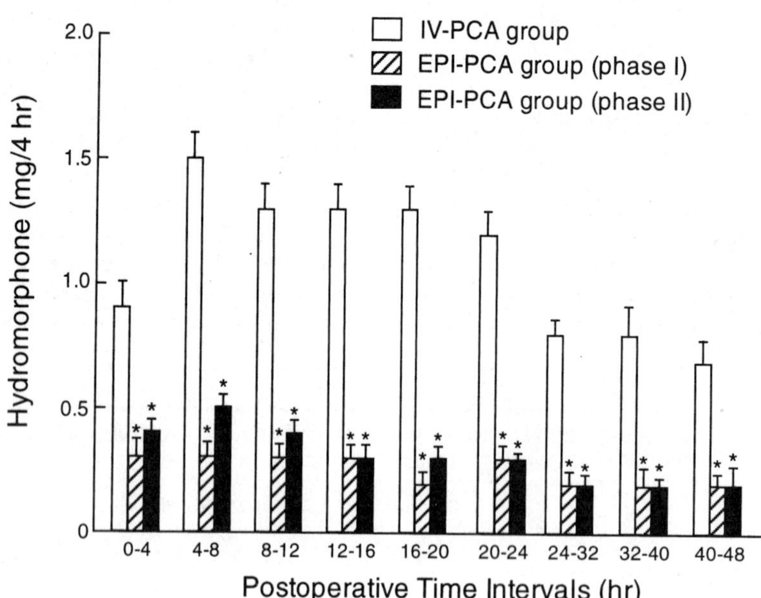

Figure 24–9 Postoperative hydromorphone use (mg/4 h interval) after either an intravenous or epidural loading dose. Results are expressed as mean ± SEM. *$P < .05$, significantly different from intravenous patient-controlled analgesia (IV-PCA) group. (From Parker R, White P: Epidural patient-controlled analgesia: an alternative to intravenous patient-controlled analgesia for pain relief after cesarean delivery. Anesth Analg 1992; 75:245–251.)

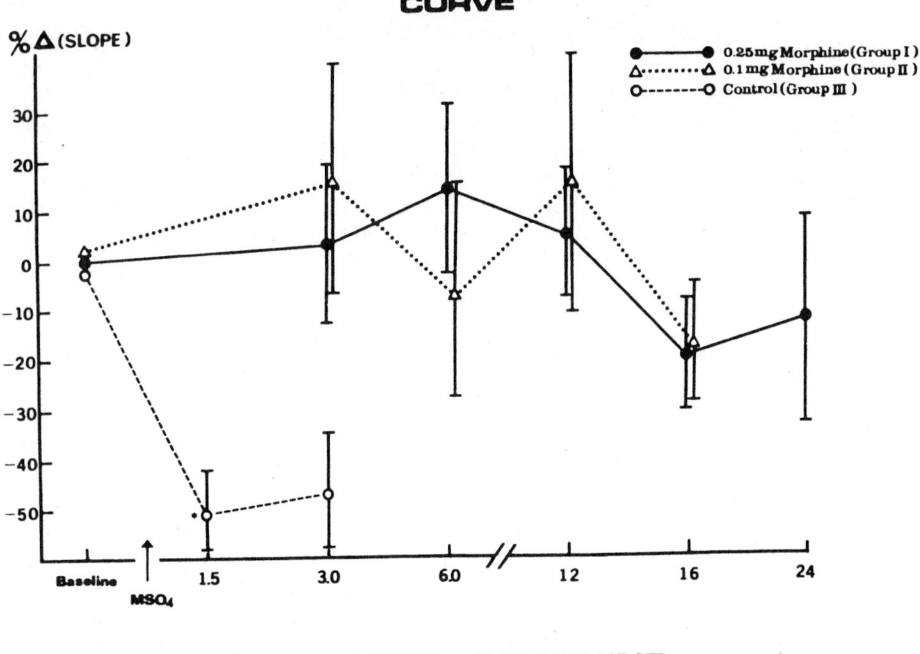

❖ **Figure 24-10** Percent change in CO_2 response slopes (L||PY|min⁻¹||PY|mm Hg⁻¹) from baseline values after patients received intrathecal or subcutaneous morphine (control). (From Abboud TK, Dror A, Mosaad P, et al: Mini-dose intrathecal morphine for the relief of post-cesarean section pain: safety, efficacy, and ventilatory responses to carbon dioxide. Anesth Analg 1988; 67:137–141.)

additional analgesia within 8 to 12 hours of morphine administration. We do not recommend administration of a second dose of epidural morphine in patients who are receiving nursing care on the postpartum ward. One option is to give an intravenous injection of a small dose of morphine (2–4 mg) or meperidine (25–50 mg).

Restricted bolus-dose IV-PCA may be safer than PRN administration of opioids when used to augment neuraxial morphine analgesia. A small dose of epidural (2–3 mg) or intrathecal (0.1–0.2 mg) morphine, combined with low-dose IV-PCA, represents an effective method of maintaining postcesarean analgesia.[87] In our experience, this regimen provides effective analgesia with less adverse events than epidural or intrathecal administration of larger doses of morphine. Benefits include uniformity of pain relief, a significant reduction in parenteral opioid dose requirements, and a reduced incidence of pruritus and other troublesome side effects. Restricted bolus-dose IV-PCA (meperidine 5 mg or morphine 0.5 mg, with a 10–15 minute lockout) maintains excellent pain control without excessive maternal sedation. Intraspinal morphine administration, followed by restricted-dose PCA, reduces parenteral opioid accumulation in breast milk and may result in a decreased likelihood of altered neonatal neurobehavior.[88]

Co-administration of α-adrenergic agonists plus opioid analgesics represents a new approach to postcesarean analgesia. α-Adrenergic agonists offer the potential of effective analgesia without the nausea, pruritus, and respiratory depression associated with intraspinal opioids.[118–121] Mogensen and coworkers[121] evaluated the quality of postoperative analgesia provided by a continuous epidural infusion of 0.125% bupivacaine and morphine, with or without clonidine. The addition of clonidine resulted in improved analgesia during cough and mobilization. However, this three-drug combination was associated with enhanced sympathetic blockade and an increased incidence of hypotension.

Nonsteroidal anti-inflammatory drugs may enhance intraspinal opioid analgesia without increasing the risk of sedation, pruritus, or respiratory depression.[122–124] In theory, these drugs may have an adverse effect on hemostasis, and they may increase the risk of postoperative bleeding. Experience suggests that limited exposure to these drugs does not result in increased postoperative bleeding. As was mentioned in the section dealing with IV-PCA, however, ketorolac is contraindicated in nursing mothers. Sun and associates[124] reported that patients treated with epidural morphine 2 mg plus intramuscular diclofenac 75 mg experienced superior postcesarean analgesia and required less supplemental meperidine than individuals who received either epidural morphine or intramuscular diclofenac alone. The pain associated with uterine cramping was better controlled in the diclofenac-morphine group. The decreased intensity of uterine cramping pain was not associated with uterine hypotonia or increased postpartum bleeding.

Many postcesarean patients are able to tolerate oral therapy 12 to 24 hours following cesarean delivery and can thus receive oral opioids or nonsteroidal anti-inflammatory drugs when supplemental analgesia following neuraxial opioids is needed.

Metoclopramide is an effective antiemetic for patients complaining of intraspinal opioid–induced nausea and vomiting. Metoclopramide also helps relieve the pain associated with uterine cramping.[125]

Epidurals and Spinal Opioid Analgesia After Cesarean Section: Current Clinical Practice at Yale-New Haven Hospital

Spinal Anesthesia for Cesarean Section

Some patients receive a single dose of preservative-free morphine (0.2–0.4 mg), which is combined with either hyperbaric bupivacaine (12.5 mg) or lidocaine (60–75 mg). Alternatively, we add two opioids to the local anesthetic solution: preservative-free meperidine (10 mg) and morphine (0.15 mg). This combination provides better analgesia than morphine alone during the first several hours after cesarean section.

All patients receive metoclopramide (10 mg) intravenously before administration of spinal anesthesia. This dose of antiemetic is readministered every 6 hours for 24 hours after surgery. Patients who complain of moderate to severe pruritus receive intravenous diphenhydramine (12.5–25 mg), naloxone (0.04–0.08 mg), or nalbuphine (5 mg).

All patients are provided restricted-dose intravenous patient-controlled analgesia (IV-PCA) morphine 0.5 mg q 8 to 10 min or meperidine (5–8 mg every 8–10 min as needed) for supplemental analgesia. Patients who receive the smaller (0.15 mg) dose of morphine are provided PCA immediately after arrival to the postpartum floor, whereas patients who receive the larger (0.25–0.4 mg) dose do not begin PCA until 8 to 12 hours after administration of spinal anesthesia. IV-PCA is continued for 24 to 36 hours, until patients can tolerate oral analgesics. Patients are followed by the Acute Pain Service. Standard orders include an hourly assessment of respiratory rate and level of sedation and intermittent use of pulse oximetry.

Epidural Anesthesia for Cesarean Section

We give most patients a small dose of epidural fentanyl (50–75 μg/mg) to augment intraoperative anesthesia. We delay epidural fentanyl administration until after the umbilical cord is clamped in cases of (1) severe fetal distress, (2) thick meconium-stained amniotic fluid, (3) preterm delivery, and (4) other conditions associated with an increased risk of neonatal respiratory depression. After delivery, we give either hydromorphone (0.5–1 mg) or a combination of preservative-free morphine (2–3 mg) and meperidine (40 mg) epidurally. We add saline so that the total volume is 10 mL. This dose of hydromorphone may be readministered every 6 hours, or the morphine-meperidine may be readministered every 12 hours for 36 hours. Alternatively, the catheter may be removed, and IV-PCA is begun 6 to 12 hours after epidural administration of opioid. Some patients receive a continuous epidural infusion of hydromorphone (10 μg/mg/mL) at a dose of 0.1 mg/h or a continuous epidural infusion of fentanyl (5 μg/mg/mL) at a dose of 40 to 60 μg/mg/h. Patient-controlled bolus doses (5–15 μg/mg of fentanyl or 5–10 μg/mg of hydromorphone every 15 minutes) may be combined with a lower background epidural infusion rate.

We administer metoclopramide for treatment of nausea and vomiting and give small doses of diphenhydramine, naloxone, or nalbuphine for treatment of pruritus. In non-nursing mothers, we give a small dose of ketorolac (15 mg slow IV bolus every 6 hours) for breakthrough pain.

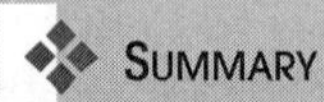

Summary

Key Points

- Poorly controlled pain following cesarean section interferes with ambulation, breast-feeding, and early maternal-infant bonding.
- Intravenous PCA allows the mother to titrate pain medication in amounts suitable for controlling excessive discomfort, while not causing undue sedation.
- Intrathecal opioid administration provides the most efficient method of activating spinal opioid receptors and provides the greatest gain in analgesic potency.
- Epidural delivery combined with a self-administration dosing regimen provides the psychologic benefits of PCA as well as the superior pain control associated with neuraxial opioids.

Key References

Parker RK, White PF: Epidural patient-controlled analgesia: an alternative to intravenous patient-controlled analgesia for pain relief after cesarean delivery. Anesth Analg 1992; 75:245–251.

Cousins MJ, Mather LE: Intrathecal and epidural administration of opioids. Anesthesiology 1984; 61:276–310.

Case Stem

A 26-year-old G2P1 undergoes a repeat cesarean section for a failed trial of labor due to a nonreassuring fetal heart rate tracing. She received combined spinal-epidural analgesia and a continuous epidural infusion of 0.125% bupivacaine with fentanyl during labor, which was converted to anesthesia for cesarean delivery using 3% chloroprocaine. Discuss the available options for postcesarean pain relief in this patient.

YALE-NEW HAVEN HOSPITAL

DOCTOR'S ORDERS

PLEASE USE BALL POINT PEN – BEAR DOWN

INSTRUCTIONS

1. EACH TIME A PHYSICIAN WRITES A MEDICATION ORDER, DETACH TOP COPY AND SEND TO PHARMACY.
2. RULE OFF UNUSED LINES AFTER LAST COPY (PINK) HAS BEEN SENT TO PHARMACY. IMPRINT NEW SET AND PLACE IN CHART.

DO NOT USE THIS SHEET UNLESS A NUMBER SHOWS ▶

YELLOW COPIES REMOVING WHILE HOLD HERE

DATE	TIME	ORDERS	DOCTOR'S SIGNATURE	NURSE'S SIGNATURE
		ACUTE PAIN SERVE/DEPARTMENT OF ANESTHESIOLOGY INTRAVENOUS OR EPIDURAL PATIENT-CONTROLLED ANALGESIA ORDERS		
1.		Drug ___		
		Concentration (mg/ml) ___ (μg/ml) ___		
		PCA dose (ml) ___		
		Continuous infusion rate (ml/hr) ___		
		4 hour limit (ml) ___		
2.		HEAD OF BED greater than ___ degrees. ACTIVITY: per surgeon.		
		VITAL SIGNS per routine, except respiratory rate q___h___ x ___ hours, then q___h___ x ___ hours, then q4h. MAINTAIN IV access while epidural catheter is in place.		
3.		PULSE OXIMETRY Yes ___; No ___. Continuous ___ for ___ hours; Intermittent ___ q ___ hours for ___ hours.		
4.		Naloxone (Narcan) two (2) ampules in patient's unit dose cassette.		
5.		NO SYSTEMIC NARCOTICS/SEDATIVES TO BE GIVEN EXCEPT AS ORDERED BY APS.		
6.		Treatment of nausea/vomiting:		
		Yes ___; No ___ droperidol (Inapsine) 0.2 ml (0.5 mg) IV q2h PRN x 2 doses		
		Yes ___; No ___ metoclopramide (Reglan) ___ mg IV q4h PRN x 2 doses		
		Yes ___; No ___ other: ___		
7.		Treatment of pruritus (itching):		
		Benadryl 12.5 mg IV q30 minutes PRN x 2 doses		
8.		Prophylactic infusion for itching/sedation: Yes ___; No ___;		
		Naloxone ___; or Nalbuphine ___. Add ___ ampule(s) per liter of maintenance IV fluid x ___ liter(s)		
9.		Ketorolac therapy: Yes ___; No ___. Loading dose ___ mg slow IV; then ___ mg q6 hours x ___ hours		
10.		Notify APS, beeper ___ for:		
		a) somnolence or confusion		
		b) respiratory rate of 10 or less		
		c) inadequate analgesia		
		d) pruritus or nausea/vomiting unresponsive to treatment		
		e) oxygen saturation less than 90%		
		f) leakage or redness around insertion site		
		Date: ___ ___ M.D.		

F-854 (Rev. 7/87)

1193 DISCHARGE DIAGNOSES IN ORDER OF DECREASING PRIORITY MUST BE SUPPLIED AT TIME OF PATIENT'S DISCHARGE.

❖ **Figure 24–11** Standardized orders for intravenous and epidural patient-controlled analgesia utilized at Yale-New Haven Hospital.

CONTROVERSIES AND RELATIVE CONTRAINDICATIONS

Most patients who qualify for either spinal or epidural anesthesia can safely receive intraspinal opioid therapy provided the nursing staff has received adequate education and close patient surveillance is maintained. Intraspinal opioid analgesia should not be used in settings where there are no standardized orders, no nursing policies and procedures, and no qualified physician available to manage complications.

There are several maternal conditions that represent relative contraindications to intraspinal opioid therapy. These include patients presenting with herpes simplex virus labialis,[126, 127] human immunodeficiency virus,[128] active asthma, multiple sclerosis,[129] and morbid obesity.[130] In these cases, the anesthesiologist should assess the risks and benefits for the individual patient before deciding whether to proceed with intraspinal opioid therapy.

EFFECTS ON OUTCOME AFTER CESAREAN SECTION

Although intraspinal opioids now represent the "gold standard" for providing effective postcesarean analgesia, it has been difficult to demonstrate that intraspinal opioid techniques improve perioperative outcome.[132] This difficulty may be attributed in part to the fact that these patients are young and most are healthy and at low risk for serious perioperative morbidity and mortality. Intraspinal opioid analgesia may improve outcome in high-risk obstetric patients.[131] Women with severe preeclampsia, cardiovascular disease, and morbid obesity may benefit from the reduction in cardiovascular stress and improved pulmonary function associated with effective analgesia.

The potential advantages of intraspinal opioid analgesia on neonatal well-being should also be considered. Reduced maternal doses of opioid should result in decreased concentrations in breast milk. In one study, a single dose of epidural morphine 4 mg significantly reduced IV-PCA morphine exposure in nursing mothers recovering from cesarean section, and this may have been responsible for the superior neurobehavioral scores observed in the breast-fed neonates in that group.[88] Current postcesarean delivery analgesic practice at Yale-New Haven Hospital is presented in Box 24–1. Standardized orders are included in Figure 24–11.

In conclusion, women recovering from cesarean delivery should not have to experience significant discomfort, as refinements in neuraxial and IV-PCA offer effective pain control with minimal side effects. These therapies can be maintained for 24 to 36 hours or until the mother can tolerate oral analgesics. The combination of neuraxial analgesia and restricted dose IV-PCA offers the benefit of reduced maternal opioid requirements and less exposure to the nursing neonate.

References

1. Marks RM, Sachar EF: Undermedication of medical inpatients with narcotic analgesics. Ann Intern Med 1973; 78:173–181.
2. Wittels B, Scott DT, Sinatra R: Exogenous opioids in human breast milk and acute neonatal neurobehavior: a preliminary study. Anesthesiology 1990; 864–869.
3. Gibbs CP, Krischer J, Peckham BM, et al: Obstetric anesthesia: a national survey. Anesthesiology 1986; 65:298–306.
4. Knapp RM, Writer DES: Obstetrical use of epidural opioids: a national survey [abstract]. Proc Soc Obstet Anesth Perinatol 1988; 20:66.
5. Chen B, Kwan W, Lee C, Cantley E: A national survey of obstetric post-anesthesia care in teaching hospitals [abstract]. Anesth Analg 1993; 76:S43.
6. Sechzer PH: Objective measurement of pain. Anesthesiology 1968; 29:209–210.
7. Bennett RL, Bradhorst RL, Bivans BA, et al: Patient-controlled analgesia: a new concept of postoperative pain relief. Ann Surg 1982; 195:700–705.
8. Sechzer PH: Patient-controlled analgesia (PCA): a retrospective. Anesthesiology 1990; 72:735–736.
9. Parker AJ, Sinatra RS, Glass PSA: Patient-controlled analgesia systems. *In* Sinatra RS, Hord AH, Ginsberg B, Preble LM (eds): Acute Pain: Mechanisms and Management. St. Louis: Mosby–Year Book; 1992: 205–224.
10. Owen H, White PF: Patient-controlled analgesia: an overview. *In* Sinatra RS, Hord AH, Ginsberg B, Preble LM (eds): Acute Pain: Mechanisms and Management. St. Louis: Mosby–Year Book; 1992: 151–164.
11. Austin KL, Stapleton JV, Mather LE: Relationship between blood meperidine concentration and analgesic response. Anesthesiology 1980; 53:460–466.
12. White PF: Use of patient controlled analgesia for management of acute pain. JAMA 1988; 259:243–247.
13. Owen H, Plummer H, Armstrong I, et al: Variables of PCA: 1. Bolus size. Anaesthesia 1989; 44:7–10.
14. Wu MYC, Purcell GJ: Patient controlled analgesia: the value of a background infusion. Anaesth Intensive Care 1990; 18:575–576.
15. Harrison DM, Sinatra RS, Morgese L, et al: Epidural narcotic and PCA for post-cesarean section pain relief. Anesthesiology 1988; 68:454–457.
16. Eisenach JC, Grice SC, Dewan DM: Patient controlled analgesia following cesarean section: a comparison with epidural and intramuscular narcotics. Anesthesiology 1988; 68:444–448.
17. Cade L, Ashley J, Ross W: Comparison of epidural and intravenous opioid analgesia after elective caesarean section. Anaesth Intensive Care 1992; 20:41–45.
18. Sinatra RS, Lodge K, Sibert K, et al: A comparison of morphine, meperidine, and oxymorphone as utilized in patient controlled analgesia following cesarean delivery. Anesthesiology 1989; 70:585–590.
19. Szeto HH, Inturrisi CE, Houde R, et al: Accumulation of normeperidine, an active metabolite of meperidine, in patients with renal failure or cancer. Ann Intern Med 1977; 86:738–741.
20. Sinatra RS, Chung KS, Silverman DG, et al: An evaluation of morphine, meperidine, and oxymorphone administered via patient-controlled analgesia (PCA) or PCA plus basal infusion in postcesarean delivery patients. Anesthesiology 1989; 71:502–507.
21. Wittels B, Sevarino FB: PCA in the obstetric patient. *In* Sinatra RS, Hord AH, Ginsberg B, Preble LM (eds): Acute Pain: Mechanisms and Management. St. Louis: Mosby–Year Book; 1992: 175–181.
22. Negre I, Gueneron JP, Jamali SR, et al: Preoperative analgesia with epidural morphine. Anesth Analg 1994; 79:298–302.
23. Weintraub SJ, Naulty JS: Acute abstinence syndrome after epidural injection of butorphanol. Anesth Analg 1985; 64:452–453.
24. Eige S: PCA opioids: common side effects and their treatment. *In* Sinatra RS, Hord AH, Ginsberg B, Preble LM (eds): Acute Pain: Mechanisms and Management. St. Louis: Mosby–Year Book; 1992: 182–193.
25. Sevarino FB, Sinatra RS, Paige D, et al: The efficacy of intramuscular ketorolac in combination with intravenous PCA morphine for postoperative pain relief. J Clin Anesth 1992; 4:285–290.
26. Ready LB, Brown CR, Stahlgren LH, et al: Evaluation of intravenous ketorolac administered by bolus or infusion for treatment of postoperative pain. Anesthesiology 1994; 80:1277.
27. Kitahata LM, Kosaka Y, Taub A: Lamina-specific suppression of dorsal horn activity by morphine sulfate. Anesthesiology 1974; 41:39–48.
28. Atweh SA, Kuhar MJ: Autoradiographic localization of opiate receptors in rat brain. I. Spinal cord and lower medulla. Brain Res 1977; 124:53–67.
29. Schmauss C, Yaksh TL: In vivo studies on spinal opiate receptor systems mediating antinociception. II. Pharmacological profiles suggesting a differential association of mu, delta, and kappa receptors. J Pharmacol Exp Ther 1984; 228:1–12.
30. Yaksh TL: Spinal opiate analgesia: characteristics and principles of action. Pain 1981; 11:293–346.
31. Wang J, Nauss LA, Thomas JE: Pain relief by intrathecally applied morphine in man. Anesthesiology 1979; 50:149–150.
32. Cousins MJ, Mather LE: Intrathecal and epidural administration of opioids. Anesthesiology 1984; 61:276–310.
33. Nordberg G, Hedner T, Mellstrand T, et al: Pharmacokinetic aspects of epidural morphine analgesia. Anesthesiology 1983; 58:545–551.
34. Nordberg G, Hedner T, Mellstrand T, et al: Pharmacokinetic aspects of intrathecal morphine analgesia. Anesthesiology 1984; 60:448–454.
35. Cousins MJ, Mather LE, Glynn CJ: Selective spinal analgesia. Lancet 1979; 1:1141–1142.
36. Rosen MA, Hughes SC, Shnider SM, et al: Epidural morphine for the relief of postoperative pain after cesarean delivery. Anesth Analg 1983; 62:666–672.

37. Carmichael EJ, Rolbin SH, Hew EM: Epidural morphine for analgesia after caesarean section. Can J Anaesth 1982; 29:359–363.
38. Leicht CH, Hughes SC, Dailey PA, et al: Epidural morphine sulfate for analgesia after cesarean section: a prospective report of 1,000 patients [abstract]. Anesthesiology 1986; 65:A366.
39. Fuller JG, McMorland GH, Douglas MJ, Palmer L: Epidural morphine for analgesia after caesarean section: a report of 4,880 patients. Can J Anaesth 1990; 37:636–640.
40. Kotelko DM, Thigpen JW, Shnider SM, et al: Postoperative epidural morphine analgesia after various local anesthetics [abstract]. Anesthesiology 1983; 59:A413.
41. Eisenach JC, Schlairet TJ, Dobson CE, et al: Effect of prior anesthetic solution on epidural morphine analgesia. Anesth Analg 1991; 73:119–123.
42. Sharar SR, Ready BL, Ross BK, et al: A comparison of postcesarean epidural morphine analgesia by single injection and by continuous infusion. Reg Anesth 1991; 16:232–235.
43. Leicht CH, Durkan WJ, Fians DH, et al: Postoperative analgesia with epidural morphine: single bolus vs. Daymate elastomeric continuous infusion technique [abstract]. Anesthesiology 1990; 73:A931.
44. Naulty JS, Datta S, Ostheimer GW, et al: Epidural fentanyl for post-cesarean delivery pain management. Anesthesiology 1985; 63:694–698.
45. Robertson K, Douglas MJ, McMorland GH. Epidural fentanyl, with and without epinephrine for post-caesarean section analgesia. Can Anaesth Soc J 1985; 32:502–505.
46. Sevarino FB, McFarlane C, Sinatra RS, et al: Epidural fentanyl does not influence intravenous PCA requirements in the post-caesarean patient. Can J Anaesth 1991; 38:450–453.
47. Youngstrom P, Hoyt M, Herman M, et al: Dose-response study of continuous infusion epidural fentanyl-epinephrine for post-cesarean analgesia. Anesthesiology 1990; 73:A984.
48. Youngstrom P, Boyd B, Rhoton F: Complaints of side effects from postcesarean epidural opioid analgesia: fewer with fentanyl-epinephrine infusion than with morphine bolus [abstract]. Anesthesiology 1992; 77:A859.
49. Loper KA, Ready LB, Sandler A: Epidural and intravenous fentanyl infusions are clinically equivalent following knee surgery. Anesth Analg 1990; 70:72–75.
50. Glass PSA, Estok P, Ginsberg B, et al: Use of patient-controlled analgesia to compare the efficacy of epidural to intravenous fentanyl administration. Anesth Analg 1992; 74:345–351.
51. Rosen MA, Dailey PA, Hughes SC, et al: Epidural sufentanil for postoperative analgesia after cesarean section. Anesthesiology 1988; 68:448–452.
52. Naulty JS, Sevarino FB, Lema MJ, et al: Epidural sufentanil for postcesarean delivery pain management [abstract]. Anesthesiology 1986; 65:A396.
53. Shnider SM: Epidural and subarachnoid opiates in obstetrics. American Society of Anesthesiologists Refresher Course Lectures, 1989:235.
54. Leight CH, Kelleher AJ, Robinson DE, et al: Prolongation of postoperative epidural sufentanil analgesia with epinephrine. Anesth Analg 1990; 70:323–328.
55. Naulty JS, Bergan W, Zurowski D, et al: Effect of diluent volume on analgesia produced by epidural sufentanil [abstract]. Anesthesiology 1989; 71:A700.
56. Rosen MA, Hughes SC, Shnider SM, et al: Continuous epidural sufentanil for postoperative analgesia [abstract]. Anesth Analg 1990; 70:S331.
57. Cheng EY, Koebert RF, Hopwood MA, et al: Continuous epidural sufentanil infusion for postoperative pain [abstract]. Anesthesiology 1987; 67:A233.
58. Coda BA, Kawata J, Ross BK: Plasma sufentanil concentration during prolonged epidural infusion for postoperative analgesia [abstract]. Anesth Analg 1993; 76:S49.
59. Paech MJ: Post caesarean section pain relief with epidural pethidine or fentanyl. Anaesth Intensive Care 1989; 17:157–165.
60. Dougherty TB, Baysinger CL, Henenberger JC, et al: Epidural hydromorphone with and without epinephrine for post-operative analgesia after cesarean delivery. Anesth Analg 1989; 68:318–322.
61. Parker R, Bottros L, Sawaki Y, White PF: Epidural PCA: use of hydromorphone versus hydromorphone-nalbuphine after cesarean delivery [abstract]. Anesthesiology 1992; 77:A1014.
62. Macrae DJ, Munishankarappa S, Burrow LM, et al: Double blind comparison of the efficacy of extradural diamorphine, extradural phenoperidine and IM diamorphine following caesarean section. Br J Anaesth 1987; 59:354–359.
63. Beeby D, MacIntosh KC, Bailey M: Postoperative analgesia after caesarean section using epidural methadone. Anaesthesia 1984; 39:61–63.
64. Abboud TK, Moore M, Zhu J, et al: Epidural butorphanol or morphine for the relief of post-cesarean section pain. Anesth Analg 1987; 66:887–893.
65. Perriss BW, Latham BV, Wilson IH: Analgesia following extradural and IM pethidine in post-caesarean section patients. Br J Anaesth 1990; 64:355–357.
66. Chestnut DH, Choi WW, Isbell TJ: Epidural hydromorphone for postcesarean analgesia. Obstet Gynecol 1986; 68:65–69.
67. Henderson SK, Matthew EB, Cohen H, et al: Epidural hydromorphone: a double-blind comparison with intramuscular hydromorphone for post–cesarean section analgesia. Anesthesiology 1987; 66:825–830.
68. Boudreault D, Brasseur L, Samii K, Lemoing JP: Comparison of continuous epidural bupivacaine infusion plus either continuous epidural infusion or patient-controlled epidural injection of fentanyl for postoperative analgesia. Anesth Analg 1991; 73:132–137.
69. Semple AJ, Macrae DJ, Munishankarappa S, et al: Effect of the addition of adrenaline to extradural diamorphine analgesia after caesarean section. Br J Anaesth 1988; 60:632–638.
70. Palacios QT, Jones MM, Hawkins JL, et al: Post-cesarean section analgesia: a comparison of epidural butorphanol and morphine. Can J Anaesth 1991; 38:24–30.
71. Barber M, Gold M, Koclanes G, et al: Epidural morphine vs butorphanol following caesarean section: comparison of PCA use post-operatively [abstract]. Proc Soc Obstet Anesth Perinatol 1991; 22:5.
72. Camann WR, Loferski BL, Fanciullo GJ, et al: Does epidural butorphanol offer any clinical advantage over the intravenous route? Anesthesiology 1992; 76:216–220.
73. Naulty JS, Ross R: Epidural fentanyl and morphine for post-cesarean delivery analgesia [abstract]. Proc Soc Obstet Anesth Perinatol 1988; 20:178.
74. Kotelko DM, Rottman RL, Wright WC, et al: Improved surgical and post-cesarean analgesia with epidural fentanyl/ morphine combination [abstract]. Anesthesiology 1987; 67:A622.
75. Naulty S, Parnet J, Pate A, et al: Epidural sufentanil and morphine for post-cesarean delivery analgesia [abstract]. Anesthesiology 1990; 73:A964.
76. Dottrens M, Rifat K, Morel DR: Comparison of extradural administration of sufentanil, morphine and sufentanil-morphine combination after caesarean section. Br J Anaesth 1992; 69:9–12.
77. Sjostrom S, Hartvig D, Tamsen A: Patient controlled analgesia with extradural morphine or pethidine. Br J Anaesth 1988; 60:358–362.
78. Chrubasik J, Wust H, Schulte-Monting J, et al: Relative analgesic potency of epidural fentanyl, alfentanil, and morphine in treatment of postoperative pain [abstract]. Anesthesiology 1988; 68:929.
79. Walmsley PNH: Patient controlled epidural analgesia. *In* Sinatra RS, Hord AH, Ginsberg B, Preble LM (eds): Acute Pain: Mechanisms and Management. St Louis: Mosby; 1992: 312–320.
80. Yarnell RW, Murphy IL, Polis T, et al: Patient-controlled analgesia with epidural meperidine after cesarean section. Reg Anesth 1992; 17:329–333.
81. Parker RK, White P: Epidural patient-controlled analgesia: an alternative to intravenous patient-controlled analgesia for pain relief after cesarean delivery. Anesth Analg 1992; 75:245–251.

82. Parker R, Sawaki Y, White PF: Epidural patient-controlled analgesia: influence of bupivacaine and hydromorphone basal infusion on pain control after cesarean delivery. Anesth Analg 1992; 75:740–746.
83. Grass JA, Zuckerman RL, Tsao H, et al: Patient controlled epidural analgesia results in shorter hospital stay after cesarean section [abstract]. Reg Anesth 1991; 15(suppl):26.
84. Grass JA, Harris AP, Sakima NT, et al: Pain management after cesarean section: sufentanil PCEA versus morphine IV-PCA [abstract]. Anesth Analg 1992; 74:S120.
85. Cohen S, Amar D, Pantuck EJ, et al: Continuous epidural analgesia post cesarean section: effect of diluent volume [abstract]. Anesthesiology 1991; 75:A860.
86. Cohen S, Amar D, Pantuck CB, et al: Adverse effects of epidural 0.03% bupivacaine during analgesia after cesarean section. Anesth Analg 1992; 75:753–756.
87. Kemper PM, Treiber N: Neuraxial morphine plus PCA: a new method of post-cesarean analgesia [abstract]. Anesth Analg 1990; 70:S198.
88. Wittels B, Glosten B, Faure E, et al: Postcesarean analgesia using both epidural morphine and intravenous patient-controlled analgesia: neurobehavioral outcomes among nursing neonates [abstract]. Anesthesiology 1992; 77:A1015.
89. Zakowski MI, Ramanathan S, Sharnick S: Uptake and distribution of bupivacaine and morphine after intrathecal administration in parturients: effects of epinephrine. Anesth Analg 1992; 74:664–669.
90. Abboud TK, Dror A, Mosaad P, et al: Minidose intrathecal morphine for the relief of post-cesarean section pain: safety, efficacy, and ventilatory responses to carbon dioxide. Anesth Analg 1988; 67:137–141.
91. Chadwick HS, Ready LB: Intrathecal and epidural morphine sulfate for postcesarean analgesia: a clinical comparison. Anesthesiology 1988; 68:925–929.
92. Abouleish E, Rawal N, Fallon K, et al: Combined intrathecal morphine and bupivacaine for cesarean section [abstract]. Proc Soc Obstet Anesth Perinatol 1987; 19:16.
93. Abouleish E, Rawal N, Rashad MN: The addition of 0.2 mg subarachnoid morphine to hyperbaric bupivacaine for cesarean delivery: a prospective study of 856 cases. Reg Anesth 1991; 16:137–140.
94. Hunt CO, Datta S, Hauch M, et al: Perioperative analgesia with subarachnoid fentanyl-bupivacaine [abstract]. Anesthesiology 1987; 67:A621.
95. Belzarena SD: Clinical effects of intrathecally administered fentanyl in patients undergoing cesarean section. Anesth Analg 1992; 74:653–657.
96. Courtney MA, Hauch M, Bader AM, et al: Perioperative analgesia with subarachnoid sufentanil administration. Reg Anesth 1992; 17:274–278.
97. Feldman JM, Griffin F, Fermo L, Raessler K: Intrathecal meperidine for pain after cesarean delivery: efficacy and dose-response [abstract]. Anesthesiology 1992; 77:A1011.
98. Naulty JS: The combination of intrathecal morphine and fentanyl for post-cesarean analgesia [abstract]. Anesthesiology 1989; 71:A864.
99. Chung JH, Sinatra RS, Sevarino FB, et al: Subarachnoid meperidine-morphine conbination: an effective postoperative analgesic adjunct for cesarean delivery. Reg Anesth 1997; 22:119–124.
100. Cohen S, Amar D, Pantuck CB: Continuous epidural-PCA post-cesarean section: buprenorphine-bupivacaine 0.03% vs. fentanyl-bupivacaine 0.003% [abstract]. Anesthesiology 1990; 73:A973.
101. Bromage PR: The price of intraspinal narcotic analgesia: basic constraints. Anesth Analg 1981; 60:461–463.
102. Kafer ER, Brown JT, Scott DD: Biphasic depression of ventilatory responses to CO_2 following epidural morphine. Anesthesiology 1987; 58:418–427.
103. Scott PV, Fischer HBJ: Intraspinal opiates and itching: a new reflex. Br Med J 1982; 284:1015–1016.
104. Zakowski MI, Ramanathan S, Khoo P, et al: Plasma histamine with intraspinal morphine in cesarean section [abstract]. Anesth Analg 1990; 70:S448.
105. Luthman JA, Kay NH, White JB: Intrathecal morphine for post caesarean section analgesia: does naloxone reduce the incidence of pruritus? Int J Obstet Anesth 1992; 1:191–194.
106. Morgan PJ, Mehta S, Kapala DM: Nalbuphine pretreatment in cesarean section patients receiving epidural morphine. Reg Anesth 1991; 16:84–88.
107. Abboud TK, Lee K, Zhu J, et al: Prophylactic oral naltrexone with intrathecal morphine for cesarean section: effects on adverse reactions and analgesia. Anesth Analg 1990; 71:367–370.
108. Borgeat A, Wilder-Smith OHG, Saiah M, et al: Subhypnotic doses of propofol relieve pruritus induced by epidural and intrathecal morphine. Anesthesiology 1992; 76:510–512.
109. Borgeat A, Saiah M, Rifat K: Does propofol relieve epidural or subarachnoid morphine-induced pruritus [letter]? Reg Anesth 1991; 16:245.
110. Evron S, Samueloff A, Simon A: Urinary function during epidural analgesia with methadone and morphine in post-cesarean section patients. Pain 1985; 23:135–140.
111. Rawal N, Mollefors K, Axelsson K, et al: An experimental study of urodynamic effects of epidural morphine and of naloxone reversal. Anesth Analg 1983; 62:641–647.
112. Durant PAC, Yaksh TL: Drug effects on urinary bladder tone during spinal morphine-induced inhibition of the micturition reflex in unanesthetized rats. Anesthesiology 1988; 68:325–334.
113. Rawal N, Schott U, Dahlstrom B, et al: Influence of naloxone infusion on analgesia and respiratory depression following epidural morphine. Anesthesiology 1986; 64:194–201.
114. Lyons HA, Antonio R: The sensitivity of the respiratory center in pregnancy and after the administration of progesterone. Trans Assoc Am Physicians 1959; 72:173–180.
115. Stienstra R, Van Poorten F: Immediate respiratory arrest after caudal epidural sufentanil. Anesthesiology 1989; 71:993–994.
116. Wells DG, Davies G: Profound central nervous system depression from epidural fentanyl for extracorporeal shock wave lithotripsy. Anesthesiology 1987; 67:991–992.
117. Labaille T, Benhamou D, Levron JC, Cohen SE: CO_2 sensitivity following epidural sufentanil in cesarean section patients [abstract]. Anesthesiology 1988; 69:A702.
118. Eisenach JC, Lysak SZ, Viscomi CM: Epidural clonidine analgesia following surgery: phase I. Anesthesiology 1989; 71:640–646.
119. Narchi P, Benhamou D, Hamza J, Bouaziz H: Ventilatory effects of epidural clonidine during the first 3 hours after caesarean section. Acta Anaesthesiol Scand 1992; 36:791–795.
120. Huntoon M, Eisenach JC, Boese P: Epidural clonidine after cesarean section. Anesthesiology 1992; 76:187–193.
121. Mogensen T, Eliasen K, Ejlersen E, et al: Epidural clonidine enhances postoperative analgesia from a combined low-dose epidural bupivacaine and morphine regimen. Anesth Analg 1992; 75:607–610.
122. Waters J, Hullander M, Kraft A, et al: Post-cesarean pain relief with ketorolac tromethamine and epidural morphine [abstract]. Anesthesiology 1992; 77:A813.
123. Mok MS, Tzeng JI: Intramuscular ketorolac enhances the analgesic effect of low dose epidural morphine [abstract]. Anesth Analg 1993; 76:269.
124. Sun HL, Wu CC, Lin MS, Chang CF: Effects of epidural morphine and intramuscular diclofenac combination in postcesarean analgesia: a dose-range study. Anesth Analg 1993; 76:284–288.
125. Rosenblatt WH, Cioffi AM, Sinatra RS, Silverman DG: Metoclopramide-enhanced analgesia for prostaglandin-induced termination of pregnancy. Anesth Analg 1992; 75:760–763.
126. Crone LAL, Conly JM, Clark KM, et al: Recurrent herpes simplex virus labialis and the use of epidural morphine on obstetric patients. Anesth Analg 1988; 67:318–323.
127. Crone LAL, Conly JM, Storgard C, et al: Herpes labialis in parturients receiving epidural morphine following cesarean section. Anesthesiology 1990; 73:208–213.
128. Hughes SC, Dailey PA, Landers D, et al: The HIV+ parturient and regional anesthesia: clinical and immunologic response [abstract]. Anesthesiology 1992; 77:A1036.
129. Berger JM, Ontell R: Intrathecal morphine in conjunction

with a combined spinal and general anesthetic in a patient with multiple sclerosis. Anesthesiology 1987; 66:400–402.
130. Stenkamp SJ, Easterling TR, Chadwick HS: Effect of epidural and intrathecal morphine on the length of stay following cesarean section. Anesth Analg 1989; 68:66–69.
131. Rawal N, Sjostrand U, Christoffersson E, et al: Comparison of intramuscular and epidural morphine for postoperative analgesia in the grossly obese: influence on postoperative ambulation and pulmonary function. Anesth Analg 1984; 63:583–588.

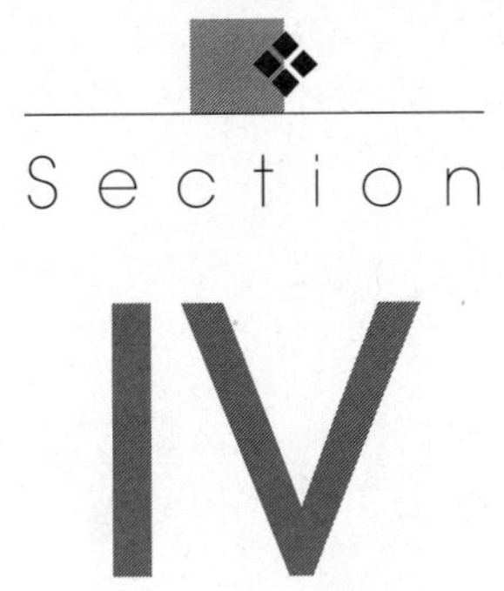

Section

IV

Obstetric and Anesthetic Complications

25

Preterm Labor

❖ Peter Gerner, MD
❖ Martin C. Haeusler, MD

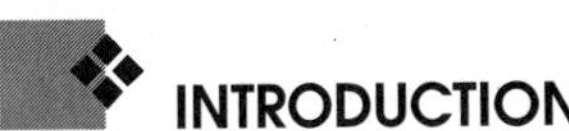

INTRODUCTION

Despite improved antenatal care, the incidence of preterm delivery in the United States has not decreased within the last 15 years and is currently approximately 10%. Although survival rates for low birthweight (LBW) infants have improved, this is not attributed to the increased incidence of cesarean section.[1] Two thirds of all infant deaths occur among infants who weigh less than 2500 g at birth. The survival rate increases as the birthweight or gestational age increases. Over the last 15 to 20 years, there has been a significant improvement in the survival rate in every very low birthweight (VLBW) subgroup, with the greatest improvement occurring in the subgroup with a birthweight of 750 to 1000 g. These infants usually have a 70% to 80% survival chance with aggressive neonatal intensive care. As neonatal survival rates improve, the issue of neonatal morbidity becomes increasingly important. Obstetricians, neonatologists, and the parents must consider the risk of morbidity and mortality when making decisions regarding the timing and method of preterm delivery. Anesthesiologists are often asked to take an active role in the overall management of the parturient with preterm labor and must therefore be aware of the obstetric and anesthetic ramifications of preterm labor and the medications used to treat this condition.

DEFINITIONS

Terminology is presented in the box. Statistics often refer to birthweight because gestational age can sometimes be difficult to determine. However, term infants can be small for gestational age and preterm infants can be large for gestational age, so this may not be a reliable correlation. Survival increases as birthweight or gestational age increases.

INCIDENCE

Preterm birth occurs in approximately 10% of all pregnancies. Delivery before 32 weeks' gestation is associated with major morbidity and mortality and most neonatal deaths and disorders occur in this group (2% of all births).

Statistics indicate that the incidence of preterm birth has not declined over the past 15 years. Preterm delivery usually occurs after spontaneous premature labor (in approximately one half of cases) or, less commonly, spontaneous rupture of the membranes (in approximately one third). Approximately one fifth of deliveries of premature infants are indicated for either the benefit of the mother or the fetus.[2] The risk factors

Terminology

Preterm labor	Regular uterine contractions producing cervical change before 37 weeks' gestation. Three criteria have to be fulfilled: 1. Gestational age from the 20th to end of the 37th week of gestation. 2. Documented uterine contractions, either 4 contractions in 20 minutes or 8 contractions in 60 minutes. 3. Documented cervical change, 80% effacement or 2-cm dilation.
Preterm infant	Infant delivered between 20 and 37 weeks' gestation, as calculated from the first day of the last menstrual period (LMP).
Stillbirth	Birth without signs of life with fetus ≥500 g, around 23–24 weeks' gestation.
Abortion	Birth without signs of life and fetus <500 g.
Low birthweight (LBW)	Weight <2500 g at birth (corresponding to approximately 35 weeks' gestation).
Very low birthweight (VLBW)	Weight <1500 g at birth (approximately 31 weeks' gestation).

for elective preterm births have been reported to be different from those associated with spontaneous preterm birth.[3]

Mortality has decreased from approximately 50% in 1960 to about 5% today among infants with a birthweight of 1000 to 1500 g, and among those with a birthweight of 500 to 1000 g mortality has decreased from approximately 95% in 1960 to about 20% today.[4, 5] This was accomplished by the use of more effective neonatal interventions (including newer modalities of mechanical ventilation, exogenous surfactant therapy, early and germ-specific antibiotic treatment) as well as appropriate electrolyte and fluid management. Obstetric interventions considered to be effective include the predelivery administration of antibiotics to reduce the incidence and severity of neonatal sepsis. The use of prenatal corticosteroids for fetal lung maturation and the prevention and aggressive treatment of fetal hypoxia have been major advances. In addition, the avoidance of oxygen toxicity has decreased morbidity that was once common in surviving infants.

Although the mortality rates are now much lower, roughly 1 out of 2 neonatal deaths occur in those infants who weigh less than 1000 g at birth. Also, the significance of an improvement in neurologic outcome[6–8] or a reduction of prematurity-associated neurologic problems has not been conclusively determined.[2]

RISK FACTORS

A history of previous preterm delivery and multiple gestation are the two most significant risk factors for preterm labor. In some cases infection such as pyelonephritis or chorioamnionitis may also cause preterm labor. In up to 50% of all cases, however, no risk factors can be identified.

In spite of recent advances in the research on the physiology of labor and delivery, the causes and mechanisms of preterm labor are not yet well understood. Also, approximately 50% of cases occur in women without apparent risk factors.

Early Identification of Preterm Labor. Fetal fibronectin, an extensively studied marker of degradation of the extracellular matrix of fetal membranes is different from the adult fibronectin of tissues. It is a glycoprotein found in the amniotic membranes, decidua, and cytotrophoblast and can be used to possibly identify women who are at risk for premature rupture of the membranes as well as preterm delivery. The production of fetal fibronectin by human amniotic cells is stimulated by release of inflammatory mediators including interleukin-1 and tumor necrosis factor-α.[9] All published studies to date have demonstrated an association between detection of cervical or vaginal fetal fibronectin and a shorter interval to delivery. Also, in patients with symptoms suggestive of preterm labor, the high negative predictive value of fetal fibronectin sampling supports less intervention for patients with this negative result.[10] On the other hand, in a meta-analysis by Chien and associates[11] the presence of fetal fibronectin in cervicovaginal mucus had limited accuracy in predicting preterm delivery. Hence further studies are necessary to determine the role of fibronectin and its possible use for the diagnosis and treatment of preterm labor.

Risk Assessment. A graded risk assessment system has been developed which includes factors that are highly associated with spontaneous preterm delivery; surprisingly this system did not identify most women who eventually had a spontaneous preterm delivery.[12] In about one half of cases, no single risk factor can be identified. Nevertheless, five groups of risk factors have been identified (Table 25–1):

- Maternal (history of preterm delivery)
- Fetoplacental (abnormal placentation)
- Uterine (multiple gestations)
- Cervical (incompetence)
- Premature rupture of membranes

Maternal risk factors (Table 25–1) include the history of preterm delivery. The risk is 35% if there is one prior preterm delivery, but increases to 70% if there are two or more. Since this is the single most important factor for predicting preterm delivery and

Table 25–1 **Risk Factors for Preterm Delivery**

Maternal Risk Factors
History of preterm delivery
Low socioeconomic status
Poor weight gain during pregnancy
History of DES exposure
History of second trimester spontaneous abortion (but not first trimester spontaneous abortion)
Extremes of age (<15 years and >40 years)
Nulliparous
Single mother
Underweight (especially if prepregnancy weight is <40 kg)
Trauma
Abdominal surgery during pregnancy (the closer to the uterus, the higher the incidence)
Physically stressful job (e.g., lifting heavy objects)
Infection (e.g., genital, urinary tract infection, pyelonephritis)
Smoking, illicit drug use
Uterine Risk Factors
Overdistention of the uterus (e.g., in multiple gestations, polyhydramnios)
Abnormal uterine cavity (e.g., fibroids, uterine anomaly, Asherman's syndrome)
Foreign body—retained intrauterine device
Cervical Risk Factors
Incompetence
Trauma
Fetoplacental Risk Factors
Abnormal placentation (e.g., placenta previa, abruptio placentae)
Genetic abnormalities
Fetal death
Premature Rupture of the Membranes

no standard protocol exists for management of prenatal care for women with a history of preterm birth, considerable efforts are directed toward clinical and laboratory development of testing to estimate the exact risk of spontaneous preterm birth.[13]

Pregnant women living in a poor social environment, and work during pregnancy are associated with increased risk for nulliparous women.[9]

Several cervicovaginal microorganisms and infections have been implicated in preterm labor and delivery; however, the various treatments have produced inconsistent results. Generally, it is accepted to screen for and treat bacterial vaginosis in patients at high risk for preterm birth but not to treat *Ureaplasma urealyticum* or group B streptococci genital colonization. The latter two and *Candida* were found not to increase the incidence of preterm labor and delivery. With preterm labor and delivery, group B streptococci infection should be treated. Antibiotics should not be given routinely to prolong pregnancy, but in patients with bacterial vaginosis and *Trichomonas vaginalis* infection, specific treatment should be administered. With preterm premature rupture of membranes, standard practices should be applied regarding group B streptococci prophylaxis, but additional antibiotics should also be given to prolong pregnancies at 24 to 32 weeks' gestation.[14]

Premature rupture of the membranes (PROM) was often thought to occur concomitant with physical stress, especially the stress associated with labor. Recently, more evidence suggests that membrane rupture is also related to biochemical processes, programmed death of cells in the fetal membranes, and disruption of collagen within the extracellular matrix of the amnion and the chorion. It is thought that the fetal membranes and the maternal uterine lining (decidua) respond to various stimuli, such as infection of the reproductive tract and membrane stretching, by producing mediators, including prostaglandins, cytokines, and protein hormones, that have a major influence on the activities of matrix-degrading enzymes.[9]

TOCOLYSIS

The initial step is a physical examination, including a sterile speculum examination to obtain a cervical culture. Ultrasound examination to estimate gestational age and fetal weight as well as a cardiotocogram is routinely performed. If necessary, an amniocentesis to determine fetal lung maturity and/or evidence of infection is performed, although this may increase uterine activity.[15] In a significant percentage of women with preterm labor, uterine contractions stop after conservative therapy alone (e.g., bed rest and hydration).

Once the diagnosis of preterm labor is established, the obstetrician must decide whether to begin tocolytic therapy. Criteria for the use of tocolytic therapy include (1) gestational age between 20 and 34 weeks' gestation; (2) fetal weight less than 2500 g; and (3) absence of "fetal jeopardy." The potential benefits of delaying delivery of the preterm infant (i.e., decreased neonatal morbidity and mortality) must be weighed against the maternal and fetal risks (i.e., maternal and/or fetal sepsis, maternal side effects of tocolytic drugs, or further compromise of a distressed fetus).

Tocolytic Drugs

About 20 years ago, ethanol was commonly used for the treatment of preterm labor. This therapy is now entirely abandoned. β-Sympathomimetics have become most popular among the different classes of tocolytic medications which are used today.

Tocolytic drugs are used in an effort to interrupt, significantly decrease, or stop uterine contractions. Although β-sympathomimetic agents have been thoroughly evaluated, the other potentially useful tocolytic drugs (e.g., magnesium, oxytocin antagonists, calcium channel blockers and nonsteroidal anti-inflammatory agents) need further investigation. Unfortunately, data from randomized trials suggest that tocolytic drugs often do not prolong pregnancy for more than 48 hours. If the goal of tocolytic therapy is to delay the delivery for more than a week or even to decrease the incidence of preterm delivery, then the effect of tocolytic therapy appears to be minimal.[2] Nevertheless, even a delay of 2 days can be beneficial since 2 days of glucocorticoid therapy can make a great difference for the preterm fetus. However, it is somewhat discouraging that the use of ritodrine in the treatment of preterm labor has had no significant beneficial effect on perinatal mortality, the frequency of prolongation of pregnancy to term, or birthweight.[16]

The widespread use of tocolytic agents has not led to a decrease in neonatal mortality. In addition, no reduction in the most common severe neonatal disease, the respiratory distress syndrome, was found, and β-adrenergic tocolytic agents have been associated with an increased risk of neonatal intraventricular hemorrhage.[2]

In a prospective study, women with preterm rupture of membranes between 34 and 37 weeks' gestation were treated with either induction of labor or expectant management. Aggressive management of preterm PROM at a gestational age of 34 or more weeks by induction of labor was found to be safe for the infant

CONTRAINDICATIONS TO TOCOLYSIS

Absolute
- Severe hemorrhage (placental abruption)
- Fetal death
- Fetal distress
- Fetal anomalies incompatible with life
- Chorioamnionitis
- Severe hypertension, either preexisting hypertension or pregnancy-induced hypertension

Relative
- Ruptured membranes
- Intrauterine growth retardation
- Cervical dilation < 4 cm
- Preeclampsia
- Severe maternal cardiac disease

and avoids maternal-neonatal infectious complications.[17] Although the delay in delivery afforded by tocolytic drugs is relatively short-lived, it allows the prenatal administration of corticosteroids to accelerate neonatal lung maturity. The combined use of maternal corticosteroid and tocolytic treatment has especially decreased the morbidity and mortality in VLBW infants by achieving a significant reduction in respiratory distress syndrome as well as intraventricular hemorrhage.[18]

β-Adrenergic Agents

β_1-Receptors are predominantly found in the heart, intestine, and adipose tissue, whereas β_2-receptors are distributed in the smooth muscle of the uterus, blood vessels, bronchioles, and also in the kidney and liver. In 1980 the Food and Drug Administration approved the first tocolytic agent, ritodrine. In Europe a variety of other agents are approved. Of these, hexoprenaline sulfate is the most popular.

The usefulness of tocolytic therapy today seems to be reserved for short-term treatment, for example, to transfer a patient to a tertiary care center, to delay delivery long enough to allow maternal administration of a glucocorticoid, and to facilitate in utero resuscitation if fetal compromise is present.

Ritodrine. The first placebo-controlled, prospective study using ritodrine was performed in the United Kingdom.[19] Ritodrine is still the only β-agonist that is approved for parenteral use in preterm labor in the United States. A very large multicenter trial concluded that although ritodrine prolonged pregnancy by 24 to 48 hours, its overall effects on perinatal mortality and morbidity were indistinguishable from those of placebo.[16] Furthermore, a meta-analysis of the effects of oral β-agonist maintenance therapy in preterm labor concluded that the data obtained do not support a role for oral β-agonist maintenance therapy after resolution of an acute episode of preterm labor.[20]

Terbutaline. This is a frequently used tocolytic agent, which is known to affect maternal metabolism. It is less expensive than ritodrine and is often the first-line β-adrenergic tocolytic agent. Decreased peripheral insulin sensitivity as well as an increased endogenous glucose production could represent the pathophysiology of abnormal glucose tolerance that is frequently seen in women who receive oral terbutaline as maintenance therapy for preterm labor. Common side effects experienced by many women on terbutaline, including tremor and tachycardia, are consistent with the finding of a significant increase in basal energy expenditure.[21]

Hexoprenaline Sulfate. Since its introduction[22] this drug has been extensively studied[23–25] and is now commonly used in Europe. Hexoprenaline sulfate has been found to have fewer side effects (tachycardia, pulmonary edema) than ritodrine. In animal studies, hexoprenaline sulfate was less toxic than ritodrine and terbutaline sulfate.[26]

Other Agents. Isoxsuprine is no longer used because of the increased risk of hypotension.

Other β-sympathomimetics, including salbutamol, clenbuterol, and fenoterol, are available but have not been found to be superior to the drugs already mentioned.

Mechanism of Action. The β-adrenergic agents predominantly bind to β_2-receptors on the outer membrane of myometrial cells. The stimulation of β_2-receptors activates adenyl cyclase which catalyzes the conversion of adenosine triphosphate to adenosine 3′, 5′-cyclic monophosphate (cAMP). An increase in cAMP causes myometrial relaxation by the mechanisms discussed earlier.

Side Effects. All β-adrenergic tocolytic agents are considered β_2-receptor selective but unfortunately also have significant β_1-receptor effects. This contributes to the undesirable side effects of these drugs.

Maternal

Cardiovascular. These are dose related and include hypotension, tachycardia, chest pain (up to 60% of patients on ritodrine), as well as arrhythmias (premature atrial contractions, premature ventricular contractions, supraventricular tachycardia), myocardial ischemia with or without electrocardiographic (ECG) changes, and palpitations (33% of patients).

Pulmonary Edema. The incidence is less than 5%, but this side effect may be a life-threatening complication of β-sympathomimetic therapy and can start within 1 to 3 days of the initiation of tocolytic therapy. Risk factors for development of pulmonary edema include multiple gestation, fluid overload, anemia, and prolonged tachycardia in a susceptible patient. The exact underlying mechanism is not known but there are several hypotheses.

Cardiogenic. Isolated left ventricular failure can cause pulmonary edema, but direct evidence supporting this mechanism is lacking.

Noncardiogenic. An increase in pulmonary vascular permeability causes pulmonary edema, especially if there is concomitant infection.[27] Reports of pulmonary edema in patients with normal or low wedge pressure support this hypothesis. β-Adrenergic stimulation may actually decrease pulmonary vascular permeability and may decrease serum albumin causing decreased colloid oncotic pressure.

Volume Overload. Pregnancy produces many physiologic changes, including increased plasma volume. During tocolysis patients may receive aggressive intravenous hydration. Excessive hydration in the presence of an increased release of aldosterone, renin, antidiuretic hormone, and antinatriuretic hormone owing to β-stimulation may cause volume overload. The risk of pulmonary edema may be decreased by limiting total fluid intake, by using the smallest effective doses of β-adrenergic tocolytics, and by keeping the duration of tocolytic therapy as short as possible. There is some concern that concurrent glucocorticoid therapy might increase the incidence of pulmonary edema, but these steroids have little mineralocorticoid activity and it is thus possible that glucocorticoid therapy administered together with ritodrine is not a risk factor for the development of pulmonary edema. The type of fluid that is for intravenous administration may also play a role in the development of pulmonary edema. Fluid overload may also occur secondary to the increased renin and aldosterone levels caused by β-adrenergic therapy. In a study comparing intravenous hydration with normal saline versus a dextrose-containing solution, more than half of patients who received isotonic saline developed pulmonary congestion requiring treatment. Therefore, the combination of ritodrine and saline should be used very cautiously, and it has been recommended that the fluid balance be monitored closely during ritodrine treatment.[28]

In general, patients who develop pulmonary edema owing to β-adrenergic therapy after open fetal surgery show a rapid resolution of symptoms except in the presence of infection or with nitroglycerin tocolysis.[29] Theoretically, therapy with high-dose nitroglycerin for tocolysis could mask initial onset of overhydration because of maximal dilation of the venous capacitance vessels.

HYPERGLYCEMIA. Stimulation of β_2-receptors of the pancreas increases glucagon which causes increases in both gluconeogenesis and glycogenolysis. Stimulation of β-receptors on hepatocytes causes increased glycogenolysis. The administration of insulin is not always required and glucose levels sometimes decrease to baseline within 24 hours of therapy. Because of this, there is some controversy regarding the use of these agents in diabetic parturients.

HYPOKALEMIA. In patients receiving β-sympathomimetic therapy, insulin is increased as a response to the hyperglycemia and also because of the direct effect of β-adrenergic stimulation of the maternal pancreas. Potassium shifts from the extracellular to the intracellular space because of the higher plasma levels of insulin. However, there is no increase in urinary excretion of potassium, so total body concentration remains stable. There is usually no need for supplemental potassium, and potassium levels usually increase to baseline within 24 hours after discontinuation of therapy.

OTHER SIDE EFFECTS. Impaired liver function (increased serum transaminase levels and hepatitis) have also been reported infrequently (< 1%) with the use of ritodrine and other β-sympathomimetics. Oral ritodrine, in 10% to 15% of patients, was associated with palpation or tremor. Nausea and jitteriness were less frequent (5–8%), while rash was observed in some patients (3–4%), and arrhythmias occurred infrequently (about 1%). There are reports of paralytic ileus, cerebral vasospasm (predominantly in patients with a former history of migraines), respiratory arrest (patients with preexisting myasthenia gravis), and severe restlessness and agitation.

FETAL. Rapid transfer of these agents across the placenta leads to increases in fetal heart rate owing to direct stimulation of fetal myocardial β_1-receptors; fetal hyperglycemia and hyperinsulinemia also occur followed by neonatal hypoglycemia caused by maternal hyperglycemia. Fortunately, there are no reports of adverse long-term effects in children exposed in utero to these tocolytic drugs.

Interaction with Anesthesia. In general, the cardiovascular effects of β-adrenergic agents continue for 60 to 90 minutes after the last administered dose. The resulting tachycardia may impact on the anesthetic and make the assessment of intravascular volume status difficult. Although many patients receiving tocolytic therapy have received anesthesia, to date there are no prospective, randomized, controlled studies of anesthesia after β-adrenergic therapy.

REGIONAL ANESTHESIA. Theoretic concerns about the prior administration of ritodrine causing a worsening of maternal hypotension during epidural anesthesia have been raised, but Chestnut and colleagues[30] evaluated this in a study of gravid ewes and concluded that these agents did not increase the incidence or severity of regional anesthesia–induced hypotension. They hypothesized that the inotropic and chronotropic activity of ritodrine helped to maintain maternal cardiac output and uterine blood flow during epidural anesthesia.

Although the administration of a prophylactic fluid bolus prior to initiation of regional anesthesia may increase the risk of pulmonary edema, the ensuing sympathectomy and decrease in preload owing to the regional technique may be protective against pulmonary edema.

In the unstable patient, continuous spinal or epidural anesthesia is advantageous as compared with a single-shot spinal block, because the slow, controlled block that is achieved via a catheter allows the patient to compensate for the sympathectomy and the anesthesiologist to titrate fluids slowly and potentially avoid use of pressors. For imminent vaginal delivery, a low spinal block provides excellent analgesia without hemodynamic perturbations. Ephedrine, an indirect sympathomimetic, is considered to be the vasopressor of choice in pregnancy because it maintains uterine blood flow. Its mechanism of action is thought to be an α-receptor–mediated uterine vasoconstriction that is offset by an increased cardiac output secondary to β-adrenergic effects. In addition, ephedrine may spare uterine perfusion during pregnancy owing to more selective constriction of systemic vessels.[31] However, in the patient who is profoundly tachycardic as a result of tocolytic therapy, hypotension may be resistant to treatment with ephedrine. In those cases, phenylephrine should be considered.

GENERAL ANESTHESIA. Tachycardia, as a result of recent tocolytic therapy, may make assessment of depth of anesthesia more difficult. Agents that might increase heart rate should be used very cautiously or avoided. They include ketamine (sympathomimetic); atropine, glycopyrrolate; and pancuronium (vagolytic properties).

If other agents are available, halothane should not be used in these patients, because it sensitizes the myocardium to catecholamine-induced arrhythmias. In addition, it is prudent to maintain normal $PaCO_2$ intraoperatively, since hyperventilation may worsen preexisting hypokalemia.

Concomitant Use of Vasopressors. As previously noted, ephedrine is an acceptable choice for therapy of regional anesthesia–induced hypotension in patients recently treated with β-adrenergic tocolytics. Phenylephrine may be used cautiously in low doses if maternal tachycardia precludes use of ephedrine, or if the administration of repeat dosages of ephedrine has been ineffective in raising the maternal blood pressure.

Magnesium Sulfate

Magnesium sulfate is used not only in preeclampsia, but is also a first-line tocolytic agent in many hospitals because it has less severe cardiovascular side effects than β-adrenergic agents and it is thought to be equally effective. In addition, it has been suggested that magnesium sulfate tocolysis is not associated with increased neonatal mortality in premature infants and is thus beneficial as a tocolytic. Therefore, any association of magnesium with reduced long-term neurologic morbidity is unlikely to be the result of selective mortality of vulnerable infants.[32] In general, its use is much more common in the United States than in Europe.

It appears that high extracellular magnesium causes an increase in intracellular magnesium, which probably inhibits calcium influx through calcium channels. Overall, magnesium seems to have similar efficacy as compared with β-adrenergic agonists for controlling preterm labor.

Mechanism of Action. It is not entirely clear, but it has been hypothesized that four major mechanisms contribute to decreased intracellular calcium and increased cAMP and therefore decreased myosin light chain activity following the administration of magnesium. They are[33]

1. Magnesium increases cAMP by activating adenylate cyclase.
2. Magnesium competes with calcium for entry into cells in the depolarization state in both the voltage-dependent and voltage-independent pathways.
3. Magnesium competes with calcium for binding sites on the sarcoplasmic reticulum which indirectly decreases intracellular calcium by inhibiting its release.
4. Magnesium sulfate attenuates peroxide-induced vasoconstriction in the human placenta. This effect is mediated by inhibition of thromboxane synthesis and antagonism of calcium.[34]

Side Effects

Maternal. Maternal side effects are determined by the plasma magnesium level:

8–10 mg/dL: Loss of deep tendon reflexes, slight respiratory depression

10–15 mg/dL: Moderate to severe respiratory depression

>15 mg/dL: Cardiac conduction defects

>20 mg/dL: Cardiac arrest

Other side effects include warmth, flushing, headache, nausea, dizziness, transient hypotension, muscle weakness, sedation, ECG changes (widened QRS, increase in PR interval), blurred vision, and chest pain.

Fetal Neonatal. A decrease in baseline fetal heart rate and variability is often observed in these patients. Neonatal flaccidity and hyporeflexia, as well as weak or absent crying can culminate in respiratory depression. These side effects, however, tend to occur after prolonged therapy with high doses of magnesium sulfate and resolve in 24 to 36 hours.

Interaction with Anesthesia. Calcium gluconate is an effective intravenous antidote for magnesium toxicity, should immediate treatment become necessary.[35] Magnesium should be cautiously used in patients with renal failure because magnesium is renally excreted. It should also be avoided in patients with myasthenia gravis and in patients with heart block.

Regional Anesthesia. Hypermagnesemia may increase hypotension during regional anesthesia because of its general vasodilating properties. Nevertheless, a slow induction of epidural or continuous spinal anesthesia is well tolerated, assuming that the level is raised slowly. In emergency situations spinal anesthesia can be safely used, provided a careful watch and aggressive treatment of maternal hypotension is established.

Concomitant Use of Vasopressors. Magnesium sulfate alters the maternal hemodynamic response to endogenous and exogenous vasopressor agents. The question arises, therefore, as to which vasopressor should be used to treat hypotension during magnesium sulfate infusion and epidural anesthesia. Sipes and coworkers[36] studied the effectiveness of ephedrine and phenylephrine in the restoration and protection of uterine blood flow and fetal oxygenation during epidural anesthesia–induced hypotension in hypermagnesemic gravid ewes. Both ephedrine and phenylephrine restored mean maternal arterial pressure to baseline. Ephedrine significantly increased cardiac output and uterine blood flow as well as pH and oxygenation when compared with the normal saline control group. In contrast to these favorable features associated with ephedrine, phenylephrine increased uterine vascular resistance and therefore did not increase uterine blood flow; it also failed to maintain fetal pH and oxygenation. Hence, it appears that ephedrine may be a better vasopressor in the presence of maternal hypotension following regional anesthesia in hypermagnesemic patients.

General Anesthesia. Minimum alveolar concentration (MAC) may be decreased in hypermagnesemic patients. Magnesium blocks the entry of Ca^+ at the neuromuscular junction and thus reduces the number of quanta released, regardless of the rate of stimulation. Therefore, it decreases the release of acetylcholine and decreases the postjunctional membrane potentials generated by acetylcholine-receptor activations. This results in potentiation of both depolarizing and nondepolarizing muscle relaxants. Therefore, one should

1. Avoid defasciculating doses of nondepolarizing neuromuscular blockers.
2. Use standard intubating dose of succinylcholine, as potentiation is variable.
3. Titrate the nondepolarizing drugs using a nerve stimulator.

Prostaglandin Synthetase Inhibitors

Prostaglandin $F_{2\alpha}$ ($PGF_{2\alpha}$) raises intracellular calcium and it is therefore not surprising that prostaglandin synthetase inhibitors are potent tocolytic agents. Indomethacin, the most commonly used prostaglandin synthetase inhibitor, has been found to be of equal tocolytic effectiveness when compared with β-agonists. However, although indomethacin is an effective oral tocolytic agent, its use is limited owing to concerns about fetal effects.

Mechanism of Action. There are two prostaglandins that are involved in preterm labor: (1) $PGF_{2\alpha}$, which stimulates release of calcium from the sarcoplasmic reticulum and entry of calcium into the cell; and (2) PGE_2, which facilitates cervical dilation. Prostaglandin synthetases convert free arachidonic acid to prostaglandins with cyclooxygenase acting as a key enzyme in this conversion. Indomethacin reversibly inhibits cyclooxygenase and thus prevents prostaglandin production.

Side Effects

MATERNAL. Prostaglandin synthetase inhibitors are generally well tolerated; however, mild side effects including nausea, heartburn, and rash do occur. An inhibition of cyclooxygenase results in a decreased production of thromboxane A_2, which plays an important role in platelet aggregation and therefore has implications for the subsequent use of regional anesthesia.

These drugs should be avoided in patients with infection, bleeding disorders, peptic ulcer disease, and renal dysfunction.

FETAL. Fetal side effects include

1. Ductus arteriosus
   a. Premature closure or narrowing
   b. Patent ductus requiring surgical ligation
2. Oligohydramnios secondary to decreased fetal urine excretion
3. Increased incidence of necrotizing enterocolitis
4. Increased incidence of intracranial hemorrhage
5. Increased respiratory distress and bronchopulmonary dysplasia

These effects may be mitigated by concomitant use of glucocorticoids.

Interaction with Anesthesia. Although theoretically a risk factor, to date there are no case reports of epidural hematoma in an obstetric patient who received indomethacin prior to placement of a catheter for regional anesthesia.

Calcium Channel Blockers

Calcium channel blockers produce an interference with slow voltage-dependent calcium channels. Nifedipine, which has been widely studied, has been found to have similar efficacy when compared with β-agonists. Nifedipine, nicardipine, and verapamil are all capable of tocolysis but nifedipine is the only one clinically used as a tocolytic agent, because it has fewer effects on cardiac conduction, more specific effects on myometrial contractility, and fewer effects on serum electrolytes.

Mechanism of Action. Calcium channel blockers block voltage-dependent calcium channels and prevent release of calcium from the sarcoplasmic reticulum. This results in a decrease in intracellular calcium and a decrease in myosin light chain activity.

Side Effects. The side effects of nifedipine include maternal facial flushing, headache, and nausea.

Interaction with Anesthesia

GENERAL ANESTHESIA. In combination with potent inhalational anesthetic agents, calcium channel blockers may cause vasodilation, hypotension, myocardial depression, and cardiac conduction defects. Therefore, close monitoring of blood pressure and ECG is necessary in parturients who have received calcium channel blocking agents.

POSTPARTUM HEMORRHAGE. Postpartum hemorrhage may occur and may be severe if uterine atony occurs after the use of nifedipine. The anesthesia team should therefore take the following precautions:

1. Oxytocin, methylergonovine maleate (Methergine), and $PGF_{2\alpha}$ may be necessary to increase uterine tone.
2. Calcium chloride may antagonize calcium channel blockers.
3. Good intravenous access is necessary before delivery.
4. Typed and crossmatched blood should be available.

Atosiban

Atosiban is an oxytocin antagonist, and initial clinical trials have been encouraging with respect to efficacy and side effect profile.[37] In subsequent trials it was found that atosiban's effect on uterine activity in preterm labor was enhanced by bolus infusion and was similar to the effect of ritodrine, but with fewer side effects.[38] Atosiban is especially interesting because it may be used in combination with other tocolytics, as its mechanisms of action are specific and different from other tocolytic drugs.

Miscellaneous Tocolytics

Ethanol was used before the 1980s; it suppresses posterior pituitary secretion of oxytocin and directly inhibits myometrial contractility. It is no longer used because of the potential for fetal alcohol syndrome and maternal complications.

Diazoxide is an effective tocolytic, but it is not widely used owing to its side effects which include decreased maternal blood pressure as well as hyperglycemia.

The *phosphodiesterase inhibitors* (e.g., aminophylline) are no longer used because of associated cardiovascular side effects.

Anesthetic agents that are still under study and should be used with caution include the progesterones and nitroglycerin, discussed subsequently.

Progesterones. Progesterones probably promote calcium storage and inhibit the transmission of impulses between myometrial cells by reducing gap junction function. They may be used in the future to augment the actions of β-mimetics while reducing their side effects or for long-term prophylaxis in women at high risk of developing preterm labor.[39]

Transdermal Nitroglycerin. Essentially, nitroglycerin forms nitric oxide, a potent smooth muscle relaxant. Nitric oxide is synthesized in the uterus and placenta and probably helps to maintain uteroplacental blood flow by decreasing the resistance in the fetoplacental and uterine circulation. The effectiveness of transdermal nitroglycerin, a donor of nitric oxide, was studied in the maintenance of uterine, umbilical, and fetal cerebral blood flow in pregnancies complicated by preeclampsia and impaired uteroplacental blood flow. It was observed that the nitroglycerin patch caused a significant fall in the mean uterine pulsatility index and resistance and authors concluded that transdermal administration of nitroglycerin may offer a potential for treatment of patients with preeclampsia who have increased uteroplacental impedance.[40] There are also observational studies showing a considerable delay of preterm labor by transdermal use of glyceryl trinitrate.[41] Nevertheless, transdermal administration is currently still in the experimental stage.[42]

Intravenous Nitroglycerin. An intravenous bolus of 50 to 100 μg of nitroglycerin has been used in cases of fetal head entrapment in breech delivery. However, nitroglycerin should be administered with great caution, since hypotension or pulmonary edema may ensue.[43] The development of pulmonary edema following nitroglycerin was attributed to an increase in vascular permeability as supported by a ratio of pulmonary edema fluid to plasma protein of 0.99.[43] Although nitroglycerin is used to provide acute tocolysis associated with tetanic uterine contractions in addition to its use to help facilitate fetal extraction, it has not been shown to be useful in gestations of more than 34 weeks.[44] Use of intravenous nitroglycerin to treat preterm labor is still speculative.

THE PRETERM INFANT

Medical Problems. Several medical problems which manifest themselves shortly after delivery are associated with preterm delivery. They include respiratory distress syndrome, intraventricular hemorrhage, sepsis, persistent ductus arteriosus, necrotizing enterocolitis, and hypoglycemia.

Fetal Heart Rate Tracing of the Premature Infant. Both antepartum and intrapartum fetal heart rate (FHR) tracings may be abnormal. In addition, a more rapid progression from a reassuring to nonreassuring FHR tracing may be observed. FHR patterns may also be difficult to interpret in extreme prematurity.

Fetal Pharmacology. A decrease in protein binding, incomplete blood-brain barrier, decreased ability to metabolize drugs, and enhanced susceptibility to myocardial depressant effects of local anesthetics may increase the preterm fetus's risk of toxicity from local anesthetics.

The cytochrome P450 monooxygenase system is especially important in the preterm fetus. The cytochrome P450 system is the major catalyst of drug biotransformation, especially local anesthetics. Although cytochrome P450 is detectable in many organ systems, the amounts are low compared with those in liver. Thus the liver is the major site of phase I drug metabolism. Consequently a premature liver as seen in a preterm fetus may be associated with a significant prolongation of the action of drugs and/or decrease in the threshold for toxicity.

Whereas the healthy term fetus tolerates the stress of labor and delivery well, the preterm fetus (especially if it is <30 weeks' gestation or has a weight of <1500 g) is much more susceptible to the trauma of delivery. Preterm infants born at less than 30 weeks' gestation have been shown to have fragile cerebral blood vessels. Because the walls of their blood vessels are composed of only one layer of endothelium without supporting smooth muscle, collagen, or elastin, the walls are prone to rupture in the event of a rapid increase in blood pressure and cerebral blood flow. The risk of rupture is aggravated by respiratory distress associated with hypoxia and hypercapnia, which cause cerebral vasodilation.[45] Both the compromised respiratory function and the low endogenous nutrient stores in preterm infants may explain the need for a postnatal increase in cerebral blood flow velocity in order to maintain the physiologically high cerebral metabolic requirements. The changes in cerebral blood flow velocities decrease with increasing maturity. Abnormalities in cerebral blood flow are one of the major factors in the etiology and pathogenesis of cerebral injury in the newborn.[46] Prevention of the factors that are known to potentially interfere with normal cerebral autoregulation (e.g., hypoxia, hypercapnia, acidosis, respiratory distress, and sepsis) may reduce the incidence of perinatal brain injury.[47] Abnormal cerebral blood flow in the fetus, which can be produced by intrauterine stress, may lead to a different setting of the autoregulation of the neonatal cerebral circulation, especially in preterm infants.

In addition, the preterm fetus has a relative deficiency of clotting factors which may increase its susceptibility to intraventricular hemorrhage and which can be exacerbated by the presence of asphyxia.

Illicit and Nonillicit Drug Abuse and Preterm Labor. Myles and coworkers[48] evaluated the effects of smoking, alcohol, and drugs of abuse on the outcome of "expectantly" managed cases of preterm babies associated with premature rupture of membranes. Interestingly, there was no association between the use of tobacco, alcohol, drugs of abuse, or cocaine and the respiratory distress syndrome, intraventricular hemorrhage, or necrotizing enterocolitis. These investigators also observed a shortened latency period for premature rupture of membranes following use of tobacco as well as cocaine. They concluded that shortened latency periods could potentially contribute to increased neonatal morbidity.[48] Delaney and colleagues[49] observed the impact of cocaine on the latency period between rupture of membranes and delivery, and reported that cocaine-positive women presented at an earlier gestational age and had a significantly longer duration of rupture of membrane to delivery than women with a urine toxicology screen that tested negative. This obviously is associated with a higher incidence of preterm deliveries and with a higher incidence of associated infections. In another study, crack cocaine use was associated with adverse pregnancy outcomes, as noted by increased risks of low birthweight and fetal growth retardation.[50] This subject is covered in greater detail in Chapter 48.

Method of Delivery. The ideal method of delivery for the preterm infant (especially the VLBW infant) remains controversial,[51] particularly before 30 weeks' gestation. Some authors favor cesarean delivery even in vertex presentation,[52] whereas others prefer vaginal delivery.[53] There is increasing evidence that cesarean delivery may not always be beneficial for preterm infants, at least in vertex presentation.[54] The obstetric management of preterm breech fetuses is also controversial. The fetal head is larger than the abdomen in these fetuses, which may lead to entrapment of the aftercoming head after delivery of the body. However, this may occur equally in cesarean delivery, even in the case of a classic uterine incision. A solution might be to deliver these infants vaginally if the cervix is soft and dilated, whereas an unfavorable cervix with urgent need for delivery would require cesarean section.

As the route of delivery is controversial, one should take into account the side effects of cesarean section. Maternal morbidity following cesarean section is related to numerous factors including infection and blood loss. Furthermore, a vertical uterine incision produces an increased risk for subsequent pregnancies.[55] Cesarean section in preterm as compared with term births carries an increased risk for endometritis (3.5 times), associated complications (3 times), severe complications (11 times), and likelihood of transfusion (14 times), thus increasing the maternal risk for morbidity 35- to 100-fold.[56]

In addition, the type of anesthesia chosen could have an impact on fetal compromise. As with advancing gestational age and increasing birthweight, the absence of fetal compromise has a major beneficial impact on the outcome of borderline viable babies that might be important when decisions are made about the appropriate level of support.[57]

The preterm fetus is at higher risk for acidosis during labor and delivery, and the preterm infant is at higher risk for intraventricular hemorrhage.[47] Therefore, obstetric management must include continuous intrapartum fetal heart rate monitoring and efforts to minimize trauma during delivery. These patients should be delivered in a tertiary care center that has a neonatal intensive care unit.

ANESTHETIC MANAGEMENT

The anesthetic team is quite often involved in the care of parturients with preterm labor, as well as in the delivery of the preterm fetus. Some of these patients may have associated systemic disease. Because of the higher incidence of abdominal delivery, a preoperative consultation regarding possible techniques for providing labor and delivery analgesia, or anesthesia for cesarean delivery, is beneficial. As most of the mothers will be receiving one or multiple tocolytic drugs, a thorough knowledge of drug interactions becomes essential. These neonates may have a higher incidence of acidosis and respiratory distress syndrome, as well as intracranial hemorrhage. Hence, if possible, a neonatologist should be present during the delivery of the premature fetus. The side effects of β-mimetic drugs can be minimized if the anesthetic management is initiated following 1 to 2 hours of discontinuation of these drugs. However, this is not possible in emergency situations.

Labor and Vaginal Delivery. If time permits, epidural analgesia or anesthesia is an ideal technique. Choosing the right anesthetic technique and agent can help to inhibit maternal expulsive efforts before full dilation of the cervix, which is especially important in parturients with a breech presentation. This technique also prevents the possibility of precipitous delivery, which can result in rapid decompression of the fetal head and increases the risk of intraventricular hemorrhage. Combined spinal-epidural or one-shot spinal analgesia and anesthesia may be the technique of choice if the delivery is imminent. As some of the tocolytic drugs may enhance the vasodilation that often occurs, proper maintenance of maternal blood pressure is essential.

Cesarean Section. In part, the choice of anesthetic technique depends on the urgency of the situation. If an epidural catheter is already in situ for labor and delivery analgesia, the anesthesia for cesarean section can be extended to higher levels (bilaterally at the T4 dermatome) with the use of 2% lidocaine with epinephrine. In the presence of severe fetal compromise, 3% 2-chloroprocaine may be an ideal choice because of rapid onset of action and very short plasma half-life. Some investigators have suggested that general anesthesia may protect the immature fetal brain; however, a retrospective comparison of epidural and general anesthesia by observing the Apgar scores did not confirm this notion.[58]

In emergency situations, in the absence of an epidural catheter, spinal anesthesia may be used; however, proper precautions must be considered during prehydration (increased incidence of maternal pulmonary edema) as well as maintenance of normal maternal blood pressure with ephedrine or phenylephrine hydrochloride in small doses if necessary, because decreased placental perfusion can significantly increase complications for the preterm fetus.

If general anesthesia becomes necessary, intravenous ketamine (unless contraindicated) may be a better induction agent. Ketamine, in the distressed fetal lamb model, was found to maintain better central nervous system perfusion by redistribution of cardiac output.[59] Succinylcholine is the neuromuscular blocker of choice to facilitate endotracheal intubation, and a nondepolarizing muscle relaxant is usually used to maintain relaxation for surgery. Magnesium sulfate, a popular tocolytic agent, can interact with depolarizing as well as nondepolarizing muscle relaxants. Maternal hyperventilation should be avoided, as it may lead to fetal acidosis because of decreased placental perfusion, and shifting of the maternal oxygen dissociation curve to the left. Finally, as all tocolytic drugs are uterine relaxants, inhalational anesthetics should be discontinued following delivery of the fetus to avoid uterine atony.

❖ Summary

Key Points

- The incidence of preterm delivery has not decreased despite other improvements.
- Tocolytic drugs are associated with several side effects. In addition, they may interact with anesthetic drugs and techniques. Pulmonary edema is the most serious side effect.
- Dexamethasone crosses the placenta and speeds lung maturation.
- The administration of tocolytic agents does not contraindicate the use of regional anesthesia. Regional anesthesia allows a more controlled delivery and thus decreases the risk of decompression of the fetal head and subsequent intracranial hemorrhage.

Key References

Goldenberg RL, Rouse DJ: Prevention of premature birth. N Engl J Med 1998; 339:313–320.

Dewan DM: Anesthesia for preterm delivery, breech presentation, and multiple gestation. Clin Obstet Gynecol 1987; 30:566–578.

Case Stem

A 24-year-old G1P0 is admitted at 31 weeks' gestation in active labor. Terbutaline was administered without success. Magnesium sulfate stopped contractions for 24 hours, but they have now returned. Membranes have been ruptured for more than 24 hours. The fetus is in breech position and the cervix is dilated 6 cm. How would you manage this patient for emergency cesarean section?

CONCLUSION

Preterm labor contributes significantly to perinatal morbidity and mortality. Many of these patients undergo cesarean delivery, thus necessitating the administration of anesthesia. An understanding of the drugs commonly used to treat preterm labor and how they interact with anesthetic agents is essential.

References

1. Ahn MO, Cha KY, Phelan JP: The low birth weight infant: is there a preferred route of delivery? Clin Perinatol 1992; 19:411–423.
2. Goldenberg RL, Rouse DJ: Prevention of premature birth. N Engl J Med 1998; 339:313–320.
3. Meis PJ, Goldenberg RL, Mercer BM, et al: The preterm prediction study: risk factors for indicated preterm births. Maternal-Fetal Medicine Units Network of the National Institute of Child Health and Human Development. Am J Obstet Gynecol 1998; 178:562–567.
4. Gray PH, Hurley TM, Rogers YM, et al: Survival and neonatal and neurodevelopmental outcome of 24–29 week gestation infants according to primary cause of preterm delivery. Aust N Z J Obstet Gynaecol 1997; 37:161–168.
5. Tin W, Wariyar U, Hey E: Changing prognosis for babies of less than 28 weeks' gestation in the north of England between 1983 and 1994. Northern Neonatal Network [see comments]. BMJ 1997; 314:107–111.
6. Improved outcome into the 1990s for infants weighing 500–999 g at birth. The Victorian Infant Collaborative Study Group. Arch Dis Child Fetal Neonatal Ed 1997; 77:F91–F94.
7. Outcome at 2 years of children 23–27 weeks' gestation born in Victoria in 1991–92. The Victorian Infant Collaborative Study Group. J Paediatr Child Health 1997; 33:161–165.
8. Changing outcome for infants of birth-weight 500–999 g born outside level 3 centres in Victoria. The Victorian Infant Collaborative Study Group. Aust N Z J Obstet Gynaecol 1997; 37:253–257.
9. Parry S, Strauss JF: Premature rupture of the fetal membranes. N Engl J Med 1998; 338:663–670.
10. Peaceman AM, Andrews WW, Thorp JM, et al: Fetal fibronectin as a predictor of preterm birth in patients with symptoms: a multicenter trial. Am J Obstet Gynecol 1997; 177:13–18.
11. Chien PF, Khan KS, Ogston S, et al: The diagnostic accuracy of cervico-vaginal fetal fibronectin in predicting preterm delivery: an overview [see comments]. Br J Obstet Gynaecol 1997; 104:436–444.
12. Mercer BM, Goldenberg RL, Das A, et al. The preterm

prediction study: a clinical risk assessment system. Am J Obstet Gynecol 1996; 174:1885–1893.
13. Iams JD, Goldenberg RL, Mercer BM, et al: The Preterm Prediction Study: recurrence risk of spontaneous preterm birth. National Institute of Child Health and Human Development, Maternal-Fetal Medicine Units Network. Am J Obstet Gynecol 1998; 178:1035–1040.
14. Gibbs RS, Eschenbach DA: Use of antibiotics to prevent preterm birth [see comments]. Am J Obstet Gynecol 1997; 177:375–380.
15. Haeusler MC, Konstantiniuk P, Dorfer M, et al: Amniotic fluid insulin testing in gestational diabetes: safety and acceptance of amniocentesis. Am J Obstet Gynecol 1998; 179:917–920.
16. Treatment of preterm labor with the beta-adrenergic agonist ritodrine: The Canadian Preterm Labor Investigators Group [see comments]. N Engl J Med 1992; 327:308–312.
17. Naef RW, Allbert JR, Ross EL, et al: Premature rupture of membranes at 34 to 37 weeks' gestation: aggressive versus conservative management. Am J Obstet Gynecol 1998; 178:126–130.
18. Atkinson MW, Goldenberg RL, Gaudier FL, et al: Maternal corticosteroid and tocolytic treatment and morbidity and mortality in very low birth weight infants. Am J Obstet Gynecol 1995; 173:299–305.
19. de Wesselius CA, Thiery M, Yo IS, et al: Results of double-blind, multicentre study with ritodrine in premature labour. BMJ 1971; 3:144–147.
20. Macones GA, Berlin M, Berlin JA: Efficacy of oral beta-agonist maintenance therapy in preterm labor: a meta-analysis. Obstet Gynecol 1995; 85:313–317.
21. Smigaj D, Roman-Drago NM, Amini SB, et al: The effect of oral terbutaline on maternal glucose metabolism and energy expenditure in pregnancy. Am J Obstet Gynecol 1998; 178:1041–1047.
22. Lipshitz J, Baillie P, Davey DA: A comparison of the uterine $beta_2$-adrenoreceptor selectivity of fenoterol, hexoprenaline, ritodrine and salbutamol. S Afr Med J 1976; 50:1969–1972.
23. McCombs J: Update on tocolytic therapy. Ann Pharmacother 1995; 29:515–522.
24. Adelwoehrer NE, Mahnert W: Hexoprenaline activates potassium channels of human myometrial myocytes. Arch Gynecol Obstet 1993; 252:179–184.
25. Lechner W: Introduction of hexoprenaline into the treatment of preterm labor [letter]. Am J Obstet Gynecol 1989; 161:1090–1091.
26. Hankins GD, Hauth JC: A comparison of the relative toxicities of beta-sympathomimetic tocolytic agents. Am J Perinatol 1985; 2:338–346.
27. Rivier G, Nicole A, Stucki D, et al: Lesional pulmonary edema associated with tocolysis by hexoprenaline sulfate [in German]. Schweiz Med Wochenschr 1992; 122:237–241.
28. Philipsen T, Eriksen PS, Lynggard F: Pulmonary edema following ritodrine-saline infusion in premature labor. Obstet Gynecol 1981; 58:304–308.
29. DiFederico EM, Burlingame JM, Kilpatrick SJ, et al: Pulmonary edema in obstetric patients is rapidly resolved except in the presence of infection or of nitroglycerin tocolysis after open fetal surgery. Am J Obstet Gynecol 1998; 179:925–933.
30. Chestnut DH, Pollack KL, Thompson CS, et al: Does ritodrine worsen maternal hypotension during epidural anesthesia in gravid ewes? Anesthesiology 1990; 72:315–321.
31. Tong C, Eisenach JC: The vascular mechanism of ephedrine's beneficial effect on uterine perfusion during pregnancy. Anesthesiology 1992; 76:792–798.
32. Grether JK, Hoogstrate J, Selvin S, et al: Magnesium sulfate tocolysis and risk of neonatal death. Am J Obstet Gynecol 1998; 178:1–6.
33. Barany M, Barany K: Dissociation of relaxation and myosin light chain dephosphorylation in porcine uterine muscle. Arch Biochem Biophys 1993; 305:202–204.
34. Walsh SW, Romney AD, Wang Y, et al: Magnesium sulfate attenuates peroxide-induced vasoconstriction in the human placenta. Am J Obstet Gynecol 1998; 178:7–12.
35. Vincent RDJ, Chestnut DH, Sipes SL, et al: Does calcium chloride help restore maternal blood pressure and uterine blood flow during hemorrhagic hypotension in hypermagnesemic gravid ewes? Anesth Analg 1992; 74:670–676.
36. Sipes SL, Chestnut DH, Vincent RDJ, et al: Which vasopressor should be used to treat hypotension during magnesium sulfate infusion and epidural anesthesia? Anesthesiology 1992; 77:101–108.
37. Shubert PJ: Atosiban. Clin Obstet Gynecol 1995; 38:722–724.
38. Goodwin TM, Valenzuela GJ, Silver H, et al: Dose ranging study of the oxytocin antagonist atosiban in the treatment of preterm labor. Atosiban Study Group. Obstet Gynecol 1996; 88:331–336.
39. Keelan JA, Coleman M, Mitchell MD: The molecular mechanisms of term and preterm labor: recent progress and clinical implications. Clin Obstet Gynecol 1997; 40:460–478.
40. Cacciatore B, Halmesmaki E, Kaaja R, et al: Effects of transdermal nitroglycerin on impedance to flow in the uterine, umbilical, and fetal middle cerebral arteries in pregnancies complicated by preeclampsia and intrauterine growth retardation. Am J Obstet Gynecol 1998; 179:140–145.
41. Rowlands S, Trudinger B, Visva-Lingam S: Treatment of preterm cervical dilatation with glyceryl trinitrate, a nitric oxide donor. Aust N Z J Obstet Gynaecol 1996; 36:377–381.
42. David M, Gungor L, Lichtenegger W: Tocolysis with a nitroglycerin patch [in German]. Zentralbl Gynakol 1998; 120:126–128.
43. DiFederico EM, Harrison M, Matthay MA: Pulmonary edema in a woman following fetal surgery. Chest 1996; 109:1114–1117.
44. David M, Halle H, Lichtenegger W, et al: Nitroglycerin to facilitate fetal extraction during cesarean delivery [see comments]. Obstet Gynecol 1998; 91:119–124.
45. Daven JR, Milstein JM, Guthrie RD: Cerebral vascular resistance in premature infants. Am J Dis Child 1983; 137:328–331.
46. Milligan DW: Failure of autoregulation and intraventricular haemorrhage in preterm infants. Lancet 1980; 1:896–898.
47. Haxhija EQ, Rosegger H: Effects of bolus tube feeding on cerebral blood flow velocity in neonates [letter; comment]. Arch Dis Child Fetal Neonatal Ed 1998; 78:F78–F79.
48. Myles TD, Espinoza R, Meyer W, et al: Effects of smoking, alcohol, and drugs of abuse on the outcome of "expectantly" managed cases of preterm premature rupture of membranes. J Matern Fetal Med 1998; 7:157–161.
49. Delaney DB, Larrabee KD, Monga M: Preterm premature rupture of the membranes associated with recent cocaine use. Am J Perinatol 1997; 14:285–288.
50. Sprauve ME, Lindsay MK, Herbert S, et al: Adverse perinatal outcome in parturients who use crack cocaine. Obstet Gynecol 1997; 89:674–678.
51. Grant A, Penn ZJ, Steer PJ: Elective or selective caesarean delivery of the small baby? A systematic review of the controlled trials. Br J Obstet Gynaecol 1996; 103:1197–1200.
52. Williams RL, Chen PM: Identifying the sources of the recent decline in perinatal mortality rates in California. N Engl J Med 1982; 306:207–214.
53. Welch RA, Bottoms SF: Reconsideration of head compression and intraventricular hemorrhage in the vertex very-low-birth-weight fetus. Obstet Gynecol 1986; 68:29–34.
54. Malloy MH, Onstad L, Wright E: The effect of cesarean delivery on birth outcome in very low birth weight infants. National Institute of Child Health and Human Development Neonatal Research Network. Obstet Gynecol 1991; 77:498–503.
55. Newton ER, Haering WA, Kennedy JLJ, et al: Effect of mode of delivery on morbidity and mortality of infants at early gestational age. Obstet Gynecol 1986; 67:507–511.
56. Evans LC, Combs CA: Increased maternal morbidity after cesarean delivery before 28 weeks of gestation. Int J Gynaecol Obstet 1993; 40:227–233.
57. Batton DG, DeWitte DB, Espinosa R, et al: The impact of fetal compromise on outcome at the border of viability. Am J Obstet Gynecol 1998; 178:909–915.
58. Boyle R: Caesarean section anaesthesia and the Apgar score. Aust N Z J Obstet Gynaecol 1993; 33:282–284.
59. Pickering BG, Palahniuk RJ, Cote J, et al: Cerebral vascular responses to ketamine and thiopentone during foetal acidosis. Can Anaesth Soc J 1982; 29:463–467.

26

Multiple Gestation and Fetal Malpresentation

❖ MANFRED G. MOERTL, MD
❖ CHRISTOPH A. BREZINKA, MD, PHD

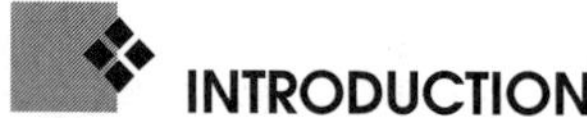

INTRODUCTION

This chapter reviews the important concepts of birth mechanics in breech and multiple pregnancies. The aim is to facilitate an understanding of these obstetric conditions, so that anesthesiologists can provide optimal conditions by combining their skills with a basic knowledge of the delivery process in these special circumstances.

The management of a breech delivery or the delivery of twins depends on successful teamwork. Optimum cooperation necessitates that all those involved in the birthing process understand the time frames and the dynamic changes of labor and delivery. Successful teamwork also requires an understanding of the possibilities and limitations of each obstetric and anesthesiologic intervention during each phase of birth. Such knowledge should not be restricted to the management interface between obstetrician and anesthesiologist—the parturient's desires and expectations should also be considered.

There are several different fetal positions for which cesarean section is routinely performed today. Such was not always the case, as illustrated by detailed descriptions of various maneuvers to be used for vaginal delivery of infants in transverse lie, primiparous breech, or shoulder presentation. With the widespread availability of safer anesthesia and surgical techniques for cesarean section, these maneuvers have become historical and only of marginal interest. In this chapter, the authors focus on two situations in which vaginal delivery still occurs, after careful consideration of the obstetric and anesthesiologic implications. These two scenarios are delivery associated with (1) breech presentation and (2) twin gestation.

The authors have concentrated on emphasizing the facts that they consider essential for the anesthesiologist to comprehend, in order to facilitate cooperation between the practitioners of obstetrics and those of anesthesiology.

BREECH PRESENTATION

In breech presentation, the fetus lies longitudinally with its buttocks in the lower pole of the uterus. All the various nomenclatures for the classification of breech presentation are based on the position of the lower extremities: basically there are three types of breech—frank, complete, and incomplete.[1]

In frank breech, also called breech with extended legs, the fetus' hips are flexed and both legs extend on the abdomen. In complete breech, both hips and knees are flexed and the feet are tucked in beside the buttocks. In incomplete breech, either a leg (also called footling breech) or a knee, or both, may present lower than the buttocks. Whereas in frank breech the presenting part is always one or both buttocks, a complete breech may at any point during birth change into an incomplete breech, and the obstetrician must be prepared to manage the delivery with the presentation of one or both legs[2] (Figs. 26–1 to 26–4).

In the general population, the frequency of breech presentation in term singletons is between 3% and 5%.[1]

Presentation of the fetus inside the uterus is dependent on several factors: tone of the uterus; tone and pressure of structures around the uterus, including the maternal abdominal wall; fetal mobility; and

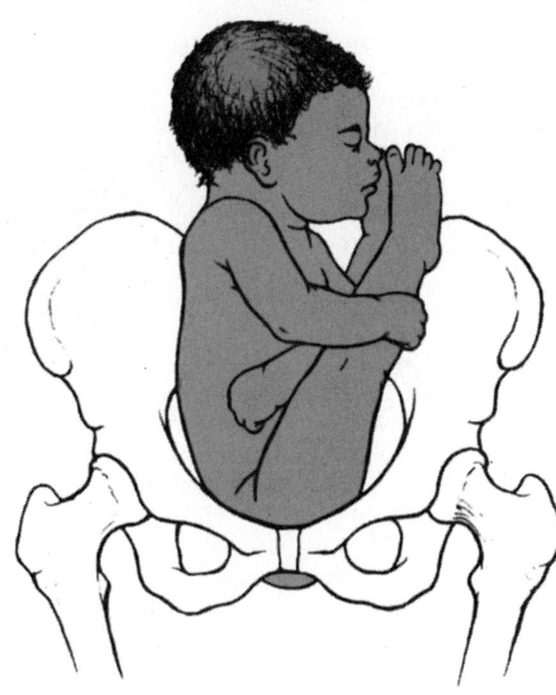

❖ **Figure 26–1** Frank breech. (From Martius G: Einteilung der Beckenendlage und Geburtsmechanismus. *In* Feige A, Krause M (eds): Beckenendlage, Vol 3. Munich: Urban & Schwarzenberg; 1998: 16; Fig. 3–1.)

the amount of amniotic fluid. It is believed that the fetal factors associated with breech presentation persist until term.[4]

"Birth Mechanics" of Breech Presentation

For the infant with breech presentation, the process of birth can be divided into five separate steps. The determining factor is the bi-trochanteric diameter, or the width of the fetal hips. Unlike birth with the fetus in the cephalic presentation, in which the head determines the process, in a breech delivery three structures of different shapes pass successively through the birth canal: (1) the hips, (2) the shoulders, and (3) the head.

- The descent of the fetus into the maternal pelvis begins with the fetal spine turned toward the maternal abdomen and the buttocks entering the oblique diameter.

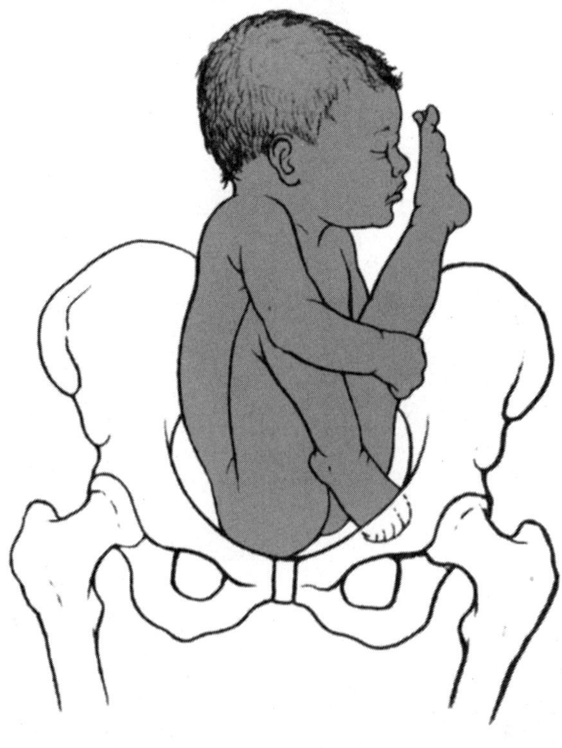

❖ **Figure 26–2** Incomplete breech. (From Martius G: Einteilung der Beckenendlage und Geburtsmechanismus. *In* Feige A, Krause M (eds): Beckenendlage, Vol 3. Munich: Urban & Schwarzenberg; 1998: 21; Fig. 3–5.)

- In order for the fetus to pass through the birth canal, several adaptive steps are necessary:
  a. descent of the fetal pole
  b. internal rotation of the buttocks
  c. shifting of the bi-trochanteric diameter into the anteroposterior diameter
- Lateral flexion of the body: While the anterior buttock acts as the lever (hypomochlion), the posterior buttock sweeps the perineum (Fig. 26–5).
- The buttocks are thus born with the lateral flexion movement. At this point, the shoulders enter the pelvis in an oblique diameter similar to that of the buttocks, easing the tension on the infant's trunk and thus enabling its rotation into the anteroposterior diameter of the outlet.

Once the trunk is delivered to the point where the lower edge of the fetal scapula is visible, the head enters the pelvis, with the sagittal suture in the transverse diameter, which is achieved with a downward movement of the fetal occiput and suboccipital region impinging on the symphysis. At this point, the lever (hypomochlion) must be the hairline of the fetal neck (Fig. 26–6).

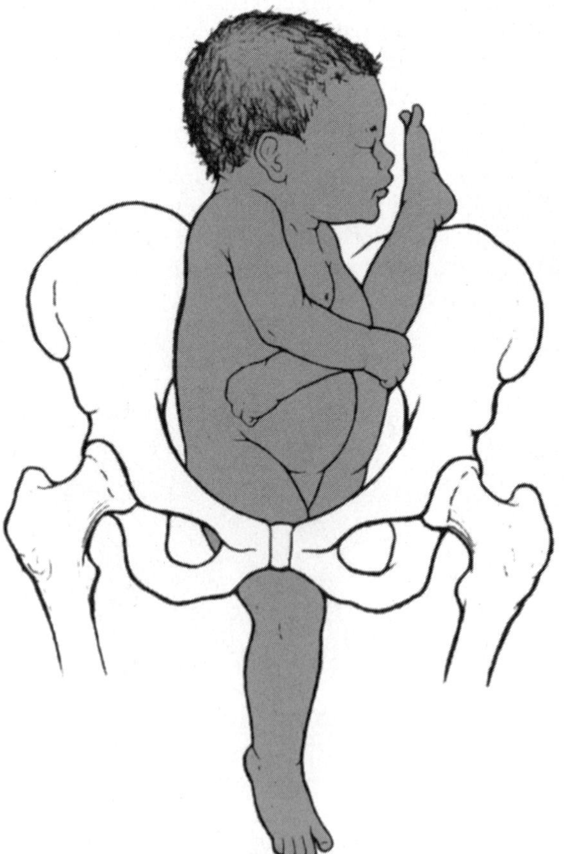

❖ **Figure 26–3** Incomplete breech: footling breech with one hip not flexed and one foot below the buttocks. (From Martius G: Einteilung der Beckenendlage und Geburtsmechanismus. *In* Feige A, Krause M (eds): Beckenendlage, Vol 3. Munich: Urban & Schwarzenberg; 1998: 18; Fig. 3–3.)

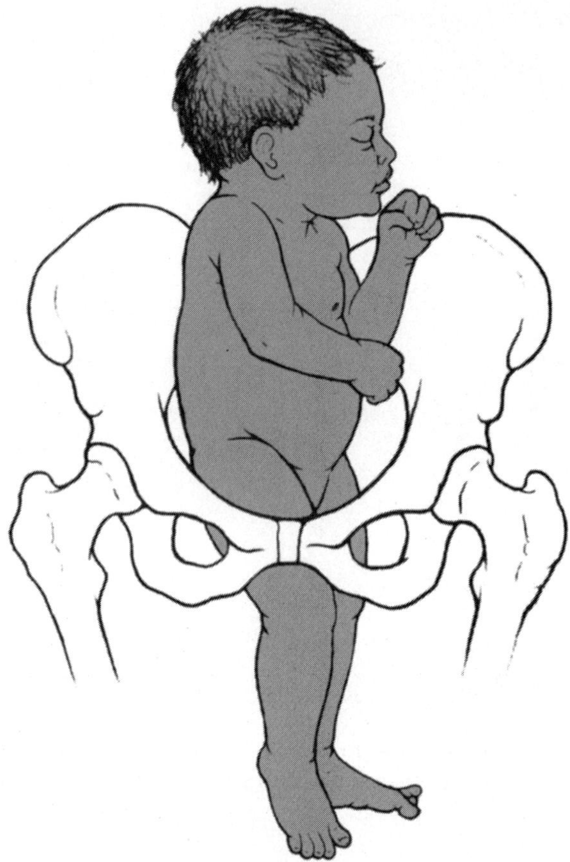

❖ **Figure 26–4** Incomplete breech: footling breech with both hips not flexed and both feet below the buttocks. (From Martius G: Einteilung der Beckenendlage und Geburtsmechanismus. *In* Feige A, Krause M (eds): Beckenendlage, Vol 3. Munich: Urban & Schwarzenberg; 1998: 17; Fig. 3–2.)

- At this stage, the body turns with the fetal spine uppermost, the chin and face sweep the perineum, and the head is born. Controlled delivery of the head is important in order to avoid sudden changes in intracranial pressures, especially in the case of premature infants (Fig. 26–7).

Any deviation from the process described earlier leads to an increase in fetal morbidity and mortality as well as an increased risk of maternal trauma.[5]

Breech Presentation and Fetal Hypoxia

Fetuses born in a breech presentation have an increased risk of intrapartum hypoxia compared with those born in a cephalic presentation.[6]

Causes of Fetal Hypoxia: Umbilical Cord

In a cephalic presentation, the distance between the umbilical cord insertion and the fetal body part lowest in the birth canal (head) is usually 28 cm[7] (Fig. 26–8),

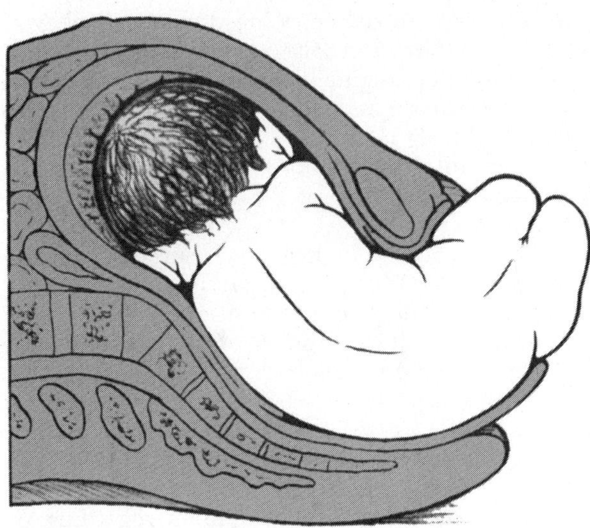

❖ **Figure 26–5** Position of the child's torso. (From Martius G: Einteilung der Beckenendlage und Geburtsmechanismus. *In* Feige A, Krause M (eds): Beckenendlage, Vol 3. Munich: Urban & Schwarzenberg; 1998: 19; Fig. 3–4.)

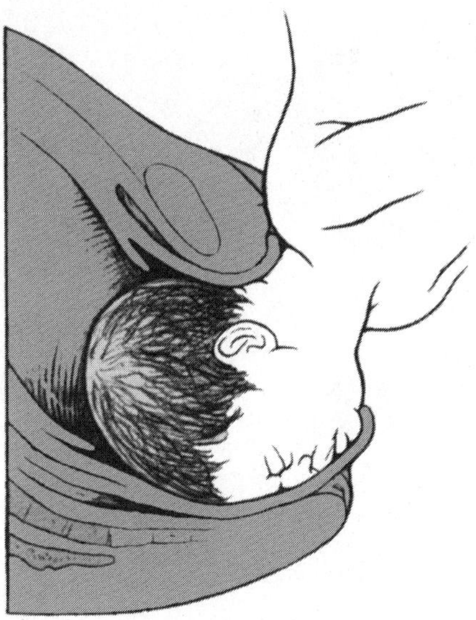

❖ **Figure 26–7** Emergence of the head. (From Martius G: Einteilung der Beckenendlage und Geburtsmechanismus. *In* Feige A, Krause M (eds): Beckenendlage, Vol 3. Munich: Urban & Schwarzenberg; 1998: 24; Fig. 3–7.)

whereas in a breech presentation the average is just 10 cm (Fig. 26–9). Thus, in breech presentation, pressure on the umbilical cord exerted by the birth canal increases with the downward movement of the fetal pelvis, leading to potential fetal hypoxia as early as the second stage of labor. This problem is virtually nonexistent in cephalic deliveries (with the possible exception of shoulder dystocia).[8]

Causes of Fetal Hypoxia: Placenta

A protracted third stage of labor is common in vaginal breech deliveries.[9]

It can lead to a significant decrease in placental perfusion during contractions. In cephalic deliveries, total uterine volume decreases by one third after delivery of the fetal head, whereas in breech deliveries uterine volume has already decreased by two thirds as soon as the fetal scapulae are visible and manual extraction can begin. In addition to this, a significant decrease of the uteroplacental exchange unit also occurs at this stage. The liberal administration of uterotonics that are commonly used at this stage can further decrease the placental perfusion. Reduction of uterine volume and placental exchange surface, together with

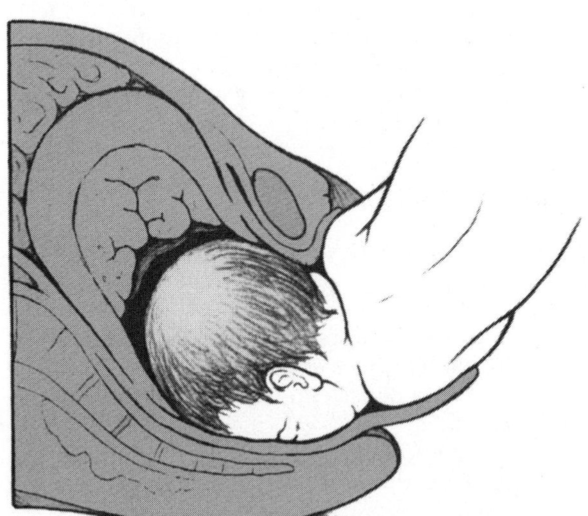

❖ **Figure 26–6** The shoulders begin to emerge (breech presentation). (From Martius G: Einteilung der Beckenendlage und Geburtsmechanismus. *In* Feige A, Krause M (eds): Beckenendlage, Vol 3. Munich: Urban & Schwarzenberg; 1998: 24; Fig. 3–6.)

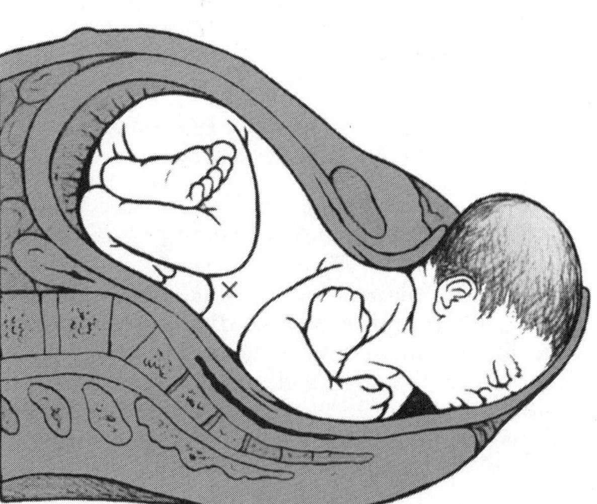

❖ **Figure 26–8** The lowest point of the navel during breech birth. (From Martius G: Einteilung der Beckenendlage und Geburtsmechanismus. *In* Feige A, Krause M (eds): Beckenendlage, Vol 3. Munich: Urban & Schwarzenberg; 1998: 27; Fig. 3–8a.)

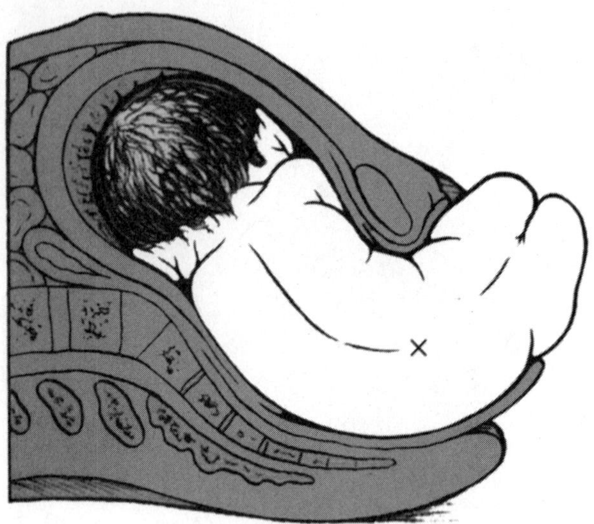

Figure 26–9 Breech birth. (After Künzel. From Martius G: Einteilung der Beckenendlage und Geburtsmechanismus. *In* Feige A, Krause M (eds): Beckenendlage, Vol 3. Munich: Urban & Schwarzenberg; 1998: 28; Fig. 3–8b.)

medication such as oxytocin, can drastically increase the risk of premature separation of the placenta.

Antenatal Management of Breech Presentation

Depending on resources and in-hospital coordination, several options are possible when a woman presents with breech at or near term:

- External cephalic version
- Planned cesarean section
- Decision to proceed with a vaginal delivery with the limitation of fetal hypoxia by assisted delivery, and with continuous fetal monitoring with the capacity of personnel to react to any sign of "fetal distress" by performing an emergency cesarean section

Obstetric and Anesthesiologic Procedures in Assisted Vaginal Breech Deliveries

A number of methods and maneuvers have been described for facilitating and shortening the final stage of a breech delivery. All are aimed at a reduction of the time interval between presentation of the fetal shoulder blades and delivery of the fetal head. At this point, the time necessary for the avoidance of hypoxia is 3 to 5 minutes; hence, a clear interdisciplinary management plan should be addressed beforehand to avoid maternal and fetal complications.

Recognition of Fetal Compromise

Continuous fetal heart rate monitoring (FHRM) cardiotocography (CTG) is still the most important technique when it comes to discerning fetal well-being. The clinical value of new technologies, such as transcutaneous fetal pulse oximetry, needs to be further assessed before they can replace continuous FHRM.[10]

No attempt at vaginal delivery of a fetus in breech presentation should be made unless continuous FHRM is available during birth.[10]

This monitoring should begin as soon as artificial or spontaneous rupture of the amniotic membranes has taken place.

All efforts should be made to ensure the presence of a continuous tracing, and any interruption (e.g., during the placement of epidural anesthesia) should be minimized. Artificial rupture of the amniotic membranes prior to the placement of an epidural anesthesia catheter should be avoided. Recurrent fetal blood sampling (FBS) should also be available, if multiple samplings become necessary during vaginal breech delivery.

There is no consensus of opinion regarding the decision to convert from vaginal to cesarean delivery. It is unlikely that clear guidelines based on clinical trials will become available. In this context, a few steps may facilitate the decision-making process.

1. Fetal pH values obtained from the presenting part should not be seen in isolation, but rather in the general trend of fetal well-being as evidenced by FHRM and by the manner in which the birthing process proceeds.
2. Interpretation and diagnosis of fetal acidosis should be based not only on pH value but also on base excess, in order to differentiate between respiratory, metabolic, and mixed acidosis.
3. When a moderate degree of acidosis is diagnosed ($pH < 7.15$, base excess < -7.0 mmol/L), a cesarean section is indicated, even when the breech has descended into the perineum. Simultaneous intrauterine resuscitation with a tocolytic agent may relieve the pressure on the umbilical cord. It is not advisable to proceed with spontaneous delivery by encouraging the woman to push when the fetus is already compromised by severe acidosis.[11]

Fetal Head Entrapment

The risks associated with breech delivery can be minimized by applying the following rules:

1. Adequate analgesia should be maintained during all stages of labor.
2. Early and conscientious risk selection should be made.
3. No active obstetric maneuvers should be performed before the infant's scapulae are visible.
4. Assisted delivery of a breech should be limited to guiding the infant's body, as determined by birth mechanics; vigorous traction or pulling should be avoided.
5. Organizational conditions must be met so that

emergency cesarean section can be performed as soon as "fetal distress" is diagnosed.

"It has been suggested that fetal head entrapment is not so much the result of an obstetrician's manual incompetence but of intellectual incompetence."[12, 13]

Should this complication arise, immediate intervention is required. The administration of medications to relax the uterus and to allay the mother's pain should improve fetal outcome. In the presence of epidural or spinal anesthesia, nitroglycerin in small doses (80 to 100 μg) can be administered intravenously for uterine relaxation—otherwise, general endotracheal anesthesia with the common volatile anesthetics may be necessary for relaxation of the uterus.[14, 15] Although fetal head entrapment is a rare complication, it should be fully discussed when one obtains an informed consent from the patient and during the planning for all eventualities in a breech delivery management plan.

Indications for Elective and Secondary Cesarean Section

Elective Cesarean Section

All the fetal and maternal conditions and pathologies that are considered indications for elective cesarean section in a cephalic presentation should also apply in a breech presentation.

A macrosomic fetus, calculated by ultrasonographic head circumference and abdominal circumference measurements, is considered an important indication for primary cesarean section in a breech presentation. Recommendations are varied, with the International Federation of Gynecology and Obstetrics (FIGO) recommending a 3500-g[16] expected fetal weight as the cutoff point above which a primary cesarean should be performed (1993), while the Nuremberg group suggests that an expected weight of at least 4500 g[17] is an absolute indication for cesarean section. The mother's wishes should be an important factor in these considerations. In the absence of sufficient communication with the mother as well as the multidisciplinary team for responding to an emergency cesarean section, an elective cesarean section may be indicated.

Prematurity as an indication for cesarean section is a topic of controversy at the present time.[18] Intact amniotic membranes, normal fetal growth, quick distention of the cervix, and rapid progress in labor are considered by some to be indications for an attempt at vaginal delivery, provided that skilled personnel are immediately available. Fetal growth retardation or premature rupture of the membranes, or both, in a premature fetus are uniformly seen as indications for cesarean section.[19]

Indications for Secondary Cesarean Section

Birth mechanics explain why vaginal birth in a frank breech presentation is usually 100 minutes longer than birth in a cephalic one. Only when more than 460 minutes have elapsed can the term "protracted delivery" be applied.[20, 21]

TWINS

In multiple pregnancy, ultrasonographic assessment of the developing fetuses at several times during gestation and prior to labor is of pivotal importance. The determination of chorionicity—whether monochorionic twins are divided by amniotic membranes—as well as fetal presentation and position prior to labor (Table 26–1) also help to determine the mode of delivery.[22]

In monoamniotic twins, primary cesarean section should always be performed.[24] Also in monochorionic-diamniotic twins, an elective cesarean section should be performed when the presenting twin is in a vertex presentation. The reason for this decision is the high incidence of acute twin-to-twin transfusion syndrome occurring during labor as well as the potential for premature separation of the placenta after the birth of the first twin[25, 26] (Fig. 26–10).

Controversies regarding vaginal delivery in cases of a twin presentation are limited to bichorionic-biamniotic twin pregnancies.

With the first twin in breech position, estimation of the size difference between the two babies is important. Only when the estimated weight difference between the two is less than 20% should an attempt at vaginal delivery be made.[27] The principles previously outlined for delivery of breech singletons similarly apply to twins with the first twin in breech. The actual position of the second twin is less important than its estimated weight. An estimated weight difference of more than 20% between the two siblings should be considered an indication for elective cesarean section.

Indications for Secondary Cesarean Section in Twins

All indications for repeat cesarean section with singletons apply equally with twins, such as presumed fetal jeopardy in one infant, umbilical cord prolapse, or premature placental separation.

Cesarean section of the second twin may be necessary in the following situations[28–32]:

1. In the presence of "fetal distress" following the successful vaginal delivery of the first infant

Table 26–1 PRESENTATIONS OF TWIN FETUSES ON ADMISSION TO DELIVERY

PRESENTATION	GERMANY (%)	UNITED STATES (%)
Cephalic/cephalic	40	42
Cephalic/breech	20	27
Breech/breech	10	5
Cephalic/transverse	8	18
Breech/transverse	2	—
Others	10	8

Data from Wernicke[22] and Divon et al.[23]

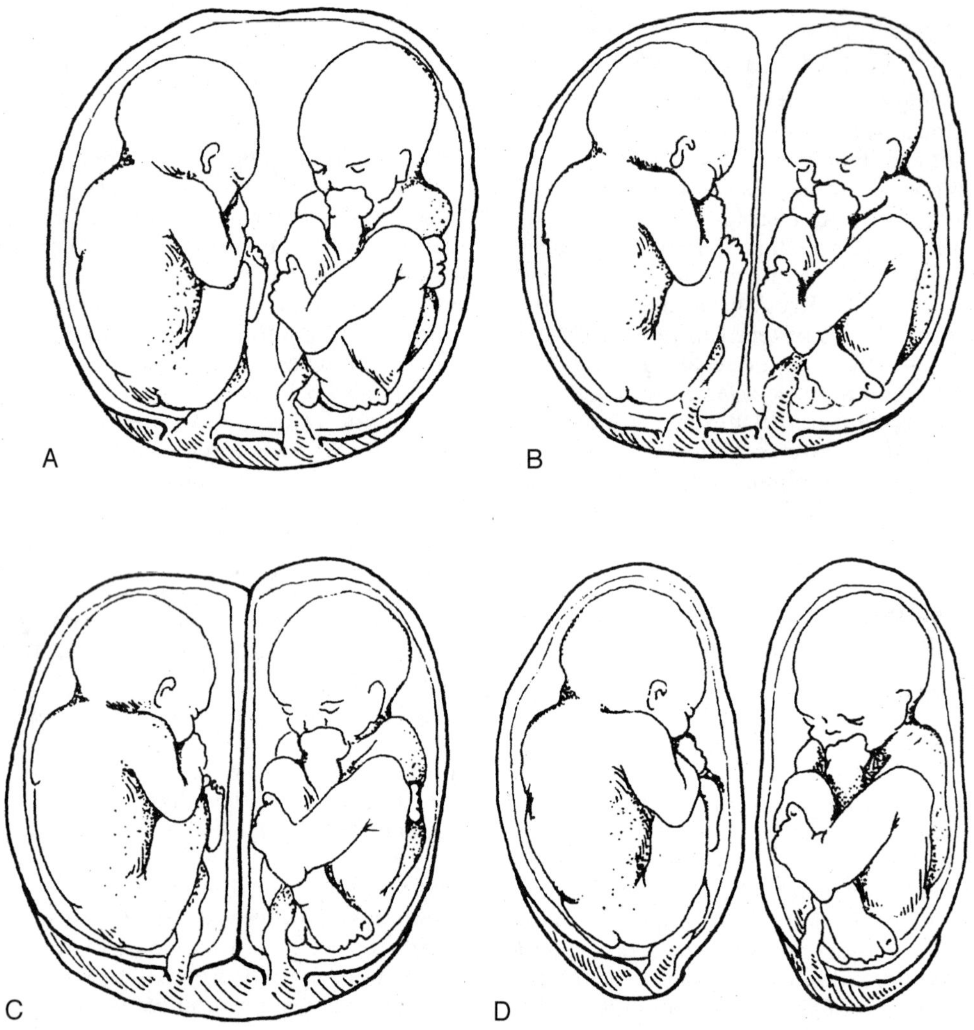

❖ **Figure 26–10** Placentation in twin pregnancies. *A*, Monochorionic; monoamniotic. *B*, Monochorionic; diamniotic. *C*, Dichorionic diamniotic (fused placenta). *D*, Dichorionic diamniotic (separate placentae). (From Hartwell BL: Fetal malpresentation and multiple birth. *In* Norris MC (ed): Obstet Anesth. 1993; 35:697; Fig. 35-3. After Gabbe SG, Niebyl JR, Simpson JL (eds): Obstetrics: Normal and Problem Pregnancies, 2nd ed. New York: Churchill Livingstone; 1991.)

2. A prolapsed cord
3. The presence of arrested labor, with the previously dilated cervix reassuming its shape
4. The presentation of the second twin in a transverse lie or a footling breech

TWINS OR BREECH PREGNANCIES

Organization and Structure of the Team Required for Dealing with Either Twins or Breech Pregnancies

- The obstetric team should be assembled and prepared to intervene at the earliest possible point in time at which a vital threat to the baby can be expected to occur. Hence, the team should be ready to address the emergency situation as soon as the breech fetus descends into the birth canal.
- The obstetric team should consist of an experienced obstetrician, with adequate assistance provided by another attending obstetrician, resident, or nurse-midwife, an anesthesiologist familiar with obstetric anesthesia, and a pediatrician with training in neonatal resuscitation. All must be present in close physical proximity.
- Conditions must be established so that an emergency cesarean section can be performed immediately.
- When the patient is informed about the possible birthing alternatives, the options should not be restricted to local practice: Also included should be the possibility of transferring her to a tertiary care center. The scheduling of the counseling is also important, with time allotted for the patient to make all necessary arrangements.

Anesthetic Management for Vaginal Delivery of Twins and Breech Presentation

The idea that the anesthesiologist needs to see the patient only minutes prior to delivery or cesarean section is still quite common worldwide. Often, this philosophy hinders the possibility of providing the best anesthesia care. Preoperative evaluation of the high-risk parturient can minimize maternal and fetal risks. In circumstances where optimal prenatal care is being practiced, a woman with a fetus in a breech position or with twins should receive care as part of a high-risk cooperative effort. Spontaneous version of a breech fetus prior to birth is possible, but this possibility should not preclude counseling of the patient about the risks and possible obstetric and anesthetic options available.

Under ideal circumstances, a woman with a high-risk pregnancy presents at the hospital 4 to 6 weeks prior to the expected date of delivery of the fetus. At this time, the anesthesiologist can inform the patient about the analgesia and anesthesia procedures available at that institution. The options of regional and general anesthesia should be discussed with the patient, and informed consent should be obtained.

The minimal preoperative evaluation should include the following:

- A family history
- The patient's history
- Information on allergies
- A history of any coagulation disorders
- The current general condition of the patient
- Information on accompanying illnesses (preeclampsia, systemic lupus erythematosus)
- Evaluation of the airway

A number of studies have evaluated the effect of regional techniques on the duration of birth from a breech presentation.[33–36] The biomechanical factors characteristic of breech presentation were not included in any of these studies. In the authors' opinion, the often-repeated statement that epidural anesthesia prolongs the expulsion period no longer holds. As described earlier, vaginal breech deliveries may last 100 minutes longer, on average, owing to birth mechanics. As of the present, whether a correctly placed and managed epidural anesthesia catheter has any influence on the duration of birth cannot be assessed on the basis of published studies. Conversely, one can argue that adequate analgesia may be the basis of successful vaginal breech delivery.

There is no specific obstetric reason for withholding regional analgesia in the woman attempting vaginal delivery of breech singletons or of twins. However, the anesthesiologist should address several facts before undertaking epidural analgesia for the vaginal delivery of breech or twins. Establishment of the necessary organizational framework is important, and such planning should include counseling of the patient at an early date.

If possible, the epidural catheter should be placed prior to the rupture of the amniotic membranes. Proper functioning of the epidural catheter should be tested by achieving the necessary level of analgesia following the administration of the initial local anesthetic without adding opiates. Once the proper placement of the catheter is verified, opiates can be used. Following this, continuous epidural anesthetic infusion and patient-controlled epidural analgesia are popular options.

Neuraxial analgesia should be managed in coordination with the progress of labor. Proper perineal analgesia and anesthesia are essential for the second stage of labor.

Even in the presence of regional analgesia and anesthesia, general anesthesia may be necessary in an extreme situation; hence, the anesthesiologist should be prepared to deal with this scenario.

An additional pudendal nerve block performed by the obstetrician at the point at which the presenting breech fetus has reached the perineum is an accepted method for optimizing perineal anesthesia.[37]

Once extensive pelvic relaxation is achieved by regional anesthesia, atraumatic delivery of the aftercoming head in breech will be facilitated.

Anesthesia for Cesarean Section

Anesthesia for cesarean section is discussed extensively in Chapters 17 and 18. This paragraph deals with the key elements that make cesarean section in a breech position or in multiple pregnancy different from the "normal" vertex singleton abdominal delivery. Both in the breech fetus and in twins, it is possible to have prolonged times from uterine incision to delivery, which may significantly affect neonatal well-being. Adequate uterine relaxation may be vital during the extraction of twins or triplets. Nitroglycerin, 50 to 100 μg IV, has been suggested to be the drug of choice because of its short half-life and its lack of serious side effects. General anesthesia is usually restricted to cases in which sudden fetal "distress" or maternal hemorrhage forces an emergency cesarean section. Because blood loss may be greater following multiple gestation, a second intravenous line should be considered and blood should be readily available if transfusion becomes necessary.

External Cephalic Version (ECV)

The recent renaissance of external cephalic version is easy to explain. In many countries, elective cesarean section is becoming the only option offered to women presenting with a breech fetus at or near term. Turning the baby around is often the only way of escaping an otherwise obligatory cesarean section.

The widespread introduction of β-sympathomimetics as tocolytic agents to relax the uterus for the purpose of external cephalic version has increased the success rate of vaginal delivery.[38, 39] With the use of Doppler ultrasonography, it is now possible to immediately verify the outcome of the external cephalic version maneuver and also to check the condition of the fetus.

The prerequisites for external cephalic version include the following:

- Term breech pregnancy: External cephalic version should be undertaken from 37 weeks of gestation onward unless it is contraindicated. In such cases, there is no upper time limit.
- Informed consent.
- Anesthesiologist on standby.

The relative contraindications for external cephalic version are as follows[40]:

- Patient's refusal of the procedure
- Previous cesarean section
- Previous uterine surgery (myomectomy, the Strassmann procedure)
- Oligohydramnios
- Compromised fetus
- Prematurity of fetus
- Placenta previa
- Placental or umbilical cord pathology, or both, as ascertained by ultrasonography
- Antepartum hemorrhage
- Preeclampsia

Several authors have observed a significant positive effect of epidural anesthesia on the success rate of external cephalic version.[41] In one study, the success rate increased from 24% to as much as 59% in the presence of epidural anesthesia.[41] Practitioners have also tried spinal anesthesia, using 10 μg of sufentanil and 2.5 mg of bupivacaine for external cephalic version. Using this technique, Dugoff and colleagues[42] did not observe any increase in the success rate. However, these authors noted that in the spinal anesthesia group the patients were more comfortable during the procedure than those in the nonspinal group. Vetter and Nierhaus[43] have described a standardized protocol for external cephalic version:

- Tocolysis with the use of fenoterol and a β-mimetic agent
- Performance of external cephalic version with the use of epidural anesthesia and the presence of an anesthesia care team for possible cesarean section
- Presence of ultrasonography to guide the procedure and the verification of fetal position
- Confirmation of fetal well-being with the use of FHRM

Changes in fetal heart rate patterns have been observed in as many as 10% of cases.[46] Several cases of fetal-maternal transfusion have also been reported. The rate of placental separation during or immediately after external cephalic version varies from 0.2% to 2%.[44] Rare cases of unexplained intrauterine death in the days following external cephalic version have been reported.[45]

When one considers a success rate of up to 60%, external cephalic version is certain to become part of management protocols for breech presentation.

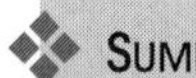

Summary

Key Points

- Multidisciplinary interactions are important in the care of the patient in this high-risk group of parturients.
- Anesthesiologists should always be prepared to deal with an emergency situation during breech delivery or external cephalic version because sudden fetal bradycardia can occur at any time during the procedure.
- The use of tocolytic agents may be associated with an increase in the success rate of external cephalic version because of the resultant relaxation of uterine muscles.
- Epidural anesthesia has also been observed to increase the success rate of the external cephalic version procedure, and the epidural catheter can also be used for cesarean section if that surgery becomes necessary.

Case Stem

A 38-year-old primigravida with a fetus at 39 weeks of gestation in a breech presentation is admitted to the obstetric unit. Her obstetrician decides to attempt external cephalic version (ECV). Discuss the anesthetic management.

Anesthetic Requirements

Most clinical protocols for external cephalic version now demand obligatory standby preparation and personnel for emergency cesarean section. Hence, the anesthesiology team should consult the woman prior to the procedure in order to discuss the proposed anesthetic management. Informed consent should also be taken at this time. However, there is controversy regarding whether neuraxial anesthesia substantially increases the success rate of external cephalic version. Ongoing and future studies will clarify this question. On the other hand, regional anesthesia is surely associated with less discomfort to the parturient.

References

1. Seeds JW: Malpresentations. *In* Gabbe SG, Niebyl JR, Simpson JL (eds): Obstetrics: Normal and Problem Pregnancies, 2nd ed. New York: Churchill Livingstone; 1991: 551.
2. Hartwell BL: Fetal malpresentation and multiple birth. Obstet Anesth 1993; 35:689–691.
3. Brown L, Karrison T, Cibilis LA: Mode of delivery and perinatal results in breech presentation. Am J Obstet Gynecol 1994; 171:28–34.
4. Rayl J, Gibson PJ, Hickok DE: A population-based case control study of risk factors for breech presentation. Am J Obstet Gynecol 1996; 174:28–32.
5. Martius G: Einteilung der Beckenendlage und Geburtsmechanismus. *In* Feige A, Krause M (eds): Beckenendlage, Vol 3. Munich: Urban & Schwarzenberg; 1998: 3:22–29.
6. Schutte MF, Van Hemel OJS, Van de Berg C, Van de Pol A:

Perinatal mortality in breech presentations as compared to vertex presentations in singleton pregnancies: an analysis based upon 57819 computer-registered pregnancies in The Netherlands. Eur J Obstet Gynecol Reprod Biol 1985; 19:391–400.
7. Künzel W, Kirschbaum M: Beckenendlage, Quer- und Schräglage. *In* Wulf KH, Schmidt-Matthiesen H (eds): Klinik der Frauenheilkunde und Geburtshilfe, 2nd ed. Vol 7/1: Künzel W, Wulf KH (eds): Physiologie und Pathologie der Geburt I. Munich: Urban & Schwarzenberg; 1990: 231.
8. Martius G: Einteilung der Beckenendlage und Geburtsmechanismus. *In* Feige A, Krause M (eds): Beckenendlage, Vol 3. Munich: Urban & Schwarzenberg; 1998: 26–27.
9. Krause M, Feige A: Darstellung der spezifischen Erfahrungen der vaginalen Beckenendlagenentbindung. *In* Feige A, Krause M (eds): Beckenendlage, Vol. 9. Munich: Urban & Schwarzenberg; 1998: 156–157.
10. Feige A, Krause M: Geburtsleitung bei Beckenendlage. *In* Feige A, Krause M (eds): Beckenendlage, Vol. 8. Munich: Urban & Schwarzenberg; 1998: 143.
11. Feige A, Krause M: Geburtsleitung bei Beckenendlage. *In* Feige A, Krause M (eds): Beckenendlage, Vol 8. Munich: Urban & Schwarzenberg; 1998: 144.
12. Robertson PA, Foran CM, Croughan-Minihane MS, Kilpatrick SJ: Head entrapment and neonatal outcome by mode of delivery in breech deliveries from 28 to 36 weeks of gestation. Am J Obstet Gynecol 1996; 174:42–49.
13. Weiss PAM: Geburtsrisiko Beckenendlage. *In* Feige A, Krause M (eds): Beckenendlage, Vol 6. Munich: Urban & Schwarzenberg; 1998: 75–99.
14. Rolbin S, Hew E, Bernstein A: Uterine relaxation can be life saving. Can J Anaesth 1991; 38:939–940.
15. Altabef KM, Spencer JT, Zinberg S: Intravenous nitroglycerin for uterine relaxation of an inverted uterus. Am J Obstet Gynecol 1992; 166:1237–1238.
16. Guidelines for the Management of Breech Delivery: Recommendations of the FIGO Committee and Perinatal Health, based upon written discussion and workshop. Rome: World Congress of Perinatal Medicine; 1993.
17. Feige A, Krause M: Geburtsleitung bei Beckenendlage. *In* Feige A, Krause M (eds): Beckenendlage, Vol 8. Munich: Urban & Schwarzenberg; 1998: 129.
18. Krause M, Feige A: Darstellung der spezifischen Erfahrungen der vaginalen Beckenendlagenentbindung. *In* Feige A, Krause M (eds): Beckenendlage, Vol 9. Munich: Urban & Schwarzenberg, 1998: 159.
19. Feige A, Krause M: Geburtsleitung bei Beckenendlage. *In* Feige A, Krause M (eds): Beckenendlage, Vol 8. Munich: Urban & Schwarzenberg; 1998: 130.
20. Krause M, Fischer TH, Feige A: Welchen Einfluss hat die Stellung der Beine bei der Beckenendlage auf den Entbindungsmodus und die neonatale Frühmorbidität. Z Geburtshilfe Neonatol (in press).
21. Martius G: Geburtshilflich—perinatologische Operationen. Stuttgart: Thieme; 1986: 147.
22. Wernicke K: Mehrlingsgeburt. *In* Wulf KH, Schmidt-Matthiesen H (eds): Klinik der Frauenheilkunde und Geburtshilfe. Vol 6: Halberstadt E, (ed): Fruhgeburt, Mehrlingsschwangerschaft. Munich: Urban & Schwarzenberg. 1987: 332.
23. Divon MY, Marin MJ, Pollack RN, et al: Twin gestation: fetal presentation as a function of gestation age. Am J Obstet Gynecol 1993; 168: 1500–1502.
24. Feige A, Krause M: Geburtsleitung bei Beckenendlage. *In* Feige A, Krause M (eds): Beckenendlage, Vol 8. Munich: Urban & Schwarzenberg; 1998: 131.
25. Feige A, Krause M: Geburtsleitung bei Beckenendlage. *In* Feige A, Krause M (eds): Beckenendlage, Vol 8. Munich: Urban & Schwarzenberg; 1998: 132.
26. Benirschke K: Twin placenta in perinatal mortality. N Y State J Med 1961; 61:1499–1508.
27. Feige A, Krause M: Geburtsleitung bei Beckenendlage. *In* Feige A, Krause M (eds): Beckenendlage, Vol 8. Munich: Urban & Schwarzenberg; 1998: 132.
28. Abu Heija AT, Ziadeh S, Abukteish F, Obeidat A: Retrospective study of outcome of vaginal and abdominal delivery in twin pregnancy in which twin I is presenting by the breech. Arch Gynecol Obstet 1998; 261:71–73.
29. Oettinger M, Ophir E, Markovitz J, et al: Is caesarean section necessary for delivery of a breech first twin? Gynecol Obstet Invest 1993; 35:38–43.
30. Queck M, Berle P: Einfluss des Geburtsintervalls auf die Sectiorate am zweiten Zwilling nach vaginaler Geburt des führenden Zwillings. Zentralbt Gynakol 1993; 115:366–369.
31. Seufert R, Casper F, Bauer H, Brockerhoff P: Schnittentbindung am zweiten Zwilling. Perinat Med 1991; 3:109–111.
32. Wessel J: Secttio am II. Zwilling. Ist dieser ungewöhnliche Geburtsmodus vertretbar? Geburtshilfe Frauenheilkd 1993; 53:609–612.
33. Confino E, Ismajovich B, Rudick V, David MP: Extradural analgesia in the management of singleton breech delivery. Br J Anaesth 1985; 57:892–895.
34. Breeson AJ, Kovacs GT, Pickles BG, Hill JG: Extradural analgesia—the preferred method of analgesia for vaginal breech delivery. Br J Anaesth 1978; 50:1227–1230.
35. Van Zundert A, Vaes L, Soetens M, et al: Are breech deliveries an indication for lumbar epidural analgesia? Anesth Analg 1991; 72:399–403.
36. Chadha YC, Mahmood TA, Dick MJ, et al: Breech delivery and epidural analgesia. Br J Obstet Gynaecol 1992; 99:96–100.
37. Datta S: Relief of labor pain by regional analgesia/anesthesia. *In* Datta S (ed): The Obstetric Anesthesia Handbook, 2nd ed, Vol 11. St. Louis: Mosby; 1995: 124.
38. Robertson AW, Kopelman JN, Read JA, et al: External cephalic version at term: is a tocolytic necessary? Obstet Gynecol 1987; 70:896–899.
39. Tan G, Jen S, Tan S, Salmon Y: A prospective randomized controlled trial of external cephalic version comparing two methods of uterine tocolysis with a nontocolysis group. Singapore Med J 1989; 30:155–158.
40. Vetter K, Nierhaus M: Die äussere Wendung des Kindes in Schädellage. *In* Feige A, Krause M (eds): Beckenendlage, Vol 7. Munich: Urban & Schwarzenberg; 1998: 108.
41. Carlan SJ, Dent JM, Huckaby T, et al: The effect of epidural anesthesia on safety and success of external cephalic version at term. Anesth Analg 1994; 79:525.
42. Dugoff L, Stamm CA, Jones OW, et al: The effect of spinal anesthesia on the success rate of external cephalic version: a randomized trial. Am J Obstet Gynecol 1999; 93:345.
43. Vetter K, Nierhaus M: Die äussere Wendung des Kindes in Schädellage. *In* Feige A, Krause M (eds): Beckenendlage, Vol 7. Munich: Urban & Schwarzenberg; 1998: 111.
44. Calhoun B, Edgeworth D, Brehm W: External cephalic version at a military teaching hospital: predictors of success. Aust N Z J Obstet Gynaecol 1995; 35:277–279.
45. Extermann P: Version cephalique externe. *In* Jahresversammlung der Schweizer Gesellschaft für Geburtshilfe. Bern: Lugano, Bäbler; 1997: 85.
46. Phelan J, Stine L, Mueller E, et al: Observations of fetal heart rate characteristics related to external cephalic version and tocolysis. Am J Obstet Gynecol 1984; 149:658.

27

Anesthesia for Vaginal Birth After Cesarean Delivery

❖ Danilo Celleno, MD
❖ Giorgio Capogna, MD
❖ Paola Dorato, MD

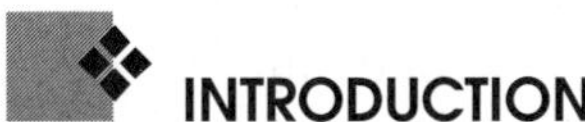

INTRODUCTION

Until one or two decades ago, all pregnant women who had undergone a previous cesarean delivery were electively scheduled for repeat cesarean section (C-section) without any attempt at vaginal delivery. This trend has been changing as clinical experience and scientific literature confirm the safety of vaginal delivery following previous C-section for both the mother and the baby. This procedure is commonly referred to as vaginal birth after cesarean section (VBAC); however, in some institutions the terminology has been changed to trial of labor after a cesarean section (TOLAC).

Although it seems appropriate to attempt a trial of labor in parturients who have previously undergone an operative delivery, proper selection of patients, knowledge of the associated risks, and proper recognition and management of the complications are keys to a successful outcome. In appropriate circumstances, the risks and complications of a trial of labor have been observed to be less when compared with elective repeat C-sections. In addition, significant cost reduction can be achieved when increasing the number of parturients who undergo vaginal birth after cesarean section.

"Once a section, always a section" had been a clinical dictum since the beginning of the 20th century.[1] Before that, too few women survived their first C-section to worry about their subsequent pregnancies. In the early 1980s, a few authors[2] had suggested that VBAC could succeed; however, such advice at that time remained just a theoretical concept, as the vast majority of these patients underwent elective repeat operative procedures. The rationale behind this widespread practice was the fear that a scarred uterus might rupture under the stress of labor, endangering the life of both mother and fetus.

Two factors led obstetricians to reexamine this practice and to consider VBAC. They are (1) the increased safety associated with the different type of uterine incision increasingly employed during C-section (transverse, lower segment) and (2) the rapid and sometimes alarming increase in the rate of cesarean deliveries throughout North America and Europe. For example, between 1970 and 1990, the rate of cesarean section in the United States increased from 5% to 25%,[3] and it was suggested that elective repeat cesarean section was responsible for two thirds of the increase in cesarean section deliveries.[4] The VBAC rate has dramatically increased and this has most likely influenced the decrease in cesarean section rate that has been occurring. This chapter discusses the rationale and evidence for the safety of VBAC and reviews the evidence for the safety of neuraxial analgesia in these patients. Although VBAC appears to be safe and is effective in 75% of women,[5] it is not without complications,[6] which are also discussed.

LOWER TRANSVERSE UTERINE SEGMENT VERSUS CLASSIC VERTICAL SCAR

The incidence and severity of uterine rupture is significantly different in relation to the types of incision as well as to the scars following C-sections. This is an important factor in selecting a patient for trial of labor.

The vertical, or classic, incision that was routinely performed before the 1980s was associated with a thicker scar and was positioned in the more contractile upper uterine segment. This incision, however, is rarely performed today unless specific indications exist. For a cephalic presentation, a transverse incision through the lower uterine segment is most often chosen because it is associated with less blood loss, is easier to repair, is located at a site least likely to rupture, and does not promote adherence of bowel or omentum to the incisional line.[7] A classic incision is sometimes performed in cases of anterior placenta previa, transverse lie with downward position of the fetal back, and dense scarring in the lower uterine segment. It is also occasionally chosen in cases of cesarean delivery for malposition in a preterm fetus or a very low birth weight nonvertex infant.[8]

The lower segment is fully formed only during labor, when it is pulled outward and thinned out by the contracting upper portion of the uterus. Since it is less vascular and it undergoes gradual stretching during labor, it is less likely to rupture. Even if it does rupture, the rupture is often incomplete and benign. Other, rarely used uterine incisions are associated with greater risk of uterine rupture. These include vertical incision of the lower uterine segment, the J incision, which also extends into the upper uterine segment, and the T incision, which is a combination of both transverse and vertical incisions in the lower uterine segment.[9]

Two types of uterine rupture, complete and incomplete, may be encountered. These differ in severity, signs, and symptoms. A complete rupture, which involves the entire thickness of the uterus (including the myometrium and the peritoneum), is most often seen after a classic scar and may produce a catastrophic event associated with significant maternal and fetal mortality or morbidity. An incomplete rupture or dehiscence does not involve the entire thickness of the uterus, is generally asymptomatic, and is not associated with increased maternal or neonatal morbidity or mortality. This type of rupture is more often observed with a lower transverse incision scar, hence more often encountered in today's practice. It is usually an incidental finding diagnosed during exploration of the uterus following vaginal delivery or at the time of C-section, as it rarely interferes with the birthing process.

Questions may be raised about the potential for endangering the mother and fetus during VBAC, when an elective cesarean section can be accomplished safely. A cesarean section is not completely devoid of risks for mother and baby, however, as is discussed in further detail in this chapter. To provide the best care to our patients, as well as to manage the ever increasing costs of health care, the risks and benefits of VBAC must be compared with those of repeat cesarean section for each patient. Rosen and colleagues[10] conducted a meta-analysis that included 31 studies with a total of 11,417 trials of labor and reported that the intended birth route made no difference in the rates of uterine dehiscence and rupture. Moreover, they reported that maternal febrile morbidity was significantly lower after a trial of labor than after an elective repeat cesarean section. Likewise, Martin and colleagues[11] reviewed obstetric literature detailing the subsequent delivery experience of patients with a prior low-segment vertical cesarean section and reported that vaginal delivery was safely accomplished in 82%. Even following a vertical incision, uterine rupture was a very rare event, and in these reports was not associated with perinatal mortality or permanent perinatal morbidity.

BENEFITS AND RISKS OF VAGINAL BIRTHS AFTER CESAREAN SECTIONS VERSUS ELECTIVE CESAREAN SECTIONS

Although studies have not been reported that randomize pregnant patients into repeat cesarean versus trial of labor groups, it has been suggested that vaginal delivery is safer for the mother than elective C-section. Maternal mortality related to C-section, due to sepsis, pulmonary embolism, hemorrhage, and complications from anesthesia, is higher than in vaginal deliveries.[10, 12, 13] Conversely, no maternal death from uterine rupture during a trial of labor was observed by Flamm and colleagues[14] who reviewed 11,000 patients from 1960 to 1990. This finding was also confirmed in a recent report by Obara et al.[15]

Maternal morbidity may also be higher in elective C-section as compared with VBAC. In particular, complications associated with cesarean deliveries that can be avoided in vaginal deliveries include injury to vital organs (especially bladder and urinary tract), increased blood loss and need for transfusions, wound infections, postoperative adhesions, and increased risk of thrombophlebitis.[16] Furthermore, it has been observed that patients delivering vaginally experience less discomfort, faster recovery, shorter hospital stays, and higher satisfaction[16, 17] and that cesarean deliveries can be associated with significant psychologic risks.[18]

Although it is true that C-section following failed TOLAC is associated with higher morbidity than elective C-section, this morbidity rate is similar to that of pregnant women who undergo primary C-section following failed labor. Since the success rate of TOLAC at the present time is high, it has been suggested that the overall maternal morbidity from VBAC is lower than when elective repeat C-section is performed.

Like mothers, babies may also benefit from VBAC, as they can avoid the risks associated with an elective C-section, such as iatrogenic prematurity and associated respiratory morbidity and mortality.[19–21] Even in the presence of documented fetal lung maturity, the absence of labor and squeezing of the fetal thoracic cage by the birth canal may prevent key physiologic changes in the fetus such as fluid reabsorption from the lungs as well as surfactant release. These factors help decrease pulmonary vascular resistance, and their absence may lead to "wet lung syndrome," which can cause pulmonary hypertension and persistent fetal circulation in the infant, thus increasing neonatal morbidity. Although rare, this does occur and can produce catastrophic outcomes. Heritage and Cunningham[21] observed this syndrome in 12 babies delivered by C-section at term. All of these infants required mechanical ventilation and three ultimately died from respiratory failure.

Other fetal complications due to C-section include asphyxia as a result of maternal hypoxia and accidental fetal lacerations.[22]

The perinatal mortality rate related to C-section has been estimated to be 4.5 per 1000,[23, 24] compared with a perinatal mortality rate of 1 per 1000 related to uterine rupture in a trial of labor.[25, 26]

UTERINE RUPTURE: INCIDENCE, SIGNS, SYMPTOMS, AND MANAGEMENT

Complete rupture of the uterus in late pregnancy is an important cause of maternal and neonatal mortality and morbidity and occurs with an overall incidence of 0.04% to 0.24%.[27] Maternal mortality is generally less than 10% following uterine rupture, but an important and somewhat underemphasized aspect of the morbidity in the mother is the undesired loss of reproductive function should a hysterectomy become necessary.

Uterine rupture can occur in a scarred uterus as well as in an intact one, but the presence of a previous scar increases the incidence of rupture. Because uterine rupture is unexpected and often uncontrolled, the consequences of spontaneous rupture of an unscarred uterus are generally more catastrophic in terms of maternal and neonatal morbidity and mortality. Unscarred uteruses may rupture following trauma, obstetric maneuvers, obstructed labor, or oxytocin use in multigravidae. A review of uterine rupture during pregnancy reported that the majority occurred in the unscarred uterus.[28]

Flamm has suggested that a woman with a prior cesarean section is at increased risk regardless of her mode of birth, and eliminating VBAC will not eliminate the risks.[29] The same conclusion was also drawn by Martin and colleagues[26] following a review of 717 patients in which 11 uterine disruptions occurred, with a similar incidence of uterine rupture regardless of the route of delivery. Meehan and Magani[23] examined the data from 2834 patients with history of previous C-section between 1972 and 1987 and reported an incidence of uterine rupture that was similar in TOLAC versus elective C-section (0.44% vs 0.37%) (Table 27–1). Complete uterine ruptures occurred in 6 of the 1350 TOLAC patients, with no maternal deaths. There were two fetal deaths and two parturients underwent gravid hysterectomies. By comparison, 4 of the 1084 patients scheduled for elective C-section sustained a complete rupture antepartum: one had a classic scar and the other three presented with abnormal placentation on the scar site. The outcome of these cases was more catastrophic, with two maternal deaths, one fetal death, and gravid hysterectomies in the two patients who survived. In this particular group, the presence of multiple scars may have caused a disorder of placentation, which led to uterine rupture; such association has also been noted by other authors.

Lao and Leung[27] reviewed 17 cases of uterine rupture that occurred over an 8-year period and also concluded that the incidence of rupture in TOLAC patients was not significantly different than in the elective repeat C-section group.

Table 27–1 INCIDENCE OF COMPLETE UTERINE RUPTURE: TRIAL OF LABOR VERSUS ELECTIVE CESAREAN SECTION

Total unit deliveries (n)	40526
Total with previous C-section (n)	2434
Scheduled for repeat C-section (n(%))	1084 (44.54)
Scar rupture in elective C-section (n(%))	4 (0.37)
Trial of labor patients (n(%))	1350 (55.46)
Successful vaginal delivery (n(%))	1097 (81.26)
Scar rupture in trial of labor (n(%))	6 (0.44)

Modified from Meehan FP, Magani IM: True rupture of a Cesarean scar (a 15-year review, 1972–1987). Eur J Obstet Gynecol Reprod Biol 1989; 30:129.

It is crucial that the diagnosis of uterine rupture be made as early as possible, but this is sometimes a difficult task. As has been described in several retrospective studies, delay in diagnosis is a major cause of catastrophic outcomes for the mother and fetus. What makes it so challenging for the clinician to recognize a true rupture of the uterus is that the classic signs and symptoms (severe abdominal pain and tenderness, cessation of labor, readily palpable fetal parts, vaginal bleeding, and shock) are not consistently present or may be completely absent (Table 27–2). This is especially the case for uterine rupture associated with low transverse segment scar, which is less dangerous compared with spontaneous or a classic incision rupture. A lower uterine segment scar is situated in a less muscular as well as less vascular part of the uterus, so rupture in this area is more gradual and insidious. Furthermore, this rupture is concealed by the bladder and may remain extraperitoneal. The subtle presentation associated with lower segment scar separation is an important concept. Although it is true that this type of scar is less prone to complete rupture, when it occurs the diagnosis may be more difficult and some of the features are easy to miss. Opponents of VBAC suggest that this is its main drawback. Abdominal pain is not a consistent finding, often being absent.[23, 30] When present, it is described as a severely painful sensation (of a tearing or shearing nature) over the lower abdomen. Intraperitoneal bleeding or amniotic fluid spillage from the ruptured uterus may produce signs of peritonitis and referred pain to the shoulder.

Table 27–2 SIGNS AND SYMPTOMS OF UTERINE RUPTURE AND THEIR INCIDENCE

Sign or Symptom	Incidence (%)
Pain	0 to 50–80
Fetal distress	50–75
Vaginal bleeding	17–67
Recession of the presenting part	25–50
Shock	0–50
Readily palpable fetal parts	17
Peritoneal signs	17

Hemorrhage and shock may also be absent, but when associated with abdominal pain, make the clinical scenario of uterine rupture similar to abruptio placentae, which is most often the first diagnosis in these cases. Unique signs of uterine rupture are extremely rare and include readily palpable fetal parts due to fetal extrusion and recession of presenting parts.

Not only is there inconsistency in the quality and intensity, the onset of symptoms can also vary from the time of the rupture and may manifest anywhere from a few minutes to many hours after the actual occurrence.[31]

The more consistent findings following uterine rupture are manifested by the fetal effects. In fact, the single most reliable sign of uterine rupture is "fetal distress," detected on continuous fetal heart rate monitoring as fetal bradycardia or late or severe variable decelerations. The use of fetal heart rate monitoring is therefore essential in the management of TOLAC parturients, as it allows close fetal surveillance during labor. Early detection of fetal heart rate changes, together with a high index of suspicion, may help establish a prompt diagnosis of uterine rupture in the absence of other classic signs and symptoms. Slowing or arrest of dilation should also be considered an important sign, since in the absence of mechanical dystocia, it may suggest ineffective uterine contractions due to a dehiscence of the uterine scar.[32, 33]

Early diagnosis and immediate intervention are essential to minimize maternal and fetal morbidity and mortality. Delay in treatment has been shown to have devastating consequences, especially for the fetus, who carries a higher mortality risk from a uterine rupture than the mother.

Treatment of complete uterine rupture includes (1) resuscitation of the patient with blood transfusion as needed while preparing for immediate laparotomy and (2) repair of the uterine rupture or hysterectomy, as indicated.

PATIENT SELECTION FOR TRIAL OF LABOR

Not all pregnant patients with a previous C-section are suitable candidates for a trial of labor, and proper patient selection is an important aspect in the management of these patients.

Absolute contraindications to TOLAC are as follows:

- Extensive uterine surgery
- T or J extension of a low transverse incision
- Patient refusal

Patients with two or more previous C-sections, low segment vertical scars, or unknown types of uterine scars are usually excluded from VBAC. There are, however, reports of successful TOLAC with good maternal and fetal outcomes in these situations.[11, 34] Although VBAC can be performed in community hospitals, it should not be attempted unless protocols are established and personnel to perform an emergency cesarean section are readily available.

Controversy still remains regarding TOLAC in the presence of a macrosomic fetus, multiple gestation, or breech presentation. Fetuses weighing more than 4000 g are considered macrosomic, and vaginal delivery for them is a concern, especially in the presence of a uterine scar. Vaginal delivery may be difficult and traumatic because of the macrosomia and shoulder dystocia with associated complications. Because many obstetricians would recommend an elective C-section in such cases, it may be appropriate to exclude this group from TOLAC. Studies have demonstrated that the success rate of TOLAC in the presence of a macrosomic fetus is indeed lower compared with the control groups (40–67% versus 81–83%, respectively).[35, 36] Patients with previous C-section due to cephalopelvic disproportion are also less likely to succeed. On the other hand, patients who are particularly motivated and present with adequate pelvis size may be allowed to attempt a vaginal delivery, especially if the fetus is estimated to weigh less than 4500 g.[36]

Multiple gestations and breech presentations are not an absolute contraindication to VBAC. In fact, there are studies that reported a greater than 70% success rate of vaginal delivery in these cases, without any significant increase in maternal or neonatal morbidity or mortality.[37–39] However, this notion is not universally accepted or practiced. Further randomized studies will be necessary before less stringent exclusion guidelines can be adopted.

SUCCESS RATE FOR VAGINAL BIRTH AFTER CESAREAN SECTION

Overall success for VBAC varies, but success rates of 75% to 90% have been reported.[5, 10, 13] The wide range of success rates is partly related to patient selection, past history, and present pregnancy conditions. Indications for previous cesarean section correlate well with the success rate. The positive result for VBAC is up to 90% if the previous cesarean section was for breech delivery, whereas it is 60% to 70% if the indication was cephalopelvic disproportion or failure to progress (Table 27–3).[40, 41] The cesarean section rate falls between these two if the indications for the previous cesarean section were for fetal distress or other reasons.

With respect to patients with two or more previous cesarean section scars, at the present time evidence suggests that vaginal delivery may be successful 45% to 80% of the time.[35, 41–43] Interestingly, the success rate is

Table 27–3 Indications for Previous Cesarean Section and Outcome of Trial of Labor

Indication for Prior Cesarean Section	Vaginal Delivery (%)
Breech	84-93
Fetal distress	70-75
Others	73-85
Cephalopelvic disproportion	65-67

high with favorable outcome if there is a history of previous successful vaginal delivery,[39] whereas positive outcome is less likely if the previous C-section was performed because of failure to progress at full cervical dilation.[44]

Recently, ultrasonography has been used to assess the potential risk for a separation of uterine scar during TOLAC. The degree of thinning of the lower segment at approximately 37 weeks has been found to correlate with the occurrence of a complete or incomplete defect in the uterine scar at the time of delivery.[45]

ROLE OF OXYTOCIN DURING TRIAL OF LABOR AFTER CESAREAN SECTION

In the past, the use of oxytocin to induce or augment labor has been incriminated as a cause of increased risk of rupture of a uterine scar, as well as a contributing factor in the failure of TOLAC. A more extensive review of the literature does not, however, confirm this opinion, as many authors now agree that oxytocin use during TOLAC is safe for both mother and fetus. The indication for use of oxytocin in TOLAC at the present time coincides with the indication for its use in any laboring patient. When used as indicated, it may increase the success rate of vaginal delivery by preventing uterine inertia and establishing regular contractions.[46] Although several studies[40, 46] have observed that oxytocin was associated with a decrease in the vaginal delivery rate in TOLAC, one may argue that this is true for every patient who required oxytocin for dysfunctional labor.

The incidence of uterine rupture is not significantly increased by oxytocin use, as confirmed by several studies.[27, 46] Horenstein and Phelan[46] described an incidence of uterine dehiscence of 3% in patients receiving oxytocin versus 2% in those who did not. The use of intracervical prostaglandin gel in TOLAC parturients has been reported to be efficacious and safe.[47, 48] Despite these encouraging findings, careful monitoring of mother and fetus is essential to detect uterine hypertonia or fetal distress when oxytocin is used in the woman attempting VBAC.

EPIDURAL ANESTHESIA IN TRIAL OF LABOR AFTER CESAREAN SECTION

With the increased incidence of TOLAC seen around the world, the involvement of anesthesiologists in the care of these women has increased significantly. Because emergency cesarean section can become necessary at any time, continuous anesthesia coverage is considered mandatory practice at many hospitals that allow VBAC. Even if analgesia is not requested, the anesthesiologist must be readily available should an emergency C-section become necessary.

The use of epidural anesthesia is not contraindicated during TOLAC, and there is now a general consensus among most anesthesiologists and obstetricians regarding this issue. When VBAC was first being attempted, epidural analgesia was considered to be relatively contraindicated because of the fear that the analgesia would mask the symptoms of uterine rupture. With the reassuring results from the literature as well as clinical practice regarding the rarity of the rupture of lower uterine transverse scar, epidural analgesia became popular for use in these women. Many studies have now confirmed the safety of epidural analgesia in women undergoing TOLAC, assuming appropriate fetal monitoring.[49–51] Abdominal pain has been observed to be an inconsistent finding in cases of separation of scar, whereas sudden fetal bradycardia or distress are common in presence of uterine rupture. With the use of newer epidural techniques that employ continuous infusions of dilute concentrations of local anesthetic with opioid, the epidural analgesia will not mask the pain of uterine rupture, sometimes termed "breakthrough pain." Johnson and Oriol[51] compared the presenting symptoms of uterine rupture in TOLAC patients with and without epidural analgesia and did not observe any significant differences between the groups. Abdominal pain was present in 21% of the patients who received epidural analgesia versus 17% who did not (Table 27–4). In the presence of low concentrations of local anesthetic, the more intense stimulation can be conducted through the blocked axons. This phenomenon was described by Crawford[52] as "epidural sieve." This may actually be helpful in the diagnosis of a complete uterine rupture, as when sudden severe pain develops unexpectedly in a previously pain-free patient with a functioning epidural block. Eckstein and coworkers[53] described an interesting case of uterine dehiscence in a laboring patient who complained of abdominal pain not relieved by adequate epidural block confirmed by pin prick test.

Pain associated with complete uterine rupture, with intraperitoneal hemorrhage or spillage of amniotic fluid, is conducted through fibers as high as T4 levels. Hence, even with adequate analgesia for labor at the T10 level, the patient will still complain of pain in the presence of peritoneal symptoms. Intraperitoneal bleeding and spillage of amniotic fluid inside the peritoneal cavity may cause diaphragmatic irritation with shoulder discomfort. Shin[54] described a case in which a patient was anesthetized with 2% lidocaine for cesarean section and still complained of shoulder pain. A complete uterine rupture was diagnosed during surgery.

Another potential hazard of epidural analgesia that has been claimed, but not supported by clinical experience, is the absence of a compensatory vasoconstrictive response in the presence of hypovolemic shock due to uterine rupture and hemorrhage. Although epidural blockade may be associated with a sympathectomy, uncontrolled hypotension does not appear to be a problem in the adequately managed parturient with epidural analgesia who develops a ruptured uterus. Adequate volume replacement with crystalloid, colloid, and treatment with vasopressors will restore hemodynamic stability, even if hemorrhage occurs following initiation of an epidural block.

To avoid the potential problems discussed earlier, it is particularly important to limit the concentration

Table 27-4 Signs and Symptoms of Uterine Rupture During Trial of Labor With or Without Epidural Analgesia

Presenting Signs and Symptoms of Rupture	Ruptures (n(%))	Epidural* (n(%))	No Epidural† (n(%))
Abdominal pain	8 (19)	3 (21)	5 (17)
Fetal distress	22 (51)	7 (50)	15 (52)
Incidental finding at cesarean section	3 (7)	1 (2)	2 (5)
Fetal distress and abdominal pain	6 (14)	2 (14)	4 (14)
Postpartum bleeding	4 (9)	1 (7)	3 (10)
Total rupture incidence	43	14 (0.76)	29 (0.28)

*Total n = 1828.
†Total n = 10,147.
Modified from Johnson C, Oriol N: The role of epidural anesthesia in trial of labor. Reg Anesth 1990; 15:304–308.

of local anesthetics to the minimum effective analgesic doses. At many institutions, including our own, the recommended dosages for patients undergoing VBAC are a bolus of 5 mL of 0.125% or 0.25% bupivacaine followed by a continuous infusion of bupivacaine 0.0625% with fentanyl 1 to 2 μg/mL at 8 to 12 mL/h. Ropivacaine may be an effective alternative to bupivacaine in a concentration of 0.1% to 0.2% combined with opioid (Fig. 27–1).[55]

There is some controversy in the literature regarding the use of neuraxial opioids in TOLAC patients. Some authors maintain that the addition of opioids to local anesthetic solutions may mask the abdominal pain from uterine rupture by abolishing the "epidural sieve" as described by Crawford.[52] This was illustrated by Tehan[56] who reported a case in which the administration of 10 mL of 0.25% bupivacaine with 50 μg of fentanyl relieved the abdominal pain from a uterine rupture that was not relieved by local anesthetic alone. Other authors, however, do not recommend that opioids be withheld in VBAC patients, since the addition of opioid to the local anesthetic mixture allows the use of more dilute concentration of local anesthetic.[57–59]

In the recent literature, there is no evidence that epidurals may decrease the likelihood of success or adversely affect either maternal or fetal outcome in

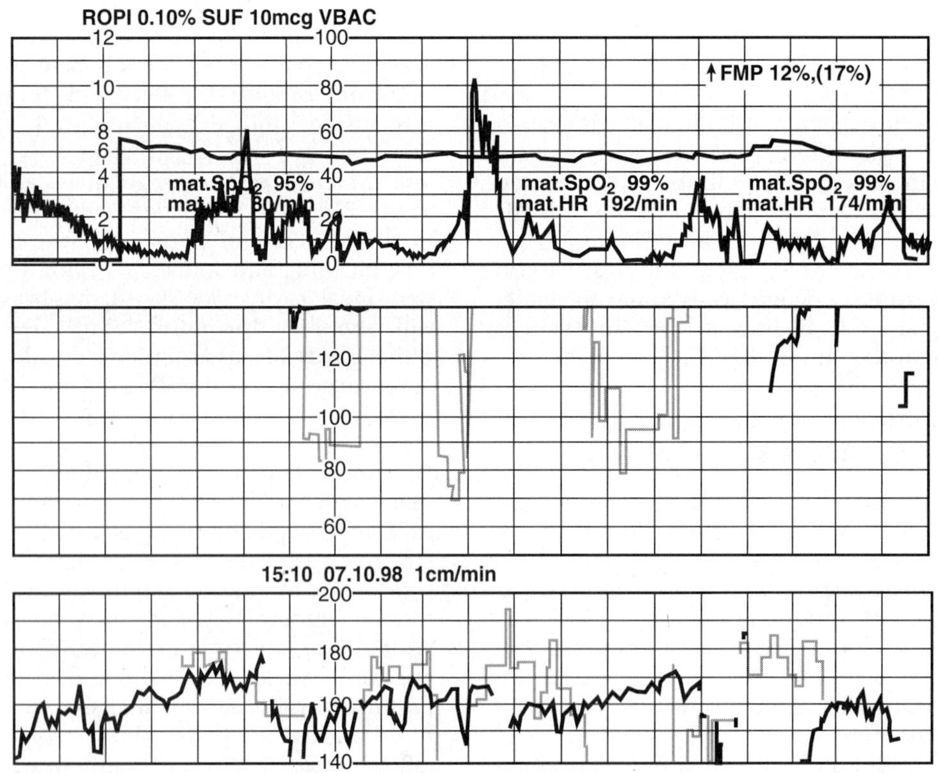

❖ **Figure 27–1** Fetal and maternal monitoring in a patient undergoing trial of labor with epidural analgesia (ropivacaine 0.10% with sufentanil 10 μg) during the second stage of labor. Noninvasive fetal oxygen saturation trace shows fetal well-being ($FSPO_2$ >30%) in the presence of second-stage mild variable decelerations.

Table 27-5 MANAGEMENT GUIDELINES FOR VAGINAL BIRTH AFTER CESAREAN DELIVERY

The following recommendations are based on good and consistent scientific evidence:

- Most women with one previous cesarean delivery with a low-transverse incision are candidates for VBAC and should be counseled about VBAC and offered a trial of labor.
- Epidural anesthesia may be used for VBAC.
- A previous uterine incision extending into the fundus is a contraindication for VBAC.

The following recommendations are based on limited or inconsistent scientific evidence:

- Women with two previous low-transverse cesarean deliveries and no contraindications who wish to attempt VBAC may be allowed a trial of labor. They should be advised that the risk of uterine rupture increases as the number of cesarean deliveries increases.
- The use of oxytocin or prostaglandin gel for VBAC requires close patient monitoring.
- Women with a vertical incision within the lower uterine segment that does not extend into the fundus are candidates for VBAC.

The following recommendations are based primarily on consensus and expert opinion:

- Because uterine rupture may be catastrophic, VBAC should be attempted in institutions equipped to respond to emergencies with physicians immediately available to provide emergency care.
- After thorough counseling that weighs the individual benefits and risks of VBAC, the ultimate decision to attempt this procedure or undergo a repeat cesarean delivery should be made by the patient and her physician.

Data from ACOG Practice Bulletin: Clinical Management Guidelines for Obstetrician-Gynecologists, Number 5, July 1999.

parturients undergoing TOLAC. On the contrary, the use of epidural analgesia seems to increase the incidence of VBAC, because of increased patient satisfaction. A parturient promised a comfortable labor may be more likely to agree to a trial of labor. Furthermore, an epidural increases the safety of the procedure, by lessening the likelihood that general anesthesia will become necessary. With an epidural in place, the level of sensory blockade can be rapidly extended to provide surgical anesthesia if C-section becomes necessary.

In conclusion, epidural analgesia is not contraindicated in patients who are attempting a vaginal delivery after a C-section. This has also been recommended in the most recent guidelines of the American College of Obstetricians and Gynecologists (1995) (Table 27–5).

Epidural analgesia is safe, provided that appropriate doses of local anesthetics with or without opioids are used, the level of the blockade is frequently checked, and continuous fetal heart monitoring with close surveillance of labor is carried out.

❖ SUMMARY

Key Points

- Trial of labor following cesarean section is becoming popular because of a high success rate.
- VBAC has been demonstrated to result in decreased costs and decreased maternal morbidity. Since most cesarean sections are now being performed with a low transverse uterine scar, the risk of uterine rupture is minimized.
- If VBAC is planned, close surveillance of labor and continuous fetal heart rate (FHR) monitoring is necessary, since FHR monitoring is sensitive for uterine rupture.
- Epidural analgesia is not contraindicated in women attempting VBAC.

Key Reference

Phelan JP, Clark SL, Diaz F, Paul RH: Vaginal birth after cesarean. Am J Obstet Gynecol 1987; 157:1510–1515.

Case Stem

A 31-year-old multigravida at term has had a previous cesarean section for breech. She has agreed to trial of labor but insists on an epidural. Her obstetrician, however, is afraid that the epidural will delay the diagnosis of uterine rupture. What information would you discuss with this obstetrician?

References

1. Cragin EB: Conservatism in obstetrics. N Y Med J 1916; 104:1–3.
2. Meier PR, Porreco RP: Trial of labor following cesarean section: A two years experience. Am J Obstet Gynecol 1982; 144:671–678.
3. Stafford R: Alternative strategies for controlling rising cesarean section rates. JAMA 1990; 263:683–687.
4. Anderson GM, Lomas J: Determinants of the increasing cesarean birth rate. N Engl J Med 1984; 311:887–892.
5. Miller DA, Diaz FG, Paul RH: Vaginal birth after cesarean: A 10 year experience. Obstet Gynecol 1994; 84:255–258.
6. Gleicher N: Mandatory trial of labor after cesarean delivery: An alternative viewpoint. Obstet Gynecol 1991; 78:727–728.
7. Cunningham FG, MacDonald PC, Gant NF, et al: Cesarean section and cesarean hysterectomy. *In* Cunningham FG, et al (eds): Williams Obstetrics, 19th ed. Norwalk, CT: Appleton & Lange; 1993.
8. Haesslein I, Goodlin RC: Delivery of the tiny newborn. Am J Obstet Gynecol 1979; 134:192–200.
9. Boyle JG, Gabbe SG: T and J vertical extensions in low transverse cesarean births. Obstet Gynecol 1996; 87:238–243.

10. Rosen MG, Dickinson JC, Westhoff CL: Vaginal birth after cesarean: A meta-analysis of morbidity and mortality. Obstet Gynecol 1991; 77:465–470.
11. Martin JN, Perry KG, Roberts WE, Meydrech EF: The case for trial of labor in the patient with a prior low-segment vertical cesarean incision. J Obstet Gynecol 1997; 177:144–148.
12. American College of Obstetricians and Gynecologists Committee on Obstetric Practice: Vaginal Delivery After a Previous Cesarean Birth. ACOG Committee Opinion No. 143. Washington DC: Author, 1994.
13. Flamm BL, Goings JR, Liu Y, Wolde-Tsadik G: Elective repeat cesarean delivery versus trial of labor. A prospective multicenter study. Obstet Gynecol 1994; 83:927–932.
14. Flamm B, Lim O, Jones C, et al: Vaginal birth after cesarean section: Results of a multicenter study. Am J Obstet Gynecol 1988; 158:1079–1084.
15. Obara H, Minikami H, Koike T, et al: Vaginal birth after cesarean delivery: Result in 310 pregnancies. J Obstet Gynecol Res 1998; 24:129.
16. Petitti DB: Maternal mortality and morbidity in cesarean section. Clin Obstet Gynecol 1985; 28:763–769.
17. Gibbs CE: Planned vaginal delivery following cesarean section. Clin Obstet Gynecol 1980; 23:507–515.
18. Fisher J, Astbury J, Smith A: Adverse psychological impact of operative obstetric interventions: A prospective longitudinal study. Aust N Z J Psychiatry 1997; 31:728–738.
19. Merrill BS, Gibbs CE: Planned vaginal delivery following cesarean section. Obstet Gynecol 1978; 52:50–52.
20. Hook B, Kiwi R, Amini SB, et al: Neonatal morbidity after elective repeat cesarean section and trial of labor. Pediatrics 1997; 100:348.
21. Heritage CK, Cunningham MD: Association of elective repeat cesarean delivery and persistent pulmonary hypertension of the newborn. Am J Obstet Gynecol 1985; 152:627–629.
22. Smith JF, Hernandez C, Wax JR: Fetal laceration injury at cesarean delivery. Obstet Gynecol 1997; 90:344–346.
23. Meehan FP, Magani IM: True rupture of a Cesarean scar (a 15-year review, 1972–1987). Eur J Obstet Gynecol Reprod Biol 1989; 30:129–135.
24. Phelan JP, Clark SL, Dias F, et al: Vaginal birth after cesarean. Am J Obstet Gynecol 1987; 157:1510–1515.
25. Lavin JP, Stephens RJ, Miodovnik M, et al: Vaginal delivery in patients with a prior cesarean section. Obstet Gynecol 1982; 59:135–148.
26. Martin JN, Harris BA, Huddleston JF, et al: Vaginal delivery following previous cesarean birth. Am J Obstet Gynecol 1983; 146:255–263.
27. Lao TT, Leung BFH: Rupture of the gravid uterus. Eur J Obstet Gynecol Reprod Biol 1987; 25:175–180.
28. Eden RT, Parker RT, Gall SA: Rupture of the pregnant uterus: A 53 year review. Obstet Gynecol 1986; 68:671–674.
29. Mastobattista JM: Vaginal birth after cesarean delivery. Obstet Gynecol Clin North Am 1999; 26:295–304.
30. Nielsen TF, Ljungblad UI, Hagberg H: Rupture and dehiscence of cesarean section scar during pregnancy and delivery. Am J Obstet Gynecol 1989; 160:569–573.
31. Schrinsky DC, Benson RC: Rupture of the pregnant uterus: A review. Obstet Gynecol Surv 1978; 33:217–232.
32. Guleria K, Dhall GI, Dhall K: Pattern of cervical dilatation in previous lower segment caesarean section patients. J Ind Med Assoc 1997; 95:131–134.
33. Khan KS, Rizvi A, Rizvi JH: Risk of uterine rupture after the partographic 'alert line' is crossed: An addition in the quest towards safe motherhood in labour following caesarean section. J Parkistan Med Assoc 1996; 46:120–122.
34. Pruett KM, Kirshon B, Cotton DB: Unknown uterine scar and trial of labor. Am J Obstet Gynecol 1988; 159:807–810.
35. Phelan JP, Eglinton GS, Horenstein JM, et al: Previous cesarean birth: Trial of labor in women with macrosomic infants. J Reprod Med 1984; 29:36–40.
36. Flamm BL, Goings J: Vaginal birth after cesarean section: Is suspected fetal macrosomia a contraindication? Obstet Gynecol 1989; 74:694–697.
37. Miller DA, Mullin P, Hou D, et al: Vaginal birth after cesarean in twin gestation. Am J Obstet Gynecol 1996; 175:194–198.
38. Odeh M, Tarazova L, Wolfson M, Oettinger M: Evidence that women with history of cesarean can deliver twins safely. Acta Obstet Gynecol Scand 1997; 76:663–666.
39. Abbassi H, Aboulfalah A, Karroumi M, et al: Accouchement des uterus cicatriciels: Peut-on enlargir l'epreuve uterine? J Gynecol Obstet Biol Reprod (Paris) 1998; 27:425–429.
40. Rosen MG, Dickinson JC: Vaginal birth after cesarean: A meta-analysis of indicators for success. Obstet Gynecol 1990; 76:865–869.
41. Flamm BL, Dunnett C, Fisherman E, et al: Vaginal delivery following cesarean section: Use of oxytocin augmentation and epidural anesthesia with internal tocodynamic and internal fetal monitoring. Am J Obstet Gynecol 1984; 149:759–763.
42. Pruett KM, Kirshon B, Cotton B, et al: Is vaginal birth after two or more C-sections safe? Obstet Gynecol 1988; 72:163.
43. Bretelle F, D'Ercole C, Cravello L, et al: Uterus bicicactriciel: La place de l'epreuve uterine. J Gyn Obst Biol Reprod 1998; 27:421–424.
44. Hoskins IA, Gomez JL: Correlation between maximal cervical dilatation at cesarean delivery and subsequent vaginal birth after cesarean delivery. Obstet Gynecol 1997; 89:591–593.
45. Rozenberg P, Goffinet F, Philippe HJ, et al: Mesure echographique de l'epaisseur du segment inferior pour evaluer le risque de rupture uterine. J Gynecol Obstet Biol Reprod (Paris) 1997; 26:513–519.
46. Horenstein JM, Phelan JP: Previous cesarean section: The risks and benefits of oxytocin usage in a trial of labor. Am J Obstet Gynecol 1985; 151:564–569.
47. Williams MA, Luthy DA, Zingheim RW, et al: Preinduction prostaglandin E2 gel prior to induction of labor in women with a previous cesarean section. Gynecol Obstet Invest 1995; 40:89–93.
48. Flamm BL, Anton D, Goings JR, et al: Prostaglandin E2 for cervical ripening: A multicenter study of patients with prior cesarean delivery. Am J Perinatol 1997; 14:157–160.
49. Kelly MC, Hill DA, Wilson DB: Low dose epidural bupivacaine/fentanyl infusion does not mask uterine rupture. Int J Obstet Anesth 1997; 6:52–54.
50. Rowbottom SJ, Tabrizian I: Epidural analgesia and uterine rupture during labour. Anaesth Intensive Care 1994; 22:79–80.
51. Johnson C, Oriol N: The role of epidural anesthesia in trial of labor. Reg Anesth 1990; 15:304–308.
52. Crawford JS: The epidural sieve and MBC (minimum blocking concentration): An hypothesis. Anesthesia 1976; 31:1277–1280.
53. Eckstein KL, Oberlander SG, Marx GF: Uterine rupture during extradural block. Can Anaesth Soc J 1973; 20:566–568.
54. Shin YK: Shoulder pain in a trial of labor after cesarean delivery. South Med J 1989; 82:1320.
55. Capogna G, Celleno D, Fusco P, et al: Relative potencies of bupivacaine and ropivacaine for labour analgesia. Br J Anaesth 1999; 82:371–373.
56. Tehan B: Abolition of the extradural sieve by addition of fentanyl to extradural bupivacaine. Br J Anaesth 1992; 69:520–521.
57. Chestnut DH, Owen CL, Bates JN, et al: Continuous infusion epidural anesthesia during labor: A randomized, double blinded comparison of 0.0625% bupivacaine/fentanyl versus 0.125% bupivacaine. Anesthesiology 1988; 68:754–759.
58. Sakala EP, Kaye S, Murray ED, Munson LJ: Epidural analgesia: Effect on the likelihood of a successful trial of labor after cesarean section. J Reprod Med 1990; 35:886–890.
59. Uppington J: Epidural analgesia and previous cesarean section. Anesthesia 1983; 38:336–341.

28

The Febrile Parturient

❖ STEPHEN H. ROLBIN, MD, FRCP(C)
❖ BEVERLY A. MORNINGSTAR, MD, FRCP(C)

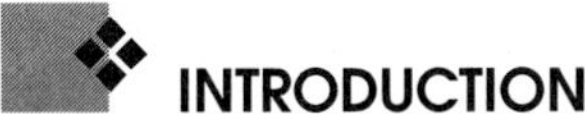

INTRODUCTION

Febrile parturients are often encountered in the labor and delivery room. At times these patients pose major problems for both the obstetrician and the anesthesiologist. Usually the illness develops shortly before or during labor. Fever can arise from a variety of microorganisms. Tissue injury (either infarction or trauma), malignancy, immunologically mediated disorders, and endocrine disorders can result in fever. Finally, fever can also be drug-induced.

This chapter briefly reviews relevant aspects of the physiology and pathophysiology of thermoregulation and relates them to the physiology of pregnancy. The effects of regional anesthesia on temperature are examined. This is followed by a discussion of febrile diseases that often complicate labor and their management. Finally, the risks and benefits of regional and general anesthesia in the febrile parturient are reviewed.

MATERNAL TEMPERATURE REGULATION

The hypothalamus normally maintains body temperature at 37°C. This norm was arrived at by measuring the axillary temperature of 25,000 people.[1] The mean oral temperature is 36.8°C ± 0.4°C (Fig. 28–1), with fluctuation from 36.2°C at 0600 hr. to 37.5°C at 1400 hr. to 1600 hr. By these criteria, a healthy person would be considered to have a fever if oral temperature is higher than 37.2°C in the morning or over 37.7°C in the afternoon. Rectal temperatures are approximately 0.6°C higher.[2]

Pregnancy is associated with an increase in the basal metabolic rate and may affect baseline temperatures.[3] Maternal temperature during labor is affected in part by the amount of hyperventilation, perspiration, and physical activity. Patients in labor who are calm and less active have higher temperatures.[4] Neonatal rectal temperature immediately after birth is best correlated with maternal vaginal temperature.[4]

The most important receptors for long-term control of body temperature are special heat-sensitive neurons located in the preoptic area of the hypothalamus.[5] Signals that arise from peripheral receptors are transmitted to the posterior hypothalamus, where they are integrated with signals from the preoptic area.[5] These cells increase their firing rate at elevated temperatures. Cold-sensitive neurons also have been found in the hypothalamus, in the septum, and in the reticular substance of the midbrain. Still other neurons change their rate of firing in response to signals coming from temperature receptors in the skin and deep tissues of the body. These signals interact in an area of the posterior hypothalamus approximately at the level of the mammary bodies and provide a very effective temperature control system. In a neutral environment, more heat is produced than is necessary to maintain body temperature. As a result, the hypothalamus controls the temperature by mechanisms of heat loss.[2]

The body has a critical temperature called the "set-point." All temperature control mechanisms continually adjust to maintain the body temperature at this level (Fig. 28–2).[2,6] Febrile conditions are characterized by body mechanisms that attempt to raise body temperature to an elevated set-point. The "thermo-

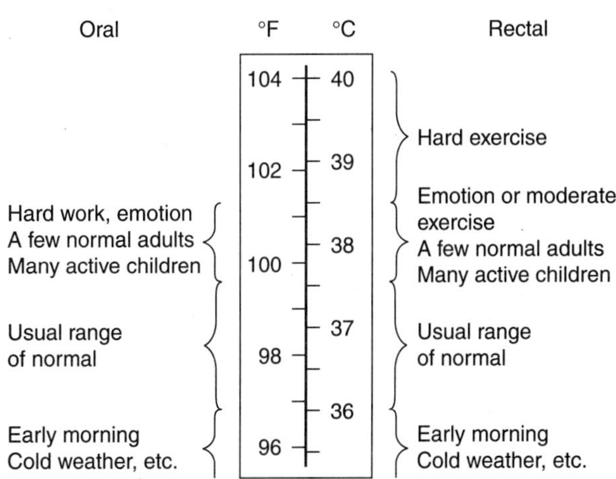

❖ **Figure 28–1** Range of normal body temperature. (From Dupois EF: Fever and the Regulation of Body Temperature. Springfield, IL: Charles C Thomas; 1948.)

stat" first responds by sending signals to the cerebral cortex, resulting in behavioral activity aimed at warming the body, such as seeking a warmer room or wearing more clothing. The patient may experience chills and feel very cold, even though body temperature is elevated. If this activity is not enough to raise body temperature to the new set-point, signals will traverse various sympathetic outflow fibers, leading to dermal vasoconstriction. Finally, shivering thermogenesis is initiated to increase heat production. Under normal circumstances, core body temperature is tightly regulated, with a variation of only 0.6°C.

After appropriate medical treatment, the set-point is lowered and the hypothalamus detects the elevated body temperature and acts to correct the temperature to the normal range. Cooling mechanisms involve both sympathetic and parasympathetic nervous systems and result in sweating and dermal vasodilation.[7] Three important mechanisms reduce body heat. Vasodilation, due to inhibition of sympathetic centers of the posterior hypothalamus, may increase the rate of heat transfer to the skin as much as eightfold. Sweating, which causes a sharp rise in heat loss by evaporation, can remove up to 10 times the basal rate of heat production. The patient feels warm, seeks out a cooler environment, and sheds coverings. Lastly, there is a strong inhibition of heat-producing mechanisms such as shivering and chemical thermogenesis.[5, 6]

PATHOGENESIS OF FEVER

The term *pyrogen* is used to describe any substance that causes fever. Pyrogens may be endogenous or exogenous. *Endogenous pyrogens* are proteins produced by cells of the immune system. Most fevers are produced by endogenous pyrogens, which trigger changes in the hypothalamus. *Exogenous pyrogens* arise from components of microorganisms such as bacteria, viruses, or parasites, or from chemical agents or drugs. They produce a fever by the release of endogenous pyrogens (Fig. 28–3).

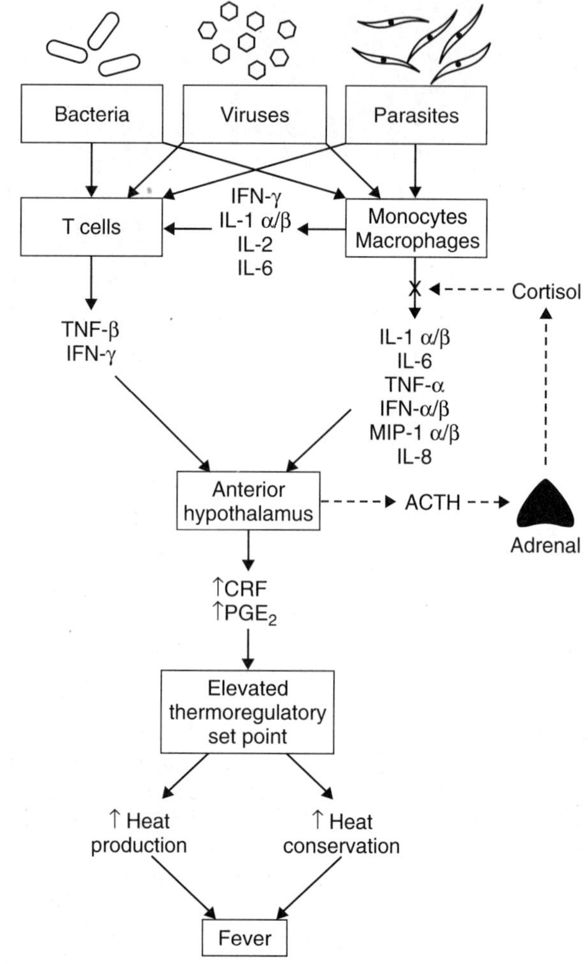

❖ **Figure 28–3** Chronology of events required for the induction of a fever. A variety of pathogens produce molecules that function as exogenous pyrogens, resulting in the release of endogenous pyrogens from mononuclear cells. Abbreviations have been defined in the text. (Adapted from Gelfand JA, Dinarello CA, Wolff SM: Fever, including fever of unknown origin. *In* Isselbacher KJ, Braunwald E, et al (eds): Harrison's Principles of Internal Medicine, 13th ed. New York: McGraw-Hill; 1994; and from Beutler B, Beutler SM: The pathogenesis of fever. *In* Wyngaarden JB, Smith LH, Bennett JC (eds): Cecil Textbook of Medicine, 19th ed. Philadelphia: WB Saunders; 1992.)

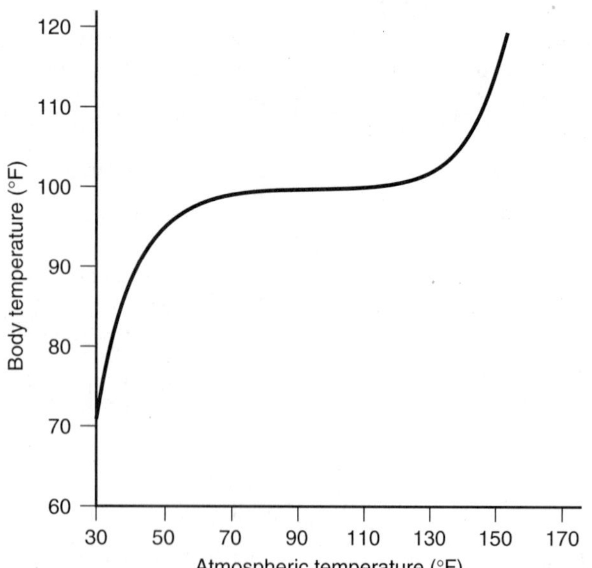

❖ **Figure 28–2** Effects of atmospheric temperature on internal body temperature. (From Guyton AC: Human Physiology and Mechanisms of Disease, 5th ed. Philadelphia: WB Saunders; 1992.)

Monocytes and tissue macrophagocytes are the main source of endogenous pyrogens. Most arise from macrophages and to a lesser extent lymphocytes. These proteins are the monokines and the lymphokines, respectively. They are often called cytokines. The same proteins may also arise from neoplastic cells. The major cytokines appear to be interleukins (IL-1α and IL-1β), interleukin-6 (IL-6), and tumor necrosis factors (TNF-α and -β). Other proteins with pyrogenic activity include interferon alpha (IFN-α) and macrophage inflammatory protein (MIP-1α,β).[8] Cytokines bind to receptors on the vascular endothelium within the preoptic/anterior hypothalamus. There is a resetting of the set-point as a result of endothelial cell production of prostaglandins PGE_2 and perhaps $PGF_{2\alpha}$.[9] Thromboxanes and lipogenase products may also change the set-point. In addition, cytokines act directly with neural tissue and may release corticotropin-releasing factor, which may trigger thermogenesis.[5] When a fever is produced, the body temperature can change in as little as 8 to 10 minutes.

Once the set-point of the hypothalamus is raised, all body mechanisms for increasing heat production are activated. Antipyretics, such as acetaminophen, impede the formation of prostaglandins from arachidonic acid and reduce or eliminate fever at the level of the hypothalamus.[5] A normal person does not have elevated cytokines, and this explains why antipyretics do not lower a normal temperature.

THE FETUS AND NEWBORN

Fetal temperature is about 0.5°C higher than maternal temperature. The fetus loses heat along this temperature gradient. Fetal-maternal temperature gradients correlate well with uterine blood flow and have been used experimentally as an indicator of fetal well-being.[10] When the maternal temperature starts to rise, the fetal-maternal temperature difference decreases. Modest increases in temperature do not cause fetal problems and may actually increase fetal blood flow.[11, 12] As the maternal temperature increases by more than 1°C, the fetal-maternal temperature difference begins to increase (Table 28–1).[10] This increased difference in temperature has been associated with distressed sheep fetuses and newborns.[11, 12] An elevation of temperature also brings about increased uterine muscle contractility in vitro.[13] Fetal heart rate may increase and fetal scalp pH will fall, resulting in depressed newborns.[11] Morishima and coworkers[14] showed more rapid deterioration of fetal baboons when their mothers became excessively pyrexic (42°C) in the absence of infection. However, the fetal consequences of epidural-related fetal tachycardia are more controversial,[15–17] and some authors wonder whether fetal compromise might occur.[15, 18]

Maternal temperature elevation (>37.4°C) is a clinical dilemma. It can be associated with an increased risk of perinatal infection.[19] Since the fetal temperature rises along with maternal temperature, and the placental function may be impaired by infection, the net result would be an increased fetal metabolic rate and oxygen consumption. This may explain the rapid fetal deterioration during hyperthermia.[20] Others have speculated that an elevated fetal temperature results in fetal tachycardia. This depletes fetal catecholamines and results in a decreased ability to adapt to stress.[15] An increase in temperature shifts the oxygen-hemoglobin dissociation curve to the right, with a resultant decrease in fetal oxygen saturation. One would expect a decrease in fetal oxygen consumption and metabolism following correction of fever.

Maternal fever during labor is associated with perinatal infection but not acidosis at birth.[19, 21] Elevated fetal heart rate precedes maternal fever in only a minority of cases and is not associated with perinatal infection.[21] Two recent small studies showed no significant differences in the acid-base status in the umbilical arteries of newborns whose mothers had chorioamnionitis.[22, 23] There was, however, a significantly increased incidence of depressed 1-minute Apgar scores in the amnionitis patients when compared with a control population.[21–23] Thus, the acid-base status may not be a sufficiently sensitive index of fetal well-being. It was recently reported that maternal fever of greater than 38°C is associated with a marked increase in cerebral palsy in infants of normal birthweight.[24] This is believed to be due to intrauterine exposure to infection.

The threshold of fetal metabolic acidosis associated with moderate or severe newborn complications is an umbilical artery base deficit of greater than 12 mmol/L.[25] Both a high base deficit (>12 mmol) and a high $Pa{CO_2}$ have been associated with Apgar scores below 7 and neonatal intensive care unit admissions.[21] As the acidosis increases, the severity of complications increases.

In conclusion, mild hyperthermia does not adversely affect the fetus. When significant pyrexia does occur, one should investigate the cause and begin appropriate therapy.

REGIONAL ANALGESIA AND MATERNAL TEMPERATURE

Core hypothermia after induction of epidural anesthesia results from both an internal core-to-periphery redistribution of body heat and a net loss of heat to the environment.[26] Redistribution of body heat to the distal legs contributes 80% to the entire 1.2°C ± 0.3°C decrease in core temperature. During regional anesthesia, the contribution of redistribution to falling temperature is greater but the actual decrease is only half when compared with the drop in temperature that occurs during general anesthesia. This is because the metabolic rate is maintained and the arms remain vasoconstricted during regional anesthesia.[26]

The extent of spinal blockade correlates with impairment of central thermoregulatory control.[27] Core temperature is lower during more extensive block. Spi-

Table 28–1 EFFECTS OF INCREASING MATERNAL TEMPERATURE ON UTERINE BLOOD FLOW AND FETAL TEMPERATURE IN THE EWE

	UTERINE BLOOD FLOW (mL/kg/min)	FETAL-MATERNAL TEMPERATURE DIFFERENCE (°C)
Control	111	0.61
+1°C	122	0.19
+2.5°C	53	1.27

From Cefalo RC, Hellegers AE: The effects of maternal hyperthermia on maternal cardiovascular and respiratory function. Am J Obstet Gynecol 1978; 131:687.

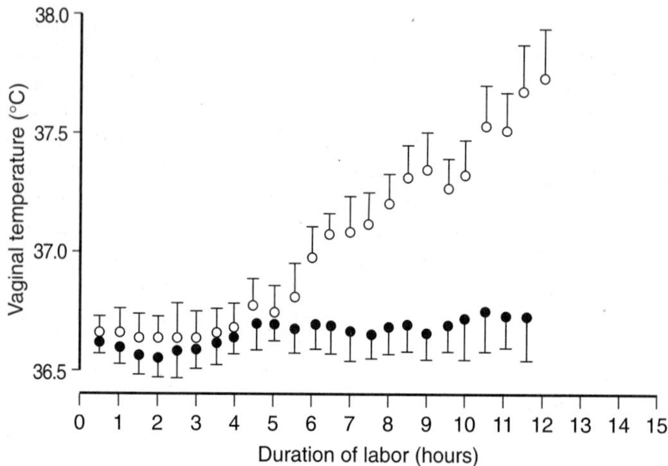

❖ **Figure 28–4** Mean vaginal temperature (°C) in two groups of patients during labor. *Closed circle*, pethidine group; *open circle*, epidural analgesia group; vertical bars, SEM. (From Fusi L, Steer PJ, Maresh MJA, et al: Maternal pyrexia associated with the use of epidural analgesia in labour. Lancet 1989; 1:1250.)

nal and epidural anesthesia probably comparably alter the thermoregulatory process.[28] Epidural anesthesia decreases the shivering threshold,[29] and shivering occurs in 30% of labors with epidural anesthesia.[30] Administering local anesthetics at room temperature also increases the incidence of shivering.[31] Shivering is thought to be the major mechanism of temperature elevation.

Fusi and coworkers[15] demonstrated a significant rise in temperature after 6 hours of labor in patients receiving epidural analgesia, when compared with a group receiving parenteral opioids only whose temperature remained constant (Fig. 28–4). This rise was not related to clinical evidence of infection. No adverse effects on the fetus or newborn were observed. Possible explanations for these findings include the following: (1) Relief of pain may decrease hyperventilation and evaporative heat loss. (2) Sympathetic blockade may reduce sweating and decrease heat loss. (3) Local anesthetic in the epidural space may alter sensory input and result in inappropriate increases in temperature. (4) During regional anesthesia there is an earlier blockade of warm sensation. Persistent cold perception by the thermoregulatory center results in increased heat production.

Camann and coworkers[16] prospectively studied the effects of epidural anesthesia on maternal temperature. One group chose parenteral opioid analgesia. The other two groups both received epidural analgesia. Patients in the epidural groups were randomly allocated to receive a continuous infusion of 0.25% bupivacaine with or without the addition of fentanyl. After 5 hours of labor, the epidural groups had a consistent and significant increase in maternal temperature, which did not exceed 1°C (Fig. 28–5). The epidural patients were not clinically febrile, and there was only a weak correlation between maternal temperature and fetal heart rate. Maternal temperature does not increase following low-dose ambulatory epidural analgesia with bupivacaine and fentanyl, but occasionally increases may occur after 10 hours.[32]

A recent retrospective chart review showed similar increases in temperature with epidural analgesia that were not clinically significant.[33] Patients receiving combined spinal epidural (CSE) analgesia had a lower incidence of temperature elevation than patients who received epidural analgesia. The authors raise the following questions: (1) Does the short duration of labor in their CSE group explain the failure to develop a fever? (2) Do spinal opioids have a lesser effect on thermoregulation?

It was suggested recently that mothers receiving epidural anesthesia have an increased incidence of fever, neonatal sepsis, and neonatal antibiotic administration.[34, 35] None of these studies have been randomized controlled trials. There has never been a study to suggest that there is an increase in infection associated with epidural anesthesia. Other investigators have concluded that regional analgesia has no significant effect on maternal core temperature or intrauterine temperature.[36]

Thermoregulatory changes are the most likely ex-

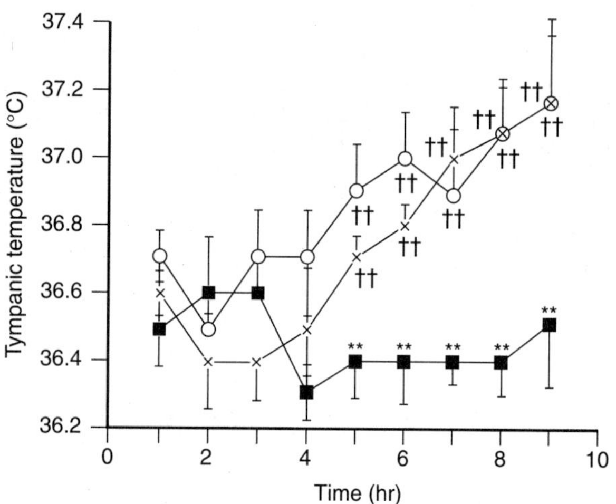

❖ **Figure 28–5** Mean tympanic temperatures during labor in three groups of patients: epidural bupivacaine-fentanyl *(open circle)*, epidural bupivacaine only *(X)*, and parenteral opioid *(closed circle)* groups. $^{**}P < .01$ compared with the epidural group. $^{\dagger\dagger}P < .01$ compared with the pre-epidural temperature. (From Camann WR, Hortvet LA, Hughes N, et al: Maternal temperature regulation during extradural analgesia for labour. Br J Anaesth 1991; 67:565.)

Table 28-2 RISK FACTORS AND CLINICAL FINDINGS IN MATERNAL INFECTION

Risk Factors[109, 120, 121]
- previous history of recent upper respiratory or urinary tract infection
- premature rupture of the membranes
- >24 hours prolonged fasting
- bimanual examination of parturient with asymptomatic bacteremia before the rupture of membranes

Clinical Findings

Minor[109]
- increased fetal heart rate
- shivering
- hyperthermia
- meconium staining
- dystocia

Absolute[120]
- temperature >38°C or <36°C
- maternal heart rate >90 beats/min
- respiratory rate >20 breaths/min or Pa_{CO_2} <32 torr
- white blood cell count >12,000 cells/mm³ or <4000 cells/mm³ or 10% immature forms (band cells)
- metabolic acidosis
- altered mental status
- oliguria

The diagnosis of sepsis requires at least two minor clinical findings in the absence of any risk factors.

Adapted from Lauretti GR: Infectious diseases. *In* Gambling DR, Douglas MJ (eds): Obstetric Anesthesia and Uncommon Disorders. Philadelphia: WB Saunders; 1998; 333–351.

planation for an elevated temperature associated with epidural use.[34] Because of this association, clinical criteria (Table 28–2), and not the sole presence of fever during labor, should be used to diagnose infections such as chorioamnionitis in patients receiving epidural analgesia.[37] The factors that are responsible for fever may also result in longer, more painful labors, with increased requests for epidural analgesia.[38]

COMMON CAUSES OF FEVER IN PREGNANCY

Chorioamnionitis

Chorioamnionitis is one of the most common causes of fever during labor. Various studies have placed the incidence of chorioamnionitis at 0.5% to 10.5% of term deliveries, with an even higher occurrence in preterm labor and delivery. It is the cause of 10% to 40% of all peripartum fever and accounts for 20% to 40% of neonatal sepsis and pneumonia.[39]

Clinical Features. Chorioamnionitis is an infection of the amniotic cavity and chorioamniotic membranes. Maternal fever of 37.8°C or higher is the hallmark of diagnosis.[40] Other clinical indicators include maternal tachycardia, uterine tenderness, and purulent or foul-smelling amniotic fluid. The fetal heart tracing shows tachycardia or decreased variability, and the biophysical profile may be low, with decreased fetal breathing activity. The maternal white blood cell count is generally greater than 20,000 cells/mm³.[41] However, both fever and leukocytosis may be a normal variant in women without obvious signs of infection (Table 28–3). The pathologic diagnosis is retrospective and based on the morphology of the placenta and membranes. Gram stain and amniotic fluid culture may be useful in confirming the diagnosis. However, chorioamnionitis should be diagnosed on clinical grounds, even in the absence of positive microbiology, and pathologic amnionitis may be detected without clinical amnionitis.

Pathogenesis. Numerous factors have been associated with the development of chorioamnionitis.[39, 42] Prolonged rupture of the membranes is the most frequent cause. When premature rupture of the membranes occurs in association with preterm labor, there is a 5- to 10-fold increase in the incidence of infection. The most significant accompanying risk factors are multiple digital vaginal examinations, longer duration of active labor, and meconium staining of the amniotic fluid.[42] The high phosphate concentration of meconium may play a role in promoting amniotic fluid infections. It inhibits a naturally occurring zinc-associated polypeptide with antibacterial properties, which is found in amniotic fluid.[43]

Several mechanisms may be responsible for intra-amniotic infection. Ascending infection from the lower genital tract in patients with prolonged rupture of the membranes is the most common route. Organisms may gain entry by hematogenous spread in mothers with bacteremia. Intra-amniotic infection may also complicate invasive procedures such as amniocentesis, intrauterine transfusion, and cervical cerclage. The usual organisms isolated in the amniotic fluid of patients with chorioamnionitis are anaerobes, genital mycoplasmas, group B streptococci, or *Escherichia coli*.

Table 28-3 INTRAPARTUM VITAL SIGNS IN ASYMPTOMATIC WOMEN

	MEAN ± SD	95TH PERCENTILE	DIAGNOSIS OF INTRA-AMNIOTIC INFECTION
Temperature (°C)	36.9±0.5	37.85	37.8
Maternal heart rate (beats/min)	85±13	110	100
Fetal heart rate (beats/min)	139±10	159	160
White blood cell count (cells/mm³)	12,500±3.9	20,100	15,000

From Newton ER: Chorioamnionitis and intraamniotic infection. Clin Obstet Gynecol 1993; 36:795.

When bacteremia is present, group B streptococci or *E. coli* is the cause of infection in 67% of women.[41]

Maternal and Neonatal Outcomes. Chorioamnionitis was a leading cause of maternal mortality in the past, due to septic shock, coagulopathy, and adult respiratory distress syndrome. Appropriate intrapartum use of broad-spectrum antibiotics has greatly improved the outcome of this condition for both mother and neonate. The main maternal consequences of chorioamnionitis today are bacteremia, dysfunctional labor, increased use of oxytocin, increased rate of cesarean delivery, and postpartum endometritis. Whether a dysfunctional labor pattern is the cause or the effect of infection remains unclear. Cesarean section in the presence of intra-amniotic infection is associated with increased blood loss (1500 mL in 12% of patients), longer duration of surgery, and a 5% to 10% incidence of postoperative wound infection.[39]

The main risks to the neonate are neonatal sepsis, pneumonia, and respiratory distress syndrome. Infection and maternal fever may lead to abruptio placentae, decreased uterine blood flow, and increased oxygen consumption. However, birth asphyxia is rarely associated with intra-amniotic infection.[22] Chorioamnionitis in pregnancies with low-birthweight infants is particularly hazardous, with a high rate of perinatal sepsis, asphyxia, intraventricular hemorrhage, and mortality. Poor outcomes may be expected when a group B streptococcus or *E. coli* is the infecting organism, or when maternal antibiotic therapy is delayed until after delivery.

Obstetric Management. Once the diagnosis is made, appropriate therapy consists of parenteral antibiotics and prompt delivery. Broad-spectrum coverage is required because of the wide variety of possible infecting organisms. Antibiotics must cross the placenta in sufficient quantity to begin treatment of the fetus. This generally consists of a penicillin such as ampicillin and an aminoglycoside such as gentamicin for treatment of group B streptococci and *E. coli* infection. Triple coverage includes clindamycin for anaerobic and gram-positive coverage if a cesarean section is performed. Bactericidal concentrations of antibiotics reach the fetus within 30 to 60 minutes.

The maternal and neonatal benefits of intrapartum antibiotic treatment outweigh the theoretic disadvantage of interference with neonatal cultures.[41] Although the neonate may require a work-up for sepsis and administration of prophylactic antibiotics if antibiotics have been given to the mother, the actual incidence of neonatal sepsis and duration of hospitalization is less. Antipyretics may make the mother feel better and may decrease the hyperthermic metabolic stress causing fetal tachycardia. Persistent fetal tachycardia despite maternal antipyretics suggests the possibility of neonatal sepsis. Continuous fetal heart rate monitoring is mandatory because of the high frequency of abnormal tracings.

Standard obstetric indications should dictate the route of delivery. In the absence of severe fetal distress, an immediate cesarean section to prevent asphyxia is not indicated.[22] There is no established time interval within which delivery must occur, provided appropriate antibiotic coverage has begun, although many obstetricians prefer to deliver the patient within 12 hours of the onset of fever. Duration of infection does not correlate with adverse fetal outcome. Dysfunctional labor, use of oxytocin, and fetal distress are frequent companions of intra-amniotic infection, however, resulting in a cesarean section rate of up to 40% in patients with chorioamnionitis.[44]

Anesthetic Management. Two recent reviews[45, 46] addressed the safety of regional anesthesia in the presence of chorioamnionitis. Although the total number of patients was small, no parturient with clinical chorioamnionitis and proven bacteremia receiving spinal or epidural anesthesia prior to antibiotic therapy developed either a spinal or epidural abscess or meningitis.

Although no evidence exists that regional anesthesia is deleterious, most anesthetists prefer to delay regional anesthesia for labor until the patient has received antibiotics and the temperature is less than 38.5°C.[47] Although septic shock is a rare event in chorioamnionitis,[40] particular attention should be paid to the state of hydration of a febrile patient in view of possible hemodynamic instability after a high sympathetic blockade.

Upper Respiratory Tract Infection

The common cold is a clinical syndrome with many viral causes. The rhinovirus is the most common pathogen. The presentation and course in pregnancy is usually similar to that in the nonpregnant state, with slight fever (less than 38°C), malaise, watery nasal discharge, sneezing, and nonproductive cough. Pharyngitis and conjunctivitis ("pink eye") may accompany adenoviral or enteroviral infection. Upper airway reactivity is increased during the acute phase of an upper respiratory tract infection, but there is little evidence that general anesthesia in adults results in an increased incidence of adverse respiratory events.[48]

Hoarseness or dyspnea may occur in up to 75% of noninfected pregnant women, due to estrogen-induced mucosal edema, capillary congestion, and hyperplastic and hypersecretory mucous glands.[49] Hoarseness and pharyngolaryngeal edema may also be the presenting feature of pregnancy-induced hypertension, preeclampsia, or fluid overload.

Pneumonia in pregnancy often begins with the common cold. Secondary bacterial infection with *Haemophilus influenzae* and *Streptococcus pneumoniae* may lead to sinusitis or otitis media. Upper airway infection with *H. influenzae* in adults may rarely present as laryngotracheobronchitis or epiglottitis. *H. influenzae* infections are six times more likely to occur in pregnant than in nonpregnant adults, with a high rate of infant mortality.[49, 50] Epiglottitis in adults is being reported with greater frequency, although there have been only three case reports of the condition occurring during pregnancy.[51] The normal reductions in cellular and humoral immunity associated with pregnancy may result in more severe forms of infections. Early recognition and aggressive airway management of both epiglottitis and laryngotracheobronchitis are critical to their successful outcome. Whereas the nonpregnant patient may tolerate a suboptimal Pao_2, the pregnant patient must receive early and optimal oxygenation to avoid any degree of fetal hypoxia.[51] Initial treatment of laryngotracheobronchitis includes intravenous antibiotics and steroids, supplemental oxygen with humidification, continuous airway monitoring, and frequent assessment of the airway. Facial and upper airway edema, stridor, dysphagia, and restlessness signal impending upper airway obstruction and hypoxia. Early intubation, while the patient can still protect her airway, is preferable to a crisis situation in an obtunded or uncooperative patient, in whom difficult intubation could increase the risk of aspiration pneumonitis or the need for an emergency surgical airway.

Pneumonia

Epidemiology. Pneumonia is one of the most serious nonobstetric infections in pregnancy. It complicates up to 1% of all deliveries[52] and is the third leading cause of indirect obstetric death.[53] Its frequency has risen in recent years, owing to an increased number of pregnant women with immunodeficiencies and illicit drug use. The recent trend to postpone childbearing until later in life, along with advances in critical care and improved survival, has resulted in more pregnant women with serious underlying illness at risk for the development of pneumonia. Anemia, prior lung disease, smoking, and alcoholism are specifically associated with antepartum pneumonia. A number of immunologic and mechanical changes that occur during normal pregnancy affect the gravida's susceptibility to pneumonia, especially in the third trimester (Table 28–4).

Etiology. The etiology of pneumonia in pregnant women is the same as in nonpregnant women. Often the infecting organism cannot be identified. Approximately two thirds of cases are bacterial in origin. *S. pneumoniae* (pneumococcus) accounts for up to 50% of cases of community-acquired infections, and approximately one quarter of these patients have positive blood cultures. *H. influenzae, Chlamydia psittaci* TWAR strain, and atypical pathogens such as *Mycoplasma pneumoniae* and *Legionella pneumophila* may also cause community-acquired pneumonia in pregnancy. Influenza is the most common viral agent causing pneumonia in pregnancy. Pneumonia caused by influenza, varicella, or measles can be particularly virulent in pregnancy, with bacterial superinfection as one of the most serious complications. Pneumonia caused by *Pneumocystis carinii,* fungi, and parasites occurs mainly in immunocompromised patients.

Clinical Presentation and Diagnosis. A mild upper respiratory tract infection precedes the onset of symptoms in 50% of cases. The major presenting features are abrupt onset of productive cough, fever, chills, and pleuritic chest pain. The atypical pneumonias usually develop over the course of several days, with myalgia, headache, dry cough, and low-grade fever. Dyspnea and tachypnea are presenting features easily overlooked when the patient is pregnant. Maternal complications include sepsis, empyema, atrial fibrillation, respiratory failure necessitating mechanical ventilation, and multiorgan damage. Preterm labor, especially in women with chronic disease, is the most common obstetric complication, occurring in 44% in one series.[54]

A chest radiograph (anteroposterior and lateral) should be considered whenever a pregnant woman has significant upper respiratory symptoms of longer than 2 weeks' duration. It may demonstrate a lobar infiltrate with air bronchograms, lobar consolidation, or multiple patchy infiltrates, depending on the causative organism. Other investigations include complete blood count with differential, arterial blood gases or pulse oximetry, sputum Gram stain and culture, blood culture, and acute and convalescent serology in cases in which atypical pathogens such as *Mycoplasma* are suspected.

Medical Management. Pneumonia in pregnancy should be treated aggressively and empirically. Because of the frequency of preterm labor and potential life-

Table 28–4 FACTORS THAT INFLUENCE THE DEVELOPMENT OF PNEUMONIA IN PREGNANCY

PHYSIOLOGIC CHANGE	EFFECT
Decreased cellular immunity	Increased susceptibility to viral and fungal infections
Altered chest wall anatomy elevation of diaphragm widened subcostal angles splayed thoracic cage	Decreased ability to clear secretions
Decreased functional residual capacity Increased oxygen consumption	Decreased tolerance of hypoxia
Capillary engorgement Hypersecretion of respiratory tract mucosa	Increased severity of respiratory infection; bacterial superinfection in viral infections

Adapted from Rigby FP, Pastorek JG II: Pneumonia during pregnancy. Clin Obstet Gynecol 1996; 39:107.

threatening complications, hospitalization of all pregnant women with radiographically confirmed pneumonia has been recommended.[55] This will ensure optimal respiratory support and determine the responsiveness of the infection to therapy. Based on clinical presentation, prior medical condition, and antibiotic usage, antibiotic therapy should be instituted while awaiting results of culture and sensitivity studies. Close monitoring and serial blood gas determinations or continuous pulse oximetry are mandatory. Appropriate oxygen therapy should aim to maintain PaO_2 above 70 mm Hg or oxygen saturation above 95%. Failure to maintain PaO_2 above 60 mm Hg despite high concentrations of oxygen, rising $PaCO_2$, and persistent metabolic acidosis are indications for mechanical ventilation.

Obstetric and Anesthetic Management. The anesthesiologist often participates in the care of obstetric patients with pneumonia, either in preterm labor or for elective induction and delivery. The pregnant woman with pneumonia is more susceptible to cardiovascular and pulmonary side effects of tocolytics such as beta-mimetics and magnesium sulfate. Damaged and inflamed pulmonary vascular membranes, mediators of the inflammatory response, and maternal fever and tachycardia, along with the normal pregnancy-associated decrease in plasma colloid oncotic pressure may all act to promote the development of pulmonary edema.[56]

Oxygen consumption increases with the increase in minute ventilation associated with painful contractions during the first and second stages of labor. Because it reduces hyperventilation and the work of breathing, effective epidural analgesia may have a beneficial effect and attenuate the increased oxygen consumption during labor.[57] However, the increase in oxygen consumption during labor is multifactorial, and oxygen delivery may be inadequate to meet the demands of the respiratory-compromised parturient in labor. Delivery of severely ill patients who require ventilatory support and who are not in labor has been recommended, with the aim of optimizing maternal hemodynamics and respiratory function.[52] However, a recent review demonstrated a 28% decrease in inspired oxygen requirements, but no dramatic improvement in other measures of respiratory function following delivery.[58] In view of the limited maternal benefit and the risks of induction of labor, extreme caution is urged in initiating elective induction of labor in these critically ill patients.

Urinary Tract Infections

Urinary tract infections are one of the most common medical complications of pregnancy. The spectrum ranges from asymptomatic bacteriuria to cystitis to pyelonephritis.

Asymptomatic Bacteriuria. The prevalence of asymptomatic bacteriuria (ASB) in pregnant women is between 4% and 7%, similar to the prevalence in other sexually active women of childbearing age. Pregnancy does not promote the development of ASB. The pathogen responsible is usually *E. coli,* or sometimes other normal vaginal and lower urethral flora. Pyelonephritis will develop in 20% to 40% of pregnant women with untreated bacteriuria.[59] Pregnancy-induced changes favoring the development of pyelonephritis include urinary stasis, caused by mechanical obstruction of the ureters by the enlarging uterus, and progesterone-induced dilation of the ureters and bladder. In addition, glucosuria and aminoaciduria provide favorable conditions for bacterial growth. The American College of Obstetricians and Gynecologists (ACOG) recommends screening of all women at the first prenatal visit to detect and treat ASB.[60] Treatment should continue for at least 10 days, and the patient should be checked regularly for recurrences.

Cystitis. Acute bacterial cystitis occurs in 0.3% to 1.3% of pregnancies. Cystitis in pregnancy does not appear to be related to ASB and usually does not progress to pyelonephritis.[61] Typical symptoms include dysuria, frequency, urgency, hematuria, and suprapubic discomfort. Urinalysis is usually positive for pus cells and bacteria, but diagnosis is confirmed with a positive urine culture. Pathogens and treatment are the same as for ASB.

Pyelonephritis. Acute pyelonephritis complicates 1% to 2% of all pregnancies. Prior pyelonephritis, structural urinary tract abnormalities, and nephrolithiasis increase the risk. It results from undetected ASB and usually develops in the second and third trimesters. A positive urine culture in the presence of fever, chills, flank pain, nausea, and vomiting is diagnostic. Right-sided pyelonephritis may be difficult to distinguish from appendicitis and cholecystitis. Renal calculi, which occur in 1 in 1500 pregnancies and produce significant fever or pain, may also pose a diagnostic dilemma.[59] Although blood cultures are not necessary to make the diagnosis, bacteremia is present in 10% to 15% of patients, most often in those patients with fever greater than 39°C. The usual organism is a coliform. Maternal complications may be life-threatening and are due to endotoxin-mediated tissue injury. They include gram-negative septic shock, adult respiratory distress syndrome, anemia, and transient or permanent renal dysfunction. Risks to the fetus include prematurity (mainly in women with underlying renal involvement) and low birthweight.[61]

Obstetric patients with pyelonephritis require immediate and aggressive treatment. These women are dehydrated from fever, anorexia, and vomiting. Although both renal dysfunction and respiratory insufficiency are potential complications, fluid restriction may cause underperfusion of vital organs, most notably the uterus.[62] Presumptive antibiotic therapy, using a cephalosporin, ampicillin, or gentamicin combined with a penicillin, should begin before culture and sensitivity results are available. Fever generally subsides within 48 hours of treatment. Failure to respond should prompt a search for underlying complications such as obstruction or a stone. Oral antibiotics may be necessary for the remainder of pregnancy, and patients should be investigated following delivery for underlying renal abnormalities.

Tuberculosis

Tuberculosis is the single leading cause of death worldwide among women of reproductive age, accounting for 9% of deaths among women aged 15 to 44 years. The decline in incidence brought about by the advent of effective antituberculous drugs and screening programs has been reversed since the mid-1980s. Much of this new epidemic is fuelled by the current spread of the human immunodeficiency virus. Other factors include increasing survival of the elderly with reactivation of old disease, increasing drug resistance, and worsening social deprivation. In developed countries, the incidence is much higher in immigrants from most countries in Africa, Asia, and Latin America, where the disease is endemic. By the end of 2000, it is projected that 10.2 million new cases and 3.5 million deaths annually will be attributable to *Mycobacterium tuberculosis.*[63]

Only about 5% of newly infected people will develop active tuberculosis. Pregnancy does not increase the risk of reactivation of prior disease,[64] but immunosuppression, debilitating disease, and extremes of age are risk factors. Tuberculosis can affect any organ, but 90% of cases are pulmonary. Infections may be primary or a reactivation. Symptoms include wheezing, cough and sputum, hemoptysis, and generalized complaints such as fatigue, anorexia, and night sweats. Pregnancy does not worsen the course of tuberculosis. In the past, there was a higher incidence of toxemia, postpartum hemorrhage, difficult labor,[65] and prematurity[66] in mothers with tuberculosis. With the development of effective treatment, today tuberculosis does not worsen the overall outcome of pregnancy.[67]

Tuberculosis is a diagnosis that will be missed unless actively investigated.[68] Patients with risk factors should be screened with a Mantoux skin test using purified protein derivative (PPD). A woman with a positive PPD who previously tested negative, with unknown time of conversion, should have a chest radiograph and three sputum samples sent for acid-fast bacilli and culture and sensitivity assays. Chemoprophylaxis can be postponed until after delivery in asymptomatic patients with normal chest radiographs. If PPD conversion is known to have occurred within the previous 2 years, prophylactic isoniazid (INH) should be started after the first trimester. For pregnant women with active tuberculosis, treatment should begin immediately with INH plus rifampin and continued for a minimum of 9 months. Ethambutol is added if INH resistance is anticipated.[69] All of these agents have been used in pregnancy without evidence of teratogenicity. Pyridoxine (vitamin B_6) should be given to decrease the incidence of INH-induced peripheral neuropathy.

There are no special management recommendations during labor apart from isolation precautions. The patient with active pulmonary tuberculosis should wear a mask, and those caring for these patients should double-mask. If general anesthesia is required, avoidance of cross-infection is mandatory. This includes the use of disposable equipment, bacterial filters inserted on the patient side of unidirectional valves and ventilator hoses, immediate disinfection or sterilization of nondisposable equipment, and removal of nonessential items from the operating room prior to the patient's arrival.

Herpes Simplex Virus

Etiology. Herpes simplex virus (HSV) belongs to a large group of human double-stranded DNA viruses, which includes herpes simplex virus type 1 (HSV-1), herpes simplex virus type 2 (HSV-2), varicella-zoster virus, cytomegalovirus, Epstein-Barr virus, and human herpesvirus 6 (associated with roseola and lymphoproliferative disorders). Herpesviruses ascend peripheral sensory nerves and reside in sensory nerve root ganglia, establishing latency with the potential for viral reactivation.[70]

Herpes simplex virus 1 has generally been associated with orolabial lesions ("cold sores") and transmission through oral contact. HSV-2 is usually associated with genital lesions and sexual contact. In fact, there is a great deal of cross-over between site of primary infection and antigenic strain. HSV-1 can account for up to one third of genital HSV.[70] The risk to the fetus and neonate is similar with both strains, although HSV-2 tends to recur more frequently in the genital area.

Epidemiology. Babies in the first few months of life are usually immune because of passive transfer of maternal antibodies. Prevalence of antibody to HSV-1 increases with advancing age, occurring in 50% of the population of the United States but up to 80% in lower socioeconomic groups. Antibody to HSV-2 is present in 50% of adults treated for sexually transmitted disease.[71] The incidence of disseminated HSV infection in the newborn has increased in the past 30 years, suggesting an increased frequency of genital herpes.

Clinical Features. In primary herpetic infections, a prodromal stage of tingling or pain for 2 days precedes the eruption of vesicular or papular lesions on the labia, vulva, urethra, vaginal mucosa, and cervix. Dysuria is frequent. Vesicles tend to be bilateral, spread rapidly to remote sites such as buttocks or thighs, ulcerate, and eventually heal without scarring after 2 to 4 weeks. Resolution of mucocutaneous lesions of a primary infection may be followed by asymptomatic shedding of the virus, hence the high rate of transmission through sexual contact. Transient viremia with systemic symptoms such as fever, headache, malaise, myalgia, and inguinal adenopathy may accompany primary attacks in two thirds of cases. Primary infections are often asymptomatic and go unnoticed.[72] Serious complications such as cauda equina syndrome, aseptic meningitis, encephalitis, hepatitis, or coagulopathy occur rarely during primary infection. Permanent antibodies are present after 4 to 6 weeks.

During recurrent infections, typical vesicular lesions usually appear on the external genitalia but antibody titers do not rise. The majority of recurrent lesions do not shed virus. Recurrent infections tend to be milder and of shorter duration, and 25% are asymptomatic.

Infection in Pregnancy. Three quarters of all pregnant women have antibodies indicating prior exposure to HSV-1, HSV-2, or both.[73, 74] Only 2% of nonimmune women acquire HSV infection during pregnancy.[74] Almost all women in late pregnancy presenting with genital HSV eruptions, systemic symptoms, and without a prior clinical history, in fact do have antibodies already, indicating recurrent and not primary infection.[74]

The major concern with HSV infections in pregnancy is the effect on the neonate. Transmission occurs either through direct contact with the virus as the infant passes through an infected birth canal, or from ascending infection after rupture of the membranes. True primary infections in the mother carry the highest risk of perinatal morbidity, such as prematurity and fetal growth retardation.[75] When primary HSV infection is acquired at or near the time of labor, the neonatal consequences can be catastrophic, with 60% mortality in the neonatal period or severe neurologic sequelae in 50% of survivors.[76] The risk of neonatal HSV infection as a consequence of recurrent genital lesions is reduced because of the less severe nature of the lesions, lesser viral shedding, and prior transplacental transfer of maternal antibodies.[77]

Obstetric management of patients known to be infected is directed at avoidance of exposure of the infant to virus in the genital tract. All pregnant women should be questioned about a history of genital HSV infection or exposure from their sexual partner. Antepartum cervical cultures are not recommended since there is little correlation between positive cultures and viral shedding in labor.[78] If there are no visible perineal lesions, the patient may deliver vaginally. The birth canal should be disinfected with povidone-iodine (Betadine).[77] In the presence of active lesions, fetal scalp electrodes should be avoided.

Current ACOG guidelines recommend that term patients who have visible lesions and are in labor or have ruptured membranes should undergo cesarean delivery.[76] However, this recommendation has become somewhat controversial for a number of reasons:

1. Most herpetic outbreaks at the time of delivery are recurrent infections with a very low rate of virus shedding.
2. The majority of neonatal infections occur in mothers with no prior clinical history of genital herpes or active lesions.[76]
3. Cesarean delivery does not guarantee prevention of neonatal transmission, and 20% to 30% of infants with neonatal herpes have been delivered abdominally.[79]
4. Neonatal herpes is rare, occurring in 1 to 5 cases per 10,000 births.[77] It has been estimated that four mothers die from cesarean-related complications for every seven babies saved from herpes-related deaths.[80]

It is unlikely that there will ever be a randomized controlled trial to objectively evaluate the value of cesarean delivery in preventing neonatal herpes. Similarly, it is improbable that many mothers would choose vaginal delivery when advised of the potential risk of transmission to their infants.

Acyclovir is used to treat primary HSV infections and to decrease the frequency of recurrent disease in nonpregnant women. Current ACOG recommendations reserve the use of acyclovir for disseminated or life-threatening infections.[60] However, investigators are currently studying the use of acyclovir in the late third trimester to prevent recurrent lesion outbreaks in patients with six or more reactivations per year.[72] Thus, acyclovir therapy may eventually decrease the rate of cesarean section. It does not, however, suppress all asymptomatic shedding of virus, so it may not decrease the incidence of neonatal herpes.

Anesthetic Management. Several recent reviews[81–83] have established the safety of both spinal and epidural anesthesia for cesarean section for recurrent HSV infection, provided the lesions are remote from the site of needle insertion. However, there have been no studies on the safety of regional anesthesia in women with primary HSV infection. The existence of fever and systemic symptoms in the presence of typical genital lesions may suggest a primary infection. HSV seroconversion (the new appearance of HSV antibodies at the time of labor) indicates a true primary infection in the parturient. The known risks of general anesthesia must be carefully weighed against the relatively low theoretic risk of regional anesthesia.[84]

The other anesthetic management issue concerns reactivation of oral HSV-1 following the use of neuraxial opioids. This recurrence has been well documented with epidural morphine[85, 86] but has also been associated with epidural fentanyl.[87] Possible mechanisms may include pruritus-induced scratching, or an excitatory effect on the spinal nucleus of the fifth cranial nerve caused by opiate receptor binding.[85] Boyle[86] found the probability of an outbreak of herpes simplex labialis following epidural narcotic to be 7.7% in patients with a prior history of mouth ulcers, and 1% with no such previous episode. On the other hand, some investigators have found no difference between parenteral and neuraxial opioids, both epidural[88] and intrathecal,[88, 89] in the rate of recurrence of oral herpes. A history of HSV infections involving less common areas should be viewed with more caution than perioral infections. A case of recurrent HSV blepharitis was reported following epidural morphine for pain control after cesarean section.[90] The author expressed concern about potentially serious sequelae such as HSV keratoconjunctivitis and meningitis. Guidelines for the use of neuraxial opioids in parturients with a "cold sore," or history of previous outbreaks, are not currently available.

Malignant Hyperthermia

Fever and tachycardia in a laboring woman may raise concerns about the development of malignant hyperthermia (MH). There have been only a handful of case reports of MH reactions during parturition.[91, 92] The number is much lower than would be predicted from the incidence of MH and estimates of the number of general anesthetics that pregnant women might have received.[93]

Although stress is frequently cited as a trigger for MH, none of these reactions occurred as a result of labor. All occurred during general anesthesia.[94] The only proven trigger agents are potent inhalational vapors and succinylcholine. Regional anesthesia, using any local anesthetic (including epinephrine) and vasopressors (such as ephedrine or phenylephrine), appears to be safe.[95] Oxytocin is considered safe in MH.[93] Routine prophylactic dantrolene is not recommended, as it causes unpleasant weakness and uterine atony with excessive blood loss for the mother.[91] It also crosses the placenta and may affect the immature neonatal neuromuscular system.[96]

In addition, one should be aware of a small number of case reports in which the newborn may develop a MH reaction.[91]

SEPTIC SHOCK

Shock is defined as the failure of organ perfusion. It may precede the onset of hypotension.[97] There are multiple causes of shock. However, in the febrile parturient we are concerned about septic shock.[97–101] Gram-negative infections cause 95% of cases of septic shock. Gram-positive aerobic or anaerobic infections cause the remainder. These organisms release toxins or substances that trigger the febrile reaction described earlier in this chapter.

Pregnant animals are more susceptible to infection or the products of infection.[102] It is unclear whether pregnant women are more susceptible to endotoxins than their nonpregnant counterparts.

In early septic shock, cardiac output increases and the systemic vascular resistance decreases as a result of dilated cutaneous vessels. The extremities remain warm and dry. Hyperventilation and oliguria are other early signs. As shock progresses, vascular permeability increases and fluids leak from the intravascular into the interstitial space. Patients in late septic shock suffer significant fluid loss. Central venous pressure and cardiac output are low, peripheral vascular resistance is increased, extremities are cold and cyanotic, and blood lactate levels are elevated. Myocardial depression or disseminated intravascular coagulation may occur.

Treatment is aimed primarily at improving the hemodynamic status and treating the infection. This includes broad-spectrum antibiotic coverage after appropriate cultures and Gram stains of specimens have been obtained. Volume expansion, vasopressors, and inotropic agents may also be needed. Invasive monitoring such as an arterial line and a pulmonary artery catheter are necessary in many patients.

Anesthesia for vaginal or cesarean delivery in hemodynamically unstable patients should be delayed up to 1 or 2 hours while appropriate monitoring devices are inserted and resuscitation is accomplished. However, the need for fluid resuscitation must be weighed against the need for rapid delivery. Sometimes prompt delivery may be the only chancc the newborn has for survival.

Regional anesthesia is usually contraindicated because of the effects of sympathetic blockade on a severely septic patient with hypovolemia. Coagulopathy would also contraindicate the use of a regional technique. If resuscitation has been successful, an epidural anesthetic may be cautiously titrated. General anesthesia is usually the method of choice for emergency delivery.

REGIONAL ANESTHESIA FOR THE FEBRILE PARTURIENT

General Considerations

The combination of febrile illness and pregnancy, especially during labor, requires a prompt evaluation. Does the fever indicate a bacterial infection? Should any other etiologies of fever be considered? What role does epidural anesthesia play in maternal fever?[34, 35, 103]

The physiologic changes of pregnancy can make it difficult to determine the etiology of fever in pregnancy. Tachypnea, urinary frequency, displacement of small bowel and appendix, and leukocytosis are all normal findings. Prostaglandins are an important mediator both in the febrile response and in the initiation of labor.[104] This is a practical concern, since maternal fever is often associated with premature labor.[105] Since uterine perfusion is not autoregulated,[106] peripheral vasodilation, shivering, or hyperemia of an infected organ may, at least theoretically, reduce the perfusion of the uterus and fetus. Regional anesthesia may further alter uterine perfusion.

Infections that are unlikely to spread to the fetus (e.g., urinary tract infection) have different implications than those that may cause fetal infection (e.g., chorioamnionitis). The former may affect the fetus only indirectly through maternal effects or premature labor. Proper treatment necessitates an accurate diagnosis, although treatment often needs to be instituted based on a presumptive diagnosis. The patient should be assessed for the presence of uterine activity and, unless contraindicated, the cervix should be examined. Many infectious diseases do cross the placenta and may cause fetal disease. This may imply the need for indirect neonatal treatment (e.g., antibiotics in maternal syphilis, zoster immunoglobulin in varicella), for direct fetal treatment via cordocentesis (toxoplasmosis), or for maternal treatment (e.g., antibiotics in chorioamnionitis, azido-thymidine if the patient tests positive for human immunodeficiency virus).

Conversely, the effect of the pregnancy on the course of the disease must be taken into account. Pregnancy is associated with decreased function of the immune system.[107] The course of some febrile illnesses such as varicella pneumonia is far worse in pregnancy.[108] However, poor outcome can often be linked to difficulties in diagnosis and delay in treatment.

Incidence of Maternal Infection

The overall incidence of maternal infection during labor has been reported as 3.1%.[109] Septicemia occurs in 0.07% to 0.8% of patients.[110] Oxytocin augmentation may be indicated in as many as 70% of these women, and cesarean sections are performed in 30% to 40%.[44, 111] In these clinical situations, there are often benefits from regional anesthesia for both mother and baby.

There is no clear consensus of opinion to guide the anesthesiologist in the use of epidural anesthesia in the presence of fever.[112, 113] In the past it was believed that regional anesthesia should be avoided in the presence of bacteremia because of concerns that a focus of infection could be initiated by the procedure.[114, 115]

The incidence of transient bacteremia, as documented in healthy patients by blood culture, is less than 1%.[110] Pregnancy may increase this incidence.[116] Ten percent of patients who are febrile for any reason are bacteremic.[110] Insertion of a urinary catheter in healthy parturients can produce a transient bacteremia in up to 60% of women even with sterile urine.[116, 117] The incidence of bacteremia is believed to be even higher in the presence of infected urine.[117, 118] Asymptomatic urinary tract infections are common in pregnancy, and bladder catheterization is commonly performed. After 4 hours of labor or ruptured membranes, bacteremia has been reported in 11% of patients following placental separation during cesarean delivery.[119] It is apparent that a transient bacteremia is very common in parturients, and certainly more so in febrile ones.

Clinical Presentation

A thorough history, physical examination, and appropriate laboratory investigations make the diagnosis of infection (see Table 28–3).[109, 120, 121] Regional anesthesia may be catastrophic in patients with late sepsis because of hypovolemia. The decision to give a regional anesthetic must be made on an individual basis. Pregnant women may be septic with few clinical signs,[99] and one must have a high degree of suspicion.

The clinical picture is confounded by several factors. Elevated temperature or rigors do not accurately correlate with bacteremia.[114, 122, 123] A patient may be hypothermic during fulminant sepsis. There is no correlation between temperature and clinical status. For example, endogenous pyrogens may produce a fever in spite of appropriate treatment of infection. Almost half of patients with documented bacteremia have a temperature of less than 38.8°C,[110] and there is no difference in the mean temperature between bacteremic and nonbacteremic patients with chorioamnionitis. In the clinical setting, blood culture and sensitivity results are not usually available.

Concerns About Regional Anesthesia

There have been several reports of central nervous system infection in association with epidural, spinal, or CSE anesthesia.[124, 125] These complications are of major severity and often result in permanent disability. Three reviews comprising over 500,000 patients found no cases of meningitis and only two cases of epidural space infection.[126–128] However, Kindler and associates[129] reported an incidence of 2 epidural abscesses in a series of 4162 obstetric epidurals. There are also two reported patients who developed an epidural abscess without any regional anesthesia for labor and delivery.[130, 131]

The rate of spontaneous epidural abscess in the general hospital population is 0.2 to 1.2 per 10,000.[132] To date, only a few anecdotal reports relating epidural abscess or meningitis with regional anesthesia have appeared in the literature.[133–135] Reports from the early days describe six caudal infections and one epidural infection.[136] It seems likely that infection resulted from nonaseptic technique, although in two cases, hematogenous spread was possible. In 1975, Baker et al.[137] reported 39 patients with epidural abscesses (20 acute and 19 chronic). Regional blockade was felt to be the probable source of infection in 3 patients. Two were lumbar punctures done in patients with vertebral osteomyelitis. Another review of 35 new and 153 previously reported epidural abscesses concluded that regional anesthesia was not a factor in any of the additional cases.[138]

Recent reviews have concluded that it may be safe to administer either spinal or epidural anesthesia to parturients with chorioamnionitis.[45, 46, 113] However, large studies are lacking. Most leading authorities have recommended that, in the presence of systemic signs of infection, antibiotics should be started before proceeding with an epidural.[45, 136, 139, 140]

Cultures from 102 patients undergoing continuous epidural catheterization found 22 catheters to be contaminated.[141] This rate of contamination should be viewed in light of the very large numbers of patients who have epidural catheters placed for labor and delivery, surgery, and pain control without clinical infections. Many of these patients are immunocompromised with malignancy. Other data point to a possible protective role local anesthetics and some narcotics may play in preventing infection.[142–144] Commonly used local anesthetics may have antimicrobial properties, which are reduced as the concentration of anesthetic decreases.[142] The incidence of epidural abscess has not risen during the past 20 years, despite the widespread and increased popularity of regional anesthesia.[145]

Septic meningitis has only rarely been reported in the past 25 years.[146] Epidural injection of foreign substances, use of a vasoconstrictor, or contaminants were possible causes in six nonobstetric patients.[147] Spinal meningitis has also been reported in five nonobstetric patients who had recently received epidural anesthesia. Antecedent factors were hematogenous spread, possible extension of a local cellulitis, and inadvertent spinal tap followed by epidural blood patch.[148, 149] Two cases of possible direct complications have been reported following spinal anesthesia.[150, 151]

The incidence of meningitis following lumbar puncture is the same as spontaneous meningitis in bacteremic patients.[152, 153] Several anecdotal reports of meningitis after subarachnoid block have cited concurrent bacteremia as a possible cause.[134, 146, 154, 155] Recently, two afebrile patients with no clinical signs of infection developed meningitis following epidural analgesia for labor.[147] There is a similar case of an afebrile patient receiving an epidural block for cesarean section who developed an epidural abscess.[135]

Tens of thousands of cases of spinal anesthetics have been reported.[124, 156] In the past, some authorities have speculated on the possibility that a lumbar puncture may create a site of diminished resistance in the blood-brain barrier, or that epidural abscess might occur for the same reason.[146] This speculation is surprising considering the frequent use of spinal anesthesia and the common occurrence of bacteremia. It is highly doubtful that a causal relationship exists between such rare events.[157]

There is evidence, however, to suggest that bacteremia may increase the risk of meningitis after subarachnoid block. A recent study[158] compared two groups of 40 chronically bacteremic rats, one which underwent percutaneous dural puncture, and one without dural puncture. Cerebrospinal fluid obtained 24 hours later grew bacteria in 12 of the rats receiving dural puncture. The non–dural puncture group all had sterile cerebrospinal fluid. Another group of bacteremic rats was pretreated with antibiotics prior to dural puncture; none of this group had infected cerebrospinal fluid. Thus, bacteremia may constitute a risk factor in the development of meningitis in patients receiving spinal anesthesia without antibiotic pretreatment, but the pertinence of these observations to humans is unknown.

Chestnut[140] states that he would administer a spinal anesthetic in the presence of fever: "Physicians often perform diagnostic lumbar puncture in patients with fever and bacteremia of unknown origin. If dural puncture during bacteremia results in meningitis, one would expect that unequivocal data should exist." Several studies do not show any association between meningitis and dural puncture.[152, 153, 159] Recently, three cases were reported of patients with meningitis following a CSE technique,[160, 161] indicating that any regional technique may rarely be associated with but not the cause of meningitis. Whenever bacteremia is a possibility, antibiotic therapy should be initiated prior to regional anesthesia to avoid serious neurologic consequences.

Suggestions for Clinical Decisions

Most epidural infections appear to result from trauma, surgical procedures, or hematogenous spread, rather than as a result of regional anesthesia.[137] There is no documented relationship between epidural vein puncture in the febrile patient and the formation of epidural abscess. Iatrogenic epidural abscesses continue to be reported, however, and are of concern.

As outlined earlier, it is often difficult to diagnose maternal infection. The severity of fever does not reflect the likelihood of bacteremia. The safest course is to begin empirical antibiotic therapy based on the likely source of infection and pathogens, replace intravascular volume, and observe an adequate clinical response prior to performing an epidural block. Although it has been stated that conduction anesthesia may be safe in parturients with chorioamnionitis without prior antibiotic therapy,[45, 46] we urge caution and prefer not to administer a spinal anesthetic to a patient without antibiotic therapy. We would also exclude the CSE technique in these circumstances, unless a similar condition is met.

The decision to use regional anesthesia should be based on the risk:benefit ratio for each individual patient. Absolute exclusion of regional anesthesia in febrile parturients may result in an excessive and unnecessary increase in morbidity and mortality from general anesthesia.[84] The avoidance or discontinuation of continuous epidural anesthesia because of theoretical concerns may expose women to unnecessary pain and risks. A case has been reported in which an epidural catheter was removed when a laboring patient became febrile. During subsequent induction of general anesthesia for cesarean section, there was unexpected gross edema of the larynx and pharynx, making tracheal intubation very difficult.[162]

Information such as the duration and severity of fever, use of antibiotics, white cell count and differential, hemodynamic status, and urine output may guide clinical decisions. There are, however, no firm criteria dictating when to proceed with regional anesthesia. Authorities recommend that an epidural anesthetic may be given to a febrile patient with localized disease and after antibiotic therapy.[1, 100]

GENERAL ANESTHESIA

Febrile parturients are more likely to receive emergency general anesthesia than their nonfebrile counterparts, either to avoid regional anesthesia or for fetal complications requiring immediate response. Although general anesthesia may result in a faster induction, there are significant risks such as maternal aspiration of gastric contents, inability to secure the airway, and the potential for newborn depression. With general anesthesia for delivery, the risk of maternal mortality is 16 times greater than with regional anesthesia.[84]

The choice of drugs used for induction of general anesthesia is dictated by the desire to maintain hemodynamic stability and uteroplacental circulation. Ketamine has been advocated, although concern has been expressed about the unpredictability of 1 to 2 mg/kg in critically ill patients.[163, 164] This is due to the myocardial depressant effect of ketamine if catecholamine levels are low. It is not clear whether the same concerns exist for patients with fevers of short duration. Sodium thiopental also causes myocardial depression in the critically ill patient. Reduced doses will diminish but not eliminate this problem. Ketamine and sodium thiopental can be used together in reduced doses to decrease the incidence of cardiovascular decompensation.[164, 165] Etomidate has also been advocated for use in these patients.

Hyperkalemia following the use of succinylcholine may be a problem in severe and prolonged sepsis (>1 week's duration).[122, 166] Pretreatment with a nondepolarizing agent may decrease but will not eliminate the release of potassium. The duration and severity of fever that would contraindicate the use of succinylcholine is unknown. Succinylcholine-induced hyperkalemia has never been reported in a patient with chorioamnionitis. If the temperature elevation is of several days' duration, we prefer to use a nondepolarizing agent for rapid sequence induction.

Some antibiotics may interact with muscle relaxants. With commonly used antibiotics, shorter acting relaxants, and use of a peripheral nerve stimulator, there is seldom a problem in adequate reversal of neuromuscular blockade.

Once the airway has been secured, the patient is maintained with a high concentration of oxygen (minimum of 50%). Low concentrations of nitrous oxide (up to 50%) may be used, but with severe fetal distress, 100% oxygen may better oxygenate the fetus. If agents such as ketamine or low-dose fentanyl are used to reduce the amount of volatile agent needed, hemodynamic stability is usually maintained. A balanced technique with small amounts of several agents is probably the key to success.

CONCLUSION

We must anticipate the problem of the febrile patient with fetal distress who is to undergo immediate delivery. A key question to be answered is whether the maternal benefits or potential fetal outcome following general anesthesia outweighs the maternal risks.[167] Sometimes fetal distress is so severe that the baby is likely to have already suffered a major deficit from asphyxia.

Epidural or spinal anesthesia has the obvious advantages of greatly reducing the risk of maternal aspiration, but no anesthetic is without risk. The slightly slower onset may be critical. The choice of anesthesia for cesarean section depends on the indication for surgery, the degree of urgency, the wishes of the patient, and the skills of the anesthesiologist. Sometimes the clinical situation can result in a distressed obstetrician or anesthesiologist. All these factors lead to an intensely emotional situation, which the anesthesiologist must anticipate. Either regional or general anesthesia can be used, but current information tends to favor regional anesthesia if time permits.

❖ Summary

Key Points

- Fever is commonly seen in laboring patients. The etiology of fever needs to be thoroughly investigated; however, low-grade maternal fever does not appear to have negative fetal implications.
- Regional anesthesia may occasionally be associated with a modest increase in maternal temperature, but this is of no clinical significance.
- Regional anesthesia can be initiated in the febrile parturient, provided that the patient is not septic. Many anesthesiologists delay the initiation of regional anesthesia until the febrile patient has received antibiotics.

Key References

Camann WR, Hortvet LA, Hughes N, et al: Maternal temperature regulation during extradural analgesia for labour. Br J Anaesth 1991; 61:565–568.

Bader AM, Gilbertson L, Kirz L, Datta S: Regional anesthesia in women with chorioamnionitis. Reg Anesth 1992; 17:84–86.

Case Stem

A 22-year-old primiparous patient who has been in labor with ruptured membranes for 12 hours requests epidural analgesia. Her temperature is 39°C. What are the considerations in the obstetric and anesthetic management of this patient?

References

1. Carp H, Chestnut DH: Fever and infection. *In* Chestnut DH (ed): Obstetric Anesthesia: Principles and Practice. St. Louis: Mosby; 1994: 686.
2. Gelfand JA, Dinarello CA: Alterations in body temperature. *In* Fauci AS, Braunwald E, Isselbacher KJ, et al (eds): Harrison's Principles of Internal Medicine, 14th ed. New York: McGraw-Hill; 1998: 84–90.
3. McMurray RG, Katz VL, Berry MG, et al: The effects of pregnancy on metabolic responses during rest, immersion, and aerobic exercise in the water. Am J Obstet Gynecol 1988; 158:481.
4. Goodlin RC, Chapin JW: Determinants of maternal temperature during labor. Am J Obstet Gynecol 1982; 143:97–103.
5. Energetics, metabolic rate, and regulation of body temperature. *In* Guyton AC, Hall JE (eds): Human Physiology and Mechanisms of Disease, 6th ed. Philadelphia: WB Saunders; 1997: 571–582.
6. Beutler B, Beutler SM: The pathogenesis of fever. *In* Wyngaarden JB, Smith LH, Bennett JC (eds): Cecil Textbook of Medicine, 19th ed. Philadelphia: WB Saunders; 1992: 1567–1571.
7. Fever and febrile syndromes. *In* Andreoli TE, Bennett JC, et al (eds): Cecil Essentials of Medicine, 4th ed. Philadelphia: WB Saunders; 1997: 663–676.
8. Dinarello CA, Wolff SM: Pathogenesis of fever and the acute phase response. *In* Mandrel GL, Bennett JE, Dolin R (eds): Principles and Practice of Infectious Diseases, 4th ed. New York: Churchill Livingstone; 1995: 530–536.
9. Body temperature, temperature regulation and fever. *In* Guyton AC, Hall JE (eds): Textbook of Medical Physiology, 9th ed. Philadelphia: WB Saunders; 1996: 911–922.
10. Morishima HO, Yeh MN, Niemann WH, et al: Temperature gradient between the fetus and mother as an index for assessing intrauterine fetal condition. Am J Obstet Gynecol 1977; 129:443–448.
11. Cefalo RC, Hellegers AE: The effects of maternal hyperthermia on maternal cardiovascular and respiratory function. Am J Obstet Gynecol 1978; 131:687–694.
12. Harris WH, Pittman QJ, Veale WL, et al: Cardiovascular

effects of fever in the fetal lamb. Am J Obstet Gynecol 1997; 128:262–265.
13. Ahlgren M, Kullander S: The influence of temperature on the motility of the human uterus in vitro. Acta Obstet Gynecol Scand 1959: 38:243–245.
14. Morishima HO, Glaser B, Niemann WH, et al: Increased uterine activity in fetal deterioration during maternal hyperthermia. Am J Obstet Gynecol 1975; 121:531–538.
15. Fusi L, Steer PJ, Maresh MJA, et al: Maternal pyrexia associated with the use of epidural analgesia in labour. Lancet 1989; 1:1250–1252.
16. Camann WR, Hortvet LA, Hughes N, et al: Maternal temperature regulation during extradural analgesia for labour. Br J Anaesth 1991; 67:565–568.
17. Macaulay JH, Bond K, Steer PJ: Epidural analgesia in labor and fetal tachycardia. Obstet Gynecol 1992; 80:665–669.
18. Gleeson NC, Nolan KM, Ford MRW: Temperature, labour and epidural analgesia. Lancet 1989; 2:861–862.
19. St. Geme J Jr, Murray DL, Carter J, et al: Perinatal bacterial infection after prolonged rupture of amniotic membranes: An analysis of risk and management. J Pediatr 1984; 104:608–613.
20. Mathews TG, Baughan B: Maternal pyrexia and the fetus. Lancet 1989; 2:284–285.
21. Herbst A, Wølner-Hanssen P, Ingemarsson I: Maternal fever in term labour in relation to fetal tachycardia, cord artery acidaemia and neonatal infection. Br J Obstet Gynaecol 1997; 104:363–366.
22. Maberry MC, Ramin SM, Gilstrap LC III, et al: Intrapartum asphyxia in pregnancies complicated by intraamniotic infection. Obstet Gynecol 1990; 76:351–354.
23. Hankins GD, Snyder RR, Yeomans ER: Umbilical arterial and venous acid-base and blood gas values and the effect of chorioamnionitis on these values in a cohort of preterm infants. Am J Obstet Gynecol 1991; 164:1261–1264.
24. Grether JK, Nelson KB: Maternal infection and cerebral palsy in infants of normal birth weight. JAMA 1997; 278:207–211.
25. Low JA, Lindsay BG, Derrick EJ: Threshold of metabolic acidosis associated with newborn complications. Am J Obstet Gynecol 1997; 177:1391–1394.
26. Matsukawa T, Sessler DI, Christensen R, et al: Heat flow and distribution during epidural anesthesia. Anesthesiology 1995; 83:961–962.
27. Leslie K, Sessler DI: Reduction in the shivering threshold is proportional to spinal block height. Anesthesiology 1996; 84:1327–1331.
28. Ozaki M, Kurz A, Sessler DI, et al: Thermoregulatory thresholds during epidural and spinal anesthesia. Anesthesiology 1994; 81:282–288.
29. Emerick TH, Ozaki M, Sessler DI, et al: Epidural anesthesia increases apparent leg temperature and decreases the shivering threshold. Anesthesiology 1994; 81:289–298.
30. Sessler DI, Ponte J: Shivering during epidural anesthesia. Anesthesiology 1990; 72:816–821.
31. Ponte J, Collett BJ, Walmsley A: Anesthetic temperature and shivering in epidural anesthesia. Acta Anaesthesiol Scand 1986; 30:584–587.
32. Thomas ML, Yentis SM, Barnes P: Maternal temperature during labour using low-dose (ambulatory) epidural analgesia with bupivacaine and fentanyl. Int J Obstet Anesth 1998; 7:108–112.
33. Birnbach DJ, Sein DJ, Hartman JK, et al: Is maternal fever associated with the administration of regional anesthesia in laboring parturients? Anesthesiology 1996; 85:A899.
34. Lieberman E, Lang JM, Frigoletto F, et al: Epidural analgesia, intrapartum fever, and neonatal sepsis evaluation. Pediatrics 1997; 99:415–419.
35. Herbst A, Wølner-Hanssen P, Ingemarsson I: Risk factors for fever in labor. Obstet Gynecol 1995; 86:790–794.
36. Wright KA, Klimek K, Compton AA: Effects of regional anesthesia on maternal temperature during labor. Society for Obstetric Anesthesia and Perinatology Annual Meeting, Vancouver, 1997, p 94.
37. Churgay CA, Smith MA, Blok B, et al: Maternal fever during labor: What does it mean? J Am Board Fam Pract 1994; 7:14–24.
38. Lewis TJ, Connelly NR: Epidural analgesia and neonatal fever [letter]. Pediatrics 1998; 101:492–494.
39. Newton ER: Chorioamnionitis and intraamniotic infection. Clin Obstet Gynecol 1993; 36:795–808.
40. Casey BM, Cox SM: Chorioamnionitis and endometritis. Inf Dis Clin North Am 1997; 11:203–222.
41. Gibbs RS, Duff P: Progress in pathogenesis and management of clinical intraamniotic infection. Am J Obstet Gynecol 1991; 164:1317–1326.
42. Seaward PG, Hannah ME, Myhr TL, et al: International multicentre term prelabor rupture of membranes study: Evaluation of predictors of clinical chorioamnionitis and postpartum fever in patients with prelabor rupture of membranes at term. Am J Obstet Gynecol 1997; 177:1024–1029.
43. Isada NB, Grossman JH III: Perinatal infections. *In* Gabbe SG, Niebyl JR, Simpson JL (eds): Obstetrics: Normal and Problem Pregnancies, 2nd ed. New York: Churchill Livingstone; 1991: 1225.
44. Duff P, Sanders R, Gibbs RS: The course of labor in term patients with chorioamnionitis. Am J Obstet Gynecol 1983; 147:391–395.
45. Bader AM, Gilbertson L, Kirz L, Datta S: Regional anesthesia in women with chorioamnionitis. Reg Anesth 1992; 17:84–86.
46. Goodman EJ, DeHorta E, Taguiam JM: Safety of spinal and epidural anesthesia in parturients with chorioamnionitis. Reg Anesth 1996; 21:436–441.
47. Beilin Y, Bodian CA, Haddad EM, et al: Practice patterns of anesthesiologists regarding situations in obstetric anesthesia where clinical management is controversial. Anesth Analg 1996; 83:735–741.
48. Nandwani N, Raphael JH, Langton JA: Effect of an upper respiratory tract infection on upper airway reactivity. Br J Anaesth 1997; 78:352–355.
49. Moses RL, Paige T, Cavalli G, et al: Laryngotracheobronchitis in pregnancy and its clinical implications. Otolaryngol Head Neck Surg 1997; 116:401–403.
50. Farley MM, Stephens DS, Brachman PS, et al: Invasive *Haemophilus influenzae* disease in adults. Ann Intern Med 1992; 116:806–812.
51. Glock JL, Morales WJ: Acute epiglottitis during pregnancy. South Med J 1993; 86:836–838.
52. Maccato ML: Pneumonia and pulmonary tuberculosis in pregnancy. Obstet Gynecol Clin North Am 1989; 16:417–430.
53. Rigby FB, Pastorek JG II: Pneumonia during pregnancy. Clin Obstet Gynecol 1996; 39:107–119.
54. Madinger NE, Greenspoon JS, Ellrodt AG: Pneumonia during pregnancy: Has modern technology improved maternal and fetal outcome? Am J Obstet Gynecol 1989; 161:657–662.
55. Bloom SL, Ramin S, Cunningham FG: A prediction rule for community-acquired pneumonia [letter]. N Engl J Med 1997; 336:1913–1914.
56. Goodrum LA: Pneumonia in pregnancy. Semin Perinatol 1997; 21:276–283.
57. Ackerman WE III, Molnar JM, Juneja MM: Beneficial effect of epidural anesthesia on oxygen consumption in a parturient with adult respiratory distress syndrome. South Med J 1993; 86:361–364.
58. Tomlinson MW, Caruthers TJ, Whitty JE, et al: Does delivery improve maternal condition in the respiratory-compromised gravida? Obstet Gynecol 1998; 91:108–111.
59. Loughlin KR: Management of urologic problems during pregnancy. Urology 1994; 44:159–169.
60. American College of Obstetricians and Gynecologists: Antimicrobial therapy for obstetric patients. ACOG Technical Bulletin No. 117. Washington, DC, 1988.
61. Millar LK, Cox SM: Urinary tract infections complicating pregnancy. Infect Dis Clin North Am 1997; 11:13–26.
62. Lucas MJ, Cunningham FG: Urinary infection in pregnancy. Clin Obstet Gynecol 1993; 36:855–868.
63. Raviglione MC, Snider DE, Koch AK: Global epidemiology of tuberculosis: Morbidity and mortality of a worldwide epidemic. JAMA 1995; 273:220–226.
64. Espinal MA, Reingold AL, Lavandera M: Effect of pregnancy on the risk of developing active tuberculosis. J Infect Dis 1996; 173:488–491.

65. Bjerkedal T, Bahna SL, Lehmann EH: Course and outcome of pregnancy in women with pulmonary tuberculosis. Scand J Respir Dis 1975; 56:245–250.
66. Ratner B, Rostler AE, Salgado PS: Care, feeding, and fate of premature and full term infants born of tuberculous mothers. Am J Dis Child 1951; 81:471–482.
67. Miller KS, Miller JM: Tuberculosis in pregnancy: Interactions, diagnosis, and management. Clin Obstet Gynecol 1996; 39:120–142.
68. Hamadeh MA, Glassroth J: Tuberculosis and pregnancy. Chest 1992; 101:1114–1120.
69. Riley L: Pneumonia and tuberculosis in pregnancy. Infect Dis Clin North Am 1997; 11:119–133.
70. Isada NB, Grossman JH: Perinatal Infections. *In* Gabbe SG, Niebyl JR, Simpson JL (eds): Obstetrics: Normal and Problem Pregnancies, 2nd ed. New York: Churchill Livingstone; 1991: 1248.
71. Shulman ST, Phair JP, Sommers HM: The Biologic & Clinical Basis of Infectious Diseases, 4th ed. Philadelphia: WB Saunders; 1992: 253–257.
72. Scott LL, Hollier LM, Dias K: Perinatal herpesvirus infections. Infect Dis Clin North Am 1997; 11:27–53.
73. Brown ZA, Selke S, Zeh J, et al: The acquisition of herpes simplex virus during pregnancy. N Engl J Med 1997; 337:509–515.
74. Hensleigh PA, Andrews WW, Brown Z, et al: Genital herpes during pregnancy: Inability to distinguish primary and recurrent infections clinically. Obstet Gynecol 1997; 89:891–895.
75. Brown ZA, Vontver LA, Benedetti J, et al: Effects on infants of a first episode of genital herpes during pregnancy. N Engl J Med 1987; 317:1246–1251.
76. American College of Obstetricians and Gynecologists: Perinatal herpes simplex virus infections. ACOG Technical Bulletin No. 122. Washington, DC, 1988.
77. Blanchier H, Huraux J-M, Huraux-Rendu C, et al: Genital herpes and pregnancy: Preventive measures. Eur J Obstet Gynecol Reprod Biol 1994; 53:33–38.
78. Arvin AM, Hensleigh PA, Prober CG, et al: Failure of antepartum maternal cultures to predict the infant's risk of exposure to herpes simplex virus at delivery. N Engl J Med 1986; 315:796–800.
79. Stone KM, Brooks CA, Guinan ME, et al: National surveillance for neonatal herpes simplex virus infections. Sex Transm Dis 1989; 16:152–156.
80. Randolph AG, Washington AE, Prober CG: Cesarean delivery for women presenting with genital herpes lesions: Efficacy, risks, and costs. JAMA 1993; 270:77–82.
81. Ramanathan S, Sheth R, Turndorf H: Anesthesia for cesarean section in patients with genital herpes infections: A retrospective study. Anesthesiology 1986; 64:807–809.
82. Crosby ET, Halpern SH, Rolbin SH: Epidural anaesthesia for caesarean section in patients with active genital herpes simplex infections: A retrospective review. Can J Anaesth 1989; 36:701–704.
83. Bader AM, Camann WR, Datta S: Anesthesia for cesarean delivery in patients with herpes simplex virus type-2 infections. Reg Anesth 1990; 15:261–263.
84. Hawkins JL, Koonin LM, Palmer SK, et al: Anesthesia-related deaths during obstetric delivery in the United States, 1979–1990. Anesthesiology 1997; 86:277–284.
85. Crone LL, Conly JM, Storgard C, et al: Herpes labialis in parturients receiving epidural morphine following cesarean section. Anesthesiology 1990; 73:208–213.
86. Boyle RK: Herpes simplex labialis after epidural or parenteral morphine: A randomized prospective trial in an Australian obstetric population. Anaesth Intensive Care 1995; 23:433–437.
87. Valley MA, Bourke DL, McKenzie AM: Recurrence of thoracic and labial herpes simplex virus infection in a patient receiving epidural fentanyl. Anesthesiology 1992; 76:1056–1057.
88. Norris MC, Weiss J, Leighton BL: The incidence of herpes simplex virus labialis after cesarean delivery. Int J Obstet Anesth 1994; 3:127–131.
89. Cascio MG, Mandell GL, Ramanathan S: Reactivation of herpes simplex labialis with intrathecal morphine in cesarean section patients. Anesthesiology 1997; 87:A868.
90. James CF: Recurrence of herpes simplex virus blepharitis after cesarean section and epidural morphine. Anesth Analg 1996; 82:1094–1096.
91. Lucy SJ: Anaesthesia for caesarean delivery of a malignant hyperthermia–susceptible parturient. Can J Anaesth 1994; 41:1220–1226.
92. Johnson C: Pregnancy and malignant hyperthermia. J Clin Anesth 1992; 4:173.
93. Longmire S, Lee W, Pivarnik J: Malignant hyperthermia. *In* Datta S (ed): Anesthetic and Obstetric Management of High-risk Pregnancy, 2nd ed. St. Louis: Mosby; 1996: 311–322.
94. Halpern S: Anaesthesia for caesarean delivery of a malignant hyperthermia–susceptible parturient [commentary]. Can J Anaesth 1994; 41:1223–1224.
95. Kaplan RF: Malignant hyperthermia. *In* 1993 Annual Refresher Course Lectures, No. 522. Washington, DC: American Society of Anesthesiologists, 1993.
96. Morison DH: Placental transfer of dantrolene [letter]. Anesthesiology 1983; 59:265.
97. Parillo JE: Shock syndromes related to sepsis. *In* Bennett JC, Plum F (eds): Cecil Textbook of Medicine, 20th ed. Philadelphia: WB Saunders; 1996: 496–501.
98. Lee W, Clark SL, Cotton DB, et al: Septic shock during pregnancy. Am J Obstet Gynecol 1988; 159:410–416.
99. Morgan PJ: Maternal death following epidural anaesthesia for caesarean section delivery in a patient with unsuspected sepsis. Can J Anaesth 1995; 42:330–334.
100. Lauretti GR: Infectious diseases. *In* Gambling DR, Douglas MJ (eds): Obstetric Anesthesia and Uncommon Disorders. Philadelphia: WB Saunders; 1998: 333–351.
101. Mabie WC, Barton JR, Sibai B: Septic shock in pregnancy. Obstet Gynecol 1989; 90:553–561.
102. Beller FK, Schmidt EH, Holzgreve W, et al: Septicemia during pregnancy: A study in different species of experimental animals. Am J Obstet Gynecol 1985; 151:967–975.
103. Pleasure JR, Stahl GE: Epidural analgesia and neonatal fever [letter]. Pediatrics 1998; 101:490.
104. Challis JR, Olson DM: Parturition. *In* Knobil E, Neill JD (eds): The Physiology of Reproduction. New York: Raven Press; 1988: 2177–2216.
105. Creasy RK: Preterm labor and delivery. *In* Creasy RK, Resnik R (eds): Maternal Fetal Medicine: Principles and Practice. Philadelphia: WB Saunders; 1989: 480.
106. Greiss FC, Anderson SG, Still JG: Uterine pressure-flow relationships during early gestation. Am J Obstet Gynecol 1976; 126:799–808.
107. Gall SA: Maternal immune system during human gestation. Semin Perinatol 1977; 1:119–133.
108. Paryani SG, Arvin AM: Intrauterine infection with varicella-zoster virus after maternal varicella. N Engl J Med 1986; 314:1542–1546.
109. Ducloy AS, Buy E, Ducloy JC, et al: Prediction of maternal infection before performing epidural analgesia in labor. Anesthesiology 1993; 100:A192.
110. Blanco JD, Gibbs RS, Castaneda YS: Bacteremia in obstetrics: Clinical course. Obstet Gynecol 1981; 58:621–625.
111. Davies JM, Thistlewood JM, Rolbin SH, et al: Infections and the parturient: Anaesthetic considerations. Can J Anaesth 1988; 35:270–277.
112. Behl S: Epidural analgesia in the presence of fever. Anaesthesia 1985; 40:1240–1241.
113. Vaddadi A, Ramanathan J, Mercer BM, et al: Epidural anesthesia in women with chorioamnionitis. Anesthesiol Rev 1992; 19:35–41.
114. Gibbs RS, Castillo MS, Rodgers PJ: Management of acute chorioamnionitis. Am J Obstet Gynecol 1980; 136:709–713.
115. Bromage PR (ed): Epidural Analgesia. Philadelphia: WB Saunders; 1978: 394–396.
116. Everett ED, Hirschmann JV: Transient bacteremia and endocarditis prophylaxis: A review. Medicine 1977; 56:61–77.
117. Sullivan NM, Mims MM, Finegold SM: Clinical aspects of bacteremia after manipulation of the genitourinary tract. J Infect Dis 1973; 127:49–55.

118. Drach GW, Cox CE: Bladder bacteria: Common but unique cause for sepsis. Post-operative endotoxic responses. J Urol 1971; 106:67–71.
119. Boggess KA, Watts DH, Hillier SL, et al: Bacteremia shortly after placental separation during cesarean delivery. Obstet Gynecol 1996; 87:779–784.
120. American College of Chest Physicians/Society of Critical Medicine Consensus Conference: Definitions for sepsis and organ failure and guidelines for the use of innovative therapies in sepsis. Crit Care Med 1992; 20:864–873.
121. Braun TI, Pinover W, Sih P: Group B streptococcal meningitis in a pregnant woman before the onset of labor. Clin Infect Dis 1995; 21:1042–1043.
122. Shelley WC, Gutsche BB: Anesthesia for the febrile parturient. *In* James FM III, Wheeler AS (eds): Obstetric Anesthesia: The Complicated Patient. Philadelphia: FA Davis; 1982: 297.
123. McHenry MC, Gavin TL, Hawk WA, et al: Gram negative bacteremia: Variable clinical courses and useful prognostic factors. Cleve Clin Quart 1975; 42:15–32.
124. Dripps RD, Vandam LD: Long-term follow-up of patients who received 10,098 spinal anesthetics. Failure to discover major neurological sequelae. JAMA 1954; 156:1486–1491.
125. Phillips OC, Ebner H, Nelson AT, et al: Neurologic complications following spinal anesthesia with lidocaine: A prospective review of 10,440 cases. Anesthesiology 1969; 30:284–289.
126. Hellman K: Epidural anesthesia in obstetrics: A second look at 26,127 cases. Can Anaesth Soc J 1965; 12:398–402.
127. Crawford JS: Some maternal complications of epidural analgesia for labour. Anaesthesia 1985; 40:1219–1225.
128. Scott DB, Hibbard BM: Serious non-fatal complications associated with extradural block in obstetric practice. Br J Anaesth 1990; 64:537–541.
129. Kindler C, Seeberger M, Siegemund M, et al: Extradural abscess complicating lumbar extradural anaesthesia and analgesia in an obstetric population. Acta Anaesthesiol Scand 1996; 40:858–861.
130. Male CG, Martin R: Puerperal spinal epidural abscess. Lancet 1973; 1:608–609.
131. Kitching AJ, Rice AS: Extradural abscess in the postpartum period [letter]. Br J Anaesth 1993; 70:703.
132. Hlavin ML, Kaminski HJ, Ross JS, et al: Spinal epidural abscess: A ten-year perspective. Neurosurgery 1990; 27:177–184.
133. Mamourian AC, Dickman CA, Drayer BP, et al: Spinal epidural abscess: Three cases following spinal epidural injection demonstrated with magnetic resonance imaging. Anesthesiology 1993; 78:204–207.
134. Loarie DJ, Fairley HB: Epidural abscess following spinal anesthesia. Anesth Analg 1978; 57:351–353.
135. Ngan Kee WD, Jones MR, Thomas P, et al: Extradural abscess complicating extradural anaesthesia for caesarean section. Br J Anaesth 1992; 69:647–652.
136. Epidural infection. *In* Bromage PR (ed): Epidural Analgesia. Philadelphia: WB Saunders; 1978: 682–690.
137. Baker AS, Ojemann RG, Swartz MN, et al: Spinal epidural abscess. N Engl J Med 1975; 293:463–468.
138. Danner RG, Hartman BJ: Update of spinal epidural abscess: 35 cases and a review of the literature. Rev Infect Dis 1987; 9:265–274.
139. Bromage PR: Neurologic complications of regional anesthesia for obstetrics. *In* Shnider SM, Levinson G (eds): Anesthesia for Obstetrics, 3rd ed. Baltimore, Williams & Wilkins; 1993: 444–446.
140. Chestnut DH: Spinal anesthesia in the febrile patient [editorial]. Anesthesiology 1992; 76:667–669.
141. Hunt JR, Rigor BM Sr, Collins JR: The potential for contamination of continuous epidural catheters. Anesth Analg 1977; 56:222–225.
142. Feldman JM, Chapin-Robertson K, Turner J: Do agents used for epidural analgesia have antimicrobial properties? Reg Anesth 1994; 19:43–47.
143. Sakuragi T, Ishino H, Dan K: Bactericidal activity of clinically used local anesthetics on *Staphylococcus aureus*. Reg Anesth 1996; 21:239–242.
144. Rota S, Kaya K, Timiodlu O, et al: Do the opioids have an antibacterial effect? Can J Anaesth 1997; 44:679–680.
145. Verner EF, Musher DM: Spinal epidural abscess. Med Clin North Am 1985; 69:375–384.
146. Berman RS, Eisele JH: Bacteremia, spinal anesthesia and development of meningitis. Anesthesiology 1978; 48:376–377.
147. Sghirlanzoni A, Marazzi R, Pareyson D, et al: Epidural anaesthesia and spinal arachnoiditis. Anaesthesia 1989; 44:317–321.
148. Ready LB, Helfer D: Bacterial meningitis in parturients after epidural anesthesia. Anesthesiology 1989; 71:988–990.
149. Berga S, Trierweiller MW: Bacterial meningitis following epidural anesthesia for vaginal delivery: A case report. Obstet Gynecol 1989; 74:437–439.
150. Bert AA, Laasberg LH: Aseptic meningitis following spinal anesthesia: A complication of the past? Anesthesiology 1985; 62:674–677.
151. Blackmore TK, Morley HR, Gordon DL: *Streptococcus mitis*-induced bacteremia and meningitis after spinal anesthesia. Anesthesiology 1993; 78:592–594.
152. Eng RHK, Seligman SJ: Lumbar puncture–induced meningitis. JAMA 1981; 245:1456–1459.
153. Smith KM, Deddish RB, Ogata ES: Meningitis associated with serial lumbar punctures and post-hemorrhagic hydrocephalus. J Pediatr 1986; 109:1057–1060.
154. Barrie HJ: Meningitis following spinal anesthesia. Lancet 1941; 1:242.
155. Roberts SP, Petts HV: Meningitis after obstetric spinal anaesthesia. Anaesthesia 1990; 45:376–377.
156. Moore DC, Bridenbaugh LD: Spinal (subarachnoid) block: A review of 11,574 cases. JAMA 1966; 195:907–912.
157. Wedel DJ, Horlocker TT: Risks of regional anesthesia: Infectious, septic. Reg Anesth 1996; 21:57–61.
158. Carp H, Bailey S: The association between meningitis and dural puncture in bacteremic rats. Anesthesiology 1992; 76:739–742.
159. Shapiro ED, Aaron NH, Wald ER, et al: Risk factors for the development of bacterial meningitis among children with occult bacteremia. J Pediatr 1986; 109:15–19.
160. Harding SA, Collis RE, Morgan BM: Meningitis after combined spinal-extradural anaesthesia in obstetrics. Br J Anaesth 1994; 73:545–547.
161. Cascio M, Heath G: Meningitis following a combined spinal-epidural technique in a labouring term parturient. Can J Anaesth 1996; 43:399–402.
162. Thomas DG: Epidural analgesia in the presence of fever [letter]. Anaesthesia 1986; 41:553–554.
163. Marx GF, Hodgkinson R: Special considerations in complications of pregnancy. *In* Marx GF, Bassell GM (eds): Obstetric Analgesia and Anesthesia. New York: Elsevier; 1980: 329–330.
164. Way WL, Trevor AJ: Ketamine. *In* Miller RD (ed): Anesthesia, 2nd ed. New York: Churchill Livingstone; 1986: 813.
165. Reich DL, Silvay G: Ketamine: An update on the first twenty-five years of clinical experience. Can J Anaesth 1989; 36:186–197.
166. Kohlschutter B, Baur H, Roth F: Suxamethonium-induced hyperkalemia in patients with severe intra-abdominal infections. Br J Anaesth 1976; 48:557–562.
167. American College of Obstetricians and Gynecologists: Anesthesia for emergency deliveries. ACOG Committee Opinion No. 104. Washington, DC, March 1992.

29

Antepartum Hemorrhage

❖ Katsuo Terui, MD

OBSTETRIC HEMORRHAGE

Obstetric hemorrhage is an age-old problem; a phrase popular among physicians is "obstetrics is a bloody business." However, at the present time it is emerging as a new problem with increasing frequency. New information continues to be reported on the epidemiology of obstetric hemorrhage, and its management continues to change. These investigations suggest that the frequency of placenta previa is increasing because of the increased cesarean section rate, and that the abruptio placentae incidence has not decreased. The incidence of uterine rupture or dehiscence appears to be increasing because of the practice of vaginal birth after cesarean section (VBAC). Emergency peripartum hysterectomy is more frequently performed for placenta accreta, which is increased because of the high cesarean section rate associated with placenta previa in recent years. These changes in obstetric hemorrhage reflect changing obstetric practice. VBAC is now an established practice in many regions of the world. Obstetric practice for placenta previa has also changed dramatically over the past three decades, from expectant inpatient management to outpatient management in selected patients, which may result in more patients requiring emergency anesthetic management.

On the other hand, there is little clinically relevant new information in the anesthesiology literature to guide our practice; although several new important studies and case reports exist. This chapter aims to review and update this important subject and discusses the anesthetic management strategy for each cause of hemorrhage. Emphasis is placed on peripartum hysterectomy, as well as modalities to reduce blood transfusion, such as uterine artery embolization and autologous blood donation.

Classification

Obstetric hemorrhage is classified as either antepartum or postpartum, depending on the timing of bleeding in relation to delivery. Antepartum hemorrhage is usually caused by placenta previa or abruptio placentae. The most frequent cause of postpartum hemorrhage is laceration to the genital tract, followed by uterine atony and retained placenta. Major causes of obstetric hemorrhage and their incidences are shown in Table 29–1.

Maternal Mortality

Maternal death due to obstetric hemorrhage has been lowered by the increased number of hospital deliveries and availability of blood products. For example, maternal mortality due to hemorrhage in Massachusetts has decreased to one tenth of its former rate, from 3.8 per 100,000 live births in the mid-1950s to 0.3 in the mid-1980s.[1] During the same period, in Japan, maternal mortality from hemorrhage has decreased from 48 per 100,000 live births in 1955 to 5.4 per 100,000 total births in 1985.[2] Maternal mortality from hemorrhage in Japan is now 1.5 per 100,000 total births.[2]

Obstetric hemorrhage remains a leading cause of maternal death, however, even in modern obstetric practice. The Centers for Disease Control and Prevention analyzed 1453 pregnancy-related maternal deaths in the United States from 1987 through 1990 and reported that hemorrhage was a direct cause in at least 29% of these deaths.[3] Hemorrhage was the leading cause of pregnancy-related mortality, followed by embolism and pregnancy-induced hypertension. This figure coincides with the hemorrhage-related mortality rate in Japan in 1996[2] (25.9% of all maternal deaths). Even now, one third to one fourth of maternal deaths are attributable to hemorrhage. The maternal mortality rate as well as the hemorrhage-related mortality rate appears to have plateaued in Japan in recent years, as shown in Figure 29–1. Further efforts to lower the hemorrhage-related mortality and morbidity rates are needed, and some of these efforts are discussed later in this chapter.

■ Table 29-1 CAUSES OF OBSTETRIC HEMORRHAGE

CAUSES	INCIDENCE PER DELIVERY
Antepartum Hemorrhage	
Abruptio placentae	1:150
Placenta previa	1:200
Vasa previa	—
Postpartum Hemorrhage	
Lacerations of vagina or cervix	1:8
Uterine atony	1:100
Retained placenta	1:160
Rupture of the uterus	1:2300
Placenta accreta	1:2500
Inversion of the uterus	1:6400

Modified from American College of Obstetricians and Gynecologists: hemorrhagic shock. ACOG Technical Bulletin 82, p.1. Washington, DC, ACOG, 1984.

Data from Shah-Hosseini R: Puerperal uterine inversion. Obstet Gynecol 1989; 73:567; Miller DA, Chollet JA, Goodwin TM: Clinical risk factors for placenta previa–placenta accreta. Am J Obstet Gynecol 1997; 177:210; Eden RD, Parker RT, Gall SA: Rupture of the pregnant uterus: a 53-year review. Obstet Gynecol 1986; 68:671.

Perinatal Outcome

Bleeding poses risk to both fetus and mothers. According to Lipitz et al.,[4] among women with uterine bleeding between 14 and 26 weeks' gestation, total fetal loss including abortions and perinatal deaths was 32%. About one fourth of the fetal loss was associated with placental abruption, and placenta previa was noted in 18% of fetal loss. In women without abruption or previa, who bled after 26 weeks' gestation, adverse perinatal outcome was noted in one third of the cases, mostly preterm delivery.[5] The impact of obstetric hemorrhage on fetal outcome is discussed in detail in each disease.

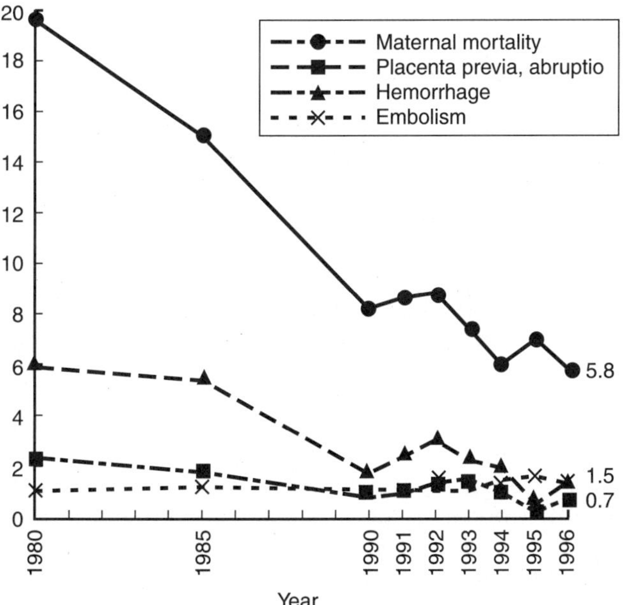

❖ **Figure 29-1** Maternal mortality in Japan (per 100,00 total births). (From Statistics and Information Department, Minister's Secretariat, Ministry of Health and Welfare: Vital Statistics of Japan, vol 1. 1996, p 310.)

MATERNAL ADAPTATIONS TO PREGNANCY AND RESPONSE TO BLOOD LOSS

Because normal delivery is accompanied by some bleeding, pregnant patients have physiologic adaptations in preparation for blood loss. These include increased blood volume and red blood cell mass, hypercoagulable state, and involution of uterus after delivery. These physiologic alterations modify patients' response to hemorrhage.

Blood Loss with Vaginal or Abdominal Delivery

Usual blood loss with different modes of delivery has been reported by several investigators.[6–8] For vaginal delivery, more than 60% of women lose less than 500 mL of blood, but about 30% lose 500 to 1000 mL. During cesarean section, mean blood loss is approximately 1000 mL for elective cesarean section, 1400 mL for elective cesarean hysterectomy,[7] and 3000 to 3300 mL for emergency cesarean hysterectomy.[7, 8] A more recent article from Hong Kong reported that blood loss with elective lower segment cesarean section was usually less than 500 mL (range 164–1438 mL), and was estimated with reasonable accuracy (60 mL difference).[9] The amount of blood loss is correlated with the degree of blood volume reduction in Table 29–2.

Physiologic Alterations During Pregnancy

Pregnancy is well known to cause various physiologic changes, and cardiovascular changes are among the most prominent. Cardiac output increases by approximately 50% at term, due to increased stroke volume and heart rate. Both of these appear to contribute almost evenly to the increased cardiac output.[10, 11] Blood volume also significantly increases during pregnancy by 45% (approximately 1.5 L) at term.[12] The increase in plasma volume exceeds the change in red cell mass, resulting in dilutional anemia of pregnancy. This increased red cell mass and blood volume protect parturients from the sequelae that might be expected to follow a blood loss of 500 mL during vaginal delivery.

■ Table 29-2 AMOUNT OF BLOOD LOSS AND REDUCTION OF BLOOD VOLUME IN PREGNANT WOMEN

CLASS	ACUTE BLOOD LOSS (mL)	% LOST
1	900	15
2	1200-1500	20-25
3	1800-2000	30-35
4	2400	40

From Baker RN: Hemorrhage in obstetrics. Obstet Gynecol Annu 1977; 6:295.

Most of the clotting factors are elevated during pregnancy, except for factors XI and XIII.[13] Although increased clotting factors may expose parturients to a higher risk of thromboembolic events, it may also be part of the protective mechanism for reducing blood loss during parturition. Fibrinolysis decreases during pregnancy, but the onset of labor results in a dramatic increase in fibrinolysis. The placenta is implicated in the reduction of fibrinolytic activity.[14]

Maternal Response to Hemorrhage

A decrease in systemic vascular resistance by 21% accompanies an increase in cardiac output during pregnancy,[10] thus maintaining blood pressure at prepregnant levels. Low-resistance placental circulation may function as an "arteriovenous fistula" and further contributes to the lowered systemic vascular resistance. Although the fetus may benefit from uteroplacental circulation that is maintained by maximal vasodilation, lack of vascular autoregulation can be hazardous to the mother when faced with hemorrhagic shock. During massive blood loss, the normal vasoconstrictor response to elevate systemic vascular resistance may be impeded by the arteriovenous fistula comprising the uteroplacental circulation. Owing to the increase in circulating blood volume, many pregnant women do not demonstrate blood pressure changes after moderate blood loss. Tachycardia as a sign of hypovolemia may be often overlooked because of the baseline increase in heart rate or frequently observed tachycardia related to tocolytic medications.

MANAGEMENT OF MASSIVE HEMORRHAGE

Management of obstetric patients with severe hemorrhage is an integral part of current anesthesia practice. In this section, the practice of fluid resuscitation and massive transfusion is reviewed briefly, with some considerations that are unique to parturients.

Assessment of Blood Loss in Parturients

Assessment of blood loss is somewhat difficult in parturients because of the increased blood volume during pregnancy and concomitant administration of a variety of vasoactive and sympathomimetic drugs. The degree of blood loss and correlating clinical signs are shown in Table 29–3. Hypotension is usually a late sign of blood loss, as heart rate increases in parturients to compensate for the blood loss. However, some patients may already have mild tachycardia due to pain from uterine contraction or from tocolytic agents. In patients with preexisting hypertension due to preeclampsia, normal blood pressure may indicate significant blood loss. In addition, it is common to underestimate the amount of the vaginal bleeding, as shown by Duthie et al.[15] They compared laboratory determination of blood loss during normal delivery with the visual estimation and found an underestimation of blood loss by 35%. The discrepancy tends to be greater as the amount of blood loss increases. All these factors make it necessary to carefully evaluate bleeding parturients from all aspects, including vital signs, subjective symptoms, presence of fetal compromise, and urine output.

Laboratory studies such as hemoglobin concentration or hematocrit are not very helpful in determining the degree of blood loss in the acute phase, because these results will not immediately decrease during acute blood loss. They will decrease only after time and after adequate fluid replacement is provided. The presence of metabolic acidosis in arterial blood gas analysis is alarming and may indicate inadequate oxygen delivery to the tissue.

Table 29–3 Clinical Staging of Hemorrhagic Shock by Volume of Blood Loss

Severity of Shock	Clinical Findings	% Blood Loss
None	None	up to 15–20
Mild	Tachycardia (<100 beats/min) Mild hypotension Peripheral vasoconstriction	20–25
Moderate	Tachycardia (100–120 beats/min) Hypotension (80–100 mm Hg) Restlessness Oliguria	25–35
Severe	Tachycardia (>120 beats/min) Hypotension (<60 mm Hg) Altered consciousness Anuria	>35

From Gonik B: Intensive care monitoring of the critically ill pregnant patient. *In* Creasy RK, Resnik R (eds): Maternal-Fetal Medicine: Principles and Practice, 3rd ed. Philadelphia: WB Saunders; 1994: 880.

Intravenous Access

When managing a hemorrhaging parturient, adequate intravenous access is the key to successful fluid resuscitation. At least two large-bore peripheral intravenous lines should be placed in the upper extremities or a jugular vein. Because of compression of the inferior vena cava by the enlarged uterus, intravenous access in lower extremities may not be helpful in restoring blood volume and venous return. The size and the length of the indwelling intravenous catheter determine the speed of fluid administration. To administer 1 L of fluid, it can take 30 minutes with an 18-gauge cannula, whereas it takes only 9 minutes with a 14-gauge cannula by gravity alone. By adding 300 mm Hg constant pressure, the time for administration can be shortened to 3.5 minutes for a 14-gauge cannula.[16] Generally, a 14- or 16-gauge cannula placed at the antecubital area, or an 8 French cordis placed at the internal jugular vein is recommended for massively bleeding parturients. Constant attention needs to be paid to avoid air injection when using pressurizing devices.

Fluid Replacement

Initial fluid replacement for hemorrhaging parturients begins with administration of crystalloid solution, which should always be readily available. The amount of crystalloid necessary to replace blood loss is approximately three times the amount lost. Lactated Ringer's solution or isotonic saline are most frequently administered. The chloride content of isotonic saline is higher than that of plasma (154 mEq/L vs. 103 mEq/L), and it may cause hyperchloremic metabolic acidosis following administration of a large volume. Although hyperchloremia has been reported, acidosis is rare.[17, 18] Lactated Ringer's or Hartmann's solution contains potassium and calcium in concentrations similar to those in plasma; however, the sodium and chloride content is lower than in isotonic saline. This results in the reduction of sodium as well as chloride concentration. There is no evidence that the lactate in Ringer's solution provides any buffer effect.[19] Acetated Ringer's solution may also be administered, but there is a possibility of peripheral vasodilation. Probably, the type of fluid is less important than the amount of volume replacement for hemorrhaging parturients. Hypertonic saline has been investigated in fluid resuscitation for hemorrhagic shock, but its safety is questionable for the fetus, and its efficacy has not been shown in parturients.

Colloid solution may be more efficacious in fluid resuscitation, because less volume is required to replace the blood loss than crystalloids. Figure 29–2 shows the effects of various crystalloid or colloid solutions on the volume of extracellular fluid compartments. One liter of 5% albumin increases plasma volume by 500 mL, whereas 1 L of isotonic saline increases it by only 275 mL. Colloid solutions currently available are listed in Table 29–4. Albumin is available in 5% or 25% solution and considered to be free of risk of infection after heat treatment. Twenty-five percent albumin increases plasma volume up to four to five times that of infused volume by drawing fluid from the interstitial space. Thus, it should not be used in volume resuscitation in hypovolemia.

Hetastarch is a synthetic colloid available as 6% solution in isotonic saline. It is composed of the amylopectin molecules of various sizes, with number-average molecular weight (Mn) similar to albumin (69,000). Its serum half-life is as long as 17 days, but the oncotic effects of hetastarch disappears within 24 hours.[17] It has the advantage of lower cost compared with albumin, but it carries the rare risk of anaphylactic reaction (0.0004%).[20] Also, it is known to interact with coagulation factor VIII and can result in prolonged partial thromboplastin time (PTT). A recent review by Warren and Durieux[21] summarizes the literature regarding its effect on coagulation. The authors concluded that, in the absence of an elaborate and large-scale study, it is reasonable to assume that hetastarch will reduce levels of the coagulation factors including fibrinogen, factor VIII, and von Willebrand's factor, and also reduce platelet function. They stated that these effects appear to be independent of the dose given, and the manufacturer's guideline of 20 mL/kg is not supported by the published data. Pentastarch is a low molecular weight derivative of hetastarch, and it is available as a 10% solution in isotonic saline. It contains smaller but more numerous starch molecules (Mn: 120,000) than hetastarch and thus has a higher colloid osmotic pressure. It is more effective as a volume expander than hetastarch and can increase plasma volume by 1.5 times the infusion volume. Pentastarch appears to have less tendency to interact with coagulation proteins than hetastarch, but the significance of this tendency is not clear.[19] Hetastarch up to 1000 mL has been administered in several studies to prevent spinal anesthesia–induced hypotension before cesarean section. There were no apparent adverse effects other than dilutional anemia in the mothers. Transplacental transfer of hetastarch was not demonstrated when studied in a sheep preparation.[22]

Dextran, another type of colloid, is a glucose polymer produced by a bacterium incubated in a sucrose medium. Dextran 40 has a Mn of 26,000, while dextran 70 has a Mn of 41,000. Dextran 40 is available in 10% solution, while dextran 70 is provided in 6% solution. They are both hyperoncotic, but the effect of dextran 40 lasts for only a few hours. The disadvantages of dextran include dose-related bleeding tendency, due to inhibition of platelet aggregation, reduction in activation of factor VIII, and promotion of fibrinolysis.[20]

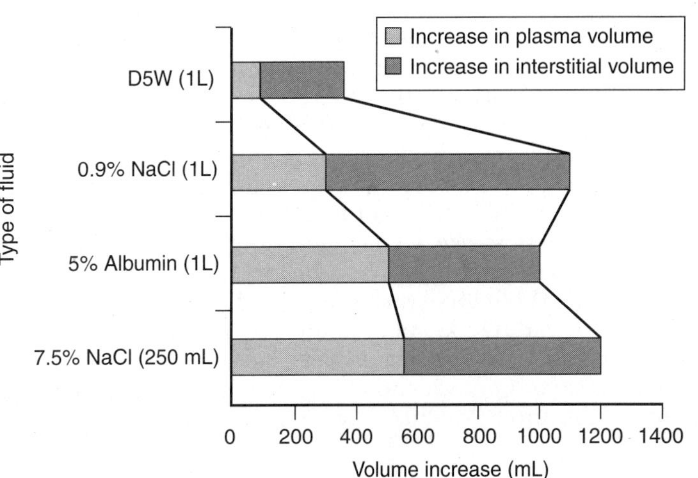

Figure 29–2 Influence of colloid and crystalloid fluids on the volume of extracellular fluid compartments. (Data from Imm A, Carlson RW: Fluid resuscitation in circulatory shock. Crit Care Clin 1993; 9:313.)

Table 29-4 Characteristics of Intravenous Colloid Fluids

Fluid	Molecular Weight (Mn)	Oncotic Pressure (mm Hg)	Plasma Volume Expansion per Infused Volume	Serum Half-Life	Side Effects
5% Albumin	69,000	20	0.7–1.3	16 h	
25% Albumin	69,000	70	4.0–5.0	16 h	
6% Hetastarch	69,000	30	1.0–1.3	17 days	coagulopathy
10% Pentastarch	120,000	40	1.5	10 h	
10% Dextran 40	26,000	40	1.0–1.5	6 h	bleeding tendency
6% Dextran 70	41,000	40	0.8	12 h	anaphylaxis acute renal failure

From Marino PL: Colloid and crystalloid resuscitation. *In* The ICU Book, 2nd ed. Baltimore: Williams & Wilkins; 1998: 234.

Data from Griffel MI, Kaufman BS: Pharmacology of colloids and crystalloids. Crit Care Clin 1992; 8:235; Imm A, Carlson RW: Fluid resuscitation in circulatory shock. Crit Care Clin 1993; 9:313.

Anaphylactic reactions were reduced from 5% in early reports to 0.032% as the current incidence.[20] Dextrans can interfere with the ability to cross-match blood by coating red blood cell surfaces. It has also been implicated as a cause of acute renal failure, presumably due to a hyperoncotic state with reduced filtration pressure. Thus, dextrans are not commonly used in fluid resuscitation of obstetric patients, although they have been tried for volume preloading before cesarean section.

Transfusion Practice

The decision to transfuse based on the conventional wisdom of an optimal hemoglobin concentration of 10 g/dL has been challenged in the era of homologous transfusion-related disease transmission and complications. The National Institute of Health Consensus Development Conference stated that "otherwise healthy patients with hemoglobin values of 100 g/L or greater rarely require perioperative transfusion, whereas those with acute anemia with resulting hemoglobin values of less than 70 g/L frequently will require red blood cell transfusions."[23] The American Society of Anesthesiologists Practice Guidelines for Blood Component Therapy[24] could not suggest a single trigger, but stated that red blood cell transfusion is usually indicated when the hemoglobin level is less than 6 g/dL.

In a recent study, however, acute isovolemic reduction of Hb concentration to 5 g/dL in conscious, healthy, resting humans did not produce evidence of inadequate systemic oxygen delivery.[25] The authors studied 11 conscious, healthy patients prior to anesthesia and 21 volunteers not undergoing surgery. They were made acutely anemic to hemoglobin concentration of 5 g/dL, but isovolemia was maintained with 5% albumin or autologous plasma or both. The authors observed an increased heart rate from 58 to 92 beats/min, increased stroke volume index from 52 to 62 mL/m^2, and increased cardiac index from 3.05 to 5.71 L/min/m^2. Although oxygen transport decreased from 13.5 to 10.7 mL O_2/kg/min, oxygen consumption did not decrease, and plasma lactate did not increase. Thus, there was no evidence of inadequate tissue oxygenation in these patients. Their result, however, cannot be directly applied to anesthetized patients with reduced compensatory increase in heart rate or cardiac output. Also, parturients with preexisting higher cardiac output may have less reserve to compensate for this degree of acute anemia. However, this study illustrates the importance of maintaining isovolemia in the setting of acute anemia. A complete recovery has been reported in a parturient with admission Hb concentration of 3 g/dL due to abruption and disseminated intravascular coagulation (DIC). Cesarean section was performed in a 1700 g fetus with distress, but both the mother and the baby survived without sequelae.[26]

If transfusion of blood is urgently necessary without sufficient time to perform a complete three-phase cross-match, type-specific, partially cross-matched blood can be given first. This procedure is fast, taking less than 5 minutes, and eliminates serious hemolytic reactions from errors in ABO typing. ABO-Rh typing alone results in a 99.8% chance of compatible transfusion, whereas complete cross-matching raises this to 99.95%.[27] When the situation is more urgent, type-specific, non–cross-matched blood may have to be transfused. Rarely, O-negative blood is used in emergency transfusion when typing or cross-matching is not available. Type O blood may be safer than non–cross-matched type-specific blood, because of laboratory error, clerical error, or patient misidentification.[28] When transfusing type O blood, O-negative packed red blood cell (PRBC) is preferred to O-negative whole blood, because PRBCs have a smaller amount of plasma containing anti-A and anti-B antibodies. If more than two units of O-negative, non–cross-matched whole blood are required during emergency transfusion, continuation with O-negative blood is recommended throughout the resuscitation of the patient, to prevent major intravascular hemolysis of subsequent donor cells of the patient's own blood type.[27] The same recommendation has been made even for O-negative PRBCs.[29] However, some patients may continue to lose large amounts of blood and take a longer time to be stabilized. It is not practical to continue O-negative blood transfusion for an extended period of time, considering the limited availability of type-O negative blood; especially in Japan, Rh-negative blood type is found in only 0.57% of the population. As the amount of anti-A and anti-B antibody transfer during PRBC transfusion is minimal, the Ministry of Health in Japan recommends switching back to the patient's original blood type as soon as it is determined. It also recommends that after a significant amount of type O PRBCs has been transfused, the decision to transfuse the patient's original blood type is made on the cross-match with the most recent blood sample from the recipient. To summarize, after type O PRBC transfusion and determination of the patient's blood type, the patient can be safely switched to the specific type needed or a compatible blood type.[30] After type O whole blood transfusion, the type-specific blood can be transfused after the anti-A and anti-B titer has fallen to low enough levels. During a time of blood shortage, one should not feel constrained to only transfuse ABO/Rh-specific blood to the patient. The use of PRBCs that are not ABO identical but are compatible is an effective means of increasing the number of available units during a shortage.[28]

If bleeding tendency is observed without clot formation during transfusion of multiple units of PRBCs, dilutional thrombocytopenia, low coagulation factors such as V and VIII, DIC, or hemolytic transfusion reaction should be suspected. For patients having massive transfusion of 10 to 15 units of PRBCs, or for those with a tendency toward clinical bleeding, prothrombin time (PT), activated PTT (aPTT), platelet counts, and fibrinogen levels need to be checked to determine the need for transfusion of fresh frozen plasma, platelets, or cryoprecipitate. Dilutional thrombocytopenia is frequently the cause of bleeding tendency following massive transfusion, but platelet levels rarely fall below 100,000/mm^3 until approximately 1.5 times the patient's blood volume has been replaced.[31] Dilution of coagulation factors during massive transfusion to a level of 30% functional activity may be associated with prolongation of PT and aPTT.[30] Obstetric patients are prone to develop DIC; therefore, laboratory determination of the cause of bleeding tendency is essential in guiding the choice of the different blood component transfusions. Commonly used blood products and their effects on blood counts and laboratory results are summarized in Table 29–5. In a few institutions, use of a thromboelastogram is becoming popular; however, further clinical studies are necessary before thromboelastography is used routinely in such situations.

Complications of Massive Transfusion

Massive transfusion can cause dilutional thrombocytopenia and dilutional coagulopathy, which can be treated by appropriate blood component transfusion. Other complications include hyperkalemia, metabolic acidosis followed by metabolic alkalosis (due to citrate load), hypothermia from infusion of inadequately warmed blood products, and citrate intoxication.

Hyperkalemia can be caused by the steady leakage from erythrocytes in stored blood products. The potassium load after 14 days of storage is 4.4 mEq per unit of whole blood and 3.1 mEq per unit of PRBC.[32] After 21 days of storage, it rises to 6.7 mEq and 3.5 mEq per unit of whole blood and PRBC, respectively (data from the Japanese Red Cross). This potassium load does not usually cause a problem because potassium reenters red cells within a few hours and the kidney rapidly clears the potassium load. However, in the presence of circulatory shock, the extra potassium from a blood transfusion can accumulate and produce hyperka-

Table 29–5 BLOOD PRODUCTS USED FOR OBSTETRIC HEMORRHAGE

BLOOD COMPONENT	CONTENT IN EACH UNIT	EFFECT
Packed red blood cell (PRBC)	Hct 70% to 80% in 300 mL volume Plasma 70 mL Total K load 5.5 mEq at expiration	Increased Hb by 1 g/dL Increased Hct by 3%
Irradiated PRBC	Total K load 5.5 mEq at 21 days	
Whole blood	450 mL donor blood 63 mL anticoagulant (CPDA-1) Total K load 15 mEq Decreased coagulation factors Lost platelets	Increased Hct Volume expansion
Irradiated whole blood	Total K load 9.3 mEq at 21 days	
Platelet concentrates	Plasma 50 mL/unit Usual adult dose 4–6 units	Increased platelet count by 7000–10,000/mm^3
Fresh frozen plasma (FFP)	Volume 200–280 mL More than 70% of procoagulant activity preserved Fibrinogen level 1–2 mg/mL	2 units raise procoagulant by about 20% and fibrinogen level by about 40 mg/dL
Cryoprecipitate	Factor VIII 80–100 U Fibrinogen 100–250 mg vWF 40–70% of original plasma	2–4 U/10 kg maintains fibrinogen level above 100 mg/dL

Modified from Terui K: Anesthesia for postpartum hemorrhage. *In* Datta S (ed): Common Problems in Obstetric Anesthesia, 2nd ed. St. Louis: Mosby; 1995: 196.

Data from Hoffman R, Benz EJ Jr, Shattil SJ, et al (eds): Hematology: Basic Principles and Practice, 2nd ed. New York: Churchill Livingstone; 1995; Japanese Red Cross, 1997.

lemia. Caution must also be exercised when administering irradiated blood products. After irradiation of blood products with 25 Gy and 21 days of storage, the potassium concentration can increase to 9.3 mEq per bag of whole blood and 5.5 mEq per bag of PRBC (data from the Japanese Red Cross). Thus, blood products containing red blood cells should be transfused soon after irradiation when used for massive transfusion. The treatments for hyperkalemia include calcium administration, glucose-insulin infusion, and sodium bicarbonate. There is no recommended dosage of these treatments specific to parturients, and the treatment may follow standard adult protocol. Although it is likely that most of the resuscitation drugs cross the placenta and may affect the fetus, stabilization of the mother is of utmost importance for antepartum resuscitation.

Citrate intoxication can be seen with massive transfusion or liver dysfunction. Citrate used for blood anticoagulation and preservation chelates calcium and may result in hypocalcemia. Signs and symptoms of hypocalcemia include central nervous system or muscle irritability, hypotension, narrow pulse pressure, and prolonged Q-T interval. Citrate intoxication rarely is observed in the healthy adult patient, in whom citrate is quickly metabolized by the liver, but it may be observed when the patient has preexisting liver disease or hypothermia, or when citrate-containing blood (fresh frozen plasma or whole blood) is quickly transfused (faster than about 1 unit of blood/5 min). Calcium administration may become necessary on these occasions. These complications of massive transfusion need to be anticipated and prevented, rather than treated after complications arise.

ABRUPTIO PLACENTAE

Abruptio placentae (placental abruption) is defined as the premature separation of the normally implanted placenta. Placental abruption can be total or partial and may result in external hemorrhage or concealed hemorrhage (Fig. 29–3). Placental abruption with concealed hemorrhage is the most problematic, because it can be associated with DIC and the extent of hemorrhage not appreciated. Maternal mortality has ranged from 0% to 3.1% but may be much higher, depending on the facilities available to physicians treating the patient.[33]

Incidence

The reported incidence of placental abruption averages 1 in 150 deliveries.[34] In the largest study from Norway during the period of 1967 through 1991, the incidence was 0.66%, or 1 in 150, among 1,446,154 births.[35] The incidence of abruption continued to increase in this report. The perinatal mortality rate in this population decreased from 25% in 1967 to 9% in 1991.[36] Saftlas et al.[37] surveyed the National Hospital Discharge Survey in the United States and also found that the incidence of abruption increased significantly in the United States from 1979 to 1987. Conversely, the frequency of severe placental abruption is decreasing at Parkland Hospital. The incidence of abruption severe enough to result in fetal death has decreased from 1 in 420 deliveries reported from 1956 through 1967 to 1 in 830 deliveries from 1974 through 1989.[38] This is likely to be the result of the availability of emergency transport and the decrease in grand multiparous women.

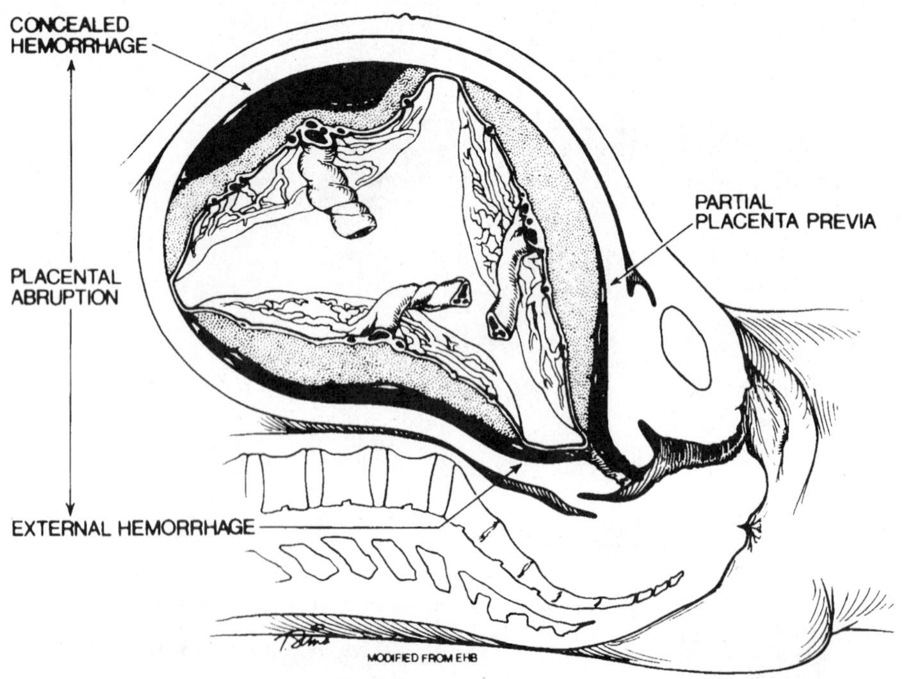

❖ **Figure 29–3** Hemorrhage from premature placental separation. (From Obstetrical hemorrhage. *In* Cunningham FG, MacDonald PC, Gant NF, et al (eds): Williams Obstetrics, 20th ed. Stamford, CT: Appleton & Lange, 1997: 747. With permission McGraw-Hill Companies.)

Risk Factors

Although the primary cause of placental abruption is unknown, there are several associated conditions, or risk factors. The most commonly associated condition is either pregnancy-induced or chronic hypertension. In the Parkland Hospital study of 408 cases of severe placental abruption causing fetal death, maternal hypertension was apparent in about half of the women once the depleted intravascular compartment was adequately refilled.[38] Also, the incidence of abruption was highest among patients with eclampsia (23%), followed by chronic hypertension (10%) and preeclampsia (2.3%).[39] In the recent meta-analysis, Ananth et al.[40] reported that the risk of abruption is strongly associated with chronic hypertension, premature rupture of the membranes, and abruption in a prior pregnancy. The association with preeclampsia was of lesser importance.[40] On the other hand, Morgan et al.[41] found that hypertensive women were more likely to suffer a more severe abruption. The University of Tokyo's experience from 1973 through 1988 showed a similar incidence of placental abruption (0.4%), and preeclampsia was noted in 22% of the cases. There was also a higher fetal demise rate (24%).[42]

Preterm premature rupture of membranes has been associated with premature placental separation. Ananth et al.[40] found a threefold risk of abruption with prematurely ruptured membranes. Sudden uterine decompression during amniocentesis may also cause placental abruption, especially in women with polyhydramnios. Other associated conditions include maternal age (younger than 25, older than 35), high parity, cigarette smoking, ethanol consumption, cocaine abuse, external trauma, and uterine leiomyoma.[34] Other etiologic determinants of abruptio placentae include severe small for gestational age birth, prolonged premature rupture of membranes, chorioamnionitis, unmarried status, and male fetal gender.[43]

Pathophysiology

In placental abruption, rupture of the spiral artery results in bleeding into the decidua basalis. The decidua is dissected and a thin layer is left adherent to the myometrium. A retroplacental hematoma then forms and may expand, further separating the placenta and involving more vessels. As the uterus is distended by the products of conception, it is unable to contract and compress the torn vessels effectively, thus persistent retroplacental bleeding ensues. As this process continues, there is progressive loss of placental function. In some cases, the maternal blood escapes into the amniotic cavity, but more frequently, it tracks between the membranes and the uterine wall, ultimately escaping via the cervix; the time for this process varies depending on the site of the placenta, the degree of separation, the adherence of the membranes, the size of the hematoma, the compliance of the uterus, and the blood pressure of the patient.[33] On some occasions, retained or concealed hemorrhage is observed when placental margin is still adherent to the myometrium, or the fetal head is so closely applied to the lower uterine segment as to prevent blood from escaping to the cervix. Chronic placental abruption can be observed when retroplacental hematoma formation somehow arrests completely.

As intrauterine pressure increases, tissue thromboplastin and amniotic debris may be forced through open venous sinuses into the maternal circulation. This may explain the increased incidence of amniotic fluid embolism and DIC seen in patients with abruptio placentae.

Placental abruption results in placental separation, maternal hemorrhage, fetal hemorrhage, and uterine hypertonus in varying degrees. All of these can cause decreased uteroplacental perfusion and contribute to the development of fetal compromise. Prompt delivery is required in most cases (Fig. 29–4).

Perinatal Outcome

Stillbirths from abruptio placentae have become especially prominent as those from other causes have decreased appreciably in recent years. For example, of all third-trimester stillbirths with over 40,000 deliveries at Parkland Hospital during the period of 1992 through 1994, 12% were the consequence of placental abruption.[35] A similar frequency was reported by Fretts et al.,[44] who studied almost 89,000 births in Montreal between 1961 and 1988. Abruptio placentae had become the leading known cause and accounted for 15% of all fetal deaths.

Diagnosis

Clinical symptoms of placental abruption vary considerably. Some cases may present with profuse external

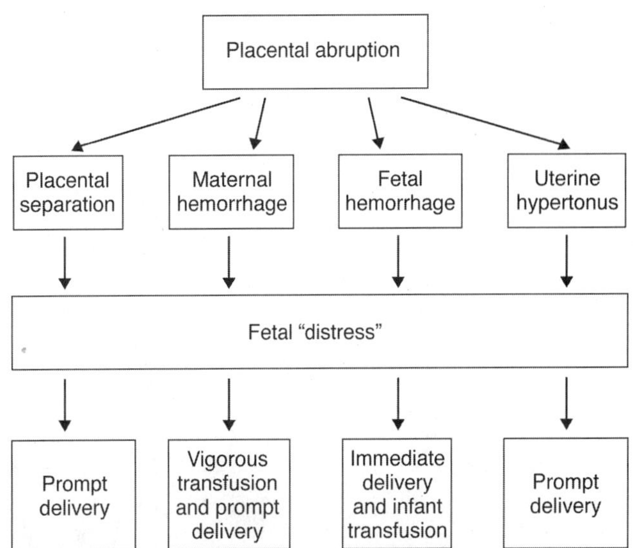

❖ **Figure 29–4** Various causes of fetal distress from placental abruption and their treatment. (From Obstetrical hemorrhage. *In* Cunningham FG, MacDonald PC, Gant NF, et al (eds): Williams Obstetrics, 20th ed. Stamford, CT: Appleton & Lange, 1997, p 752. With permission McGraw-Hill Companies.)

Table 29–6 SIGNS AND SYMPTOMS OF ABRUPTIO PLACENTAE

SIGN OR SYMPTOM	FREQUENCY (%)
Vaginal bleeding	78
Uterine tenderness or back pain	66
Fetal distress	60
High frequency contractions (17%)	34
Hypertonus (17%)	
Idiopathic preterm labor	22
Dead fetus	15

From Hurd WW, Miodovnik M, Hertzberg V, et al: Selective management of abruptio placentae: a prospective study. Obstet Gynecol 1983; 61:467.

bleeding but with minimal placental separation and a well fetus. Some may present with concealed hemorrhage and total placental separation, resulting in fetal demise. The classic signs and symptoms of abruptio placentae include abdominal pain, hemorrhage, uterine irritability or tenderness, coagulopathy, and fetal distress or death. Hurd et al.,[45] in a prospective study, identified the frequency of a variety of pertinent signs and symptoms (Table 29–6). It is important to note that they were able to recognize a retroplacental hematoma sonographically in only 1 of 59 cases. Thus, a negative finding with ultrasonographic examination does not exclude potentially life-threatening placental abruption.[34]

A clinical classification of abruptio placentae has been proposed by Page and colleagues and is shown in Table 29–7. As concealed hemorrhage is detected at the time of delivery in most cases, the clinical usefulness of this classification is limited.

There are neither laboratory tests nor diagnostic methods that accurately detect lesser degrees of placental separation. As stated earlier, ultrasonography is not reliable in detecting abruptio placentae. The cause of vaginal bleeding sometimes remains obscure even after delivery.[34] Some serum markers have been proposed as a diagnostic tool in placental abruption. Witt et al.[46] reported observations on the utility of maternal serum CA-125 antigen levels as a marker for placental abruption. They reported a sensitivity of 70% and specificity of 94% in the diagnosis of abruption. Thrombomodulin, an endothelial cell marker, was reported to be significantly elevated in women with placental abruption in a preliminary report.[47]

Obstetric Management

Treatment for placental abruption will vary depending on gestational age and the status of the mother and fetus. When external hemorrhage is massive, intensive resuscitation with blood or an electrolyte solution, or both, and prompt delivery are necessary to control hemorrhage. Stabilization and prompt delivery are lifesaving for the mother and maximize the chance of fetal survival. When the blood loss is occurring at a much slower rate, fetal gestational age and condition will become the main focus. If the fetus is alive and there is no evidence of fetal compromise, and if maternal hemorrhage is not causing serious hypovolemia or anemia, delivery can be delayed with very close observation in a facility where immediate intervention can be provided. When the fetus is immature, this conservative management may prove beneficial to the fetus. If the fetus is close to term, prompt delivery is usually most beneficial to both mother and fetus.

Cesarean section is reserved for usual obstetric indications. Fetal compromise with an unfavorable cervix necessitates cesarean section. Severe hemorrhage or worsening coagulopathy developing at a time remote from term can be an indication for urgent cesarean section. In one report, the cesarean section rate was 56% in hypertensive patients with abruption, whereas the rate was 35.6% in a nonhypertensive group.[39] Judicious use of abdominal delivery may well reduce surgery or anesthesia-related maternal morbidity. As long as the fetus is not distressed, cesarean section is generally reserved for situations in which bleeding is heavy and cervical dilation is not advanced. The physician should balance the risks of surgery against the risks of continued labor. With stable maternal hemodynamics in active labor with no fetal compromise, vaginal delivery can be pursued. Continuous electronic fetal monitoring is essential. However, lack of ominous decelerations does not guarantee the safety of the intrauterine environment for any period of time. The placenta may further separate at any instant and can seriously compromise the placental circulation, causing fetal death unless delivery is performed immediately. It is therefore mandatory to have adequate resources including personnel and blood products readily available if attempting vaginal delivery in these patients. Early notification of and consultation by the anesthesiologist are most helpful in case emergency cesarean section becomes necessary.

Table 29–7 CLASSIFICATION OF ABRUPTIO PLACENTAE BY PAGE

GRADE	CONCEALED HEMORRHAGE	UTERINE TENDERNESS	MATERNAL SHOCK	COAGULOPATHY (OVERT)	FETAL DISTRESS	COMMENTS
0	No	No	Absent	No	No	No symptoms
1	No	No	Absent	No	No	Blood loss variable
2	Yes	Yes	Absent	Rare	Yes	Usually progress to grade 3
3	Extensive	Yes	Present	Common	Fetal death	Major maternal complication

From Page EW, King EB, Merril JA: Abruptio placentae: dangers of delay in delivery. Obstet Gynecol 1954; 3:385.

If placental separation is severe enough to cause fetal death, vaginal delivery is preferred unless hemorrhage is so brisk that it cannot be successfully managed even by vigorous blood replacement, or there are other obstetric complications that prevent vaginal delivery.[34] Serious coagulation defects are especially troublesome with cesarean delivery. However, the best treatment for DIC is to deliver the fetus and placenta. The delivery should be accomplished within a reasonably short time, although there is no evidence that establishing an arbitrary time limit for delivery is necessary.

Anesthetic Management

Anesthetic management of bleeding parturients largely depends on the hemodynamic and coagulation status of the patient, as well as the fetal status. In evaluating these patients, one needs to keep in mind that normal blood pressure can be misleading, as pregnancy-induced or chronic hypertension is associated with abruption. Severity of hemorrhage is also difficult to evaluate, because of the possibility of concealed hemorrhage. Intravascular volume status of the patient can be estimated by following vital signs and urine output. Central venous pressure (CVP) monitoring may be helpful in adjusting fluid replacement, but it is often impractical to place the CVP catheter preoperatively. Invasive blood pressure monitoring is very helpful in severe or moderately severe cases. The presence of a coagulation abnormality often dictates the choice of anesthetic management, and it is therefore very important to detect coagulopathy preoperatively. This evaluation should be performed while fluid replacement and transfusion are being instituted.

When a bleeding patient is transferred from another institution, anesthesiologists usually do not have enough time to thoroughly evaluate the patient. The parturient may be rushed into the operating room as soon as the diagnosis of abruption is confirmed and blood products are sent for. Anesthesiologists as well as operating room staff need to be notified as soon as the transfer request is accepted by the obstetrician. Upon arrival of the patient to the labor and delivery suite, the anesthesiologist should evaluate the patient (especially her volume status and airway). Her medical and surgical history can be obtained while the patient is being evaluated by the obstetrician and prepared for cesarean section. Efficient and systematic evaluation in a short period, a concise explanation of the anesthetic management, and reassurance are helpful to these mothers who are often in abdominal pain and very anxious concerning the well-being of the baby.

Anesthesia for Vaginal Delivery

Vaginal delivery of a viable fetus is possible only in mild abruption without fetal compromise, uteroplacental insufficiency, hypovolemia, or coagulopathy. Anesthetic management should include avoidance of hypotension for maternal and fetal safety. After laboratory confirmation of the absence of coagulopathy, continuous epidural analgesia can be provided, if requested. The fetus may already have somewhat compromised uteroplacental blood flow, so judicious use of epidural local anesthetic and avoidance of hypotension are recommended. Close attention to fetal monitoring is also important.

Anesthesia for Cesarean Delivery

The urgency of cesarean delivery may vary considerably. Thus, good communication with the obstetrician is the key to successful outcome. The urgency of the situation can be appreciated by the anesthesiologist through exchanging information on the severity of abruption and fetal distress. "Fetal distress" can include a variety of fetal conditions, and not all of them require immediate cesarean section. It is very important to obtain information regarding the time frame within which the obstetrician wants to deliver the baby. Stat cesarean section with inadequate evaluation of the cardiovascular and airway status of the mother can compromise her safety.

If cesarean section is indicated for fetal jeopardy, and the patient is hemodynamically stable without coagulopathy, spinal anesthesia can usually be provided. Severe coagulopathy such as DIC is likely to be absent for several hours after the onset of abruptio placentae if the fetus is alive. Aspiration prophylaxis with an oral antacid is recommended regardless of the anesthetic method. Technical proficiency is required for spinal anesthesia in these situations. Helping hands are beneficial to preoxygenate the parturient during initiation of the regional anesthetic, so that one can switch to general anesthesia if difficulty in placement of spinal anesthesia or fetal bradycardia is encountered during the performance of the block. If the patient has previously received epidural analgesia and then develops abdominal pain and fetal bradycardia, the decision to extend the level of anesthesia via the epidural catheter or to proceed with general anesthesia depends on each anesthesiologist and patient. It is prudent to provide general anesthesia if a massive abruption is suspected, but the anticipation of difficult intubation may influence this decision. Conversely, a functioning epidural catheter can be used to extend the block with higher concentrations of local anesthetic mixed with bicarbonate. Regardless of technique, avoidance of hypotension is absolutely necessary.

When the fetus is severely compromised (such as in prolonged bradycardia), general endotracheal anesthesia is indicated, so that the time interval between the decision for cesarean section and delivery can be shortened. General anesthesia is also indicated for hemodynamically unstable patients. Clear antacid such as sodium citrate 30 mL should always be given orally prior to induction. Metoclopramide and an H_2 blocker should also be given intravenously, which will help decrease the risk of aspiration at the time of extubation. An arterial line is essential in the hemodynamically unstable hemorrhaging parturient. CVP monitoring may be helpful, but insertion may be too time consuming before induction of anesthesia and commencement of surgery. Induction with thiopental warrants caution to prevent precipitous hypotension and it should be used sparingly or avoided. Ketamine 1 mg/kg may be the better induction agent because of its sympathomimetic effect. However, ketamine is a direct myocardial depressant and this effect may predominate if the patient is severely hypovolemic with maximum sympathetic activity. Also, doses greater than 1.5 mg/kg may result in increased uterine tone, jeopardizing the fetal condition further. Etomidate 0.3 mg/kg IV can provide stable hemodynamics, owing to minimal cardiac depression.[48]

Endotracheal intubation is generally facilitated with intravenous succinylcholine in rapid-sequence induction for cesarean section. Rocuronium or high-dose vecuronium may be an alternative to achieve rapid onset of muscle relaxation, but the duration of action may be too long for a routine cesarean section. Maintenance of anesthesia is provided with nitrous oxide and a low concentration of a volatile agent if the patient tolerates it. A nitrous oxide–opioid–muscle relaxant technique may be better in some situations. A small dose of benzodiazepine is strongly recommended in this technique to avoid intraoperative awareness. Extubation is performed after adequate hemostasis when the patient is fully awake and hemodynamically stable. The patient may come back to the operating room when bleeding persists from uterine atony or coagulopathy. Reintubation in a hemodynamically unstable patient can be avoided by careful decision-making regarding extubation. For the same reason, the existing epidural catheter may be kept until the patient is discharged from the recovery or critical care room.

Especially in abruption, the risk of uterine atony is high and one should be prepared to provide pharmacologic treatment of uterine atony, as discussed in the following section. Acute renal failure is rare with lesser degrees of placental abruption but may be seen in severe forms including those in which treatment of hypovolemia is delayed or incomplete. Adequate perfusion of the kidneys must be maintained and should be monitored by urine output. Terao et al.[49] suggested that acute renal failure is likely to be prevented by the delivery of the fetus (and hysterectomy if necessary) within 5 hours of the onset of abruption.

Management of Uterine Atony

Uterine contraction and constriction of uterine blood vessels are vital to stop hemorrhage after delivery of the placenta. In placental abruption, especially with uteroplacental apoplexy (Couvelaire uterus), uterine contraction may be impaired and result in persistent bleeding. In Couvelaire uterus, widespread extravasation of blood into the uterine musculature and beneath the uterine serosa is found, thus impairing adequate contraction of the uterine musculature. Retained placenta, retained blood clot, and disruption of the uterine wall may all cause inadequate uterine contraction. Exploring the uterine cavity eliminates these possibilities. Anticipation of uterine atony in these patients with abruption facilitates prompt and aggressive treatment.

Nonpharmacologic treatment of uterine atony includes uterine massage, removal of intrauterine clot, and cooling of the uterus and abdomen.

Pharmacologic treatments include oxytocin, ergot alkaloids, and prostaglandins. Oxytocin is the first line of therapy, and can be given both intravenously and intramyometrially. Continuous infusion of oxytocin (20 U/L) following a 2- to 3-unit bolus is our routine. Intramuscular methylergonovine 0.2 mg is also effective. Ergot alkaloid should be avoided in patients with hypertension, preeclampsia, or connective tissue disorders, as it can precipitate severe hypertensive crisis and result in central nervous system complications. Some prostaglandin derivatives are effective in treating postpartum uterine atony if other modalities fail. Intramyometrial administration of prostaglandin F_2 alpha ($PGF_{2\alpha}$) is preferred to both intravenous or intramuscular injection.[50] A 15-methyl analogue of $PGF_{2\alpha}$ is more potent than $PGF_{2\alpha}$, and 0.25 mg is recommended intramuscularly or intramyometrially. This agent can cause bronchospasm, as well as transient arterial desaturation due to intrapulmonary shunting.[51] If all these nonpharmacologic and pharmacologic treatments fail, hysterectomy is the definitive treatment.

Management of Disseminated Intravascular Coagulation

Placental abruption is the most common cause of consumptive coagulopathy in pregnancy. The major mechanisms for consumptive coagulopathy are DIC and, to a lesser degree, retroplacental bleeding. DIC complicates approximately 10% of all abruptions but is more common in those cases in which fetal death has occurred.[52] Overt hypofibrinogenemia (plasma concentration less than 150 mg/dL), elevated levels of fibrin degradation products, D-dimer, and variable decreases in other coagulation factors occur in 30% of women with placental abruption that is severe enough to cause fetal demise.[34]

Disseminated intravascular coagulation produces a dramatic decrease in coagulation factors and platelets. It results from the release of a thrombogenic substance, thought to be thromboplastin, into the circulation. Thromboplastin triggers extrinsic coagulation pathway activation. Thrombin converts fibrinogen to fibrin and initiates intravascular clotting. DIC ends in consumption of factors I, II, V, and VIII and of platelets. The resultant fibrin deposits and thrombi in the microcirculation compromise blood flow to vital organs. DIC develops rapidly in obstetric patients, especially with placental abruption or amniotic fluid embolism. Laboratory evidence of prolonged PT and PTT, hypofibrinogenemia, thrombocytopenia, and elevated fibrin degradation products confirms DIC. The half-life of fibrin degradation products is long (5 to 7 hours), and thus it is not very useful for following the clinical course of DIC.[31] Another test for DIC is antithrombin III levels, which are lower in most patients with DIC. The diagnosis of DIC in obstetric patients should be suspected from underlying disease such as abruption, and treatment should not be delayed until laboratory confirmation of DIC.

Treatment of DIC is aimed at removing the underlying pathologic process and supplementation of clotting factors and platelets. In abruptio placentae, delivery of the fetus within 5 hours of onset is likely to prevent acute renal failure as a result of DIC and decreased organ perfusion.[49] However, there is no evidence that establishing an arbitrary time limit for delivery is necessary when the fetus is dead or previable.[34] Replacement of coagulation factors is provided by transfusion of fresh frozen plasma or cryoprecipitate or both. Platelet transfusion is often necessary. Anticoagulation to block the generalized intravascular coagulation is a controversial therapy. Although it can be effective in certain forms of hematologic malignancy-related DIC, there is no evidence that this therapy is beneficial in obstetric patients. In Japan, antithrombin III is often administered for these patients as well as protease inhibitors such as gabexate mesilate or nafamostat mesilate, but there is no convincing study to document their efficacy in obstetrics except for antithrombin III.[53] The infusion of heparin to block DIC could result in bleeding complications in these patients with placental abruption or other situations in which the integrity of the vascular system is compromised.

PLACENTA PREVIA

Placenta previa is defined as an abnormal location of the placenta over or very near the internal os of the uterus. It is presumed to be the result of irregularity or damage of the endometrium, causing the fertilized egg to implant at an unusual site. The incidence is rather high, approximately 1 in 200 deliveries. Reported incidence varies from 0.3 to 0.5%[34, 52] in the United States, and 0.57 to 0.85% in Japan.[42] It is the leading cause of third-trimester bleeding and results in considerable maternal and fetal morbidity.[54–56]

Risk Factors

Risk factors of placenta previa include increased maternal age, high parity, previous cesarean section, prior abortion, and cigarette smoking. Cocaine use,[57] as well as Asian origin,[58] were recently added to this list. Interestingly, patients with placenta previa have been shown to have a decreased frequency of pregnancy-induced hypertension (relative risk, 0.5).[59] In contrast to the modest association of maternal age with abruptio placentae, the risk of placenta previa increases dramatically with advancing maternal age. Women older than 40 years have a nearly ninefold greater risk than women under the age of 20.[60] Maternal age-adjusted relative risk is 2.6 among women with more than two parities compared to nulliparous women.[60] Clark et al.[61] assessed the relationship between increasing numbers of previous cesarean sections and the subsequent development of placenta previa and placenta accreta. The risk of placenta previa was 0.26% with an unscarred uterus, and the incidence increased linearly with the number of prior cesarean sections (up to 10% with four or more cesarean sections). Placenta previa itself is associated with the development of placenta accreta, secondary to the poor desidual development at the lower uterine segment. The incidence of placenta accreta in patients with placenta previa but without previous cesarean section was 5%. A history of cesarean section with the scar at this segment further increases the risk of placenta accreta by allowing trophoblastic invasion into the scar when the placenta lies over it. The incidence of placenta accreta in patients with placenta previa and one previous cesarean section was 24%. This incidence increases to 67% with placenta previa and four or more previous cesarean sections.[61]

Classification

Placenta previa is classified as follows (Fig. 29–5):

1. Total placenta previa. The internal cervical os is covered completely by placenta.
2. Partial placenta previa. The internal os is partially covered by placenta.
3. Marginal placenta previa. The edge of the placenta is at the margin of the internal os.
4. Low-lying placenta. The placenta is implanted in the lower uterine segment such that the placental edge actually does not reach the internal os but is in close proximity to it.

Low-lying placenta is not clearly defined regarding how close to the internal os it should be for the diagnosis. It is often considered to be a rather benign condition, because the placenta often "migrates" upward as gestation progresses and the cervix dilates. However, Oppenheimer et al. found that low-lying placenta is associated with frequent cesarean section due to bleeding characteristic of a placenta previa when it is located within 2 cm of the internal os.[62] Obata and Ishihara[62a] in Japan also reported 13 patients whose placenta was located within 2 cm of the internal os out of 1771 pregnancies, examined within 1 week before delivery. In five of eight patients, emergency operative deliveries were needed due to abnormal first-stage bleeding. Two patients of five who had vaginal deliveries lost 1200 to 1500 mL of blood during delivery. They concluded that a placenta that is within 2 cm of the internal os at 1 week before delivery should be considered abnormal and may be associated with higher incidence of obstetric complications.

Pathophysiology and Perinatal Outcome

In placenta previa, the progress of pregnancy results in a shearing force between the uterine wall and the rather nonelastic placenta. Bleeding is inevitable as pregnancy advances and with cervical dilation. Bleeding is usually noted vaginally with fresh red blood. With repeated bleeding, the mother may become anemic, sometimes requiring blood transfusion.

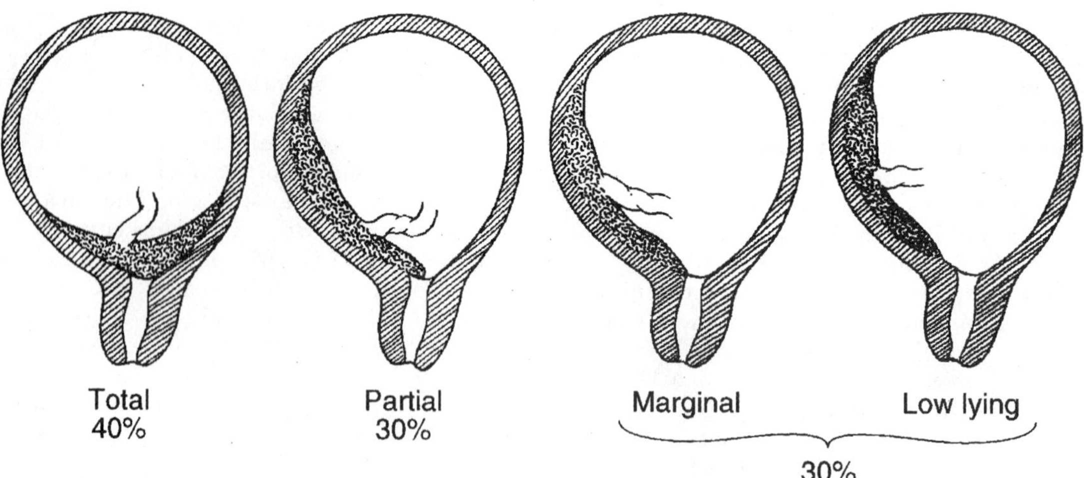

❖ **Figure 29-5** Classification of placenta previa. (From Suresh MS, Belfort MA: Antepartum hemorrhage. *In* Datta S (ed): Anesthetic and Obstetric Management of High Risk Pregnancy, 2nd ed. St. Louis: Mosby; 1996: 93. Illustration copyright 1995, Baylor College of Medicine.)

Preterm delivery and respiratory distress syndrome is a major cause of perinatal death, even though expectant management of placenta previa is practiced. McShane et al.[56] reported a perinatal mortality rate of 81 out of 1000. Nearly two thirds of the patients delivered before term. The incidence of respiratory distress syndrome was 22%. Serious fetal malformations are also somewhat more common. Fetal growth retardation is increased with placenta previa,[63] but this is not conclusive.

Diagnosis

The most characteristic event in placenta previa is **painless** bleeding. Hemorrhage usually does not appear until near the end of the second trimester or after. The initial bleeding is usually not very profuse. It may accompany uterine contraction and pain, which sometimes makes it difficult to differentiate from abruptio placentae. The diagnosis is best confirmed by transabdominal sonography, which requires adequate identification of the uterine cervix. The average accuracy is about 95%, and rates as high as 98% have been observed.[34] In Japan as well as the United States, most cases of placenta previa are diagnosed by routine prenatal ultrasonography before the onset of symptoms.

Vaginal examination is never permissible unless the woman is in an operating room, prepped and draped and ready for immediate cesarean section, because even the gentlest examination of this sort can cause severe hemorrhage.[34] This preparation should involve anesthesiologists who are ready to perform general anesthesia for emergency cesarean section. This is called "double set-up," but it is seldom necessary, as placental location can almost always be discovered by careful sonography.

Recently, transvaginal sonography has been used to diagnose placenta previa. It can provide better visualization of the uterine cervix and internal os and helps differentiate low-lying placenta from placenta previa. In theory it may carry a similar risk of probe-related trauma as digital vaginal examination, but this does not appear to be the case with careful application.

Obstetric Management

Patients with complete or partial placenta previa require cesarean delivery to ensure maternal safety. The timing of cesarean section is largely determined by the fetal lung maturity or degree of bleeding. Upon initial bleeding that is usually self-limited, patients are evaluated and observed for 1 or 2 days in the hospital with bedrest. If the bleeding ceases and if the fetus is considered to be healthy, the patient can often be followed as an outpatient. With outpatient management, significant reduction in hospital costs without compromising maternal and fetal outcome has been shown in retrospective studies[64, 65] and in one randomized clinical trial[66] that compared inpatient with outpatient management. It is important to note, however, that a significant percentage (62%) of patients had recurrent bleeding and most of them required expeditious cesarean delivery in that trial. To avoid increased emergency cesarean sections due to bleeding in outpatients, it is very important to select suitable patients for outpatient management and instruct them about their condition and possible need for quick transport to the hospital before significant blood loss ensues.

Tocolysis may be beneficial for some patients when the bleeding accompanies uterine contraction with a preterm fetus. Magnesium sulfate is usually chosen, but beta-sympathomimetics have been used. The latter may worsen hypotension from bleeding and may mask the signs of blood loss. The benefit of tocolysis in prolonging pregnancy in symptomatic placenta previa patients has been shown in a retrospective study.[67] The prolongation resulted in a weight gain of 400 g in 2-kg neonates. Considering the surprisingly improved mortality of premature neonates in the modern neonatal intensive care unit, especially with the installation of surfactant replacement therapy and nasal continuous positive airway pressure, there seems to be less need to wait until full term. In Kobe Children's Hospital in Japan during the period of 1995 through 1997, 25% of babies born at 30 or 31 weeks' gestational age did not require mechanical ventilation, and 62% of the 32 or 33 weeks' gestational age neonates did not. Neonatologists at this institution are comfortable in elective delivery of preterm infants after 32 weeks. Although it is true that neonates whose condition is complicated with placenta previa may be more likely to have intrauterine growth restriction and other problems, the benefit of elective delivery by cesarean section may be greater than emergency cesarean delivery in later gestation because of significant bleeding. Serial amniocentesis for a fetal lung maturity test has been advocated to determine the timing of delivery for these infants. However, amniocentesis itself carries some risks. Instead of relying on this evaluation heavily, it is mandatory to follow the patient closely and determine the appropriate timing of cesarean section on an individual basis. In a recent report[68] on placenta previa and placenta accreta, the preterm birth rate was 65% for placenta previa-accreta, which is similar to that of placenta previa alone (63%). It is encouraging to know that mean gestational age at delivery was almost 35 weeks.

Cesarean delivery of patients with placenta previa may be complicated with more maternal and fetal blood loss during uterine incision. A transverse uterine incision can be made in most cases. In some cases, however, a vertical incision may be necessary to avoid cutting through the placenta. The lower uterine segment in which the placenta implants has poor contractile nature, thus placenta previa may result in more bleeding after removal of the placenta, even without placenta accreta. In cases of placenta accreta or other abnormally adherent placenta, bleeding may continue and immediate treatment is required. The treatments include sewing the placenta implantation site, uterine artery or internal iliac artery ligation, and hysterectomy. These treatment modalities are discussed in the following section.

Anesthetic Management

Anesthetic management of patients with placenta previa varies, depending on the urgency of cesarean section and the severity of hemorrhage. If the brisk bleeding continues, general endotracheal anesthesia following rapid sequence induction will provide hemodynamic stability. If cesarean section is performed electively, regional anesthesia may be the preferred method, depending on the anesthesiologist's choice and the availability of support staff.

Emergency Cesarean Section

Some patients come to the operating room directly from the emergency room owing to hemorrhage, especially when they are managed as outpatients. Anesthesiologists have a limited amount of time before initiating anesthesia. To decrease the possibility of anesthetizing a pregnant patient without prior knowledge about her and the baby, it is helpful to evaluate all the patients with placenta previa after 22 weeks upon the first bleeding episode and hospitalization. Pertinent medical history and anesthesia-related problems, if present, should be known to the anesthesia team beforehand. When the patient shows persistent hemorrhage, one has to assess the degree of blood loss quickly as well as the ease of intubation (by physical examination). Blood should be sent for, and at least two large-bore (16-gauge or larger) intravenous lines are placed. Fluid resuscitation and management of massive emergency transfusion must be undertaken as already discussed. Management of general anesthesia for bleeding parturients is the same as discussed in relation to abruptio placentae. If the patient is hemodynamically stable with minimum bleeding when she is brought to the operating room, spinal anesthesia may be cautiously performed with adequate fluid replacement.

Elective Cesarean Section

Anesthesia for elective cesarean section for a patient with placenta previa can be provided with regional anesthesia while keeping in mind the possibility of cesarean hysterectomy. If the patient is known to have placenta accreta, increta, or percreta, it may be safer to begin with general anesthesia rather than to convert from regional anesthesia to general anesthesia during the operation (especially in a situation of limited help) because of intraoperative bleeding or prolonged procedure.

Spinal or epidural anesthesia is appropriate for uncomplicated placenta previa without a prior history of cesarean section. However, the risk of placenta accreta increases as the number of previous cesarean sections increases.[61] For those patients with one or two previous cesarean sections but without known accreta, 2 to 4 units of PRBCs should be cross-matched and kept for the patient either in the operating room or designated area nearby. At least two intravenous cannulae are recommended by Chestnut et al.,[69] but one large-bore intravenous catheter may be sufficient at the beginning. The authors reported in a multi-institutional study that none of the patients with epidural anesthesia for cesarean section required conversion to general anesthesia when cesarean hysterectomy became necessary. They also suggested that they would not withhold epidural anesthesia from normovolemic patients undergoing elective, repeat cesarean section for placenta previa, despite the high risk for placenta accreta and emergency hysterectomy in these patients. Combined spinal epidural anesthesia may be beneficial in extending the duration of anesthesia for these patients in whom the procedure may take a longer time, while providing rapid onset of block with good sacral anesthesia.

PLACENTA ACCRETA/INCRETA/PERCRETA

Infrequently, the placenta is unusually adherent to the implantation site, with scanty or absent decidua, so that

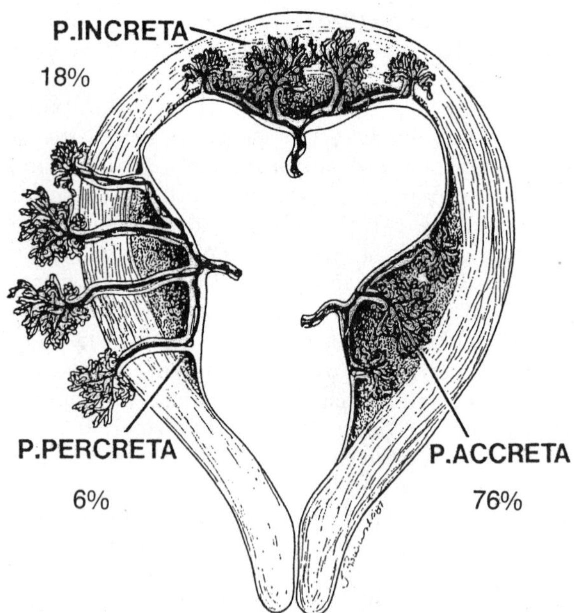

❖ **Figure 29–6** Classification of placenta accreta, increta, and percreta. (From Kamani AAS, Gambling DR, Christilaw J, et al: Anesthetic management of patients with placenta accreta. Can J Anaesth 1987; 34(6):613; data from Miller DA, Chollet JA, Goodwin TM: Clinical risk factors for placenta previa-placenta accreta. Am J Obstet Gynecol 1997; 177(1):210.)

the physiologic line of cleavage through the decidual spongy layer is lacking. As a consequence, one or more cotyledons are firmly bound to the defective decidua basalis or even to the myometrium. This condition is called placenta accreta, and it is one of the most challenging problems to obstetric anesthesiologists. It is the cause of hemorrhage at the time of delivery, but it is discussed in this chapter because of its close relation to placenta previa.

Abnormally adherent placenta is defined as follows (Fig. 29–6):

1. Placenta accreta. Placenta is firmly attached to the implantation site, but it does not invade the myometrium.
2. Placenta increta. Placenta invades the myometrium.
3. Placenta percreta. Placenta penetrates through the myometrium, sometimes further invading adjacent organs such as bladder or intestine.

The incidence of placenta accreta is increasing. Read et al.[70] reported the incidence of about 1 per 2500 deliveries, and concluded that there is a higher reported incidence and a greater incidence of associated placenta previa (63%), as well as decreasing maternal and perinatal mortality. They reported 1 maternal mortality out of 22 patients in their series in the late 1970s. Although maternal mortality has decreased significantly, it is still a major cause of maternal morbidity, such as massive hemorrhage and infectious complications.

Risk Factors

The associated conditions include implantation in the lower uterine segment, over a previous cesarean section scar or other previous uterine incisions, or after repeated uterine curettage (Asherman's syndrome). In the most recent report on placenta previa and placenta accreta, Miller et al.[68] reported the risk of placenta accreta among 155,670 deliveries in 10 years from 1985 to 1994 in one institution in California. There were 127 cesarean hysterectomies performed due to the clinical diagnosis of placenta accreta, but in only 62 cases (48%) was the diagnosis confirmed histologically. This illustrates the importance of histologic confirmation in diagnosing placenta accreta. Among these 62 cases, 76% were placenta accreta, 18% were placenta increta, and 6% were placenta percreta. Among 590 women with placenta previa, 55 (9.3%) had placenta accreta. By comparison, placenta accreta occurred in 44 of 155,080 women (0.005%) without placenta previa (relative risk, 2065; 95% CI: 944 to 4516). With the increase of previous cesarean section numbers, the incidence of placenta accreta increased dramatically, as shown in Figure 29–7. Maternal mortality was reported to be 9.5% by Fox[71] in a review of 622 cases of placenta accreta between 1945 and 1969. A recent study by Miller et al.[68] reported no maternal deaths, which reflects significant improvement in the management of this condition. Fetal mortality also decreased from 9.6% reported by Fox to 0% by Miller. However, maternal morbidity due to hemorrhage and surgical complications was significant even in Miller's study. Estimated blood loss exceeded 2000 mL in 66% of cases of accreta, 5000 mL in 15%, 10,000 mL in 6.5%, and 20,000 mL in 3%. Blood transfusion was required in 55% of patients. Five percent of patients received more than 70 units of blood products. Other complica-

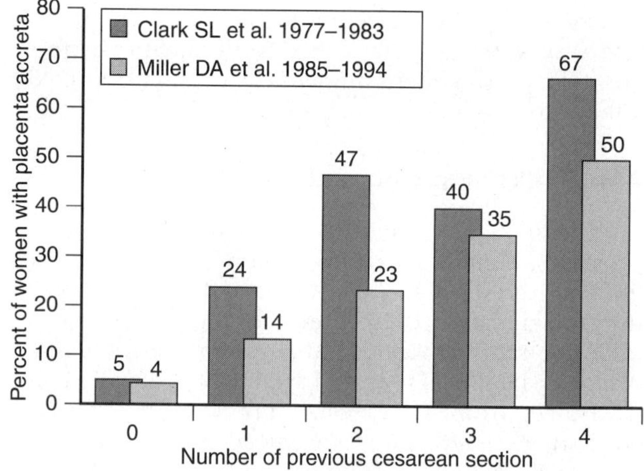

❖ **Figure 29–7** Incidence of placenta accreta in patients with placenta previa in relation to the number of previous cesarean sections. (Data from Clark SL, Koonings PP, Phelan JP, et al: Placenta previa/accreta and prior cesarean section. Obstet Gynecol 1985; 66(1):89; Miller DA, Chollet JA, Goodwin TM: Clinical risk factors for placenta previa-placenta accreta. Am J Obstet Gynecol 1997; 177(1):210.)

tions included ureteral transection, DIC, hypotensive shock, enterotomy, and reoperation for hemostasis.

Diagnosis

Placenta accreta is noted at the time of delivery or cesarean section with difficulty in separating the placenta from the uterine wall. However, recent utilization of transvaginal ultrasonography has made it possible to diagnose placenta accreta in 78% to 100% of cases when used in the third trimester.[72, 73] By screening high-risk patients, one can better identify patients with placenta accreta. Then, the extent of trophoblast invasion can be evaluated by magnetic resonance imaging in some patients.[74]

Obstetric Management

For a patient with known placenta accreta, the desired approach is to deliver by elective cesarean section, recognizing the high probability of cesarean hysterectomy. Patients may donate autologous blood beforehand in anticipation of significant blood loss at the time of delivery. There have been several reports of this technique without significant fetal effect.[75] Recombinant erythropoietin has also been used in parturients. These modalities to minimize homologous blood transfusion are discussed later.

When placenta accreta or other abnormally adherent placenta is first noted at the time of delivery, the bleeding continues and immediate treatment is required. The treatment options include sewing the placenta implantation site, uterine artery or internal iliac artery ligation, and hysterectomy. Zelop et al.[76] reported that placenta accreta was the most frequent indication for emergency peripartum hysterectomy. Prompt hysterectomy may be lifesaving for these patients. In other patients with relatively stable hemodynamics with adequate hemostasis, conservative management may be attempted. There have been several reports of methotrexate use to facilitate necrosis of retained placenta to preserve fertility. However, this treatment carries the increased risk of delayed hemorrhage and infection. Thus, its indication is limited to hemodynamically stable patients who strongly desire fertility preservation. Other conservative treatments such as uterine artery ligation or internal iliac artery embolization may also preserve fertility.

Considering the significant maternal morbidity associated with placenta accreta/increta/percreta, it is very important to increase the likelihood of antenatal diagnosis and elective cesarean delivery with better preparation for cesarean hysterectomy. Autologous blood can be harvested and used efficiently. There is a case report[77] of preoperative catheterization of abdominal aorta via axillary artery for subsequent uterine artery embolization in the operating room in case of significant hemorrhage refractory to local measures. Modalities to reduce morbidity or homologous blood transfusion continue to be tried for patients with placenta accreta. Recent information[69] regarding the high-risk group of placenta accreta confirmed the report by Clark et al.[62] These data will help in the selective application of transvaginal ultrasonography and magnetic resonance imaging for these high-risk patients, and in the diagnosis of placenta accreta antenatally.

Anesthetic Management

Anesthetic management of patients with placenta accreta is required for elective cesarean hysterectomy for known placenta accreta, and for emergency cesarean hysterectomy for undiagnosed placenta accreta.

Elective Cesarean Hysterectomy

Cesarean hysterectomy is not a frequent procedure. The incidence of obstetric hysterectomy, excluding those due to malignancy, ranged between 0.08% and 0.20% depending on institutions.[70] Zelop et al.[76] reported the incidence of 0.155% from 1983 to 1991 at Brigham and Women's Hospital in Boston. Thus anesthesiologists encounter peripartum hysterectomy infrequently. As a result, there are not many reports regarding anesthetic management in cesarean hysterectomy.

In an earlier report by Chestnut and Redick,[78] between 1972 and 1984, 7 of 25 patients required intraoperative general anesthesia. The causes were patient discomfort and inadequate operating conditions. Three factors precipitate inadequate epidural anesthesia. First, the operative time for cesarean hysterectomy is twice that required for cesarean section only. This predisposes the patient to fatigue and restlessness. Second, intraperitoneal manipulation, dissection, and traction are excessive during cesarean hysterectomy, compared with cesarean section. This surgical manipulation may result in pain, nausea, and vomiting. Third, the engorged edematous vasculature requires careful dissection.

The subsequent prospective study by Chestnut et al.[69] tried to overcome this problem of infrequent cesarean hysterectomy by involving five institutions and answering several clinically important questions. They reported that, among 46 obstetric hysterectomies performed between 1984 and 1987, 25 were elective and 21 were emergent. Eleven of the 21 emergency hysterectomies were due to placenta previa or accreta or both. Continuous epidural anesthesia was performed in 8 elective and 4 emergency cesarean sections, and none of them required conversion to general anesthesia intraoperatively. The authors concluded that continuous epidural anesthesia is not contraindicated for elective cesarean hysterectomy.

On the other hand, there is always a possibility that immediate conversion from regional anesthesia to general anesthesia will be required in the middle of an acute hemorrhagic crisis. To have the airway secured beforehand might make anesthetic management simpler on these occasions, allowing the anesthesiologist to focus on hemodynamic management. It is important to have adequate personnel available when one proceeds with continuous epidural anesthesia for elective cesarean hysterectomy.

Another issue of continuous epidural anesthesia for elective cesarean hysterectomy includes the possibility of perioperative coagulation disorders such as DIC. Chestnut et al.[69] reported the intraoperative and postoperative complications of cesarean hysterectomy. DIC was found in 19% of emergency obstetric hysterectomies, but none of the elective hysterectomies were complicated with DIC. DIC becomes an issue more often in emergency hysterectomies. When the patient develops a bleeding diathesis after the initiation of epidural anesthesia, the question of when to remove the epidural catheter arises. Several cases of epidural hematoma have been reported at the time of catheter removal, especially in the setting of anticoagulation with low molecular weight heparin.[79] If possible, the epidural catheter should be removed when the patient's coagulation status is normal, or back to baseline. The reasonable approach for recently developed coagulopathy in a parturient with an indwelling epidural catheter is summarized by Sprung[80] as follows:

1. If there is no evidence of intraspinal bleeding, the catheter must be removed as early as possible because of the potential for intravascular catheter migration and initiation of bleeding. (Although this could result in hematoma formation, it may be better than to wait for an indeterminate time in the setting of worsening coagulopathy.)
2. If bleeding is present around the catheter insertion site and possibly in the epidural/subarachnoid space, the catheter must be left in place for tamponading effect.
3. Frequent assessment of neurologic status is important until the underlying cause of the coagulopathy is treated and the bleeding is resolved.
4. If intraspinal hematoma leading to neurologic deficit occurs, immediate neurologic consultation and decompression surgery is needed.

As stated earlier, continuous epidural anesthesia can be provided for patients undergoing elective cesarean hysterectomy for placenta accreta. However, for those requiring more extensive intra-abdominal manipulation due to placenta increta or percreta, general anesthesia may be better tolerated. On the other hand, epidural analgesia is helpful for excellent postoperative pain control which may be very important for these patients as well. However, timing of epidural catheter removal warrants caution if the patient develops coagulopathy.

Emergency Cesarean Hysterectomy

When cesarean hysterectomy becomes necessary intraoperatively because of uncontrollable hemorrhage, anesthetic management starts with the evaluation of airway and oxygenation, and establishment of large-bore intravenous access. As discussed earlier, conversion to general anesthesia is not always necessary. When the ongoing blood loss is significant, however, securing the airway with endotracheal intubation and conversion to general anesthesia may be appropriate. Restoring hemodynamic stability and adequate organ perfusion are of paramount importance. Management of fluid resuscitation and transfusion were discussed in an earlier section of this chapter. It is important to reemphasize that the rapid fluid infusion is more important than the choice of fluid or immediate hemodynamic monitoring.[81]

The estimated blood loss in emergency cesarean hysterectomies was 2526 ± 1240 mL (mean ± SD) in the study by Chestnut et al.,[69] which is significantly more than in cases of elective cesarean hysterectomies (1319 ± 396 mL). Placenta accreta was the most frequent indication for emergency peripartum hysterectomy and accounted for more than half of the cases in studies by Chestnut et al and Zelop et al.[76] It is also worth mentioning that the estimated blood loss among patients varies significantly, as shown in large standard deviation in the study by Chestnut et al. Zelop et al. reported their experience of placenta accreta requiring emergency cesarean hysterectomy. One patient required a large amount of transfusion and became hypothermic and then sustained cardiac arrest. Cardiopulmonary bypass was initiated and the patient was rewarmed and resuscitated without major neurologic sequelae. No maternal death was reported in these two studies, illustrating that aggressive and efficient care increases the likelihood of good outcome.

Although no maternal deaths were reported in these two studies, maternal perioperative morbidity was quite prevalent. Table 29–8 lists the complications of peripartum hysterectomy as reported in previous studies.

VASA PREVIA

Vasa previa is uncommon and has a very high rate of fetal mortality. It is the velamentous insertion of the cord in the lower uterine segment. The umbilical vessels run through the membranes between the fetal presenting part and the cervix. The vessels are unsupported and very vulnerable to tearing or occlusion during labor. Vaginal bleeding that occurs immediately after membrane rupture, as well as immediate fetal heart rate abnormalities, are suggestive of vasa previa. The bleeding is from the fetal circulation in this condition, and thus a relatively small amount of bleeding may cause fetal demise. The only choice is immediate cesarean section to save the fetus.

Recently, color-Doppler sonography has been successfully used for antenatal diagnosis of vasa previa. It is hoped that more frequent antenatal diagnosis will facilitate prompt intervention, thus improving fetal survival.

UTERINE RUPTURE

Definition

Uterine rupture is defined as a full thickness defect of the uterine wall. It may be spontaneous, secondary to

Table 29-8 COMPLICATIONS ASSOCIATED WITH PERIPARTUM HYSTERECTOMY

	ELECTIVE (%)	EMERGENCY (%)
Maternal death	0	0-1
Cardiac arrest	0	4
Estimated blood loss (mL)	1100-1300	2500-3500
Infection	42	49
Febrile morbidity	14-27	33-61
Wound infection	0-5	3-12
Pneumonia	0	0.8-1.7
Sepsis		3.4
Urinary tract infection	10-11	0-18
Hepatitis B		0.8
Infected hematomas		0.8
Septic thrombophlebitis		0.8-3
Vaginal cuff infection	0-9.6	18
Respiratory		18-21
ARDS		3.4
Prolonged intubation		10
Pulmonary edema		4.3
Atelectasis	0-8	1.7-10
Chest tube placement		1.7
Urologic		8.5
Cystostomy	4-5	0-8
Ureteral injury	0-5	2-4
Neurologic		2.6
Coma		0.8
Seizure		0.8
Stroke	0	0.8
Thromboembolic	0	0-9
Deep venous thrombosis	0	0-1.7
Pulmonary embolus	0	0-0.8
Gastrointestinal	0	0-2.6
Ileus		2.6
Hemorrhagic		87
Disseminated intravascular coagulation	0	19-27
Loss of adnexa because of bleeding	5-6.8	4.5-17
Transfusion requirement	45-66	79-100
Reexploration because of bleeding	0	2.3-5
Other		1.7
Compartment syndrome		0.8
Transfusion reaction		0.8

Data from Zelop CM, Harlow BL, Frigoletto FD Jr, et al: Emergency peripartum hysterectomy. Am J Obstet Gynecol 1993; 168:1443; Chestnut DH, Eden RD, Gall SA, et al: Peripartum hysterectomy: a review of cesarean and postpartum hysterectomy. Obstet Gynecol 1985; 65:365; Clark SL, Yeh SY, Phelan JP, et al: Emergency hysterectomy for obstetric hemorrhage. Obstet Gynecol 1984; 64:376; Chestnut DH, Dewan DM, Redick LF, et al: Anesthetic management for obstetric hysterectomy: a multi-institutional study. Anesthesiology 1989; 70:607.

trauma, or it may result from rupture of a previous uterine scar. It can occur either antepartum or postpartum, so it is discussed briefly in this chapter. Prolonged or obstructed labor is thought to be the predominant causative factor of uterine rupture.[82]

If it occurs at the previous cesarean section scar, it is important to differentiate between rupture and dehiscence of the scar. Rupture refers to separation of the old uterine incision throughout most of its length, with rupture of the fetal membranes so that the uterine cavity and the peritoneal cavity communicate.[35] In these circumstances, all or part of the fetus is usually extruded into the peritoneal cavity. Bleeding from the edges of the scar is usually significant. There may be an extension of the rent into previously uninvolved uterus. On the other hand, with dehiscence of a cesarean section scar, the fetal membranes are not ruptured and the fetus is not extruded into the peritoneal cavity, and bleeding tends to be insignificant.

The incidence of uterine rupture is not very rare, about 1 in 2300. The incidence did not decrease appreciably in a study by Eden et al.[83] from Duke University over a period of 53 years. The incidence of uterine rupture was 1 in 1280 from 1931 to 1950, whereas it was 1 in 2250 from 1973 to 1983. The most recent report by Miller et al.[84] from Los Angeles County showed that, in nearly 190,000 deliveries, the incidence of uterine rupture was 1 in 1234. Among women with previous cesarean section, the incidence was 0.7%, whereas women without previous cesarean section had an incidence of 0.007%. At Parkland Hospital from 1990 through 1994, only 4 cases of uterine rupture out of nearly 74,000 deliveries were noted when scar dehiscence is excluded.[35]

Etiology

The most common cause of uterine rupture is separation of a previous cesarean section scar.[35] This risk is increasing with the developing trend of allowing a trial of labor following prior transverse cesarean section. In the study by Miller et al.,[84] from 1983 through 1994, only 11 of 153 cases of uterine rupture were not associated with prior cesarean section. Other common predisposing factors to uterine rupture are previous uterine surgery or manipulations, such as uterine curettage or perforation.

Classic vertical scar of the uterus is associated with several times greater probability of rupture compared with lower-segment horizontal scar. Classic scars can result in rupture before labor in about one third of cases. Classic incision is still utilized to deliver a depressed fetus expeditiously, or to gently deliver a very premature fetus with breech presentation when the uterine musculature is very thick and noncompliant. Delivery by cesarean section in subsequent pregnancy will not prevent all such ruptures.

Maternal and Perinatal Outcome

A considerable number of studies have been conducted that observe the benefits and safety of VBAC.[85] It has been the experience of many practitioners that separation of the transverse uterine incision that develops antepartum or during early labor is usually limited to dehiscence without an appreciable increase in maternal or perinatal mortality, if prompt response to the event is ensured. Scar separation following a trial of labor in a woman with a prior transverse incision has not been associated with maternal death.[86, 87] Eden et al.[83] reported one maternal death and a 46% perinatal loss. Although maternal mortality is rare, significant morbidity still may occur to both mother and fetus, even with prior low transverse incision. Specifically, Jones et al.[88] and Scott[89] described a total of 20 cases of uterine rupture associated with a previous low-segment cesarean scar. Among these 20 women, there were three perinatal deaths, at least two infants had long-term neurologic sequelae, and three women required hysterectomy. Thus, while complete rupture of the uterus is uncommon when a trial of labor is allowed after a previous low transverse cesarean section, when it occurs, the results may be disastrous for mother, fetus, or both. Unfortunately, such catastrophes are generally unpredictable. The fact remains that VBAC patients are at higher risk for complications, and prompt response to rupture is vital in managing these patients.

Diagnosis

Some patients may complain of symptoms of impending uterine rupture, such as anxiety, tachycardia, and respiratory distress. The uterus may become hard and tender. Upon uterine rupture, abdominal pain is considered to be the classic sign of this condition. However, recent studies reported that pain does not always accompany uterine rupture, as illustrated in a review by Johnson and Oriol.[90] Also, loss of uterine contraction is not a reliable indicator of uterine rupture. Rodriguez et al.[91] described data from 39 women with uterine rupture in whom an intrauterine pressure catheter was placed. Four women had increased baseline pressure associated with severe variable decelerations. An intrauterine catheter is not useful nor prerequisite in performing VBAC. Instead, the most common finding in all of these 76 cases was sudden, severe fetal heart rate decelerations, seen in almost 80% of cases.

Anesthetic Management for Vaginal Birth After Cesarean Section

Lumbar epidural analgesia was once considered to be contraindicated in VBAC, for fear that it might mask the pain from uterine rupture. However, abdominal pain is not the most frequent symptom of rupture, as stated earlier. In addition, with the use of low concentration local anesthetic combined with opioid, the patient may complain of breakthrough pain, or at least an uncomfortable sensation. Epidural analgesia is not considered contraindicated for VBAC at the present time. The success rate of VBAC does not appear to be affected by epidural analgesia, as summarized by Glassenberg et al.[92] Oxytocin augmentation can be used in a previously scarred uterus with epidural analgesia. This topic is discussed in greater detail in Chapter 27.

Anesthetic Management for Emergency Cesarean Section

The presenting symptom of uterine rupture may well be sudden fetal "distress," which necessitates urgent cesarean section. If the patient does not appear to be hypovolemic, labor epidural analgesia can be extended quickly by 3% 2-chloroprocaine mixed with bicarbonate. Even spinal anesthesia may be chosen in selected patients with stable hemodynamics, since the patient may have only dehiscence of a previous cesarean section scar. However, if the patient is hemodynamically unstable, or in the presence of severe fetal compromise, general endotracheal anesthesia may be preferable.

EMERGENCY PERIPARTUM HYSTERECTOMY

Peripartum hysterectomy includes elective cesarean hysterectomy, emergency cesarean hysterectomy, and emergency postpartum hysterectomy. Emergency peripartum hysterectomy is one of the most critical and difficult situations that obstetric anesthesiologists face.

Zelop et al.[76] reviewed the 117 emergency peripartum hysterectomies at the Brigham and Women's Hospital in Boston from 1984 through 1991. The annual incidence was 1.55 per 1000 deliveries. They found that abnormal placentation was the most common cause preceding gravid hysterectomy (64%). Uterine atony accounted for 21% of cases. Although no maternal deaths occurred, maternal morbidity remained high, including postoperative infection in 58 patients (50%), intraoperative urologic injury in 10 patients (9%), and need for transfusion in 102 patients (87%). Median blood loss was 3000 mL. The frequency of maternal complications in peripartum hysterectomy is shown in Table 29–8. Twenty percent of patients had regional anesthesia. This study illustrates the current clinical scenario of emergency obstetric hysterectomy.

There are few studies of anesthetic management for emergency gravid hysterectomy. LaPlatney and O'Leary[93] reported a series of 60 patients who underwent either elective (83%) or emergency (17%) cesarean hysterectomy between 1961 and 1966. Eighteen of the women received spinal anesthesia and none received epidural anesthesia. Four (22%) of those 18 women required "augmentation with inhalation anesthesia because of prolonged surgery," and two of those four developed aspiration pneumonia. The authors concluded that "prolonged surgery, increased intraoperative complications, excessive blood loss, and need for multiple transfusions all serve as relative contraindications to spinal anesthesia."[93]

Chestnut et al.[69] focused on anesthetic management of obstetric hysterectomy in a study involving Wake Forest University, Duke University, University of Florida, University of North Carolina, and University of Iowa between 1984 and 1987. There were 46 obstetric hysterectomies in 41,107 deliveries, an incidence of 0.11%. Of the 46, 21 were emergency hysterectomies, among which 11 were due to placenta previa or accreta or both. The authors reported that women in the emergency group had greater intraoperative blood loss, were more likely to have intraoperative hypotension, and were more likely to receive donor blood than women in the elective group. Four of 21 in the emergency group received epidural anesthesia, and none of them required conversion to general anesthesia intraoperatively.

The effect of epidural anesthesia initiated before hemorrhage on uterine blood flow and maternal and fetal response to hemorrhage were investigated in an animal study by Vincent et al.[94] They showed that epidural anesthesia significantly worsened maternal hypotension, uterine blood flow, and fetal oxygenation during hemorrhage (20 mL/kg) in gravid ewes. This study suggested that epidural anesthesia may adversely affect the compensatory response to untreated hemorrhage in pregnant women. Although their study primarily tried to investigate the risk of initiating labor epidural analgesia for those patients at high risk for hemorrhage (e.g., abnormal placentation, partial placental abruption, or intrauterine hemangioma), the result may be applicable to the situation in which emergency cesarean hysterectomy becomes necessary because of intraoperative refractory hemorrhage. It is easily conceivable that managing hemorrhage during epidural anesthesia requires more aggressive treatment of hemorrhage and continuous attention to the airway and maternal oxygenation.

The same group later investigated the effects of epidural anesthesia on uterine vascular resistance and renin activity during hemorrhage in gravid ewes.[95] They observed that uterine vascular resistance increases due to hemorrhage and was attenuated with epidural anesthesia, and that vasopressin and renin activity were lower in the epidural group. However, fetal hypoxemia and acidosis during hemorrhage is closely related to the reduction in maternal mean arterial pressure regardless of the etiology (i.e., sympatholytic and hemorrhage versus hemorrhage alone). Thus, we cannot be comfortable by noting that hypotension is partly due to epidural anesthesia. General anesthesia is thus chosen for actively bleeding patients with unstable hemodynamics. The management strategy has already been discussed.

Treatment of hypotension should be achieved by volume replacement or transfusion if necessary. Management of massive hemorrhage and transfusion is discussed earlier in this chapter. A vasopressor is often required until adequate volume replacement is achieved. Any vasopressor, including pure α-adrenergic agonist can be given if indicated, based on maternal condition. For example, some patients may have been given magnesium sulfate. These clinical scenarios include patients who receive tocolysis for placenta previa, or seizure prophylaxis in preeclamptic patients who subsequently present with abruptio placentae. Magnesium has been shown to attenuate the maternal compensatory response to hemorrhage in gravid ewes, perhaps by decreasing the response to endogenous vasopressors.[96] Magnesium was shown also to alter the maternal cardiovascular response to vasopressor agents in gravid ewes by Sipes et al.[97] Magnesium antagonizes the effect of α_1-adrenergic agonists, α_2-adrenergic agonists, and angiotensin II on the uterine vasculature, thus potentially providing a level of protection for the fetus in situations of maternal stress. Magnesium has variable effects on systemic circulation and uterine circulation in response to a variety of vasopressors. This finding may be of importance when maternal hypotension develops while the fetus is alive in utero, so that preservation of uteroplacental circulation is desired. In case of cesarean hysterectomy, any vasopressor may be given after delivery of the infant; the choice depends primarily on maternal hemodynamics. Calcium is usually recommended to counteract magnesium toxicity. However, it is only briefly effective in restoring hypotension due to magnesium and hemorrhage in gravid ewes.[98] Magnesium may increase the pressor requirement in treating hypotension during gravid hysterectomy, but it is not difficult to compensate its effect unless the patient is overtly hypermagnesemic.

CONSERVATIVE METHODS FOR HEMOSTASIS

Internal Iliac Artery Ligation

Ligation of the internal iliac artery (hypogastric artery) is sometimes performed for two purposes. One is to stop hemorrhage so that hysterectomy is avoided. The second is to decrease obstetric hemorrhage prior to hysterectomy, so that bleeding vessels are better identified and intraoperative blood loss is decreased.

The uterus has abundant collateral blood supply. The major blood supply is provided by uterine arteries via internal iliac arteries, as well as ovarian arteries via the abdominal aorta. The localization of the internal iliac artery is shown in Figure 29–8. The rationale for internal iliac artery ligation is an 85% reduction in pulse pressure distal to the ligated artery, thus turning an arterial pressure system into those in the venous circulation, which is more amenable to hemostasis via simple clot formation.[99] The reduction in blood flow by internal iliac artery ligation is only 48%. This is the reason for the relatively low success rate of this technique. Evans and McShane[100] reported 18 cases of obstetric hypogastric ligations from 1966 to 1982, revealing a 43% success rate in avoiding hysterectomy. Clark et al.[101] reported a similar success rate (42%) in the same year after reviewing 19 patients who underwent bilateral hypogastric artery ligation. The most frequent indication for this technique was uterine atony (78%). Among the patients with uterine atony, the success rate of this method was 40%. In cases of placenta accreta or uterine rupture, this technique is rarely attempted. There was an increased complication rate of both ureteral injury and cardiac arrest secondary to hypovolemia in patients undergoing internal iliac artery ligation, compared with those with hysterectomy only. Two patients who suffered hypovolemic cardiac arrest were in the group undergoing unsuccessful internal iliac artery ligation for uterine atony. The observed ureteral injuries appeared to be due to ensuing hysterectomy rather than being associated with ligation of the artery itself. Clark et al. subsequently stated that "the high rate of complications and the low rate of success suggests that hypogastric artery ligation for the control of obstetric hemorrhage should be reserved for hemodynamically stable patients of low parity in whom future childbearing is of paramount concern."[101]

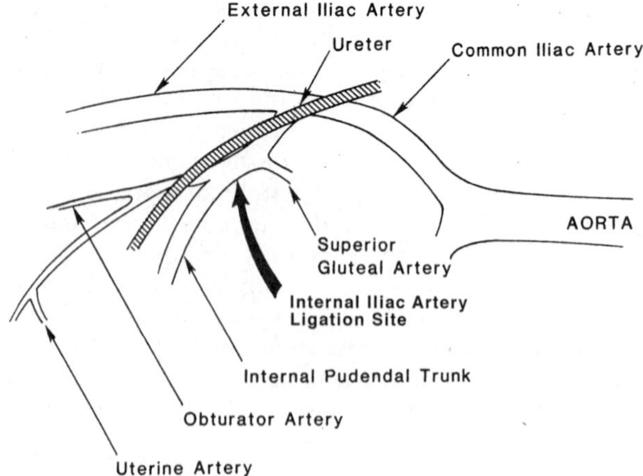

Figure 29–8 Localization of the internal iliac artery along the right pelvic sidewall. (Modified from Gonik B: Intensive care monitoring of the critically ill pregnant patient. *In* Creasy RK, Resnik R [eds]: Maternal-Fetal Medicine: Principles and Practice, 3rd ed. Philadelphia: WB Saunders; 1994: 882.)

On the contrary, Chattopadhyay et al.[102] compared 29 patients with bilateral internal iliac artery ligation as the initial approach for severe postpartum hemorrhage (45%) with those with hysterectomy (55%). Internal iliac artery ligation was successful in controlling hemorrhage in 65%, and it failed in 35% in whom hysterectomy was required as a lifesaving procedure. Failure of hypogastric artery ligation was more evident in atonic postpartum hemorrhage patients than in other situations. Complications were more frequent in patients undergoing hysterectomy. Those complications included reexploration and two cases of death. Contrary to the report by Clark et al., the mean estimated blood loss was higher with hysterectomy. Chattopadhyay et al. concluded that hypogastric artery ligation was found to be a relatively easy, safe, and successful procedure that ought to be attempted as an initial surgical approach for all severe postpartum hemorrhage. They did not provide a detailed description of maternal deaths, but it is conceivable that these women suffered from more intractable bleeding, necessitating hysterectomy as an initial intervention. To increase the chance of maternal survival, not too much time should be wasted in this procedure. In performing this procedure, care must be taken to avoid inadvertent ligation of the external iliac artery. Pulsation in the external iliac artery must be ascertained before and after ligation. Careful dissection up to the common iliac artery may be necessary to avoid this complication.

Because of the abundant collateral blood supply to the uterus, successful term pregnancies have been reported after bilateral ligation of both ovarian and internal iliac arteries.[103]

Uterine Artery Embolization

Transcatheter arterial embolization has recently emerged as a highly effective percutaneous technique for controlling acute and chronic genital bleeding in a wide variety of obstetric and gynecologic disorders. In a recent review by Vedantham et al.,[104] the authors concluded from their comprehensive literature review and clinical experience that embolization should be used before surgical treatment of nonmalignant pelvic bleeding in many clinical settings, including postpartum, postcesarean, and postoperative bleeding. It has been used for uterine atony, or persistent hemorrhage due to placenta accreta. There are not many reported cases of radiologic uterine artery embolization to date. So far, the success rate is 16 of 18 (89%) for postcesarean hemorrhage.[105–109] The largest report from Japan includes 15 patients after vaginal delivery and 17 patients with vaginal bleeding from neoplasms.[109] Among those patients after vaginal delivery, hysterectomy had been performed in two, but failed to control the bleeding. All of them reportedly responded to the embolization therapy.

The technique involves the identification of a bleeding vessel or uterine artery by angiography, then the injection of gelfoam pledgets or placement of coils. The procedure is less invasive than laparotomy and may be beneficial in patients who have developed coagulopathy. It may be easier to maintain hemodynamic stability than during laparotomy. The complications of the pelvic embolization procedure have been extremely uncommon. The reported incidence of complications is low (6% to 7%) with no deaths. The complications fall into three categories: complications of angiography, pelvic infection, and ischemic phenomena. In the postpartum-postcesarean setting, reported angiographic complications consist of a single technical error (external iliac artery perforation) and one groin hematoma but potentially include groin infection and contrast-related nephrotoxicity. Two postembolization pelvic abscesses have developed. A third case of abscess occurred in the anterior abdominal wall 18 days after postcesarean embolization of both hypogastric and uterine arteries. It is unclear whether the embolization procedure was a contributing factor. Low-grade postprocedure fever has been noted in many patients, warranting the use of antibiotics. The failure has been due to previous ipsilateral internal iliac artery ligation, resulting in difficulty in identifying the bleeding vessel. The drawbacks or limitations of implementing this technique are the need for transfer of potentially unstable patients to the radiology suite and the unfamiliarity of radiologists with this technique in many institutions.

The technique has also been used prophylactically before elective cesarean hysterectomy for placenta accreta. Mitty et al.[77] reported prophylactic and emergency arterial catheterization and embolotherapy in 18 patients. Among nine patients who underwent emergency embolization, three had placenta accreta as the primary cause of hemorrhage. Among the other nine patients who had prophylactic arterial catheter placement for anticipated perioperative risks of bleeding, three had placenta previa alone, and two had placenta accreta. These patients were brought to the radiology room just prior to cesarean section. The gravid uterus was shielded with a lead apron. A catheter was passed from the left axillary artery to the level of the first lumbar vertebra, just above the shielded uterus. The axillary approach was preferred in the operating room, because the patient's groin is near the draped incision site. The axillary artery catheter was infused with normal saline solution, and the patient was transported to the operating room and positioned on an operating room table that allowed fluoroscopic examination. The radiologist, radiologic technician, and a special procedure nurse were present in the operating room. In all, two patients with placenta accreta required bilateral uterine artery embolization, whereas none of the patients with placenta previa alone required embolization. It is evident that better patient selection is needed before the use of prophylactic arterial catheterization and more frequent use of embolotherapy. However, the emergency angiographic embolization for obstetric hemorrhage may become popular in the future. Mitty et al. stated, "A team approach in the angiography suite with the obstetrician and anesthesiologist actively involved to ensure adequate blood replacement and ventilation provides the radiologist with the best opportunity for an efficient and successful procedure." Obstetric anesthesiologists may be asked to be involved in patient care in these new settings more often.

BLOOD CONSERVATION TECHNIQUES

To protect parturients from the risks of homologous blood transfusion, several methods have been tried. Those include preoperative autologous blood donation, acute hemodilution, erythropoietin administration, and intraoperative blood salvage with cell saver.

Autologous Blood Donation

Autologous blood donation has become a routine in selected patients in some institutions in Japan, the United States, and other countries. Multiple reports document its safety.[75, 110, 111] Droste et al.[75] studied the hemodynamic effect of a 450-mL blood donation in 16 pregnant women and found that neither orthostasis nor blood loss caused significant changes in the umbilical systolic:diastolic ratio.[75] Kuromaki et al.[110] studied 34 pregnant patients who were at high risk for peripartum hemorrhage. Each patient donated 300 mL of blood three times every week. The hemoglobin concentration decreased by 0.6 g/dL on average. Erythropoietin levels and reticulocyte counts both increased soon after blood donation. Twelve of the 34 women received the autologous blood transfusion during or after cesarean delivery, and homologous blood transfusion was avoided. McVay et al.[111] found no adverse effect on the mothers or infants in their series of 273 patients in the third trimester.

The difficulty of autologous blood donation in parturients stems from the fact that there are not many patients who require blood transfusion during parturition. Camann and Datta[112] reviewed the transfusion of red cells from 1984 to 1987 and found that the transfusion rate declined from 6.2% to 3.2% during the study period. In addition, Andres et al.[113] reviewed 2265 deliveries in 6 months in their institution and identified 251 patients who had traditionally accepted risk factors, such as repeat cesarean section, multiple gestation, placenta previa, and grand multiparity. Only 4 of these 251 patients received transfusion. From this result, the authors concluded that autologous blood donation may not be beneficial or cost-effective when considering the low frequency of blood transfusions in this high-risk obstetric population and the difficulty in accurately predicting those likely to require transfusions.[113] However, the authors only reviewed their status of blood transfusion in obstetrics retrospectively. They did not institute autologous blood transfusion practice, nor did they simulate a cost and benefit comparison when a certain autologous blood transfusion program is implemented. If one is able to better identify very high risk patients for significant blood loss during cesarean section, for example those with documented placenta percreta, it is possible that autologous blood donation may become beneficial. Risks of autologous blood transfusion, such as bacterial contamination and clerical errors, need to be appreciated to compare the risks and benefits of such programs.

Acute Normovolemic Hemodilution

The first report of acute normovolemic hemodilution for cesarean section was recently made by Grange et al.[114] It includes 38 healthy parturients who are at high risk for hemorrhage (placenta previa, 33 patients; placenta accreta, 1 patient). Two thirds of the patients pre-donated autologous blood, and prehemodilution hemoglobin concentration was 10.9 g/dL. After 750 to 1000 mL of blood collection that was replaced by an equal amount of 10% pentastarch, the hemoglobin level decreased to 8.3 g/dL (range 6.7–9.5) with a hematocrit of 25% (range, 20–30%). All the blood was reinfused at the end of operation or before. The hemoglobin level and hematocrit before blood reinfusion were 7.3 g/dL and 22%, respectively. Regarding anesthetic methods of these patients, 19 patients had spinal anesthesia, 15 had epidural anesthesia, 3 had general anesthesia, and 1 had combined spinal-epidural anesthesia. Hypotension requiring vasopressor occurred in 13 patients with spinal anesthesia, 3 patients with epidural anesthesia, and none with general anesthesia. There was only one patient with placenta previa who required perioperative homologous blood transfusion, who had not donated autologous blood, and who lost 3000 mL intraoperatively. On the contrary, another patient with a surgical blood loss of 5000 mL required 2 units of preoperative autologous donation and 2 units of acute normovolemic hemodilution but no homologous blood. Apparently, there were no adverse effects on the fetus as judged by fetal heart rate monitoring, Apgar score, and umbilical venous blood gases.

The authors summarized the potential advantages of acute normovolemic hemodilution over preoperative autologous donation as follows[114]:

1. Reduction of red blood cell mass lost for a given volume lost during surgery.
2. Limited processing of blood with little risk of storage or clerical error.
3. Collected blood is always reinfused, avoiding wastage.
4. Collected blood is reinfused fresh, ensuring adequate function of clotting factors and platelets.
5. Possible use in patients who are hepatitis carriers.

This method appears promising, and further evaluation of its effects on fetal safety is desired.

Erythropoietin

Erythropoietin may be administered to pregnant patients to compensate for loss of blood by autologous blood donation. The permeability of erythropoietin across the placenta is very low,[115] and it has been used without significant maternal or fetal side effects.[116] However, the clinical experience of human recombinant erythropoietin in pregnancy is still very limited, and its safety needs to be established.

Intraoperative Blood Salvage

The concern over intraoperative blood salvage during cesarean section stems from the potential of fetal or amniotic substances to cause amniotic fluid embolism or DIC. A recent report found that cell savers can effectively separate amniotic fluid from blood and can be used in cases of massive obstetric hemorrhage.[117] Subsequently, Jackson et al. reported the use of intraoperative blood salvage in 109 parturients. Sixty of these patients received a total of 127 salvaged units. Thus, the previous concern about cardiovascular collapse or DIC was not substantiated by this report. If the safety of these blood conservation modalities can be established, the perioperative morbidity of parturients may be reduced, so that we can better serve these patients.

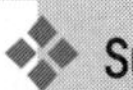

SUMMARY

Key Points

- Obstetric hemorrhage remains a leading cause of maternal death.
- Visual assessment of blood loss is often misleading, and hypotension is usually a late sign of blood loss in the pregnant patient.
- Owing to the increase in circulating blood volume, many pregnant women do not demonstrate blood pressure changes, even after moderate blood loss.
- If transfusion of blood is urgently needed, type-specific, partially cross-matched blood can be made ready within minutes; provision of such blood eliminates serious hemolytic reactions due to errors in ABO typing. When the situation is more urgent, type-specific non–cross-matched blood may be used.

Key References

Kramer MS, Usher RH, Pollack R, et al: Etiologic determinants of abruptio placentae. Obstet Gynecol 1997; 89:221.

Chestnut DH, Dewan DM, Redick LF, et al: Anesthetic management for obstetric hysterectomy: a multi-institutional study. Anesthesiology 1989; 70:607.

Case Stem

A 28-year-old woman at 36 weeks' gestation is admitted to L&D with painless vaginal bleeding of approximately 800 mL. She has had two previous cesarean sections. She is in active labor and is to undergo an emergent repeat cesarean section. An ultrasound demonstrates a low-lying anterior placenta previa. Describe the obstetric and anesthetic implicatons and your proposed anesthetic management.

CONCLUSION

Obstetric hemorrhage remains the leading cause of maternal mortality in many regions of the world. The incidence of some of the obstetric hemorrhages are increasing at the present time, mainly due to long-term effects of our high cesarean section rate[119] and to changing obstetric practice. Although anesthesia-related maternal mortality decreased by 47% from early 1980s to late 1980s, the hemorrhage-related mortality rate decrease has reached a plateau.[4] Further reduction in the rates of hemorrhage-related maternal and perinatal mortality and morbidity should be achieved by the better identification of high-risk parturients with antenatal diagnosis, prompt and intensive care for emergency situations, and appropriate anesthetic management and by combining modalities to reduce blood loss and homologous blood transfusion.

References

1. Sachs BP, Brown DAJ, Driscoll SG, et al: Maternal mortality in Massachusetts: trends and prevention. N Engl J Med 1987; 316:667–672.
2. Statistics and Information Department, Minister's Secretariat, Ministry of Health and Welfare: Vital Statistics of Japan, Vol 1. 1994.
3. Berg CJ, Atrash HK, Koonin LM, et al: Pregnancy related mortality in the United States, 1987–1990. Obstet Gynecol 1996; 88:161–167.
4. Lipitz S, Admon D, Menczer J, et al: Midtrimester bleeding: variables which affect the outcome of pregnancy. Gynecol Obstet Invest 1991; 32:24–27.
5. Ajayi RA, Soothill PW, Campbell S, et al: Antenatal testing to predict outcome in pregnancies with unexplained antepartum haemorrhage. Br J Obstet Gynaecol 1992; 99:122–125.
6. Pritchard JA, Baldwin RM, Dickey JC, et al: Blood volume changes in pregnancy and the puerperium: II. Red blood cell loss and changes in apparent blood volume during and following vaginal delivery, cesarean section, and cesarean section plus total hysterectomy. Am J Obstet Gynecol 1962; 84:1271–1282.
7. Clark SL, Yeh SY, Phelan JP, et al: Emergency hysterectomy for obstetric hemorrhage. Obstet Gynecol 1984; 64:376–380.
8. Chestnut DH, Eden RD, Gall SA, et al: Peripartum hysterectomy: a review of cesarean and postpartum hysterectomy. Obstet Gynecol 1985; 65:365–370.
9. Duthie SJ, Ghosh A, Ng A, et al: Intraoperative blood loss during elective lower segment caesarean section. Br J Obstet Gynaecol 1992; 99:364–367.
10. Clark SL, Cotton DB, Lee W, et al: Central hemodynamic assessment of normal term pregnancy. Am J Obstet Gynecol 1989; 161:1439–1442.
11. Conklin KA: Physiologic changes of pregnancy. *In* Chestnut DH (ed): Obstetric Anesthesia: Principles and Practice. St. Louis: Mosby; 1994: 21.
12. Pritchard JA: Changes in the blood volume during pregnancy and delivery. Anesthesiology 1965; 26:393.
13. Coopland A, Alkjaersig N, Fletcher AP: Reduction in plasma factor (fibrin stabilization factor) concentration during pregnancy. J Lab Clin Med 1969; 73:144–153.
14. Astedt B: Significance of placenta in depression of fibrinolytic activity during pregnancy. J Obstet Gynaecol Br Commw 1972; 79:205–206.
15. Duthie SJ, Ven D, Yung GLK, et al: Discrepancy between laboratory determination and visual estimation of blood loss during normal delivery. Eur J Obstet Gynecol Reprod Biol 1991; 38:119–124.
16. Plumer MH: Bleeding problems. *In* James FM, Wheeler AS, Dewan DM (eds): Obstetric Anesthesia: The Complicated Patient, 2nd ed. Philadelphia: FA Davis; 1988: 309–344.
17. Griffel MI, Kaufman BS: Pharmacology of colloids and crystalloids. Crit Care Clin 1992; 8:235–253.
18. Lowery BD, Cloutier CT, Carey LC: Electrolyte solutions in resuscitation in human hemorrhagic shock. Surg Gynecol Obstet 1971; 133:273–284.
19. Marino PL: Colloid and crystalloid resuscitation. *In* ICU Book, 2nd ed. Baltimore: Williams & Wilkins; 1998: 231.
20. Nearman HS, Herman ML: Toxic effects of colloids in the intensive care unit. Crit Care Clin 1991; 7:713–723.
21. Warren BB, Durieux ME: Hydroxyethyl starch: safe or not? Anesth Analg 1997; 84:206–212.
22. Marcus MA, Vertommen JD, Van-Aken H: Hydroxyethyl starch versus lactated Ringer's solution in the chronic maternal-fetal sheep preparation: a pharmacologic and pharmacokinetic study. Anesth Analg 1995; 80:949–954.
23. Office of Medical Applications of Research, National Institute of Health: perioperative red blood cell transfusion. JAMA 1988; 260:2700–27003.
24. American Society of Anesthesiologists Task Force on Blood Component Therapy: practice guidelines for blood component therapy. Anesthesiology 1996; 84:732–747.
25. Weiskopf RB, Viele MK, Feiner J, et al: Human cardiovascular and metabolic response to acute, severe isovolemic anemia. JAMA 1998; 279:217–221.
26. Kimura T, Watanabe S, Takeshima R, et al: Critical cases treated in the Ibaraki Perinatal Center. J Japan Soc Clin Anesth 1995; 15:83.
27. Miller RD: Transfusion therapy. *In* Miller RD (ed): Anesthesia, 3rd ed. New York: Churchill Livingstone; 1990: 1472.
28. Shulman IA, Spence RK, Petz LD: Surgical blood ordering, blood shortage situations, and emergency transfusions. *In* Petz LD, Swisher SN, Kleinman S, Spence R, Strauss RG (eds): Clinical Practice of Transfusion Medicine, 3rd ed. New York: Churchill Livingstone: 1996: 509–520.
29. Murray DJ: Blood component therapy: indications and risks. *In* Rogers MC, Tinker JH, Covino BJ, et al (eds): Principles and Practice of Anesthesiology. St. Louis: Mosby; 1993: 2490.
30. Ross S, Jeter E: Emergency surgery-trauma and massive transfusion. *In* Petz LD, Swisher SN, Kleinman S, et al (eds): Clinical Practice of Transfusion Medicine, 3rd ed. New York: Churchill Livingstone; 1996: 563–579.
31. Counts RB, Haish C, Simon TL, et al: Hemostasis in massively transfused trauma patients. Ann Surg 1979; 190:91–99.
32. Michael JM, Dorner I, Bruns D, et al: Potassium load in CPD-preserved whole blood and two types of packed red blood cells. Transfusion 1975; 15:144–149.
33. Suresh MS, Belfort MA: Antepartum hemorrhage. *In* Datta S (ed): Anesthetic and Obstetric Management of High Risk Pregnancy, 2nd ed. St. Louis: Mosby; 1996: 76–109.
34. Obstetrical hemorrhage. *In* Cunningham FG, MacDonald PC, Gant NF, et al (eds): Williams Obstetrics, 20th ed. Stamford, CT: Appleton & Lange; 1997: 746.
35. Rasmussen S, Irgens LM, Bergsjo PB, et al: The occurrence of placental abruption in Norway 1967–1991. Acta Obstet Gynecol Scand 1996; 75:222–228.
36. Rasmussen S, Irgens LM, Bergsjo PB, et al: Perinatal mortality and case fatality after placental abruption in Norway 1967–1991. Acta Obstet Gynecol Scand 1996; 75:229–234.
37. Saftlas AF, Olson DR, Atrash HK, et al: National trends in the incidence of abruptio placentae, 1979–1987. Obstet Gynecol 1991; 78:1081–1086.
38. Pritchard JA, Cunningham FG, Pritchard SA, et al: On reducing the frequency of severe abruptio placentae. Am J Obstet Gynecol 1991;165:1345–1351.
39. Abdella TN, Sibai BM, Hays JM, et al: Relationship of hypertensive diseases to abruptio placentae. Obstet Gynecol 1984; 63:365–370.
40. Ananth CV, Savitz DA, Williams MA: Placental abruption and its association with hypertension and prolonged rupture of membranes: a methodologic review and meta-analysis. Obstet Gynecol 1996; 88:309–318.
41. Morgan MA, Berkowitz KM, Thomas SJ, et al: Abruptio placentae: perinatal outcome in normotensive and hypertensive patients. Am J Obstet Gynecol 1994; 170:1595–1599.

42. Sakamoto S, Mizuno, Taketani Y (eds): Principles of Obstetrics and Gynecology. Tokyo: Medical View; 1998: 361.
43. Kramer MS, Usher RH, Pollack R, et al: Etiologic determinants of abruptio placentae. Obstet Gynecol 1997; 89:221–226.
44. Fretts RC, Boyd ME, Usher RH, et al: The changing pattern of fetal death, 1961–1988. Obstet Gynecol 1992; 79:35–39.
45. Hurd WW, Miodovnik M, Hertzberg V, et al: Selective management of abruptio placentae: a prospective study. Obstet Gynecol 1983; 61:467–473.
46. Witt BR, Miles R, Wolf GC, et al: CA 125 levels in abruptio placentae. Am J Obstet Gynecol 1991; 164:1225–1228.
47. Magriples U, Chan DW, Copel JA, et al: Thrombomodulin: a novel marker for abruptio placentae [abstract]. Am J Obstet Gynecol 1996; 174:364.
48. Downing JW, Buley RJR, Brock-Utne JG, et al: Etomidate for induction of anaesthesia at caesarean section: comparison with thiopentone. Br J Anaesth 1979; 51:135–140.
49. Terao T, Maki M, Ikenoue T: A prospective study in 38 patients with abruptio placentae of 70 cases complicated by DIC. Asia-Oceania J Obstet Gynaecol 1987; 13:1–13.
50. Takagi S, Yoshida T, Togo Y, et al: The effects of intramyometrial injection of prostaglandin F2-alpha on severe postpartum hemorrhage. Prostaglandins 1976; 12:565–579.
51. Hankins GDV, Berryman GK, Scott RT Jr, et al: Maternal arterial desaturation with 15-methyl prostaglandin F2-alpha for uterine atony. Obstet Gynecol 1988; 72:367–370.
52. Green JR: Placental abnormalities: placenta previa and abruptio placentae. *In* Creasy RK, Resnik R (eds): Maternal Fetal Medicine: Principles and Practice, 3rd ed. Philadelphia: WB Saunders; 1994: 592–612.
53. Maki K, Terao T, Ikenoue T, et al: Clinical evaluation of antithrombin III concentrate (BI6.013) for disseminated intravascular coagulation in obstetrics: well-controlled multicenter trial. Gynecol Obstet Invest 1987; 23:230–240.
54. Iyasu S, Saftlas AK, Rowley DL, et al: The epidemiology of placenta previa in the United States, 1979 through 1987. Am J Obstet Gynecol 1993; 168:1424–1429.
55. Sauer M, Parsons M, Sampson M: Placenta previa: an analysis of three years experience. Am J Perinatol 1985; 2:39–42.
56. McShane PM, Heyl PS, Epstein MF: Maternal and perinatal morbidity resulting from placenta previa. Obstet Gynecol 1985; 65:176–182.
57. Macones GA, Sehdev HM, Parry S, et al: The association between maternal cocaine use and placenta previa. Am J Obstet Gynecol 1997; 177:1097–1100.
58. Taylor VM, Peacock S, Kramer MD, et al: Increased risk of placenta previa among women of Asian origin. Obstet Gynecol 1995; 86:805–808.
59. Ananth CV, Bowes WS Jr, Savitz DA, et al: Relationship between pregnancy-induced hypertension and placenta previa: a population-based study. Am J Obstet Gynecol 1997; 177:997–1002.
60. Ananth CV, Wilcox AJ, Savitz DA, et al: Effect of maternal age and parity on the risk of uteroplacental bleeding disorders in pregnancy. Obstet Gynecol 1996; 88:511–516.
61. Clark SL, Koonings P, Phelan JP, et al: Placenta previa/accreta and prior Cesarean section. Obstet Gynecol 1985; 66:89–92.
62. Oppenheimer LW, Farine D, Ritchie JWK, et al: What is low-lying placenta? Am J Obstet Gynecol 1991; 165:1036–1038.
62a. Obata S, Ishihara K: Ultrasonographic study of low-lying placenta and its clinical significance. Nippon Sanka Fujinka Gakkai Zasshi 1993; 45:1101–1108.
63. Brar HS, Platt DL, DeVore GR, et al: Fetal umbilical velocimetry for the surveillance of pregnancies complicated by placenta previa. J Reprod Med 1988; 33:741–744.
64. Droste S, Keil K: Expectant management of placenta previa: cost-benefit analysis of outpatient treatment. Am J Obstet Gynecol 1994; 170:1254–1257.
65. Mouer JR: Placenta previa: antepartum conservative management, inpatient versus outpatient. Am J Obstet Gynecol 1994; 170:1683–1685.
66. Wing DA, Paul RH, Millar LK: Management of symptomatic placenta previa: a randomized, controlled trial of in-patient versus out-patient expectant management. Am J Obstet Gynecol 1996; 175:806–811.
67. Besinger RE, Moniak CW, Paskiewicz LS, et al: The effect of tocolytic use in the management of symptomatic placenta previa. Am J Obstet Gynecol 1995; 172:1770–1775.
68. Miller DA, Chollet JA, Goodwin TM: Clinical risk factors for placenta previa–placenta accreta. Am J Obstet Gynecol 1997; 177:210–214.
69. Chestnut DH, Dewan DM, Redick LF, et al: Anesthetic management for obstetric hysterectomy: a multi-institutional study. Anesthesiology 1989; 70:607–610.
70. Read JA, Cotton DB, Miller FC: Placenta accreta: changing clinical aspects and outcome. Obstet Gynecol 1980; 56:31–34.
71. Fox H: Placenta accreta, 1945–1969. Obstet Gynecol Surv 1972; 27:475.
72. Lerner JP, Deane S, Timor-Tritsch IE: Characterization of placenta accreta using transvaginal sonography and color Doppler imaging. Ultrasound Obstet Gynecol 1995; 5:198–201.
73. Finberg HJ, Williams JW: Placenta accreta: prospective sonographic diagnosis in patients with placenta previa and prior cesarean section. J Ultrasound Med 1992; 11:333–343.
74. Thorp JM Jr, Councell RB, Sandridge DA, et al: Antepartum diagnosis of placenta previa percreta by magnetic resonance imaging. Obstet Gynecol 1992; 80:506–508.
75. Droste S, Sorensen T, Price T, et al: Maternal and fetal hemodynamic effects of autologous blood donation during pregnancy. Am J Obstet Gynecol 1992; 167:89–93.
76. Zelop CM, Harlow BL, Frigoletto FD Jr, et al: Emergency peripartum hysterectomy. Am J Obstet Gynecol 1993; 168:1443–1448.
77. Mitty HA, Sterling KM, Alvarez M, et al: Obstetric hemorrhage: prophylactic and emergency arterial catheterization and embolotherapy. Radiology 1993; 188:183–187.
78. Chestnut DH, Redick LF: Continuous epidural anesthesia for elective cesarean hysterectomy. South Med J 1985; 78:1168–1169.
79. Horlocker TT, Wedel DJ: Spinal and epidural blockade and perioperative low molecular weight heparin: smooth sailing on the Titanic. Anesth Analg 1998; 86:1153–1156.
80. Sprung J, Cheng EY, Patel S: When to remove an epidural catheter in a parturient with disseminated intravascular coagulation. Reg Anesth 1992; 17:351–354.
81. Owen MD: Anesthesia for the bleeding obstetric patient. *In* Dewan DM, Hood DD (eds): Practical Obstetric Anesthesia. Philadelphia: WB Saunders; 1997:160.
82. Golan A, Sandbank O, Rubin A: Rupture of the pregnant uterus. Obstet Gynecol 1980; 56:549–550.
83. Eden RD, Parker RT, Gall SA: Rupture of the pregnant uterus: a 53-year review. Obstet Gynecol 1986; 68:671–674.
84. Miller DA, Goodwin TM, Gherman RB, et al: Rupture of the unscarred uterus [abstract]. Am J Obstet Gynecol 1996; 174:345.
85. Rosen MG, Dickinson JC, Westhoff CL: Vaginal birth after cesarean: a meta-analysis of morbidity and mortality. Obstet Gynecol 1991; 77:465–470.
86. Flamm BL, Lim OW, Jones C, et al: Vaginal birth after cesarean section: results of a multicenter study. Am J Obstet Gynecol 1988; 158:1079–1084.
87. Rachagan SP, Raman S, Balasundram G, et al: Rupture of the pregnant uterus: a 21-year review. Aust N Z J Obstet Gynaecol 1991; 31:37–40.
88. Jones RO, Nagashima AW, Hatnett-Goodman MM, et al: Rupture of low transverse cesarean scars during trial of labor. Obstet Gynecol 1991; 77:815–817.
89. Scott JR: Mandatory trial of labor after cesarean delivery: an alternative viewpoint. Obstet Gynecol 1991; 77:811–814.
90. Johnson C, Oriol N: The role of epidural anesthesia in trial of labor. Reg Anesth 1990; 15:304–308.
91. Rodriguez MH, Masaki DI, Phelan JP, et al: Uterine rupture: are intrauterine pressure catheters useful in the diagnosis? Am J Obstet Gynecol 1989; 161:666–669.
92. Glassenberg R, Vaisrub N, Rodino KL, et al: Vaginal delivery after a previous cesarean section. *In* Datta S (ed): Common Problems in Obstetric Anesthesia, 2nd ed. St. Louis: Mosby; 1995: 175.

93. LaPlatney DR, O'Leary JA: Anesthetic considerations in cesarean hysterectomy. Anesth Analg 1970; 49:328–330.
94. Vincent RD, Chestnut DH, Sipes SL, et al: Epidural anesthesia worsens uterine blood flow and fetal oxygenation during hemorrhage in gravid ewes. Anesthesiology 1992; 76:799–806.
95. Vincent RD, Chestnut DH, McGrath JM, et al: The effects of epidural anesthesia on uterine vascular resistance, plasma arginine vasopressin concentrations, and plasma renin activity during hemorrhage in gravid ewes. Anesthesiology 1994; 78:293–300.
96. Chestnut DH, Thompson CS, McLaughlin GL, et al: Does intravenous infusion of ritodrine or magnesium sulfate alter the hemodynamic response to hemorrhage in gravid ewes? Am J Obstet Gynecol 1988; 159:1467–1473.
97. Sipes SL, Chestnut DH, Vincent RD, et al: Does magnesium sulfate alter maternal cardiovascular response to vasopressor agents in gravid ewes? Anesthesiology 1991; 75:1010–1018.
98. Vincent RD, Chestnut DH, Sipes SL, et al: Does calcium chloride help restore maternal blood pressure and uterine blood flow during hemorrhagic hypotension in hypermagnesemic gravid ewes? Anesth Analg 1992; 74:670–676.
99. Burchell RC: Physiology of internal iliac artery ligation. J Obstet Gynaecol Br Commonw 1968; 75:642–651.
100. Evans S, McShane P: The efficacy of internal iliac artery ligation in obstetric hemorrhage. Surg Gynecol Obstet 1985; 160:250–253.
101. Clark SL, Phelan JP, Yeh S, et al: Hypogastric artery ligation for obstetric hemorrhage. Obstet Gynecol 1985; 66:353–356.
102. Chattopadhyay SK, Deb Roy B, Edrees YB: Surgical control of obstetric hemorrhage: hypogastric artery ligation or hysterectomy? Int J Obstet Gynecol 1990; 32:345–351.
103. Mengert WF, Burchell RC, Blumstein RW, et al: Pregnancy after bilateral ligation of the internal iliac and ovarian arteries. Obstet Gynecol 1969; 34:664–666.
104. Vedantham S, Goodwin SC, McLucas B, et al: Uterine artery embolization: an underused method of controlling pelvic hemorrhage. Am J Obstet Gynecol 1997; 176:938–948.
105. Joseph JF, Mernoff D, Donovan J, et al: Percutaneous angiographic arterial embolization for gynecologic and obstetric pelvic hemorrhage: a report of three cases. J Reprod Med 1994; 39:915–920.
106. Rosenthal DM, Colapinto R: Angiographic arterial embolization in the management of postoperative vaginal hemorrhage. Am J Obstet Gynecol 1985; 151:227–231.
107. Feinberg BB, Resnik E, Hurt WG, et al: Angiographic embolization in the management of late postpartum hemorrhage. J Reprod Med 1987; 32:929–931.
108. Shweni PM, Bishop BB, Hansen JN, et al: Severe secondary postpartum hemorrhage after caesarean section. S Afr Med J 1987; 72:617–619.
109. Yamashita Y, Harada M, Yamamoto H, et al: Transcatheter arterial embolization of obstetric and gynaecological bleeding: efficacy and clinical outcome. Br J Radiol 1994; 67:530–534.
110. Kuromaki K, Takeda S, Seki H, et al: Clinical study of autologous blood transfusion in pregnant women. Acta Obstet Gynaecol Jpn 1994; 46:1213–1220.
111. McVay PA, Hoag RW, Hoag MS, et al: Safety and use of autologous blood donation during the third trimester of pregnancy. Am J Obstet Gynecol 1989; 9160:1479–1486.
112. Camann WR, Datta S: Red cell use during cesarean delivery. Transfusion 1991; 31(1):12–15.
113. Andres RL, Piacquadio KM, Resnick R: A reappraisal of the need for autologous blood donation in the obstetric patient. Am J Obstet Gynecol 1990; 163:1551–1553.
114. Grange CS, Douglas J, Adams TJ, et al: The use of acute hemodilution in parturients undergoing cesarean section. Am J Obstet Gynecol 1998; 178:156–160.
115. Schneider H, Malek A: Lack of permeability of the human placenta for erythropoietin. J Perinat Med 1995; 23:71–76.
116. McGregor E, Stewart G, Junor BJR, et al: Successful use of recombinant human erythropoietin in pregnancy. Nephrol Dial Transplant 1991; 6:292–293.
117. Bernstein HH, Rosenblatt MA, Gette S, Lockwood C: The ability of the haemonetics and cell saver system to remove tissue factor from blood contaminated with amniotic fluid. Anesth Analg 1997; 85:831–833.
118. Hemminki E, Merilainen J: Long-term effects of cesarean sections: ectopic pregnancies and placental problems. Am J Obstet Gynecol 1996; 174:1569–1574.

30

Postpartum Hemorrhage

❖ ANDREW D. L. WARMINGTON, MBChB, FANZCA

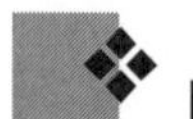

INTRODUCTION

Postpartum hemorrhage (PPH) remains a major cause of maternal morbidity and mortality worldwide including New Zealand, where intrapartum and postpartum hemorrhage has accounted for 8.9% of maternal deaths attributable to an obstetric cause over the years 1969 to 1991.[1] A massive sudden PPH can be a terrifying event for the medical and nursing staff, as well as the parturient and her family. A good outcome requires a cooperative approach from anesthetic, obstetric, medical, and nursing teams. Particularly important is the recognition that a problem exists.

INCIDENCE AND DEFINITION

All births are at some risk of PPH. At a low-risk birthing center at which patients considered at risk for PPH were excluded, the incidence of PPH was still 3.1%.[2] PPH contributes to about 80% of the postpartum complications that occur in 4% to 7% of all deliveries in Australian secondary and tertiary units.[3, 4] Cesarean section increases the risk of PPH markedly, with the incidence rising from 3.9% in a vaginal delivery to 15.4% for a cesarean section. The definition of what constitutes a postpartum hemorrhage is variable. Studies using an accurate estimation of blood loss show that a normal vaginal delivery has an average loss of 500 mL.[5]

Many studies use estimates of blood loss that rely on visual estimation, which is inaccurate.[6] Often a blood loss of 500 to 600 mL is used as a defining volume for PPH, but clearly this volume falls within the normal physiologic range of hemorrhage. However, in most of the world literature, primary postpartum hemorrhage is defined as a blood loss of 500 to 600 mL occurring within 24 hours of birth. Hemorrhage occurring more than 24 hours after delivery until 6 weeks postpartum is variously called delayed, late, or secondary hemorrhage, and it is a condition that appears to have been given little attention in the anesthetic literature. This is probably due to its association with morbidity rather than with mortality.

PHYSIOLOGY AND ANATOMY OF PREGNANCY

Changes in maternal physiology associated with pregnancy (as described in Chapter 2) have equipped the expectant mother to cope with a mandatory blood loss associated with delivery. The changes in maternal physiology that result in an increase in blood volume, increase in cardiac output, and changes in the distribution in blood flow affect the response to and seriousness of a bleed from the uterus and lower genital tract.

Cardiovascular Changes of Pregnancy. The greatest change in the maternal cardiovascular system is the development of the placental circulation, effectively a shunt in the maternal circulation. Cardiac output begins to increase from the 13th week of pregnancy and reaches a plateau at around 27 weeks, at which time output is 30% to 40% above nonpregnant levels. Rise in cardiac output is caused by an increase in stroke volume and a rise in the heart rate. Despite these changes, except in pathologic conditions, pregnancy is associated with a fall in blood pressure caused by a fall in total peripheral resistance and the placental shunt.[7] During labor, the cardiac output increases by a further 50%, with a maximal increase immediately postpartum.

With the growth of the uterus and fetus, blood flow to the uterus increases from only 2% of cardiac output in the nonpregnant woman to 17% at term. Blood flow through the maternal circulation of the placenta is over 600 mL/min, hence the potential for massive blood loss. Every minute of hemorrhage from the placental site represents the loss of 1 unit of blood.

Maternal blood volume begins to increase from the 20th week of gestation, and at a time just prior to delivery is 30% above the nonpregnant level. The increase in blood volume of 1 to 2 L over and above the mother's usual blood volume affords a considerable safety margin for the usual blood losses of up to 500 to 600 mL.[7]

Pregnancy is associated with a physiologic anemia and a hemoglobin of less than 100 g/L is common. Increased hepatic production of coagulation factors produces a hypercoagulable state associated with a rise in most coagulation factors and in particular a rise in the fibrinogen level. A normal pregnancy may, however, show a slight fall in platelet numbers at term. This hypercoagulable state acts to protect against hemorrhage at delivery.

Anatomy. Blood supply to the uterus is via two main arteries; predominantly supply is from the uterine artery, itself derived from the internal iliac artery and secondarily from the ovarian artery via the abdominal aorta. The maternal placental circulation is composed of 8 to 10 spiral endometrial arteries that propel blood into the intervillous space of the placenta, in jetlike streams. Maternal blood flows around and over the villi of the placenta allowing metabolic and gaseous exchange to take place, eventually reaching the floor of the intervillous space to reenter the maternal circulatory system via the endometrial veins.[8]

Separation and Delivery of the Placenta. Postpartum contractions cause the uterus to contract to a smaller size producing a shearing effect between the placenta itself and the walls of the uterus. This shearing effect causes the separation of the placenta. Separation of the placenta opens the placental sinuses causing bleeding. Uterine smooth muscle is arranged in a "figure-of-eight" pattern around the supplying blood vessels as they pass through the uterine wall; contraction of the uterus simultaneously produces constriction of the vessels that previously supplied the placenta. Prostaglandins formed at placental separation may cause additional vessel spasm.[7]

CAUSES AND RISKS

The causes of PPH are divided into uterine and nonuterine (Table 30–1). The most frequent uterine cause of hemorrhage is atony, and is easily diagnosed when the bleeding is associated with a boggy and flaccid uterus. Retained placental products are a further cause of uterine bleeding and requires that examination and curettage of the uterus occurs to ensure complete removal of the placenta. Retained placental fragments are the most frequent cause of delayed PPH.[9] Uterine causes of bleeding also include uterine rupture, which should be considered when other causes of hemorrhage are not obvious, and uterine inversion. The occurrence of uterine rupture is rare, reported as 0.086% in an Australian study, but the consequences are catastrophic, with maternal mortality ranging from nil to as high as 13%.[10] The clinical presentation may be severe hypotension and bradycardia, but the common presentation is usually atypical abdominal pain, failure to progress, vaginal bleeding, and fetal heart rate abnormalities.[10, 11] Scar dehiscence may not be diagnosed until operation for fetal distress. Uterine scars account for the majority of uterine ruptures; scar dehiscence is associated with less blood loss than a de novo uterine rupture.[11]

Abnormal placentation occurs when the protective barrier of the endometrial decidua is deficient, allowing the placenta to attach directly to the myometrium (placenta accreta); in placenta increta the placenta extends into the myometrium, and in placenta percreta it invades the surrounding organs. While these abnormalities are rare in the overall obstetric population, occurring with an incidence of about 1:3000, uterine scarring from previous cesarean sections predisposes to both placenta previa and placenta accreta. In patients with placenta previa (overall risk 1:300) the risk of placenta accreta is 5%, while in patients presenting with placenta previa and a history of previous cesarean section the incidence may be 1:4.[12] Placenta previa in a woman with a history of previous cesarean section should ring alarm bells. Blood loss can be massive, and hysterectomy is usually required.

At cesarean section, placenta previa is associated with heavy bleeding because of both the possible incision through an anterior placenta previa and the poorly developed musculature in the lower uterine segment which is unable to contract firmly. Uterine inversion is classified by both its duration and extent and is usually caused by traction on the cord during the third stage of labor. The usual clinical presentation is major hemorrhage and abdominal pain. The fundus cannot be palpated and the uterus may fill the vault or protrude from the vagina.[13]

Bleeding from a cervical laceration is a common cause of early bleeding sometimes occurring spontaneously after vaginal delivery and often associated with operative vaginal procedures. If there is no uterine atony or significant retained products, the most common cause of major postpartum bleeding is from the lower genital tract, including an episiotomy.

Postpartum hemorrhage may occasionally present as a puerperal hematoma. This condition can be a cause of both morbidity and mortality, and may frequently require a transfusion.[14] A puerperal hematoma can be vulval, vaginal, or subperitoneal. The presenting symptom may be agonizing pain in the presence of a vulval mass. Vaginal and subperitoneal hematoma is more insidious. Symptoms may include pain, fever, anemia, shock, ileus, and leg edema. Subperitoneal hematoma can result in a significant loss of blood from retroperitoneal dissection in all directions, and may show few signs or symptoms other than shock.

Predictors of Potential Postpartum Hemorrhage. Although any birth carries a small risk of PPH, a large number of medical and obstetric conditions are associated with PPH. Awareness of potential at-risk patients in a delivery unit should allow anesthetic input from an early stage. If help has not already been sought, timely anesthetic intervention may prevent potential disasters.

Good communication about high-risk patients is vital. The on-call anesthetic team should always make

Table 30-1 Etiology of and Risk Factors for Postpartum Hemorrhage

Causes

Uterine
- Immediate causes
  - Atony
  - Disruption: tear, rupture, inversion, surgical
  - Retained products
  - Abnormal placentation
- Delayed causes
  - Retained products
  - Disruption or involution/subinvolution of placental vessels
  - Endometritis

Nonuterine
- Vaginal tear
- Perineal hematoma/tear
- Coagulopathy
- Nonpregnancy trauma

Risk Factors

- Antepartum hemorrhage
  - Placenta previa
  - Placental abruption
- Atony
  - Induction of labor
  - Augmentation of labor
  - Multiple gestation
  - Nulliparous labor
  - Prolonged first stage
  - Prolonged second stage
  - Large baby >4000 g
  - Arrest of descent
  - Use of magnesium sulfate
- Primary coagulopathy
  - Von Willebrand factor deficiency
  - Platelet dysfunction
- Induced coagulopathy
  - Heparin
  - Warfarin
  - Low molecular weight heparin
  - Aspirin/NSAIDs
- Pregnancy-related coagulopathy
  - Preeclampsia
  - Thrombocytopenia of pregnancy
  - Amniotic fluid embolism
  - Sepsis
- Intervention
  - Cesarean section; further risk with classic incision
  - Cesarean section before 37 weeks' and after 42 weeks' gestation
  - Cesarean section under general anesthesia
  - Instrumental delivery
  - Episiotomy
  - Epidural anesthesia
- Antepartum factors
  - Ethnicity (Hispanic, Asian, and/or American Indian)
  - Obesity (in cesarean section)
  - Previous postpartum hemorrhage
  - Congenital medical syndromes—many medical syndromes may be associated with coagulopathies, connective tissue disorders and vessel fragility, and disorders of uterine function

NSAIDs, nonsteroidal anti-inflammatory drugs.
Data from references 4–6, 15–17.

themselves aware of potential problems on the delivery unit, and any known or potential problems should be clearly identified beside the patient's name on the unit's admission board, or on the operating room (OR) schedule.

Increased risk of PPH appears to have its strongest association with the augmentation of labor.[3, 4, 6] Induction of labor with amniotomy or oxytocin infusion increased the risk of PPH over that found with vaginal prostaglandins.[6] PPH should be considered a complication of induction.

Nulliparity, epidural anesthesia, and instrumental delivery are also risk factors for PPH. Grand multiparous patients were at no greater risk than that of a group of age-matched control patients (the control patients were multiparous).[15]

While the association of epidural anesthesia with PPH may be due to a higher incidence of instrumental delivery in this group, a retrospective analysis has shown that PPH is increased in association with epidural anesthesia even in normal deliveries.[4] The incidence of PPH in vaginal delivery with an epidural catheter in situ was found to be twice that in vaginal delivery without an epidural catheter. These findings have not been seen in other studies, however.

Cesarean section is associated with a greater degree of hemorrhage than vaginal delivery, and blood losses of up to 600 to 1000 mL can be considered as "normal." At cesarean section the factors most strongly associated with PPH are general anesthesia, amnionitis, prolonged active phase of labor, and second-stage arrest of labor. Amnionitis is associated with dysfunctional labor and has a similar association with hemorrhage in vaginal deliveries.[16] Ethnic origin may have an association with PPH, as does operation before 37 and after 42 weeks' gestation.[17]

Preeclampsia has a frequent association with PPH. Patients with HELLP (hemolysis, elevated liver enzymes, and low platelets) syndrome who maintain a platelet count of greater than 40,000/μL are unlikely to have clinically significant postpartum bleeding.[18] Significant PPH may be more frequent when the platelet count, fibrinogen level, or both were low in early pregnancy.[19]

IMMEDIATE MANAGEMENT

The hallowed concept in trauma of the "golden hour," with excellent outcomes associated with expeditious treatment in successfully resuscitated trauma patients, has its parallel in obstetrics. In PPH the most important factor in the early successful management of bleeding is the recognition by the obstetric team that significant blood loss is occurring. Rapid transfer to the OR in a few minutes can be lifesaving because excessive resuscitation in the delivery unit is time-consuming and delays definitive surgical treatment while bleeding continues. Any bleed associated with hypotension and not responsive to 500 to 1000 mL of resuscitation fluid (colloid or crystalloid) should be in the hands of the anesthetic team with early consideration of transport to an appropriate OR (Table 30–2).

Initial management in any resuscitation must attend to the cardinals of primary resuscitation: airway, breathing, and circulation (ABC) with the appropriate use of drug therapy. Simultaneously, a rapid primary survey of the PPH must occur. Factors also to be taken into consideration are the history of pregnancy and labor, timing of delivery, timing and completion of the third stage of labor, medical history and relevant conditions, medications, allergies, and anesthetic history. A protocol for PPH should be available at all delivery sites, and the staff involved in direct patient management should be aware of its content (Fig. 30–1).

The usual steps in the obstetric management of PPH are[20]:

1. Palpation of the abdomen is done; if the uterus is well contracted the cause of bleeding is not atony but likely to be a laceration that requires repair.
2. The atonic uterus is manually stimulated to contract. If it fails to contract after "rubbing up," the bladder is emptied.
3. Intravenous ergometrine or Syntometrine (a combination of ergometrine plus Oxytocin) is given.
4. Bimanual compression is performed to stimulate the uterus and compress it. This process may also reduce the amount of bleeding. Bimanual compression is performed by placing one hand in the vagina which elevates the uterus, keeping the uterine vessels on a "stretch," decreasing the bore of the vessels and reducing blood flow, while the other hand is palpating the abdomen.[21]
5. Intramuscular injection of a prostaglandin analogue is given.
6. Failure of an intramuscular injection at this stage, combined with a failure of evacuation of the uterus, should result in the use of an intramyometrial injection of prostaglandin in the operating room environment.
7. Continuing failure of the uterus to contract and ongoing PPH requires more active therapy.

A lifesaving maneuver in the delivery unit or the OR in the presence of significant and unresolved hemorrhage may be the use of external abdominal aortic compression. Aortic compression is performed by firmly pressing the clenched fist into the abdomen in the midline just above the umbilicus with the palmar aspect of the hand facing caudad. Firm pressure is applied directly backward compressing the aorta against the vertebral column. In a prospective study aortic compression was able to produce an unrecordable lower limb blood pressure and absent femoral pulse in 55% of patients and significantly reduced lower limb pressure in another 10%.[22] The difficulty with this procedure in the actively bleeding patient is that most cases of PPH are secondary to an atonic uterus, and the fundus of the large floppy uterus is likely to be above the umbilicus.

This is a technique that should be considered in any situation in which control of hemorrhage is difficult or active management of bleeding is not occurring, such as in the transport of the bleeding patient to the OR, during induction of anesthesia, or while waiting for a drug response.

Table 30–2 OPERATING ROOM FLOW FOR A MAJOR POSTPARTUM HEMORRHAGE (PPH)

Significant PPH ± hypotension ± surgical indication

Initial Assessment

1. Send for blood.
2. Rapid scan (seconds) to evaluate clinical anemia, poor perfusion, early shock.
3. Rapid evaluation of situation, review proposed surgical cause and operation, check last BP/HR/JVP if visible.
4. Anesthetic immediate intervention: obtain large-bore IV access, preferably in upper limbs; give IV H_2 blocker/prokinetic agent.
   a. Administer antacid.
   b. Consider placement of arterial line.
   c. Consider placement of central line for CVP monitoring, inotropes, and as best IV access.
5. If CVS are unstable prepare for general anesthesia. If CVS are stable and further bleeding is unlikely, consider the use of an existing epidural catheter when adequate assistance is available.

BP, blood pressure; CVP, central venous pressure; CVS, cardiovascular signs; HR, heart rate; IV, intravenous; JVP = jugular venous pressure.

Uterine Packing. Uterine packing was common until the 1950s when it fell out of favor, because it was considered to be not physiologically sound. A concern with packing is the risk of concealed and ongoing bleeding; however, this is probably not warranted.[23] Uterine packing can be considered for control of bleeding in uterine atony, placenta previa, and placenta accreta. Packing of the uterus needs to be complete and uniform. The pack can be safely left in place for 24 to 36 hours. Packing has at times been performed using specific packing devices such as the Torpin packer or the Holmes packer.[23] Proponents of packing would consider it unusual for a uterus to bleed once the packing is removed. If control of bleeding with packing is unsuccessful, it is usually immediately obvious.

Uterine packing is not always popular but a quote attributed to a Charleston obstetrician may be timely:

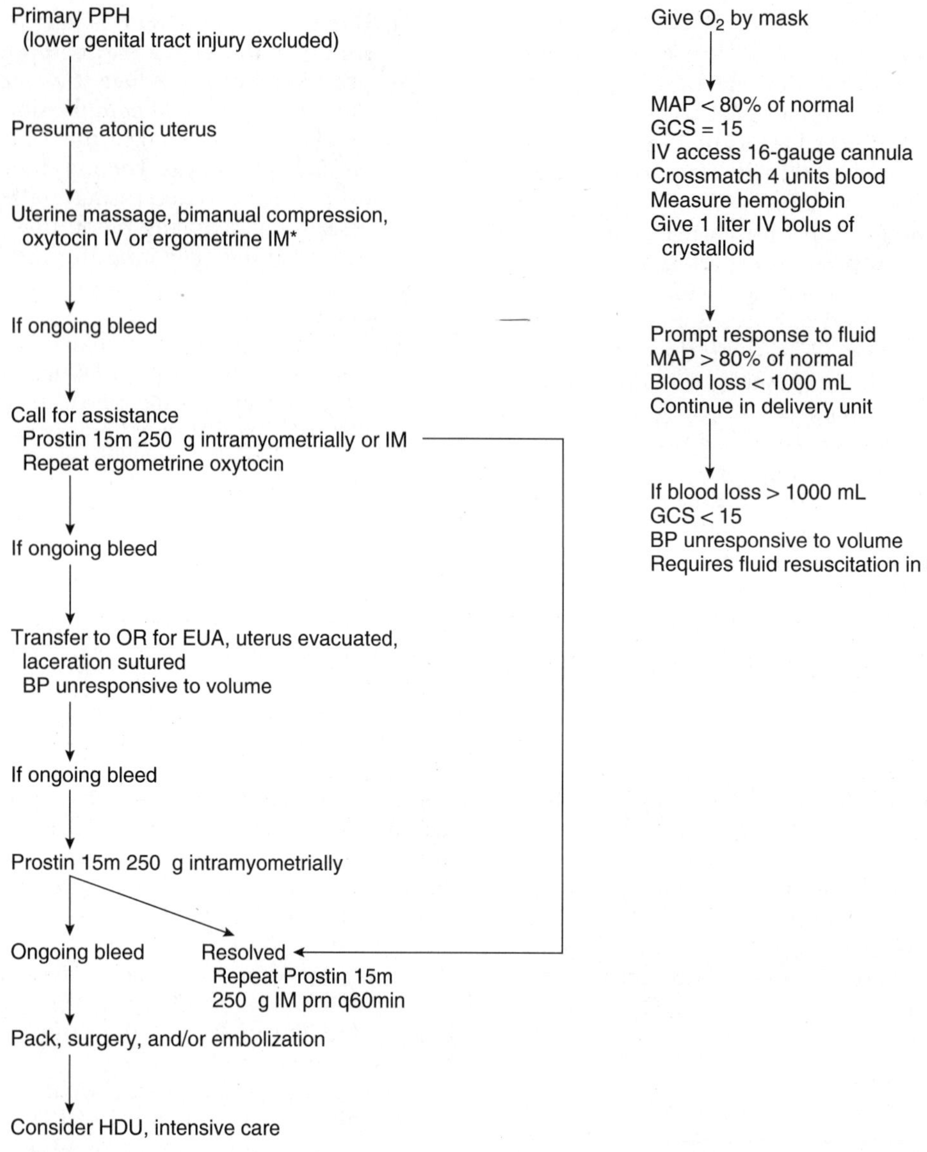

Figure 30-1 The immediate management of postpartum hemorrhage (PPH). **Note:* ergometrine and ergometrine-oxytocin combination is contraindicated in cardiac disease. BP, blood pressure; EUA, examination under anesthesia; GCS, Glasgow Coma Scale; HDU, high dependency unit; MAP, mean arterial pressure; OR, operating room; Prostin 15m, 15 methyl-$PGF_{2\alpha}$. (Modified from Harrison K, McCowan L: National Women's Hospital Protocols: Post Partum Haemorrhage. National Women's Hospital, Auckland, NZ 1996.)

"When blood is flowing in rivers, it will make packers out of non-packers in a hell of a hurry!"[24] Uterine packing with a "thrombogenic pack" maybe a useful option. Iodoform gauze soaked in thrombin solution (5000 units in 5 mL of sterile saline) is packed into the lower uterine segment.[25] Thrombin can be used topically, that is, directly on to bleeding vessels; its primary action is to convert fibrinogen to fibrin. Tranexamic acid as an intravenous infusion, 3 g over 24 hours, has also been described in the management of obstetric hemorrhage in which its use successfully avoided hysterectomy in combination with the use of plasma and ongoing transfusion. Tranexamic acid is a synthetic fibrinolytic inhibitor.[26]

Similarly, control of persistent hemorrhage has been achieved by the placement of urinary-type Foley catheters in the uterus with the catheters inflated and tamponading the hemorrhage for 24 to 36 hours.[27] The Sengstaken-Blakemore tube has been similarly used, whereby the gastric balloon of the Sengstaken tube was inflated to 300 mL and then after 24 hours was slowly deflated.[28] The Sengstaken-Blakemore tube is usually used for the tamponade of esophageal varices.

Angiographic Embolization. Angiographic embolization of vessels can be used for persistent uterine bleeding.[29] Uterine embolization is a nonsurgical method of uterine devascularization with less potential for the development of collateral circulation than surgical ligation and theoretically reduces the incidence of rebleeding from collaterals, while it avoids the need to evacuate hematoma that may be tamponading bleeding vessels. Embolization allows easy identification of the bleeding site, and allows the angiographer to visualize, catheterize, and occlude vessels that continue to bleed. Importantly, it preserves the uterus and fertility.[30] The advent of digital angiographic technology has reduced the average time for the procedure to around 2 hours with hemostasis achieved in less time.

Prophylactic embolectomy catheters can be placed in the identified high-risk patient prior to surgery and in the case of a nonviable fetus embolization can occur preoperatively.[31] In an acute situation with large blood loss, it is likely that embolectomy is of benefit only if there is the capacity for digital mapping. It is suggested that angiographic embolization should occur before ligation of the vessels as, once ligation is performed, access to the pelvic vessels for embolectomy is lost. The success rate for embolization in a postpartum setting is high and ranges from over 40% to 100%.[29, 30]

Surgical Options. Surgery is the final and definitive treatment in the management of continuing PPH; it includes the option of internal iliac artery ligation (also known as the hypogastric artery in some literature) or direct ligation of the uterine vessels. Ligation of the internal iliac artery or uterine vessels reduces distal pulse pressure in the uterine arterial tree, transforming it into a venous-like system allowing normal clot formation to proceed.[29] Internal iliac artery ligation is successful in approximately 50% of cases.[30] The vascular occlusion produced is only temporary, since recanalization occurs and normal uterine circulation is reestablished. Stepwise uterine devascularization follows a pathway of ligation from initially unilateral uterine artery ligation, followed, if unsuccessful, by bilateral uterine artery ligation, then low uterine artery ligation, unilateral ovarian vessel ligation, and finally bilateral ovarian vessel ligation. This was effective in 100% of cases with hysterectomy avoided in all cases, and this technique may be a viable alternative to hysterectomy.[32]

For an anesthetist, definitive treatment would be a timely hysterectomy. Maternal morbidity and mortality is high enough to suggest that early hysterectomy is indicated in a situation of profuse bleeding. In a patient who is unwilling to accept blood or blood products, a discussion of hysterectomy should have occurred with the patient earlier in her pregnancy. A decision to perform a hysterectomy should then occur as an early treatment. Timely hysterectomy may avoid the need for high-volume blood transfusion, avoid the complication of disseminated intravascular coagulation, and avoid the risks of intensive care and prolonged hospitalization. Although it renders the woman infertile, the choice of serious morbidity and mortality versus infertility is worth considering.

The decision to perform a hysterectomy should be made by an obstetrician and should be performed by an obstetric attending who has experience with cesarean hysterectomy.[33] Because of the potential difficulties, in some institutions the gyn-oncologist is called for assistance. Any decisions beyond the failure of bolus oxytocin (Syntocinon) or ergometrine/Syntocinon (Syntometrine) to arrest hemorrhage should be made under the guidance of an experienced obstetrician.

The Use and Pharmacology of Prostaglandins and Oxytocics

Oxytocic drugs can be divided into four categories: (1) the ergot alkaloids (ergometrine); (2) the oxytocins (e.g., Syntocinon); (3) Syntometrine (ergometrine/Syntocinon); and (4) prostaglandins. As uterine atony is the most frequent cause of PPH and may complicate other possible causes of postpartum hemorrhage, routine administration of an oxytocin bolus or infusion after first-stage labor is common practice. This "active management of the third stage of labor" helps prevent PPH, the routine administration of oxytocin after delivery reducing the risk of PPH by 40%.[34] It is established that the known benefits of routine oxytocic administration outweigh the likely risks of vascular complications in women without cardiovascular risk factors.

A review of 27 trials involving oxytocics concluded that there was no strong evidence that oxytocin and ergot alkaloids differ in their ability to reduce the risk of PPH. Oxytocin is less likely than an ergot alkaloid to cause hypertension, although the effects on nausea and vomiting are variable. There was no significant difference between Syntometrine and ergot alkaloids in the rate of PPH. Syntometrine is less likely to cause the 20 mm Hg elevation of diastolic blood pressure associated with the ergot alkaloids. It was found that Syntometrine is superior to the use of oxytocin alone in reducing the risk of PPH and that central pressure is likely to rise after the use of Syntometrine.[35]

Uterine smooth muscle has a high degree of spontaneous electrical and contractile activity. Gap junctions, which provide a low-resistance pathway between cells, enabling the spread of excitable electrical activity, increase in pregnancy in response to hormonal activity. The influx of sodium ions is the major cause of depolarization. The availability of calcium ions (and therefore the presence of calcium channel blockers) influences the response of uterine smooth muscle to physiologic and pharmacologic stimuli. Calcium ions crossing the plasma membrane act to release further calcium ion from the sarcoplasmic reticulum and, as with skeletal muscle, the interaction of actin and myosin is dependent on calcium. Both α_1-adrenergic (excitatory) and β_2-adrenergic (inhibitory) receptors are found in the myometrium. Excitatory receptors for oxytocin have been found. Toward the end of pregnancy, the number of myometrial oxytocin receptors increases. Prostaglandin E_2 and $F_{2\alpha}$ increase uterine activity.[36]

Oxytocin. Oxytocin is synthesized in distinct neurones in the supraoptic and paraventricular nuclei of the hypothalamus, separate from antidiuretic hormone. Stimuli from the cervix, vagina, and breast initiate the secretion of oxytocin. Oxytocin stimulates the force and frequency of uterine contraction, and its effects require the presence of estrogen. Oxytocin produces a decrease in systolic and diastolic blood pressures; it also produces flushing, a reflex tachycardia, and an increase in blood flow in the peripheries. It is a weak arterial vasoconstrictor in the renal, splanchnic, and skeletal muscle circulations in in vitro studies.

Oxytocin is amnestic when injected into the cerebral ventricles (this may explain the number of women who go through further pregnancies despite major complications in their earlier pregnancies). The half-life of oxytocin is from 5 to greater than 12 minutes.[36] The use of oxytocin has been associated with pulmonary edema, subarachnoid hemorrhage, cardiac arrhythmias, and anaphylactic reaction.[37]

Ergot Alkaloids. Ergot, a contaminant of edible grain, has been known for centuries and was known as an obstetric herb before it was identified as the cause of St. Anthony's fire (gangrene of the feet and hands). The first pure ergot alkaloid discovered was ergotamine, later followed by ergonovine (also called ergometrine).

The action of ergot alkaloids[36, 38, 39] on the uterus is probably via α-adrenergic receptors, tryptaminergic receptors, or both. Effects of all ergot alkaloids appear to be as the result of their actions as partial agonists or antagonists at adrenergic, dopaminergic, and tryptaminergic receptors. The spectrum of effect depends on the specific agent, the tissue, and experimental or physiologic conditions.

The effect of all the natural alkaloids is to increase the motor activity of the uterus, increasing both the force and frequency of contraction. Sensitivity of the uterus to ergot alkaloids varies according the degree of uterine maturity and the stage of gestation. Ergonovine is the most active of the ergot uterine stimulants and is less toxic than ergotamine. Ergonovine is also effective after oral use. The ergot alkaloids produce constriction of arteries and veins, raising the blood pressure and decreasing blood flow in the extremities when administered in therapeutic dosage. The intensity of the pressor response is enhanced when the blood pressure is already elevated. Ergotamine and the other ergot alkaloids can produce coronary vasoconstriction, often associated with anginal pain and ischemic electrocardiographic (ECG) changes in patients with a history of ischemic heart disease. The ergot alkaloids usually produce a bradycardia even when the blood pressure is not elevated. This is due to a direct reduction in sympathetic tone and possible direct myocardial depression.

Prostaglandins. The prostaglandins (PGs)[36] tend to exert their effect locally and are usually inactivated in the tissues in which they are synthesized. Prostaglandins predominantly found in the uterus are those of the E and F types. Prostacyclin (PGI_2) is found in the uterus but tends to be confined to the uterine umbilical and fetal vasculature. It may have a role in promoting adequate blood flow. Both PGE_2 and $PGF_{2\alpha}$ cause strong uterine contractions. As pregnancy progresses, the sensitivity of the uterus to the effects of the prostaglandins increases. In the nonpregnant condition contractile strength is greatest prior to menstruation. $PGF_{2\alpha}$ consistently produces uterine contraction in both the pregnant and nonpregnant uterus. In late pregnancy, however, $PGF_{2\alpha}$ and PGE are effective at producing uterine contractions.[36]

The side effects associated with the administration of these drugs are related to their stimulatory effects on smooth muscle, causing diarrhea and vomiting. PGE_2 and 15-methyl-$PGF_{2\alpha}$ (a synthetic derivative) may produce pyrexia owing to effects on the hypothalamus. Large doses of $PGF_{2\alpha}$ or 15-methyl-$PGF_{2\alpha}$ can cause hypertension through constriction of vascular smooth muscle. PGE produces a fall in blood pressure caused by vasodilatation, but flow to vital organs tends to be increased.[40] The effects in the hypertensive patient can be exaggerated.[36] Both PGE and PGF are able to increase cardiac output,[40] through both a weak inotropic effect and vasodilatation. Prostaglandins may have a role in modulating coronary resistance in response to sympathetic stimulation, PGE_2 and PGI_2 producing coronary vasodilatation.[41]

PGFs contract the bronchial smooth muscle, and asthmatic patients are particularly sensitive to $PGF_{2\alpha}$. The PGEs can produce relaxation of the bronchial muscle.[40] The use of prostaglandins for the control of PPH is well described. The use of 15-methyl-$PGF_{2\alpha}$ as an intramyometrial injection has an onset of action of 5 minutes, while its intramuscular use has an onset of action of 45 minutes before maximal effect is seen.[42] Prostaglandins can also be given orally as prophylactic therapy for the prevention of PPH.[43]

The inadvertent use of PGE_1 instead of $PGF_{2\alpha}$ has been described resulting in severe and unremitting hypotension, disseminated intravascular coagulation, and ventricular tachycardia.[44] The possible influence of prostaglandins on coronary artery flow has already been alluded to, and a case report of myocardial infarction associated with the use of PGE_2 in an otherwise well 32-year-old woman has been described.[45] Severe hypertension with arterial spasm has been associated with PGE_2 (usually associated with hypotension).[46] This may possibly be due to a central effect of the prostaglandin.

The anesthesiologist should always be aware of which drugs the attending obstetrician is using. The use of prostaglandins can be associated with disastrous consequences, particularly if a process of checking and cross-checking is not in place. An emergency situation requires no less meticulous care.

ANESTHETIC MANAGEMENT

(Tables 30–3 and 30–4)

In any serious postpartum bleed, the anesthesiologist's involvement, as stated previously, should have begun in the delivery unit. The range of patients for whom assistance is called extends from the patient with a slow trickle requiring a curettage and examination for retained placental products to the patient requiring an urgent examination and treatment for ongoing heavy bleeding associated with cardiovascular changes. There are also those patients predicted to have a higher risk for a potential PPH; these cases may be handled as an elective, emergent, or urgent procedure.

In each case the anesthesiologist must be prepared for possible catastrophic bleeding. Even the sim-

Table 30-3 GENERAL ANESTHESIA MANAGEMENT OF MAJOR POSTPARTUM HEMORRHAGE

1. Aggressive fluid resuscitation.
2. Consider blood transfusion in terms of ASA guidelines.
3. Encourage rapid definitive surgery if possible, e.g., may need to consider hysterectomy.
4. Optimize hemodynamics to reduce venous and arterial bleeding.
   a. MAP >60 mm Hg but not >90 mm Hg
   b. CVP > 0 cm H_2O but not >15 cm H_2O
5. Optimize physiology/hematology by frequent checks of ABG/PCV/coagulation screens.
6. Use pharmacologic adjuvants:
   Oxytocin IV bolus/infusion
   Syntometrine IV/IM
   Ergometrine IM/IV
   Prostaglandins IV/intrauterine
7. Avoid uterine relaxants.
   a. Avoid inhalational agents >0.5%.
   b. Avoid β_2-agonists/GTN.

ABG, arterial blood gases; CVP, central venous pressure; GTN, glyceryl trinitrate (also known as nitroglycerin); MAP, mean arterial pressure; PCV, packed cell volume.

plest dilatation and curettage can turn into a case involving major blood loss.

The Potentially Simple Postpartum Curettage

The usual anesthetic assessment of the patient should also look for factors that may indicate a potential for substantial blood loss. An estimation of the quantity of blood already lost at delivery and after delivery should be made by observing swabs, blood loss in the bed, blood in any buckets or containers, the amount of blood on the floor; the amount of blood on the patient as well as the degree of ongoing bleeding should also be assessed. A lying and sitting blood pressure combined with resting heart rate can give a good indication of blood loss, as does the appearance of the patient, particularly evident as shortness of breath, confusion, characteristics of the pulse (e.g., full or weak and thready), and clamminess of the skin.

In any pregnant or postpartum woman, particular note should be made of the airway, especially after delivery since the strain of bearing down combined with intravenous fluids may have contributed to quite marked airway edema.

Anesthesia can be straightforward, providing that the potential for major blood loss is recognized. It is not uncommon in my institution for this procedure to be carried out under a regional anesthesia technique, and often this may be at the request of the patient. This is probably not controversial, providing there is no evidence of coagulopathy or evidence of major blood loss. The woman should be warned that if there are any difficulties with ongoing blood loss, she may receive general anesthesia. My personal preference in this situation is to use general anesthesia: most women are tired, the procedure is usually short, and in the hands of a practicing obstetric anesthetist the risk of an unexpected intubation difficulty is small.

Blood should at least be grouped so that if it is required, it is rapidly available. In a situation in which there are known antibodies, at least 2 units should be crossmatched so that there is no delay in obtaining group-specific blood. If one is working in a small institution with an off-site blood bank, blood should be crossmatched and available in the operating room before starting the procedure. Good intravenous access should be obtained with at least one size-16 cannula and further intravenous access equipment must be immediately available.

If general anesthesia is used, a rapid-sequence induction with cricoid pressure, preoxygenation, and intubation using a rapidly acting muscle relaxant, usually suxamethonium because of its rapid onset and short duration, should be chosen because of the risk of aspiration in the immediately postpartum patient. The patient should be given a histamine type 2 (H_2) blocker or similar agent as early as possible, and a nonparticulate antacid should be given before induction.

In the stable patient there is really a free choice of induction agent: maintenance of anesthesia may be with an intermittent bolus of an intravenous agent or a volatile agent, although there is the potential for uterine relaxation with volatile anesthetics (see later).

The High-Risk Delivery: Abnormal Placentation

There is a high risk of PPH in cesarean section for placenta previa, because the placental incision results in blood loss to both the baby and mother when the placenta is anteriorly placed and because the lower segment is unable to adequately contract and ensure hemostasis. Any patient with abnormal placentation is at high risk for placenta accreta, percreta, or increta, and the risk is substantially increased with a history of previous cesarean section.

In my institution, common practice in the presence of an anterior placenta previa is to use general anesthesia. Some may disagree with this method of management and suggest that epidural or spinal anesthesia is a legitimate and appropriate anesthetic. Emergency cesarean hysterectomies have successfully been carried out under continuous epidural anesthesia without an increase in intraoperative complications or any significant difference in blood loss or incidence of blood transfusion compared with the same procedure using general anesthesia, and the authors of this multi-institutional study concluded that epidural anesthesia was not contraindicated in this high-risk group.[47] My belief is that the anesthetic technique chosen is very dependent on the resources available and the patient population. Chestnut and coworkers[47] did hypothesize in their report that epidural anesthesia was appropriate in selected patients.

Any consideration of anesthetic technique should look at the consequences of a large blood loss. While a blood loss of 500 to 1000 mL is well tolerated, with

Table 30-4 A Checklist for the Anesthetic Management of Postpartum Hemorrhage

Preoperative history of underlying medical complications, obstetric complications, history of previous anesthesia, history of medication and allergy	
Assessment of blood loss, drapes, buckets/bowls, surgeon/delivery room floor	
Patient appearance, tachycardia, lying/sitting blood pressure, confusion, tachypnea	
Level of resuscitation, volume given, response to volume, ongoing hemorrhage	
Decision to transfer	Inform OR Blood crossmatched, blood bank informed of high volume requirements Transfer monitors High-flow oxygen Patent intravenous lines with running fluids Running oxytocic Further resuscitation fluid for transport available Consider abdominal compression for transfer
Theater	Second anesthetist with role defined, assistance to anesthetists available Dedicated orderly Roles for ancillary staff, checking blood, administration of volume Calling for results, etc
Induction	Antacids/H_2-blockers/gastric emptying-prokinetic agents Preoxygenation/cricoid pressure "rapid sequence induction" Wide range of intubation equipment, including small endotracheal tubes Available range of IV equipment available (including large-bore lines) Percutaneous dilational IV system Central access equipment (including large-bore lines) Blood warmers High-pressure infusion system preprimed Range of IV fluids available and prewarmed Crossmatched blood available in theater
Monitoring	Standard monitoring Initial NIBP on 1–3 min blood pressures Arterial monitoring readily available Ongoing bleeding—placement of central line Method of rapid hemoglobin determination available
Postinduction	Blood taken for coagulation screen Review of anesthesia method, e.g., volatile vs. IV Consider early inotropes
Situation controlled	Consider optimal postoperative placement for the patient, i.e., a standard postoperative ward vs. a high-dependency unit vs. an intensive care unit.

only minor hypotension, blood loss above this level can result in marked hypotension leading to nausea and restlessness in the mother, which distracts from the management of blood loss and its consequences. The use of a regional technique in patients in whom communication is limited can make the discussion of ongoing events difficult, especially the need to convert to general anesthesia. The use of large-volume infusions can be painful, the situation can be alarming for medical staff, and this fear adds to the patient's worries and those of her partner. A major blood loss situation is not a time for discussing the pleasantries of birth. If general anesthesia needs to be induced, the patient is already hemodynamically compromised, and large volumes of intravenous fluids already transfused may have exaggerated pharyngeal and glottic edema in tissues already edematous because of pregnancy.

Sympathectomy produced by epidural anesthesia may reduce the patient's ability to maintain adequate blood pressure without the use of inotropes. In the case of massive blood loss and transfusion, often resulting in disseminated intravascular coagulation, an epidural catheter in situ is a source of worry over both epidural hematoma and its potential as a nidus for infection.

The advantage of a regional anesthetic technique is the mother's ability to partake in the birthing process and the avoidance of potential airway difficulties, still a major cause of maternal morbidity and mortality. It must also be accepted that not all placenta previa results in massive blood loss and many women have an epidural or possibly a spinal anesthetic and are unaware of anything other than a straightforward procedure. At my institution we believe that while anesthetic backup should be available at all times in placenta previa, epidural anesthesia for placenta previa requires two experienced anesthetists in the operating room at all times—one to attend to the patient, the other to attend to the management of blood loss. Such a level of manpower is not available in all institutions. Each institution should introduce a policy consistent with its style of practice and be prepared to regularly evaluate and update the policy.

At my institution we believe that general anesthesia is a safe option, providing that the risk of difficult airway anatomy is not high. Unfortunately, one of the biggest fears in modern obstetric practice appears to be the use of general anesthesia even in its appropriate place.

In a case of suspected placenta accreta, increta, or percreta we believe there is no place for an "awake" cesarean section, as the risk in these cases is for massive blood loss even in the best of surgical hands. This will, however, always remain a controversial issue.

Monitoring

The monitoring requirements to a large extent are governed by the needs of any preexisting medical conditions. In my institution, monitoring for a known placenta previa is the locally and internationally accepted standard of continuous ECG, Spo_2, carbon dioxide, oxygen, and volatile gases, but with the use of intra-arterial blood pressure monitoring. In a posterior placenta previa the use of an arterial line may be superfluous. All cases of cesarean section have a urinary catheter in place, and in a case of suspected high blood loss, a means of measuring hourly urine output is useful. We place a central line, either as a simple central venous catheter or as a Swan-Ganz catheter, when a preexisting cardiac condition indicates its use or there is limited intravenous access. Two large-bore intravenous catheters, usually 14 gauge, are indicated, with one attached to a blood warmer and an infusion set capable of being pressurized and being able to "pump" fluids. The second intravenous line should have its patency checked and can then be used as required, again with the use of a blood warmer.

Routine practice is to crossmatch a minimum of 4 units of type-specific, or type O blood, which should be kept available in the operating unit. A method of warming the patient should be available. This is most commonly and effectively accomplished through the use of a forced-air warming blanket.

The Call to a Massive Ongoing Hemorrhage

Massive hemorrhage should be managed in the operating room as soon as it is possible to transfer the patient. If the distance to the surgical suite is too great, such as in another hospital, the viability of the obstetric unit should be reviewed.

Intravenous access should initially be secured peripherally, usually using two 14-gauge cannulas. The use of a percutaneous dilatational system can be very helpful, allowing the conversion of an earlier-placed small intravenous line into a useful large-bore (12-gauge or larger) intravenous line. The use of dilatational systems is particularly helpful, as it is unlikely that a patient with significant uncompensated and ongoing bleeding will have easy intravenous access. Both intravenous lines should be connected to a running infusion given through a blood warmer, and at least one line should be a high-pressure infusion set. A technique for warming the patient should be available; an upper-body forced-air blanket covering both the torso and arms is useful.

Monitoring initially should be standard, but with an early attempt at intra-arterial monitoring of blood pressures, as this allows not only measurement of beat-to-beat blood pressure but also the early withdrawal of blood for baseline studies of a full blood count, coagulation profile, and arterial blood gas. Induction should not be delayed for the want of an arterial line. An automated noninvasive blood pressure cuff set to inflate every 1 to 2 minutes can adequately give information on vital trends in blood pressure. Consideration of central access at the time of initial resuscitation should only be given when peripheral access is not available.

Induction of Anesthesia

There is no place in the cardiovascularly unstable patient for a regional anesthetic technique, nor is there in a situation of likely coagulopathy.

In the initial examination of the patient, one should have checked for suitability of existing intravenous access and sites for further intravenous lines, Mallampati score and potential difficulties with intubation, and evidence of heart failure possibly secondary to high-dose tocolytics or infused fluids, plus a brief and relevant medical and anesthetic history.

Preparation of the operating room should be ongoing while the patient is initially evaluated.

The operating room should have a range of intravenous access equipment and arterial monitoring available. There should be a difficult airway trolley immediately accessible, and induction drugs and inotropes should be available. A good supply of warmed intravenous fluids should be in the operating room and blood should have been crossmatched, the blood bank should be alerted to an ongoing requirement for blood and blood products, and an orderly should be specially assigned to the operating room to take blood samples to the laboratory and retrieve products from the blood bank.

Staff should be assigned to specific tasks such as checking blood labels, mixing intravenous fluids such as freeze-dried plasma, and checking and communication of blood results. Individuals should be assigned to assist with fluid replacement. There should be at least two anesthetists: as in any resuscitative effort, someone must direct the situation from a global perspective, while a colleague gives the anesthetic.

As in any rapid-sequence induction, the patient should be preoxygenated with 100% oxygen and cricoid pressure must be used at induction. An H_2 blocker and nonparticulate antacid should be given prior to induction. Too often in obstetric practice little time is taken to position a patient correctly for intubation, probably because of the high incidence of regional anesthesia techniques for operative deliveries (in my institution this is >95%). The rate of difficult intubation in obstetric practice is higher than that in the nonobstetric population and is probably on the order of 1 in 500 patients.[48] In the patient with gestational proteinuria or hypertension, glottic edema may increase the risk of difficult intubation. The airway should be secured with a cuffed endotracheal tube. The availability of a range of tube sizes is useful, as airway edema caused by resuscitation fluids or gestational hypertension may have narrowed the glottis. Choice of induction agent varies, but ketamine and etomidate are both proven agents in the presence of hypovolemia. The alternative is a "cardiac" induction with a high-dose narcotic; this, however, tends to preclude a rapid wakeup, but since many of these patients require postoperative ventilation this may not be an issue. An argument against a high-dose narcotic induction is the potential for failed intubation and subsequent loss of ability to "wake the patient up." In the postpartum situation with no baby on board, if there is a difficult airway, it would be more prudent to attempt oral fiberoptic technique or a surgical airway. Midazolam in combination with a narcotic or a small dose of propofol may be suitable. Significant blood loss means that very little of any agent is required. Initial maintenance should be with oxygen only and intermittent bolus administration or infusion of the induction agent of choice. Nitrous oxide should be added only as oxygenation and blood pressure allow.

With ongoing hemorrhage, anesthetic maintenance should be with an intravenous agent and not with a volatile anesthetic. Although this may risk awareness, there is a major risk of perpetuating uterine atony through the use of a volatile agent.

A low-dose propofol infusion is useful in this situation; usually an infusion at a rate of 4 to 12 mg/kg/h is appropriate. An alternative that provides analgesia as well as anesthesia is the addition of alfentanil to the mix, 1 mg of alfentanil to 200 mg of propofol, infused at a rate of 0.5 to 1 mL/kg/h. The use of nitrous oxide depends on the degree of cardiovascular stability and can be added as the situation dictates. Ketamine can also be used as an intravenous maintenance agent in the dose range of 5 to 30 mg/kg/h, usually in combination with a benzodiazepine. Good muscle relaxation is essential to aid the surgeon. I don't believe that there is any major indication or contraindication to the use of any of the modern muscle relaxants in this situation, excepting that a rapidly acting agent should be used at induction. Suxamethonium would still be my choice, although high-dose rocuronium, 0.6 to 0.9 mg/kg, produces rapid intubating conditions and provides good cardiovascular stability.

Intravenous Agents

Ketamine. Ketamine use in obstetrics is well accepted and outside of First World countries it is probably one of the most common anesthetic agents. Ketamine use in emergency situations is also well described, in which its maintenance of blood pressure combined with its analgesic effects are used to good effect. The use of ketamine in the situation of a postpartum bleed would appear more than reasonable. In this situation there does not appear to be any contraindication to its use.[49] The usual induction dose is 1 to 2 mg/kg intravenously.

Propofol. While not an ideal agent for induction in an emergency situation associated with cardiovascular instability, propofol is an ideal agent in a situation in which the volatile agents may be associated with possible uterine relaxation. There does not appear to be any available evidence for propofol contributing to uterine relaxation and hence aggravation of bleeding. It should be remembered, however, that in a serious state of hemodynamic instability only a low-dose propofol infusion is required, probably on the order of 2 to 5 mg/kg/h.

Etomidate. At my institution etomidate is probably the induction agent of choice in a situation of critically unstable hemodynamics. Used in an induction dose of 0.3 mg/kg, etomidate is not associated with a fall in blood pressure. We most often use etomidate in association with a dose of narcotic at induction since etomidate has no analgesic properties. This agent can be used as an infusion, but its inhibition of the hypopituitary axis has made it an unpopular choice for this use.

The Use of Volatile Agents for Maintenance. In 1970, Cullen and colleagues[50] showed that blood loss at abortion was significantly affected by the type of anesthesia chosen. The depressant effects of halothane on the uterine muscle is well accepted; however, the degree of depression produced is frequently forgotten. Naftalin and coworkers,[51] using isolated strips of pregnant and nonpregnant human uterus showed that in the pregnant uterus 0.5% halothane reduced the peak developed tension by 25% while having no effect in the nonpregnant uterus. At a concentration of 2%, peak developed tension was reduced by 60% in the pregnant uterus and 44% in the nonpregnant uterus.

A similar study using isolated muscle strips from rat uteruses has shown that isoflurane, halothane, and enflurane all produce depression of uterine contractile force at levels as low as a 0.5% minimum alveolar concentration (MAC) equivalent. The level of inhibition ranged from 23.1% with isoflurane to 40.3% with halothane. In this study the influence of verapamil was also reviewed and was shown to produce dose-related depression of contractile force that was additive with the effects of the volatile agents. Altering the calcium concentration could partially reverse the trends. These authors concluded that interference with Ca^{2+} homeostasis, particularly intracellular Ca^{2+} availability, affects the contractile activity of the myometrium.[52]

Decrease in uterine contractility has also shown similar results using isolated human uterine strips, with concentrations as low as 0.5% MAC producing uterine depression.[53] Halothane concentrations of 0.5% and less are not associated with significantly increased blood loss compared with a regional anesthesia technique in elective cesarean sections.[54]

Equianesthetic concentrations of sevoflurane and isoflurane produce comparable results, including those for blood loss and uterine relaxation in the gravid uterus at cesarean section,[55] and hence should not be used in the face of uterine atony.

It is common for the hypertensive pregnant patient to be placed on calcium channel blockers, often as an acute therapy. The possible aggravation of postpartum atony in the presence of calcium channel blockers and volatile anesthetic agent should not be overlooked. In the presence of a large blood loss and subsequent transfusion, the use of Ca^{2+} supplementation may not only enhance cardiac performance, but also may aid in uterine contractility.

HEMATOLOGIC CONSIDERATIONS

Blood Transfusion and Volume Replacement

With the potential for massive blood loss, there should always be prompt and immediate access to blood banking facilities. The blood bank should be notified as soon as a problem has been identified and a warning given that large volumes of blood and blood products will be required. Informing a hematologist of the situation can be helpful in guiding the use of coagulation factors and blood products.

As in any resuscitation, attention should be given first to the preservation of circulating volume and maintenance of the microcirculation, then to the type of fluid used. The debate over crystalloid versus colloid solution is still ongoing, and the best practice is to follow the institution's guidelines. We, like many centers, follow the middle ground and use a combination of crystalloid and colloid. Once blood loss is significant, at least half of the estimated blood volume, there is little choice but to use blood and blood products. Transfusion should be based on frequent measurement of hemoglobin and the coagulation profile unless the blood loss is so phenomenal that it is intuitive that blood is required. The value of intraoperative coagulation tests in the face of large-volume transfusions has been questioned and the use of the thromboelastograph in their place suggested.[56] Consideration must always be that there is the potential for the development of a consumptive coagulopathy and at my institution we still rely on frequent (every 30 to 60 minutes) coagulation screens of an activated partial thromboplastin time, prothrombin ratio, platelets, fibrinogen, and hemoglobin.

Owing to the risk of human immunodeficiency virus transmission via the use of transfused blood, interest in the use of autologous blood has increased. Common methods are the use of predonation, immediate preoperative hemodilution, and the use of various cell-saving techniques.

Pregnancy is not a contraindication to the use of predonation but the latter is not considered to be cost-effective.[57] The difficulty is, of course, that not all obstetric patients are going to require transfusion but, as described earlier, there are a large number of factors that may predict the patient at high risk for PPH, and for these patients there should be early consideration of preoperative donation. The use of hemodilution preoperatively (with withdrawal of cells) (e.g., in cesarean section for placenta previa) may be more controversial, as the pregnant patient is already subject to the hemodilution of pregnancy. The use of intraoperative blood salvage in obstetrics has been suggested.[58] The use of blood salvage in PPH, however, must be considered in face of the causes of hemorrhage and the site of salvage. Salvage from the peritoneal cavity or uterine cavity may run the risk of contamination by amniotic fluid and meconium. It is difficult to find reference in the literature to the use of intraoperative salvage in an acute obstetric situation. The use of intraoperative salvage in massive bleeding with a ruptured ectopic pregnancy has been considered efficacious.[57]

The Use of Blood and Blood Products
(Table 30-5)

The rationale for the appropriate use of transfusion of products must be considered in any case and many institutions have their own guidelines. The American Society of Anesthesiologists (ASA) Task Force on Blood Component Therapy[59] developed evidence-based guidelines for the transfusion of blood products. A summary of their recommendations follows in subsequent text.

Packed Cells. Transfusion is rarely indicated when the hemoglobin is greater than 10 g/dL, and almost always indicated when the hemoglobin is less than 6 g/dL. At hemoglobin levels between 6 and 10 g/dL, transfusion should be based on the risk of complications of inadequate oxygenation. The use of a single trigger figure (hemoglobin level) without consideration of all parameters is not recommended. Transfusion of 1 unit of packed cells increases the hematocrit by 3% or the hemoglobin by 1 g/dL in a 70-kg adult.

Table 30-5 NORMAL BLOOD INVESTIGATION VALUES IN PREGNANCY (NATIONAL WOMEN'S HOSPITAL NORMAL RESULTS)

Hb	100–140 g/L
Hct	0.28–0.41
Coagulation	
APTT	23–37 sec
PR/INR	0.8–1.2
Platelets	150–400 × 10^9/L
WBC	5.0–15.0 × 10^9/L
Fibrinogen	>4.0 g/L
D-dimer	<200 μg/L
Haptoglobins	0.72–3.8 g/L

APTT, activated partial thromboplastin time; Hb, hemoglobin; Hct, hematocrit; PR/INR, prothrombin ratio/International Normalized Ratio; WBC, white blood cells.

Platelets. Obstetric patients with microvascular bleeding usually require platelet transfusion if the platelet count is less than 50 × 10^9/L. Therapy is rarely required if the platelet count is greater than 100 × 10^9/L. At intermediate counts the determination should be based on the risk for more significant bleeding. Transfusion may be indicated despite an apparently adequate platelet count if there is known platelet dysfunction and microvascular bleeding. Transfusion of 1 unit of platelet concentrate increases the platelet count by 5 × 10^9 in an average adult.

Fresh-Frozen Plasma. Fresh-frozen plasma (FFP) should be used for the correction of microvascular bleeding in the presence of an elevated (>1.5 times normal) prothrombin time (PT) or partial thromboplastin time (PTT). It is used in the correction of microvascular bleeding secondary to coagulation factor deficiency in patients transfused with more than one blood volume *and* when activated partial thromboplastin time (APTT) and PT cannot be obtained in a short time. FFP should be given in a dose to achieve a minimum of 30% of plasma factor concentration (usually achieved with administration of 10–15 mL/kg). Four to 5 platelet concentrates give a similar quantity of coagulation factors as that in 1 unit of FFP. FFP is contraindicated for the augmentation of plasma volume.

Cryoprecipitate. Cryoprecipitate[59] is indicated in the correction of microvascular bleeding in massively transfused patients with fibrinogen concentrations less than 80 to 100 mg/dL (*or* when fibrinogen concentration cannot be measured in a timely fashion). One unit of cryoprecipitate per 10 kg body weight raises the plasma fibrinogen level by 50 mg/dL in the absence of continued bleeding or consumptive coagulopathy.

It is fortunate (from a physiologic and resuscitative point of view) that PPH occurs in young patients with sound physiology and little pathology. These patients can tolerate low hemoglobin concentrations with little likelihood of a significant adverse outcome. In major PPH we routinely make frequent measurements of hemoglobin and we use these figures as a base to drive the indication for transfusion of red cells. We tolerate hemoglobin to a level of 60 to 70 before transfusing with red cells, and this appears to be an acceptable figure in the obstetric literature[58]; however, it is important that indications for transfusion are more than hemoglobin level alone. The degree of ongoing blood loss, cardiovascular stability (judged via heart rate, blood pressure, and, where used, central pressures including cardiac output measurements), respiratory complications, the level of hemodilution, and preexisting pathology must be considered. It is possible to calculate blood requirements based on oxygen extraction, using invasive monitoring[60]; it is unlikely, however, that in any serious ongoing PPH there is a place for this degree of perfection.

Complications of Transfusion. Blood transfusion is not without risk and these have been well documented previously (Table 30–6).

Disseminated Intravascular Coagulation

Disseminated intravascular coagulation (DIC) may be a frequent accompaniment to the large PPH and this may be due to several mechanisms:

1. DIC is the inciting cause of the hemorrhage, for example, amniotic fluid embolism, placental abruption, sepsis, and fetal death.
2. It is a result of hemorrhage, for example, shock, excessive surgical trauma.
3. It is a result of treatment of the PPH, for example, massive transfusion, transfusion reaction.

While DIC is not common during a normal gestation, pregnant women are at risk for developing DIC because of pregnancy-related complications.[61]

The laboratory tests used to screen for DIC are the APTT, PT, D-dimer and fibrinogen, platelets, and a full blood count. There may be evidence of hemolysis, such as fragmented cells on a slide and discoloration of the urine.

Treatment of DIC requires the treatment of the underlying and precipitating cause, as DIC is not in itself a disease. In PPH treatment involves control of the hemorrhage, management of the circulation, and replacement of coagulation factors. Hypofibrinogenemia (usually from placental abruption) is the most common cause of consumptive coagulopathy in pregnancy,[61] and hence the early use of cryoprecipitate may be helpful. The use of heparin in the treatment of DIC is controversial but well described; heparin has been considered useful in amniotic fluid embolism[62] and intra-uterine death.[61]

Inotropes

Frequently during the resuscitative process large fluid shifts, hypovolemia, hypothermia, and other factors require the use of inotropes to maintain sufficient cardiac output to ensure adequate perfusion levels. Once bleeding is controlled and volume is adequately replaced, there may be no need to continue with inotropic support. I usually start with low-dose dopamine and increase the rate of infusion as required with a low threshold to change to epinephrine as required. Choice of inotropes is usually guided by institutional protocols.

Postoperative Placement (Table 30–7)

Early consideration needs to be given to the postoperative placement and care of the patient following a postpartum hemorrhage. This could range from observation in the ward in the case of a small hemorrhage, to intensive care management in the case of a massive transfusion. In all but the smallest of hemorrhages (i.e., less than 1000 mL in a case of PPH associated with atony) we would place a patient in at least a high dependency unit, where the patient can be monitored for both ongoing blood loss (return of uterine atony) and evidence of complications associated with volume

Table 30-6 BLOOD TRANSFUSION COMPLICATIONS

PROBLEM	COMMENTS
Infection transmission viruses	
Hepatitis C	USA 1:5000 units transfused; UK 1:6000 units transfused.[57]
Hepatitis B	USA 1:200,000 units transfused.[57]
HIV	The window period when HIV antibody test remains negative in infectious blood continues to be a problem. Risk of transmission in the USA is 1:420,000.[60] In the UK it is estimated that HIV risk may be approaching 1:3 million units transfused.[58]
HTLV I and II	USA 1:200,000 units transfused.[60] These retroviruses are rare but may be important in endemic areas or in drug addicts who share needles. HTLV-I has been linked with adult T-cell leukemia/lymphoma; HTLV-II has been linked with hairy cell leukemia.
Cytomegalovirus, Epstein-Barr virus	In the UK transfer has been as high as 2.5–12.5% of individual units. Both have been transmitted via blood transfusions; blood can be irradiated to avoid CMV.
Bacteria	Rates between 1:2,500 and 1:1 million for combined bacterial and parasitic infection.[57,60] Mortality from transfusion-acquired septicemia may be as high as 35%.[58]
Syphilis	*Treponema pallidum* is not viable after 72 h at 40°C. The test can be used as a marker for high-risk-category donors.
Protozoa: malaria, toxoplasmosis, babesiosis	
Immunologic suppression: renal transplant survival	Statistically improved.
Malignancy	About 30 retrospective studies: ⅓ show worse survival; ⅓ show similar nonsignificant trend; ⅓ show no difference.
Postoperative infection	May be increased.
Alloimmunization	Reactions differ from mild fever to fatal hemolysis if ABO-incompatible blood has been transfused.
Transfusion-related lung injury	Noncardiac acute pulmonary edema within 2–4 h of transfusion. Possibly caused by leukoagglutinin reactions. Patients often have a history of obstructive airway disease, multiple transfusions, or multiple pregnancies. May require mechanical ventilation; lungs usually clear in 48 h.
Hyperkalemia	High potassium level in old blood may be important if infusion rate is >1.5–2 mL/kg/min. ECG changes occur. Peaked T waves, wide PR and QRS intervals with ultimate loss of P waves, and ST elevation may be seen with ventricular fibrillation or cardiac standstill in diastole. If ECG signs of hyperkalemia occur, the transfusion should be stopped and IV Ca^{2+} given. After warming and redistribution, K^+ reenters cells, and potassium level may be subnormal.
Hypocalcemia	Caused by the citrate chelating circulating ionized calcium. The effect is transient, lasting about 10 min with rapid transfusion (>1.5–2 mL/kg/min). ECG may show prolonged QT intervals, widened QRS, and flat T waves associated with a decrease in blood pressure. Treatment is IV calcium.
Acid-base	The initial metabolic acidosis becomes an alkalosis as citrate is metabolized to bicarbonate. Bicarbonate should not be given routinely.
Hypothermia	Blood should be warmed.
Oxygen dissociation	With CPDA stored blood, the oxygen-carrying capacity of transfused blood normalizes in a few hours.
Microembolism	Microfilters are no more effective than standard 170-μm blood filters.
Dilutional thrombocytopenia	Unusual if less than 2 blood volume replacements are given; 1 blood volume replacement lowers platelet levels only 30–40%. Generalized microcapillary bleeding from all cut surfaces after a massive transfusion is more likely due to thrombocytopenia than clotting factors.
Hyperglycemia	

CMV, cytomegalovirus; CPDA, citrate-phosphate-dextrose-adenine; ECG, electrocardiogram; HIV, human immunodeficiency virus; HTLV, human T-cell lymphotropic virus.

Modified from Gordon A, Gordon I: Peri-operative blood and blood component therapy. Can J Anaesth 1992; 39:1105–1115.

Table 30–7 Indications for High Dependency and Intensive Care in Postpartum Hemorrhage

1. Ongoing disseminated intravascular coagulation
2. Continued hemorrhage
   - Likely requirement for further surgery; pack in situ
   - Monitoring of blood loss, maintenance of high-dose oxytocic
3. Ventilation
   - Airway obstruction due to airway edema; previously noted difficult airway
   - Cardiac (heart failure, fluid overload, leaky capillaries)
   - Early development of adult respiratory distress syndrome
   - Respiratory depression secondary to narcotic and/or anesthesia
   - Amniotic fluid embolism, pulmonary embolism

Criteria for Ventilation*

Parameter	Ventilation Indicated	Normal Range
Mechanics		
Respiratory rate (breath/min)	>35	10–20
Tidal volume (mL/kg body weight)	<5	5–7
Oxygenation		
$Pa{O_2}$ (mm Hg)	<60 ($FI{O_2}$ 0.6)	75–100 (air)
$PA{O_2} - Pa{O_2}$ (mm Hg)	>350	25–65 ($FI{O_2}$ 1.0)
Ventilation		
$Pa{CO_2}$ (mm Hg)	>60	35–45

Blood Gas on Air

pH	7.36	
$P{CO_2}$	4.6–6.0 kPa	35–45 mm Hg
HCO_3	20–27 mmol/L	
$P{O_2}$	10.6–13.0 kPa	80–98 mm Hg
Base excess	−2–+2	
Sat O_2	95–100%	

4. Hypothermia
5. Inotropic therapy, any indication (including for renal or cardiac cause)
6. Sepsis
7. Cardiac
   - Failure secondary to fluid therapy, or oxytocin, or ß-agonists
   - Amniotic fluid embolism
   - Sepsis
   - Infarction or arrhythmia secondary to metabolic shifts (hypocalcemia, hyperkalemia, or hypothermia), shock
8. Renal failure (pending or actual)
   - Prerenal
   - Renal

*Modified from Tan IKS, Oh TE: Mechanical ventilatory support. *In* Oh TE (ed): Intensive Care Manual, 4th ed. Oxford, England: Butterworth-Heinemann; 1997: 247.

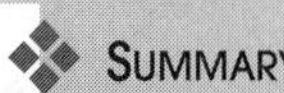

SUMMARY

Key Points

- The most frequent cause of acute postpartum hemorrhage is uterine atony, whereas delayed postpartum hemorrhage is most often caused by retained placental fragments.
- Nonsurgical techniques, such as angiographic embolization of uterine vessels, have been successfully used to treat postpartum hemorrhage.
- Ligation of the internal iliac or uterine vessels reduces the distal pulse pressure in the uterine arterial tree, thus allowing normal clot formation to occur, and may be effective in terminating postpartum hemorrhage without the need to resort to hysterectomy.
- Patients with placenta previa who are undergoing repeat cesarean section are at an increased risk for placenta accreta, which may result in massive hemorrhage.

Key References

Clark SL, Koonings PP, Phelan JP: Placenta previa/accreta and prior cesarean section. Obstet Gynecol 1985; 66:89–92.

Vedantham S, Goodwin SC, McLucas B, et al: Uterine artery embolization: an underused method of controlling pelvic hemorrhage. Am J Obstet Gynecol 1997; 176:938–948.

Case Stem

A 22-year-old primiparous patient undergoes a cesarean section after a failed 24-hour induction of labor with oxytocin. Intraoperative EBL is 1600 mL, and bleeding continues. The obstetrician states that the uterus appears to be atonic. What are the obstetric and anesthetic implications and options?

replacement. If the PPH was associated with a laceration, it is easier to be sure that there is little chance of a rebleed and the patient can be placed on the ward. Some patients may require ongoing intensive care for the provision of ventilatory therapy,[63] management of renal complications, or treatment of an ongoing coagulopathy.

CONCLUSION

Postpartum hemorrhage is a serious obstetric complication that requires a team approach to its management. For the anesthetic team this requires a high level of preparation, suitable trained assistance, and the availability of institutional guidelines.

References

1. Maternal Mortality Newsletter, Issue 13. New Zealand Maternal Deaths Assessment Committee, 25 May 1996 Wellington, NZ.
2. Stern C, Permezel M, Petterson C, et al: The Royal Womens' Hospital Family Birth Centre: the First 10 years reviewed. Aust N Z J Obstet Gynaecol 1992; 32:291–296.
3. St. George L, Crandon AJ: Immediate postpartum complications. Aust N Z J Obstet Gynaecol 1990; 30:52–56.
4. Allen DG, Correy JF, Marsden DE: Primary postpartum haemorrhage in Tasmania, 1982–1986. Aust N Z J Obstet Gynaecol 1988; 28:279–283.
5. Combs CA, Murphy EL, Laros RK Jr: Factors associated with postpartum hemorrhage with vaginal birth. Obstet Gynecol 1991; 70:69–76.
6. Gilbert L, Porter W, Brown VA: Postpartum haemorrhage—a continuing problem. Br J Obstet Gynaecol 1987; 94:67–71.
7. Pregnancy and lactation. *In* Guyton AC, Hall JE (eds): Textbook of Medical Physiology, 9th ed. Philadelphia: WB Saunders; 1996: 1033–1046.
8. Moore KL: The placenta and fetal membranes. *In* Before We Are Born: Basic Embryology and Birth Defects. Philadelphia: WB Saunders; 1977: 68–87.
9. Kong TY, Khong TK: Delayed postpartum hemorrhage: a morphologic study of causes and their relation to other pregnancy disorders. Obstet Gynecol 1993; 82:17–22.
10. Lynch JC, Pardy JP: Uterine rupture and scar dehiscence: a five-year survey. Anaesth Intensive Care 1996; 24:699–704.
11. Biehl DR: The anesthetic management of obstetrical hemorrhage. Int Anesthesiol Clin 1990; 28:52–57.
12. Clark SL, Koonings PP, Phelan JP: Placenta previa/accreta and prior cesarean section. Obstet Gynecol 1985; 66:89–92.
13. Druelinger L: Postpartum emergencies. Emerg Med Clin North Am 1994; 12:219–235.
14. Ridgway LE: Puerperal emergency: vaginal and vulval haematomas. Obstet Gynecol Clin North Am 1995; 22:275–282.
15. Toohey JS, Keegan KA Jr, Morgan MA, et al: The "dangerous multipara": fact or fiction? Am J Obstet Gynecol 1995; 172(2 Pt 1):683–686.
16. Combs CA, Murphy EL, Laros RK Jr: Factors associated with hemorrhage in cesarean deliveries. Obstet Gynecol 1991; 77:77–82.
17. Naef RW III, Chauhan SP, Chevalier SP, et al: Prediction of hemorrhage at cesarean delivery. Obstet Gynecol 1994; 83:923–926.
18. Roberts WE, Perry KG Jr, Woods JB, et al: The intra partum platelet count in patients with HELLP (hemolysis, elevated liver enzymes, and low platelets) syndrome: is it predictive of later haemorrhagic complications? Am J Obstet Gynecol 1994; 171:799–804.
19. Simon L, Santi TM, Sacquin P, et al: Pre-anaesthetic assessment of coagulation abnormalities in obstetric patients: usefulness, timing, and clinical implications. Br J Anaesth 1997; 78:678–683.
20. Drife J: Management of primary postpartum haemorrhage. Br J Obstet Gynaecol 1997; 104:275–277.
21. Roberts WE: Emergent obstetric management of postpartum hemorrhage. Obstet Gynecol Clin North Am 1995; 22:283–302.
22. Riley DP, Burgess RW: External abdominal aortic compression: a study of a resuscitation manoeuvre for postpartum haemorrhage. Anaesth Intensive Care 1994; 22:571–576.
23. Maier RC: Control of postpartum hemorrhage with uterine packing. Am J Obstet Gynecol 1993; 169(2 Pt 1):317–323.
24. Horger E: Quoted in Maier RC: Control of postpartum hemorrhage with uterine packing. Am J Obstet Gynecol 1993; 169(2 Pt 1):317–323.
25. Bobrowski RA, Jones TB: A thrombogenic uterine pack for postpartum hemorrhage. Obstet Gynecol 1995; 85(5 Pt 2): 836–837.
26. Alok K, Hagen P, Webb JB: Tranexamic acid in the management of postpartum haemorrhage. Br J Obstet Gynaecol 1996; 103:1250–1251.
27. De Loor JA, van Dam PA: Foley catheters for uncontrollable obstetric or gynecologic hemorrhage. Obstet Gynecol 1996; 88(4 Pt 2):737.
28. Katesmark M, Brown R, Raju KS: Successful use of a Sengstaken-Blakemore tube to control massive postpartum haemorrhage. Br J Obstet Gynaecol 1994; 101:259–260.
29. Duggan PM, Jamieson MG, Wattie WJ: Intractable postpartum haemorrhage managed by angiographic embolisation: case report and review. Aust N Z J Obstet Gynaecol 1991; 31:229–233.

30. Vedantham S, Goodwin SC, McLucas B, et al: Uterine artery embolization: an underused method of controlling pelvic hemorrhage. Am J Obstet Gynecol 1997; 176:938–948.
31. Mitty HA, Sterling KM, Alvarez M, et al: Obstetric hemorrhage: prophylactic and emergency arterial catheterisation and embolotherapy. Radiology 1993; 188:183–187.
32. Abd Rabbo SA: Stepwise uterine devascularisation: a novel technique for management of uncontrollable postpartum hemorrhage with preservation of the uterus. Am J Obstet Gynecol 1994; 171:694–700.
33. Chestnut DH, Eden RD, Gall ST, et al: Peripartum hysterectomy: a review of cesarean and postpartum hysterectomy. Obstet Gynecol 1985; 65:365–370.
34. Prendiville W, Elbourne D, Chalmers I: The effects of routine oxytocic administration in the management of the third stage of labour: an overview of the evidence from controlled trials. Br J Obstet Gynaecol 1988; 95:3–16.
35. Elbourne D, Prendiville W, Chalmers I: Choice of oxytocic preparation for routine use in the management of the third stage of labour: an overview of the evidence from controlled trials. Br J Obstet Gynaecol 1988; 95:17–30.
36. Graves CR: Agents that cause contraction or relaxation of the uterus. *In* Hardman JG, Limbird LE (eds): Goodman and Gilman's The Pharmacological Basis of Therapeutics, 9th ed. New York: McGraw-Hill; 1996: 939–949.
37. Reynolds JEF (ed): Hypothalamic and pituitary hormones. *In* Martindale's The Extra Pharmacopoeia, 31st ed. London: Royal Pharmaceutical Society; 1996;1290–1291.
38. Peroutka SJ: Drugs effective in the therapy of migraine. *In* Hardman JG, Limbird LE (eds): Goodman and Gilman's The Pharmacological Basis of Therapeutics, 9th ed. New York: McGraw-Hill; 1996:487–502.
39. Hoffman BB, Lefkowitz RJ: Catecholamines, sympathomimetic drugs, and adrenergic receptor antagonists. *In* Hardman JG, Limbird LE (eds): Goodman and Gilman's The Pharmacological Basis of Therapeutics, 9th ed. New York: McGraw-Hill; 1996: 199–248.
40. Campbell WB, Halushka PV: Lipid-derived autocoids, eicosanoids and platelet-activating factor. *In* Hardman JG, Limbird LE (eds): Goodman and Gilman's The Pharmacological Basis of Therapeutics, 9th ed. New York: McGraw-Hill; 1996: 601–616
41. Serneri GG, Gensini GF, Abbate R, et al: Physiologic role of coronary PGI_2 and PGE_2 in modulating coronary vascular response to sympathetic stimulation. Am Heart J 1990; 19:848–854.
42. Bigrigg A, Chui D, Chissell S: Use of intramyometrial 15-methylprostaglandin $F_{2\alpha}$ to control atonic postpartum haemorrhage following vaginal delivery and failure of conventional therapy. Br J Obstet Gynaecol 1991; 98:734–736.
43. El-Refaey H, O'Brien P, Morafa W, et al: Use of oral misoprostol in the prevention of postpartum haemorrhage. Br J Obstet Gynaecol 1997; 104:336–339.
44. Reedy MB, McMillion JS, Engvall WR, et al: Inadvertent administration of prostaglandin E_1 instead of prostaglandin $F_{2\alpha}$ in a patient with uterine atony and hemorrhage. Obstet Gynecol 1992; 79(5 Pt 2):890–894.
45. Fliers E, Düren DR, van Zwieten PA: A prostaglandin analogue as a probable cause of myocardial infarction in a young woman. BMJ 1991; 302:416.
46. Verber B, Gauthé M, Michel-Cherqui M, et al: Severe hypertension during postpartum haemorrhage after I.V. administration of prostaglandin E_2. Br J Anaesth 1992; 68:623–624.
47. Chestnut DH, Dewan DM, Redic LF, et al: Anesthetic management for obstetric hysterectomy: a multi-institutional study. Anesthesiology 1989; 70:607–610.
48. Davies JM, Crone LA: Difficult intubation in the parturient. Can J Anaesth 1989; 36:668–674.
49. Oats JN, Vasey DP, Waldron BA: Effects of ketamine on the pregnant uterus. Br J Anaesth 1979; 51:1163–1166.
50. Cullen BF, Margolis AJ, Eger EI II: The effects of anesthesia and pulmonary ventilation on blood loss during elective therapeutic abortion. Anesthesiology 1970; 32:108–113.
51. Naftalin NJ, McKay DM, Phear WPC, et al: The effects of halothane on pregnant and nonpregnant human myometrium. Anesthesiology 1977; 46:15–19.
52. Laszlo A, Buljubasic N, Zsolnai B, et al: Interactive effects of volatile anesthetics, verapamil, and ryanodine on contractility and calcium homeostasis of isolated pregnant rat myometrium. Am J Obstet Gynecol 1992; 67:804–810.
53. Munson ES, Embro WJ: Enflurane, isoflurane, and halothane and isolated human uterine muscle. Anesthesiology 1977; 46:11–14.
54. Hood DD, Holubec DM: Elective repeat cesarean section: effect of anesthesia type on blood loss. J Reprod Med 1990; 35:368–372.
55. Gambling DR, Sharma SK, White PF, et al: Use of sevoflurane during elective cesarean birth: a comparison with isoflurane and spinal anesthesia. Anesth Analg 1995; 81:90–95.
56. Irving GA: Perioperative blood and blood component therapy. Can J Anaesth 1992; 39:1105–1115.
57. Santoso JT, Lin DW, Millar DS: Transfusion medicine in obstetrics and gynecology. Obstet Gynecol Surv 1995; 50:470–481.
58. Ekeroma AJ, Ansari A, Stirrat GM: Blood transfusion in obstetrics and gynaecology. Br J Obstet Gynaecol 1997; 104:278–284.
59. Practice guidelines for blood component therapy: a report by the American Society of Anesthesiologists Task Force on Blood Component Therapy. Anesthesiology 1996; 84:732–747.
60. Greenburg AG: New transfusion strategies. Am J Surg 1997; 173:49–52.
61. Richey ME, Gilstrap LC III, Ramin SM: Management of disseminated intravascular coagulopathy. Clin Obstet Gynecol 1995; 38:514–520.
62. Isbister JP: Haemostatic failure. *In* Oh TE (ed): Intensive Care Manual, 4th ed. Oxford, England: Butterworth-Heinemann; 1997: 767–778.
63. Tan IKS, Oh TE: Mechanical ventilatory support. *In* Oh TE (ed): Intensive Care Manual, 4th ed. Oxford, England: Butterworth-Heinemann; 1997: 246–255.

31

Air and Amniotic Fluid Embolism

❖ Alfredo N. Cattaneo, MD

AIR EMBOLISM IN OBSTETRICS

Historical Aspects

Air embolism has been recognized as a pathophysiologic condition since at least the time of the Napoleonic Wars. It was at that time, in the 18th century, that Baron Larre first observed that cavalry officers suffering saber wounds of the head and neck frequently died, not as a result of blood loss, but because of air bubbles in the right heart and pulmonary circulation.[1] The first clinical documentation of arterial gas embolism in humans is probably one by Morgagni, in his treatise "The Seats and Causes of Disease," published in 1769.[2]

Intraoperative venous air embolism as a consequence of surgery was first reported in 1818, in a case describing a young blacksmith having a supraclavicular tumor excised while in the seated position. The patient suddenly cried out, lost consciousness, and died within a few minutes. Instead of finding air in the pleural space, as the surgeon had expected, the surgeon found air in the right heart, vena cava, and pulmonary artery.[3]

Cormack[4] presented the first report of gas embolism associated with obstetrics in 1837, in his thesis "The Presence of Air in the Organs of Circulation." It was not until 1839, however, that Amussat, in his presentation to the French Academy of Medicine,[5] suggested that a hole in a vein could cause a venturi effect to entrain room air into the venous system. By 1885, Senn[6] had described the pathophysiology of air entrainment in great detail, observing that whenever an animal's head was elevated above the level of the heart, air would enter the circulation, and that this process would stop only when the head was lowered. He also noted that air could be removed from the heart by aspiration through rubber catheters inserted into the right heart via the neck veins.

Introduction

Today, venous air embolism is generally associated with neurosurgical procedures performed on patients in the sitting position. As this chapter will demonstrate, however, venous air embolism can occur during many other procedures, and in many different positions.

Venous air embolism can occur in any surgical patient in whom the operative field is 5 cm or more above the right heart. In obstetrics, there are numerous situations in which venous air embolism can develop, including vaginal delivery, cesarean section, manual extraction of the placenta, and after the insertion, disconnection, or removal of central venous catheters. In addition, several reports have suggested that the injection of air, as part of the loss of resistance technique, during insertion of an epidural anesthetic may also precipitate air embolism.[7, 8]

It has been suggested that venous air embolism can be recognized by the onset of an audible hissing sound in the surgical field, followed, in the awake patient, by the patient's expressing a sense of impending doom.[9] Obviously, not all patients present in this way. Morbidity and mortality related to venous air embolism depend on the size of the embolus, the rate of air entry, the possible development of paradoxical air embolism, and the monitoring being used at the moment of the event. With increasing volumes of air into the venous system, greater compromise of cardiovascular function may occur. Doses of air greater than 1 mL/kg cause hypotension and cardiac arrhythmias; 5 mL/kg of air entraining rapidly can be lethal. It has been suggested that 100 mL of air can enter the circulation through a 14-gauge catheter in 1 second.[10]

During an episode of venous air embolism, the cardiovascular, pulmonary, and central nervous systems may all be affected, with severity ranging from no symptoms to immediate cardiovascular collapse and death. According to Matjasko et al.,[11] the incidence of severe morbidity or mortality from venous air embolism, even as a consequence of neurosurgery, is only about 1% when patients are treated adequately and in a timely fashion.

Incidence of Venous Air Embolism

The true incidence of venous air embolism is unknown and, for numerous reasons, is probably underestimated. As is discussed later in this chapter, subclinical air embolism in hospitalized patients, obstetric cases included, may occur quite commonly. Figures related to clinically significant venous air embolism, despite their association with significant morbidity and mortality, are very difficult to obtain, since most cases of embolism are reported under the general heading of "pulmonary embolism," without the embolus type being specified.

Venous air embolism is a well-recognized cause of sudden death arising due to a variety of causes. The causes during neurosurgical procedures and their incidence are as follows:

1. Posterior fossa craniotomy (sitting position): 45–55%[12, 13]
2. Posterior fossa craniotomy (other positions): 10–15%[13]
3. Cervical laminectomies (sitting position): 5–15%[14]
4. Transsphenoidal pituitary resection (horizontal position):12%[15]
5. Lumbar spine procedures: three cases reported[16]

Many other procedures, however, may be associated with venous air embolism. These include liver transplantation, cardiopulmonary bypass, open or blunt chest trauma, angiography, laparoscopic procedures, radical hysterectomy, hysteroscopy, orthopedic procedures, and dental implants. The most common non-neurosurgical causes of intraoperative venous air embolism and their incidence are as follows:

1. Cesarean section: 11–97%[17–22]
2. Total hip replacement: 67%[23]
3. Hysteroscopy: although possible, no figures reported
4. Central venous catheter placement and removal: <2%[24]

Even though central venous catheters are commonly used in the treatment of critically ill patients, they may be the cause of air embolism. The mortality rate following symptomatic venous air embolism associated with central venous catheterization may be as high as 30%.

Among the 2475 maternal deaths that occurred in the United States between 1974 and 1978, 25 were attributed to air embolism.[25] Likewise, a summary of maternal mortality in New York City, between the years 1981 and 1983, reported that pulmonary embolism was one of the leading causes of maternal mortality. Although only one case of embolic death was specifically attributed to air embolism, other cases could not be excluded because of incomplete reporting and incorrect diagnosis.[26]

Air embolism is a rare life-threatening complication of obstetric procedures. Predisposing factors in pregnancy include uterine surgery, uterine manipulation, hypovolemia, and certain maternal positions.[19] The actual incidence of venous air embolism in the pregnant patient is closely related to the means of detection employed. Fong et al.,[21] using ultrasonic Doppler and two-dimensional echocardiography, determined an incidence of 29% of venous air embolism during cesarean sections. Lew et al.,[22] however, employing more sophisticated monitors such as expired nitrogen concentrations and precordial Doppler, detected an incidence of venous air embolism of 97% in patients undergoing cesarean delivery.

Venous Air Embolism in Obstetrics

During Pregnancy

- Vaginal insufflation of powder, liquid, or gas may precipitate an embolism. When used in pregnant women, the substance insufflated under pressure may dissect the membranes and enter the uterine sinuses. Fortunately, these treatments are rarely, if ever, used.
- In countries where abortion is illegal, cases of air embolism and maternal death have been related to illicit attempts to induce abortion. The feature common to most of the cases of air embolism related to abortion is the introduction into the uterus of a mixture of air and a solution under pressure, with the resultant separation of the membranes and entry of air into the dilated uterine sinuses.[26]
- Therapeutic air embolism may be employed for the selective termination of a multiple pregnancy. In these cases, a small volume of air is injected into one fetus, either intracardially or through the umbilical vein. Although there are no reports of maternal air embolism associated with this practice, the air is introduced under pressure, and therefore maternal air embolism is theoretically possible.
- There is one reported case of proven paradoxical air embolism following cervical cerclage.[27]
- Several reports have described the occurrence of gas embolism resulting from orogenital sex during pregnancy.[28]

During Labor and Delivery

- Air embolism during normal labor and delivery has been reported.[29] Although the exact mechanism could not be determined, it has been theorized that partial separation of the placental edge allowed air to enter the uterine sinuses, and uterine contractions forced air into the systemic circulation.[26]
- There are numerous case reports describing air embolism during delivery, including during manual removal of retained placenta, in cases of placenta previa or accreta, in placental abruption, in forceps and vacuum delivery, in a case of a ruptured uterus, and after breech delivery.[26]
- Cesarean section has been implicated as a cause of venous air embolism, with an incidence of 11% to 97%. The majority of

these cases are subclinical, but anesthesiologists must be aware that patients undergoing cesarean section are at risk of developing air embolism. The introduction of a previously exteriorized uterus is considered to be a major risk factor.[19, 30] In addition, both prolonged rupture of membranes and prolonged interval between uterine incision and fetal extraction were found to predispose to air embolism in cesarean sections.[26]

During the Puerperium

- One case of venous air embolism following postpartum sterilization has been reported.[31]
- A number of publications have described venous air embolism as a consequence of the "knee-chest" position, recommended in the past for puerperal women to prevent and treat the retroversion and subinvolution of the uterus.[32]

Pathophysiology

Air can enter the venous system as a passive process, when the pressure gradient is created by patient position and hemodynamics; or as an active process, in which the gas enters the venous system forced under pressure into a body cavity. In cases of passive air embolism, it is recognized that room air can enter the venous system through any open vein, when the intraluminal pressure is negative, or below atmospheric pressure.

The following are required conditions for development of passive venous air embolism:

1. An open, noncollapsible vein in the operative field.
2. A hydrostatic pressure gradient between the operative site and the right heart.

During cesarean section, especially when the uterus is exteriorized, a pressure gradient often develops because the operative site is above the level of the right atrium. A height difference as small as 5 cm is all that is necessary to allow air entrance. A contracted blood volume and low central venous pressure also augment gradients between an open vessel and the right heart.

In cases of active venous embolism, a gas is insufflated into a cavity during surgery and high intracavitary pressures can force gas into any noncollapsible vein that has been opened during the surgery. This event is seen most commonly during laparoscopy or arthroscopic procedures,[33] when a pressurized infusion system for fluids or blood is used. But active venous embolism can also occur in a patient undergoing a routine cesarean section. For example, during repositioning of a previously exteriorized uterus, air that has been trapped inside the uterus may be squeezed and can be embolized into the venous system. In addition, spontaneous respiration during regional anesthesia creates a negative intrathoracic pressure, which could potentially increase the pressure gradient, and thus the possibility of air embolism. Doppler studies have clearly demonstrated that putative signs of embolization were significantly more common when the uterus was exteriorized than when it was left inside the abdomen.[30]

Generally, when a vein is opened, either bleeding occurs or the vein collapses. In some operative procedures, however, veins remain open, supported by surrounding tissues so that even if venous pressure is very low, the vein cannot collapse.[33] This may occur in the pregnant patient, in whom veins in the gravid uterus are actually within another vascular structure and may not collapse. In the obstetric setting, air most commonly enters the venous system through the pelvic venous plexus. Free-flowing blood in an opened vein produces a venturi effect, allowing room air to enter the vein and permitting air to pass, as a stream of bubbles, to the right heart. This fact, combined with a large negative hydrostatic gradient between the operative site and the right heart, provides a perfect setting for the room air entrance. Since there is no bleeding from the lacerated vein that is aspirating room air, it is very difficult for the surgeon to identify the responsible vein, which must be closed immediately to control the situation.

The access of air into the venous system (venous air embolism) produces signs and symptoms due to effects on the right ventricle, the pulmonary circulation, or the systemic circulation. The severity of symptoms is related to the degree of air entry. Small amounts of air do not generally produce symptoms, and air bubbles are quickly removed from the circulation. It has been determined in animal studies of the lung's capacity to act as a filter that a bolus 0.05 mL/kg/min, infused directly into the right ventricle, is completely filtered and remains undetected by transesophageal echocardiography.[34] Intermediate amounts of air (less than 3 mL/kg) end up in the pulmonary circulation, producing a vascular injury manifested by capillary pulmonary reaction. Large amounts of air (more than 3 mL/kg) will cause severe and potentially fatal effects. Human data, although limited to accidental circumstances, show that oxygen given intravenously at flow rates of 0.1 to 0.4 mL/kg/min have not been fatal.[35]

Once in the venous system, air travels rapidly through the heart to the lungs. Having arrived in the lungs, air in the pulmonary circulation obstructs precapillary arterioles, thereby decreasing pulmonary blood flow. The predominant pathophysiologic changes induced by the majority of episodes of air venous embolism occur in the pulmonary vasculature. The presence of nitrogen in the air bubble (because nitrogen is the principal component of air) plays a major role in the evolution of an air embolism. Because nitrogen is a relatively insoluble gas, the consequences of a nitrogen embolus are more severe than when the embolism is produced by soluble gases such as CO_2 and N_2O.[36]

When massive venous air embolism occurs, a large and rapidly entrained bolus of air can fill the right

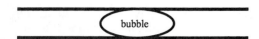

Figure 31–1 An air bubble interposed in a liquid column (blood), into a thin tube (vein), is limited by two meniscuses.

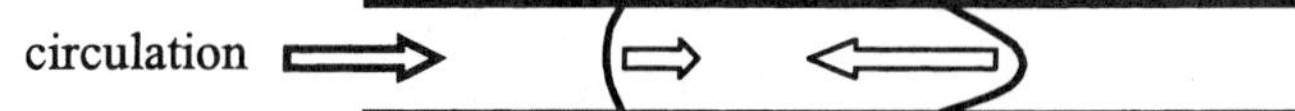

Figure 31–3 If we exert pressure on the bubble (circulation), trying to push it in the direction of the circulation, the meniscus will be deformed, and the combination of both forces (different radius of the meniscuses) is opposite to the circulation of the liquid column.

atrium, causing an outflow obstruction of the right ventricle, better known as an "air lock." This complication leads to obstruction of the right ventricular outflow tract, with a consequent increased right heart afterload; increased preload, as measured by central venous pressure; decreased venous return, and decreased cardiac outflow, which result in an acute right ventricular failure and cardiovascular collapse, which could lead to a fatal outcome. The primary mechanism for cardiac dysfunction appears to be the combination of increased right ventricular afterload and arterial hypotension, possibly due to subsequent right ventricular ischemia rather than right ventricular outflow obstruction.[37] In many postmortem examinations following fatal venous air embolism, the right heart and pulmonary outflow tract have been noted to be obstructed by frothy bloody foam.[38] Recent studies have likewise indicated that when a large enough bolus of air enters the right heart, an immediate cessation of forward blood flow into the pulmonary vasculature occurs.[39] The resistance to pulmonary blood flow interferes with alveolar gas exchange, decreasing end-tidal CO_2, and PaO_2, and causing reflex tachypnea in spontaneously ventilating patients.

The laws of physics can help to explain the "air lock" phenomenon that occurs during air embolism. An air bubble interposed in a liquid column in a thin tube is limited by two meniscuses, as is shown in Figure 31–1. Because of the superficial tension of the bubble, the forces exerted by the two meniscuses are directly proportional to the radius of each hemisphere forming the air bubble (Fig. 31–2). If we exert some pressure on the bubble, trying to push it in the direction of the circulation, the meniscus will be deformed, as is shown in Figure 31–3. The result of these changed forces is opposite to the circulation of the liquid column.[40] If the bubbles are numerous, or a very big one is present, the circulation of the liquid could be stopped, as can occur in the hearts of patients following an air embolism episode.

In most cases of air embolism, however, small volumes of entrained air quickly pass through the right heart and are distributed within the pulmonary arterial blood flow, primarily to the alveolar capillaries. At this site, most of the air apparently traverses the alveolar-capillary membrane and can be measured in exhaled gas as an increase in end-tidal nitrogen concentration,[9] without any other physiologic consequences. If venous air embolism continues, however, the small bubbles lead to a pulmonary microvascular occlusion, with a consequent increase in pulmonary vascular resistance, due both to mechanical obstruction of the pulmonary vasculature and to release of endogenous vasoactive substances.[33] The pathogenesis of the pulmonary endothelial injury is not fully understood but is associated with platelet fibrin thrombi, cytokine release, and neutrophil, platelet, and component activation at the microvascular air-blood interface. Lipid peroxidation and oxygen radicals may also mediate injury. One of the hallmarks of pulmonary air embolism is a marked increase in pulmonary vascular resistance, with a subsequent increase in pulmonary arterial pressure. This increase of the pulmonary vascular resistance will further compromise right ventricular function, which could manifest through an elevation of the right ventricular and central venous pressures. Pulmonary microvascular compromise also results in a coexistent ventilation-perfusion mismatch that produces a considerable increase in the dead space and intrapulmonary shunt, causing slightly raised arterial CO_2, and substantially decreased arterial oxygen tension. In other words, alveoli without circulation are ventilated. Bronchoconstriction may also occur as a result of the release of endothelial mediators, complement production, and the presence of other mediators, causing an increase in the airway pressure.

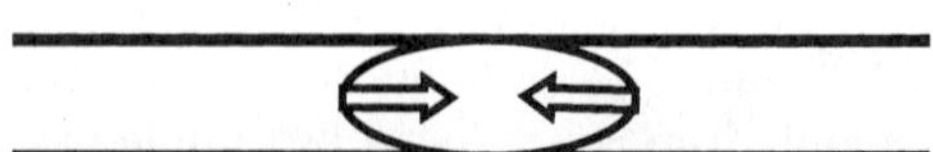

Figure 31–2 Because of the superficial tension of the bubble, the forces exerted by the two meniscuses of the bubble are directly proportional to the radius of each hemisphere (meniscus).

Occasionally, there may be multiple small episodes of air embolism during surgery, so that although the patient remains hemodynamically stable intraoperatively, signs and symptoms of air embolism become obvious in the postoperative period, when decreases in cardiac output and hypotension lead to cardiovascular compromise, cardiovascular dysrhythmias, and collapse.

In some patients, pulmonary edema and acute respiratory distress syndrome may develop after venous air embolism.[33, 41] This complication could be the result of air bubble–induced disruption of the alveolar capillary membrane. The production and release of toxic oxygen metabolites by leukocytes may cause endothelial damage.[41] Pulmonary edema may occur rapidly, or several hours later, but usually it is present only after multiple episodes of air trapping.[41] This condition may not be appreciated during surgery, because of the support of positive pressure during mechanical ventilation. When spontaneous ventilation is restored, serious hypoxemia may appear.[42]

Paradoxical Air Embolism

Paradoxical air embolism as a result of venous air embolism is a rare occurrence but can result in serious morbidity and mortality. It occurs when air from a venous air embolism embolizes into arterial vessels. Next to total cessation of cardiac output from an "air lock" at the right side of the heart, the most dangerous aspect of air embolism is the risk of having air bubbles entering the arterial circulation, where they may produce devastating consequences.

Venous air bubbles may gain access to the systemic circulation by passing through a cardiac defect, most frequently in obstetric patients, a patent foramen ovale. Patent foramen ovale is reported to be present in 25% to 34% of asymptomatic adults.[43, 44] The incidence is higher in younger patients. The average size of a patent foramen ovale defect is 4.5 mm in diameter.[43] Commonly, blood flow through a patent foramen ovale is minimal because left atrial pressure is higher than right atrial pressure. This tends to keep the flap-like septum primum and septum secundum in a closed position.[9] If left atrial pressure, measured as pulmonary artery occlusion pressure, is less than right atrial pressure, the patient must be considered to be at an increased risk of paradoxical embolism. The atrial pressure gradient and its direction together are a prognostic indicator of whether venous air embolism will become a dangerous paradoxical air embolism.[33] There are some patients in whom a patent foramen ovale is demonstrated preoperatively during a cardiac evaluation; there are others who have a known right-to-left shunt. It seems that these patients might be at risk for paradoxical air embolism if an episode of venous air embolism occurs. Nevertheless, preoperative determinations of atrial pressure gradients do not appear to be reliable predictors of paradoxical air embolism risk during a venous air embolism episode. When administering anesthesia to these patients, it seems prudent to prevent every possible cause of air entrance into the venous system.

Transpulmonary passage of air bubbles can also occur.[45] In these cases, air bubbles may enter the arterial circulation in the absence of cardiac septal defects. Presumably, air bubbles are able to traverse the pulmonary capillary bed. Intrapulmonary shunts may also serve as a route for air passage into the arterial circulation.[9, 46] If this occurs, it may result in an overloading of the pulmonary system's capacity to remove air from the central circulation, resulting in transpulmonary passage of air to the arterial circulation. The ability of the lungs to inhibit transpulmonary air passage has been quantified in a canine model, which demonstrated a finite limit to pulmonary filtering ability.[47] The protective filtering properties of the human lung against paradoxical air embolism during episodes of venous air embolism appear to be substantial. The lungs are not, however, impenetrable. It has been suggested that some pathways become functionally open for air passage only during episodes of venous air embolism in which significant elevations of pulmonary artery pressure occur.[45]

Currently, paradoxical air embolism can be accurately diagnosed with transesophageal echocardiography. However, during most clinical episodes of venous air embolism, this monitoring modality is not readily available and does not allow one to discriminate between right-to-left interatrial shunting and transpulmonary passage of air emboli.[45]

Once air has entered the arterial circulation, the bubble of gas follows the blood flow until it is eventually blocked by smaller caliber vessels. The progressive diffusion of the air reduces the size of the embolus, which then migrates into smaller vessels. Air bubbles in the arterial circulation will tend to be distributed to areas of highest flow, particularly the coronary and cerebral vascular beds. Once bubbles are lodged in small arteries or arterioles, subsequent pathologic manifestations result from mechanical obstruction, leading to ischemia and inflammatory reactions to air, acting as a foreign body.[48] The bubbles prevent distal blood flow and thus induce ischemic tissue damage by preventing delivery of oxygenated blood.[9] In the case of cerebral air embolism, these episodes will result in stroke. Computed tomography of the brain has demonstrated multifocal discrete ischemic areas in the cerebral hemispheres.[49] Coronary artery embolism is likely to occur if the patient remains supine. In these cases, even 0.5 mL of air may cause a fatal arrhythmia.[26] Gas bubbles, trapped in the microcirculation, may cause late manifestations, such as disseminated intravascular coagulation, tissue ischemia and necrosis, and gastrointestinal bleeding due to mucosal damage, all of which are caused by blockage of blood vessels and destruction of adjacent tissue.[26]

It is not clear what volume of paradoxical air embolism can safely be considered insignificant. Therefore, it should be assumed that any amount of paradoxical air embolism can place the patient at real risk for serious morbidity or mortality. Therefore, when paradoxical air embolism is suspected, aggressive treatment must be promptly initiated.

Delayed Air Embolism

In a limited number of cases, some of them after cesarean section for placenta previa, symptoms of venous air embolism occurred some hours after air entered the circulation. This phenomenon is known as delayed air embolism.[50]

Diagnosis and Monitoring

Clinical presentation of the patient following venous air embolism is highly dependent on numerous factors, including the following:

1. Patient's position
2. Flow rate of the air entering
3. Total volume of gas embolized
4. Size of the bubbles
5. Weight of the patient
6. Anesthesia technique the patient is receiving
7. Physical status of the patient prior to the event

Acute respiratory failure and cardiovascular instability in pregnancy are important causes of maternal and fetal morbidity and mortality. **Venous air embolism** is one of the possible diagnoses. Other differential diagnoses include the following:

- Acute respiratory distress syndrome (due to sepsis, pneumonia, aspiration, or amniotic fluid embolism)
- Anaphylaxis
- Side effects of β-adrenergic tocolysis
- Asthma
- Thromboembolism
- Heart disease
- Pneumothorax
- Pneumomediastinum[51]

Frequently noted symptoms in the rare cases of clinically obvious venous air embolism in awake patients depend on the amount of embolized air and include dyspnea, faintness, chest pain or chest discomfort, cough, nausea and vomiting, and fear of death. Clinical findings include deep inspirations, tachypnea, tachycardia, coughing, gasping, wheezing, cyanosis, hypotension, altered sensorium, and circulatory collapse.[52]

Clinicians originally made the diagnosis of air embolism by hearing the hissing sound of the air entering venous circulation and by recognizing the peculiar lapping sound created by air in the right heart.[1, 3] Traditionally, it was believed that the sudden intraoperative appearance of a cardiorespiratory event, and a "mill wheel" murmur on cardiac auscultation, was pathognomonic for venous air embolism, but today we know that this is a very late finding in the diagnosis of unexpected air embolism. The prognosis is particularly grim when the diagnosis is made very late, as by the operating surgeon seeing air bubbles in the arteries of the surgical field.[53]

With the advent of modern technology, making or confirming the diagnosis of venous air embolism has substantially improved. Today, the key to preventing major morbidity or mortality from venous air embolism is its early detection. Monitoring for venous air embolism includes some elements not routinely found in the obstetric clinical setting. These monitors include precordial Doppler, right atrial catheter, pulmonary arterial catheter, transesophageal echocardiography, expired nitrogen analyzer or mass spectrometer, and the standard monitors including capnograph, esophageal stethoscope, electrocardiograph, pulse oximeter, and blood pressure monitors. The most sensitive of these modalities are transesophageal echocardiography and precordial Doppler ultrasonography, followed by measurement of expired nitrogen, and end-tidal carbon dioxide, and examination by right atrial catheter. The least sensitive is examination by esophageal stethoscope (Fig. 31–4).[33] The sensitivity of each method depends on the sensitivity itself of each monitor and on the time that has elapsed since the air has entered the venous system. The first warning that an air embolism has occurred is the sound of hissing from the air entering the vein. Later, the precordial Doppler and transesophageal echocardiographic findings will change, and finally, classic sounds will be heard with the esophageal stethoscope. Once the air reaches the

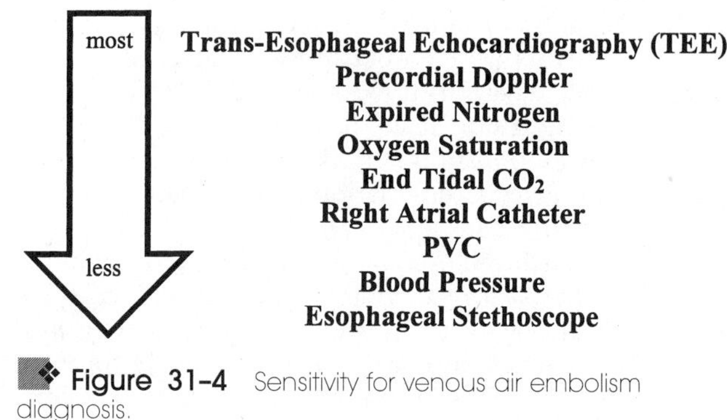

Figure 31–4 Sensitivity for venous air embolism diagnosis.

pulmonary vasculature, changes to the pulmonary artery pressure and the central venous pressure will occur. Because of pulmonary effects of the embolism, the anesthesiologist will observe changes in expired nitrogen and end-tidal carbon dioxide. Finally, depending on the size of the embolism, it will cause a decrease in cardiac output, and ultimately, a fall in the systemic blood pressure (Fig. 31–5).

The clinical signs and symptoms of a venous air embolism include the following:

- Sudden development of hypotension
- Hypoxia
- Drop in end-tidal CO_2
- Chest tightness or pain
- Deterioration of mental status (this can be assessed only in the awake patient)

Precordial Doppler

The introduction of the Doppler ultrasonography into clinical practice has revolutionized the awareness of venous air embolism as an intraoperative hazard.[54] The Doppler monitor uses ultrahigh frequency sound waves (commonly between 2 and 3 megahertz) to measure blood flow velocity and changes in the density of the blood. All the information obtained is converted to a characteristic sound. The distinctive sound of venous air embolism, lasting 15 seconds or longer,[55] is easily identifiable, thus allowing the anesthesiologist to attend to other tasks during the surgery while monitoring for air embolism. To gain familiarity with precordial Doppler sounds, anesthesiologists can visit the following Internet web site: http://gasnet.org/gta/vae.html. The correct position of the probe over the right heart can be achieved by positioning the transducer parasternally over the fourth intercostal space. The clinician can verify correct positioning by rapidly injecting saline into a central venous pressure or large-bore peripheral intravenous line and listening for the typical sounds. In some cases, especially in obstetric patients, it may be difficult to correctly position the probe.

Precordial Doppler ultrasonography is one of the most sensitive, but nonspecific methods for detecting air emboli. Although it is not routinely used by anesthesiologists in obstetrics, it should be considered for use, especially in high-risk cases. It is noninvasive and

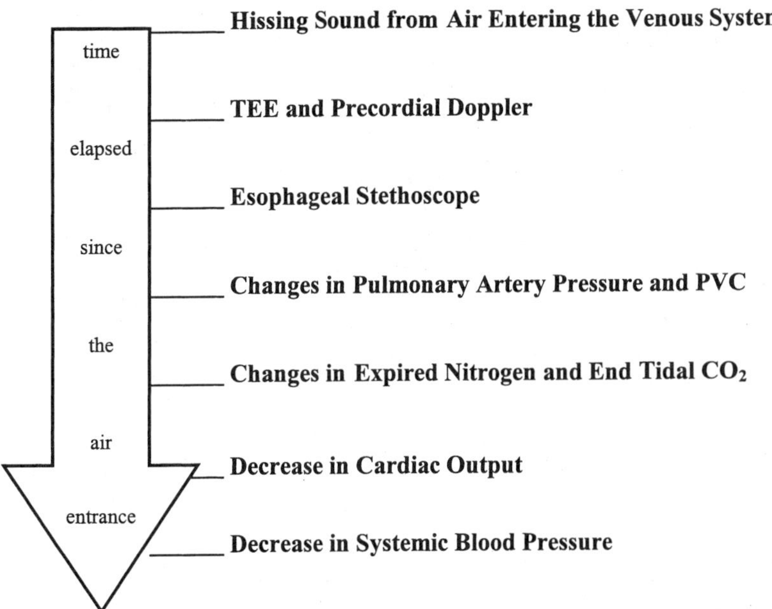

❖ **Figure 31-5** Relative time necessary for detecting an episode of venous air embolism in relation to the monitoring method.

easy to use. If one is not available, a Doppler monitor can usually be borrowed from the obstetricians, as this is typically the method used for external fetal heart rate monitoring. Doppler ultrasonography is particularly useful because it detects air before it enters the pulmonary circulation. Although a correctly positioned precordial Doppler probe is considered by many to be the "gold standard," it is by no means foolproof.[9] The Doppler monitor is sensitive, but it is not quantitative, and it does not differentiate between a massive air embolism and a pathophysiologically insignificant embolism. False-positive results may occur during a fast intravenous injection, with a crystallized manitol dose, and during the compression of retroperitoneal structures.[22] It can be argued that such sensitivity is precisely the early warning needed to identify the occurrence of venous air embolism early, thus preventing severe complications.[33] Precordial Doppler is, however, associated with a 10% incidence of false-negative detection of episodes. Other disadvantages are related to radiofrequency interference; the Doppler monitor does not function during electrocautery.

Right Atrial Catheter

Rapid injection of saline through the right atrial catheter can help to confirm that the Doppler probe is properly placed over the right heart. Air from the right atrium can frequently be aspirated through the right atrial catheter when detected on Doppler. Suspected venous air embolism can be confirmed by aspiration of air. The right heart catheter may be positioned by pressure recordings, radiographs, or ECG control.[56] The tip of the multiorifice catheter must be placed where the air will most likely collect, and this position depends on the position of the patient. Although proper right atrial catheter position has been specified for the patient undergoing sitting craniotomy, the optimal position for cesarean section has not yet been determined. Whenever air embolism is suspected, an attempt should be made to confirm the diagnosis by recovery of air from the right heart by aspirating through a central venous catheter, if one is in place.[9] In addition, this will allow measurement of the central venous pressure, which is typically elevated in symptomatic venous air embolism. Double-lumen multiorifice catheters may offer advantages over single-lumen catheters. Animal studies have confirmed that multiorifice catheters have been effective in resuscitating swine from experimental venous air embolism.[57]

Transesophageal Echocardiography

Transesophageal echocardiography (TEE) is the most sensitive monitor for venous air embolism. Although it is more sensitive than Doppler monitoring, it is also more invasive and technically more difficult to place and to interpret. Its major benefit is that, unlike other commonly used techniques, it can distinguish between air and other emboli. The use of TEE to monitor for air embolism is work-intensive compared with Doppler, which allows the anesthesiologist to attend to other activities while listening for its characteristic sounds. If echocardiography is chosen, the echocardiographer needs to observe the screen continuously. In the practical obstetric anesthesia sense, TEE is not used because most obstetric patients are under regional anesthesia and not sedated. Under these conditions, TEE is almost impossible to perform. But in the theoretic situation of having TEE available and having a high-risk patient under general anesthesia, TEE may be worth the extra effort since it not only allows the visualization of air bubbles but also allows a determination of the volume of aspirated air and the localization of air within cardiac chambers and will show air passing through a patent foramen ovale into the left atrium and into the systemic circulation.[45] It can also be used for the precise placement of a right atrial air aspiration catheter.[58]

Pulmonary Artery Catheter

Although increases in pulmonary artery pressure are not specific for air embolism, the pulmonary artery catheter is a sensitive monitor that can be helpful for both diagnosis of air embolism and assessment of treatment once the diagnosis has been made. Air entering the pulmonary circulation may cause mechanical obstruction and reflex vasoconstriction due to pulmonary hypoxemia, causing an increase of the pulmonary artery pressure. Increases in pulmonary artery pressure and decreases in end-tidal CO_2 concentration are approximately equal in detection sensitivity to end-tidal nitrogen monitoring.[33] If the pulmonary artery pressure increases during venous air embolism, and the Doppler normalizes, a return of pulmonary artery pressure to previous levels suggests that air obstructing the pulmonary circulation has moved distally, probably being excreted through the lungs.[59] A major advantage of pulmonary artery pressure monitoring is its ability to observe changes in the relationship between right and left atrial pressures. Thus, by noting right atrial pressures that consistently exceed left atrial pressures,[9] it is possible to identify patients who are prone to paradoxical air embolism. Pulmonary artery catheter monitoring is not perfect, however. In experienced hands, the pulmonary artery catheter is relatively easy to place, but it is an invasive monitor and associated with numerous complications. In addition, its small lumen may make the aspiration of air very difficult (see Fig. 31–5).

End-Tidal Nitrogen

Increases in end-tidal nitrogen are seen when a venous air embolism is excreted through the lungs. The determination of end-tidal nitrogen concentration is highly specific for air embolism, with evidence of an increase in expired nitrogen concentration of 0.1 vol% from the baseline.[22] Unfortunately, these types of monitors can only be used in patients who are receiving general endotracheal anesthesia. In addition, in these conditions the concentration of exhaled nitrogen is usually less than 2%, and this value is below the threshold of some commercial nitrogen analyzers (e.g., mass spectrometers) (see Figs. 31–4 and 31–5).

End-Tidal Carbon Dioxide

The use of capnography demonstrates a decrease in end-tidal carbon dioxide during venous air embolism. End-tidal carbon dioxide ($ETCO_2$) monitoring is widely available, commonly used, and has a sensitivity that is intermediate. It is not a specific monitor for venous air embolism, because hyperventilation, low cardiac output, and other types of emboli can also decrease $ETCO_2$. One can expect to see changes in $ETCO_2$ after Doppler changes occur, but before hemodynamic changes occur (see Fig. 31–5).[33] If $ETCO_2$ decreases during an air embolism, it is indicative of a significant degree of air embolism, and when the $ETCO_2$ increases again, the situation has generally improved (Fig. 31–6).

Oxygen Saturation

Pulse oximetry is routinely used in all patients undergoing cesarean section under both regional and general anesthesia but is not a sensitive method for determining air embolism. The development of hypoxia, as evidenced by desaturation, must be considered a very late sign of venous air embolism, especially in those patients receiving supplemental oxygen. Since there are many causes of maternal hypoxemia during cesarean section, the diagnosis of air embolism should not be made in exclusion of other signs and without considering the other differential diagnoses.[20]

Precordial or Esophageal Stethoscope

The least sensitive monitor for determination of air embolism is the precordial or esophageal stethoscope. A "mill wheel murmur" is a very late sign that indicates a massive air embolism. This finding is of limited benefit to the anesthesiologist, however, since cardiovascular collapse is imminent once a mill wheel murmur is heard (see Fig. 31–5).

Less specific signs of air embolism include the sudden appearance of systemic arterial hypotension, due to decreased left heart filling, and ventricular irritability, related to acute right heart strain.[9] An increase in end-tidal oxygen content because of less oxygen extraction in the lungs, and a decrease in dynamic lung compliance detected by side-stream spirometry have also been advocated as sensitive monitors for the detection of venous air embolism.[60]

Laboratory Studies

Arterial blood gases usually demonstrate hypoxemia, hypercapnia, and metabolic acidosis. Mild cases may demonstrate only mild hypoxemia and hypocapnia.

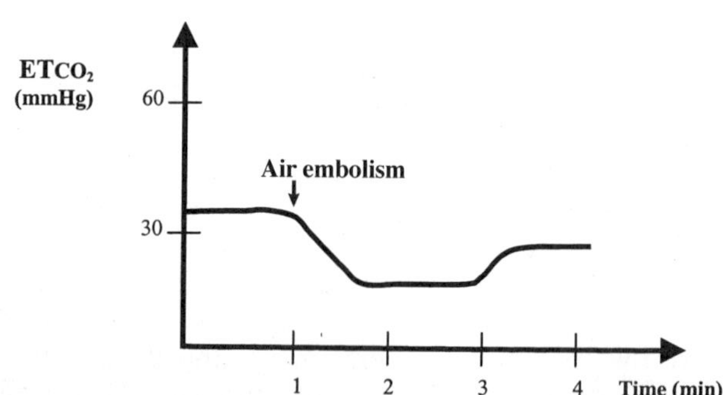

❖ **Figure 31–6** End tidal carbon dioxide tendency tracing showing sudden decrease in a minor venous air embolism episode.

Other laboratory studies are nonspecific and are obtained as indicated by associated conditions.

Chest Radiograph

The finding of the chest radiograph may be normal or may demonstrate air in the pulmonary arterial system. Other radiographic signs that may be present include pulmonary arterial dilatation, focal oligemia (Westermark's sign), and pulmonary edema.[24]

Electrocardiography

Nonspecific electrocardiographic findings that may accompany air embolism include tachycardia, bradycardia, right axis deviation, right ventricular strain, and ST depression. Because of the likelihood of some degree of venous air embolism during operative obstetric procedures, some type of monitoring for air embolism should be considered.

As has been previously discussed, anesthesiologists cannot rely on changes in vital signs for detection of air embolism in the obstetric patient. With appropriate monitoring and treatment of venous air embolism, related morbidity and mortality are rare.[12, 13]

Although embolic phenomena can cause sudden cardiorespiratory collapse in an obstetric patient, other possible differential diagnoses must also be considered. These other causes include total spinal or high epidural block, accidental intravascular injection of local anesthetics, allergic reactions, amniotic fluid embolism, myocardial infarction, massive blood loss, sepsis, pulmonary aspiration, and ruptured intracranial aneurysm.[61] A definitive diagnosis of air embolism may be obtained by demonstrating gas bubbles in the heart or circulation by aspiration or on postmortem examination by opening the heart under water to detect gas bubbles.[26]

Therapy

When the sudden onset of the previously described signs and symptoms leads to a presumed diagnosis of venous air embolism, treatment must be undertaken immediately. Tasks should be distributed so that all available help is being effectively utilized. As soon as the anesthesiologist determines that the patient may be experiencing an air embolus, it is imperative that this be communicated to the surgeon. Rarely, the surgeon can confirm the diagnosis by observing that an open vein is entraining air instead of bleeding. The primary goal of the treatment of air embolism is to stop the air entrance, with the source of air identified and removed. As soon as the surgeon has been informed that the diagnosis is suspected, the surgical site should be flooded with fluid or packed with a wet dressing, and open veins cauterized or stitched. Although this is sometimes difficult in obstetric cases, the surgeon should also apply pressure to the inferior vena cava, to increase the venous pressure at the wound site. If N_2O is being administered, it must be discontinued immediately, and the patient ventilated with 100% oxygen. Administration of 100% oxygen serves two functions. It treats hypoxemia and it allows reduction in the partial pressure of nitrous oxide and nitrogen. Whenever possible, the operative site should be immediately positioned below the level of the heart. This is particularly true if the uterus has been exteriorized following delivery by cesarean section. In addition, tilting the table or bed more than 10 degrees head-up (reverse Trendelenburg) may help bring the operative site below the heart. This maneuver may also increase venous pressure at the operative site so as to cause the lacerated vein to bleed rather than entrain air. Although these changes to patient position may help in the treatment of air embolism, it does not appear to prevent the occurrence of air embolism. It has been demonstrated, for example, that a modest 5 to 10 degree head-up position does not appear to influence the occurrence of venous air embolism in patients undergoing cesarean section.[18] Further treatment of the patient with suspected air embolism includes administration of intravenous fluids to counteract hemoconcentration. If a large volume of air has been entrained, and surgical conditions permit, patients should be positioned in the left lateral decubitus position (Durant's position[62]). Cardiovascular collapse during venous air embolism can result from outflow obstruction of the right ventricle by a large air embolus, and this position has been suggested as a means of relieving the outflow obstruction. With the patient in this position, the buoyancy of the air embolus would theoretically cause it to float away from the outflow tract of the right ventricle, relieving the obstruction, and relocating intracardiac air to nondependent areas of the right heart. In practice, few anesthesiologists have used this maneuver in recent years,[33] and others do not support the recommendation of repositioning into the left lateral recumbent position for the treatment of venous air embolism.[63] The effectiveness of this maneuver has been questioned, since in animal studies it has been found that body repositioning after venous air embolism provided no hemodynamic benefits, although relocation of intracardiac air was demonstrated.[37]

In addition to the above-mentioned functions, the principal role of the anesthesiologist during the management of a patient with air embolism is to support the patient's cardiorespiratory system, which often requires the initiation of cardiopulmonary resuscitation. Most of the treatment of the venous air embolism is supportive. The blood pressure should be supported with fluids and vasopressors. Increasing preload and cardiac output will not only support hemodynamics but will also aid in pushing the air through the heart and into the peripheral pulmonary circulation. If a right catheter or pulmonary arterial catheter is in place, aspiration of air from the right heart should be attempted. Aspiration of air will confirm the presumed diagnosis of air embolism and will also help the situation, since the aspirated air is removed before it enters the pulmonary circulation. However, it has been suggested that the recovery of air from the right heart has only limited therapeutic value, and there is no evidence that this treatment changes outcome. Although there are numerous case reports describing the removal of large volumes of air from the right atrium using standard central venous catheters,[64] there are no such reports using a Swan-Ganz catheter.[9] It has been suggested that the aspiration of air from the right atrium during venous air embolism is lifesaving only in the rare situations of massive entrance of air.[33]

As previously mentioned, morbidity and mortality during a venous air embolism may also occur due to arterial spread of air, a phenomenon termed "paradoxical" air embolism. In these cases, even small volumes of air may result in significant complications. If air emboli lodge in the coronary arteries, myocardial ischemia will occur; treatment should include inotropic agents, usually epinephrine. The goals are to support the patient's hemodynamics, increase ventricular contractility, and attempt to break up the emboli, thus relieving coronary artery obstruction.

Although all of the above-mentioned measures serve to stabilize and improve the patient's condition, the single most effective therapy for gas embolism is hyperbaric oxygenation.[26] Hyperbaric oxygen therapy is based on Boyle's law: the volume of a gas is inversely proportional to the pressure to which it is subjected.

Should air emboli lodge in the cerebral circulation, leading to symptomatic cerebral ischemia, hyperbaric oxygen along with supportive therapy is the best therapeutic option. Hyperbaric oxygenation acts by reducing bubble size, allowing the bubbles to pass more distally and to be eliminated from the cerebral circulation, and thus improving oxygen delivery to tissues distal to the obstructed vessels. Although it is assumed that hyperbaric oxygen therapy offers the best results, randomized controlled trials demonstrating the efficacy of this treatment modality have not been performed. If a hyperbaric chamber is available, it is advisable to arrange for immediate transportation of the patient to that facility. Unfortunately, hyperbaric medicine centers are usually located in diving centers and are seldom available close to labor and delivery suites.

Serious neurologic consequences of paradoxical air embolism have been described. Bacha et al.[48] estimated this number at 19% to 50% of the patients. In a controlled prospective study, they described a 14% mortality rate even if hyperbaric oxygen therapy was given within 12 hours of the accident. In a retrospective analysis of patients treated with hyperbaric oxygen therapy, however, the authors reported a complete recovery in 69% of cases, sequelae in 26%, and death in 5% of cases. According to these authors, prognosis differs greatly, depending on the etiology of the embolism and the existence of neurologic disorders related to the embolism. Venous air embolism has better improvement than arterial emboli.[65]

Induced hypertension can also be considered for treatment, but its efficacy in this situation has not been clearly demonstrated.[33]

Summarizing, therapeutic interventions related to venous air embolism include mechanical measures, such as positioning, withdrawal of air from the right heart, and measures aimed at reducing bubble size. Air will find its way to the pulmonary circulation, where it will be exhaled, provided cardiac output and alveolar ventilation are maintained. Therefore, the supportive treatment should be based on the use of vasopressors (dopamine), inotropic agents (ephedrine, phenylephrine, epinephrine, dopamine, amrinone), antiarrhythmics (lidocaine), infusion of fluids, and maintenance of an appropriate ventilation. In critical cases, cardiopulmonary resuscitation should be initiated immediately. External cardiac compression may help to expel air from the pulmonary outflow tract and disperse it into the peripheral pulmonary venous system.

Anesthetic Management

It has been suggested that patients undergoing procedures with a high risk for venous air embolism should have preoperative echocardiography performed to detect cardiac defects that would indicate a risk for paradoxical air embolism.[33] Preoperative testing of obstetric patients, however, almost never occurs. Most episodes of paradoxical air embolism occur via a patent foramen ovale,[66] but when echocardiography fails to detect a patent foramen ovale, the risk of paradoxical air embolism cannot be excluded. To diminish the risk of venous air embolism, the pressure gradient between the operative site and the right heart should be increased. This can be achieved by lowering the operative site relative to the right atrium, as often occurs when the pregnant patient is placed in a reverse Trendelenburg position. In addition, these patients should be well hydrated, which will increase their central venous pressure and thus decrease the risk of embolism. Hydration will also decrease the pressure gradient at the wound level and increase left atrial pressure, which will minimize the risk of paradoxical air embolism to the left side of the circulation. Although this therapy appears prudent, its efficacy in terms of reducing the magnitude of the venous air embolism has not been evaluated.

When venous air embolism occurs in the presence of nitrous oxide, the air bubbles increase in size because nitrous oxide is many times more soluble than nitrogen and thus nitrous oxide diffuses in faster than nitrogen can diffuse out. Munsen and Merrick found that breathing 50% nitrous oxide rapidly doubled the volume of an air embolus, whereas breathing 70% nitrous oxide caused a tripling of the size of the embolus.[64] Because of this phenomenon, inhalation of nitrous oxide may turn an otherwise innocuous volume of embolized air into a lethal event. All the symptoms and signs related to venous air embolism are increased when nitrous oxide is used.[67] If nitrous oxide is being administered during a cesarean section in which air embolism is suspected, the nitrous oxide must be discontinued immediately and the patient ventilated with 100% oxygen. It has also been suggested that even if the patient returns to baseline condition, if air embolism was suspected, nitrous oxide should not be readministered during the case.[68] On the other hand, it has been suggested that the use of nitrous oxide in patients who are at risk for venous air embolism may actually be beneficial. Because the use of nitrous oxide during venous air embolism will cause the air bubbles to increase their size, it could increase the sensitivity of monitors for venous air embolism.[69] However, animal data comparing monitor sensitivity during venous air embolism with and without nitrous oxide have demonstrated that the use of nitrous oxide did not alter the sensitivity of sensitive monitors, but it did increase the sensitivity of less sensitive monitors.[33, 70] In addition, hemodynamic effects of a given volume of venous air embolism were unchanged by the administration of nitrous oxide, as long as the nitrous oxide was discontinued once venous air embolism was detected.[69]

Although small amounts of positive end-expiratory pressure (PEEP) may reduce the risk of air entrance, the use of PEEP in these circumstances is controversial. An amount of 5 to 10 cm of PEEP has been advocated to decrease the incidence of venous air embolism or to help in identifying the site of air entry.[71] However, studies examining the effectiveness of clinically applicable levels of PEEP have demonstrated that it was ineffective in increasing central venous pressure and would be of little help in the prevention of venous air embolism.[72] In addition, if sufficient PEEP is used to produce an increased right atrial pressure, it has been suggested that this application may result in an increased risk for the development of paradoxical air embolism during venous air embolism in the presence of a patent foramen ovale.[69] This fact was not demonstrated in laboratory animals. However, at the moment of releasing of PEEP, an increase in right-to-left passage of the embolus could occur.[73] This occurrence could be explained because at the moment of releasing PEEP, the venous return to the right heart and its pressure increase so that for a brief period pressure of the right heart exceeds pressure of the left heart.[33] Although controversy still exists regarding the use of PEEP, most current evidence suggests that the potential risks outweigh potential benefits.[33]

Conclusion

The sudden development of hypotension and hypoxia and a decrease in $ETCO_2$ are typical signs of venous air embolism. With the development of current monitoring and treatment modalities, venous air embolism is rarely a cause of mortality, with most morbidity and mortality from venous air embolism currently occurring during procedures in which the possibility of venous air embolism was not anticipated. Although most of the studies related to venous embolism have been performed under specific conditions of monitoring, this is not the reality of the obstetric setting in most hospitals around the world. In addition, much of our current knowledge regarding anesthetic management of patients with venous air embolism has been derived from studies of patients under general anesthesia. In obstetrics, however, most of our patients receive regional anesthesia and thus have different pulmonary pressures, ventilation patterns, gradients of venous pressure, and hemodynamics.

Serious venous air embolism is an unusual complication in obstetric anesthesia. But, with the use of sensitive monitors for venous air embolism, such as precordial Doppler ultrasonography and measurement of end-tidal nitrogen concentration, we have realized that less important episodes are as frequent as 97%[22] and probably occur at most cesarean sections. Since the clinical presentation of gas embolism has many faces, it is important to identify it as early as possible, because timely treatment may be lifesaving and a delay may have serious consequences.[74]

AMNIOTIC FLUID EMBOLISM

Historical Aspects

The earliest report of amniotic fluid embolism (AFE) was that of Meyer in 1926.[75] However, this entity, as a syndrome, was not recognized until 1941, when fatal pulmonary embolism due to components of amniotic fluid was first described by Steiner and Luschbaugh,[76] pathologists at the University of Chicago. In their classic article, they described anatomic and pathologic findings that consisted of mucin, amorphous eosinophilic material, and, in some cases, squamous cells in the maternal pulmonary vasculature found at the autopsy of eight women who suffered unexplained and sudden death during pregnancy. This picture, occurring in multiparous patients after tumultuous or hyperstimulated labor, became the classic "amniotic fluid embolism syndrome." Before this description, the most common clinical diagnosis in patients suffering these signs and symptoms was "postpartum hemorrhage." In 1969, Liban and Raz[77] reported similar observations in 14 cases of peripartum death. These investigators also reported the detection of squamous cells throughout the systemic circulation of their patients, including the kidneys, liver, spleen, pancreas, and brain. The purported pathway of fetal squamous cells from the uterine veins to the maternal systemic circulation was not described at that time. Interestingly, Liban and Raz,[77] and later Thompson and Budd,[78] described the appearance of squamous cells in the uterine veins of pregnant patients without clinical AFE.

Introduction

Although the syndrome of AFE has been known for more than 50 years, during the last decade the knowledge related to this potentially devastating condition has increased, and necessitated a reevaluation of many classic beliefs regarding this condition. Many old concepts regarding the pathogenesis of AFE are based on early animal models, which have unfortunately been inadequately extrapolated to humans. Most of these animal studies have been poorly designed and evaluated. Although Steiner and Luschbaugh initially showed that rabbits and dogs could be killed by an intravenous injection of amniotic fluid and meconium, this only tells us that it is possible to kill animals by a systemic injection of large boluses of foreign material from another species.[75] In most of these animal studies, male animals and pregnant and nonpregnant female animals were injected with high volumes of previously collected and stored heterologous amniotic fluid. It was obvious that these studies could not be easily extrapolated to humans because significant interspecies differences exist in the physiologic response to experimental AFE.[75] In fact, a primate model suggests that the infusion of even large amounts of normal autologous amniotic fluid is not necessarily pathogenic and may have no effect on blood pressure, pulse, or respiratory rate.[79, 80] Thus the clinical and pathophysiologic profiles of AFE are very complex and, despite recent advances, still remain poorly understood. Much of the research related to AFE syndrome has been published by Clark and colleagues, who have established a National Registry of AFE in the United States.[75, 81–87] The relationship between amniotic fluid and AFE syndrome is just one of the many unanswered questions.

Amniotic fluid embolism, although rare, remains the most lethal and unpredictable complication of pregnancy, with a mortality rate as high as 80%.[82] There is now growing evidence to support the idea that the classic picture of AFE represents only the lethal end of a continuum, which also includes much less dramatic and less lethal presentations of the syndrome, and perhaps even some subclinical or asymptomatic cases. There are probably unnoticed cases in our daily practice, and it is probable that many cases of AFE have actually gone undiagnosed, because in the past, fatal outcome was considered essential for the diagnosis, and thus less severe and atypical cases may have been excluded from the correct diagnosis. On the other hand, it is also probable that in the past other causes of maternal death, including thromboembolism and placental abruption, have been misdiagnosed as AFE. Even in 1948, Eastman[88] exhibited a great understanding of this problem when he said, "Let us be careful not to make the diagnosis of AFE a waste basket for all cases of unexplained death in labor, especially cases without autopsy confirmation."

Incidence and Maternal Mortality

It is almost impossible to know the precise incidence of AFE. The most significant problem related to gathering this information is the lack of a frequent correlation between clinical and laboratory criteria. Nevertheless, AFE, along with pulmonary thromboembolism, remains the leading cause of maternal mortality in the United States,[25] being responsible for roughly 10% of all maternal deaths.[87] In a large series from Australia evaluating a 27-year period, AFE was found to be the cause of obstetric death in 7.5% of the cases.[89] It was also the fifth most common cause of direct maternal mortality in the United Kingdom between 1985 and 1990.[90, 91] According to another large study by Burrows and Khoo,[89] the incidence of AFE is 15.2 cases per 100,000 pregnancies. Other authors, however, have suggested that AFE occurs from 1 in 8000 to 1 in 80,000 pregnancies.[76, 92]

The AFE syndrome has a very high mortality rate, varying between 22% and 86%,[75, 87, 89, 92, 93] with deaths attributable to cardiopulmonary collapse or uncontrolled hemorrhage related to disseminated intravascular coagulation (DIC) (Table 31–1). Half of all deaths occur within the first hour of the start of symptoms. As previously mentioned, because it is often difficult to diagnose AFE, different studies have reported very dissimilar outcomes.

Intact maternal survival following AFE is rare. Data from Clark et al.[87] and Morgan[92] suggest that only 15% of patients survive AFE without consequences, which means that 85% of women either died or sustained permanent neurologic damage following documented AFE. Recent studies have suggested a lower incidence of neurologic deficit in survivors,[87, 92] and there are currently more nonfatal cases being reported. This apparently improved survival rate, with a recent report suggesting that only 36% of these patients had died in the first 2 hours, may reflect improved care of the critically ill pregnant woman.[87]

Predisposing Factors

It has traditionally been suggested that precipitating factors for AFE include increasing maternal age, overactivity of the uterus and overuse of oxytocic drugs, multiparity, a large fetus, prolonged gestation, meconium-contaminated liquor, placental abruption, uterine rupture, and intrauterine fetal demise.[76, 77, 89, 93, 95–99] Today, however, there are well designed studies reporting that no such identifiable risk factors for AFE exist.[89] An analysis of the data from the National Registry of AFE, for example, reveals no demographic maternal risk factors. Age, race, parity, obstetric history, weight gain, and blood pressure have not been found to be risk factors for AFE.[87] The only irrefutable predisposing factor that remains unquestionable is pregnancy.

Clinical Presentation

The AFE syndrome can present before, during, or after delivery, with the majority of the cases reported during labor. Analysis of data from the National Registry[87] demonstrated that 70% of the cases of AFE syndrome occurred during labor (66% of them during the first stage of labor and 33% during the second stage), 11% after vaginal delivery, and 19% during cesarean section. The route of delivery does not appear to affect the risk of AFE.

Sudden death attributable to this syndrome has been reported under widely varying circumstances, including first and second trimester induced abortion, during an uncomplicated second trimester of preg-

Table 31–1 Mortality Rate Due to Amniotic Fluid Embolism

	Deaths per 100,000 Births
Australia 1984–1993[89]	3.37
Australia 1964–1990[89]	1.03
Irish Republic 1989–1991[94]	1.28

nancy, and following abdominal trauma and amniocentesis. There are also cases of AFE that occurred as late as 48 hours following delivery.[75] It is worth mentioning that a majority of patients experienced AFE after rupture of membranes,[87] with a striking temporal association, in which AFE developed within minutes of artificial rupture of membranes. Other cases have been reported to have occurred during or after positioning of intrauterine pressure catheters.[87] In the previously mentioned series from Burrows and Khoo,[89] 44% of the patients who developed AFE did so after an intravenous bolus of an oxytocic drug for delivery of the placenta.

The classic presentation of AFE is a pregnant patient experiencing sudden and unexpected dyspnea and restlessness, followed by desaturation, hypotension, cardiac dysrhythmias, and often by cardiorespiratory arrest. The initial disturbances involve profound alterations in oxygenation and hemodynamics, and in 40% of the cases this is followed by laboratory or clinical evidence of consumptive coagulopathy, clinically manifested by persistent bleeding from venipuncture sites or surgical incisions. Massive vaginal bleeding may also occur.

Signs and symptoms of AFE are as follows:

- Sudden desaturation, cyanosis
- Hypotension
- Tachycardia
- Dyspnea, wheezing, bronchospasm, cough, respiratory distress
- Chest pain, cardiac dysrhythmias, cardiac arrest
- Headache, loss of consciousness, convulsions
- Coagulopathy

Fetal "distress" generally accompanies this maternal catastrophe. All mothers who are undelivered at the time of AFE experience the abrupt onset of fetal bradycardia or of severe variable decelerations leading, within minutes, to fetal jeopardy.[87] Cardiac dysrhythmias include bradycardia, wide QRS complex tachycardia, ventricular tachycardia or fibrillation, electromechanical dissociation, and asystole.[87] Because of the profound hypoxia, an altered neurologic status and coma frequently ensue. If the patient survives the initial hemodynamic collapse, a noncardiogenic pulmonary edema develops in 24% to 70% of cases.[75, 100] Not all cases of AFE, however, are exactly like those previously mentioned. In fact, there have now been reports of less severe cases, with patients surviving an "incomplete" AFE.

Etiology

Despite many attempts to develop a valid animal model, the cause of AFE remains an enigma, even when considering only those cases with an autopsy-proven diagnosis. For embolism of amniotic fluid to occur, it is obvious that there must be a disruption of the normal barriers between amniotic fluid and maternal venous circulation. This may involve rupture of the fetal membranes and open or disrupted cervical or uterine veins (as occurs with vaginal delivery, cesarean section, or placental abruption) and a pressure gradient allowing the entrance of amniotic fluid into maternal circulation.[100, 101]

Steiner and Luschbaugh[76] postulated that uterine tetany, observed in some of their patients, may force amniotic fluid into the maternal circulation. But, when intrauterine pressure is increased to values above the mean pressure of maternal venous blood flow, the maternal-fetal exchange should cease. Thus, far from acting as a pump for amniotic fluid from fetus to mother, uterine contractions appear to be a highly effective barrier to uterine venous blood flow and embolism. There is thus no evidence supporting the old belief that a major risk of AFE is a short and tumultuous labor that is augmented with oxytocin. While in the past a pattern of vigorous labor or hypertonic uterine contractions have been implicated in the pathogenesis of AFE, evidence for this association is entirely anecdotal.[75] Morgan[92] has summarized this by stating, "In view of the very wide use of accelerated labor and the rarity of AFE, it must be concluded that there is no direct association between the two." In the large series of 69 AFE patients analyzed by Clark et al.,[87] there was only one patient with evidence of a hyperstimulated contraction pattern at the time of the acute AFE event. However, uterine tetany did develop in 10% of the patients either simultaneously with the onset of maternal cardiovascular collapse or immediately thereafter. Uterine hypoxia appears to induce myometrial hypertonus. Thus, hypertonus of the uterus may be the result, rather than the cause, of the insult.

Amniotic fluid embolism may be related to other thromboembolic conditions, as there have been reports of pulmonary embolism in which clots contained amniotic fluid elements.[102–105] The amount of particulate matter found in the pulmonary vasculature has not been consistently related to the clinical presentation of the syndrome in both animal and human studies;[82, 83] however, the effects appear to be more important when meconium is involved.[87, 106] Among those women with AFE associated with meconium-stained fluid, none survived neurologically intact, as compared with 16% who survived neurologically intact following AFE with clear amniotic fluid.[87] These observations confirm that substances in meconium may be more likely to initiate a severe reaction than when clear fluid is involved.[75, 107] Interestingly, there are three animal trials, with monkeys and rabbits, in which autologous clear amniotic fluid injections were well tolerated, with no manifestation of AFE syndrome.[79, 80] Thus, AFE may not be caused by the entrance into the maternal circulatory system of normal amniotic fluid but may occur following entrance of even small amounts of meconium-containing amniotic fluid. This presumably occurs because "abnormal" amniotic fluid entering the maternal circulation evokes a more serious maternal response in a susceptible mother.

The syndrome of AFE shares many characteristics with anaphylactoid reactions and septic shock. The ensuing clinical, hematologic, and hemodynamic derangements are virtually identical,[87] suggesting similar pathophysiologic mechanisms. Moreover, amniotic fluid contains prostaglandins, prostacyclins, thromboxane, leukotrienes, and other metabolites from arachidonic acid. Most of these are present in growing amounts during the evolution of pregnancy, are especially elevated during labor, and produce many of the hemodynamic and hematologic effects associated with AFE. Experimental infusion of leukotrienes C_4 and D_4 causes transient pulmonary and systemic hypertension, with a severe reduction in cardiac output and prolonged systemic hypotension. It also causes a major alteration of capillary permeability.[81, 86, 100, 108, 109] Pretreatment with a leukotriene inhibitor has now been demonstrated to decrease the likelihood of cardiovascular collapse and death in rabbits encountering AFE caused by the injection of heterologous amniotic fluid.[89, 109] In addition, endothelin-1, a potent vasoconstrictor and bronchoconstrictor, may also play a role in the early and transient pulmonary hypertension seen in AFE. Using immunohistologic techniques to identify endothelin-1 presence in the lungs, Khong[110] found a substantial presence in two cases of AFE. This indirect evidence suggests that the clinical symptoms of AFE may not be sequelae of an abnormal volume of amniotic fluid entering the maternal circulation or a direct physical effect in pulmonary capillaries, but rather may be related to a qualitatively abnormal substance within amniotic fluid.[81] Since the entrance of abnormal amniotic fluid into maternal circulation and the onset of clinical symptoms of AFE are not always temporally related, there may be, in some cases, a delay of many hours between the two events.[75]

Recent human, animal, and laboratory investigations have added substantially to our current understanding of AFE. At the same time, these studies have raised new questions that challenge traditional beliefs regarding AFE.[75] That the syndrome of AFE exists is irrefutable, but the exact relationship of this syndrome to amniotic fluid remains somewhat obscure.

Pathogenesis

Following exposure to "abnormal amniotic fluid," the principal maternal response involves hemodynamic changes, pulmonary capillary injury, and coagulopathy.[75] Early animal studies suggest that right ventricular failure played a key role in the hemodynamic perturbations. In a study by Reis et al.,[111] the intravenous injection of amniotic fluid resulted in a prompt 90% increase in mean pulmonary artery pressure, a 69% rise in central venous pressure, and a 150% increase in pulmonary vascular resistance, without a rise in pulmonary capillary wedge pressure. Pulmonary artery pressure rapidly returned to normal within 30 minutes. Because of these findings, many anesthesiologists have erroneously concluded that the pathophysiology of AFE principally involves severe pulmonary hypertension secondary to occlusive or vasospastic changes in the pulmonary vasculature leading to acute cor pulmonale.[75] Available hemodynamic data from humans with AFE, however, present a much different hemodynamic picture. Most cases of AFE in humans, in whom central hemodynamic monitoring was utilized, have demonstrated findings of mild to moderate elevations in pulmonary artery pressure, variable increases in central venous pressure, elevated pulmonary capillary wedge pressure, and, most importantly, clear evidence of left ventricular dysfunction or failure.[84, 112, 113] For example, during a confirmed episode of AFE in a patient with an indwelling pulmonary artery catheter, Shah et al.[114] found a transient elevation of the pulmonary pressure followed by ventricular tachycardia. In all human cases, hemodynamic monitoring has demonstrated that left ventricular failure is a constant. In the presence of this condition, moderate elevations of pulmonary artery pressure cannot be interpreted as indicating intrinsic pulmonary arterial vasospasm.[115] Pulmonary artery diastolic pressure in humans primarily reflects left ventricular end-diastolic pressure. Elevations of pulmonary capillary wedge pressure, secondary to left ventricular failure, cause a rise in pulmonary artery diastolic pressure of similar magnitude.[115] Thus, in patients with left ventricular dysfunction, elevations of pulmonary artery pressure may be solely a reflection of elevated left heart pressures.[75] If the patient presents with intrinsic pulmonary vascular disease, pulmonary artery diastolic pressure should exceed the pulmonary capillary wedge pressure by 6 to 10 mm Hg, and pulmonary vascular resistance should exceed 300 dyne/sec/cm^2.[115] To explain these hemodynamic changes, Clark and colleagues have postulated a biphasic pattern for AFE pathophysiology that includes initial and secondary phases.

Initial Phase. The "abnormal" amniotic fluid that enters into the maternal circulation causes a transient pulmonary vasospasm, with acute pulmonary hypertension, profound hypoxia, and dramatic fall in cardiac output. This initial pulmonary hypertension is believed to be caused by physical obstruction of the pulmonary vasculature and functional vasoconstriction,[109] and is quite transient (15–30 minutes in the animal model). During this initial phase, respiratory failure due to embolism in the pulmonary system occurs. This inevitably results in a ventilation/perfusion mismatch and hypoxemia.[116] Partial oxygen pressures of these patients reflects a profound shunting, exacerbated by the increased dead space. This initial period of hypoxemia, which is often intense, may account for the roughly 50% of patients who die within the first hour after the onset of clinical symptoms. Hypoxia may also account for the many patients who survive, but with severe central nervous system damage or brain death, despite eventual successful resuscitation.[75, 112] The rapidity with which patients develop brain damage after the onset of symptoms is alarming.[87]

Secondary Phase. Those patients who survive the initial phase may experience a secondary phase of hemodynamic compromise, with right ventricular function appearing normalized, and with a preponderant characteristic of left ventricular failure. With or without evidence, vascular resistance may be decreased. The secondary elevation of the pulmonary artery pressure is variable. Most of the hemodynamic effects found in this phase could be due to the left ventricular failure secondary to the hypoxic or direct myocardial depressant effect of amniotic fluid on the myocardium.[75] It is this secondary phase that is the typical hemodynamic picture described in most human clinical cases. Because of a lack of detailed early hemodynamic data from patients with AFE syndrome, the initial phase of transient pulmonary vasospasm in humans remains a matter of speculation. There are no reported cases in which invasive monitoring was established before AFE.[75, 87]

Based on clinical observation, it has been suggested that the hemodynamic profile observed in animals is not applicable to humans. For example, while pulmonary edema is absent in the animal model, it occurs in up to 70% in humans with AFE.[82] Based on current literature, it appears that AFE syndrome presents mild to moderate increases in mean pulmonary arterial pressure, with a variable increase in central venous pressure, an increased pulmonary capillary wedge pressure, and, in most cases, a decreased left ventricular stroke work index. These findings exclude acute cor pulmonale, as was traditionally supported.[84]

Coagulation derangements related to AFE syndrome range from minor disturbances in platelet count or coagulation profile to DIC. Forty percent of the patients surviving the initial hemodynamic event may develop DIC.[100] Bleeding may be the initial presentation in 10% to 15% of the AFE cases,[92, 93] and even if bleeding is the only symptom, may still be associated with a 75% mortality rate.[106] Four different elements have been hypothesized as responsible for this coagulopathy: (1) Amniotic fluid has been shown to contain a direct factor-X activator; however, the total amount of this procoagulant in amniotic fluid is probably not enough by itself to cause DIC.[100] (2) The trophoblast releases potent thromboplastin-like substances that could also precipitate the coagulopathy.[75] (3) Leukotrienes and other arachidonic acid metabolites that are present have been shown to have procoagulant activity. (4) Humoral elements related to tissue damage, caused by the effects of hypoxemia and low cardiac output, can also be related to the development of platelet aggregation and DIC.[61] Nevertheless, the exact nature of the coagulopathy observed in humans with AFE syndrome is not completely understood. In patients who develop a significant coagulopathy, the clinical hemorrhage is often compounded by the simultaneous occurrence of uterine atony attributable to the myometrial depressant effect of amniotic fluid.[117]

As previously mentioned, clinical and hemodynamic manifestations of AFE are very similar to those seen in anaphylaxis. A significant relationship between AFE syndrome and a history of allergy or atopy has been described and suggests a common pathophysiologic mechanism. In a large series presented by Clark et al.,[87] 41% of patients with AFE had a known history of allergy or atopy. Variations in the nature and severity of the clinical AFE syndrome may thus be dependent on variations in antigenic exposure and in individual response, consistent with other anaphylactoid reactions in humans.[87] Amniotic fluid may routinely enter the venous circulation of many pregnant women[75] and potentially sensitize the mother this way. This has been demonstrated by an animal study that showed that an initial intravenous bolus of homologous amniotic fluid caused minimal effects, but 1 month later, identical doses caused profound hypotension and alterations in coagulation.[118] Benson and Lindberg[119] have proposed that to support this anaphylactic hypothesis, serum tryptase levels need to be obtained within a few hours of the appearance of symptoms of AFE. The term *amniotic fluid embolism* thus appears to be a misnomer that has led to confusion and possibly hindered our understanding of the syndrome. Clark et al.[87] have suggested that the name "amniotic fluid embolism" should be changed into "anaphylactoid syndrome of pregnancy." This new point of view may allow better understanding of this disease and allow for more innovative research and development of new therapies, such as the use of high doses of corticosteroids or epinephrine.[87]

Fetal Outcome

Intact survival of fetuses in utero at the time of an AFE event is rare. Profound acidemia develops in fetuses of mothers with AFE who have cardiac arrest. In these cases, neonatal survival is inversely related to the interval between cardiac arrest and delivery.[87, 120] Earlier delivery appears to improve prognosis, although fetal neurologic injury may occur even when delivery occurs within 5 minutes of the arrest. It has been suggested that the perinatal mortality rate approximates 21%, but half of the survivors presented with permanent neurologic damage,[87] leaving less than 40% of surviving fetuses neurologically intact.

Diagnosis

To assist in the understanding of the AFE syndrome, a National Registry for Amniotic Fluid Embolism was established in 1988 in the United States.[84] The criteria for acceptance into this registry include the following[87]:

1. Acute hypotension or cardiac arrest
2. Acute hypoxia, defined as dyspnea, cyanosis, or respiratory arrest
3. Coagulopathy, defined as laboratory evidence of intravascular consumption, or fibrinolysis, or severe clinical hemorrhage in the absence of other explanations
4. Onset of the above-mentioned signs and symptoms during labor, cesarean section, or dilatation and evacuation, or within 30 minutes post partum
5. Absence of any other significant confounding condition or potential explanation for the signs and symptoms observed

Diagnosis of AFE is difficult and controversial and is normally made clinically. Because of the short time characteristic of its presentation, the diagnosis must be made initially on clinical grounds, with later confirmation from results of other investigations. The characteristic hemodynamic findings may help to make the diagnosis of AFE, and the laboratory abnormalities indicative of coagulopathy usually support the final diagnosis. The extent of laboratory evaluations that become necessary varies greatly, principally depending on the length of patient survival and degree of clinical coagulopathy. Laboratory abnormalities include decreased fibrinogen and elevated levels of fibrin split products or d-dimer, prolonged partial thromboplastin and prothrombin times, and thrombocytopenia. The laboratory detection of fetal debris within the maternal pulmonary vasculature has been regarded as the basis of the definitive diagnosis, but this element is very difficult to determine unless the patient dies and an autopsy is performed. The antemortem detection of fetal squames, fetal hair, or mucin in a central venous or pulmonary artery blood sample can support the clinical diagnosis of AFE, but it cannot be considered pathognomonic, because it has been demonstrated that small amounts of such elements can enter the maternal circulation in the absence of AFE.[121] Indeed, there are a variety of cases in which the detection of squamous cells within the pulmonary artery circulation is a common finding. For example, any type of venipuncture may result in the introduction of squames into the venous system, thus confusing the diagnosis of AFE. Moreover, samples from the pulmonary vessels are often difficult to obtain,[83] and in several published reports, fetal elements were detected only after the use of special stains or immunostaining methods not routinely used in clinical practice.[87] Thus the detection of cellular or acellular debris of presumed fetal origin in the central maternal circulation may, in some cases, be only a marker of fetal tissue exposure, but is neither sensitive nor specific for the diagnosis of the AFE syndrome.[87] The characteristic debris of presumed fetal origin can include squamous cells, hair, fat droplets, nonspecific cellular debris, and nonspecific proteinaceous, keratinaceous, or mucinous material in the pulmonary vessels. In addition to these distinctive constituents, placental and decidual tissue fragments, as well as isolated trophoblastic cells and megakaryocytes are also potentially detectable within pulmonary vessels.[122] Some of these elements have also been found in the uterus, kidneys, heart, and central nervous system in postmortem confirmed cases of AFE. Although several options exist, the most likely route of passage is via a patent foramen ovale.

The impact of fetal debris in the maternal circulation is variable. For example, in autopsies performed in animals following AFE, pulmonary findings ranged from massive vascular plugging with fetal debris to minimal plugging with extensive pulmonary hemorrhage to entirely normal, despite the antecedent of hemodynamic collapse.[75] Likewise, in 46 patients with AFE syndrome analyzed by Clark et al.,[87] only one patient, a woman with meconium-stained amniotic fluid, presented with histologic findings described as "vessels occluded with squames." Autopsies performed in mothers in whom the cause of death was not AFE have also found elements of amniotic fluid.[123] Thus, finding elements of amniotic fluid in maternal pulmonary artery blood during the peripartum period is not synonymous with the diagnosis of AFE.[83, 124–126] Amniotic thrombi of squamous cells have been found in uterine venous and myometrium without the clinical diagnosis of AFE.[127] Attwood and Park[128] found evidence of trophoblastic embolism to the lungs in 43% of patients who died in the peripartum period, but that of AFE in less than 1%.

New methods for the noninvasive diagnosis of AFE have been proposed. Kobayashi and colleagues[129, 130] have described the use of TKH-2, a monoclonal antibody clearly directed to a characteristic component in amniotic fluid called sialyl Tn. This method is very sensitive for the detection of meconium and meconium fluid–derived mucin in serum and in lung sections of patients with AFE syndrome. Kanayama et al.[131] have also reported maternal plasma levels of zinc coproporphyrin-1 as a characteristic component of meconium. Lunetta and Penttilä[122] proposed an immunohistochemical analysis for identification of syncytiotrophoblastic cells and megakaryocytes to provide more precise data on the incidence and distribution in physiologic and pathologic conditions of AFE.[122] Other investigations, including electrocardiography, thoracic radiography, and pulmonary arteriography have not been shown to be particularly helpful in the diagnosis of AFE. Today, there is no single clinical or laboratory finding that, by itself, can either diagnose or exclude AFE syndrome.[75]

Differential Diagnosis

Because there is no specific and fast diagnostic test for AFE, clinical signs of AFE can be confused with many other conditions. The differential diagnosis is as follows:

- Eclampsia
- Pulmonary aspiration
- Pulmonary thromboembolism
- Air embolism
- Septic shock
- Acute myocardial infarction
- Anaphylaxis
- Coagulopathy
- Uterine rupture
- Uterine atony
- Cerebrovascular accident
- Anesthetic toxicity
- Medication error

Early exclusion of other differential diagnoses may allow the diagnosis of AFE and thus potentially improve the treatment and outcome for these patients.

Treatment

Care of the mother with AFE is primarily supportive. The goal of treatment is principally to maintain oxygenation, restore normal blood pressure and cardiac output, and correct the coagulopathy. Once the diagnosis is suspected, cardiopulmonary resuscitation must be initiated as soon as indicated, without delay. Maternal survival without sequelae following cardiac arrest is rare, and prompt delivery may benefit not only the fetus, but also the mother, by improving the success of cardiopulmonary resuscitation.[89] Therefore, it is highly recommended that perimortem cesarean section be initiated as soon as possible after maternal cardiac arrest in cases of AFE.[87]

Since left heart failure is usually observed, inotropic support is indicated. Treatment of hypotension, which is usually secondary to cardiogenic shock, involves optimization of cardiac preload with rapid volume infusion and subsequent dopamine infusion if the patient remains hypotensive.[75] After correction of hypotension, fluid therapy should be restricted to maintenance levels to minimize the risk of pulmonary edema. The use of a pulmonary artery catheter may be of great value in resuscitative fluid management, especially to minimize the possibilities of pulmonary edema. In a report from Clark et al.,[84] five patients with AFE syndrome, whose therapy was guided by central hemodynamic monitoring, had 100% survival.

It is essential to ventilate the patient with the highest concentration of oxygen possible. If the patient is conscious, oxygen in high concentration should be administered by mask. If unconscious, the patient should be intubated and ventilated with 100% oxygen. To correct the coagulopathy, the use of blood products such as fresh whole blood, packed cells, and fresh frozen plasma must be readily available. Such component replacement is often successful. There are still insufficient data to warrant routine heparinization.[75]

Despite optimal care, most patients with AFE syndrome die, and many of the survivors are neurologically impaired.[87] Nevertheless, we must be prepared to deal with this sudden, unheralded, and potentially catastrophic event in any pregnant patient.[61] Early aggressive measures to correct hypoxemia and return other hemodynamic parameters to normal not only can prevent early deaths and permanent neurologic defects but possibly also abort progression of the syndrome.[88]

Prevention

At the present time, with our current state of knowledge, AFE cannot be predicted or prevented. Nevertheless, it is possible that the routine use of maternal pulse oximetry in the peripartum period may help to detect "asymptomatic" or preclinical cases of the syndrome at an early stage. This hypothesis has not been studied, however, and few centers now routinely monitor all parturients with pulse oximetry.

Prognosis

Amniotic fluid embolism is a very rare clinical syndrome and, if massive, is associated with little chance of successful treatment. Even if appropriate supportive care is initiated in a timely manner, the prognosis remains poor for mother and fetus. Interestingly, Burrows et al.[89] described a patient who survived AFE and had a subsequent pregnancy that resulted in a healthy baby at term by normal vaginal delivery with no consequences.

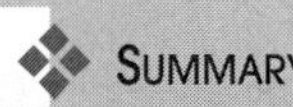

SUMMARY

Key Points

- Embolism in the pregnant patient is a common cause of maternal morbidity and mortality.
- The vascular structure of the gravid uterus allows air entrance during cesarean section, and air embolism is a frequent subclinical finding, especially on exteriorization of the uterus.
- Prevention of repeat embolism is key to the management of the pregnant patient with pulmonary embolism.
- Amniotic fluid embolism should be considered if a parturient experiences sudden dyspnea or cardiovascular collapse. AFE can occur at any time during labor and delivery, and remains unpredictable, unpreventable, and often untreatable.

Key Reference

Clark SL: New concepts of amniotic fluid embolism: a review. Obstet Gynecol Surv 1990; 45:360–368.

Case Stem

A healthy 27-year-old parturient is undergoing cesarean section under epidural anesthesia. Immediately following delivery, the patient suddenly complains of dyspnea. Within seconds, the pulse oximeter reading is <80, and she is unresponsive, cyanotic, and bradycardic. Discuss the differential diagnosis and anesthetic management.

Conclusions

The last decade has shown dramatic changes in our understanding of the AFE syndrome. To achieve further improvement, it will be necessary to develop better experimental animal models that will ultimately allow the extrapolation of results to humans. In the meantime, anesthesiologists should maintain a low threshold for diagnostic consideration of AFE because immediate and appropriate management is critical to survival.[89] It has been said that "while much has been learned, AFE remains unpredictable, unpreventable and for the most part untreatable."[75] Despite the ensuing chaos that follows AFE, treatment of these patients requires a disciplined approach in which teamwork is the cornerstone.

References

1. Lesky E: Notes on the history of air embolism. Germ Med Monthly 1961; 6:159–161.

2. Morgagni J: The Seats and Causes of Disease. Translated by Benjamin Alexander. London, 1769.
3. Magendie F: Physiologic Researches on Life and Death. Boston, Bichat X, 1827, p187. 1821; 1:192.
4. Cormack J: The entrance of air by the open mouths of the uterine veins, considered as a cause of danger and death after parturition. London J Med 1850; 2:928–934.
5. Amussat J: Recherches sur l'introduction accidentale de l'air dans les veins. Paris, Germer Bailliere 1839; 225.
6. Senn N: An experimental and clinical study of air embolism. Ann Surg 1885; 3:197–302.
7. Saberski L, Kondamuri S, Osinubi O: Identification of the epidural space: Is loss of resistance to air a safe technique? A review of the complications related to the use of air. Reg Anesth 1997; 22:3–5.
8. Jaffe R, Siegel L, Schnittger I, et al: Epidural air injection assessed by transesophageal echocardiography. Reg Anesth 1995; 20:152–155.
9. Bedford R: Perioperative air embolism. Semin Anesth 1987; VI:163–170.
10. Jensen Bundy P: Pathophysiology and treatment of air embolism. *In* Faust R (ed): Anesthesiology Review, 2nd ed. New York: Churchill Livingstone; 1994:403.
11. Matjasko J, Petrozza P, Cohen M, et al: Anaesthesia and surgery in the seated position: Analysis of 554 cases. Neurosurgery 1985; 17:695–702.
12. Matjaskoo J, Petrozza P, Cohen M, et al: Anaesthesia and surgery in the seated position: Analysis of 554 cases. Neurosurgery 1985; 17:695–702.
13. Black S, Ockert D, Oliver W, et al: Comparison of outcome following posterior fossa craniectomy done in either a sitting or horizontal position. Anesthesiology 1988; 69:49–56.
14. Losasso T, Muzzi D, Dietz N, et al: Fifty percent nitrous oxide does not increase the risk of venous air embolism in neurosurgical patients operated upon in the sitting position. Anesthesiology 1992; 77:21.
15. Newfield P, Albin MS, Chestnut JS, et al: Air embolism during transsphenoidal pituitary operations. Neurosurgery 1978; 2:39.
16. Albin M, Ritter R, Pruett C, et al: Venous air embolism during lumbar laminectomy in the prone position: report of three cases. Anesth Analg 1991; 73:346–349.
17. Fong J, Gadalla F, Gimbel A: Precordial Doppler diagnosis of hemodynamically compromising air embolism during caesarean section. Can J Anaesth 1990; 37:262–264.
18. Karuparthy V, Dowing J, Husain F, et al: Incidence of venous air embolism during caesarean sections unchanged by the use of a 5 to 10° head-up tilt. Anesth Analg 1989; 69:620–623.
19. Lowenwirt I, Chi D, Handwerker S: Nonfatal venous air embolism during cesarean section: A case report and review of the literature. Obstet Gynecol Surv 1994; 49:72–76.
20. Kawahito S, Kimura H, Kohyama A, et al: Hypoxemia during cesarean section: Evaluation of venous air embolism by transesophageal echocardiography. Masui 1995; 44:10–14.
21. Fong J, Gadalla F, Pierri M, et al: Are Doppler detected venous emboli during cesarean section air emboli? Anesth Analg 1990; 71:254–257.
22. Lew T, Tay D, Thomas E: Venous air embolism during cesarean section: More common than previously thought. Anesth Analg 1993; 77:448–452.
23. Evans R, Palazzo M, Ackers J: Air embolism during total hip replacement: Comparison of two surgical techniques. Br J Anaesth 1989; 62:243–247.
24. Conrad SA: Venous air embolism. *http://emedicine.com/emerg/topic787.htm.*
25. Kaunitz A, Hughes J, Grimes D, et al: Causes of maternal mortality in the United States. Obstet Gynecol 1985; 65:605–612.
26. Weissman A, Shahar K, Bezalel A: Gas embolism in obstetrics and gynecology. J Reprod Med 1996; 42:103–111.
27. Mitterschiffthaler G, Bertchtold J, Andrel P, et al: Letale "paradoxe Luftembolie" bei geburtshilflicher Routineoperation (Zervixcerclage). Anaesthesist 1989; 38:29–31.
28. Fyke F, Kazmier F, Harms R: Venous air embolism: Life-threatening complication of orogenital sex during pregnancy. Am J Med 1985; 78:333–336.
29. Milks G Jr, Brown A, Robinson C: Air embolism during labor. Can Med Assoc J 1947; 56:427–429.
30. Epps S, Robbins A, Marx G: Complete recovery after near-fatal venous air embolism during cesarean section. IJOA 1998; 7:131–133.
31. McCullough K, Morales E: Air embolism following postpartum surgical sterilization: Report of a case. Md Med J 1955; 4:273–274.
32. Redfield R, Bodine H: Air embolism following the knee-chest position. JAMA 1939; 113:671–673.
33. Black S: Venous air embolism. Probl Anesth 1997; 9(1):113–124.
34. Vik A, Brubakk A, Hennessy T, et al: Venous air embolism in swine: Transport of gas bubbles through the pulmonary circulation. J Appl Physiol 1990; 69:237–244.
35. Nelson P: Pulmonary gas embolism in pregnancy and the puerperium. Obstet Gynecol Surv 1960; 15:449–481.
36. Roberts M, Mathiesen K, Ho H, et al: Cardiopulmonary responses to intravenous infusion of soluble and relatively insoluble gases. Surg Endosc 1997; 11:341–346.
37. Geissler H, Allen S, Mehlhorn V, et al: Effect of body repositioning after venous air embolism: An echocardiographic study. Anesthesiology 1997; 86:710–717.
38. Larson C: Venous air embolism. Am J Clin Pathol 1951; 21:247–250.
39. Adornato D, Gildeberg P, Ferrario C, et al: Pathophysiology of intravenous air embolism in dogs. Anesthesiology 1978; 49:120–127.
40. Frumento S: Fenómenos de superficie. *In* Frumento S (ed): Biofísica, 3rd ed. Madrid, Mosby/Doyma Libros, 1995: 237–238.
41. Lam K, Hutchinson R, Gin T: Severe pulmonary oedema after venous air embolism. Can J Anaesth 1993; 40:964–967.
42. Chandler W, Dimsheff D, Taren J: Acute pulmonary edema following venous air embolism during neurosurgical procedures. Neurosurg 1974; 40:400–402.
43. Hagen P, Scholz D, Edwards W: Incidence and size of patent foramen ovale during the first 10 decades of life: An autopsy study of 965 normal hearts. Mayo Clin Proc 1984; 59:997–1004.
44. Butler B, Robinson R, Sutton T, et al: Cardiovascular pressures with venous gas embolism and decompression. Aviat Space Environ Med 1995; 66:408–414.
45. Bedell E, Berg K, Losasso T: Paradoxic air embolism during venous air embolism: Transesophageal echocardiographic evidence of transpulmonary air passage. Anesthesiology 1994; 80:947–949.
46. Suriani R, Losasso T, Berge K: Echocardiographic identification of paradoxical air embolism. Anesthesiology 1994; 81:1548.
47. Butler B, Hills B: Transpulmonary passage of venous air emboli. J Appl Physiol 1985; 59:543–547.
48. Bacha S, Annane D, Gajdos P: Iatrogenic air embolism. Presse Med 1996; 25:1466–1472.
49. Tommasino C, Rizzardi R, Beretta L, et al: Cerebral ischemia after venous air embolism in the absence of intracardiac defects. J Neurosurg Anesthesiol 1996; (1):30–34.
50. Cluroe A: Delayed paradoxical air embolism following caesarean section for placenta previa: A case history. Pathology 1994; 26:209–211.
51. Hollingsworth H, Irwin R: Acute respiratory failure in pregnancy. Clin Chest Med 1992; 13:723–740.
52. Tucker W Jr: Symptoms and signs of syndromes associated with mill murmurs. N C Med 1988; 49:569–572.
53. Albin M: The paradox of paradoxical air embolism: PEEP, Valsalva and patent foramen ovale. Should the sitting position be abandoned? Anesthesiology 1984; 61:222.
54. Michenfelder J, Miller R, Gronert G: Evaluation of an ultrasonic device (Doppler) for the diagnosis of venous air embolism. Anesthesiology 1972; 36:164–168.
55. Malinow A, Naulty J, Hunt C, et al: Precordial ultra-sonic monitoring during cesarean delivery. Anesthesiology 1987; 66:816–819.

56. Artru A, Colley P: The site of origin of the intravascular electrocardiogram recorded from multiorificed intravascular catheters. Anesthesiology 1988; 69:44–48.
57. Mongan P, Hinman J: Evaluation of a double-lumen multiorifice catheter for resuscitation of swine from lethal venous air embolism. Anesthesiology 1995; 83:1104–1111.
58. Reeves S, Bevis L, Bailey B: Positioning a right atrial air aspiration catheter using transesophageal echocardiography. J Neurosurg Anesthesiol 1996; 8:123–125.
59. Perkins-Pearson N, Marshall W, Bedford R: Atrial pressures in the seated position: Implications for paradoxical air embolism. Anesthesiology 1982; 57:493.
60. Kyttä J, Randell T, Tanskanen P, et al: Monitoring lung compliance and end-tidal oxygen content for the detection of venous air embolism. Br J Anaesth 1995; 75:447–451.
61. Noble W, St-Amand J: Amniotic fluid embolus. Can J Anaesth 1993; 40:971–980.
62. Durant T, Long J, Oppenheimer M: Pulmonary (venous) air embolism. Am Heart J 1947; 33:269–281.
63. Mehlorn U, Burke E, Butler B, et al: Body position does not affect the hemodynamic response to venous air embolism in dogs. Anesth Analg 1994; 79:734–739.
64. Campkin T: Air embolism: Placement of central venous catheters. Anesthesiology 1982; 56:406.
65. Boussuges A, Blanc P, Moleant F, et al: Prognosis on iatrogenic gas embolism. Minerva Med 1995; 86:453–457.
66. Gazzaniga A, Dalen J: Paradoxical embolism: Its pathophysiology and clinical recognition. Ann Surg 1970; 171:137.
67. Kyttä J, Tanskanen P, Randell T: Comparison of the effects of controlled ventilation with 100% oxygen, 50% oxygen in nitrogen, and 50% oxygen in nitrous oxide on responses to venous air embolism in pigs. Br J Anaesth 1996; 77:658–661.
68. Sibai A, Baraka A, Moudawar A: Hazards of nitrous oxide administration in presence of venous air embolism. Middle East J Anesthesiol 1996; 13:565–571.
69. Cucchiara R, Seward J, Nishimura R, et al: Identification of patent foramen ovale during sitting position craniotomy by transesophageal echocardiography with positive airway pressure. Anesthesiology 1985; 63:107.
70. Losasso T, Black S, Muzzi D, et al: Detection and hemodynamic consequences of venous air embolism. Does nitrous oxide make a difference? Anesthesiology 1992; 77:148–152.
71. Voorthies R, Fraser R, Poznak A: Prevention of air embolism with positive end expiratory pressure. Neurosurgery 1983; 12:503.
72. Toung T, Ngeow Y, Long D, et al: Comparison of the effects of positive end-expiratory pressure and jugular venous compression on canine cerebral venous pressure. Anesthesiology 1984; 61:169–172.
73. Black S, Cucchiara R, Nishimura R, et al: Parameters affecting occurrence of paradoxical air embolism. Anesthesiology 1989; 71:235–241.
74. Weissman A, Kol S, Peretz B: Gas embolism in obstetrics and gynecology. A review. J Reprod Med 1996; 41:103–111.
75. Clark SL: New concepts of amniotic fluid embolism: A review. Obstet Gynecol Surv 1990; 45:360–368.
76. Steiner P, Luschbaugh C: Maternal pulmonary embolism by amniotic fluid as a cause of obstetric shock and unexpected deaths in obstetrics. JAMA 1941; 117:1341–1345.
77. Liban E, Raz S: A clinicopathological study of fourteen cases of amniotic fluid embolism. Am J Obstet Gynecol 1969; 51:477–486.
78. Thompson W, Budd J: Erroneous diagnosis of amniotic fluid embolism. Am J Obstet Gynecol 1963; 91:606.
79. Adamsons K, Mueller-Heubach E, Myers RE: The innocuousness of amniotic fluid infusion in the pregnant rhesus monkey. Am J Obstet Gynecol 1971; 109:977–984.
80. Stolte L, Van Kessel H, Seelen J, et al: Failure to produce the syndrome of amniotic fluid embolism by infusion of amniotic fluid and meconium into monkeys. Am J Obstet Gynecol 1967; 98:694–697.
81. Clark SL: Arachidonic acid metabolites and the pathophysiology of amniotic fluid embolism. Semin Reprod Endocrinol 1985; 3:253–257.
82. Clark SL: Amniotic fluid embolism. Clin Perinatol 1986; 13:801.
83. Clark SL, Pavlova Z, Horenstein J, et al: Squamous cells in the maternal pulmonary circulation. Am J Obstet Gynecol 1986; 154:104–106.
84. Clark SL, Cotton DB, Gonik B, et al: Central hemodynamic alterations in amniotic fluid embolism. Am J Obstet Gynecol 1988; 158:1124–1126.
85. Clark SL: Amniotic fluid embolism. Crit Care Clin 1991; 7:877–882.
86. Clark SL: Successful pregnancy outcomes after amniotic fluid embolism. Am J Obstet Gynecol 1992; 167:511–512.
87. Clark SL, Hankins GDV, Dudley DA, et al: Amniotic fluid embolism: Analysis of the national registry. Am J Obstet Gynecol 1995; 172:1158–1167.
88. Eastman N: Editorial: Comment. Obstet Gynecol 1970; 106:1201.
89. Burrows A, Khoo S: The amniotic fluid embolism syndrome: 10 years' experience at a major teaching hospital. Aust N Z Obstet Gynaecol 1995; 35:245–250.
90. Department of Health: Report on Confidential Enquiries into Maternal Deaths, 1985–87; 46–51.
91. Department of Health: Report on Confidential Enquiries into Maternal Deaths, 1988–90; 55–60.
92. Morgan M: Amniotic fluid embolism. Anaesthesia 1979; 34:20–32.
93. Courtney L: Amniotic fluid embolism. Obstet Gynecol Surv 1974; 29:169–187.
94. Jenkins D, Carr C, Stanley J, et al: Maternal mortality in the Irish Republic 1989–1991. Ir Med J 1996; 89:140–141.
95. Price T, Baker V, Cefalo R: Amniotic fluid embolism. Three case reports with a review of the literature. Obstet Gynecol Surv 1985; 40:462–473.
96. Petersen E, Taylor H: Amniotic fluid embolism. An analysis of 40 cases. Obstet Gynecol 1970; 35:787–793.
97. Smibert J: Amniotic fluid embolism: A clinical review of twenty cases. Aust N Z J Obstet Gynaecol 1967; 7:1.
98. Aguillon A, Andjus T, Grayson A, Race G: Amniotic fluid embolism: A review. Obstet Gynecol Surv 1962; 98:336.
99. Anderson D: Amniotic fluid embolism: A re-evaluation. Am J Obstet Gynecol 1967; 98:336.
100. Dudney T, Elliott C: Pulmonary embolism from amniotic fluid, fat, and air. Prog Cardiovasc Dis 1994; 36:447–474.
101. Masson R: Amniotic fluid embolism. Clin Chest Med 1992; 13:657–665.
102. Bauer P, Lelarge P, Hennequin L, et al: Thrombo-embolism during amniotic fluid embolism [letter]. Intensive Care Med 1995; 21:384–388.
103. Esposito RA, Grossi EA, Coppa G, et al: Successful treatment of postpartum shock caused by amniotic fluid embolism with cardiopulmonary bypass and pulmonary artery thromboembolectomy. Am J Obstet Gynecol 1990; 163:572–574.
104. Kern SB, Duff P: Localized amniotic fluid embolism presenting as ovarian vein thrombosis and refractory postoperative fever. Am J Clin Path 1981; 76:476–480.
105. Turner R, Gusack M: Massive amniotic fluid embolism. Ann Emerg Med 1984; 13:359–361.
106. Porter TF, Didly GA, Blanchard J, et al: Normal values for amniotic fluid index during uncomplicated twin pregnancy. Am J Obstet Gynecol 1996; 87:699–702.
107. Hankins GDV, Snyder RR, Clark SL, et al: Acute hemodynamic and respiratory effects of amniotic fluid embolism in the pregnant goat model. Am J Obstet Gynecol 1993; 168:1113–1130.
108. Maher J, Wenstrom K, Hauth J, Meis P: Amniotic fluid embolism after saline amnioinfusion: Two cases and review of the literature. Obstet Gynecol 1994; 83:851–854.
109. Azegami M, Mori N: Amniotic fluid embolism and leukotrienes. Am J Obstet Gynecol 1986; 155:1119–1124.
110. Khong T: Expression of endothelin-1 in amniotic fluid embolism and possible pathophysiological mechanism. Br J Obstet Gynaecol 1998; 105:802–804.
111. Reis R, Pierce W, Behrendt D: Hemodynamic effects of amniotic fluid embolism. Surg Obstet Gynecol 1965; 129:45.

112. Clark SL, Montz F, Phelan J: Hemodynamic alterations associated with amniotic fluid embolism: A reappraisal. Am J Obstet Gynecol 1985; 151:617.
113. Girard P, Mal H, Laine J, et al: Left heart failure in amniotic fluid embolism. Anesthesiology 1986; 64:262.
114. Shah K, Karlman R, Heller J: Ventricular tachycardia and hypotension with amniotic fluid embolism during cesarean section. Anesth Analg 1986; 65:533–535.
115. Harvey R, Enson Y, Ferrer M: A reconsideration of the origins of pulmonary hypertension. Chest 1971; 59:82.
116. Koegler A, Sauder P, Marolf A, Jaeger A: Amniotic fluid embolism: A case with noncardiogenic pulmonary edema. Intensive Care Med 1994; 20:45–46.
117. Courtney L: Coagulation failure in pregnancy. Br Med J 1970; 1:691.
118. Stefanini M, Turpini RA: Fibrinogenopenic accident of pregnancy and delivery: a syndrome with multiple etiological mechanisms. Ann N Y Acad Sci 1959; 75:601–625.
119. Benson M, Lindberg R: Amniotic fluid embolism, anaphylaxis, and tryptase. Am J Obstet Gynecol 1996; 175:737.
120. Katz VJ, Dotters DJ, Droegemueller W: Perimortem cesarean delivery. Obstet Gynecol 1986; 68:571–576.
121. Fava S, Caruana Galizia A: Amniotic fluid embolism. Br J Obstet Gynaecol 1993; 100:1049–1050.
122. Lunetta P, Penttilä A: Immunohistochemical identification of syncytiotrophoblastic cells and megakaryocytes in pulmonary vessels in a fatal case of amniotic fluid embolism. Int J Legal Med 1996; 108:210–214.
123. Thurlbeck W, Miller R: *In* Rubin E, Farber JL (eds): Pathology. Philadelphia: JB Lippincott, 1988:620.
124. Kuhlman K, Hidvegi D, Tamura R, et al: Is amniotic fluid material in the central circulation of peripartum patients pathologic? Am J Perinatol 1985; 4:295–299.
125. Lee K, Catalano P, Ortiz-Giroux S: Cytologic diagnosis of amniotic fluid embolism. Report of a case with a unique cytologic feature and emphasis on the difficulty of eliminating squamous contamination. Acta Cytol 1986; 30:177–182.
126. Plauche W: Amniotic fluid embolism. Am J Obstet Gynecol 1983; 147:982–983.
127. Craven C, Ward K: Premature rupture of the amniotic membranes diagnosed by placental bed biopsy. Arch Pathol Lab Med 1997; 121:167–168.
128. Attwood H, Park W: Embolism to the lungs by trophoblast. J Obstet Gynaecol Br Commonw 1961; 68:611–617.
129. Kobayashi H, Ohi H, Terao T: A simple, noninvasive, sensitive method for diagnosis of amniotic fluid embolism by monoclonal antibody TKH-2 that recognizes NeuAc2-6GalNAc. Am J Obstet Gynecol 1993; 168:848–853.
130. Kobayashi H, Ohi H, Hayakawa H, et al: Histological diagnosis of amniotic fluid embolism by monoclonal antibody TKH-2 that recognizes NeuAc alpha 2-6GalNAc epitope. Hum Pathol 1997; 28:428–433.
131. Kanayama N, Yamazaki T, Naruse H, et al: Determining zinc coproporphyrine in maternal plasma: A new method for diagnosing amniotic fluid embolism. Clin Chem 1992; 38:33–35.

32

Difficult and Failed Intubation

SEIJI WATANABE, MD, PHD

FUMI HANDA, MD

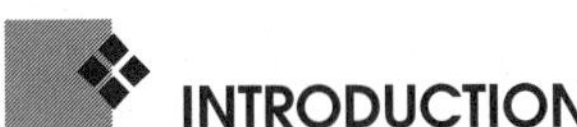

INTRODUCTION

In the enthusiasm for teaching the principles of anesthesia, the fact that much of medicine depends on the acquisition of technique is overlooked. Technique can be critical in many situations in which academic knowledge is useless. The importance of shifting from a knowledge-based to a performance-based education and assessment system is recommended.[1] It is sheer lack of skill that kills.[2]

SAFETY IN ANESTHESIA

The possibility of surgical failure seems to be accepted, albeit reluctantly, by both patient and surgeon. The anesthetist enjoys no such luxury, and anesthetic failure is all too often assumed to be negligence. The public expects anesthesia to be a safe adjunct to operation; yet, anesthesia is inherently dangerous. The latitude of understanding that anesthetists can expect from a damaged patient is slight. Failed intubation may lead to death and subsequently to litigation.

One of the first reviews of deaths caused by anesthesia suggested that the rate was about 3 per 10,000.[3] In an early study in the three regions making up the United Kingdom, there were 4000 deaths in over half a million anesthetic inductions.[4] Of these, 3 deaths (0.1%) were the direct result of anesthesia, and in 72 deaths (1.8%) the anesthetic was contributory. The death rate of 0.054 per 10,000 anesthetic inductions calculated in the British study compares favorably with that in other reports. Eichorn[5] reported a death rate of 0.066 per 10,000 from 1976 to 1985. An older French study described a mortality of 0.76 per 10,000.[6]

Gannon[7] found 10 cases ascribable to failed intubation and 2 to total spinal anesthesia and failure to intubate among 25 anesthetic deaths that were reported between 1982 and 1986.

The 10 most common critical incidents during anesthesia as reported by Cooper and associates[8] are related to failure to ventilate (70%), malfunction of the laryngoscope (11%), premature extubation (10%), and problems with the tracheal tube (7%). Obvious adverse events related to tracheal extubation accounted for 7% (35 of 522) of the respiratory-related claims in the American Society of Anesthesiologists (ASA) Closed Claims Study.[9]

These data serve as an admonition to anesthesiologists, particularly regarding the checking of equipment in emergency procedures. If minimum standards of monitoring are implemented, the risk of hypoxic injury is considerably lessened because the anesthetist will have been alerted to trouble early enough to do something about it. An anesthetist working without adequate monitoring is like a pilot flying an airliner without any instruments or warning devices.

Mishaps can be minimized by thorough preparation for all contingencies. In a review of anesthetic-related malpractice claims between 1974 and 1988, Tinker and coworkers[10] suggest that a third of negative outcomes would have been prevented by additional monitors such as pulse oximetry and capnometry. Of special importance is their use in the recovery area where (1) one half the cases of death and cerebral damage occur and (2) progressive respiratory failure causing postoperative difficulties is linked with aspiration pneumonia.

Over the past few years, since the adoption of minimum standards in the United States, the cost of malpractice claims against anesthesiologists has decreased by about two thirds, and in Boston, Massachusetts, insurance premiums for anesthesiologists have been reduced by 40%.[11] Needless to say, good communication with patients, the acquisition of informed consent, and accurate anesthetic record keeping are essential for anesthetic safety and avoidance of litigation.

INCIDENCE OF DIFFICULT AND FAILED INTUBATION

Difficult or failed intubation is encountered in approximately 5% of obstetric general anesthesia.[12] In one retrospective study undertaken over a 6-year period, the incidence of failed intubation is 1 in 300 pregnant patients,[13] that is, eight times higher than in other surgical patients (1:280 vs. 1:2230).[14] The same ratio is observed between obstetric and nonobstetric patients (7:1980 vs. 6:13,380).[15]

In England and Wales, from 1979 to 1981, 24% of maternal deaths related to anesthesia were directly related to difficulties with tracheal intubation.[16] In 1985 to 1987, 4 of 6 deaths directly attributable to anesthesia were associated with failed tracheal intubation,[17] but in 1988 to 1990, only 1 of 4 deaths was a result of problems related to tracheal intubation.[18] In one nongovernmental report covering the period 1978 to 1994 published in the United Kingdom, there were 23 (0.4%: 13, white; 5, Asian; and 5, African/Afrocaribbean) intubation failures.[19]

Historically, the United States[20] and Japan rely heavily for failed intubation data on the British triennial Confidential Enquiry into Maternal Deaths (CEMD) reports. Maternal mortality in England and Wales in 1982 was 7 per 100,000 live births, compared with 18 per 100,000 in Japan. This difference was attributable to the fact that 50% of anesthetics for cesarean section in district general hospitals were given by obstetricians in Japan. Currently, the obstetric hospital/anesthetist ratio is 2.7 to 3.0 for England and Wales, 4.9 for the United States, and 0.2 for Japan. The first analysis of the Japanese-government report on maternal deaths in 1997 shows that there were 197 maternal deaths during 1991 to 1992. Among them, there were 4 failed intubation deaths during cesarean section in the 72 cases that were retrospectively assessed as being "preventable."[21] Anesthesia-related death is the sixth leading cause (at approximately 7%) of pregnancy-related mortality in the United States.[22, 23] In this group, failed intubation and aspiration are recognized as two major causes of mortality. In the North American Closed Claims Study, difficult tracheal intubation and esophageal intubation constituted 23% of damaging events associated with obstetric general anesthesia.[24] Anesthesia-related deaths occur primarily during cesarean section. At least 82% of maternal deaths occur during general anesthesia for cesarean section as reported in a study conducted recently in the United States.[20] According to an African analysis of 1500 patients undergoing emergency and elective cesarean section under general anesthesia, the incidence of difficult intubation and failed intubation was 2.1% and 0.1%, respectively.[25] Hasty surgical intervention, either tracheostomy or cricothyrotomy, during failed intubation is dangerous. Three of the 10 anesthesia-related deaths in the 1982 to 1984 CEMD report were associated with failed tracheostomy.[26]

Maternal mortality related to anesthesia has probably reached its nadir. This decrease could be tentatively ascribed to the declining use of general anesthesia. Despite this, there is an impression that failure to intubate is no less common than it was in 1985 (from 1 in 300 patients in 1985 to 1 in 250 patients for 1990).[19] The CEMD report for 1991 to 1993 suggests that there is no appreciable abatement of the number of deaths directly related to anesthesia. Rather, it indicated that most deaths would have been avoidable in the presence of senior staff and appropriate monitoring.[27] An improvement in disaster statistics in obstetrics, if any, appears to be due to the marked decrease in the use of general anesthesia in the last decade. The number of deaths secondary to complications of general anesthesia, although small, is not decreasing in the United States.[20] A recent study indicates that the case-fatality risk ratio for regional anesthesia for obstetrics is 16.7 times less than for general anesthesia, primarily because of a decreased number of complications associated with regional anesthesia. About one fourth of the 129 deaths from anesthesia-related complications were associated with problems that occurred during the administration of regional anesthesia, mainly (and equally) from either high epidural anesthesia or local anesthetic toxicity.[20] However, recent fiscal constraint in the United States may result in a backward step toward greater use of general anesthesia (inherently with higher rates of complications than regional anesthesia) for cesarean section.[28]

PHYSIOLOGIC CHANGES RELATED TO THE AIRWAY DURING PREGNANCY AND LABOR

Weight Gain and Breast Enlargement. Large breasts can be an obstacle when a laryngoscope is inserted. This can be solved by using a laryngoscope blade with a short handle such as the Datta-Briwa short-handled laryngoscope.[29] If necessary, breasts may be lifted further when a pillow is placed under the parturient's shoulder, making surgical airway procedures in the neck easier. Data from a recent meeting suggest that pregnancy increases the incidence of Mallampati class IV airway (Fig. 32–1) and is associated with suboptimal laryngoscopic views following induction of general anesthesia. A weight gain greater than 15 kg during pregnancy decreases the probability of optimal visualization of the larynx during rigid laryngoscopy.[30]

Airway Edema. Edema of the upper airway could develop, especially in parturients with preeclampsia and/or during prolonged labor. It was concluded in a case report in 1977[31] that preeclamptic toxemia might be associated with laryngeal edema. Stridor or other evidence of upper airway obstruction may not occur at rest. The presence of swollen pharynx, epiglottis, and larynx may ultimately result in failed intubation.[32] Strenuous "bearing down" efforts in the second stage of labor may cause upper airway edema with or without any external manifestations. Pilkington and colleagues[33] have concluded that although pharyngeal edema causes some hindrance to tracheal intubation in obstetrics it is not enough to explain the high failure rate reported. They suggest that more research on neck extension as an evaluator of difficult intubation in obstetrics is needed. Heretofore, the Mallampati test has been used to evaluate airway difficulty, although its sensitivity and specificity are not compellingly high (Fig. 32–1). The incidence of Mallampati class IV cases at the end of pregnancy varies widely from 5%[34] to 56%.[33] The increased incidence of higher grade of

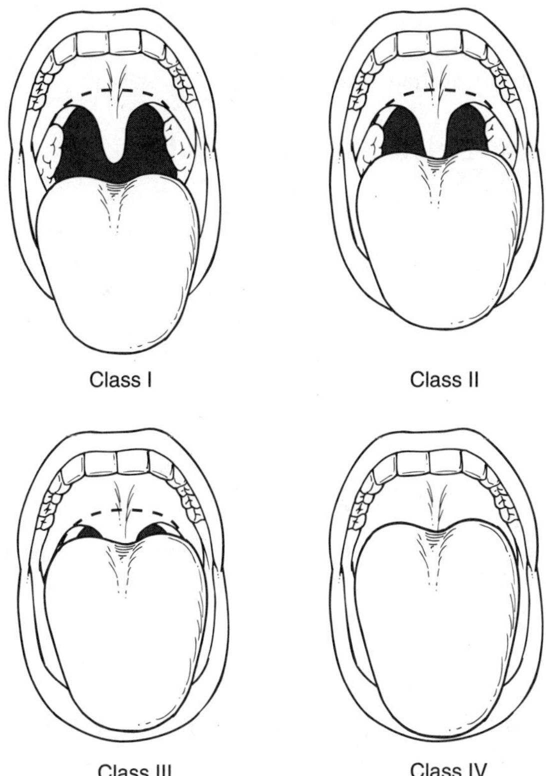

❖ **Figure 32–1** Classification of the upper airway in terms of the size of the tongue and the pharyngeal structures that are visible on the mouth opening. In Mallampati class I patients, the soft palate, fauces, uvula, and anterior and posterior tonsillar pillars can be seen. In Mallampati class II patients, all of the above can be seen except the tonsillar pillars, which are hidden by the tongue. In Mallampati class III patients, only the soft palate and the base of the uvula can be seen. In Mallampati class IV patients, not even the uvula can be visualized. (From Mallampati SR, Gatt SP, Gugino LD, et al: A clinical sign to predict difficult tracheal intubation: a prospective study. Can J Anaesth 1985; 32:429–434.)

Mallampati class is associated with an increase in worse laryngeal visualization, by about 34%.[34] Ethnic difference might account for this variance; this may, on the contrary, not be of undue importance, because the frequency of difficult laryngoscopy is very similar in the white population (1.7%) and black population (1.6%). The risk of edema development increases in the presence of eclampsia and preeclampsia, regardless of the severity of the toxicity triad. Edema is thought to be caused by the effect of estrogen on the ground substance of connective tissue. The mucous membranes become friable in late pregnancy. The risk of bleeding is particularly high in the parturient and should be elicited in the preoperative assessment.

Reduction of Functional Residual Capacity (FRC). Oxygen requirement increases as a result of increase in maternal muscle work and fetal metabolic requirement. The FRC is decreased, especially in a supine position. These factors may result in a sudden onset of hypoxia during apnea, and therefore a much shorter time is allowed for induction of obstetric general anesthesia than in nonobstetric patients. Rosen[35] suggests that intubation should be limited to two attempts of 1 minute each, separated by 30 seconds of ventilation. An unusual benefit of decrease in FRC may be a hastening of inhalation induction of general anesthetic using sevoflurane in case of dire emergency during cesarean section in a parturient with no intravenous access.[36]

Delayed Gastric Emptying. Gastric emptying is delayed in obstetric patients.[37] Preventive antacid and antiemetic therapy are mandatory. The antiemetic efficacy of ondansetron and/or droperidol for cesarean section patients under epidural anesthesia has been confirmed.[38] Gastric emptying may be delayed by drugs administered neuraxially (e.g., extradural fentanyl), and this may increase the chance of vomiting and aspiration of gastric contents.[39] Metoclopramide may increase lower esophageal sphincter tone and thereby may help prevent regurgitation.

PREDICTION AND PREVENTION OF THE DIFFICULT INTUBATION

Prevention or avoidance of foreseeable airway difficulty is important. If a patient is suspected of having a difficult airway, the situation should be discussed with both obstetrician and patient early in labor. Rapid-sequence induction should be avoided because it can result in an anesthetized, paralyzed patient who cannot be intubated. No matter how urgent the situation, repeated checks of equipment should be done and preoperative information should be collected including history of previous surgery and time of last food intake (every emergency patient should be managed as a full stomach case). The presence of senior doctors who have experience, skill, and education in handling a difficult airway and who are also familiar with obstetric anesthesia is indispensable.

It is difficult, or sometimes impossible, to implement well-recognized (but time-consuming) airway assessment in parturients who are writhing with labor pain or in distress and, therefore, not cooperative. Although there are various methods to predict difficult intubation, there is large interobserver variability in performing the same tests on the same patient. Poor visualization of the glottis is not always associated with a difficult intubation.[40] Cormack-Lehane grade 1 laryngoscopy (Fig. 32–2) is not synonymous with easy intubation.[41] According to a recent report, only in one third of the patients in whom failure to intubate occurred was difficulty anticipated by the finding of a Mallampati class II or III transoral visualization.[19, 42] For an extremely difficult intubation final outcome is often dependent on the experience and skill of the anesthesiologist. Previous experience and daily practice may be rewarding. The anesthesiologist's body posture,[43] proper external laryngeal pressure by a skilled assistant, full extension of the patient's head, an appropriate pillow with the neck fully flexed (Fig. 32–3) all make successful intubation more likely.

The presence of carbon dioxide in the exhaled gas is the only absolute diagnostic test of correct placement of a tracheal tube. "When in doubt, take it out."

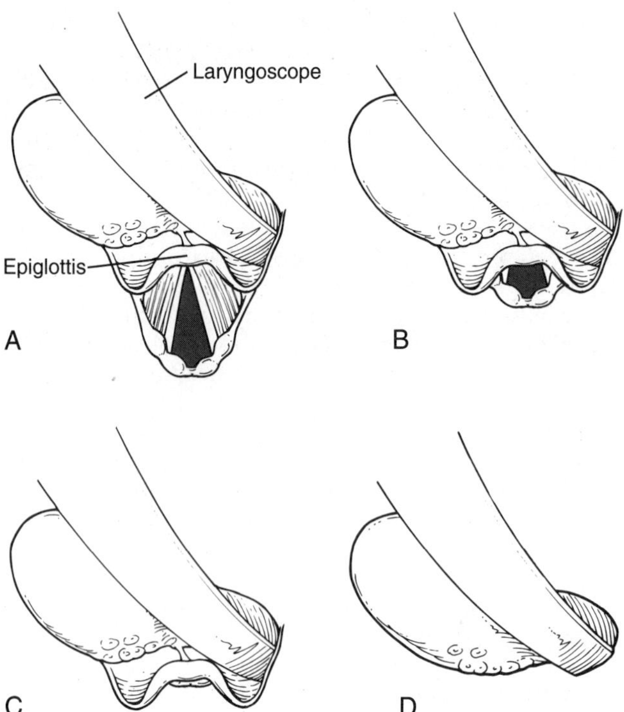

❖ **Figure 32–2** The best views obtainable at laryngoscopy, assuming correct technique. Frequencies apply to patients without neck pathology. Cormack-Lehane grade 1 laryngoscopy is not always indicative of an easy intubation. Severe pathology may produce Cormack-Lehane grade 4 laryngoscopy, but otherwise this occurs rarely. Approximate frequencies are grade 1 *(A)*, 99%; grade 2 *(B)*, 1%; grade 3 *(C)*, 1 per 2000; grade 4 *(D)*, less than 1 per 10^5. (From Cormack RS, Lehane J: Difficult tracheal intubation in obstetrics. Anaesthesia 1984; 39:1105–1111.)

A simulated Cormack-Lehane grade 3 view achieved by lowering the blade and thereby producing descent of the epiglottis (hiding the cords) is a good method to train difficult intubation on a daily basis.[44] Logistic preparation for difficult airway management is also important (Table 32–1). Limited time prior to and/or during emergency cesarean section renders such training inappropriate and impractical.

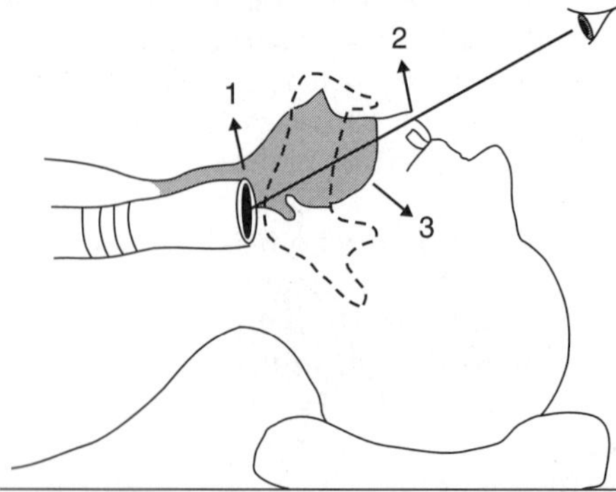

❖ **Figure 32–3** Anatomic factors relevant to difficult intubation. At laryngoscopy the line of vision to the cords must be cleared. Difficulty may occur if the cords (1), the upper teeth (2), or the tongue (3) are displaced in the direction of the arrows. Even with no pathology, this may occur owing to variation in the normal anatomy. (From Cormack RS, Lehane J: Difficult tracheal intubation in obstetrics. Anaesthesia 1984; 39:1105–1111.)

MANAGEMENT: PREDICTION AND PREVENTION

Preanesthetic Assessment. Simple methods of airway evaluation are more practical even if they are somewhat subjective. Rocke studied airway difficulty in obstetric patients using subjective and objective factors. There was no significant correlation between difficulty at tracheal intubation and facial edema and/or swollen tongue (which are regarded as signs suggesting difficulty in obstetric patients). Objectively determined factors showed that unexpected difficulty arose even in those with Mallampati class I and II. Mallampati class III or IV patients with short neck, protruding maxillary incisors, and receding mandible suggested extreme difficulty.[28]

Anesthetists, irrespective of their experience, must be aware there are some obstetric patients whom they may never be able to intubate. Despite optimal preanesthetic evaluation and planning, failed intubation can occur.

The following are useful to elicit in determining whether intubation is likely to be easy or difficult:

1. Airway history: previous surgery, trauma, inborn anomalies
2. Physical examination
   a. Dentition: full, missing, protruding, overbite, buckteeth

Table 32–1 Suggested Contents of the Portable Storage Unit for Difficult Airway Management

IMPORTANT: The items listed in this table represent suggestions. The contents of the portable storage unit should be customized to meet the specific needs, preferences, and skills of the practitioner and health care facility.

1. Rigid laryngoscope blades of alternate design and size from those routinely used.
2. Endotracheal tubes of assorted size.
3. Endotracheal tube guides. Examples include (but are not limited to) semirigid stylets with or without a hollow core for jet ventilation, light wands, and forceps designed to manipulate the distal portion of the endotracheal tube.
4. Fiberoptic intubation equipment.
5. Retrograde intubation equipment.
6. At least one device suitable for emergency nonsurgical airway ventilation. Examples include (but are not limited to) a transtracheal jet ventilator, a hollow jet ventilation stylet, the laryngeal mask, and the esophageal-tracheal Combitube.
7. Equipment suitable for emergency surgical airway access (e.g., cricothyrotomy).
8. An exhaled CO_2 detector.

From Practice guideline for management of difficult airway: a report by the American Society of Anesthesiologists Task Force on Management of the Difficult Airway. Anesthesiology 1993; 78:597–602.

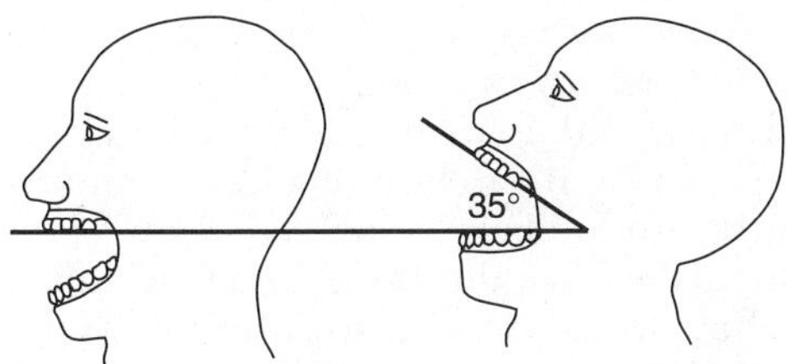

❖ **Figure 32–4** Clinical method for quantitating atlanto-occipital joint extension. When the head is held erect and faces forward, the plane of the occlusal surface of the upper teeth is horizontal and parallel to the floor. When the atlanto-occipital joint is extended, the occlusal surface of the upper teeth will form an angle with the plane parallel to the floor. The angle between the erect and the extended planes of the occlusal surface of the upper teeth quantitates the degree of atlanto-occipital joint extension. A normal person can produce 35 degrees of atlanto-occipital joint extension. (From Bellhouse CP, Doré C: Criteria for estimating likelihood of difficulty of endotracheal intubation with MacIntosh laryngoscope. Anaesth Intensive Care 1988; 16:329–337.)

b. Neck: thick and/or short
c. Thyromental distance: > 7 cm is normal[45]
d. Mobility of the mandible: interincisor distance >2 fingerbreadths. Calculate an interincisor distance of ≥2 cm for the intubating laryngeal mask airway (ILMA) (Fastrack Euromedical, U.S.A.)
e. Receding mandible: 3 finger breadths between the mentum and the upper edge of the thyroid cartilage is normal
f. Mallampati grading (see Fig. 32–1)
g. Atlanto-occipital joint extension (Fig. 32–4)
h. Mandibular space: line of vision (Fig. 32–5; see Fig. 32–3)

3. Simulation laryngoscopy
   a. The silhouette of a laryngoscope blade is superimposed on a lateral view film of the face and neck. The patient's head is placed on a 10-cm-high intubation pillow to obtain full flexion of the neck. The mouth is opened as fully as possible. A marker is placed on the mentum. The anesthesiologist applies cricoid pressure using one hand and simultaneously tries to keep the patient's head extended as much as possible using the other hand. A laryngoscope blade is photocopied and adjusted for magnification using the change in size of a marker. The laryngoscope photocopy is then superimposed on the x-ray film.
   b. This procedure can foretell whether direct laryngoscopy will be able to allow visualization of the glottis.[46, 47]

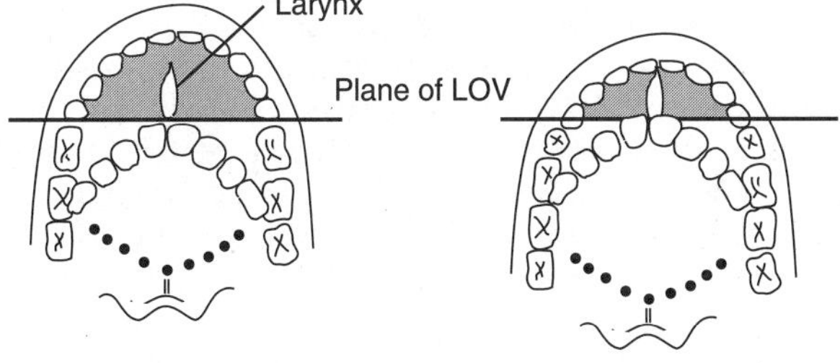

❖ **Figure 32–5** The mandibular space. If the line of vision (LOV) to the larynx were made perfectly horizontal and the observer was standing behind the top of the patient's head, the most posterior structure along the LOV would be the upper teeth, the most anterior structure would be the lower incisors, and the tongue and larynx would be between the upper and lower incisors. The mandibular space *(shaded area)* is the area bounded by the plane of the LOV and the part of the mandibular arch in front of this plane. (From Bellhouse CP, Doré C: Criteria for estimating likelihood of difficulty of endotracheal intubation with MacIntosh laryngoscope. Anaesth Intensive Care 1988; 16:329–337.)

Management of the Difficult Intubation

(Table 32–2)

I. Awake Intubation: If time and situation permit, awake intubation should be chosen (see Table 32–1).[48] If the larynx can be visualized by direct laryngoscopy following topical spray, the patient should be intubated, or intubation can be performed after induction of general anesthesia.

II. Ancillary Techniques
   A. Transoral approaches:
      1. External laryngeal pressure is applied backward, upward, and rightward.
      2. Bimanual cricoid pressure should be the initial technique during rapid-sequence in-

Table 32–2 TECHNIQUES FOR DIFFICULT AIRWAY MANAGEMENT

IMPORTANT: This table displays commonly cited techniques. It is not a comprehensive list. The order of presentation is alphabetical and does not imply preference for a given technique or sequence of use. Combinations of techniques may be employed. The techniques chosen by the practitioner in a particular case will depend upon specific needs, preferences, skills, and clinical constraints.

I. Techniques for Difficult Intubation
- Alternative laryngoscope blades
- Awake intubation
- Blind intubation (oral or nasal)
- Fiberoptic intubation
- Intubating stylet/tube changer
- Light wand
- Retrograde intubation
- Surgical airway access

II. Techniques for Difficult Ventilation
- Esophageal-tracheal Combitube
- Intratracheal jet stylet
- Laryngeal mask
- Oral and nasopharyngeal airways
- Rigid ventilating bronchoscope
- Surgical airway access
- Transtracheal jet ventilation
- Two-person mask ventilation

From Practice guideline for management of difficult airway: a report by the American Society of Anesthesiologists Task Force on Management of the Difficult Airway. Anesthesiology 1993; 78:597–602.

duction, but in a minority of cases, switching to a single-handed technique may improve the laryngoscopic view.[49]
3. Introducer: Over the past decade, a consensus has emerged internationally that the most effective method of handling difficult intubation (Mallampati grade II and III) is to use a flexible introducer of either gum elastic or soft wire.
4. Light wand[50]
5. Standard/intubating LMA (Fastrack)[51–54]

B. Transtracheal approaches:
1. Retrograde wire (or equivalent) introduced into the oropharynx via cricothyroid puncture

C. Transnasal approaches:
1. The blind nasal approach is the most frequently used, but it almost invariably precipitates troublesome bleeding and should not be used without prior intranasal vasoconstriction.

III. Fiberoptic Technique
A. This is the "gold standard" for difficult intubation. A fiberscope is placed either directly through the mouth or indirectly through the LMA.
B. Transnasal fiberoscopy during mask ventilation or transnasal fiberoscopy through one nostril and transnasal ventilation through the tube placed through the other nostril with the mouth closed tight. The latter is not as useful in the pregnant woman at term because of the potential for nasal bleeding.

IV. Cesarean Section: Whenever possible, cesarean section should be performed under regional anesthesia. If time does not permit (in the presence of "fetal distress" or acute hemorrhage) or if the patient is unhappy with regional anesthesia and/or there is no strong contraindication to general anesthesia then general anesthesia with tracheal intubation can be used. To avoid general anesthesia, epidural analgesia should be vigorously encouraged in those classified as Mallampati grades III and IV.

V. Prophylactic Epidural Catheter: Morgan and coworkers[55] recommended that a "prophylactic" epidural catheter be placed in all patients in whom intubation is judged to be potentially difficult. Regional anesthesia can then be used if emergency delivery is needed. Continuous spinal anesthesia may also be used as an alternative with an anticipated difficult airway.[56]

Delivery of the neonate should be expedited if maternal cardiac arrest is imminent, as this provides the best chance of neonatal survival. Maternal resuscitation is usually impossible in the presence of a term fetus in utero.[19]

Management of the Failed Intubation Oxygenation Without Aspiration in Nonfasted Parturient

(Table 32–2)

"Can't intubate and can't ventilate." Appropriate application of cricoid pressure. Thorough familiarity with several ancillary techniques, instruments, and maneuvers for this critical situation is essentially important.

Cormack and Lehane[44] contend that, based on their experience, if three intubation attempts fail further efforts are unlikely to succeed. Scott[57] has argued that patients do not die from failure to intubate but from failure to stop trying to intubate. Repeated attempts at intubation are contraindicated in two situations: (1) ineffective cricoid pressure and (2) progressive hypoxia.

Anesthesia for the Difficult Airway. In the presence of a difficult airway it is important to maintain an adequate level of anesthesia. Sevoflurane and/or propofol could be indicated because they are less irritating to the airway[58] and less likely to induce nausea and vomiting.[36] Repeated attempts at intubation may provoke retching, vomiting, and, possibly, aspiration of gastric contents. A short-acting muscle relaxant (e.g., suxamethonium) is strongly recommended. It wears off rapidly should the securing of an airway prove impossible.

Cricoid Pressure. Cricoid pressure (CP) should be maintained whenever possible during difficult intubation. The pressure should be exerted on the cricoid ring cartilage by the index finger with the neck fully extended. This occludes the esophagus by backward pressure on the cricoid.[59] In pregnancy, the higher intragastric pressure requires more effective upper esophageal counterpressure.

Since CP was first advocated by Monro in the 1770s, no report has confirmed its clinical benefits. It has been reported to be ineffective even when applied by experienced personnel. Justification for the continued use of the maneuver is based, in part, on audit of maternal deaths, which shows a reduction in aspiration-related mortality since its widespread introduction.[60] According to a French report, only 52% of anesthetists were able to describe the technique of CP correctly.[61] Flexion of the head at the atlanto-occipital joint should not be decreased by CP. CP should be applied gently to the awake patient simultaneously with the injection of the induction agent and should be increased when the patient has become unconscious.

There are many reports that question the safety and efficacy of CP, but no better maneuver is presently available. A survey from France, where CP is rarely used, showed a lower rate of aspiration than did another large survey.[6] An anesthesiologist performing laryngoscopy should guide the hand of his or her assistant to the place where the optimal view of the larynx has been obtained and should ask the assistant to decrease or increase CP.

Assistants should be taught how to apply supportive cricoid pressure by asking them to press on an infant-weighing scale as if they were applying CP until the scale registers 3 to 4 kg. This approximates the pressure one must apply clinically to obtain a good seal of the esophagus.[62]

In difficult ventilation, holding a mask and squeezing the bag should be performed separately by two persons. The anesthetist should ask the surgeon and the nurse to stop and help with airway management. When pulmonary ventilation is difficult, CP is ineffective, and regurgitation and/or vomiting occurs, cuff inflation of the "endo-esophageal tube" and suction through it may help prevent aspiration.[63] Mask ventilation with airtight fit, prevention of gastric regurgitation, gastric acidity neutralization, and pharyngeal suctioning may be simultaneously obtained by using the modified "failed intubation" mask developed by Sivaneswaran.[64]

The logical next step is to check that the pharynx is dry. If CP is being applied correctly but is not working (i.e., regurgitation is obvious with fluid filling the throat), then not even one attempt at intubation should be made. The patient should be put head down or in a lateral position and the failed intubation drill should be started.[65] Similarly, if hypoxia is developing and the patient's lungs cannot be ventilated while maintaining CP, attention must focus on restoring oxygen supply.

Laryngeal Mask Airway. Recently, the laryngeal mask airway (LMA) has been regarded as the first step in failed intubation. LMA does not reliably protect against aspiration. However, ventilation and oxygenation takes precedence over measures to prevent aspiration at this juncture.

The incidence of aspiration of 2.3 per 10,000 with the LMA in low-risk patients is comparable to that found for elective anesthesia (2.6 per 10,000) or even for outpatient anesthesia using the face mask or tracheal tube.[66] In emergency cesarean section, patients should be treated as nonfasted and difficult to intubate (Fig. 32–6).

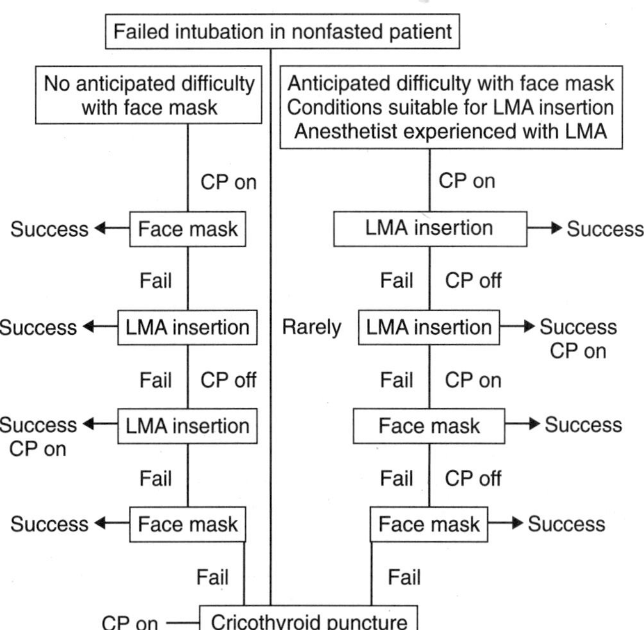

Figure 32–6 Proposed algorithm for laryngeal mask airway (LMA) use in the nonfasted patient. CP, cricoid pressure. (From Brimacombe J: An algorithm for use of the laryngeal mask airway during failed intubation in the patient with a full stomach. Anesth Analg 1993; 77:398–399.)

Although the LMA is contraindicated in patients "at risk" for regurgitation, several anecdotal accounts exist in which it proved lifesaving in cesarean section when tracheal intubation or ventilation with a face mask was unsuccessful.[67] Passage of a fiberoptic bronchoscope through the LMA, the gold standard in cases of airway difficulty, is nearly 100% successful in most series.[68] However, a fiberscope is not universally available and its use requires some training. Furthermore, blind tracheal intubation through the LMA may be worthwhile attempting, especially if an intubating laryngeal mask (ILMA Fastrack) is available. This can be rewarding but may itself cause obstruction of an otherwise patent airway (Fig. 32–7).

Tracheal Intubation Through LMA. When the ILMA is used as an aid to intubation with or without muscle relaxant, the manufacturer recommends that a particular endotracheal tube be used.[69] This particular tube, however, can be substituted with other commercially available tracheal tubes that have a standard reinforced-type tracheal tube; with other soft tubes with a curved or round, less traumatic tip (such as Endotrol, Mallinckrodt Medical); or with a Linder-cuffed (naso) tracheal airway with an Airguide introducer (Polamedco, Los Angeles, CA).[70] These tubes are less likely to cause epistaxis, which is a very real hazard in difficult intubation patients. Hard polyvinyl chloride tubes with a bevel tip should not be used in these circumstances.

"Last-Resort" Choices. It is possible to complete general anesthesia in a cesarean section patient using only an LMA with cricoid pressure applied. Several reports support that the presence of an LMA does not compromise CP,[71] and that it does reduce the incidence of gastric insufflation. CP does not dislodge an LMA correctly placed, but it may impede ventilation, particularly if the neck is unsupported.[72]

There is compelling evidence that the LMA can be successfully inserted in those with the worse grades of Mallampati classification and Cormack-Lehane visualization. A substantial number of cases of known difficult intubation (Mallampati class III or IV; Cormack-Lehane grade 3) have been successfully "intubated" using the LMA.[73]

An important disadvantage of the ILMA is that it cannot be inserted through a less than 20-mm interdental gap.[74] When a lateral position is indicated during anesthesia induction the LMA copes nicely with this situation.

Every anesthetist should become accustomed to neonatal resuscitation using the LMA in case of unavailability of a neonatalogist. Neonatal airway management just after delivery can be difficult, even for those with advanced airway control skills.

An Esophagotracheal Combitube (Sheridan, U.S.A.) can be an alternative because LMA does not protect the parturient from aspiration of gastric contents,[75] and the Combitube esophageal airway may offer an advantage over the laryngeal mask. The Combitube, however, can cause esophageal rupture.[76] An advantage of the Combitube is that it can be placed by

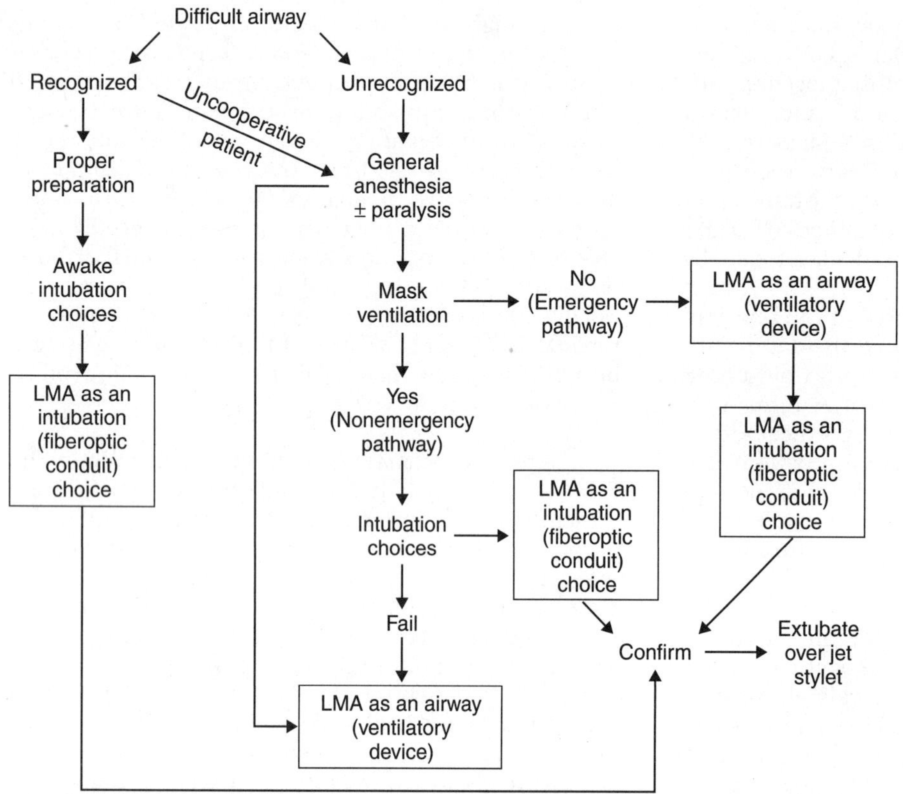

Figure 32–7 The laryngeal mask airway (LMA) fits into ASA algorithm on the management of the difficult airway in five places, as an airway (ventilatory device) or as a conduit for a fiberscope. (From Anesthesiology 1996; 84:686–689.)

anesthetic assistants with relatively little formal training. A laryngoscope blade should be used to assist placement if the first attempt is not successful.[77]

If neither LMA/ILMA (with or without attempts at trans-LMA intubation with tracheal tube) nor Combitube intubation is successful, transtracheal approaches such as cricothyroidotomy, transtracheal jet ventilation (TTJV) or tracheostomy need to be attempted.

The most definitive option should be resolutely taken without losing any time. Sometimes, these alternatives do not protect the airway from aspiration (Fig. 32–7). It has been an accepted policy since 1980[65] to have the equipment needed for this in all maternity operating suites. The use of these techniques has been reviewed.[78]

A modified TTJV system can be quickly assembled using a 14-gauge intravenous catheter, a three-way stopcock, oxygen tubing, 5-mL syringe barrel, and the fresh gas flow from the anesthesia machine.

Difficulties with cricothyroidostomy are usually understated in the literature.[79] We should bear in mind that during emergency cesarean section it is not an easy task to successfully approach the trachea promptly in a limited time. The head and neck space is usually cramped. At the cephalad end, anesthesiologists are usually battling with the oral space and move caudad, while the obstetricians are doing their "jobs" in the abdomen. Even an experienced surgeon may have difficulty performing a tracheostomy or identifying the larynx for cricothyroid puncture. This is particularly difficult in an obese patient, especially when the neck is not fully extended by using a pillow under the shoulders.

A relatively inexperienced anesthetist's chance of placing a transtracheal airway correctly is slim, thus prolonging the period of hypoxia.

The transtracheal approach should be attempted only when an LMA or a Combitube is in place. Mallick and coworkers[80] have reported on the use of the Combitube for airway maintenance during percutaneous tracheostomy.

Puncture of the cricothyroid membrane should be achieved with a 16-gauge (or larger) intravenous catheter. This should be large enough for minimal oxygenation by insufflation or jet ventilation. It should be remembered that any cannula may kink or become misplaced. Insufflation through a cannula improperly placed can be devastating. Smooth expiration has to be confirmed following every insufflation.

EXTUBATION

In emergency cesarean section patients with a difficult airway, extubation should only be undertaken when the mother is fully awake. The stomach should be emptied as much as possible using the orogastric sound. SpO_2 values should be above 95% without additional oxygen when spontaneous respiration is established. It is best to place the patient head down.

When upper airway edema signs, such as swollen tongue and oropharyngeal mucosal edema, are apparent at intubation or if multiple intubation attempts were necessary, extubation over a jet stylet is advisable.

Rocke and Scoones[81] recommend that a cuff deflation test be performed prior to extubation. The cuff is deflated and the tracheal tube lumen occluded digitally to assess whether the patient is able to breathe around the tube. Air moving past the tube confirms

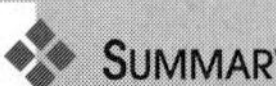

SUMMARY

Key Points

- Anesthesiologists should be aware that there are some parturients whom they may not be able to intubate, regardless of their experience, optimal preanesthetic evaluation, or planning. Careful preanesthetic evaluation, however, will identify many of the patients with "difficult" airways.
- Patients do not generally die from failure to intubate, but they do die from failure to stop trying to intubate. If there is no fetal or maternal "distress," the patient who cannot be intubated can be awakened, at which point regional anesthesia or awake intubation can be performed.
- If a difficult airway is expected, every effort should be made to initiate an early regional anesthetic via a catheter technique.
- If failed intubation occurs, the operator must focus his or her attention on maintaining and/or restoring oxygen supply while minimizing the risk of aspiration.

Key Reference

Pilkington S, Carli F, Dakin MJ: Increase in Mallampati score during pregnancy. Br J Anaesth 1995; 74:638–642.

Case Stem

A 24-year-old patient is scheduled for cesarean section owing to severe preeclampsia. Her weight is 86 kg (2 weeks ago, wt = 70 kg), her blood pressure is 170/110 mm Hg, and she has edema of the lower extremities, face, and neck. At laryngoscopy, the cords are not visualized and intubation is not possible. Discuss the anesthetic management.

that the airway is patent. If the patient is unable to do this, laryngeal edema is present and fiberoptic evaluation or gentle direct laryngoscopy are suggested before extubation. The anesthesiologist should inform the patient or her next of kin of the airway difficulty encountered. The anesthetist should record the presence of a difficult airway, the apparent reasons for difficulty, and any implications for future care. It is best to follow the patient for potential complications, such as edema, bleeding, tracheal and esophageal perforation, pneumothorax, and aspiration.[82]

Anesthesiologists who care for those with a difficult airway must also guarantee communication of this difficult airway to future caretakers. The letter given to the patient should include both a description of the airway difficulties that were encountered and a description of the various airway management techniques that were employed.

References

1. Dykes MHM: Comment on the American Board of Anesthesiology's "Quality Anesthesia Care." A question of learning objectives. Anesthesiology 1980; 53:237–241.
2. Rosen M: Comment on mortality studies in obstetrics. *In* Lunn JN (ed): Quality Care in Anaesthetic Practice. London: The Macmillan Press; 1994.
3. Beecher HK, Todd DP: A study of the deaths associated with anaesthesia and surgery based on a study of 599,428 anaesthesias in 10 institutions, 1948–1952 inclusive. Ann Surg 1954; 140:2–35.
4. Buck N, Devlin HB, Lunn JN: Report of a Confidential Enquiry into Perioperative Deaths. London: Nuffield Provincial Trust and King's Fund; 1987.
5. Eichorn JH: Prevention of intraoperative anaesthesia accidents and related severe injury through safety monitoring. Anesthesiology 1989; 70:572–577.
6. Tiret L, Desmonts J-M, Hatton F: Complications associated with anaesthesia—a prospective survey in France. Can Anaesth Soc J 1986; 33:336–344.
7. Gannon K: Mortality associated with anesthesia practice. Anaesthesia 1991; 46:962–966.
8. Cooper JB, Newbower RS, Kitz RJ: Analysis of major errors and equipment failure in anesthesia management: consideration for prevention and detection. Anesthesiology 1984; 60:34–42.
9. Caplan RA, Posner KL, Ward RJ: Adverse respiratory events in anesthesia: a closed claims analysis. Anesthesiology 1990; 72:828–833.
10. Tinker JH, Dull DL, Caplan RA: Review of 1175 anesthesia related malpractice claims between 1974 and 1988. Anesthesiology 1989; 71:541–546.
11. Taylor TH, Goldhill DR: Standards and audit. *In* Standards of Care in Anaesthesia. Oxford, England: Butterworth-Heinemann; 1992.
12. Gibbs CP: Gastric aspiration: prevention and treatment. Clin Anesthesiol 1986; 4:47–52.
13. Lyon G: Failed intubation: six years' experience in a teaching maternity unit. Anaesthesia 1985; 40:759–762.
14. King TA, Adams AP: Failed tracheal intubation. Br J Anaesth 1990; 65:400–414.
15. Samsoon GLT, Young JRB: Difficult tracheal intubation: a retrospective study. Anaesthesia 1987; 42:487–509.
16. Turnbull AC, Tindall VR, Robson G: Report on Confidential Enquiry into Maternal Deaths (CEMD) in England and Wales, 1979–1981. London: Her Majesty's Stationery Office; 1986.
17. Report on Confidential Enquiry into Maternal Deaths in the United Kingdom in 1984–1987. London: Her Majesty's Stationery Office; 1991.
18. Report on Confidential Enquiry into Maternal Deaths in the United Kingdom in 1988–1990. London: Her Majesty's Stationery Office; 1994.
19. Hawthorne L, Wilson R, Lyon G: Failed intubation revisited: 17-yr experience in a teaching maternity unit. Br J Anaesth 1996; 76:680–684.
20. Hawkins JL, Koonin LM, Palmer SK: Anesthesia-related deaths during obstetric delivery in the United States, 1979–1990. Anesthesiology 1997; 86:277–284.
21. Maternal and Child Health Statistics of Japan. Statistics and Information Department, Minister's Secretariat, Ministry of Health and Welfare, Tokyo, Japan 1997.
22. Berg JC, Atrash HK, Koonin LM: Pregnancy-related mortality in the United States, 1987–1990. Obstet Gynecol 1996; 88:161–167.
23. Koonin LM, Atrash HK, Lawson HW: Maternal mortality surveillance, United States, 1979–1986. MMWR Morb Mortal Wkly Rep 1991; 40:1–13.
24. Chadwick HS, Posner K, Caplan R: A comparison of obstetric and nonobstetric malpractice claims. Anesthesiology 1991; 74:242–249.
25. Rocke DA, Murray WB, Rout CC: Relative risk analysis of factors associated with difficult intubation in obstetric anesthesia. Anesthesiology 1992; 77:67–73.
26. Report on Confidential Enquiry into Maternal Deaths in England and Wales, 1982–1984. London: Her Majesty's Stationery Office; 1987.
27. Report on Confidential Enquiry into Maternal Deaths in the United Kingdom, 1991–1993. London: Her Majesty's Stationery Office; 1997.
28. Chestnut DH: Anesthesia and maternal mortality [editorial views.] Anesthesiology 1997; 86:273–276.

29. Datta S, Briwa J: Modified laryngoscope for endotracheal intubation of obese patient. Anesth Analg 1981; 10:120–121.
30. Shanker KB, Krishna S, Moseley HSL: Airway changes during pregnancy. ASA abstract A 895 87. Anesthesiology No. 3 A, 1997.
31. Brock-Utne JG, Downing JW, Seedat F: Laryngeal edema associated with pre-eclamptic toxaemia. Anaesthesia 1977; 32:556–558.
32. Jouppilla R, Jouppilla P, Hollmén A: Laryngeal edema as an obstetric anaesthesia complication: case reports. Acta Anaesthesiol Scand 1980; 24:97–98.
33. Pilkington S, Carli F, Dakin MJ: Increase in Mallampati score during pregnancy. Br J Anaesth 1995; 74:638–642.
34. Carli F, Williams KN, Cormack RS: Difficult laryngoscopy. Br J Anaesth 1992; 68:117–118.
35. Rosen M: Difficult and failed intubation in obstetrics. *In* Latto IP, Rosen M (eds): Difficulties in Tracheal Intubation. London: Baillière Tindall; 1984:152–155.
36. Schaut DJ, Khona R, Gross JB: Sevoflurane inhalation induction for emergency Cesarean section in parturient with no intravenous access. Anesthesiology 1997; 86:1392–1394.
37. Jayaram A, Bowen MP, Deshpande S: Ultrasound examination of the stomach contents of women in the postpartum period. Anesth Analg 1997; 84:522–526.
38. Pan PH, Moore CH: Intraoperative antiemetic efficacy of prophylactic ondansetron versus droperidol for Cesarean section patients under epidural anesthesia. Anesth Analg 1996; 83:982–986.
39. Kelly MC, Carabine UA, Hill DA: A comparison of the effect of intrathecal and extradural fentanyl on gastric emptying in laboring women. Anesth Analg 1997; 85:834–838.
40. Williams KN, Carli F, Cormack RS: Unexpected difficult laryngoscopy: a prospective survey in routine general surgery. Br J Anaesth 1991; 66:38–44.
41. Benumof JL: Difficult laryngoscopy: obtaining the best view. Can J Anaesth 1994; 41:361–365.
42. Cooper DS, Benumof JL, Reisner LS: The difficult airway: risk, prophylaxis, and management. *In* Chestnut DH (ed): Obstetric Anesthesia: Principles and Practice. St. Louis: CV Mosby; 1989:577–605.
43. Matthewes AJ, Johnson CHJ, Goodman NW: Body posture during simulated tracheal intubation. Anaesthesia 1998; 53:331–334.
44. Cormack RS, Lehane J: Difficult tracheal intubation in obstetrics. Anaesthesia 1984; 39:1105–1111.
45. Freneck CM: Predicting difficult intubation. Anaesthesia 1991; 46:1005–1008.
46. Watanabe S, Takeshima R, Taguchi N: Simulation laryngoscopy using a X-ray film taken during a laryngoscopic position and an isometric size blade silhouette. Anesth Analg 1997; 84:S1–S599.
47. Taguchi N, Watanabe S, Kumagai M: Radiographic documentation of increased visibility of the larynx with a Belscope laryngoscope blade. Anesthesiology 1994; 81:773–775.
48. Benumof JL: Management of the difficult adult airway with special emphasis on awake tracheal intubation. Anesthesiology 1991; 75:1087–1110.
49. Yentis SM: The effect of single-handed and bimanual cricoid pressure on the view at laryngoscopy. Anaesthesia 1997; 52:332–335.
50. Ellis DG, Jakymec A, Kaplan MR: Guided orotracheal intubation in the operating room using a lighted stylet: a comparison with direct laryngoscopic technique. Anesthesiology 1986; 64:823–826.
51. Brimacombe JR: Difficult airway management with the intubating laryngeal mask. Anesth Analg 1997; 85:1173–1175.
52. Kapila A, Addy EV, Vergese C: The intubation laryngeal mask airway. I. An initial assessment of performance. Br J Anaesth 1997; 79:710–713.
53. Brain AIJ, Vergese C, Addy EV: The intubation laryngeal mask. II. A preliminary clinical report of a new means of intubating the trachea. Br J Anaesth 1997; 79:710–713.
54. Parr MJA, Gregory M, Basket PJF: The intubating laryngeal mask. Anaesthesia 1998; 53:343–348.
55. Morgan BM, Magni V, Goroszenuik T: Anaesthesia for emergency cesarean section. Br J Obstet Gynaecol 1990; 97:420–424.
56. Malan TP, Johnson MD: The difficult airway in obstetric anesthesia: technique for airway management and the role of regional anesthesia. J Clin Anesth 1988; 1:104–111.
57. Scott DB: Endotracheal intubation: friend or foe? BMJ 1986; 292:157–158.
58. Mostafa SM, Atherton AMJ: Sevoflurane for difficult tracheal intubation. Br J Anaesth 1997; 79:392–393.
59. Sellick BA: Cricoid pressure to control regurgitation of stomach contents during induction of anaesthesia. Lancet 1961; 2:404.
60. Brimacombe JR, Berry AM: Review article: cricoid pressure. Can J Anaesth 1997; 44:414–425.
61. Benhamon D: French obstetric anaesthetist and acids aspiration prophylaxis. Eur J Anaesthesiol 1993; 10:27–32.
62. Dodge C, Blike G: Aspiration in obstetrics. *In* Datta S (ed): Common Problems in Obstetric Anesthesia, 2nd ed. St. Louis: CV Mosby; 1995:27–38.
63. Boys JE: Failed intubation in obstetric anaesthesia. Br J Anaesth 1983; 55:187–188.
64. Sivaneswaran N, McGuinness JJ: Modified mask for failed intubation at emergency Caesarean section. Anaesth Intensive Care 1984; 12:279–280.
65. Tunstall ME: Anesthesia for obstetric operations. Clin Obstet Gynecol 1980; 7:665–694.
66. Benumof JL: Laryngeal mask airway and the ASA difficult airway algorithm. Anesthesiology 1996; 84:686–699.
67. Gatature PS, Hughes JA: The laryngeal mask airway in obstetrical anaesthesia. Can J Anaesth 1995; 42:130–133.
68. Benumof JL: The pharyngeal mask airway: indications and contraindications [editorial]. Anesthesiology 1992; 77:843–846.
69. Brimacombe JR, Brain AIJ, Berry AM: The Laryngeal Mask Airway: A Review and Practical Guide. Chap. 17, Future Direction. London: WB Saunders; 1997:227–247.
70. Watanabe S, Yaguchi Y, Suga A: A "bubble-tip" (Airguide ™) tracheal tube system: its effects on incidence of epistaxis and ease of tube advancement in the subglottic region during nasotracheal intubation. Anesth Analg 1994; 78:1140–1143.
71. Strang TL: Does the laryngeal mask airway compromise cricoid pressure? Anaesthesia 1992; 47:829–831.
72. Asai T, Barcley K, McBeth D: Cricoid pressure applied after placement of the laryngeal mask prevents gastric insufflation but inhibits ventilation. Br J Anaesth 1996; 76:772–776.
73. Brimacombe J: Analysis of 1500 laryngeal mask uses by one anaesthetist in adults undergoing routine anaesthesia. Anaesthesia 1996; 51:76–80.
74. Watanabe S, Suga A, Asakura N: Determination of the distance between the laryngoscope blade and the upper incisor during direct laryngoscopy: comparison of a curved, an angulated straight, and two straight blades. Anesth Analg 1994; 79:638–641.
75. Brimacombe J, Berry A, Brain A: The laryngeal mask airway. Anesthesiol Clin North Am 1995; 13:411–437.
76. Klein H, Williamson M, Sue-Ling HM: Esophageal rupture associated with the use of the Combitube™. Anesth Analg 1997; 85:937–939.
77. Bishop MJ, Kharash ED: Is the Combitube™ a useful emergency airway device for anesthesiologists? Anesth Analg 1998; 86:1141–1142.
78. Benumof JL, Scheller MS: The importance of transtracheal jet ventilation in the management of the difficult airway. Anesthesiology 1989; 71:769–778.
79. Dob DP, McLure HA, Soni N: Case report: failed intubation and emergency percutaneous tracheostomy. Anaesthesia 1998; 53:69–78.
80. Mallick A, Quinn AC, Bodenham AR: Apparatus: use of Combitube for airway maintenance during percutaneous dilational tracheostomy. Anaesthesia 1998; 53:249–255.
81. Rocke DA, Scoones GP: Rapidly progressive laryngeal oedema associated with pregnancy induced hypertension. Anaesthesia 1992; 47:141–143.
82. Practice guideline for management of difficult airway: a report by the American Society of Anesthesiologists Task Force on Management of the Difficult Airway. Anesthesiology 1993; 78:597–602.

33

Pulmonary Aspiration

❖ Y. K. Chan, MD

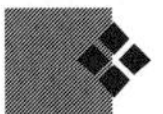

INTRODUCTION

The obstetric patient is predisposed to aspiration of gastric contents because of the anatomic and physiologic changes of pregnancy. Measures taken in labor to relieve pain, anxiety, and the process of delivery, especially operative delivery under anesthesia, also contribute to an increased risk of aspiration. Gastric emptying is delayed and the gastroesophageal barrier pressure is reduced because of a reduction in the lower esophageal sphincter pressure. Narcotics further delay the gastric emptying, and general anesthesia depresses protective laryngeal reflexes.

The mainstay of management of pulmonary aspiration involves supportive oxygen therapy with close monitoring for respiratory failure. Immediate suctioning of the gastric contents when seen in the airway is advocated, but subsequent bronchoscopy or lavage may have minimal effect. Ventilation is required in approximately 17% of cases,[1] and various modes of positive pressure ventilation have been advocated for optimizing lung function to increase pulmonary alveolar recruitment, optimize gas exchange, minimize cardiovascular instability, and maximize oxygen delivery. Fluids lost through the lungs need to be replaced, and hydration has to be monitored. Steroids and prophylactic antibiotics have not been found to be useful.

Pulmonary aspiration is largely preventable, and strategies have been developed to minimize the occurrence of this condition. Steps to reduce the volume and acidity of stomach contents include fasting, emptying the stomach by the use of orogastric tubes and metoclopramide, and using antacids and H_2 receptor blockers. The gastroesophageal barrier pressure may be increased with metoclopramide. Correct application of cricoid pressure prevents esophageal contents from reaching the oropharynx. Use of regional anesthesia allows the retention of protective airway reflexes and eliminates the risk of pulmonary aspiration considerably, but aspiration may still occur in situations of local anesthetic toxicity. General anesthesia for emergency cesarean sections increases the risk of pulmonary aspiration. In an effort to reduce aspiration during general anesthesia, a number of maneuvers can be undertaken to increase safety. These include adequate acid aspiration prophylaxis, proper evaluation of the parturient's airway, rapid-sequence induction with correct application of cricoid pressure, the use of functioning equipment, having a preplanned rational approach to difficult or failed intubation, and ensuring that the stomach is emptied preoperatively in a parturient who has recently eaten.

These preventive strategies have collectively resulted in a reduction in the incidence of aspiration since the 1950s. The exact role of each of the strategies in preventing pulmonary aspiration may never be known. There is pressure from certain quarters to be less stringent about the implementation of some of these strategies, but leniency must be weighed against the consequences of aspiration pneumonitis.

Pulmonary aspiration in the obstetric patient is still a much feared complication because it contributes significantly to patient morbidity[1, 2] and mortality.[2–5] It is a potential threat to every parturient, but more so to those undergoing operative deliveries under anesthesia,[5, 6] eclamptic patients,[7] and those obtunded[8] by excessive narcotics for pain relief. The mortality is estimated to be approximately 30% of identified cases.[5, 9] It is one of the two leading causes of maternal death under general anesthesia and frequently aspiration and failure of airway management occur together.[10]

Since Mendelson's[11] classic description of this entity in 1946, there have been remarkable strides made in an attempt to prevent the condition in the obstetric population.

INCIDENCE

The incidence of pulmonary aspiration in the general population undergoing elective surgery has been quoted as 1:2131 to 1:3216.[1, 12] It occurs more frequently in patients undergoing emergency surgery and has been quoted[12] as 1:895. In the obstetric patient presenting for cesarean section, a study in Sweden[1] found an incidence of 1:661. There has been a progressive decline in the rate of pulmonary aspiration as a cause of maternal death.[6, 13] While this may indirectly indicate a decrease in incidence, it may also reflect improved survival among those afflicted.[1, 4] In the United Kingdom, there were 32 deaths (2.3 deaths from pulmonary aspiration per 100 maternal deaths) from aspiration documented in the *Report on Confidential Enquiries into Maternal Deaths* in the 1952 to 1954 triennium.[6] In the 1991 to 1993 triennium[13] there was only one mortality (0.3 death from pulmonary aspiration per 100 maternal deaths) resulting from aspiration.

The declining incidence is also seen in the contribution of pulmonary aspiration anesthetic-associated maternal deaths. Previously 65% of anesthetic-related maternal deaths[6] were due to aspiration. In developing countries where the level of anesthetic care may be less evenly distributed, it constitutes only 20%[14] of anesthetic-related mortality in obstetrics.

PREDISPOSING FACTORS

For pulmonary aspiration of gastric contents to occur, three components of the process must be present together.[15] These are the presence of an "at-risk"[16] stomach, reflux or regurgitation of gastric contents into the oropharynx, and the inhalation of these contents into the lungs. The first two occur more frequently in the pregnant patient.[16–19] This is due to anatomic and physiologic changes that occur as pregnancy progresses. During labor, the risk is further increased by pharmacologic agents administered for the relief of pain[20–22] and the process of delivery itself, especially if the patient undergoes operative delivery under general anesthesia.[5]

As pregnancy progresses, the enlarging intra-abdominal uterus increases intragastric pressure.[23] There is a concomitant decrease in lower esophageal sphincter pressure, which becomes more marked toward term as a result of increased progesterone.[17] The lowered esophageal sphincter pressure in the presence of increased intragastric pressure decreases gastroesophageal barrier pressure, which predisposes the pregnant patient at term to a higher incidence of reflux.[18] Vanner[19] demonstrated gastric reflux in 17 out of 25 women near term compared with an incidence of only 5 in the same group of women more than 36 hours after delivery.

Gastric emptying is delayed in pregnancy.[24] Labor itself slows gastric emptying.[21, 25] Narcotics for pain relief whether administered by the parenteral[20, 21] or epidural route[21, 22] further delay the process and allow a massive increase in gastric volume.[21, 26] A volume of greater than 25 mL and a pH of less than 2.5 present in the stomach have been accepted as criteria for increased risk of aspiration pneumonitis.[16] Contrary to popular belief, there is no evidence that the acidity is increased in pregnancy or during labor compared with nonpregnant controls,[17] but Taylor[26] demonstrated that as many as 55% of parturients at term presenting for cesarean section had a pH of 2.5 or below.

The mother at term is at higher risk for difficult intubation[27] when subjected to general anesthesia. The difficulty has been estimated to be 1:300, that is, 10 times more often than the general population. It is in the circumstances of a difficult or failed intubation, when the airway is unprotected, that aspiration is most likely to occur.[10]

Parturients with eclampsia have a high risk of aspiration.[7] Episodes of eclampsia and the anticonvulsants used in their management depress the patient's state of consciousness and laryngeal reflex, exposing the parturient with eclampsia to pulmonary aspiration.

PATHOLOGY

The pulmonary damage following aspiration of gastric contents has been extensively studied, but much of the current body of knowledge is based on experimental animal studies. The injury is dependent on the pH[28, 29] of the gastric contents, gastric volume,[16, 30, 31] and the presence of solids or liquids.[29]

Mendelson[11] was the first to focus on the acids in the stomach contents as being responsible. He found that the damage was very much reduced when he instilled neutralized gastric contents into the airway of rabbits. Teabeaut[28] extended this finding and found that the degree of tissue damage corresponded to the acidity of the aspirated solution between pH 1.5 and 2.4. Aspiration of solution with pH greater than 2.5 produced the same tissue reaction as isotonic saline solution.[28]

Histologic findings in the lung after aspiration with gastric acid show damage to alveolar and endothelial cells, with alveolar exudate consisting of edema, hemorrhage, fibrin, polymorphonuclear leukocytes, and macrophages.[29, 32] Electron microscopy reveals necrosis of type 1 and type 2 alveolar cells.[33] The lungs on gross examination[33] show areas of atelectasis, edema, and hemorrhage and usually weigh 2 to 3 times more than the average normal lungs.[34] Kennedy and colleagues[32] also demonstrated a time course to the damage. The inflammatory response is minimal at 1 hour but becomes maximal at 4 hours.

An unpublished study on rhesus monkeys, cited by Roberts and Shirley,[16] suggested that a critical volume of greater than 0.4 mL/kg produced significant changes in the lungs. Subsequent work by Raidoo and coworkers[30] revealed that a gastric volume greater than 0.8 mL/kg was required to produce significant damage leading to death. James and colleagues[31] in their studies on rats demonstrated that the critical volume for lethal lung damage depended on the pH of the aspirate. A volume of 0.3 mL/kg was lethal 90% of the time when liquid aspiration at a pH of 1.0 occurred. The global mortality was 14% for rats that aspirated 1 or 2 mL/kg of a solution with a pH of 1.8 or greater.

Mendelson[11] also differentiated between aspiration of solids and liquids. Autopsy of his two patients who died of suffocation revealed complete obstruction of the major respiratory passages. In aspiration of gastric contents with smaller food particles, Schwartz and associates[29] demonstrated that the histologic findings were similar to those seen with liquid acid aspiration, but the inflammatory response also affected respiratory bronchioles and alveolar ducts. In aspiration of gastric contents containing food particles, the mortality depends on the acidity of the food particles. Schwartz[29] demonstrated 100% mortality in his dogs who aspirated food particles with a pH of 1.8.

PHYSIOLOGY

Hypoxia[29, 32–35] occurs very rapidly after pulmonary aspiration of gastric contents because of the various changes that occur as a result of the aspiration. Surfactant production is decreased[33] as a result of the destruction of type 2 cells, and this results in atelectasis. Intra-alveolar edema, hemorrhage, and fibrin formation further contribute to the shunting. Pulmonary vasoconstriction, seen in arterioles[36] after aspiration, probably contributes to ventilation-perfusion imbalance. The hypoxemia is closely related to the degree of lung damage and is worst with aspiration of gastric contents of low pH–containing food particles.[29] In experimental studies,[29] the hypoxemia peaked at about 10 minutes after the episode of aspiration and by 24 hours there was already a fair amount of resolution, although baseline values were not reached.

Pulmonary aspiration induces an acute chemical pneumonitis[32] which increases pulmonary capillary permeability and allows transudation of large amounts of plasma-like fluid into the pulmonary interstitium and alveoli. The hematocrit rises if the fluid volume deficit is not corrected,[34] and hypovolemia results in hypotension.

The increase in lung water, atelectasis, and reduction in surfactant reduce pulmonary compliance, the latter reflected by a flattening in the pressure-volume curves of lungs affected by pulmonary aspiration of gastric contents.[35]

CLINICAL FEATURES

In the obstetric patient, aspiration of gastric contents is likely to occur in an unfasted patient undergoing emergency cesarean section under general anesthesia.[5] The risk is increased in association with difficult intubation,[10] in eclamptic patients,[7] and when the mother is obtunded owing to the excessive use of sedatives or narcotics[8] or to overdose of other drugs such as local anesthetics.

A definite diagnosis of aspiration can be made if gastric contents are seen in the airway at the time of intubation or recovered from the tracheobronchial tree after the event.[12] Most of the time, however, a presumptive diagnosis has to be made in a patient with predisposing factors to aspiration and clinical signs suggestive of aspiration. Postoperative chest radiographs[12] showing pulmonary infiltrates not seen before the suspected episode may further strengthen the diagnosis.

Aspiration of large particulate matter leads immediately to complete or partial airway obstruction. In fact, 2 of Mendelson's[11] 5 patients who aspirated solid food particles died immediately.

The physical signs present fairly immediately, and in Bynum's series[37] of 50 patients all had some pulmonary derangement within 2 hours of the incident. The fulminant onset of this condition distinguishes it from other forms of pulmonary dysfunction.[37] The clinical findings[11, 37, 38] are typically hypoxemia, tachypnea, bronchospasm, and diffuse crepitations in the lungs. Cough and apnea may also be seen in some patients. Shock complicates the clinical course in approximately 20% to 30% of patients.[37] Patients with severe hypoxemia and shock are more likely to have a fatal outcome in the course of the disease.[37] In Bynum's series,[37] those patients with arterial-alveolar oxygen ratio of 0.5 or less (normal is greater than 0.8) had a mortality of 48%, whereas in those with ratios greater than 0.5, the mortality was 14%.

The initial chest radiograph findings[2] are extremely variable and noncharacteristic. Infiltrates are seen with mainly radial or perihilar distribution or distribution into the lower right or left zones.[2] Immediate chest radiographs may not reveal any abnormality, but all show some abnormality within 24 to 36 hours.[37]

The majority of patients show rapid clinical improvement and recovery, but 10% to 15% rapidly deteriorate[2, 37] and die within 24 hours as a result of respiratory failure. The remainder develop various complications including superimposed nosocomial pneumonia, acute respiratory distress syndrome, and multiple organ failure.

Hospitalization is prolonged by an average of 8 to 21 days,[4, 37] and most of these are spent in the intensive care unit. The overall mortality in the nonobstetric population of patients with significant aspiration has been variously estimated to be around 30%.[2, 9, 37] This probably also applies to the obstetric patient, since there is no evidence to indicate that the mortality following aspiration of acidic stomach contents is significantly higher in patients who are pregnant compared with the general population.[39]

PREVENTION

In a condition in which the mortality has been seen in many series to be unacceptably high, prevention is the better alternative. Since the 1950s, the preventive strategies shown in Table 33–1 have collectively served to reduce the incidence of pulmonary aspiration. The significance of each of these in individually reducing the risk of pulmonary aspiration, however, is unknown.

Strategies to Reduce the "At-Risk" Stomach Contents

Fasting. Fasting has traditionally been the mainstay of acid aspiration prophylaxis management. Roberts and Shirley[16] showed that there is a fall in mean volume of gastric contents as the time between meal and delivery or meal and onset of labor lengthens. The risk of not fasting the obstetric patient for cesarean section under general anesthesia was clearly demonstrated by Lewis and Crawford.[40] They showed significantly increased volume of gastric contents and a low pH in their patients allowed to eat and drink within 4 hours of cesarean section compared with con-

Table 33-1 Prevention of Pulmonary Aspiration

Strategies to Reduce "At-Risk" Stomach Contents
Reduction of gastric volume
Fasting
Emptying by nasogastric tube
H_2 receptor blocker
Metoclopramide
Omeprazole
Increasing gastric pH
Antacids
H_2 receptor blockers
Omeprazole
Strategies to Prevent Reflux/Regurgitation
Increasing gastroesophageal barrier pressure
Metoclopramide
Preventing reflux of esophageal/gastric contents entering the pharynx
Cricoid pressure
Strategies to Protect the Airway
Preserving integrity of laryngeal reflex
Use of regional anesthesia
Competent handling of airway
Rapid-sequence induction with cricoid pressure
Rational approach to difficult/failed intubation
Awake intubation with fiberoptic bronchoscopy

trols who fasted overnight. In their 11 patients given toast, 2 had recognizable food particles. Regardless of the period of fasting, patients may still have volumes exceeding 50 mL[16] or even solids in the stomach.[25] Conversely, when fasting is prolonged[16] (over 20 hours), the gastric volume increases with time.

Currently, however, there is much pressure to liberalize oral intake in labor.[15, 41] The fasting practice is fairly variable, as exemplified in the survey done by Michael and Reilly[42] of fasting practices during labor in the United Kingdom. Of the obstetric units surveyed, 3.6% did not allow any form of oral intake, 64.7% allowed drinks only, and 31.7% allowed drinks and food. Of the 96.4% of obstetric units that allowed oral intake (whether drinks only or drinks and food), 68.3% had policies regarding selection of mothers according to risk categories.

Obstetric care providers seem divided on the issue of fasting. The exact contribution of fasting in reducing the incidence of pulmonary aspiration will never be known. The American College of Obstetricians and Gynecologists[43] has advised all mothers in labor not to ingest anything except for small sips of water, ice chips, and preparations to moisten the mouth and lips. Obstetric units that allow feeding in labor should incorporate consideration of operative risk in their feeding policy,[15] and in mothers with a high risk of operative delivery they should be allowed only water intake during labor.

Emptying by Nasogastric Tube. A wide-bore orogastric or nasogastric tube seems ideal to empty stomach contents preoperatively to reduce the risk of aspiration. However, this may not significantly reduce the number of patients at risk of acid aspiration.[44, 45] Solids may not be removable, and in an awake patient the procedure is very unpleasant.[45] Despite this, and the risk of nasopharyngeal trauma and epistaxis, some authors still recommend that the stomach be emptied via a gastric tube before emergency cesarean section in those who have just eaten.[5] Most obstetric anesthesiologists, however, do not place gastric tubes in awake obstetric patients. A multilumen nasogastric tube with an air vent facilitates emptying of the stomach.[46] Effective cricoid pressure can be maintained in the presence of a nasogastric tube.[47] Pulmonary aspiration can also occur following extubation, and the gastric tube should be drained before the patient is extubated.[48]

Current Chemoprophylaxis. In the 1970s the majority of obstetric units gave their patients antacid prophylaxis during labor.[49] With the greater use of regional analgesia both for labor as well as for cesarean section, many obstetric units have discontinued their policies of routine pharmacologic acid aspiration prophylaxis. Burgess and Crowhurst[50] found that only 22.4% of Australian hospitals administered routine antacid prophylaxis during labor. In a survey of 202 obstetric units in the United Kingdom,[51] only 57% of the units carry out routine acid aspiration prophylaxis in all parturients in labor. Antacid prophylaxis was provided for women in the high-risk category and for those who were likely to undergo instrumental or operative delivery.[51] Parturients undergoing elective cesarean section received acid aspiration prophylaxis in 98% of the units surveyed, and sodium citrate and oral ranitidine was the preferred option.[51] Sodium citrate and intravenous ranitidine with or without metoclopramide were given for emergency cesarean section.[51]

Antacids. The use of an alkali to neutralize stomach contents was discussed by Mendelson[11] in his paper. The use of antacids for acid aspiration prophylaxis became widespread only following Taylor's study[26] on the effectiveness of magnesium trisilicate in raising the gastric pH of mothers in labor requiring general anesthesia for cesarean section.

Antacids are used to neutralize existing stomach acids. Various agents have been used through the years. Most obstetric units now use nonparticulate antacids. Particulate antacids have been reported[52] to cause lung damage when aspirated. Nonparticulate antacids mix better than particulate antacids with stomach contents.[53] The most commonly used antacid today is sodium citrate, which has been shown to be effective in increasing the gastric pH to greater than 2.5 in all parturients.[54–56] Others have demonstrated that when sodium citrate is used alone, as many as 37% to 40% of parturients may have a pH less than 2.5.[57, 58] There is also concern that repeated doses may in effect add to the volume of gastric contents.[59]

H_2 Receptor Blockers. H_2 receptor blockers obliterate the histamine-mediated secretion of hydrochloric acid. The ability of these drugs to reduce gastric volume and improve pH is mainly dependent on prevention of further secretion of hydrochloric acid and hence they cannot be expected to neutralize existing acids in the stomach.[46] Timing of dosage is, therefore, important[60] and better results are obtained when H_2 receptor blockers are combined with antacids.[58, 59]

Cimetidine and ranitidine are both used, but ranitidine is the preferred choice in most obstetric units.[51] There is limited experience with famotidine for acid aspiration prophylaxis in the general population[61] or in the obstetric patient.[62] Ten percent of parturients given an oral dose of 40 mg of famotidine before elective cesarean section under regional anesthesia had a pH less than 2.5.[62] Oral ranitidine is the most frequently used agent for acid aspiration prophylaxis for mothers in active labor.[51] Intravenous ranitidine is frequently given for emergency cesarean section[51] and should be administered slowly because rapid injection has been associated with the development of serious arrhythmias in the form of severe bradycardia.[63]

Metoclopramide. Metoclopramide, a procainamide derivative, has diverse effects on the gastrointestinal tract. It increases lower esophageal sphincter tone,[64] and increases gastric peristalsis and relaxation of the pylorus leading to improved gastric emptying.[65] Howard and Sharp[66] found that 10 mg intramuscularly significantly reduce the volume of a 750-mL test meal of water during established labor even when meperidine had been given. Gastric volume is decreased, but metoclopramide has no effect on the pH.[67]

Single-dose metoclopramide has no demonstrable side effects and is safe for the fetus.[66, 68] It is frequently used in combination with sodium citrate and ranitidine prior to induction of general anesthesia for emergency cesarean section.[51]

Omeprazole. Omeprazole is a proton pump inhibitor that prevents further production of acids. Four different studies[69–72] in obstetric patients showed that omeprazole alone or in combination with ranitidine and/or sodium citrate was successful in putting 70% to 95% of parturients into the "not at risk" category with respect to stomach contents. Hence it offers no more advantage than the more established regimen of ranitidine and sodium citrate. Omeprazole is three times more expensive[70] than ranitidine, and it is therefore unlikely to become popular for acid aspiration prophylaxis for the obstetric patient.

Strategies to Prevent Regurgitation

Regurgitation is a passive process that occurs in the presence of relaxed upper and lower esophageal sphincters.[73] The process allows gastric contents to enter the esophagus and also the oropharynx.

Strategies to prevent regurgitation can thus be directed at either preventing reflux of gastric contents into the esophagus or preventing the gastric or esophageal contents from reaching the oropharynx.

Preventing Reflux at the Gastroesophageal Junction. Brock-Utne and coworkers[64] using 10 mg of intravenous metoclopramide significantly increased the lower esophageal sphincter tone and barrier pressure in late pregnancy. This effect may be negated by the simultaneous use of atropine.[74] No study has evaluated the effect of metoclopramide on the lower esophageal sphincter pressure of mothers in established labor or during anesthesia.

Mechanically preventing reflux at the gastroesophageal junction with the use of a cuffed esophageal catheter placed in the stomach[75] and more recently with nasogastric balloon catheters has been described.[76] Although not studied in the obstetric population, it is unlikely to gain much popularity, as Holdsworth[45] reported that more than 50% of his awake parturients found the insertion of a stomach tube "very unpleasant."

Cricoid Pressure. Cricoid pressure is a maneuver whereby digitally applied pressure on the cricoid cartilage posteriorly against the cervical vertebral body temporarily occludes the upper end of the esophagus. This was first described in 1961 by Sellick[77] and has been advocated as a means of preventing gastric or esophageal contents from reaching the oropharynx and also of preventing gastric distention[78] when the lungs are ventilated by intermittent positive pressure.

Using this maneuver Sellick[77] was able to prevent regurgitation even with esophageal pressure up to 100 cm H_2O. There are reports, however, of pulmonary aspiration even when cricoid pressure was applied.[79, 80] These were attributed to wrong technique or inadequate force during the application.[81] The force required has been determined[82] as equivalent to 44 N, although Vanner and colleagues[83] in more recent studies have found that 40 N was more than adequate to induce an upper esophageal sphincter pressure of 38 mm Hg (median awake upper esophageal sphincter pressure). There is no regurgitation when upper esophageal sphincter pressure is greater than 35 mm Hg.[83] The Triennial Report on Maternal Deaths[8] recommends the use of two hands, one to press on the cricoid cartilage and the other to maintain the head in the proper position for intubation. Sellick[84] also recommends that the onset of unconsciousness, the achievement of muscle relaxation, and the application of cricoid pressure be timed to occur simultaneously. The teaching of proper application of cricoid pressure with the correct force is advocated,[81] so that it can be used as a second line of defense against stomach contents entering the oropharynx.

It may sometimes be necessary to apply cricoid pressure in the presence of nasogastric tubes inserted in an attempt to empty the stomach to reduce the risk of regurgitation. Salem and coworkers[47] found that cricoid pressure is effective under such situations in sealing the esophagus around the nasogastric tube even when the intraesophageal pressure has been increased to 100 cm H_2O. Therefore some suggest that it is unnecessary to withdraw the nasogastric tube before induction of anesthesia, and if the tube is left vented it may limit the increase of intragastric pressure.[47]

Cricoid pressure is known to distort the upper

airway[8, 85] making laryngoscopy and intubation difficult. Brimacombe and Berry[85] suggest that if a Cormack and Lehane Grade 3 (only epiglottis visible) or Grade 4 (even epiglottis not visible) laryngoscopic view is seen, cricoid pressure should be reduced to 20 N for a few seconds under direct vision and with suction ready for a repeat attempt at intubation.

Strategies to Protect the Airway

Use of Regional Anesthesia. Regional anesthesia is considered safer than general anesthesia in the obstetric patient. This has been borne out by most of the anesthetic mortality figures in the Triennial Report since the 1980s[5, 8, 13, 86–88] when regional anesthesia for obstetric patients became popular. Most of the deaths associated with anesthesia occurred in patients undergoing general anesthesia. In the triennium 1988 to 1990 there were 15 deaths associated (either directly or indirectly) with anesthesia in the United Kingdom; 11 of these were due to general anesthesia and only 4 were due to regional anesthesia. None of the 4 regional anesthesia deaths had pulmonary aspiration as a cause of death, while 6 of the 11 general anesthesia deaths were variously suspected or confirmed to have had aspiration as a complication.[5]

The obvious advantage of regional anesthesia is the awake patient, in whom protective upper airway reflexes are maintained, minimizing the risk of aspiration. However, aspiration may still occur in the conduct of regional anesthesia in the presence of local anesthetic toxicity, high or total blockade, and if associated with severe hypotension.

Competent Administration of General Anesthesia. General anesthesia is still the most common mode of anesthesia for the emergency cesarean section worldwide.[51, 89] In the Triennial Report of 1988 to 1991 there were 6 deaths in which aspiration of gastric contents was suspected, and all these cases were done under emergency general anesthesia.[5] Similarly, in the 1981 survey of the Society of Obstetric Anesthesia and Perinatology in which 21 cases of pulmonary aspiration were reported, all the patients had undergone general anesthesia, of which 15 inductions were for emergency cesarean section.[10] If the incidence of pulmonary aspiration of gastric contents is to be reduced, competent administration of general anesthesia, especially under emergency situations, must be sought for.

General anesthesia for emergency cesarean section must therefore be of the same standard as that for elective cesarean section. Some considerations for the safe provision of general anesthesia for the obstetric patient include having a proper evaluation of the parturient's airway,[90] the administration of acid aspiration prophylaxis, having functioning equipment,[91] the correct maintenance of cricoid pressure by a skilled assistant,[77] rapid-sequence induction and intubation with properly cuffed[92] endotracheal tubes, having a preplanned approach to the management of difficult and failed intubation,[10] making an attempt to empty the stomach before induction[5] or at least before extubation in nonfasted parturients,[48] and having a trained or closely supervised anesthetic trainee of adequate experience to administer the anesthetic.[93]

General anesthesia if used for surgery during the second and third trimester,[94, 95] as well as for immediate postpartum surgery,[96, 97] should follow the same standard as for general anesthesia for cesarean section. James and colleagues[98] found that 60% of his postpartum patients had gastric contents that, if aspirated, would cause significant aspiration pneumonitis.

Rational Approach to Difficult or Failed Intubation. Aspiration is noted to occur more frequently in the presence of a difficult or failed intubation.[10] Thus, in 1976 when Tunstall[99] provided some direction in the management of failed intubation with his failed intubation drill, it was rapidly adopted by most obstetric units. This protocol was useful, as his drill emphasized how to oxygenate the mother without exposing her to aspiration under such circumstances. The practicalities of ensuring oxygenation without aspiration, however, remained elusive. The failed intubation drill has since been revised[100] and modified.[101, 102]

The latest modification by Harmer[102] gives a chronologic approach to both difficult and failed intubation. It emphasizes oxygenation but also rationally defines the limits of the urgency of proceeding when the mother is ventilated without an adequately protected airway. His grading system[102] for when to commit the parturient to continued anesthesia when the airway is unprotected provides a very clear approach on how to minimize the risk of aspiration in the event of a difficult or failed intubation, two events that have been known to often occur together.[10]

In a parturient with a known "difficult airway" with a contraindication to regional anesthesia, fiberoptic awake intubation[103] should be considered for securing the airway.

MANAGEMENT

Suction. When aspiration is witnessed, as when it occurs during laryngoscopy and endotracheal intubation, suctioning should be attempted.[104] Suctioning aids in reducing the amount of material that causes lung damage. As pulmonary damage is almost instantaneous,[38] within 12 to 18 seconds of exposure of the lung to the gastric contents, it is important to suction before ventilating in order to minimize the dispersal of the inhaled material distally.

Bronchoscopy. Bronchoscopy is useful to remove solid material that causes significant obstruction in the airway[105, 106]; otherwise it has no role in the management of liquid aspiration.

Bronchial Lavage. Similarly, lavage with saline or alkali solution is not helpful to manage aspiration. Experimental studies on lavage in animals[107] have shown no improvement but rather worsening of lung damage. Gibbs and Modell[105] believe that lavage is useful only for removing inspissated secretions or particulate matter obstructing the conducting airway.

Improving Lung Function. Changes in pulmonary function following aspiration are related to the quantity and acidity of aspirated gastric contents and evolve with time, reaching a peak at 4 hours.[32] It is imperative to monitor respiratory function frequently for signs of tachypnea, crepitations, wheezing, atelectasis, consolidation, and arterial oxygen desaturation. The patient should be admitted to a high dependency area. There is a time lag between the fall of arterial oxygen tension (PaO_2) and the arterial oxygen saturation measured by pulse oximetry. Pulse oximetry may be insufficient to reveal worsening shunting or widening alveolar-arterial oxygen tension difference in the presence of atelectasis, consolidation, and interstitial or alveolar edema. It should not be relied on as the major method of respiratory monitoring.

In mild cases with minimal clinical and radiologic evidence of atelectasis, consolidation, and interstitial pulmonary edema, gas exchange is usually preserved. In the absence of signs of respiratory distress or arterial desaturation, oxygen therapy via a face mask in addition to continued respiratory monitoring may be sufficient.

If atelectasis or consolidation is present in the dependent lung zones, alveolar recruitment is necessary to optimize ventilation-perfusion matching and to prevent a widening alveolar-arterial oxygen gradient and progression of acute lung injury. This can be achieved with the use of continuous positive airway pressure up to 12 to 14 mm Hg via a tightly fitting mask.[105] Optimal results are obtained in patients who are alert, cooperative, and have an unobstructed airway.[105]

Ventilation. Experimental studies by Chapman[108] and Cameron[109] and their colleagues indicated that immediate positive-pressure ventilation even for a few hours improved survival. Toussaint and coworkers[110] noted improved survival even on air in animals receiving positive-pressure ventilation. The common factor of positive airway pressure may be important in the recruitment of alveoli for optimal lung function following the damage.

The patient who is unable to maintain a patent airway, is not alert or cooperative, and has clinical and radiologic evidence of significant pulmonary aspiration, or worsening gas exchange in response to the previously mentioned therapy requires intubation and mechanical ventilation.[105] In Olsson's series[1] 17% of his patients required ventilation. The mode chosen must be individualized[105, 111] to meet the needs of the patient in the process of alveolar recruitment,[109] minimize the effects on the cardiovascular system, and minimize the risk of ventilator-associated lung injury.

Repeated opening and closing of alveoli in the dependent lung region during mechanical ventilation has been recognized as an important contributor to maintaining and aggravating the lung injury.[112] Animal studies have demonstrated that a ventilation approach limiting peak inspiratory pressures, using positive end-expiratory pressure (PEEP) to maintain an open lung and limiting tidal volumes, minimizes lung injury with acceptable gas exchange.[113] A similar strategy of limitation of peak inspiratory pressure and reduction of regional lung overdistention by the use of low tidal volumes with permissive hypercapnia has reduced ventilator-induced lung injury and improved outcome in humans.[114] A recent randomized clinical study from Amato[115] and colleagues has demonstrated that using an open lung approach with volume- and pressure-limited strategy markedly improves lung function in patients with acute respiratory distress syndrome, with earlier weaning and improved chances of lung recovery as well as a decrease in mortality.

Close monitoring of the oxygenation, keeping the inspired oxygen as low as possible to maintain acceptable alveolar-arterial oxygen gradient or PaO_2/FIO_2 ratio, and the avoidance of pulmonary oxygen toxicity is important. Djalal and colleagues[116] in their experimental studies on rats with induced acid aspiration demonstrated worse lung injury in rats exposed to unnecessarily high levels of oxygen after injury.

Fluid Therapy. Large volumes of fluid are lost in the lungs because of pulmonary aspiration,[32, 34] and these must be replaced. Monitoring of the fluid status with central venous pressure monitoring and even pulmonary artery occlusion pressure monitoring may be warranted in more severe cases to guide hydration.

Use of Steroids. Steroids have been used in the past as part of the treatment regimen for pulmonary aspiration of gastric contents.[38] This was based mainly on the theoretical consideration that steroids could reduce the inflammatory response. The studies suggesting that steroids may be useful in reducing the pulmonary effects of gastric aspiration[38, 107] were not conducted in a controlled manner. In addition, there was no improvement in the survival rate of animals given steroids.[107]

From the 1970s onward, properly controlled studies showed no difference in the physiologic and pathologic consequences of pulmonary aspiration[117, 118] as well as the survival between animals treated with steroids compared with those not treated. There was no demonstrable beneficial effect of steroids even when the severity of the pulmonary aspiration was varied.[117, 118] Steroid therapy suppresses neutrophil and macrophage activation and increases the risk of secondary bacterial infection. Steroids are currently not recommended as part of the treatment regimen for pulmonary aspiration of gastric contents.[105]

Use of Antibiotics. In experimental models of pulmonary aspiration of gastric contents, infection is not a feature of the acute lung injury.[11, 34] In Lewis's series[119] of 18 patients who had aspiration pneumonitis, only 3 of 15 patients (whose sputum culture was available at the onset of the illness) had positive sputum culture. In addition, his series[119] contained subgroups of patients who had been hospitalized for prolonged periods. In spite of prophylactic antibiotics, 13 of his 15 patients developed infection, and in 4 of

❖ SUMMARY

Key Points

- Pulmonary aspiration of gastric contents is a potential threat to every parturient.
- Failed intubation and aspiration continue to cause morbidity and mortality. Aspiration most often occurs during emergency cesarean section with the patient under general anesthesia, especially in situations in which difficult or failed intubation is encountered.
- Measures for preventing aspiration focus on the reduction of the use of general anesthesia, administration of a clear antacid, and restriction of oral intake during labor.
- PEEP is the treatment of choice for aspiration-induced hypoxia.

Key References

Mendelson CL: The aspiration of stomach contents into the lungs during obstetric anesthesia. Am J Obstet Gynecol 1946; 52:191–205.

Olsson GL, Hallen B, Hambraeus-Jonzon K: A computer-aided study of 185,358 anaesthetics. Acta Anaesthesiol Scand 1986; 30:84–92.

Case Stem

A 30-year-old obese primigravida was admitted to the labor ward in active labor after eating a large meal. One hour later, the obstetrician requests an urgent cesarean section for fetal bradycardia. Following induction of general anesthesia, the cords could not be visualized and several attempts at intubation failed. The anesthesiologist tries again and observes vomitus in the airway. Discuss the anesthetic management of the "failed intubation" and aspiration.

these, the organisms were resistant to the antibiotics that had been administered.

The more rational approach would be to avoid the use of prophylactic antibiotics[104, 119]; to monitor for signs of fever, tachycardia, leukocytosis, and sputum production; and to initiate antibiotic therapy based on positive cultures or significant worsening in clinical status and radiologic findings.

References

1. Olsson GL, Hallen B, Hambraeus-Jonzon: Aspiration during anaesthesia: a computer-aided study of 185,358 anaesthetics. Acta Anaesthesiol Scand 1986; 30:84–92.
2. Landay MJ, Christensen EE, Bynum LJ: Pulmonary manifestations of acute aspiration of gastric contents. Am J Roentgenol 1978; 131:587–592.
3. Kaunitz AM, Hughes JM, Grimes DA, et al: Causes of maternal mortality in the United States. Obstet Gynecol 1985; 65:605–612.
4. Cameron JL, Mitchell WH, Zuidema GD: Aspiration pneumonia: clinical outcome following documented aspiration. Arch Surg 1973; 106:49–52.
5. Report on Confidential Enquiries into Maternal Deaths in the United Kingdom, 1988–1990. London: Her Majesty's Stationery Office; 1994.
6. Report on Confidential Enquiries into Maternal Deaths in England and Wales, 1952–1954. London: Her Majesty's Stationery Office; 1957.
7. Douglas KA, Redman CWG: Eclampsia in the United Kingdom. BMJ 1994; 309:1395–1400.
8. Turnbull AC, Tindall VR, Beard RW, et al: Report on Confidential Enquiries into Maternal Deaths in England and Wales, 1982–1984. London: Her Majesty's Stationery Office; 1989.
9. Arms RA, Dines DE, Tinstman TC: Aspiration pneumonia. Chest 1974; 65:136–139.
10. Gibbs CP, Rolbin SH, Norman P: Cause and prevention of maternal aspiration. Anesthesiology 1984; 61:111–112.
11. Mendelson CL: The aspiration of stomach contents into the lungs during obstetric anesthesia. Am J Obstet Gynecol 1946; 52:191–205.
12. Warner MA, Warner ME, Weber JG: Clinical significance of pulmonary aspiration during the perioperative period. Anesthesiology 1993; 78:56–62.
13. Hibbard BM, Anderson MM, Drife JO, et al: Report on Confidential Enquiries into Maternal Deaths in the United Kingdom, 1991–1993. London: Her Majesty's Stationery Office; 1996.
14. Dalina AM, Inbasegaran K: Anaesthetic related maternal deaths in Malaysia—a review. Med J Malaysia 1996; 51:52–63.
15. Smith ID, Bogod DG: Feeding in labour. *In* Bogod DG (ed): Baillieres Clin Anaesthesiol 1995; 9:735–747.
16. Roberts RB, Shirley MA: Reducing the risk of acid aspiration during cesarean section. Anaesth Analg 1974; 53:859–868.
17. Van Thiel DH, Gavaler JS, Shobha AB, et al: Heartburn of pregnancy. Gastroenterology 1977; 72:666–668.
18. Hey VMF, Cowley DJ, Ganguli PC, et al: Gastro-oesophageal reflux in late pregnancy. Anaesthesia 1977; 32:372–377.
19. Vanner RG, Goodman NW: Gastro-oesophageal reflux in pregnancy at term and after delivery. Anaesthesiology 1989; 44:808–811.
20. Nimmo WS, Wilson J, Prescott LF: Narcotic analgesics and delayed gastric emptying during labour. Lancet 1975; 1:890–893.
21. Holdsworth JD: Relationship between stomach contents and analgesia in labour. Br J Anaesth 1978; 50:1145–1148.
22. Wright PMC, Allen RW, Moore J, et al: Gastric emptying during lumbar extradural analgesia in labour: effect of fentanyl supplementation. Br J Anaesth 1992; 68:248–251.
23. Spence AA, Moir DD, Finlay WEI: Observations on intragastric pressure. Anaesthesia 1967; 22:249–256.
24. Simpson KH, Stakes AF, Miller M: Pregnancy delays paracetamol absorption and gastric emptying in patients undergoing surgery. Br J Anaesth 1988; 60:24–27.
25. Carp H, Jayaram A, Stoll M: Ultrasound examination of the stomach contents of parturients. Anesth Analg 1992; 74:683–687.
26. Taylor G, Pryse-Davies J: The prophylactic use of antacids in the prevention of the acid-pulmonary-aspiration syndrome (Mendelson's syndrome). Lancet 1966; 1:288–291.
27. Lyons G: Failed intubation: six years' experience in a teaching maternity unit. Anaesthesia 1985; 40:759–762.
28. Teabeaut JR: Aspiration of gastric contents: an experimental study. Am J Pathol 1952; 28:51–67.
29. Schwartz DJ, Wynne JW, Gibbs CP: The pulmonary consequences of aspiration of gastric contents at pH values greater than 2.5. Am Rev Respir Dis 1980; 121:119–126.
30. Raidoo DM, Rocke DA, Brock-Utne JG, et al: Critical volume for pulmonary acid aspiration: reappraisal in a primate model. Br J Anaesth 1990; 65:248–250.
31. James CF, Modell JH, Gibbs CP, et al: Pulmonary aspiration—effects of volume and pH in the rat. Anaesth Analg 1984; 63:665–668.
32. Kennedy TP, Johnson KJ, Kunkel RG, et al: Acute acid aspiration lung injury in the rat: biphasic pathogenesis. Anesth Analg 1989; 69:87–92.
33. Greenfield LJ, Singleton RP, McCaffree DR, et al: Pulmonary effects of experimental graded aspiration of hydrochloric acid. Ann Surg 1969; 170:74–86.

34. Awe WC, Fletcher WS, Jacob SW: The pathophysiology of aspiration pneumonitis. Surgery 1966; 60:232–239.
35. Cameron JL, Caldini P, Toung JK, et al: Aspiration pneumonia: physiologic data following experimental aspiration. Surgery 1972; 72:238:245.
36. Booth DJ, Zuidema GD, Cameron JL: Aspiration pneumonia: pulmonary arteriography after experimental aspiration. J Surg Res 1972; 12:48–52.
37. Bynum LJ, Pierce AK: Pulmonary aspiration of gastric contents. Am Rev Respir Dis 1976; 114:1129–1136.
38. Hamelberg W, Bosomworth PP: Aspiration pneumonitis: experimental studies and clinical observations. Anaesth Analg 1964; 43:669–677.
39. Crawford JS: Maternal mortality from Mendelson's syndrome. Lancet 1986; 1:920–921.
40. Lewis M, Crawford JS: Can one risk fasting the obstetric patient for less than 4 hours? Br J Anaesth 1987; 59:312–314.
41. Elkington KW: At the water's edge: where obstetrics and anaesthesia meet. Obstet Gynecol 1991; 77:304–308.
42. Michael S, Reilly CS: Policies for oral intake during labour: a survey of maternity units in England and Wales. Anaesthesia 1991; 46:1071–1073.
43. Hauth JC, Merenstein GB (eds): Guidelines for Perinatal Care, 4th ed. Elk Grove Village, IL: American Academy of Pediatrics and American College of Obstetricians and Gynecologists; 1997.
44. Brock-Utne JG, Rout C, Moodley J, et al: Does pre-operative gastric emptying decrease the risk of acid aspiration in obstetrical anesthesia? (A study of gastric acidity and volume at emergency cesarean section) [abstract]. Anesth Analg 1989; 68:S39.
45. Holdsworth JD, Furness RMB, Roulston RG: A comparison of apomorphine and stomach tubes for emptying the stomach before general anaesthesia in obstetrics. Br J Anaesth 1974; 46:526–529.
46. Macdonald AG: The gastric acid problem. *In* Atkinson RS, Adams AP (eds): Recent Advances in Anaesthesia and Analgesia, No. 15. Edinburgh: Churchill Livingstone; 1985:107–131.
47. Salem MR, Joseph NJ, Heyman HJ, et al: Cricoid compression is effective in obliterating the esophageal lumen in the presence of a nasogastric tube. Anesthesiology 1983; 63:443–446.
48. May AE: The Confidential Enquiry into Maternal Deaths, 1988–1990. Br J Anaesth 1994; 73:129–131.
49. Crawford JS: The anaesthetist's contribution to maternal mortality. Br J Anaesth 1970; 40:70–73.
50. Burgess RW, Crowhurst JA: Acid aspiration prophylaxis in Australian obstetric hospitals—a survey. Anaesth Intens Care 1989; 17:492–495.
51. Grieff JMC, Tordoff SG, Griffiths R, et al: Acid aspiration prophylaxis in 202 obstetric anaesthetic units in the UK. Int J Obstet Anesth 1994; 3:137–142.
52. Gibbs CP, Schwartz DJ, Wynne JW, et al: Antacid pulmonary aspiration in the dog. Anesthesiology 1979; 51:380–385.
53. Holdsworth JD, Johnson K, Mascall G, et al: Mixing of antacids with stomach contents. Anaesthesia 1980; 35:641–650.
54. Lahiri SK, Thomas TA, Hodgson RMH: Single-dose antacid therapy for the prevention of Mendelson's syndrome. Br J Anaesth 1973; 45:1143–1146.
55. Viegas OJ, Ravindran RS, Stoops CA: Duration of efficacy of sodium citrate as an antacid [abstract]. Anaesth Analg 1982; 61:220.
56. Viegas OJ, Ravindran RS, Shumacker CA: Gastric fluid pH in patients receiving sodium citrate. Anaesth Analg 1981; 60:521–523.
57. Hester JB, Heath ML: Pulmonary acid aspiration syndrome: should prophylaxis be routine? Br J Anaesth 1977; 49:595–599.
58. Chan YK: A comparison of sodium citrate and sodium citrate–ranitidine combination for acid aspiration prophylaxis. Med J Malaysia 1992; 47:27–30.
59. Colman RD, Frank M, Loughnan BA, et al: Use of I.M. ranitidine for the prophylaxis of aspiration pneumonitis in obstetrics. Br J Anaesth 1988; 61:720–729.
60. Durrant JM, Strunin L: Comparative trial of the effect of ranitidine and cimetidine on gastric secretion in fasting patients at induction of anaesthesia. Can Anaesth Soc J 1982; 29:446–451.
61. Gallagher EG, White M, Ward S, et al: Prophylaxis against acid aspiration syndrome. Anaesthesia 1988; 43:1011–1014.
62. Lin CJ, Huang CL, Hsu HW, et al: Prophylaxis against acid aspiration in regional anaesthesia for elective caesarean section: a comparison between oral single-dose ranitidine, famotidine and omeprazole assessed with fiberoptic gastric aspiration. Acta Anaesthesiol Sin 1996; 34:179–184.
63. Camarri E, Chirone E, Fanteria G, et al: Ranitidine induced bradycardia [letter]. Lancet 1982; 2:160.
64. Brock-Utne JG, Dow TGB, Welman S, et al: The effect of metoclopramide on the lower oesophageal sphincter in late pregnancy. Anaesth Intens Care 1978; 6:26–29.
65. Schulze-Delrieu K: Drug therapy: metoclopramide. New Engl J Med 1981; 305:28–33.
66. Howard FA, Sharp DS: Effect of metoclopramide on gastric emptying during labour. BMJ 1973; 1:446–448.
67. Olsson GL, Hallen B: Pharmacological evacuation of the stomach with metoclopramide. Acta Anaesth Scand 1982; 26:417–420.
68. Cohen SE, Jasson J, Talafre ML, et al: Does metoclopramide decrease the volume of gastric contents in patients undergoing cesarean section? Anaesthesiology 1984; 61:604–607.
69. Orr DA, Bill KM, Gillon KRW, et al: Effects of omeprazole, with and without metoclopramide, in elective obstetric anaesthesia. Anaesthesia 1993; 48:114–119.
70. Yau G, Kan AF, Gin T, et al: A comparison of omeprazole and ranitidine for prophylaxis against aspiration pneumonitis in emergency caesarean section. Anaesthesia 1992; 47:101–104.
71. Moore J, Flynn RJ, Sampaio M, et al: Effect of single-dose omeprazole on intragastric acidity and volume during obstetric anaesthesia. Anaesthesia 1989; 44:559–562.
72. Rocke DA, Rout CC, Gouws E: Intravenous administration of the proton pump inhibitor omeprazole reduces the risk of acid aspiration at emergency cesarean section. Anesth Analg 1994; 78:1093–1098.
73. Cotton BR, Smith G: Regurgitation and aspiration. *In* Kaufman L (ed): Anaesthesia: Review 2. Edinburgh: Churchill Livingstone; 1984:162.
74. Brock-Utne JG, Rubin J, Dowing JW, et al: The administration of metoclopramide with atropine. Anaesthesia 1976; 31:1186–1190.
75. Zohairy AFM: Prevention of regurgitation during induction of anaesthesia with a cuffed oesophageal catheter. BMJ 1967; 1:545–546.
76. Roewer N: Can pulmonary aspiration of gastric contents be prevented by balloon occlusion of the cardia? A study with a new nasogastric tube. Anesth Analg 1995; 80:378–383.
77. Sellick BA: Cricoid pressure to control regurgitation of stomach contents during induction of anaesthesia. Lancet 1961; 2:404–406.
78. Lawes EG, Campbell I, Mercer D: Inflation pressure, gastric insufflation and rapid sequence induction. Br J Anaesth 1987; 59:315–318.
79. Whittington RM, Robinson JS, Thompson JM: Fatal aspiration (Mendelson's) syndrome despite antacids and cricoid pressure. Lancet 1979; 2:228–230.
80. Schwartz DJ, Matthay MA, Cohen NH: Death and other complications of emergency airway management in critically ill adults. Anesthesiology 1995; 82:367–376.
81. Howells TH, Chamney AR, Wraight WJ, et al: The application of cricoid pressure: an assessment and a survey of its practice. Anaesthesia 1983; 38:457–460.
82. Wraight WJ, Chamney AR, Howells TH: The determination of an effective cricoid pressure. Anaesthesia 1983; 38:461–466.
83. Vanner RG, O'Dwyer JP, Pryle BJ, et al: Upper oesophageal sphincter pressure and the effect of cricoid pressure. Anaesthesia 1992; 47:95–100.
84. Sellick BA: Rupture of the oesophagus following cricoid pressure? Anaesthesia 1982; 37:213–214.
85. Brimacombe JR, Berry AM: Cricoid pressure. Can J Anaesth 1997; 44:414–425.

86. Tomkinson J, Turnbull A, Robson G, et al: Report on Confidential Enquiries into Maternal Deaths in England and Wales, 1976–1978. London: Her Majesty's Stationery Office; 1982.
87. Turnbull A, Tindall VR, Robson G, et al: Report on Confidential Enquiries into Maternal Deaths in England and Wales, 1979–1981. London: Her Majesty's Stationery Office; 1986.
88. Tindall VR, Beard RW, Sykes MK, et al: Report on Confidential Enquiries into Maternal Deaths in the United Kingdom, 1985–1987. London: Her Majesty's Stationery Office; 1991.
89. Russell IF: Anaesthesia for emergency caesarean section. Curr Anaesth Crit Care 1995; 6:202–205.
90. Chestnut DH: Anesthesia for fetal distress. *In* Chestnut DH (ed): Obstetric Anaesthesia: Principles and Practice. St. Louis: CV Mosby; 1994:487.
91. Moir DD: Maternal mortality and anaesthesia. Br J Anaesth 1980; 52:1–3.
92. Bernhard WN, Cottrell JE, Sivakumaran C, et al: Adjustment of intracuff pressure to prevent aspiration. Anesthesiology 1979; 50:363–366.
93. Thomas TA: Anaesthesia and Maternal Mortality. Curr Anaesth Crit Care 1991; 2:85–91.
94. Cohen SE: Nonobstetric surgery during pregnancy. *In* Chestnut DH (ed): Obstetric Anaesthesia: Principles and Practice. St. Louis, CV Mosby; 1994:273.
95. Peterson HB, DeStefano F, Rubin GL, et al: Deaths attributable to tubal sterilization in the United States, 1977 to 1981. Am J Obstet Gynecol 1983; 146:131–136.
96. Hawkins J: Postpartum tubal sterilisation. *In* Chestnut DH (ed): Obstetric Anaesthesia: Principles and Practice. St. Louis, CV Mosby; 1994:443.
97. Bogod DG: The postpartum stomach—when is it safe? Anaesthesia 1994; 49:1–2.
98. James CF, Gibbs CP, Banner T: Postpartum perioperative risk of aspiration pneumonia. Anesthesiology 1984; 61:756–759.
99. Tunstall ME: Failed intubation drill. Anaesthesia 1976; 31:850.
100. Tunstall ME, Geddes C: Failed intubation in obstetric anaesthesia: an indication for use of the "esophageal gastric tube airway." Br J Anaesth 1984; 56:659–661.
101. Davies JM, Weeks S, Crone LA: Difficult intubation in the parturient. Can J Anaesth 1989; 36:668–674.
102. Harmer M: Review: Difficult and failed intubation in obstetrics. Int J Obstet Anesth 1997; 6:25–31.
103. Edwards RM: Fibreoptic intubation: a solution to failed intubation in a parturient? Anaesth Intens Care 1994; 22:718–719.
104. Bartlett JG, Gorbach SL: The triple threat of aspiration pneumonia. Chest 1975; 68:560–566.
105. Gibbs CP, Modell JH: Pulmonary aspiration of gastric contents: pathophysiology, prevention and management. *In* Miller RD (ed): Anesthesia, 4th ed, Vol 2. New York; Churchill Livingstone; 1994:1437–1464.
106. Wynne JW, Modell JH: Respiratory aspiration of stomach contents. Ann Intern Med 1977; 87:466–474.
107. Bannister WK, Sattilaro AJ, Otis RD: Therapeutic aspects of aspiration pneumonitis in experimental animals. Anesthesiology 1961; 22:440–443.
108. Chapman RL, Modell JH, Ruiz BC, et al: Effect of continuous positive-pressure ventilation and steroids on aspiration of hydrochloric acid (pH 1.8) in dogs. Anaesth Analg 1974; 53:556–562.
109. Cameron JL, Sebor J, Anderson RP, et al: Aspiration pneumonia: results of treatment by positive-pressure ventilation in dogs. J Surg Res 1968; 8:447–457.
110. Touissant GPM, Chiu CJ, Hampson LG: Experimental aspiration pneumonia: hemodynamics, ventilator and membrane oxygenator support. J Surg Res 1974; 16:324–329.
111. Van Hook JW: Acute respiratory distress syndrome in pregnancy. Semin Perinatol 1997; 21:320–327.
112. Dreyfuss D, Soler P, Basset G, et al: High inflation pressure pulmonary edema: respective effects of high airway pressure, high tidal volume and positive end-expiratory pressure. Am Rev Respir Dis 1988; 137:1159–1164.
113. Muscedere JG, Mullen JBM, Gan K, et al: Tidal ventilation at low airway pressures can augment lung injury. Am J Respir Crit Care Med 1994; 149:1327–1334.
114. Hickling KG, Walsh J, Henderson S, et al: Low mortality rate in adult respiratory distress syndrome using low-volume, pressure-limited ventilation with permissive hypercapnia: a prospective study. Crit Care Med 1994; 22:1568–1578.
115. Amato MBP, Barbas CSV, Medeiros DM, et al: Beneficial effects of the "open lung approach" with low distending pressures in acute respiratory distress syndrome. Am J Respir Crit Care Med 1995; 152:1835–1846.
116. Djalal NN, Knight PR, Davidson BA, et al: Hypoxia exacerbates microvascular lung injury following acid aspiration. Chest 1997; 112:1607–1614.
117. Chapman RL, Downs JB, Modell JH, et al: The ineffectiveness of steroid therapy in treating aspiration of hydrochloric acid. Arch Surg 1974; 108:858–861.
118. Downs JB, Chapman RL, Modell JH, et al: An evaluation of steroid therapy in aspiration pneumonitis. Anesthesiology 1974; 40:129–135.
119. Lewis RT, Burgess JH, Hampson LG: Cardiorespiratory studies in critical illness. Arch Surg 1971; 103:335–340.

34

Allergic Reactions

❖ PAMELA J. MORGAN, MD, CCFP, FRCPC

IMMUNOLOGY OF ALLERGIC REACTIONS

Allergy to an antigenic challenge may manifest as an immediate or a delayed reaction. The management of immediate-type allergic reactions may be challenging for the anesthesiologist since the nature and severity of the reaction requires instant recognition and treatment. Anaphylaxis, an immediate hypersensitivity reaction, produces secondary physiologic changes including upper airway obstruction secondary to edema; bronchoconstriction, which may be associated with dyspnea and wheezing; hypotension; and cardiovascular collapse. Cutaneous manifestations include pruritus, urticaria, and possibly angioedema. For a reaction to be considered allergic, it must be reproducible with antigen rechallenge and must involve antigen-antibody–effector cell interaction. Immediate hypersensitivity reactions develop within minutes of exposure, the reaction being initiated by humoral antibodies produced by B lymphocytes. This contrasts with delayed reactions, in which symptoms may not appear for hours or even days. Humoral antibodies are not involved in delayed reactions, in which the manifestations are initiated instead by T lymphocytes.[1]

Immediate Hypersensitivity Reaction. Host exposure to a polyvalent antigen, one capable of binding two or more adjacent immunoglobulin E (IgE) molecules, initiates the immediate hypersensitivity response.[2] IgE antibodies, located on mast cells and basophil surface membranes, undergo stereochemical changes and subsequently cause the release of vasoactive amines. These amines increase vascular permeability and open gaps between endothelial cells of postcapillary venules leading to edema formation. Exocrine gland secretion and smooth muscle contraction are also stimulated in the process.[1] Other reservoirs such as platelets and circulating basophils also react by the release of vasoactive amines (Fig. 34–1).

Mast cells are found in cutaneous tissue and in the mucosa of the gastrointestinal and respiratory tracts and contain histamine granules that are released in response to the offending antigen. The contribution of basophils to the hypersensitivity reaction has been well established. It is of interest to note that extracellular calcium concentration appears to play a significant role in the secretory mediator release by basophils and mast cells in the hypersensitivity response.[3, 4] The cellular influx of calcium initiates a cascade response (Fig. 34–2).

Pathophysiology. Immediate hypersensitivity reactions affect three main organ systems: respiratory, cardiovascular, and integumentary. The severity of the reaction may vary between individuals and the explanation for the differences is complex. The general physiologic condition of the host along with antigen concentration, mode of contact, the amount of cell-bound IgE, and the presence of inhibiting factors may all play a role.[5]

Polymorphonuclear leukocyte function is impaired during pregnancy, which may explain the increased incidence of infection.[6] Pregnancy by itself has not been demonstrated to be associated with suppression of autoantibody production.[7] Levels of IgA, IgG, and IgM are unchanged, and there is no evidence that pregnancy alters the host response to antigen exposure.[8]

Respiratory System. Respiratory changes that develop during pregnancy are important considerations for the obstetric anesthesiologist. Mucosal engorgement occurs in all parts of the respiratory tract. Swelling of the airway may ultimately involve the larynx and trachea, and this situation may worsen with respiratory infection or the edema associated with preeclampsia. Airway obstruction occurs more readily after induction of general anesthesia, and rapid and severe hypoxemia can occur. Owing to laryngeal swelling, endotracheal intubation using a small endotracheal tube is recommended to avoid trauma. The airway edema that is associated with an immediate allergic reaction in a parturient can cause life-threatening airway obstruction necessitating definitive and rapid tracheal intubation. The combination of a 20% decrease in functional residual capacity and a 40% to 60% increase in oxygen consumption places the parturient at risk for the rapid development of hypoxemia if the patency of the airway and maintenance of ventilation is threatened.[9] Apnea on induction of anesthesia results in a twofold faster fall in PaO_2 in a pregnant versus a nonpregnant woman.[10] Other respiratory changes include dilatation

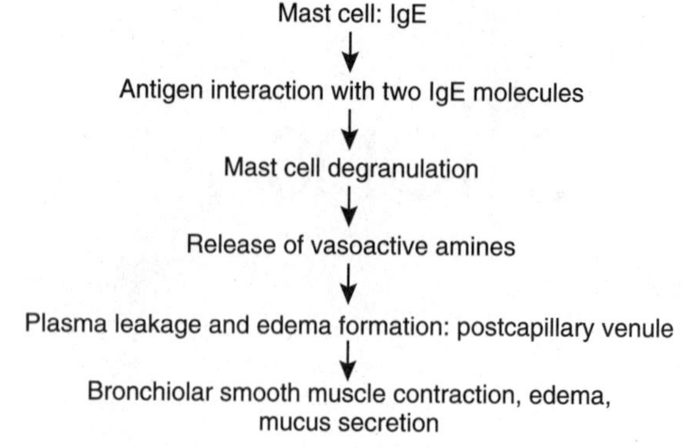

Figure 34–1 Cellular activation in the immediate hypersensitivity reaction.

of the large airways below the larynx as well as a 45% increase in minute and alveolar ventilation.[11]

Airway obstruction and edema are the hallmark respiratory effects of an anaphylactic reaction. Multiple mediators are responsible for the development of smooth muscle constriction, edema, and mucus formation. Histamine (H_1 effect), leukotrienes C_4, D_4, and E_4, prostaglandin $F_{2\alpha}$, thromboxane A_2, bradykinin, and platelet-activating factor (PAF) are responsible for the hypersensitivity-associated bronchospasm.[12] Airway inflammation results from the effect of chemotactic factors, leukotriene B_4, and PAF, and mucosal edema mediators include histamine, leukotrienes, prostaglandin E_2, bradykinin, and PAF.[12] It is important to understand the mediators involved since the process may be reversible if mediator-directed pharmacotherapy is initiated.

Cardiovascular System. The physiologic changes in the cardiovascular system during normal pregnancy are an attempt to accommodate the needs of the fetus and the associated maternal blood loss at delivery. Significant increases occur in blood volume (35%), cardiac output (50%), stroke volume (25%), and heart rate (25%). Further increases in cardiac output occur with labor and delivery, with increases of 80% over prepregnancy values occurring during the second stage of labor. Systemic vascular resistance falls by about 15%, which may be reflected by lower systemic arterial blood pressure during pregnancy.[13] One of the most significant findings in the parturient is the development of hypotension associated with pallor, diaphoresis, nausea, vomiting, dizziness, or confusion when the mother adopts the supine position. Compression of the inferior vena cava and its branches by the gravid uterus may impair venous return from the lower half of the body. Some blood is shunted through the epidural veins to the azygos system and then to the heart, reducing the amplitude of the associated hypotension. However, the combination of an elevated venous pressure and compression of the aorta leads to a fall in uterine perfusion pressure. Events that cause vasodilation further decrease venous return producing further deterioration in an already compromised uteroplacental unit. The presence of a sympathetic block with regional anesthesia (epidural or spinal) prevents maternal compensation through peripheral vasoconstriction. It is imperative, therefore, to avoid the development of the supine hypotensive syndrome by ensuring that the patient is placed in the lateral position or that 15 to 30 degrees of left uterine displacement is implemented.

The same mediators involved in the respiratory effects of the allergic response play a part in the cardiovascular system changes. In addition to the previously mentioned mediator substances, mediators such as prostacyclin, histamine (H_2), kallikrein, and substance P cause vasodilation leading to the catastrophic cardiovascular effects.[2]

Indirect and direct effects of released mediators lead to pronounced vasodilation. The interaction of the endothelium and specific mediators produces endothelium-derived relaxing factor, and this in combination with the direct effects on vascular smooth muscle causes a significant fall in systemic vascular resistance and venous return. Factors responsible for the cardiovascular changes are summarized in Table 34–1.

Hemodynamic monitoring, specifically transesophageal echocardiography, has allowed a closer look at the immediate cardiovascular changes during an anaphylactic reaction. Increases in cardiac output, stroke volume, and ejection fraction were noted in a patient who developed an anaphylactic reaction to cefazolin.[14] The initial rise in these parameters may reflect the activation of the sympathetic response to histamine release and hypotension. Later in the course of the anaphylactic process, a fall in cardiac output (caused by the mechanisms described in Table 34–1) may occur and result in the classic shock syndrome associated with the allergic response. Ultimately, the effect of the complex interaction of vasoactive mediators depends on the physiological well-being of the

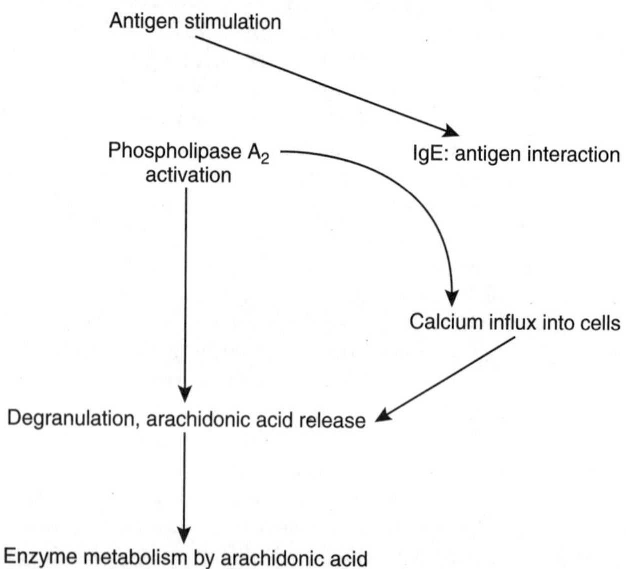

Figure 34–2 Role of calcium in mediator release.

Table 34-1 CARDIOVASCULAR CHANGES IN ANAPHYLAXIS

FACTOR	EFFECT
↓ Venous return, arrhythmias, hemoconcentration, right heart failure, ↑ PVR, hypotension leads to fall in coronary blood flow	↓ Cardiac output
Bronchospasm	↑ PVR
Hypotension	Myocardial ischemia
↑ PVR	RV failure
Thromboxane A_2	Coronary, pulmonary vasoconstriction
Increased capillary permeability	Pulmonary edema

PVR, pulmonary vascular resistance.

host and the variables that contribute to cardiac output.

Sympathetic blockade as produced by regional anesthetic techniques in labor and delivery can impair the parturient's response to vasodilation secondary to an allergic reaction. All of the cardiovascular changes occurring during an anaphylactic reaction may be significantly aggravated in the presence of a sympathetic block. It is crucial, therefore, to initiate aggressive resuscitation measures in a suspected hypersensitivity reaction in this situation. Further compromise of the uteroplacental unit must be offset by ensuring left uterine displacement to avoid compromise of venous return by the gravid uterus.

CUTANEOUS MANIFESTATIONS. Characteristic eruptions of well-circumscribed, discrete cutaneous wheals with erythematous, raised borders should alert the clinician to the development of an allergic reaction. Cutaneous mast cells located in the dermis are responsible for the typical wheal-and-flare eruption.[15] As the process begins to involve underlying tissue, edema results leading to a nonpitting, localized reaction known as angioedema. Periorbital, pharyngeal, and perioral areas may be involved in an asymmetric distribution. Gastrointestinal involvement also occurs, and significant loss of intravascular volume owing to the increased permeability of the vasculature in these areas may occur. Flushing, pruritus, tingling, or a feeling of warmth may accompany the cutaneous manifestations.

ALLERGY TO LOCAL ANESTHETICS

Local anesthetics are classified into two broad chemical groups, amides and esters. Ester agents such as procaine, cocaine, and tetracaine are derivatives of *p*-aminobenzoic acid (PABA). PABA occurs as a metabolite of these compounds and has been implicated as the agent responsible for allergic reactions to ester local anesthetics.[16] The amide group, which includes lidocaine, mepivacaine, prilocaine, and bupivacaine among others, is not metabolized to PABA and is therefore less likely to cause hypersensitivity reactions. True allergic reactions to local anesthetics are rare, and allergy to amides have been estimated to constitute less than 1% of all reactions to local anesthetic drugs.[17] It is important for the anesthesiologist to recognize other possible causes of reactions to local anesthetic agents. Patients who describe an "allergy" to these drugs may have experienced reactions to vasoconstrictor, methylparaben, or metabisulfite additives; a systemic toxic effect; or simply a vasovagal response. Without the accompanying hallmarks of a hypersensitivity reaction including skin, respiratory, and cardiovascular symptoms, the diagnosis of true local anesthetic allergy should be questioned.

Despite the fact that anaphylactic reactions to local anesthetic agents are unusual, there continue to be case reports in the literature describing reactions to these drugs.[18–23] Allergic reactions have occurred with the use of bupivacaine and prilocaine used as agents for infiltration, and with the use of intravenous regional anesthesia (Bier block), as well as epidural and spinal anesthesia for labor and delivery.[18–23] Erkkola and coworkers[20] reported a case of an allergic reaction to bupivacaine administered epidurally for labor analgesia. After incremental boluses of 0.5% bupivacaine totaling 8 mL given over a period of 1 hour and 45 minutes, hypotension, blood pressure of 60/40 mm Hg, tachycardia, and facial erythema were noted. Owing to severe fetal bradycardia, emergency cesarean section was performed. Immunologic studies demonstrated a rise in C3 activation products and a decrease in IgE. Serum bupivacaine levels were normal. Thomas and Caunt[21] reported on a patient who gave a past history of an allergic rash following cesarean section under epidural anesthesia with bupivacaine. The earlier allergic reaction had not been attributed to a local anesthetic allergy. Twenty-five minutes after receiving a total dose of 18 mL of epidural 0.5% bupivacaine for repeat cesarean section, the patient became hypotensive with a systolic blood pressure of 70 mm Hg and developed erythema and itchiness, with obvious swelling of the lips, eyelids, fingers, and toes. At birth, the infant was edematous and limp with cyanosis. Pulmonary edema was diagnosed. Plasma levels of IgE were moderately elevated. Skin testing in both of these cases proved negative for bupivacaine allergy. The second patient, however, was positive for lidocaine allergy.

A similar case is described by Allman.[22] An otherwise healthy woman developed urticaria, nausea, and edema during an elective cesarean section under epidural anesthesia with 0.5% bupivacaine. Follow-up included intradermal testing that was negative for bupivacaine and lidocaine. Forty minutes after spinal anesthesia was administered with 0.5% heavy bupivacaine for a repeat cesarean section, the patient became hypotensive, nauseated, itchy, and developed marked edema and erythema of the face and body. Immunoglobulin testing was performed but was unremarkable. The case reports cited here suggest local anesthetic allergy as the cause for the signs and symptoms that developed in each patient despite the fact that skin testing was negative for local anesthetic allergy. Whether these cases represent "true" local anesthetic allergic responses is unclear. Latex allergy may have been a causative factor.

In situations in which patients give a convincing history of allergic reactions to local anesthetics, it is suggested that another amide agent be used for subsequent procedures. There is, however, some recent evidence that cross-sensitivity may exist between local anesthetic agents in the amide group.[23] Further study is warranted to determine the validity of these findings.

Local Anesthetic Additives: Parabens and Metabisulfites. Parabens are used as bacteriostatic and fungistatic agents in a variety of products, among which are multidose parenteral preparations including local anesthetic drugs.[24] Hypersensitivity to these 1- to 4-carbon alkyl esters of *p*-hydroxybenzoic acid has been reported as early as 1940. Delayed hypersensitivity reactions to paraben esters were demonstrated in 3% of patients in a multicenter study of 1200 individuals.[25] PABA and parabens differ in their chemical structure only in that the parabens have a hydroxyl rather than an amino group in the *para* position.[24] Table 34–2 illustrates the chemical composition of some of the congeners of benzoic acid.

Recognition of hypersensitivity reactions to parabens and other additives such as sodium benzoate has led to the exclusion of these compounds from many local anesthetic preparations. Careful attention to drug labeling is necessary before use of local anesthetic agents for major regional anesthesia. Avoidance of preservative-containing drugs in these situations is prudent.

Metabisulfites are antioxidant agents used in many pharmaceutical compounds including some local anesthetic solutions. Sulfites have been reported to cause asthma, anaphylaxis, urticaria, hypotension, angioedema, and respiratory distress.[26] Previously documented "allergic" reactions to local anesthetic agents may well have represented hypersensitivity reactions to sulfite additives. Soulat and colleagues[27] reported a case of anaphylactoid shock during cesarean section under epidural anesthesia with 0.5% bupivacaine containing a metabisulfite additive. Systolic blood pressure fell to 60 mm Hg accompanied by a tachycardia of 120 beats/min. Generalized erythema and periorbital edema were also noted. Intravenous administration of epinephrine (100 μg), etilefrine infusion, and hydrocortisone resulted in return of cardiovascular stability. Subsequent skin testing proved positive for metabisulfite and negative for bupivacaine, latex, and oxytocin.

Table 34–2 CONGENERS OF BENZOIC ACID

Benzoic acid	H	C_6H_4	CO	OH
Methylparaben	HO	C_6H_4	CO	OCH_3
p-Aminobenzoic acid	NH_2	C_6H_4	CO	OH
Benzocaine	NH_2	C_6H_4	CO	OC_2H_5
Procaine	NH_2	C_6H_4	CO	$OC_2H_4N(C_2H_5)_2$

Modified from Nagel JE, Fuscaldo JT, Fireman P: Paraben allergy. JAMA 1977; 237:1594–1595.

Preservative-free local anesthetic solutions are available and recommended for use for epidural and spinal anesthesia. Again, close inspection of the drug label and its contents ensure the use of metabisulfite-free solutions.

Testing for Local Anesthetic Allergy. It is important to confirm the diagnosis of a true local anesthetic allergy so that the patient is not denied the beneficial aspects of local anesthetic use. In the pregnant population, the use of local anesthetic agents for regional anesthetic techniques is standard practice. To withhold pain management with these techniques because of an unclear reaction to previous local anesthetic exposure is unnecessary. Administration of general anesthesia for cesarean delivery to avoid local anesthetic exposure is fraught with danger.

The reliability of skin testing in the detection of "safe" and "unsafe" local anesthetic agents is confusing. Skin reactions to the intradermal injection of local anesthetics are typically graded according to the size of the wheal-and-flare response. Strongly positive reactions are characterized by larger wheals with surrounding erythema and pseudopods, and less positive reactions by smaller wheal size.[28] The actual size of the wheal in a "positive" reaction is variable, as is the volume of intradermal injectate. False-positive reactions occur with some frequency and various etiologies, with needle trauma, tissue distention, histamine release from skin puncture, and injectate additives all implicated.

Immediate-type allergic reactions appear to involve IgE-mediated mechanisms. However, there is some evidence to suggest the involvement of immune complex mechanisms in some local anesthetic reactions.[18, 29, 30] In two case reports, the patients also had evidence of an autoimmune disorder as evidenced by a positive antinuclear factor in one and rheumatoid arthritis in the other.[18, 29] Although this association has not been proved, antigen-antibody complex mechanisms may play a role in some local anesthetic reactions.[31]

Incremental subcutaneous or intramuscular challenge testing has been advocated as a more reliable test than intradermal skin testing for the evaluation of possible local anesthetic allergy.[31] If skin testing has proved negative in a patient with a strong history, a challenge test could then be performed. If the drug to which the patient reacted is known, a non–cross-reacting drug should be chosen, specifically the drug that may be used in the future. If prior drug exposure is unknown, lidocaine is generally used. Vasoconstrictors should be avoided and preservative-free solutions should be employed. One protocol for subcutaneous challenge involves five steps using 0.1 mL of a 1:100 dilution, 1:10 dilution, and undiluted drug (steps 1 to 3). Steps 4 and 5 follow with 0.5 mL and 1.0 mL of undiluted drug administered at 20- to 30-minute intervals.[31] Facilities to deal with potential adverse reactions to skin testing should be present. Other protocols exist involving different dilutions and injectate volumes and often in conjunction with a histamine control test. There appears to be general agreement that local anesthetic use is safe after negative incremental subcutaneous testing has been confirmed.[32–36] Safe clinical use of local anesthetic agents in patients with a prior history of allergic response has occurred, including the uneventful use of bupivacaine for episiotomy repair in a patient with two previous adverse reactions to local anesthetics.[32] In one case report, positive incremental skin challenge reactions occurred with several amide local anesthetic agents, suggesting the possibility of cross-reactivity between drugs in this group.[23] Further study is required to determine if such a relationship exists.

Lidocaine itself has been reported to inhibit allergic reactions. Yanagi and coworkers[37] examined the effect of lidocaine on histamine release from in vitro mast cells and basophils. Intracellular calcium concentrations were also assessed. In this study, lidocaine was found to directly inhibit histamine release from rodent mast cells and human basophils, and was associated with parallel decreases in Ca^{2+} mobilization. If these mechanisms are discovered to exist in vivo, it would be highly unlikely that allergic reactions to lidocaine exist.

Summary. Allergic reactions to local anesthetics are rare. The use of preservative-free amide local anesthetic solutions eliminates the possibility of a reaction to a benzoic acid derivative or antioxidant agents such as metabisulfite. Careful questioning of the patient about prior adverse local anesthetic reactions should help elucidate whether or not a true allergy exists. Classic findings on history taking include the development of urticaria, angioedema, hypotension, and respiratory distress and should alert the clinician to the possibility of true hypersensitivity. Incremental subcutaneous challenge testing should be undertaken by a qualified individual, and drugs specifically anticipated to be used in future procedures should be tested. Results of the allergy testing should be sent to physicians who are involved in the clinical management of a patient with a documented allergy, including the anesthesiologist. If challenge testing has been negative, the local anesthetic may be safely used. The parturient should not be put at risk for general anesthesia for cesarean section or be denied the benefit of epidural or spinal analgesia for labor and delivery in the absence of substantial confirmatory evidence of a true local anesthetic allergy.

LATEX ALLERGY

Latex allergy has emerged as a relatively new phenomenon, although isolated cases of reaction to rubber products date back to the 1930s. In the earlier case reports, contact dermatitis to gloves was noted, but in the following years reactions to equipment resulted in serious anaphylactic reactions. Both immediate hypersensitivity reactions (IgE mediated) and delayed hypersensitivity reactions (T lymphocyte mediated) have been demonstrated. Immediate-type hypersensitivity reactions require sensitization from previous exposure during which no clinical manifestations were observed. Certain populations of individuals are at risk for latex allergy and they include (1) patients with severe congenital urologic disorders or myelodysplasia; (2) health care workers; (3) rubber product workers; and (4) patients with specific food allergies.[38] Repeated exposure of mucous membranes to latex-containing products may account for the susceptibility to latex allergy in patients with spina bifida, myelomeningocele, paraplegia, quadriplegia, and major urologic abnormalities.[38–40] Gloves appear to be the sensitizing factor in the delayed hypersensitivity reactions experienced by health care workers. Powder in latex gloves dispersed in the atmosphere contains latex allergens and may cause reactions when inhaled by sensitized individuals.[41] It is unclear whether a person who has a demonstrated type IV, or delayed allergic response, is at risk for the development of a type I, or immediate hypersensitivity reaction.

Diagnosis of Latex Allergy. A careful clinical history of previous exposure to latex-containing products is crucial in the diagnosis of latex allergy in high-risk groups. Specific questioning about reactions to equipment used in prior surgical procedures, condoms, or the inflation of rubber balloons may help elucidate hypersensitivity. Classic symptoms of anaphylaxis, such as the development of bronchospasm, wheezing, urticarial eruptions, edema, hypotension, or cardiovascular collapse, are highly indicative of latex allergy. Other symptoms may include rhinoconjunctivitis or atopic eczema. A history of atopy increases the risk of latex allergy fourfold.[42] Fruit allergies, specifically allergy to papaya, avocados, or bananas, may also predispose patients to an increased risk of latex allergy.[39, 43, 44]

An important distinguishing feature of latex allergy is the time of onset of the reaction after exposure. Most intraoperative anesthetic-related hypersensitivity reactions occur within minutes of administration of the offending agent. Reactions from latex contact in the operating room are delayed 40 minutes or more after exposure.[45] Time for systemic absorption from the responsible vehicle may account for this delay.

Subcutaneous and intradermal skin testing to latex formed the basis of diagnosis in the early years of study of this phenomenon. However, there was no standardization of extract concentrations, and reports of anaphylaxis to the testing appeared.[38] Although Europe and Canada still allow skin testing to be performed, the Food and Drug Administration of the United States no longer approves any latex extract for general skin testing. Other methods of diagnosis include in vitro tests, such as the radioallergosorbent test, which measures the amount of IgE antibody to latex in the patient's serum. Sensitivity and specificity of the test are variable but appear to range between 60% to 90% for specificity and 80% to 90% for sensitivity.[45, 46] Histamine levels rise immediately after the reaction is initiated but fall quickly. In contrast, serum levels of tryptase, a protease found only in mast cells, are elevated for hours later and may be a more reliable indicator of latex allergy.[45]

A summary of recommended guidelines for latex allergy testing and care of these patients has been published by the American Academy of Allergy and Immunology.[47] These recommendations are summarized in Table 34–3.

Latex Allergy in the Obstetric Population. A number of reports in the obstetric literature have implicated local anesthetic agents and fentanyl as triggers for hypersensitivity reactions. A case report by Zucker-Pinchoff[48] published in the journal *Anesthesiology* in 1989 outlined the author's personal experience during cesarean section. The author developed orbital pruritus, nasal congestion, erythema, hypotension, and edema following the injection of epidural fentanyl. Subsequent skin testing proved positive for allergy to fentanyl. Four years later, the author retracted the case report and indicated that the reaction was most likely related to latex allergy.[49] Suspicion of latex allergy, especially in high-risk groups such as health care workers, should cause the clinician to aggressively pursue testing specifically if an implicated drug has rarely been identified as an allergic trigger. If local anesthetic allergy is not supported by testing or clinical presentation, latex allergy should be considered.[21, 50–52]

Allergic reactions to latex have been reported during cesarean section and vaginal delivery.[53–57] Surgical gloves were implicated, and in all cases the patients tested positive for latex allergy. Positive histories of previous contact dermatitis, atopy, or allergic reactions to fruit were retrospectively identified in these patients. A report by Konrad and associates[58] described an urticarial reaction to the tape of the cardiotocograph used for fetal monitoring. The patient was a health care worker and subsequently tested positive for latex allergy.

Table 34–3 AMERICAN ACADEMY OF ALLERGY AND IMMUNOLOGY GUIDELINES FOR LATEX ALLERGY

High-risk patient groups should be identified.
All patients, regardless of risk status, should be questioned about a history of latex allergy.
All high-risk patients should be offered latex allergy testing.
All patients with spina bifida, regardless of their history, should be treated in a latex-free environment.
Any patients with a positive history of latex allergy, regardless of risk status, should be treated in a latex-free environment.
Equipment including gloves, catheters, adhesives, tourniquets, and anesthesia equipment that come into contact with the patient should be free of latex.
Low-risk patients with negative histories are extremely unlikely to react to latex.
If a patient has been positively identified as latex-allergic either by history or testing, he or she should be advised to wear a Medic Alert bracelet and carry self-injectable epinephrine. Medical records should be labeled appropriately.

Modified from Task Force on Allergic Reactions to Latex: Committee report. J Allergy Clin Immunol 1993; 92:16–18.

The obstetric patient experiences repeated exposure to latex gloves during vaginal examinations in the prenatal period and during labor and delivery. Careful history of previous exposure, allergies, atopy, and delivery experiences assists the anesthesiologist in the prevention of subsequent reactions to latex products. In cases in which local anesthetic allergy is suspected but not proved on follow-up testing, latex allergy should be suspected and confirmed or denied.

Equipment. Many medical supplies contain latex. Surgical gloves, urinary catheters, intravenous injection ports, plastic syringe plungers, medication vial stoppers, tourniquets, airway masks, ventilator bellows, blood pressure cuffs, breathing circuits, and elastic bandages are some examples of anesthetic equipment containing latex. Generally speaking, the following items do *not* contain latex: suction catheters, disposable endotracheal tubes, disposable face masks, esophageal stethoscopes, airways, nasogastric tubes, electrocardiographic pads, laryngeal masks, and temperature probes.[38] There are a large number of non–latex-containing examination and sterile gloves that should be used in situations in which a patient has been identified as being allergic to latex.[59] Although by no means complete, Table 34–4 summarizes the content of some commonly used regional anesthesia equipment. Since the publication of this table, many regional anesthesia kits are now latex-free.

Many operating rooms and obstetric wards have assembled "latex carts" containing latex-free equipment for use in sensitive individuals. An accompanying booklet listing the latex content of the equipment specifically used in these areas should be attached to the cart for easy reference by the user.

Summary. Latex allergy is now a well-recognized entity. High-risk groups such as health care workers, patients with spina bifida or congenital urologic problems, rubber workers, and individuals with a history of contact dermatitis to latex-containing materials or allergies to exotic fruits should be carefully questioned about a history of latex allergy. The absolute avoidance of latex-containing equipment and materials is necessary if there is any suggestion of previous reactions. Latex carts with an accompanying list of products and their contents will assist the anesthesiologist in the avoidance of latex-containing equipment in sensitized individuals.

OTHER AGENTS

Syntocinon and Oxytocin. A few case reports in the literature have described anaphylactoid reactions to Syntocinon (synthetic oxytocin).[60–65] Although rare, consideration of the possibility of oxytocin as an allergic trigger must be kept in mind by obstetric anesthesiologists. Physical signs of an allergic reaction include hypotension, bronchospasm, facial erythema, and edema. If the uterus has been evacuated, it has been suggested that resuscitation should be initiated with

Table 34-4 LATEX CONTENT OF REGIONAL ANESTHESIA EQUIPMENT

EQUIPMENT	MANUFACTURER	CONTENT	LATEX
Epidural Trays			
	Abbott Abbott Park, IL	Latex in catheter adaptor sleeve and syringe plungers; none in drape or prep sponge adhesives	Yes
	Arrow International Reading, PA	Syringe plunger seal contains latex; snap lock adaptor (ethylenediene propylene monomer), drape adhesive, and prep sponge adhesive do not contain latex components	Yes
Durasafe Epidural Tray	Becton Dickinson Franklin Lakes, NJ	Latex in adaptor gland (no contact with fluid path), and syringe plunger tips	Yes
Curity Continuous Epidural Anesthesia Tray	Kendall Health Care Products	Latex in wrapper paper on Curad bandage; none in adaptor or adhesives	Yes
Combined Spinal-Epidural Trays			
Espocan Combined Spinal/Epidural Trays	B. Braun/Burron Medical, Inc.	Latex in catheter connector, syringes, and drape adhesive	Yes
Epidural Catheters			
Perifix Epidural Catheter	B. Braun/Burron Medical, Inc. Bethlehem, PA	Latex in catheter connector, syringes, and drape adhesive	Yes
Spinal Trays			
Spinoscan/Sprotte/Atraucan/Pencan	B. Braun/Burron Medical, Inc.	Latex in syringes and drape adhesive	Yes
Portex	Smiths Industries Medical Systems (Portex) Keene, NH	Latex in syringe plunger tips; none in adaptor or adhesives	Yes
Spinal Needles			
Whitacre	Becton Dickinson		No
Sprotte, Spinoscan, Atraucan, Pencan	B. Braun/Burron Medical, Inc.		No
Monojet Spinal Needle	Sherwood Medical		No
Glass Syringes		Without rubber plungers; wash and sterilize	No

Adapted from Schlais RA, Skit J, Newman LM, et al: Latex Allergy Management and Latex Content of Anesthesia Equipment. Department of Anesthesiology, Rush-Presbyterian–St. Luke's Medical Center, Chicago, IL.

epinephrine because of a variable response to ephedrine.[62, 64] Skin testing may not necessarily confirm the diagnosis, and laboratory evidence such as elevated tryptase levels may assist in diagnosis.[65]

Colloid Volume Expanders. Colloid solutions have a longer half-life than crystalloid solutions and have been used extensively for this reason. Specifically in obstetric anesthesia, colloids have been administered before spinal or epidural anesthesia for cesarean section in an attempt to prevent the hypotension associated with regional block.[66–68] In a multicenter prospective study, Ring and Messmer[69] reported the incidence of allergic reactions to colloids as follows: human serum albumin, 0.011%; gelatin, 0.115%; dextran, 0.32%; and hydroxyethyl starch, 0.085%. In another review, Ring[70] reported a 15% incidence of cardiac arrest in patients who developed a dextran-induced anaphylactoid reaction.

Dextrans are among the most commonly used colloid volume expanders and have the added advantage of being antithrombotic agents.[71] In a prospective study by Paull,[71] severe reactions to dextrans occurred in a combined gynecologic-obstetric population with an incidence of 1:383, or 0.26%. One neonatal death occurred secondary to a maternal cardiac arrest following the administration of a dextran 70 solution. The author suggests that there is a higher incidence of a severe reaction from the prophylactic use of dextran than from the development of a serious consequence related to pulmonary embolism. The routine use of dextran as an antithrombotic agent was therefore questioned.

Other colloid expanders such as polygelatin (Haemaccel) have also been implicated in anaphylactoid reactions in the obstetric population.[72–76] It appears that polygelatin exposure results in a direct histamine release in the host leading to an anaphylactoid reaction.[72, 77]

The use of colloid volume expanders carries a significant risk for the development of anaphylactoid reactions. The routine use of these solutions as antithrombotic agents in the obstetric population has been seriously questioned.[71] A neonatal death was reported by Barbier and coworkers,[68] who described the use of dextran given as a volume expander before epidural anesthesia for cesarean section. It appears that the routine use of these solutions in either of the aforementioned situations may cause catastrophic outcomes in both mother and fetus. The management of hypotension associated with regional anesthesia, especially that associated with anesthesia given for cesarean section, should be managed with prophylactic crystalloid infusion and timely treatment of hypotension with vasopressor agents.

Blood Products. Transfusion reactions are common and range in severity from minor febrile reactions to major ABO incompatibility reactions. The development of the classic physical signs of an allergic response that begins shortly after the intravenous administration of blood products should be cause for discontinuation of the blood product and suspicion of an anaphylactic reaction.

General Anesthetic Agents. A 20-year review (1964–1984) of the French and English literature revealed 975 cases of immediate-type allergic reactions to intravenous anesthetic agents.[78] The triggering agents implicated were as follows: hypnotic agents (42.3%), muscle relaxants (50%), opioids (3.2%), benzodiazepines (2.3%), and neuroleptic agents (1.0%).[78] Induction agents such as propanidid (Eponatol) and alfaxalone/alfadolone (Althesin) have been removed from clinical use because of the high incidence of allergic reactions secondary to the cremophor component of the solution. Anaphylactic reactions to thiopental can also occur, and propofol may be a suitable substitute if allergic reactions to thiopental are documented.

Muscle relaxants account for the majority of intravenous anesthetic agent allergic reactions.[78–81] In a study of 51 patients referred for investigation of allergic reactions during anesthesia, 29 of 36 patients reacted to muscle relaxants.[79] Responsible agents are listed in Table 34–5. It also appears that cross-reactivity occurs in patients with muscle relaxant allergies when exposed to other quaternary ammonium molecules of similar structure.[82, 83]

Table 34–5 Muscle Relaxants Identified as Definite or Probable Causes of Allergic Reactions

	Totals	Causal	Contributory with Succinylcholine
Alcuronium	1	1	
Atracurium	8	6	2
Gallamine	3	2	1
Pancuronium	1	1	
Succinylcholine (Suxamethonium)	18	18	
Vecuronium	1	1	
Tubocurarine	2	1	1

Modified from Pepys J, Pepys EO, Baldo BA, et al: Anaphylactic/anaphylactoid reactions to anaesthetic and associated agents. Anaesthesia 1994; 49:470–475.

Opioids cause a dose-related release of histamine from cutaneous mast cells with subsequent physiologic responses resembling anaphylactic reactions. Meperidine was the first opioid to be responsible for a true confirmed allergic reaction.[84] Morphine has not been identified as the cause of an allergic reaction despite the use of high doses. Scattered case reports have described allergic reactions to fentanyl.[85, 86]

Other Drugs. Antibiotics are commonly administered to parturients during labor and delivery. Prophylaxis of infection from premature rupture of the membranes or treatment of ongoing bacterial processes account for the majority of patients who receive antibiotics. Penicillin, vancomycin, and sulfonamides are responsible for the majority of anaphylactic reactions that occur with antibiotic therapy.[87] Although the thiazolidine ring of the cephalosporins differs from that of the penicillin group, there is a cross-reactivity between the drugs. Anaphylactic reactions to cefazolin in pregnancy have been reported but are much less common than reactions to penicillin.[88] Antihistamines or H_2 blockers are often given to obstetric patients prior to cesarean section. Although rare, an allergic reaction to ranitidine has been described in a patient undergoing emergency cesarean section.[89]

MANAGEMENT OF THE PATIENT WITH AN ALLERGIC HISTORY

Preoperative Considerations. Patients with a history of atopy are more likely to develop an anaphylactic reaction to intravenous anesthetic agents.[90–92] Any patient who gives a history of previous allergic reactions to an individual drug should not be given that drug during a subsequent anesthesia induction. Questionable reactions should be investigated by an allergist. Often obstetric anesthesiologists have not had the luxury of meeting the parturient before a request for anesthesia during labor and delivery. This may limit the ability to obtain detailed information of previous drug reactions.

A careful and detailed history of exposure and drug reactions as well as the temporal sequence of the reaction is crucial. All identified causative agents should be avoided. If a history of latex reaction is elicited, all precautions for latex-free management should be undertaken. Explicit information about the nature of a previous reaction to local anesthetics should be obtained, and regional anesthesia should not be avoided because of a vague history of an unknown reaction to a local anesthetic agent. If the patient has had a positive skin test to ester local anesthetics, amide drugs may be used.

Patients with a history of allergic responses to drugs should be referred to an allergist for identification of the causative agent. This is especially important in patients who will require repeated surgical procedures and exposure to multiple drugs. Strict protocols for skin testing are necessary to obtain accurate and useful information. Fisher[93] has described a detailed method for intradermal testing of a series of anesthetic agents.

Pretreatment. The administration of drugs may attenuate the cardiovascular and respiratory responses that occur with an anaphylactic reaction. There is no definitive evidence in the literature that prophylactic pharmacologic therapy is useful. Nonetheless, many physicians would opt to give the patient some therapy in advance. H_1 and H_2 blockers and steroids have been used. It appears that the histamine blocking drugs blunt the physiologic response to histamine but do not prevent secondary mediator release after mast cell activation.[94] Although commonly administered, steroids have not been proved to be of value in the pretreatment of anaphylaxis, and reactions have occurred despite a single-dose administration of steroids.[95]

Treatment of Anaphylactic Reactions. Establishing the diagnosis of an anaphylactic reaction is not always straightforward, requiring the clinician to maintain a high degree of suspicion. The importance of noting the temporal sequence of events assists in ruling out other potential causes of cardiovascular collapse. Prompt and definitive treatment is crucial since the mortality, estimated by retrospective studies to be 3% to 4%, increases with delay in management.[96–98]

Potential causes of sudden, severe hypotension are summarized in Table 34–6. If the signs and symptoms are suggestive of an anaphylactic reaction, the treatment plan outlined in Table 34–7 should be followed.

It is important to note that if the patient has received a spinal or epidural anesthetic, higher doses of epinephrine may be required to overcome the sympatholytic effects of these two regional anesthetic techniques. Secondary effects of epinephrine on uteroplacental perfusion may adversely affect fetal well-being. The obstetrician should be informed and consultation between the anesthesiologist and obstetrician will decide on the best course of delivery in this situation.

Table 34–6 DIFFERENTIAL DIAGNOSIS OF SEVERE HYPOTENSION

Complications of Regional Anesthesia	*Embolic Phenomena*
Total spinal	Thromboembolism
Subdural injection of local anesthetic	Amniotic fluid embolism
Intravascular injection	Venous air embolism
Cardiac Complications	*Obstetric Complications*
Ischemia, infarction	Abruptio placentae
Cardiomyopathy	Placenta previa
Arrhythmia	Uterine rupture
Valvular disease	
Other Causes	
Hemorrhage (nonobstetric)	
Septic shock	
Drug effects	
Anaphylaxis	

Table 34–7 TREATMENT OF ANAPHYLACTIC REACTIONS

Initial Therapy

1. Stop the offending agent (if applicable).
2. Assess ABCs—airway, breathing, and circulation.
3. Ensure patent airway, deliver 100% oxygen.
4. Give fluid resuscitation: 25–50 mL/kg of a balanced salt solution (2–4 L).
5. Administer epinephrine:
   a. 5–10 μg IV for treatment of hypotension
   b. 0.5–1.0 mg IV for treatment of cardiovascular collapse

Secondary Treatment

1. Catecholamine infusions with starting doses:
   a. Epinephrine, 4–8 μg/min (0.05–0.1 μg/kg/min)
   b. Norepinephrine, 4–8 μg/min (0.05–0.1 μg/kg/min)
   c. Isoproterenol, 0.05–0.1 μg/min
2. Antihistamines (0.5–1.0 mg/kg of diphenhydramine)
3. Corticosteroids (0.25–1.0 g of hydrocortisone; alternately, 1–2 g of methylprednisolone)
4. Bicarbonate (0.5–1.0 mEq/kg with persistent hypotension or acidosis)
5. Airway evaluation before extubation

From Levy JH: Management of anaphylaxis. *In* Levy JH (ed): Anaphylactic Reactions in Anesthesia and Intensive Care, 2nd ed. Boston: Butterworth-Heinemann; 1992:162–174.

Difficult intubation is more likely in the parturient than in the nonpregnant population with an incidence of 1:280.[99] The associated angioedema with anaphylactic reactions can further compromise the airway of the parturient experiencing an allergic event. Early intubation, at the first sign of respiratory distress, should be performed. Difficulty with endotracheal intubation should be anticipated, and appropriate airway equipment should be available to deal with this problem.[100] The identification of an air leak, or direct laryngoscopy and assessment of the soft tissues of the larynx, is necessary before extubation of the trachea occurs.

In some cases, patients may be refractory to the initial and secondary treatment listed in Table 34–7. In these cases, more invasive hemodynamic monitoring may be necessary and transfer to an intensive care unit setting may be required.[101]

CONCLUSION

The recognition and management of an anaphylactic reaction may present a challenge to the anesthesiologist. The associated cardiovascular collapse, airway edema, and bronchospasm require prompt airway intervention and pharmacotherapy. Mortality from these reactions occurs, especially with delay in management. The obstetric patient presents a more challenging situation, since the fetus must also be considered during the course of treatment.[102, 103] In addition, the airway may be extremely difficult to manage and if a regional anesthetic has been used, resuscitation may require higher doses of epinephrine to achieve a satisfactory effect.

A careful history, especially detailing previous ad-

❖ Summary

Key Points

- A careful history is key for identification of patients who are at risk for allergic reactions. Preoperative skin testing should be performed when drug allergy is suspected.
- A history of contact dermatitis, atopy, or allergic reactions to fruit in a healthcare worker should alert the clinician to the possibility of latex allergy.
- Early tracheal intubation during an anaphylactoid reaction in the parturient is advisable.
- The administration of epinephrine for the treatment of anaphylaxis may have effects on the uterine vasculature.

Key Reference

Levy JH: Initiation and clinical manifestations of anaphylaxis. *In* Levy JH (ed): Anaphylactic Reactions in Anesthesia and Intensive Care, 2nd ed. Boston: Butterworth-Heinemann; 1992: 13–27.

Case Stem

A G1P0 with a history of contact dermatitis to surgical gloves is undergoing an elective cesarean section under spinal anesthesia for breech presentation. Five minutes after delivery, the patient complains of shortness of breath. Oxygen saturation on 40% face mask has decreased from 99 to 90. Discuss the differential diagnosis and management.

verse reactions to drugs, is necessary to avoid allergic reactions during anesthetic management. Patients at high risk for latex allergy should be appropriately treated. Blood products should be given only when indicated. Patients suspected of having an allergy to an anesthetic agent (local or general) should have a consultation with an allergist and receive appropriate skin testing. Although pretreatment with H_1 or H_2 blockers and corticosteroids is often used in the patient with an allergic history, these drugs will not prevent the development of an anaphylactic reaction. In all situations in which drugs are parenterally administered, resuscitative equipment and drugs should be readily available if an allergic reaction occurs. Allergy to local anesthetic agents is rare, as are anaphylactic reactions to anesthetic agents in general. Recognition of the signs and symptoms of these reactions and knowledge of the management should result in a favorable outcome.

Acknowledgment

The author would like to acknowledge the excellent assistance of J. Lam-McCulloch in the preparation of this manuscript.

References

1. Lindquist RR: Immediate hypersensitivity. *In* Thomas BA (ed): Immunology: A Scope Monograph. Kalamazoo, MI: The Upjohn Company; 1975:33–45.
2. Levy JH: Initiation and clinical manifestations of anaphylaxis. *In* Levy JH (ed): Anaphylactic Reactions in Anesthesia and Intensive Care, 2nd ed. Boston: Butterworth-Heinemann; 1992:13–27.
3. Tedeschi A, Miadonna A, Lorini M, et al: Receptor-operated, but not voltage-operated, calcium channels are involved in basophil leukocyte activation and histamine release. Int Arch Allergy Appl Immunol 1989; 90:109–111.
4. Benyon RC, Robinson C, Church MK: Differential release of histamine and eicosanoids from human skin mast cells activated by IgE-dependent and nonimmunological stimuli. Br J Pharmacol 1989; 97:898–904.
5. Terr AI: Anaphylaxis. Clin Rev Allergy 1985; 3:3–23.
6. Krause PJ, Ingardia CJ, Pontius LT, et al: Host defense during pregnancy: neutrophil chemotaxis and adherence. Am J Obstet Gynecol 1987; 157:274–280.
7. Patton PE, Coulam CB, Bergstrahl E: The prevalence of autoantibodies in pregnant and nonpregnant women. Am J Obstet Gynecol 1987; 157:1345–1350.
8. Mendenhal HW: Serum protein concentrations in pregnancy. I. Concentrations in maternal serum. Am J Obstet Gynecol 1970; 106:388–389.
9. Spätling L, Fallenstein F, Huch A, et al: The variability of cardiopulmonary adaptation to pregnancy at rest and during exercise. Br J Obstet Gynaecol 1992; 99(suppl 8):1–40.
10. Archer GW, Marx GF: Arterial oxygen tension during apnoea in parturient women. Br J Anaesth 1974; 46:358–360.
11. Gee JBL, Packer BS, Millen JE, et al: Pulmonary mechanics during pregnancy. J Clin Invest 1967; 46:945–952.
12. White MV: The role of histamine in allergic diseases. J Allergy Clin Immunol 1990; 86:599–605.
13. Conklin KA: Physiologic changes of pregnancy. *In* Chestnut DH (ed): Obstetric Anesthesia: Principles and Practice. St. Louis: Mosby; 1994:17–43.
14. Beaupre PN, Roizen MF, Cahalan MK, et al: Hemodynamic and two-dimensional transesophageal echocardiographic analysis of an anaphylactic reaction in man. Anesthesiology 1984; 60:482–484.
15. Austen KF: Diseases of immediate type hypersensitivity. *In* Thorn GW, Adams RD, Braunwald E, et al (eds): Harrison's Principles of Internal Medicine, 8th ed, Vol I. New York: McGraw-Hill; 1977:391–396.
16. Covino BG, Vassallo HG: Chemical aspects of local anesthetic agents. *In* Kitz RJ, Laver MB (eds): Local Anesthetics: Mechanisms of Action and Clinical Use. New York: Grune & Stratton; 1976:1–11.
17. Verrill PJ: Adverse reactions to local anaesthetics and vasoconstrictor drugs. Practitioner 1975; 214:380–387.
18. Brown DR, Beamish D, Wildsmith JAW: Allergic reaction to an amide local anaesthetic. Br J Anaesth 1981; 53:435–437.
19. Ruiz K, Stevens JD, Train JJA, et al: Anaphylactoid reactions to prilocaine. Anaesthesia 1987; 42:1078–1080.
20. Erkkola R, Kanto J, Mäenpää J, et al: Allergic reaction to an amide local anesthetic in segmental epidural analgesia. Acta Obstet Gynecol Scand 1988; 67:181–184.
21. Thomas AD, Caunt JA: Anaphylactoid reaction following local anaesthesia for epidural block. Anaesthesia 1993; 48:50–52.
22. Allman KG: Anaphylactoid reaction following spinal anaesthesia for Caesarean section [correspondence]. Anaesthesia 1993; 48:545.
23. Cuesta-Herranz J, de las Heras M, Fernández M, et al: Allergic reaction caused by local anesthetic agents belonging to the amide group. J Allergy Clin Immunol 1997; 99:427–428.
24. Nagel JE, Fuscaldo JT, Fireman P: Paraben allergy. JAMA 1977; 237:1594–1595.
25. Epidemiology of contact dermatitis in North America: 1972. North American Contact Dermatitis Group. Arch Dermatol 1973; 108:537–540.
26. Schwartz HJ, Sher TH: Bisulfite sensitivity manifesting as

allergy to local dental anesthesia. J Allergy Clin Immunol 1984; 75:525–527.
27. Soulat JM, Bouju PH, Oxeda C, et al: Choc anaphylactoïde aux métabisulfites au cours d'une césarienne sous anesthésie péridurale. Cah Anesth 1991; 39:257–259.
28. Aldrete JA, Johnson DA: Evaluation of intracutaneous testing for investigation of allergy to local anesthetic agents. Anesth Analg 1970; 49:173–183.
29. Tannenbaum H, Ruddy S, Schur PH: Acute anaphylaxis associated with severe complement depletion. J Allergy Clin Immunol 1975; 56:226–234.
30. Stefanini M, Hoffman MN: Studies on platelets. XXVIII. Acute thrombocytopenic purpura due to lidocaine (Xylocaine)-mediated antibody: report of a case. Am J Med Sci 1978; 275:365–371.
31. Schatz M: Skin testing and incremental challenge in the evaluation of adverse reactions to local anesthetics. J Allergy Clin Immunol 1984; 74:606–616.
32. Fisher MM, Pennington JC: Allergy to local anaesthesia. Br J Anaesth 1982; 54:893–894.
33. Chandler MJ, Grammer LC, Patterson R: Provocative challenge with local anesthetics in patients with a prior history of reaction. J Allergy Clin Immunol 1987; 79:883–886.
34. Fisher MM, Graham R: Adverse responses to local anaesthetics. Anaesth Intensive Care 1984; 12:325–327.
35. Wasserfallen J-B, Frei C: Long-term evaluation of usefulness of skin and incremental challenge tests in patients with history of adverse reaction to local anesthetics. Allergy 1995; 50:162–165.
36. deShazo RD, Nelson HS: An approach to the patient with a history of local anesthetic hypersensitivity: experience with 90 patients. J Allergy Clin Immunol 1979; 63:387–394.
37. Yanagi H, Sankawa H, Saito H, et al: Effect of lidocaine on histamine release and Ca^{2+} mobilization from mast cells and basophils. Acta Anaesthesiol Scand 1996; 40:1138–1144.
38. Vassallo SA: Perioperative care of latex-allergic patients. *In* Lake CL, Rice LJ, Sperry RJ (eds): Advances in Anesthesia. St. Louis: CV Mosby; 1998:107–131.
39. Slater JE: Latex allergy. J Allergy Clin Immunol 1994; 94:139–149.
40. Birmingham PK, Dsida RM: Latex precautions should be used in all spina bifida patients. Pediatr Neurosurg 1992; 18:224.
41. Walls RS: Latex allergy: a real problem [editorial]. Med J Aust 1996; 164:707–708.
42. Lagier F, Vervloet D, Lhermet I, et al: Prevalence of latex allergy in operating room nurses. J Allergy Clin Immunol 1992; 90:319–322.
43. Laxenaire MC, Moneret-Vautin DA: L'allergie au latex. Chirurgie 1994; 120:526–532.
44. Leynadier F, Dry J: Allergy to latex. Clin Rev Allergy 1991; 9:371–377.
45. Hirshman CA: Latex anaphylaxis. Anesthesiology 1992; 77:223–225.
46. Ownby DR, McCullough J: Testing for latex allergy. J Clin Immunoassay 1993; 16:109–113.
47. Task Force on Allergic Reactions to Latex: Committee report. J Allergy Clin Immunol 1993; 92:16–18.
48. Zucker-Pinchoff B, Ramanathan S: Anaphylactic reaction to epidural fentanyl. Anesthesiology 1989; 71:599–601.
49. Zucker-Pinchoff B, Chandler MJ: Latex anaphylaxis masquerading as fentanyl anaphylaxis: retraction of a case report. Anesthesiology 1993; 79:1152–1153.
50. Lee JJ: Anaphylactoid reaction following epidural block: local anaesthetic or latex? [Correspondence]. Anaesthesia 1994; 49:263.
51. Rae SM, Milne MK, Wildsmith JAW: Anaphylaxis associated with, but not caused by, extradural bupivacaine. Br J Anaesth 1997; 78:224–226.
52. Seigne R: Allergies and anaesthesia [correspondence]. Br J Anaesth 1997; 78:778.
53. Turjanmaa K, Reunala T, Tuimala R, et al: Allergy to latex gloves: unusual complication during delivery. Anaesthesia 1988; 297:1029.
54. Laurent J, Malet R, Smiejan JM, et al: Latex hypersensitivity after natural delivery. J Allergy Clin Immunol 1992; 89:779–780.
55. Díaz T, Antépara I, Usandizaga JM, et al: Latex allergy as a risk during delivery. Br J Obstet Gynaecol 1996; 103:173–175.
56. Santos R, Hernández-Ayup S, Galache P, et al: Severe latex allergy after a vaginal examination during labor: a case report. Am J Obstet Gynecol 1997; 177:1543–1544.
57. Leynadier F, Pecquet C, Dry J: Anaphylaxis to latex during surgery. Anaesthesia 1989; 44:547–550.
58. Konrad C, Fieber T, Schüpfer G, et al: Latex allergy to the tape of the cardiotocograph [correspondence]. Anesth Analg 1997; 84:230.
59. Schlais RA, Skit J, Newman LM, et al: Latex Allergy Management and Latex Content of Anesthesia Equipment. Department of Anesthesiology, Rush-Presbyterian–St. Luke's Medical Center, Chicago, IL.
60. Giuffrida JG, Singh S, Bizzarri D: Anaphylaxis to thiopental or oxytocin—a case report. Anesthesiol Rev 1981; 8:30–33.
61. Slater RM, Bowles BJM, Pumphrey RSH: Anaphylactoid reaction to oxytocin in pregnancy. Anaesthesia 1985; 40:655–656.
62. Kawarabayashi T, Narisawa Y, Nakamura K, et al: Anaphylactoid reaction to oxytocin during cesarean section. Gynecol Obstet Invest 1988; 25:277–279.
63. Emmott RS: Recurrent anaphylactoid reaction during caesarean section [correspondence]. Anaesthesia 1990; 45:62.
64. Maycock EJ, Russell WC: Anaphylactoid reaction to Syntocinon. Anaesth Intensive Care 1993; 21:211–212.
65. Morriss WW, Lavies NG, Anderson SK, et al: Acute respiratory distress during caesarean section under spinal anaesthesia: a probable case of anaphylactoid reaction to Syntocinon. Anaesthesia 1994; 49:41–43.
66. Mathru M, Rao TLK, Kartha RK, et al: Intravenous albumin administration for prevention of spinal hypotension during cesarean section. Anesth Analg 1980; 559:655–658.
67. Rout CC, Rocke DA: Prevention of hypotension following spinal anesthesia for cesarean section. Int Anesthesiol Clin 1994; 32:117–135.
68. Barbier P, Jonville A-P, Autret E, et al: Fetal risks with dextrans during delivery. Drug Saf 1992; 7:71–73.
69. Ring J, Messmer K: Incidence and severity of anaphylactoid reactions to colloid volume substitutes. Lancet 1977; 1:466–469.
70. Ring J: Anaphylactoid reactions to plasma substitutes. Int Anesthesiol Clin 1985; 23:67–95.
71. Paull J: A prospective study of dextran-induced anaphylactoid reactions in 5745 patients. Anaesth Intensive Care 1987; 15:163–167.
72. Lund N: Anaphylactoid reaction to infusion of polygelatin (Haemaccel): a study in pregnant women. Anaesthesia 1980; 35:655–659.
73. Laxenaire MC, Moeneret-Vautrin DA, Mouton C, et al: Réactions anaphylactoïdes en anesthésie-réanimation. Cah Anesth 1990; 38:11–14.
74. Duffy BL, Harding JN, Fuller WR, et al: Cardiac arrest following Haemaccel. Anaesth Intensive Care 1994; 22:90–92.
75. Rosewarne F, Davidson A: Anaphylactoid reaction to Haemaccel. Anaesth Intensive Care 1994; 22:317–318.
76. Fenwick DG, Andersen GJ, Munst PS: Anaphylactoid reaction to Haemaccel [correspondence]. Anaesth Intensive Care 1995; 23:521.
77. Lorenz W, Doenicke A, Messmer K, et al: Histamine release in human subjects by modified gelatin (Haemaccel) and dextran: an explanation for anaphylactoid reactions observed under clinical conditions? Br J Anaesth 1987; 48:151–164.
78. Levy JH: Common anaphylactic and anaphylactoid reactions. *In* Levy JH (ed): Anaphylactic Reactions in Anesthesia and Intensive Care, 2nd ed. Boston: Butterworth-Heinemann; 1992:83–120.
79. Pepys J, Pepys EO, Baldo BA, et al: Anaphylactic/anaphylactoid reactions to anaesthetic and associated agents. Anaesthesia 1994; 49:470–475.
80. Matthews MD, Ceglarski JZ, Pabari M: Anaphylaxis to suxamethonium—a case report. Anaesth Intensive Care 1977; 5:235–238.

81. Galletly DC, Treuren BC: Anaphylactoid reactions during anaesthesia. Anaesthesia 1985; 40:329–333.
82. Harle DG, Baldo BA, Fisher MM: Assays for, and cross-reactivities of, IgE antibodies to the muscle relaxants gallamine, decamethonium and succinylcholine (suxamethonium). J Immunol Methods 1985; 78:293–305.
83. Harle DG, Baldo BA, Fisher MM: Cross-reactivity of metocurine, atracurium, vecuronium and faxadinium with IgE antibodies from patients unexposed to these drugs but allergic to other myoneural blocking drugs. Br J Anaesth 1985; 57:1073–1076.
84. Levy JH, Rockoff MR: Anaphylaxis to meperidine. Anesth Analg 1982; 61:301–303.
85. Lowenstein E, Hallowell P, Levine FH, et al: Cardiovascular response to large doses of morphine in man. N Engl J Med 1969; 281:1389–1394.
86. Bennett MJ, Anderson LK, McMillan JC, et al: Anaphylactic reaction during anaesthesia associated with positive intradermal skin test to fentanyl. Can Anaesth Soc J 1986; 33:75–78.
87. Kraft D: Other antibiotics. *In* de Weck AL, Bundgaard H (eds): Allergic Reactions to Drugs. Berlin: Springer-Verlag; 1983:483–520.
88. Konno R, Nagase S: Anaphylactic reaction to cefazolin in pregnancy. J Obstet Gynaecol Res 1995; 21:577–579.
89. Powell JA, Maycock EJ: Anaphylactoid reaction to ranitidine in an obstetric patient. Anaesth Intensive Care 1993; 21:702–703.
90. Clarke RSJ, Dundee JW, Garrett RT, et al: Adverse reactions to intravenous anaesthetics: a survey of 100 reports. Br J Anaesth 1975; 47:575–585.
91. LaForest M, More D, Fisher M: Predisposing factors in anaphylactoid reactions to anesthetic drugs in an Australian population: the role of allergy, atopy and previous anaesthesia. Anaesth Intensive Care 1980; 8:454–459.
92. Watkins J, Clarke RSJ, Fee JPH: The relationship between reported atopy or allergy and immunoglobulins: a preliminary study. Anaesthesia 1981; 36:582–585.
93. Fisher MM: Intradermal testing after anaphylactoid reaction to anaesthetic drugs: practical aspects of performance and interpretation. Anaesth Intensive Care 1984; 12:115–120.
94. Levy JH: Allergic reactions and the intraoperative use of foreign substances. *In* Barash P (ed): Refresher Course in Anesthesiology, Vol 13. Presented at Annual Meeting Course Lectures. 1985:129–141.
95. Levy JH, Zaidan JR, Faraj B: Prospective evaluation of risk of protamine reactions in NPH insulin–dependent diabetics. Anesth Analg 1986; 65:739–742.
96. Fisher MM, More DG: The epidemiology and clinical features of anaphylactic reactions in anaesthesia. Anaesth Intensive Care 1981; 9:226–234.
97. Mantz JM, Gauli G, Meyer P, et al: Le choc anaphylactique. Rev Med Interne 1982; 3:331–338.
98. Barnard JH: Studies of 400 *Hymenoptera* sting deaths in the United States. J Allergy Clin Immunol 1973; 52:259–263.
99. Samsoon GLT, Young JRB: Difficult tracheal intubation: a retrospective study. Anaesthesia 1987; 42:487–490.
100. Edwards RM, Hunt TL: Blind nasal intubation in an awake patient for Caesarean section. Anaesth Intensive Care 1982; 10:151–153.
101. Levy JH: Management of anaphylaxis. *In* Levy JH (ed): Anaphylactic Reactions in Anesthesia and Intensive Care, 2nd ed. Boston: Butterworth-Heinemann; 1992:162–174.
102. Baraka A, Sfeir SL: Anaphylactic cardiac arrest in a parturient: response of the newborn. JAMA 1980; 243:1745–1746.
103. Warner JA, Jones AC, Miles EA, et al: Maternofetal interaction and allergy. Allergy 1996; 51:447–451.

35

Post–Dural Puncture Headache

❖ MARKUS C. SCHNEIDER, MD
❖ MICHAEL SCHMID, MD

HISTORY

More than a century ago, in August 1898, the German surgeon August Bier decided to evaluate the potential of the local anesthetic cocaine to numb the spinal nerves following injection into his own subarachnoid space.[1] His pioneering studies were based on accumulating experimental and clinical experience with this alkaloid that had been isolated in 1860 from leaves of the coca plant *(Erythroxolon cocae)* by Albert Niemann. Crystalline cocaine soon received a lot of attention from surgeons who seeking alternative anesthetic techniques to operate on patients without relying solely on the still rather risky inhalational anesthesia, the reputation of which was tarnished by a high rate of often lethal complications. Thus, the ophthalmologist Karl Koller used cocaine successfully for topical anesthesia of the cornea and conjunctiva,[2] and Carl Ludwig Schleich for local infiltration anesthesia.[3] Obviously, the local anesthetic effect of spinally injected cocaine observed by Bier and his teammate Hildebrandt was expected, in contrast to the occurrence of an incapacitating headache that persisted for days in all subjects included in this early experimental series. Typically, it was a headache that was described as being postural because it disappeared when the patient was in the supine position whereas it worsened in the upright position and was accompanied by nausea and vomiting. Bier reasoned that post–dural puncture headache (PDPH) was unlikely to be related to cocaine but rather in some way to the dural breach caused by the large-bore needles used and the loss of cerebrospinal fluid (CSF) increased by poor fit of the syringes. However, MacRobert[4] is usually credited with the initial suggestion that continuous CSF leakage into the epidural space was the mechanism responsible for PDPH. Such equivocal experience did not cause Oskar Kreis,[5] a first-year resident in obstetrics at the Basel Women's Hospital, to waver in his enthusiasm for evaluating this method of pain relief for women in labor. According to his report on six cases, 10 mg of spinally administered cocaine induced analgesia up to a midabdominal level, allowing for pain-free obstetric manipulations during delivery and even surgical repair of a perineal tear. In two of these women, nausea was observed for a short period.

PATHOPHYSIOLOGY

Age, Gender, Disposition

Although deliberate or unanticipated puncture of the dura mater is clearly related to the occurrence of PDPH, a variety of independent factors influence and modulate both the frequency and the severity of this syndrome. Thus, the frequency of PDPH decreases with increasing age and is uncommon in elderly subjects,[6–10] whereas both female gender and pregnancy are considered to represent important risk factors for developing this bothersome side effect.[6, 10–13] Furthermore, alterations in hormonal states occurring during menstruation, pregnancy, and menopause have been shown to trigger migraine attacks and change its incidence.[14] A fall in estrogen level associated with menstruation or delivery has been established as a factor precipitating headaches in women with a previous history of migraine or premenstrual migraine.[15, 16] Obviously, several elements predisposing to PDPH are present in pregnant women. This may explain, to some extent, why this field of anesthetic practice has also been identified as a high risk area in this respect. Finally, psychological influences cannot be disregarded, as they appear to be important cofactors in modulating the consequences of a dural tap resulting in headache, unexpected distress, and, subsequently, loss of cooperation on the part of otherwise healthy subjects.[17, 18] Ultimately, a psychosomatic component may also come into play. In 1967, Kaplan[19] made a surprising observation related to PDPH that, unfortunately, was never reproduced. In a study in healthy volunteers presenting for real (22-gauge needle) or sham lumbar punctures, a similarly high incidence of PDPH was observed (28% vs. 22%, respectively). The frequency of headache was even four times higher in those volunteers in the sham puncture group who expressed concern about this complication as compared to those who did not express such a concern (46% vs. 11%).

Central Nervous System and Cerebrospinal Fluid

The central nervous system is surrounded by approximately 150 mL of CSF that is equally distributed between the cranial cavity and the spinal canal. Most of CSF is produced and absorbed by the choroid plexus at an average rate of 0.35 mL/min, or 500 mL per day. The formation of CSF is in equilibrium with CSF absorption during steady-state conditions. While CSF production remains constant over a wide range of intracranial pressure values, CSF absorption increases with increasing intracranial pressure. According to the Monroe-Kelly doctrine, CSF volume and intracranial blood volume inversely correlate, as evidenced by vasodilation observed during a state of CSF deficiency.[20] Using transcranial Doppler ultrasonography in 45 patients undergoing diagnostic lumbar puncture, investigators identified higher flow velocities and asymmetry in interhemispheric cerebral hemodynamics as risk factors for PDPH.[21] Associated with a significant reduction in flow velocity of the right middle cerebral artery, asymmetry in flow velocity disappeared in those subjects complaining about PDPH, indicating some vasodilation.

When there is a clinically significant CSF loss across a dural hole, physiologic compensatory mechanisms may be unable to meet CSF demand, which results in a reduction of intracranial CSF volume as demonstrated by magnetic resonance imaging (MRI) 24 hours after lumbar puncture with an 18-gauge needle.[22] Interestingly, natural variations and physiologic changes of intracranial CSF volume have been described using MRI. Whereas total CSF volume increased premenstrually in the majority of women with a normal menstrual cycle, no such changes were observed on repeat examination in postmenopausal females and in males.[23] In both sexes, total intracranial CSF volume increases steeply with advancing age.[24] Notwithstanding all of these biologic variables, we can assume that CSF leaking will persist for some time and contribute to a loss of intracranial CSF volume as long as the dural hole remains unsealed. In consequence, definitive cure of PDPH results from spontaneous closure of the dural rent or from any therapeutic intervention sealing off the leaking site and thus preventing further loss of CSF.[25]

Cerebrospinal Fluid Leakage

For almost a century, the theory of CSF volume depletion has been embraced by the vast majority of the medical community to explain PDPH, in spite of the growing evidence for a more complex mechanism. Fifty years ago, accumulations of large amounts of epidural fluid were observed during endoscopy in completely asymptomatic subjects who underwent lumbar puncture 2 to 4 days previously.[26] This finding is in agreement with observations in patients that did not indicate any correlation between the occurrence of PDPH and the volume of CSF leakage into the paraspinal area as calculated from T2-weighted MR images.[27] Nevertheless, as removal of 20 mL of CSF in volunteers reliably produces severe headache that is immediately relieved by subarachnoid injection of normal saline,[28] CSF volume alterations appear to be intimately associated with mechanisms related to PDPH.[26]

Any change in CSF volume may be reflected by a concomitant change in intracranial, subarachnoid, and epidural pressures and in pressure gradients that become more clinically important in the upright as compared with the supine position.[18] In the sitting or standing position, a marked change appears in the pressure difference between the base of the brain, with its roughly atmospheric intracranial pressure, and the lumbar subarachnoid space, where a value exceeding 40 cm H_2O can be measured while the subatmospheric epidural pressure persists. These barometric conditions favor further CSF loss, occasionally leading to sagging of the brain, that results in traction on and stretching of pain-sensitive intracranial structures such as cerebral vessels, venous sinuses, the tentorium, and the falx cerebri.[22] This may explain differences in manifestations of PDPH that, on the one hand, is transferred to the frontal region via the first division of the trigeminal nerve, which supplies virtually all pain-sensitive supratentorial structures,[29] and, on the other hand, is transferred to the occiput, neck, and shoulders via the glossopharyngeal, vagus, and upper three cervical nerves that supply the posterior fossa.[30] We hypothesize that changes in intracranial CSF volume status may have differential effects on these nerves as suggested by variable patterns and localization of PDPH. It is noteworthy that both primary intracranial hypotension resulting in orthostatic headache[31] and benign intracranial hypertension[32] may be associated with similar symptoms of headache and visual impairment, although the underlying etiology is completely different. This again emphasizes that the origins of headache, in general, and PDPH, in particular, are multifactorial.

CLINICAL FINDINGS

Definition

By definition, PDPH always occurs in association with intentional or unintentional breach of the dura mater, such as following diagnostic lumbar puncture during myelography and spinal anesthesia or accidental dural puncture in association with epidural anesthesia. This causal prerequisite is complementary to a number of typical clinical features allowing the differentiation between PDPH and other forms of headache. Such a differentiation is important insofar as rational therapeutic management is concerned. The hallmark of PDPH is the postural nature of the headache, which is aggravated in the upright position and relieved by adopting the supine posture. Classically, the headache is throbbing in nature. If a headache cannot be triggered by this change in position, the diagnosis should be questioned.

Clinical Features

The severity of PDPH may vary, it often radiates to the forehead and the occiput, and it may also involve neck and shoulders. According to some observational communications, pain sensation has been found to be localized to the frontal or occipital areas in 50% and 25% of cases, respectively, whereas a more generalized pattern was observed in another 25%.[33] In a more recent trial, a similar pattern of pain localization was found: 28% and 27% of patients reported pain in the frontal and occipital areas, respectively, whereas 45% of patients complained of pain in both regions.[34] Some authors suggest that aggravation of headache by coughing or sneezing should be used as an inclusion criterion for diagnosis of PDPH.[35] Neck stiffness and scapular pain may be present and mimic meningitis. PDPH is often associated with nausea and vomiting, dizziness, ataxia, and loss of appetite. In addition, PDPH may include signs suggestive of cranial nerve involvement, such as diplopia and other visual disturbances. Although very rare, abducens nerve paresis should be considered whenever diplopia occurs.[36] Abducens nerve paresis may coincide with oculomotor nerve paresis[37] and is believed to be caused by mechanical traction of the nerve related to a reduction of intracranial CSF volume. Changes in hearing acuity and tinnitus are among the rare observations occurring in association with PDPH. They are related to vestibulocochlear dysfunction ranging from minor auditory losses unaccompanied by PDPH to major hearing deficit and even deafness usually in association with PDPH. These complications have been mainly reported in elderly patients scheduled for transurethral resection of the prostate under spinal anesthesia and attributed to the presence of an endolymphatic hydrops resulting from a lower than normal CSF pressure that is transmitted to the inner ear by the cochlear aqueduct.[38] One does not know whether increasing age represents a risk factor for this complication, as no studies exist demonstrating these complications in younger subjects. Finally, there are extremely rare complications of PDPH such as the development of an intracranial subdural hematoma.[39]

It is of paramount importance to adopt strict criteria when diagnosing PDPH, to establish a common basis that allows the generalization of findings on the incidence of this common side effect. Depending on the set of inclusion criteria used in different institutions, underreporting as well as overreporting may occur, further hampering comparisons and common steps in therapeutic strategies.[40] A common database founded on prospective randomized controlled trials would certainly contribute a great deal to further improving patient outcome.[41]

Severity

The severity of PDPH may vary, and only a few investigations have used a 10-cm visual analog scale (VAS) for quantification.[10, 40, 42, 43] Descriptive grading has not been used in the large body of available literature, making valid comparisons between different trials extremely difficult if not impossible. Because PDPH interferes with daily activities, a functional grading system was suggested recently[43] that comprises three categories:

Functional grading (FG) categories of PDPH:

- FG 1: headache not interfering with normal activity
- FG 2: periodic bedrest necessary to relieve headache
- FG 3: incapacitating headache rendering it impossible to sit up and eat

This functional grading can be combined with the VAS scoring to form the following more comprehensive PDPH grading system[43]:

PDPH grades:

- Grade I: VAS score 1 – 3 and FG category 1
- Grade II: VAS score 4 – 7 and FG category 2
- Grade III: VAS score 8 – 10 and FG category 3

A similar classification of PDPH was utilized in a large prospective study in 873 patients undergoing a total of 1021 spinal anesthetic procedures.[34] In this classification, a three-point scoring system is used:

PDPH scores:

- Score I: mild PDPH restricting daily activities; patient not bedridden at any time during the day, no other symptoms
- Score II: moderate PDPH significantly restricting daily activities; patient is bedridden part of the day, associated symptoms may or may not be present
- Score III: severe PDPH resulting in the patient's desire to stay in bed all day; associated symptoms always present

These authors arranged additional symptoms associated with PDPH according to the following system:[34]

PDPH-associated symptoms:

- vestibular symptoms: nausea, vomiting, vertigo, dizziness
- cochlear symptoms: hearing loss, hyperacusis, tinnitus
- ocular symptoms: photophobia, diplopia, difficulty in accommodation
- musculoskeletal symptoms: stiffness of neck, scapular pain

Time of Onset and Duration

The chronology of PDPH is characterized by some typical features. In a series of 1134 nonobstetric patients receiving spinal anesthesia, PDPH was reported within 24 hours in 38% of cases and in another 53% within the next 48 hours; that is, in the vast majority of cases, PDPH manifested during the first 3 days after lumbar puncture.[33] According to another large prospective study in patients with a median age of 52 years (range, 16–90) for males and 52 years (range, 15–93) for females presenting for orthopedic or genitourinary surgery, PDPH occurred in 65% of cases within 24 hours and in 92% of cases within 48 hours following lumbar puncture.[34] There are some indications that a later onset of symptoms may be associated with a decreased severity and duration of PDPH. Such conclusions concerning late onset do not always take into account the relatively short duration of PDPH, which commonly is a self-limiting complication. Obstetric patients are at high risk for PDPH because of their gender and relatively young age. Accidental dural puncture while using an epidural needle for labor analgesia led ultimately to PDPH with a frequency of 73% on the first postpartum day, and, by the third day, typical symptoms were present in all of those who developed PDPH, provided no therapy had been instituted.[44] A similar pattern of onset of PDPH was also observed in those parturients in whom an elective forceps delivery was performed, suggesting that the mode of delivery did not modify its natural course.

The duration of PDPH is an important point for both the patient and the attending physician and often has an influence on therapeutic management options. In an early study, PDPH subsided within 3 days in 70% of the affected patients.[33] In only 18% of the subjects, a duration of more than 5 days was observed. Comparable results were obtained in the more recent trial in which spontaneous recovery was allowed to occur under a conservative therapeutic regimen that included nonsteroidal anti-inflammatory drugs (NSAIDs), antiemetics, tranquilizers, and hypnotics: for mild, moderate, and severe PDPH, a median duration of 5 days (range, 2–10, 1–12, and 1–11 days, respectively) was observed.[34] However, there are several case reports that indicate that PDPH may occasionally persist for weeks, months, or even years.[45, 46] Therefore, the results of the 20-year survey from the Birmingham Maternity Hospital are particularly interesting.[44] Regardless of whether there was treatment or not, the mean durations of PDPH presenting on the first or second day after delivery were very similar (4.6 to 6 days), ranging between 1 and 10 days. The duration of PDPH with a very late onset tended to be much shorter, as evidenced by five mothers who experienced typical symptoms only on the fifth postpartum day, followed by complete recovery on the subsequent day.

DIFFERENTIAL DIAGNOSIS

Migraine, Tension Headache

Anesthetic practice appears to be full of paradoxes. Thus, headaches after childbirth do not necessarily signify PDPH, even with a history of an epidural or spinal anesthetic.[14–16, 47] The importance of a complete medical history and a thorough examination have already been stressed. During the first postpartum week with a peak on days 4 to 6, headache unrelated to anesthesia was observed in 39% of mothers.[15] In these women, headache was significantly associated with a previous or family history of migraine and premenstrual migraine. Remarkably, such headaches were not described by these women as being one of their typical migraines, as they were considerably milder. Apparently, tension may have played an important role in some of these women who were found to be anxious and depressed. It is well known that sleep deprivation, fatigue, and stress in anticipation of new tasks as a mother have a deep impact on self-esteem and impinge on personal well-being, thereby predisposing for troublesome psychological effects. Although epidemiologic studies show that migraine sufferers report less headache activity during pregnancy, this trend is abruptly reversed in the week of childbirth and migraine often recurs.[16] In a large-scale survey performed in France a decade ago, a headache rate of 12% was reported in women who had an epidural analgesia during labor that was not complicated by dural puncture.[47] Surprisingly, in mothers who did not receive epidural labor analgesia, the incidence of postpartum headache tended to be higher, a finding without statistical significance owing to the small number of patients who complained of headache.

Hypertension and Pregnancy-Related Hypertensive Disorders

There are many causes for non-PDPH postpartum headaches. They may or may not be related to an anesthetic procedure or lumbar puncture. In obstetric practice, late-onset preeclampsia or as yet undiagnosed preeclampsia should always be considered in women presenting with a headache that may be associated with visual disturbances and restlessness. It has been noted that as many as 44% of eclamptic seizures occur postpartum without other premonitory signs. More importantly, according to the observation of a prospective descriptive study conducted in the United Kingdom in 1992, prodromal symptoms did not predate intrapartum or postpartum eclampsia in 50% of cases.[48]

Caffeine Withdrawal Headache

Interruption of caffeine consumption can cause a withdrawal syndrome characterized by headache, fatigue, irritability, and, in some instances, nausea and vomiting. In severe cases, neurologic signs may be present that can lead to further radiologic investigations.[49] In a prospective randomized study, 50% of patients with a regular daily caffeine intake averaging approximately 400 mg, which is the equivalent of four cups of coffee or tea, reported headache in the evening of the day of operation related to caffeine withdrawal for more than 24 hours.[50] No patient in whom caffeine was substituted during the perioperative period complained of headache following surgery. As caffeine is among the most widely used behaviorally active substances, the possibility of caffeine withdrawal syndrome should always be excluded.

Infectious Disease

Both chronic or acute sinusitis and meningitis can present with headaches. Septic bacterial meningitis is extremely rare in current anesthetic practice, provided that strict aseptic techniques and appropriate hygiene standards are implemented. Nonetheless, cases of meningitis following obstetric epidural anesthesia still appear in the literature.[51–55] Such infectious complications are not only related to the skin flora but may be caused by a bloodborne spread of infectious organisms from the vaginal or urinary tract. Alternatively, a more benign form of meningitis, the aseptic chemical meningitis, should be excluded by appropriate laboratory tests. Inadvertent contamination of the subarachnoid space by substances used for disinfection[56] or local anesthetic additives or preservatives have also been suggested as causative factors.

Dural Venous Sinus Thrombosis

Dural venous sinus thrombosis is an unusual complication of pregnancy that occurs commonly during the first 7 postpartum days with an incidence in the range of 1 in 10,000 to 1 in 20,000.[57, 58] MRI is a sensitive test for detection of dural venous sinus thrombosis and can easily be supplemented by MRI angiography. Computed tomography (CT) scan was reported to be inadequate, but angiography was recommended only for the very difficult cases.[58]

Intracranial Pathology

Persistent headache may be present in the event of a space-occupying intracranial lesion or tumor. In a literature overview covering almost 30 years, 32 patients were identified who reportedly developed an intracranial hematoma following spinal anesthesia or accidental dural puncture.[59] Six of these subjects were pregnant and received spinal (n = 2) or epidural anesthesia (n = 4). In a rare event, a subdural bleed presented as puerperal psychosis.[60] Interestingly, a patient who presented with postspinal headache had an associated unverified pineal body tumor producing obstructive hydrocephalus.[61] Recurrent spinal headache was the presenting feature associated with another rare malformation, the Chiari I malformation, defined as displacement of the tonsils of the cerebellum through the foramen magnum.[62] In this case, an epidural blood patch could not prevent recurrence of severe headache, which was only relieved by prednisone.

Pneumocephalus

Pneumocephalus resulting from subarachnoid air injection can cause sudden onset of severe headache. Nowadays, pneumoencephalography has been largely replaced by more up-to-date techniques, thereby eliminating the inconvenience of its dire side effects. However, air is still popular in certain places for use in localization of the epidural space by applying the loss of resistance technique to air (LORA). In a recent review, the safety of this approach was scrutinized.[63] Numerous complications associated with this technique were discovered, including pneumocephalus in at least 13 cases. Therefore, the authors concluded that potential complications associated with LORA may outweigh disputable benefits. This conclusion is corroborated by findings from another study comparing the incidence of PDPH in patients receiving epidural anesthesia after localization of the epidural space using either LORA or loss-of-resistance to saline (LORS).[64] With an equal accidental dural puncture rate of 2.6% in a total of 2720 blocks, the incidence of PDPH was more than six times higher in the LORA group (67% vs. 10%). Furthermore, supraspinal intrathecal air bubbles were detected in almost all patients in the LORA group on a brain CT scan, which was performed immediately after onset of PDPH. Onset of PDPH was more rapid in the LORA group than in the LORS group, and in two thirds of the cases symptoms appeared within 1 hour. However, the ultimate decision of using either air or saline for LORS will depend on individual success and experience. (At one of the editors' institutions, LORA has been used for more than 40 years and, based on the institution's data, there is no reason to discontinue this practice.)

NEEDLES AND DURAL PUNCTURE

Needle Type, Needle Size, and Tip Configuration

Manufacturers of equipment for epidural and spinal procedures have engaged in a fierce competition to win the largest market shares. There is still ongoing research in development of needles with improved qualities that are easy to handle and position, safe to use, and also inexpensive. Anesthesiologists should not only keep abreast of important quality standards but should also strive for a balance between skyrocketing expenditures and growing economic constraints.

The number of different epidural and spinal needles on the market is legion (Fig. 35–1). However, they all can be traced back to two archetypal needles, a large-bore needle for epidural anesthesia and a small-bore needle for spinal anesthesia. They differ considerably in size and needle design. Whereas epidural needles have not changed a lot during the past decade, there have been major advances in spinal needle manufacturing. For epidural anesthetics, the 17- or 18-gauge Tuohy needles are very popular and can be considered as standard cannulae, although alternative makes are in use, such as the Hustead needle[65] and the Weiss needle.[66] We have used the 18-gauge model successfully for many years.

The situation is somewhat more complicated in the realm of spinal anesthesia. As the incidence and severity of PDPH is clearly related to the tear in the dura mater produced by the puncturing needle, manu-

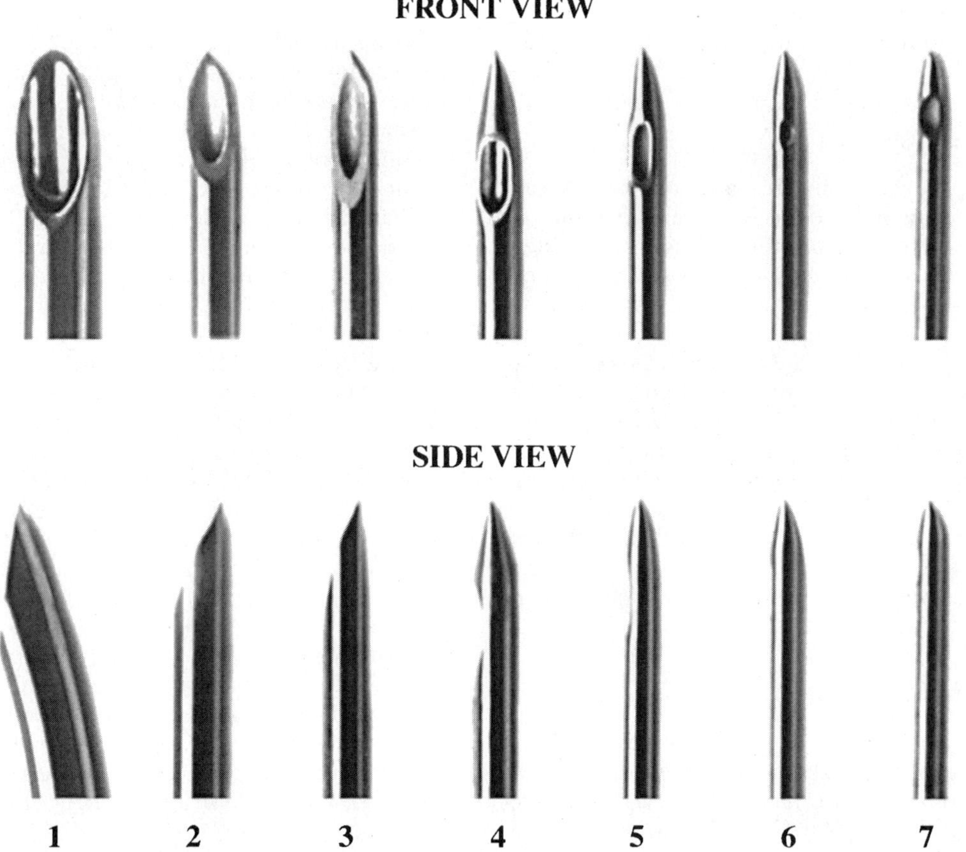

❖ **Figure 35–1** Front *(upper line)* and side view *(lower line)* of the following needles: 1 = 18-gauge Tuohy; 2 = 20-gauge Quincke; 3 = 22-gauge Quincke; 4 = 24-gauge Sprotte; 5 = 25-gauge Polymedic; 6 = 25-gauge Whitacre; 7 = 26-gauge Gertie Marx. Magnification is shown as seven times the original size.

facturers increasingly concentrated on developing less traumatizing cannulae. Thus, for almost half a century, there was a growing interest in producing so-called atraumatic needles with a rounded tip instead of a cutting bevel, as in the case of Quincke-type needles. As far back as 1926, the use of a needle with such a tip was advocated by Greene.[67] In 1951, the use of a 20-gauge pencil-point needle with a conical tip in which the orifice was on the shaft in proximity to the tip was advocated; this design eventually became known as the Whitacre-type needle, which was the name of the second author of the study.[68] In 1987, the interest in less traumatizing needles was boosted by Sprotte's report on a spinal needle with a 0.02% associated incidence of PDPH, which was also recommended for a variety of other regional anesthetic procedures.[69] In contrast to the Whitacre needle, the Sprotte needle has a larger lateral orifice with a diameter at least equal to the internal diameter of the cannula. This may be the reason that fluids injected through a Sprotte needle tend to distribute more homogeneously within the spinal fluid space, because the fluid jet is less lateralized than with a Whitacre needle. In current practice, the needle choice depends on a variety of factors and may be influenced to some extent by observations made during experimental testing for differences in qualitative properties of needles.

Similar to automotive bumper tests that are used to determine the relative stability of bumpers after a low-speed impact, the vulnerability of spinal needles can be assessed by inspection under light microscopy (LM) and scanning electron microscopy (SEM) following spinal anesthesia associated with a bone contact. In such a study, contact with bone resulted in clearly bent tips in 7% of 22-gauge to 29-gauge Quincke-type needles, indicating that damage still occurs in modern thin spinal needles.[70] However, there was no SEM evidence that such a damaged needle caused any additional tearing destruction in the dural membranes of cadavers. In some of the dural holes, an "open tin can" configuration was observed. In another investigation, a total of 220 spinal needles (Quincke, Sprotte, and different makes of pencil-point needles) were compared following routine use.[71] Although this investigation provided evidence that spinal needles may be damaged during their use, it came as a surprise that damage was not related to the number of impacts with bone or the number of attempts. In Sprotte and pencil-point needles, blunting, chipping, and roughening of the tip were observed. All of these findings were flawed by a very inhomogeneous case mix. In another study on cadavers submitted to spinal puncture using three different needle types, LM showed that fluorescein used with the disinfectant and tissue particles were attached to currently used types of needles following dural puncture.[72] Only pencil-point needles (27-gauge Pencan) were superior in withstanding adherence of foreign material and, even more importantly, in tip stability than Quincke-type needles (27-gauge Spinocan and 26-gauge Atraucan).

The risk of spinal anesthetic failure is increased with placement failure as a result of deflection and bending.[73] As repeat dural puncture significantly increases the risk of PDPH,[74] needle shaft deviation from its axis of insertion is undesirable. In Sitzman and Uncles' study[73] using a porcine paraspinal muscle preparation, needle deflection was inversely related to its gauge, increased with the degree of tip bend, and was dependent on the type of needle. The 22- and 25-gauge Whitacre needles were superior to 22- and 25-gauge Sprotte needles and the latter again superior to 22- and 25-gauge Quincke needles in resistance to deflection during insertion, even when there was a bend in the needle tip of 5 to 10 degrees.[73] Similar findings were reported by others who found that needle deviation was least with pencil-point spinal needles (Whitacre, Sprotte), more with needles used for epidural anesthesia (Tuohy, Hustead, Crawford), and most with beveled spinal needles (Quincke, Atraucan).[75] Such observations are likely to influence many practitioners' needle choice.

Effects of Needles on Dura Mater

Before potential effects of dural puncture on the dura mater are described, the gross anatomic structural features should be summarized. In fresh preparations of dura mater from cadavers, low-power LM revealed that the tissue is composed of lamellae branching irregularly and arranged concentrically relative to the spinal cord.[76] These lamellae consist mainly of bundles of collagen fibers that pursue wavy courses in various directions. SEM reveals elastic fibers directed longitudinally and gaps devoid of structured elements representing ground substance. Such a texture may enhance retraction forces that contribute to rapid closure of holes produced by needle puncture. Some authors observed a "tin-lid" phenomenon when using 20- to 29-gauge Quincke needles that was capable of sealing the dural hole after a short time.[77] Histologic findings also confirm that dural trauma is different according to needle type and is correlated directly with the gauge of the needle utilized.[78] With 22- to 29-gauge Quincke needles, an ellipsoidal hole was produced, surrounded by compressed and sectioned fibers as assessed under LM, whereas a more rounded hole without evidence of cut fibers was observed quite frequently with the pencil-point needles (24-gauge Sprotte and 22-gauge Whitacre).

The controversy about the impact of spinal needle bevel direction has subsided to a large extent with the advent of pencil-point needles, as they are devoid of any cutting bevel. Nevertheless, we would like to list some references concerning this topic. According to two already quoted studies,[77, 78] rotation of the bevel by 90 degrees did not have a marked effect on the morphology of the dural hole. In another investigation evaluating lesions produced by Quincke needles in the human dura mater by SEM, parallel and perpendicular bevel directions produced similar holes appearing as V-shaped or half-moon-shaped lesions.[79] In contrast, transdural fluid leaks across human dura were significantly increased when the bevel of a 22-gauge Quincke needle was oriented so as to be perpendicular and not parallel to the long axis of the dura.[80] This leak was reduced when using a 22-gauge Whitacre needle and by reducing the angle of needle insertion from 90 degrees to 30 degrees, as in the case of a paramedian approach. In another study, leakage rate was related only to the needle size, progressively decreasing for 22-, 26-, and 29-gauge needles, not to bevel alignment parallel to the longitudinal direction of the fibers.[81] In this in vitro study, fluid loss across the human dura decreased in all cases and ceased within 5 minutes in 10% of punctures made with a 22-gauge needle and in 28% and 65% of the punctures produced by the smaller needles.

As to epidural anesthesia, the problem of needle rotation is somewhat different. In a study using dura mater from cadavers, it was demonstrated that rotation of a Tuohy needle significantly reduced the force required to puncture the dura.[82] This observation was the reason for recommending that Tuohy needles not be rotated once they have been inserted into the epidural space. This recommendation has certainly influenced our own policies and those of other institutions. However, it should be noted that the force required to pierce bovine dura with a 16-gauge Tuohy needle is almost twice as high as with 25- or 26-gauge pencil-point needles.[83] According to this in vitro model, pencil-point needles required significantly more force to puncture the dura than Quincke needles of the same size. At the same time, pencil-point needles caused a lesser CSF leakage than their Quincke equivalents, an indication of their superiority in terms of PDPH. Finally, we refer to some caveats mentioned with regard to laboratory reports of spinal needles, as they may be misleading and improper for identifying the best buy, a lesson more readily learned in practice.[84]

Human Factors

Any risk analysis would fall short of being complete without including human beings as a risk factor. In the case of accidental dural puncture, lack of training and practice are important contributory factors. A large-scale prospective analysis of 10,995 epidural anesthetics collected between 1989 and 1994 in a tertiary referral obstetric unit in Australia showed that trainees were twice as likely to accidentally puncture the dura compared with the specialists.[85] In another 10-year survey on women who had suffered from accidental puncture during obstetric epidural analgesia, 59 of 63 cases involved trainees.[86] These findings are in contrast to those of a 20-year survey from the Birmingham Maternity Hospital reviewing the incidence of dural taps.[44] Paradoxically, the highest rate of accidental dural punctures was observed for consultants (2.1%), while senior registrars had the lowest rate (1%), and the overall incidence was 1.3%. As the rank of an anesthesiologist is not necessarily related to any specific experience in epidural anesthesia, such findings are not too startling.

INCIDENCE

Related to Spinal Anesthesia

The advent of fine gauge and pencil-point spinal needles has enhanced the popularity of spinal anesthesia in patient groups characterized by a higher than average susceptibility to PDPH. Thus, in women presenting for operative delivery or asking for labor pain relief, both spinal and combined spinal epidural anesthesia are a part of current anesthetic practice. Each of these techniques can be largely justified, as the incidence of PDPH may be even lower than that linked to inadvertent dural puncture in the course of epidural anesthesia. Additionally, as PDPH associated with deliberate spinal puncture is less severe compared with accidental dural puncture using an epidural needle, the indication for performing an epidural blood patch for its cure is very rare.

In recent years, a few randomized controlled trials have been performed prospectively to evaluate the risk of PDPH in the obstetric population, whereas a large body of evidence regarding PDPH exists in nonobstetric subjects, a field of practice that is not the topic of this review. The most pertinent findings on PDPH related to obstetric anesthesia practice are briefly summarized in Table 35–1.

In 1990, Barker[87] published results from a prospective randomized study including 100 obstetric patients given spinal anesthesia using a 25- or 26-gauge Quincke needle. He drew attention to a marked and significant reduction in incidence of PDPH from 17.6% to 2% when the finer needle was used.

Concomitantly, Cesarini et al.[88] observed in a prospective randomized study of 110 patients undergoing cesarean section under spinal anesthesia that the incidence of PDPH was significantly reduced (14.5% vs. 0%) by using a 24-gauge Sprotte instead of a 25-gauge Quincke-type needle. In the Quincke group, five of eight patients required a blood patch.

In a similar randomized, prospective, blinded study, again using either a 24-gauge Sprotte or a 25-gauge Quincke-type needle in 194 patients requiring cesarean delivery, Devcic et al.[89] could not confirm the absence of PDPH in the Sprotte group, but the incidence of 4.2% was lower than that in the Quincke group (7.1%). In both study groups, two patients required an epidural blood patch. A further point made in this study was that the addition of 20 μg of fentanyl to the local anesthetic did not reduce the risk of PDPH.

Mayer et al.[90] evaluated the risk of PDPH in a large obstetric population undergoing cesarean section. In this study, 298 women were randomly assigned to spinal anesthesia using either a 24-gauge Sprotte or 27-gauge Quincke needle. There was no significant difference in the incidence of PDPH between the two groups, which was 0.7% in the Sprotte and 3.5% in the Quincke group. There was no need for blood patch therapy, as all PDPHs resolved quickly with conservative treatment. The authors of this study hypothesized that the trend toward a lower incidence of PDPH in the Sprotte group might have become significant if a much larger sample size with 800 to 1000 subjects per group had been included. Thus, the possibility of a type II error could not be excluded, as indicated by the erroneous conclusion of lack of effect when using the Sprotte instead of the Quincke needle.

Shutt et al.[91] investigated the incidence of PDPH after spinal anesthesia for cesarean delivery, comparing 22- and 25-gauge Whitacre needles with 26-gauge

Table 35–1 Influence of Needle Design and Diameter on the Incidence of Post–Dural Puncture Headache After Cesarean Section

Reference	Year	Needle Size and Type	Sample Size	PDPH (%)	Statistical Significance
Cutting Versus Noncutting Needles					
Cesarini[88]	1990	24 S/25 Q	55/55	0/14.5	S
Mayer[90]	1992	24 S/27 Q	151/147	0.7/3.4	NS
Shutt[91]	1992	22 W/26 Q	49/48	1.1/10.4	NS
		25 W	47	0	
Devcic[89]	1992	24 S/25 Q	96/98	4.2/7.1	S
Lambert[66]	1997	25 W/26 Q	1000/2265	1.2/5.2	S
		25 W/27 Q	1000/860	1.2/2.7	S
Noncutting Needles, Different Designs and Diameters					
Campbell[92]	1993	25 W/24 S	150/150	0.7/4	NS
Smith[94]	1994	25 W/27 W	104/108	3.8/0	NS
Hopkinson[95]	1997	25 W/25 P	170/170	0/0.6	NS
		24 S/24 P	173/168	1.2/1.2	NS
Herbstmann[97]	1998	27 W/27 DS	103/102	0/1	NS
		25 DS/26 GM	102/100	1/0	NS

Spinal needle types: Q, Quincke; S, Sprotte; W, Whitacre; DS, Durasafe; GM, Gertie Marx; P, Polymedic. The gauge size is indicated by the numbers. NS, nonsignificant, S, significant.

Quincke needles. Although the use of pencil-point needles was associated with a low incidence of PDPH (22- and 25-gauge Whitacre, 2% vs. 0%, respectively), a much higher incidence was found for the 26-gauge Quincke cannula (10.4%). Although this difference was not statistically significant compared with the other groups, the authors concluded that the balance of favor was definitely against using a 26-gauge cutting needle, which certainly represents a change in thinking within less than a decade.

In a prospective, randomized double-blind trial in 304 women undergoing elective cesarean delivery, the 25-gauge Whitacre needle was compared with the 24-gauge Sprotte needle with respect to the incidence of PDPH.[92] Not surprisingly, the frequency of PDPH tended to be higher in the Sprotte group (4%) than in the Whitacre group (0.7%), but with one subject in each group requiring a blood patch for severe PDPH, there was no difference in this regard. However, patients in the Sprotte group needed significantly more intraoperative analgesic supplementation than those in the Whitacre group (17.3% vs. 3.3%, respectively). This incidental finding was not related to the sensory block level but, hypothetically, to the possibility that only a part of the local anesthetic solution reached the spinal fluid space due to the considerably larger side hole of the Sprotte needle allowing some extradural drug disposition.

Extremely low rates of PDPH were observed in another prospective, randomized study in obstetric patients receiving spinal anesthesia using either a 22- or a 24-gauge Sprotte needle.[93] In these 375 women, the frequency of PDPH was 1.6% in each group and all headaches resolved within 72 hours with conservative treatment.

A randomized comparison of 25- and 27-gauge Whitacre needles in 212 women undergoing cesarean section showed that PDPH was prevented by using the smaller needle, whereas an incidence of 4% was reported for the larger needle and one patient even required a blood patch.[94] On the other hand, 23% of anesthesiologists categorized the 27-gauge Whitacre needle as excessively flexible, thus rendering its use difficult and contributing to some anesthetic failures.

More recently, a large-scale multicenter trial was completed evaluating four different pencil-point needles for cesarean section under spinal anesthesia in 681 patients.[95] The incidence of severe headache with the typical features of PDPH was very low, but nevertheless a number of patients subsequently were treated with an epidural blood patch (24-gauge Sprotte 1.2%, 25-gauge Whitacre 0%, 24-gauge and 25-gauge Polymedic 1.2% and 0.6%, respectively). Patient outcome and needle performance were judged to be comparably satisfactory, although a surprisingly high overall incidence of headache prior to discharge (11.1%) was observed.

A much larger sample size was provided by another nonrandomized, nonblinded study that still may fall short of the number needed to show a further reduction in very low incidences of PDPH. A series from the Brigham and Women's Hospital covering the period between 1987 and 1991 included 4125 spinal anesthetics, and both cutting bevel and pencil-point bevel needles were utilized.[66] The incidences of PDPH were significantly different, being 5.2% for 25-gauge and 2.7% for 27-gauge Quincke needles, but an even lower incidence of 1.2% was observed following the use of a 25-gauge Whitacre needle. As the frequency of accidental dural puncture occurring occasionally during initiation of epidural analgesia fluctuated between an average of 1.1% and 1.7%, the use of Whitacre needles was consequently associated with the lowest absolute requirement for epidural blood patch therapy, judged necessary in 13% to 39% in the spinal group in relation to 75% in the epidural group.

Two studies evaluated different spinal needles in association with combined spinal epidural for cesarean delivery. Lesser et al.[96] used a 30-gauge needle in conjunction with a regular Tuohy needle. In only 74% of 49 subjects, spinal anesthesia alone was adequate despite appropriate dosing. The authors blamed technical difficulties for the high failure rate and argued that in half of these cases, there was an obvious doubt about correct needle placement. Moreover, 11% of patients admitted to a mild and transient headache, but in only one of these women an accidental dural puncture with a Tuohy needle was suspected. In conclusion, an extremely small needle is not always the best solution to obviate PDPH and "a balance has to be struck between practicality, on the one hand, and a reduced incidence of side effects on the other."[96]

More recently, four different pencil-point needles were randomly selected for use in 407 consecutive obstetric patients to provide combined spinal epidural during labor or for cesarean delivery.[97] The incidence of PDPH was inconsequential, as it was similar for the four types of pencil-point needles (27-gauge Whitacre and 26-gauge Gertie Marx needles had 0%, and 25- and 27-gauge Durasafe needles had 1% incidence of PDPH).

Related to Accidental Dural Puncture

In the early 1970s, the Birmingham Maternity Hospital had a database of 27,000 cases of epidural block, showing the rate of PDPH as 77.5%.[98] Crawford had set up the obstetric epidural service in 1968 and introduced a standardized record chart for documentation the following year.[44] Twenty years later, an incidence of PDPH of 86% was reported when conservative management was practiced; 34,819 epidural blocks performed over the period of 1969 through 1988 had an incidence of 1.3% dural taps.[44]

The same incidence of PDPH (86%) was reported by Costigan and Sprigge[86] based on a 10-year analysis of cases at a district hospital maternity unit. These authors emphasized that their rate of inadvertent dural puncture was only 0.8% and thus below the 1% to 2% threshold of rare and remote risks established in England as the legal cutoff point obliging doctors to inform patients of the risk. It is noteworthy that patients suffering from PDPH did not share that position at all and believed that all pregnant women should be aware of this specific risk.[86] For England, an average dural puncture rate of 0.85% was calculated on the basis of a questionnaire covering the years 1991 through 1995, with a total of 294,268 epidural blocks.[99] Although underreporting cannot be excluded with certainty, this survey pointed out that the risk of accidental dural puncture was significantly increased from 0.7% to 1.1% if the epidural space was identified by implementing the LORA instead of the LORS technique. Similar observations regarding the risk of testing with air versus saline were also made in the Birmingham survey.[44]

As in Birmingham, at the Brigham and Women's Hospital of Boston there is also an impressive database of women receiving epidural anesthesia.[66] In 21,578 cases, in which a 17-gauge Huber-tipped Weiss needle was used, accidental dural puncture occurred with an average rate between 1.1% and 1.7%, resulting in a 75.3% incidence of PDPH requiring an epidural blood patch. Although poorly understood, the incidence of PDPH after accidental dural puncture in morbidly obese parturients with a body mass index in excess of 30 was lower than in women with a body mass index of less than 30.[100]

ECONOMIC IMPLICATIONS

The occurrence of PDPH may have significant economic effects because hospital stay is extended and patients are unable to return to work owing to persisting malaise. Such considerations are important in the current climate of growing economic constraints. An analysis of closed claims cases revealed that among injuries associated with obstetric regional anesthesia, headache was the second most common, accounting for 18% of the total claims.[101] In terms of payment, despite the relatively minor nature of headache, 56% of these cases were settled by awarding a median amount of $5000 (range, $1000 to $20,000) according to an estimate published in the early 1990s.[102] In comparison with the cost of such settlements, the costs of spinal and epidural needles are negligible. In Switzerland, the costs of different needles are as follows (converted to US dollars): $1 for a 25-gauge Quincke needle, $5.40 for a 25-gauge Sprotte needle, $5.70 for a 25-gauge pencil-point needle (Pencan), and $6.10 for an 18-gauge Tuohy needle set (Perifix).

PREVENTION

Prevention is better than cure, an admonition that is particularly applicable to PDPH. Although the "therapeutic approach is often a hit-or-miss affair with unpredictable results,"[103] this does not necessarily apply as much to preventive measures such as careful technique and appropriate equipment; these measures are imperative and should always be implemented.

Selecting the Best Needle

With reference to the data mentioned earlier, which are largely gathered from prospective randomized studies, there is little doubt that small-sized pencil-point needles should be used in all patients at increased risk for developing PDPH after spinal anesthesia, such as in obstetric anesthesia. Certainly, a similar benefit might also accrue from using extremely fine Quincke-type cutting needles. Unfortunately, the risk of technical failure is often enhanced by the inherent difficulties in handling and placing such needles and by slowing or even absence of CSF backflow.[96]

As far as epidural anesthesia is concerned, such considerations are irrelevant as long as an accidental dural puncture does not complicate the procedure. However, in the case of accidental dural puncture, little or no information is available on differences in frequency, severity, and duration of PDPH in relation to the size of the epidural needle used for the anesthetic. Nonetheless, it is reasonable to believe that larger needles are more likely to increase both the probability and the severity of PDPH.

Orientation of the Needle Bevel

Among practitioners still using Quincke-type needles in patients at increased risk for PDPH, the controversy about the effect of the orientation of the bevel of the needle tip has been settled, although laboratory and clinical evidence is far from conclusive. It has become a standard technique to insert cutting needles with the bevel parallel to the longitudinal axis of the dural fibers.[43]

In 482 patients of a wide age range alternately assigned to receive spinal anesthesia with the use of either a 22- or a 25-gauge needle, a significantly lower incidence of PDPH was observed in those in whom the needle bevel was inserted parallel to the longitudinal dural fibers (0.24%) as opposed to vertical insertion (16.1%).[104] Lybecker et al.[8] confirmed this observation in a prospective study including 873 consecutive patients undergoing 1021 spinal anesthetic procedures: the frequency was reduced by almost 50%, from 10.2% with perpendicular insertion to 5.5% with the bevel parallel to the longitudinal axis of the dural fibers. In a recent article, Corbey et al.[43] stressed another point as they observed that PDPH also occurred in patients in whom the needle was removed with the bevel perpendicular to the dural fibers following parallel insertion. They stated that they did not observe any PDPH except in those subjects in whom Quincke needles had been inserted and removed with the bevel parallel to the dural fibers. This conclusion certainly deserves further analysis. Just recently, another intriguing observation was made by neurologists showing that the incidence of PDPH was reduced significantly by reinserting the stylet (mandrin) before removing the 21-gauge Sprotte spinal needle used for diagnostic lumbar puncture.[105] In this prospective, randomized trial involving 600 patients, PDPH developed in 5% of the patients in whom the stylet was reinserted to the tip of the needle before removing the needle as opposed to 16% of the patients in whom the stylet was not reinserted.

Even in the case of inadvertent dural puncture,

the PDPH rate may be reduced by inserting the 17- or 18-gauge epidural needle with the needle bevel oriented parallel to the longitudinal fibers. Thus, Norris et al.[65] observed that both the incidence and the severity of PDPH were significantly reduced despite similar frequencies of accidental dural punctures of 2.6%; in 1558 parturients, only 31% vs. 73% of subjects developed moderate to severe PDPH and the requirement for therapeutic blood patch was significantly decreased from 50% to 19%.[65] In a subsequent study from the same institution, continuous spinal anesthesia using a macro–epidural catheter via the hole made by accidental dural puncture did not reduce the incidence or severity of PDPH.[106]

Bedrest

In the first controlled study on the preventive effect of 24-hour bedrest on the incidence of PDPH in 100 neurologic patients following diagnostic lumbar puncture with an 18-gauge needle, PDPH occurred in 40% of those mobilized immediately and in 42% of those kept in bed for 24 hours.[107] In another study in 129 elderly patients allocated randomly to bedrest for 4 or 24 hours after spinal anesthesia (22-gauge spinal needle) for urologic or gynecologic surgery, the lack of efficiency of prolonged recumbency in preventing PDPH was corroborated.[108] In a third study in 202 young male patients immobilized in a random order for 6 or 24 hours after spinal anesthesia using a 25-gauge needle, PDPH was observed in 3.1% of patients immobilized for 24 hours as opposed to 3.8% in those allowed to get up early.[109]

The same results were found for 80 obstetric patients after spinal anesthesia for cesarean section who were randomly allocated to a 24-hour period of bedrest or mobilization after 6 hours[110]; there was even a significantly greater incidence of severe PDPH in the group confined to bed for a day (20.5% vs. 2.4%, respectively). Moreover, three of eight women with severe PDPH required a blood patch for pain relief. All of these findings confirmed a previous publication in which the author stated that "there was no predictable pattern relating the time spent recumbent to the occurrence of postspinal headaches, but once headache occurs, recumbency aids in pain relief."[33]

Volume Therapy

In an effort to restore the volume of CSF lost into the epidural space, intravenous volume administration may be required in patients unable or unwilling to take oral fluids because of nausea and malaise. Otherwise, caffeine-containing fluids such as coffee, tea, or cola soft drinks are especially recommended, as they may also produce beneficial effects through an additional pharmacologic effect of caffeine (see later discussion). To date, there is no convincing evidence that hyperhydration should be recommended, because there is autoregulation of CSF production. There was no difference in the incidence and severity of PDPH in subjects receiving either 1.5 L or 3 L of oral fluids per day over a period of 5 days after diagnostic lumbar puncture.[111] On the other hand, it is obvious that aggressive hydration of patients will enhance urine production and, as a consequence, the need to get up more frequently to go to the bathroom, which is a real inconvenience for sombody suffering from PDPH.

In modern therapeutic concepts, subarachnoid saline infusion is not utilized, although its effectiveness has been known for many years.[112] This approach was originally based on the immediate relief of PDPH observed by replacement of CSF volume removed in an experimental setting.[28]

The epidural route seems to be much more acceptable for volume therapy, although the association with risks and limitations in efficiency exist. Crawford[113] was among the pioneers who presented convincingly favorable data for this approach. Using an infusion regimen consisting of an epidural drip administered for 24 hours, only 5 of 16 patients developed a remarkably mild PDPH. But the efficiency of such a therapy is limited; the Birmingham database shows that the frequency of PDPH was reduced from 86% in those managed conservatively to 70% for those receiving epidural volume therapy.[44] The risk associated with bolus injections of 40 to 60 mL of saline was eliminated by the use of an infusion. Intraocular and retinal hemorrhages related to an abrupt rise in epidural and subarachnoid pressures are among the risks reported in the literature, as these changes in pressure are transmitted to the optic nerve.[114]

A novel regimen advocates the use of dextran 40 instead of saline or blood to prevent PDPH.[115] In this small study, 17 patients, including 3 pregnant women who suffered accidental dural puncture with a 17- or 18-gauge Tuohy needle, received a bolus of 20 mL dextran 40 once the surgical procedure or labor was finished. With no other preventive measures, all subjects remained asymptomatic. Although dysesthesia or burning sensations may be produced at the injection site, such side effects were not noted by these women, probably because of residual local anesthetic effects. In this short communication, there is no indication that intravenous dextran 1 was given prior to dextran 40 administration, a measure recommended to reduce the risk of an anaphylactoid reaction.[116]

Prophylactic Blood Patch

In 1985, the somewhat provocative question was asked: "Extradural blood patch: why delay?"[117] In seven nonobstetric patients, a prophylactic epidural blood patch (EBP) of 15 to 17 mL administered within 15 minutes of accidental dural puncture with 16-, 17-, and 18-gauge Tuohy needles did not interfere with subsequent anesthesia and prevented PDPH in all subjects.

Prophylactic EBP was also demonstrated to be effective in seven obstetric patients.[118] In this study, 17 to 20 mL of autologous blood obtained by an aseptic technique was injected via the epidural catheter as rapidly as possible, over 2 to 3 minutes. In a prospective sequentially randomized study, Colonna-Romano and Shapiro[119] assessed the effectiveness of a prophylactic EBP using 15 mL autologous blood given through the epidural catheter to 39 parturients and compared the success of conservative measures in preventing PDPH. In the control group, 80% of patients developed PDPH and almost one half of these eventually received an EBP. In the study group, only 21% suffered from PDPH, which was successfully treated in three of four subjects with another EBP. Using the same epidural catheter for the EBP can be advantageous in terms of eliminating the risk of another dural tap and, furthermore, may even allow confirmation in some cases that the PDPH was due to an unrecognized dural puncture.[120]

Because an EBP is not devoid of risks and complications that may persist for months, such as a lumbovertebral syndrome,[121] the value of EBP prophylaxis still remains controversial.[86] In addition, prophylaxis may fail in some instances, particularly if the volume of autologous blood necessary for EBP therapy has been underestimated. In an early trial, a blood volume ranging between 5 and 10 mL was associated with a failure rate of 54%.[122] Therefore, it is our practice to wait until PDPH develops and not to proceed to a therapy that could be completely unnecessary.

Local Anesthetics

The influence of spinally administered local anesthetic solutions on the incidence of PDPH is an interesting finding that is difficult to explain, as no such observation was ever made in patients receiving epidural anesthesia. According to Naulty et al.,[123] the frequency of PDPH was 9.5% in patients who received hyperbaric lidocaine for spinal anesthesia, whereas those receiving hyperbaric bupivacaine or an isobaric mixture of tetracaine and procaine had rates of 7.6% and 5.8%, respectively. Hypothetically, the osmotic effect of glucose was considered to be a key factor in producing some sort of cerebral irritation, although this hypothesis is difficult to prove.

THERAPY

Because PDPH is usually a self-limiting problem and often does not last for more than a few days (see previous discussion), many therapeutic regimens have been suggested, although the success rates are often questionable. Fifty different remedies have been proposed in a monograph to solve the problem of PDPH, the majority of which are without any scientific background.[124] We will focus only on treatment modalities that are in use in current anesthetic practice.

Psychological Support

A PDPH interferes with ambulation and independence and makes breast-feeding and infant-bonding more difficult for mothers. Therefore, anxiety and malaise often are mixed with anger about a bothersome side effect. In this context, supportive psychological care represents an important component of a multimodal therapeutic approach. When explaining the etiology of PDPH to the patient, we should emphasize that by its nature the condition is expected to subside within a limited period of time.

Bedrest

If the patient avoids the upright position, PDPH symptoms disappear and the patient will feel more comfortable.[33] There is no evidence that other maneuvers such as the head-down prone position or the application of abdominal binders are of any therapeutic value.[18] If the patient is given some advice on how to relax, painful muscular contractions causing tension pain may be relieved via biofeedback mechanisms.

Analgesics

An analgesic therapy based on nonsteroidal anti-inflammatory drugs or paracetamol, or both, should be prescribed on a regular basis until symptoms of PDPH vanish. There is almost no indication to include narcotics in analgesic regimens, as they may exacerbate nausea and thus impinge additionally upon the patient's well-being.

Another avenue of therapy implements drugs that are useful in the management of migraine headaches, such as dihydroergotamine or methysergide. Because these ergot alkaloids have many other effects, they are not recommended for breast-feeding mothers. Sumatriptan, however, belongs to a new class of drug used in patients with migraine and cluster-type headaches. Like serotonin, sumatriptan activates the serotonin type-1d receptor, thus causing cerebral vasoconstriction and reversal of cerebral vasodilation occurring during migraine and cluster headache attacks.[125] Its ability to relieve PDPH was tested in six patients. In four parturients with incapacitating PDPH following a wet tap, a subcutaneous injection of 6 mg of sumatriptan resulted in pain relief within half an hour, allowing the patients to resume normal activities and caring for their babies.[125] However, there is the risk of recurrence due to the rather short plasma half-life of approximately 2 hours, a feature that may limit the usefulness of this drug, which appears particularly promising in patients in whom EBP therapy is contraindicated.

Caffeine

Since PDPH results in part from cerebral vasodilation, caffeine and caffeine-containing drinks and food may reduce the severity of symptoms by promoting vasoconstriction. In a double-blind, placebo-controlled trial, a single oral dose of 300 mg caffeine provided satisfactory pain relief within 4 hours in 90% of 20 patients.[126] Although pain relief was only transient in 30% of subjects, the magnitude of the decrease in VAS score was more than three times greater than in the placebo group and persisted in 70% of the patients. In another randomized, controlled study, 500 mg of intravenous caffeine administered in combination with sodium benzoate relieved PDPH in 75% of patients, and a repeat dose 2 hours later provided pain relief in an additional 10% of patients.[127] Yet large doses of intravenous caffeine may be risky, as central nervous system activation can result in overt grand mal seizures.[128]

Epidural Infusion Therapy

Epidural saline infusion can provide permanent pain relief in patients in whom EBP therapy has failed.[129, 130] As an alternative, a patient-controlled continuous epidural infusion of saline can be instituted to avoid or at least reduce the risk of low back pain, orbital pain, and retinal hemorrhages that may complicate the administration of too large volume loads.[114] This form of therapy does not appear to be as successful as EBP and is not often used.

Dextran 40 may be used as an alternative for saline or blood as an epidural patch.[116] To augment its efficacy, a dextran bolus of 20 mL may be followed by an infusion of 3 mL per hour until PDPH is resolved.[131] There is no evidence that such a therapy deserves priority over others with an established safety record.

Epidural Blood Patch

The EBP represents the most invasive technique for treating PDPH and, therefore, should be reserved for patients with severe or incapacitating symptoms or when more conservative treatment options have failed. The typical procedure is performed by two physicians. While one is performing an epidural puncture at the level of or one level below the original puncture site, the other collects, in a sterile fashion, about 20 to 25 mL of venous blood from the patient's antecubital fossa, which is subsequently injected epidurally by the first physician. It is of paramount importance to use strictly aseptic techniques. Optionally, a further blood sample can be withdrawn for a bacteriologic culture. The 15 to 25 mL of autologous blood should be injected slowly until the patient reports pressure in the back. If paresthesia occurs, injection should be stopped immediately. After the EBP, the patient should be left supine for approximately 1 hour. Then mobilization should be encouraged and discharge allowed, provided that PDPH has subsided and the patient feels well. The patient should be discharged with some guidelines.

In 1960, Gormley[132] reported on the first epidural injection of autologous blood. With a blood volume of only 2 to 3 mL, he claimed a 100% success rate in eight subjects, including himself as he suffered from PDPH after myelography. In the 1970s, DiGiovanni and colleagues[25, 103] described their experience with EBP using larger blood volumes. In these two studies, which included 108 patients, a blood volume averaging 5 to 10 mL was injected. Immediate and permanent pain relief was observed in 90% of subjects and partial relief in another 8% within 24 hours. As early as 1974, a large-scale prospective study was undertaken by the Society for Obstetric Anesthesia and Perinatology (SOAP) that included 185 patients in whom PDPH was first noticed about 1 day after accidental dural puncture.[133] EBP was performed approximately 4 days after the onset of symptoms when conservative treatment failed. Complete and permanent pain relief was achieved in 98% of patients given an EBP with an average blood volume of about 10 mL. Three therapeutic failures were attributed to inadequacy of EBP blood volume consisting of only 6 mL. There were no severe or permanent complications. A similarly high overall success rate of 97.5% was reported by Abouleish et al.,[134] who evaluated the long-term effectiveness of EBP in 118 patients.

There is still some controversy about the most effective volume of autologous blood in EBP therapy and the optimal timing. As to the most effective volume, there seems to be a direct relationship between the volume injected and the success rate. Crawford[135] pointed out that in his experience a blood volume of 20 mL should be used whenever performing an EBP, unless the patient complains of pain or discomfort during the injection. With less than 20 mL, complete and permanent pain relief was provided in 83% of subjects, whereas an injection of at least 20 mL was successful in 91% of the patients.[136] In a recent prospective study in 81 nonobstetric subjects, the efficacy of different volumes of blood for EBP was evaluated.[137] With a volume of 10 mL in the first part of the study and 10 to 15 mL in the second part, only 61% of patients reported permanent pain relief, although after 2 hours EBP was considered to be successful in 88% and 96% of the cases, respectively. This observation casts doubt on the magic bullet status of EBP in the treatment of PDPH. One might wonder how many recurrences of PDPH were missed in earlier studies.

The optimal moment to perform an EBP also remains a topic of controversy. It is a common belief that efficiency increases with an interval of more than 24 hours from accidental dural puncture. In one study, the failure rate of an EBP done less than 24 hours after dural puncture was 71%; that of EBP done after 24 hours was only 4%.[138] As the authors mentioned, the mechanism of greater success of late EBP is a matter of speculation. Failure of the first EBP is not necessarily related to timing, as it occurs with a frequency of 68% to 90%.[44, 133, 135] As failure may be due to inadequte volume or wrong level of injection, a repeat EBP can be safely administered if the initial patch fails to provide satisfactory or permanent pain relief.[136] If headache still persists, alternative diagnoses should be excluded (see earlier discussion) before performing another EBP or proceeding to alternative therapies.

Administration of an EBP is associated with a number of side effects and risks. Transient side effects include severe backache, pain in the neck, and paresthesia radiating down both legs. The risk of infection should be minimal provided a strictly aseptic technique was achieved. The occurrence of a long-lasting lumbovertebral syndrome[121, 134] or permanent neurologic complications is extremely rare.[139, 140] It is stressed that a previous wet tap, with or without EBP, does not reduce the success of subsequent epidural anesthesia.[141] However, based on these retrospective data, the chances of another accidental dural puncture tended to be slightly increased.

New imaging techniques have been employed to investigate the distribution of EBP, assess the volume effect, and follow the fate of the injectate over time. Using technetium-labeled red cells for marking an EBP administered in 10 patients with PDPH, blood spread was studied using a gamma camera during injection and after 30 minutes and 3 hours.[142] The average volume injected was 15 mL (range, 12–18 mL), which resulted in a spread over nine spinal segments (range, 7–14 segments). Blood spread more readily in the cephalad than in the caudad direction. In conclusion, the authors deemed a volume of 15 mL sufficient to seal the dural rent. They found it advisable to inject either at the same interspace or at one interspace below the place of dural puncture to bring the EBP as close to the dural leak as possible. By using MRI, the authors confirmed predominant cephalad spread of the EBP, which was accompanied by a marked compression of the intradural space present at 30 minutes and 3 hours after application.[143] By 7 hours, however, the blood clot had resolved, leaving only a thick layer of mature clot over the dorsal part of the dural membrane. As some blood was seen leaking from the injection site into the subcutaneous tissues and occasionally compressing nerve roots, a potential factor that could account for backache was identified. Tamponade at the site of dural puncture was also suggested as the probable mechanism underlying the action of an EBP.[144] Such findings are supported by animal studies performed in goats, which showed that an EBP per se is innocuous and that clot organization with early fibroblast activity and collagen deposition occurred in a regular way.[103] As far as histologic findings are concerned, there was no difference between animals receiving an EBP and control animals submitted to an epidural puncture alone.

There are some instances in which an EBP is contraindicated. They are similar to those of regional anesthesia and include localized or systemic infection, sepsis, coagulation disorder, and patient refusal (as with Jehovah's Witnesses). EBP in subjects with human immunodeficiency virus infection is somewhat controversial, although there is a report of successful administration without untoward sequelae in six seropositive patients.[145]

Surgical Treatment

Surgical repair of a cerebrospinal fluid leak with dorsolumbar fascia has been reported to result in almost complete alleviation of longstanding PDPH.[146] In this case, a 58-year-old woman experienced incapacitating headache and occipital paresthesia that could not be cured by conservative methods of treatment for 5 years, following a lumbar myelography.

CONCLUSIONS

A thorough knowledge of the factors affecting the incidence of PDPH is important. Since PDPH is an entirely iatrogenic complication, it can result in strong emotional reactions by the patient as well as the physician. It is of paramount importance that the patient be informed about this potential problem. Substandard care should be banned to avoid injury to patients who are, in fact, consumers and therefore expect to obtain the best possible service. As the "therapeutic approach to the problem is often a hit-or-miss affair," it is far better to prevent PDPH than to treat it.[103] There are many controversial as well as a few substantiated therapeutic methods. Before resorting to invasive treatments such as EBP, noninvasive conservative therapeutic modalities should always be utilized, unless early invasive treatment of severe PDPH is indicated.

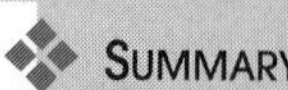

SUMMARY

Key Points

- Headaches after childbirth are multifactorial and do not necessarily signify PDPH, even after an intentional or unintentional dural puncture.
- PDPH is aggravated in the upright position and relieved in the supine position.
- The risk of PDPH is decreased by implementing careful technique and "atraumatic" spinal needles.
- Conservative therapy for PDPH should precede administration of an epidural blood patch, if symptoms allow.
- Epidural blood patch is safe and highly effective for the treatment of PDPH.

Key Reference

Paech MJ, Godkin R, Webster S: Complications of obstetric epidural analgesia and anaesthesia: A prospective analysis of 10,995 cases. Int J Obstet Anesth 1998; 7:5–11.

Case Stem

A 24-year-old G2P1 had an unintentional dural puncture during placement of epidural analgesia for labor. Twenty-four hours after vaginal delivery, the woman complains of severe headache when sitting up or standing. Her symptoms resolve when she is recumbent. Discuss the differential diagnosis and therapeutic modalities.

References

1. Bier A: Versuche über Cocainisierung des Rückenmarks. Dtsch Z Chir 1899; 51:361.
2. Koller K: Vorläufige Mitteilung über locale Anaesthesierung am Auge. Klin Monatsbl Augenheilkd 1884; 22:Beilageheft 60.
3. Schleich CL: Die Infiltrationsanästhesie (lokale Anästhesie) und ihr Verhältnis zur allgemeinen Narkose (Inhalationsanästhesie). Verh Dtsch Ges Chir 1892; 1:121.
4. MacRobert RG: The cause of lumbar puncture headache. J Am Med Assoc 1918; 70:1350.
5. Kreis O: Über Medullarnarkose bei Gebärenden. Centrlbt Gyn 1900; 28:724.
6. Kortum K, Nolte H, Kenkmann HJ: Sex difference related

complication rates after spinal anaesthesia [German]. Reg Anesth 1982; 5:1.
7. Rasmussen BS, Blom L, Hansen P, et al: Postspinal headache in young and elderly patients. Two randomised, double-blind studies that compare 20- and 25-gauge needles. Anaesthesia 1989; 44:571.
8. Lybecker H, Møller JT, May O, et al: Incidence and prediction of postdural puncture headache. A prospective study of 1021 spinal anesthesias. Anesth Analg 1990; 70:389.
9. Sarma VJ, Boström U: Intrathecal anaesthesia for day-care surgery. A retrospective study of 160 cases using 25- and 26-gauge spinal needles. Anaesthesia 1990; 45:769.
10. Kang SB, Goodnough DE, Lee YK, et al: Comparison of 26- and 27-G needles for spinal anesthesia for ambulatory surgery patients. Anesthesiology 1992; 76:734.
11. Vandam LD, Dripps RD: Long-term follow-up of patients who received 10,098 spinal anesthetics. Syndrome of decreased intracranial pressure (headache and ocular auditory difficulties). J Am Med Assoc 1956; 161:586.
12. Tourtellotte WW, Henderson WG, Tucker RP, et al: A randomized, double-blind clinical trial comparing the 22- versus 26-gauge needle in the production of the post-lumbar puncture syndrome in normal individuals. Headache 1972; 12:73.
13. Vilming ST, Schrader H, Monstad I: The significance of age, sex, and cerebrospinal fluid pressure in post-lumbar-puncture headache. Cephalalgia 1989; 9:99.
14. Silberstein SD: The role of sex hormones in headache. Neurology 1992; 42(Suppl):37.
15. Stein G, Morton J, Marsh A, et al: Headaches after childbirth. Acta Neurol Scand 1984; 69:74.
16. Scharff L, Marcus DA, Turk DC: Headache during pregnancy and in the postpartum: A prospective study. Headache 1997; 37:203.
17. Daniels AM, Sallie R: Headache, lumbar puncture, and expectation. Lancet 1981; 1:1003.
18. Brownridge P: The management of headache following accidental dural puncture in obstetric patients. Anaesth Intensive Care 1983; 11:4.
19. Kaplan G: The psychogenic etiology of headache post lumbar puncture. Psychosom Med 1967; 29:376.
20. Sechzer PH: Post-spinal anesthesia headache treated with caffeine. Part II: Intracranial vascular distension, a key factor. Curr Ther Res 1979; 26:440.
21. Gobel H, Klostermann H, Lindner V, et al: Changes in cerebral haemodynamics in cases of post–lumbar puncture headache: A prospective transcranial Doppler ultrasound study. Cephalalgia 1990; 10:117.
22. Grant R, Condon B, Hart I, et al: Changes in intracranial CSF volume after lumbar puncture and their relationship to post-LP headache. J Neurol Neurosurg Psychiatry 1991; 54:440.
23. Teasdale GM, Grant R, Condon B, et al: Intracranial CSF volumes: Natural variations and physiological changes measured by MRI. Acta Neurochir Suppl 1988; 42:230.
24. Grant R, Condon B, Lawrence A, et al: Human cranial CSF volumes measured by MRI: Sex and age influences. Magn Reson Imaging 1987; 5:465.
25. DiGiovanni AJ, Dunbar BS: Epidural injections of autologous blood for postlumbar-puncture headache. Anesth Analg 1970; 49:268.
26. Raskin NH: Lumbar puncture headache: A review. Headache 1990; 30:197.
27. Iqbal J, Davis LE, Orrison WW Jr: An MRI study of lumbar puncture headaches. Headache 1995; 35:420.
28. Kunkle C, Ray BS, Wolff H: Experimental studies on headache. Analysis of the headache associated with changes in intracranial pressure. Arch Neurol Psychiatry 1943; 49:323.
29. Feindel W, Penfield W, McNaughton F: The tentorial nerves and localization of intracranial pain in man. Neurology 1960; 10:555.
30. Kimmel DL: Innervation of spinal dura mater and dura mater of the posterior cranial fossa. Neurology 1961; 11:800.
31. Khurana RK: Intracranial hypotension. Semin Neurol 1996; 16:5.
32. Lussos SA, Loeffler C: Epidural blood patch improves postdural puncture headache in a patient with benign intracranial hypertension. Reg Anesth 1993; 18:315.
33. Jones RJ: The role of recumbency in the prevention and treatment of postspinal headache. Anesth Analg 1974; 53:788.
34. Lybecker H, Djernes M, Schmidt JF: Postdural puncture headache (PDPH): Onset, duration, severity, and associated symptoms. An analysis of 75 consecutive patients with PDPH. Acta Anaesthesiol Scand 1995; 39:605.
35. Lynch J, Krings-Ernst I, Strick K, et al: Use of a 25-gauge Whitacre needle to reduce the incidence of postdural puncture headache. Br J Anaesth 1991; 67:690.
36. Richer S, Ritacca D: Sixth nerve palsy after lumbar anesthesia. Optom Vis Sci 1989; 66:320.
37. Whiting AS, Johnson LN, Martin DE: Cranial nerve paresis following epidural and spinal anesthesia. Trans Pa Acad Ophthalmol Otolaryngol 1990; 42:972.
38. Fog J, Wang LP, Sundberg A, et al: Hearing loss after spinal anesthesia is related to needle size. Anesth Analg 1990; 70:517.
39. Bjärnhall M, Ekseth K, Boström S, et al: Intracranial subdural haematoma: A rare complication following spinal anaesthesia. Acta Anaesthesiol Scand 1996; 40:1249.
40. Corbey MP, Berg P, Quaynor H: Classification and severity of postdural puncture headache. Comparison of 26-gauge and 27-gauge Quincke needle for spinal anaesthesia in day-care surgery in patients under 45 years. Anaesthesia 1993; 48:776.
41. Halpern S, Preston R: Postdural puncture headache and spinal needle design. Anesthesiology 1994; 81:1376.
42. Lynch J, Kasper SM, Strick K, et al: The use of Quincke and Whitacre 27-gauge needles in orthopedic patients: Incidence of failed spinal anesthesia and postdural puncture headache. Anesth Analg 1994; 79:124.
43. Corbey MP, Bach AB, Lech K, et al: Grading of severity of postdural puncture headache after 27-gauge Quincke and Whitacre needles. Acta Anaesthesiol Scand 1997; 41:779.
44. Stride PC, Cooper GM: Dural taps revisited. A 20-year survey from Birmingham Maternity Hospital. Anaesthesia 1993; 48:247.
45. Levine MC, White DW: Chronic postmyelographic headache. A result of persistent cerebrospinal fluid fistula. J Am Med Assoc 1974; 229:684.
46. Abouleish E: Epidural blood patch for the treatment of chronic post–lumbar puncture cephalalgia. Anesthesiology 1978; 49:291.
47. Benhamou D, Hamza J, Ducott B: Post-partum headache after epidural analgesia without dural puncture. Int J Obstet Anesth 1995; 4:17.
48. Douglas KA, Redman CWG: Eclampsia in the United Kingdom. Br Med J 1994; 309:1395.
49. Hampl KF, Stotz G, Schneider MC: Postoperative transient hemihypaesthesia and severe headache associated with caffeine withdrawal [letter]. Anaesthesia 1994; 49:266.
50. Hampl KF, Schneider MC, Rüttimann U, et al: Perioperative administration of caffeine tablets for prevention of postoperative headaches. Can J Anaesth 1995: 42:789.
51. Ready LB, Helfer D: Bacterial meningitis in parturients after epidural anesthesia. Anesthesiology 1989; 71:988.
52. Roberts SP, Petts HV: Meningitis after obstetric spinal anaesthesia. Anaesthesia 1990; 45:376.
53. Lee JJ, Parry H: Bacterial meningitis following spinal anaesthesia for Caesarean section. Br J Anaesth 1991; 66:383.
54. Davis L, Hargreaves C, Robinson PN: Postpartum meningitis. Anaesthesia 1993; 48:788.
55. Liu SS, Pope A: Spinal meningitis masquerading as postdural puncture headache [letter]. Anesthesiology 1996; 85:1493.
56. Gurmarnik S: Skin preparation and spinal headache. Anaesthesia 1988; 43:1057.
57. Gewirtz EC, Costin M, Marx GF: Cortical vein thrombosis may mimic postdural puncture headache. Reg Anesth 1987; 12:188.
58. Borum SE, Naul LG, McLeskey CH: Postpartum dural venous sinus thrombosis after postdural puncture headache and epidural blood patch. Anesthesiology 1997; 86:487.
59. Schmidt A, Nolte H: Subdural and epidural haematomas following spinal, epidural, or caudal anaesthesia [German]. Anaesthesist 1992; 41:276.

60. Campbell DA, Varma TRK: Chronic subdural haematoma following epidural anaesthesia, presenting as puerperal psychosis. Br J Obstet Gynaecol 1993; 100:782.
61. Dutton DA: A 'postspinal headache' associated with incidental intracranial pathology. Anaesthesia 1991; 46:1044.
62. Hullander RM, Bogard TD, Leivers D, et al: Chiari I malformation presenting as recurrent spinal headache. Anesth Analg 1992; 75:1025.
63. Saberski LR, Kondamuri S, Osinubi OYO: Identification of the epidural space: Is loss of resistance to air a safe technique? Reg Anesth 1997; 22:3.
64. Aida S, Taga K, Yamakura T, et al: Headache after attempted epidural block. The role of intrathecal air. Anesthesiology 1998; 88:76.
65. Norris MC, Leighton BL, DeSimone CA: Needle bevel direction and headache after inadvertent dural puncture. Anesthesiology 1989; 70:729.
66. Lambert DH, Hurley RJ, Hertwig L, et al: Role of needle gauge and tip configuration in the production of lumbar puncture headache. Reg Anesth 1997; 22:66.
67. Greene HM: Lumbar puncture and the prevention of postpuncture headache. J Am Med Assoc 1926; 86: 391.
68. Hart JR, Whitacre RJ: Pencil-point needle in prevention of postspinal headache. J Am Med Assoc 1951; 147:657.
69. Sprotte G, Schedel R, Pajunk H, et al: An atraumatic needle for single-shot regional anesthesia [German]. Reg Anesth 1987; 10:104.
70. Jokinen MJ, Pitkänen MT, Lehtonen E, et al: Deformed spinal needle tips and associated dural perforations examined by scanning electron microscopy. Acta Anaesthesiol Scand 1996; 40:687.
71. Benham M: Spinal needle damage during routine clinical practice. Anaesthesia 1996; 51:843.
72. Rosenberg PH, Pitkänen MT, Hakala P, et al: Microscopic analysis of the tips of thin spinal needles after subarachnoid puncture. Reg Anesth 1996; 21:35.
73. Sitzman BT, Uncles DR: The effect of needle type, gauge, and tip bend on spinal needle deflection. Anesth Analg 1996; 82:297.
74. Seeberger MD, Kaufmann M, Staender S, et al: Repeated dural punctures increase the incidence of postdural puncture headache. Anesth Analg 1996; 82:302.
75. Kopacz DJ, Allen HW: Comparison of needle deviation during regional anesthetic techniques in a laboratory model. Anesth Analg 1995; 81:630.
76. Fink BR, Walker S: Orientation of fibers in human dorsal lumbar dura mater in relation to lumbar puncture. Anesth Analg 1989; 69:768.
77. Dittmann M, Schäfer H-G, Ulrich J, et al: Anatomical re-evaluation of lumbar dura mater with regard to postspinal headache. Effect of dural puncture. Anaesthesia 1988; 43:635.
78. Celleno D, Capogna G, Costantino P, et al: An anatomic study of the effects of dural puncture with different spinal needles. Reg Anesth 1993; 18:218.
79. Reina MA, Lopez-Garcia A, de Andres-Ibanez JA, et al: Electron microscopy of the lesions produced in the human dura mater by Quincke beveled and Whitacre needles [Spanish]. Rev Esp Anestesiol Reanim 1997; 44:56.
80. Ready LB, Cuplin S, Haschke RH, et al: Spinal needle determinants of rate of transdural fluid leak. Anesth Analg 1989; 69:457–460.
81. Cruickshank RH, Hopkinson JM: Fluid flow through dural puncture sites: An in vitro comparison of needle point types. Anaesthesia 1989; 44:415.
82. Meiklejohn BH: The effect of rotation of an epidural needle. An *in vitro* study. Anaesthesia 1987; 42:1180.
83. Westbrook JL, Uncles DR, Sitzman BT, et al: Comparison of the force required for dural puncture with different spinal needles and subsequent leakage of cerebrospinal fluid. Anesth Analg 1994; 79:769.
84. Lyons G, Lesser P, Bembridge M: Lessons from *in vitro* testing of spinal needles. Anaesthesia 1995; 50:964.
85. Paech MJ, Godkin R, Webster S: Complications of obstetric epidural analgesia and anaesthesia: A prospective analysis of 10,995 cases. Int J Obstet Anesth 1998; 7:5.
86. Costigan SN, Sprigge JS: Dural puncture: The patient's perspective. A patient survey of cases at a DGH maternity unit 1983–1993. Acta Anaesthesiol Scand 1996; 40:710.
87. Barker P: Are obstetric spinal headaches avoidable? Anaesth Intensive Care 1990;18:553.
88. Cesarini M, Torrielli R, Lahaye F, et al: Sprotte needle for intrathecal anaesthesia for Caesarean section: Incidence of postdural puncture headache. Anaesthesia 1990; 45:656.
89. Devcic A, Sprung J, Patel S, et al: PDPH in obstetric anesthesia: Comparison of 24-gauge Sprotte and 25-gauge Quincke needles and effect of subarachnoid administration of fentanyl. Reg Anesth 1993; 18:222.
90. Mayer DC, Quance D, Weeks SK: Headache after spinal anesthesia for cesarean section: A comparison of the 27-gauge Quincke and 24-gauge Sprotte needles. Anesth Analg 1992; 75:377.
91. Shutt LE, Valentine SJ, Wee MYK, et al: Spinal anaesthesia for Caesarean section: Comparison of 22-gauge and 25-gauge Whitacre needles with 26-gauge Quincke needles. Br J Anaesth 1992; 69:589.
92. Campbell DC, Douglas J, Pavy TJG, et al: Comparison of the 25-gauge Whitacre with the 24-gauge Sprotte spinal needle for elective Caesarean section: Cost implications. Can J Anaesth 1993; 40:1131.
93. Sears DH, Leeman MI, Jassy LJ, et al: The frequency of postdural puncture headache in obstetric patients: A prospective study comparing the 24-gauge versus the 22-gauge Sprotte needle. J Clin Anesth 1994; 6:42.
94. Smith EA, Thorburn J, Duckworth RA, et al: A comparison of 25 G and 27 G Whitacre needles for Caesarean section. Anaesthesia 1994; 49:859.
95. Hopkinson JM, Samaan AK, Russell IF, et al: A comparative multicentre trial of spinal needles for Caesarean section. Anaesthesia 1997; 52:998.
96. Lesser P, Bembridge M, Lyons G, et al: An evaluation of a 30-gauge needle for spinal anaesthesia for Caesarean section. Anaesthesia 1990; 45:767.
97. Herbstman CH, Jaffee JB, Tuman KJ, et al: An *in vivo* evaluation of four spinal needles used for the combined spinal-epidural technique. Anesth Analg 1998; 86:520.
98. Crawford JS: Lumbar epidural block in labour: A clinical analysis. Br J Anaesth 1972; 44:66.
99. Gleeson C, Scrutton M, Reynolds F: Accidental dural puncture in UK obstetric practice (abstract). Int Monitor 1997; 9:124.
100. Faure E, Moreno R, Thisted R: Incidence of postdural puncture headache in morbidly obese parturients (letter). Reg Anesth 1994; 19:361.
101. Chadwick HS: An analysis of obstetric anesthesia cases from the American Society of Anesthesiologists closed claims project database. Int J Obstet Anesth 1996; 5:258.
102. Chadwick HS, Posner K, Caplan RA, et al: A comparison of obstetric and nonobstetric anesthesia malpractice claims. Anesthesiology 1991; 74:242.
103. DiGiovanni AJ, Galbert MW, Wahle WM: Epidural injection of autologous blood for postlumbar-puncture headache. II. Additional clinical experiences and laboratory investigation. Anesth Analg 1972; 51:226.
104. Mihic DN: Postspinal headache and relationship of needle bevel to longitudinal dural fibers. Reg Anesth 1985; 10:76.
105. Strupp M, Brandt T: Should one reinsert the stylet during lumbar puncture? N Engl J Med 1997; 336:1190.
106. Norris MC, Leighton BL: Continuous spinal anesthesia after unintentional dural puncture in parturients. Reg Anesth 1990; 15:285.
107. Carbaat PAT, Van Drevel H: Lumbar puncture headache: Controlled study on the preventive effect of 24 hours' bed rest. Lancet 1981; 2:1133.
108. Cook PT, Davies MJ, Beavis RE: Bed rest and postlumbar puncture headache. The effectiveness of 24 hours' recumbency in reducing the incidence of postlumbar puncture headache. Anaesthesia 1989; 44:389.
109. Frenkel C, Altscher T, Groben V, et al: Incidence of post–dural puncture headache in a young patient population [German]. Anaesthesist 1992; 41:142.

110. Thornberry EA, Thomas TA: Posture and post–spinal headache. Br J Anaesth 1988; 60:195.
111. Dieterich M, Brandt T: Incidence of post–lumbar puncture headache is independent of daily fluid intake. Eur Arch Psychiatry Neurol Sci 1988; 237:194.
112. Pickering GW: Lumbar puncture headache. Brain 1948; 71:274.
113. Crawford JS: The prevention of headache consequent upon dural puncture. Br J Anaesth 1972; 44:598.
114. Clark CJ, Whitwell J: Intraocular haemorrhage after epidural injection. Br Med J 1961; 1:1612.
115. Salvador L, Carrero E, Castillo J, et al: Prevention of post–dural puncture headache with epidural-administered dextran 40 [letter]. Reg Anesth 1992; 17:357.
116. Stevens DS, Peeters-Asdourian C: Treatment of postdural puncture headache with 'epidural dextran patch' [letter]. Reg Anesth 1993; 18:324.
117. Quaynor H, Corbey M: Extradural blood patch—why delay? Br J Anaesth 1985; 57:538.
118. Cheek TG, Banner R, Sauter J, et al: Prophylactic extradural blood patch is effective. Br J Anaesth 1988; 61:340.
119. Colonna-Romano P, Shapiro BE: Unintentional dural puncture and prophylactic epidural blood patch in obstetrics. Anesth Analg 1989; 69:522.
120. Shah JL, Veness AM: Epidural blood patch using a catheter. Diagnosis of an unrecognised dural tap. Anaesthesia 1985; 40:1120.
121. Seeberger MD, Urwyler A: Lumbovertebral syndrome after extradural blood patch. Br J Anaesth 1992; 69:414.
122. Palahniuk RJ, Cumming M: Prophylactic blood patch does not prevent post–lumbar puncture headache. Can Anaesth Soc J 1979; 26:132.
123. Naulty JS, Hertwig L, Hunt CO, et al: Influence of local anesthetic solution on postdural puncture headache. Anesthesiology 1990; 72:450.
124. Tourtellotte WW, Haerer AF, Heller GL, et al: Post–Lumbar Puncture Headaches. Springfield, IL: Charles C Thomas; 1964:87, 98.
125. Carp H, Singh PJ, Vadhera R, et al: Effects of the serotonin-receptor agonist sumatriptan on postdural puncture headache: report of six cases. Anesth Analg 1994; 79:180.
126. Camann WR, Murray S, Mushlin PS, et al: Effects of oral caffeine on postdural puncture headache. A double-blind, placebo-controlled trial. Anesth Analg 1990; 70:181.
127. Sechzer PH, Abel L: Post–spinal anesthesia headache treated with caffeine. Evaluation with demand method. Part I. Curr Ther Res 1978; 24:307.
128. Bolton VC, Leicht CH, Scanlon TS: Postpartum seizure after epidural blood patch and intravenous caffeine sodium benzoate. Anesthesiology 1989; 70;146.
129. Baysinger CL, Menk EJ, Harte E, et al: The successful treatment of dural puncture headache after failed epidural blood patch. Anesth Analg 1986; 65:1242.
130. Stevens RA, Jorgensen N: Successful treatment of dural puncture headache with epidural saline infusion after failure of epidural blood patch. Acta Anaesthesiol Scand 1988; 32:429.
131. Aldrete JA: Epidural dextran for PDPH [letter]. Reg Anesth 1993; 18:325.
132. Gormley JB: Treatment of postspinal headache. Anesthesiology 1960; 21:565.
133. Ostheimer GW, Palahniuk RJ, Shnider SM: Epidural blood patch for post–lumbar-puncture headache [letter]. Anesthesiology 1974; 41:307.
134. Abouleish E, de la Vega S, Blendinger I, et al: Long-term follow-up of epidural blood patch. Anesth Analg 1975; 54:459.
135. Crawford JS: Experience with epidural blood patch. Anaesthesia 1980; 35:513.
136. Crawford JS: Epidural blood patch [letter]. Anaesthesia 1985; 40:381.
137. Taivainen T, Pitkänen M, Tuominen M, et al: Efficacy of epidural blood patch for postdural puncture headache. Acta Anaesthesiol Scand 1993; 37:702.
138. Loeser EA, Hill GE, Bennett GM, et al: Time vs. success rate for epidural blood patch. Anesthesiology 1978; 49:147.
139. Mantia AM: Clinical report of the occurrence of an intracerebral hemorrhage following post–lumbar puncture headache. Anesthesiology 1981; 55:684.
140. Sperry RJ, Gartrell A, Johnson JO: Epidural blood patch can cause acute neurologic deterioration. Anesthesiology 1995; 82:303.
141. Blanche R, Eisenach JC, Tuttle R, et al: Previous wet tap does not reduce success rate of labor epidural analgesia. Anesth Analg 1994; 79:291.
142. Szeinfeld M, Ihmeidan IH, Moser MM, et al: Epidural blood patch: Evaluation of the volume and spread of blood injected into the epidural space. Anesthesiology 1986; 64:820.
143. Beards SC, Jackson A, Griffiths AG, et al: Magnetic resonance imaging of extradural blood patches: Appearances from 30 min to 18 h. Br J Anaesth 1993; 71:182.
144. Griffiths AG, Beards SC, Jackson A, et al: Visualization of extradural blood patch for post–lumbar puncture headache by magnetic resonance technique. Br J Anaesth 1993; 70:223.
145. Tom DJ, Gulevich SJ, Shapiro HM, et al: Epidural blood patch in the HIV-positive patient. Review of clinical experience. Anesthesiology 1992; 76:943.
146. Harrington H, Tyler HR, Welch K: Surgical treatment of post–lumbar puncture dural CSF leak causing chronic headache. Case report. J Neurosurg 1982; 57:703.

36

Complications of Regional Anesthesia

❖ Clive Bourn Collier, MBBS, MD, MRCP, FRCA, FANZCA

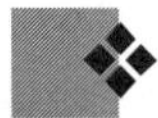

INTRODUCTION

This chapter describes many of the complications of epidural and subarachnoid block that may occur in the course of labor and delivery, or in the postpartum period. There have been several recent advances in the equipment, analgesic solutions, and anesthetic techniques employed for regional anesthesia and a seemingly corresponding increase in the number of reports of complications appearing in the anesthetic literature, or as anecdotal information. Whether the true incidence of complications is indeed growing remains to be determined.

Some of the complications to be discussed are unique to one technique or the other, but there is considerable overlap, and the use of combined techniques may cause diagnostic confusion. Each complication is discussed in approximately chronologic order under the three types of regional anesthesia—epidural block (EPB), subarachnoid block (SAB), and combined spinal-epidural block (CSE)—as applicable.

COMPLICATIONS ARISING DURING NEEDLE OR CATHETER INSERTION

Paresthesias

In epidural block, transient paresthesias frequently follow contact between incoming epidural catheters and adjacent nerve roots, with an incidence as high as 44% in one series.[1] Contact between epidural needles and the laterally placed nerve roots is extremely rare. With soft catheters a brief episode of shooting pain, similar to an electric shock down one leg, is usually the only complaint, and sequelae are extremely rare.[2] However, if paresthesias persist, the catheter should be removed and inserted in another intervertebral space. The use of fairly rigid catheters, particularly those incorporating stylets, appears to be associated with the highest incidence of paresthesias and the definite possibility of a subsequent traumatic mononeuropathy with the development of an area of sensory loss or hyperesthesia, lasting several weeks or months.[3] Soft flexible-tip catheters are associated with the lowest incidence of paresthesias on insertion and appear ideal, but the pliant catheter tips may be easily diverted from their ideal position in the epidural space and unsatisfactory blocks may result.

In SAB, paresthesias resulting from contact between cutting-point spinal needles and the nerve roots in the subarachnoid space were rarely reported prior to 1990. However, an incidence of 6% when Quincke cutting-point needles were used has recently been published.[4] Pencil-point needles have become a popular innovation in the last few years, but they have recently been associated with a higher incidence of paresthesias (12%).[5] A relationship between paresthesias on spinal needle insertion and subsequent nerve damage has been recognized for many years, but is not clear-cut, although repeated episodes of paresthesias constitute a known risk factor.[6]

An even higher incidence of paresthesias (27%) has been reported following spinal needle insertion during the relatively new CSE technique using a single-space approach.[7] The reason for this may be related to both the unusual acute angle of approach to the nerve roots adopted by the spinal needle point as it emerges from the epidural needle and also possible fixation of the dura and the underlying cauda equina by the tip of the epidural needle. There are published reports and anecdotal accounts of unexplained neurologic deficits after CSE block,[8, 9] although no direct correlation with prior occurrence of paresthesias has been detected. Close scrutiny of future results will be mandatory.

Venous Puncture

Puncture of epidural veins by either the epidural needle or more commonly the epidural catheter is a fairly frequent complication with epidural and CSE block in the obstetric patient, with a reported incidence ranging between 3% and 16%.[10] The incidence may be reduced by several methods. These include not advancing the needle or catheter into the epidural space when the patient is straining and raising her epidural venous pressure during a contraction, "lubricating" the epidural space with a small volume of fluid prior to catheter insertion,[11] and the use of smaller gauge (18 gauge or less) catheters. Also, the use of softer, more pliable catheters may be advantageous. Blood vessel trauma may lead to hematoma formation, but compression of spinal cord or nerve roots is extremely unlikely to follow in fit, young obstetric patients.[12]

Single-shot spinal anesthesia (SAB) is associated with the lowest incidence of spinal hemorrhage of all the techniques. Bleeding usually arises from subdural vessels.

Accidental Dural Puncture

Accidental puncture of the dura by epidural needles, or more rarely by epidural catheters, is unfortunately a fairly common complication in epidural block. The quoted figures for incidence vary widely, from 0.19% to 4.4% in recent surveys.[12] Figures above 1% would appear largely to reflect the lack of experience and possibly poor technique of trainee operators as well as an insufficient degree of supervision, and are difficult to justify in view of the serious nature of the recognized sequelae. These include the development of excessively high levels of block following inadvertent local anesthetic injection and the late onset of headache and associated morbidity.

Immediate Management of Dural Puncture. The loss of cerebrospinal fluid (CSF) should be minimized by immediately replacing the stylet of the epidural needle, or alternatively, removing the needle completely. Partial removal of the epidural needle until its tip is outside the dura and CSF flow has stopped is not recommended, as the subdural rather than the epidural space may be entered, and a high block may follow local anesthetic injection.[13]

If it is decided to proceed with SAB, then caution should be exercised as, again, there is risk of a high block, especially if any fluid has been injected into the epidural space.[14] The mechanism underlying this is believed to be increased hydrostatic pressure in the epidural space, which compresses the contents of the subarachnoid space and encourages the spread of intrathecal local anesthetic solutions.

Epidural puncture may be repeated in an adjacent interspace, although there appears to be an increased risk of a second dural puncture. The volume of epidural local anesthetic injected should be decreased by about 25% and given in small increments following a satisfactory test dose, because it is possible that the tip of the catheter or part of the epidural dose of local anesthetic may enter the subarachnoid space through the hole in the dura.[15] It is fairly common to observe an unusual degree of motor block in the legs following the epidural injection of solutions such as 0.25% bupivacaine in the presence of a dural puncture. Postcesarean section infusions of more dilute solutions may be ineffective in the presence of copious volumes of CSF.[16] Figure 36–1 demonstrates large filling defects produced by CSF in the body of contrast which would normally fill the lumbar epidural space. Figure 36–2 shows a normal epidurogram for comparison. As much as 200 mL of CSF per day may flow through the dural hole.[17]

The conduct of labor is not altered following dural puncture, despite earlier recommendations that forceps delivery be encouraged, in order to avoid strenuous pushing and straining activity which might have increased the CSF loss.[18]

After delivery, the epidural catheter may be left in place for the injection of saline or blood in an attempt to prevent the onset of headache. Both these injection techniques have met with only limited success when used for prophylaxis rather than treatment of headache.[19] Similarly, bed rest (with one pillow) is not effective in the prevention of headache, although it may delay the onset of symptoms; however, bed rest almost certainly relieves headache once the symptoms occur.[20] One disadvantage of early energetic mobilization is the increased incidence of temporary abducent nerve (cranial nerve VI) palsy with diplopia, which is not uncommon, with two cases being seen at my institution (Royal Hospital for Women, Sydney) in our last 100 patients with dural puncture. A previous report recorded an incidence of diplopia of only 1 in 5000 to 8000 dural punctures,[21] but these patients were probably maintained on bed rest for a few days.

Post–Dural Puncture Syndrome. It seems more accurate to call the clinical picture that may follow dural puncture the post–dural puncture syndrome (PDPS), rather than to categorize it as just a headache (or post–dural puncture headache [PDPH]), since the classic symptoms consist of photophobia, nausea, neck stiffness, backache, and dizziness in addition to the often severe headache which is usually frontal in origin, radiates to the occiput, and is exacerbated by sitting or standing. The main diagnostic criterion is the dramatic improvement on assuming the supine position, although the occasional accompanying hearing loss, tinnitus, and diplopia are more slow to resolve. Occasionally, a headache may develop at the same moment as dural puncture or shortly after, and persist for several hours or throughout labor, but usually the onset of symptoms is delayed for at least 24 to 36 hours, and sometimes longer.

In general, the larger the gauge of the needle breaching the dura, the more likely it is for symptoms to appear, and for their intensity to be greater. The symptoms seem to result from traction on pain-sensitive cerebral blood vessels and meningeal and tentorial structures as the brain shifts in relation to the dura, following the loss of pressure in the spinal subarachnoid compartment. The incidence of headache following dural puncture with a 17-gauge epidural needle has been reported to be in the range of 76% to 85%,[22] whereas in using 24- or 25-gauge pencil-point spinal needles a figure as low as 0.75% has been reported for subarachnoid block.[5] It should be remembered that in

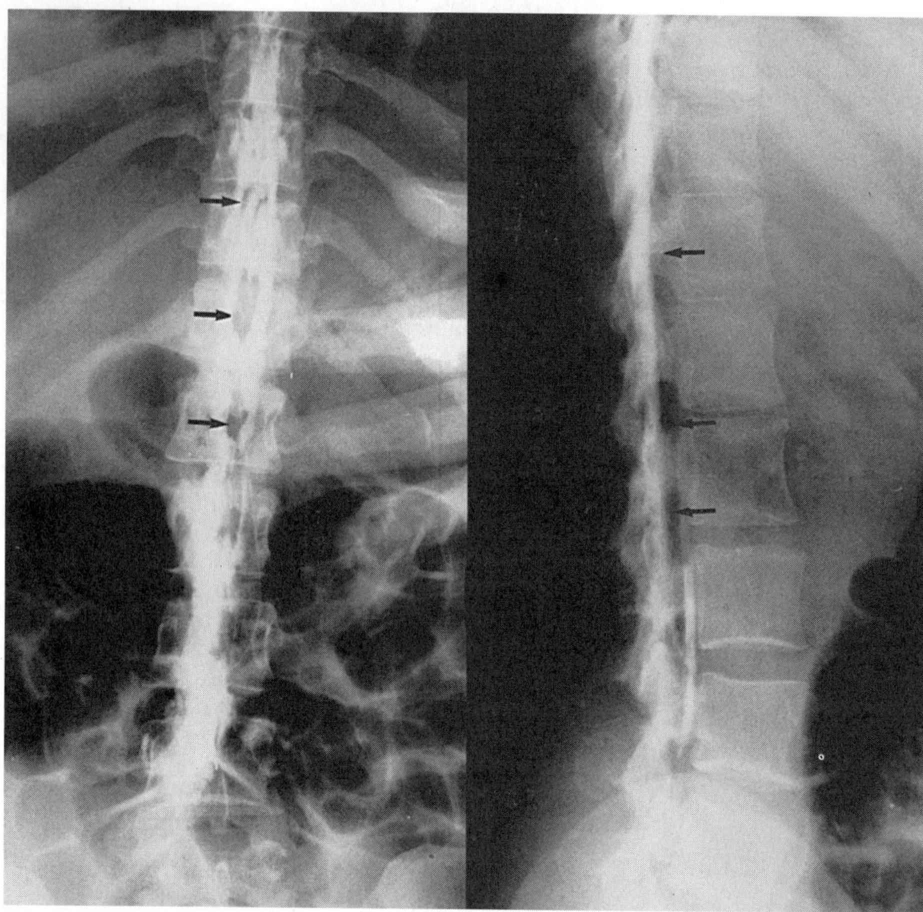

❖ **Figure 36–1** Anteroposterior *(left)* and lateral views on an epidurogram *(right)*, following inadvertent dural puncture, showing large filling defects *(arrows)* occupied by cerebrospinal fluid. The contrast is mostly posterior, and there is little flow into the intervertebral foramina or nerve root spaces.

about one third of cases of PDPS following attempted epidural block, dural puncture goes unrecognized or unrecorded.[23]

Several authors have reported a very low or zero incidence of PDPS using 26- to 29-gauge spinal needles in the CSE technique, probably reflecting meticulous puncture of the dura, as the epidural needle serves as an excellent introducer.[24] Other workers report that their incidence of accidental dural puncture by the epidural needle was also reduced when the CSE technique was used.[25]

Whatever the cause of PDPS, as soon as significant complaints are made by the patient, effective treatment should be offered. Without question, epidural blood patching is the most efficient and rapid form of treatment, for all but the mildest of headaches and for neck stiffness. Although it was previously thought that PDPS would invariably get better of its own accord within 1 week,[26] such a view is now regarded as erroneous. Subdural hematoma and tentorial coning are two of the rare but recognized major complications of neglected PDPS,[27] but unhappy patients with uncomplicated long-term headache are also becoming a regular source of litigation.[28]

Epidural Blood Patch. The simple procedure of injecting 15 to 20 mL of freshly drawn autologous blood into the patient's epidural space should be undertaken as soon as conveniently possible after the first complaint of significant headache, or neck stiffness. Some patients are naturally reluctant to suffer another "needle in the back," and these individuals should be offered the option of intravenous sedation during the procedure.

Blood patching is a remarkably efficient therapy, with some workers reporting well over 90% success rates at the first attempt.[21] Although some failures result from errors in diagnosis, injection of the blood outside the epidural space, or an inability of the blood to clot, it appears that a correctly performed technique is usually successful. In rare cases, in which symptoms persist or recur after the patch "blows off," a repeat blood injection is required. It is not essential to inject the blood in exactly the same space as that in which the dural puncture occurred, for a large volume of blood is used and the posterior lumbar epidural space is relatively narrow with a mean diameter of approximately 7 mm.[29] It has been found that injection of 15-mL volumes of blood is sufficient to cover an area of 8 to 10 spinal segments.[30] However, it should be noted that epidural solutions tend to flow preferentially in a cephalic direction,[30] so that the blood should not be injected at a higher vertebral level than the dural puncture site if known. The incidence of side effects

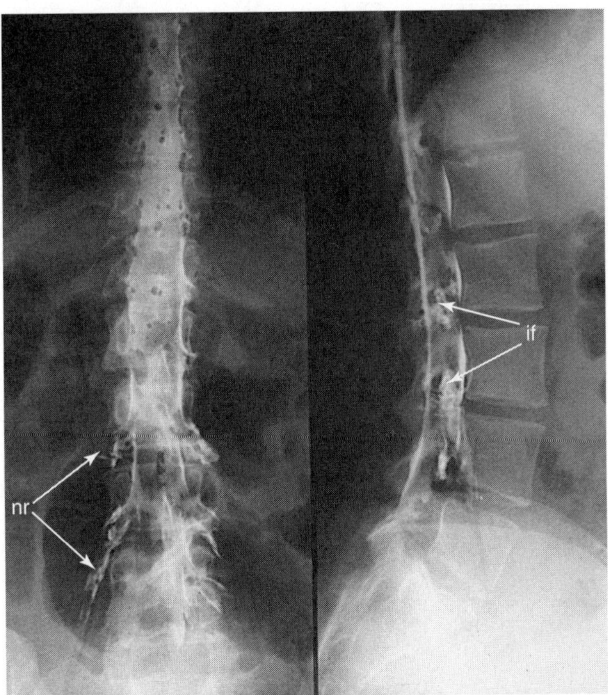

Figure 36–2 A typical anteroposterior *(left)* and lateral view on an epidurogram *(right)*, showing contrast spreading across the width of the epidural space and filling several intervertebral foramina (if) and nerve root spaces (nr).

after blood patch is low, with minor complications including backache and transient paresthesias being occasionally reported.

Catheter Breakage

Catheter breakage is discussed here, as it appears that in several recent cases the catheter has been damaged and weakened at the time of insertion rather than removal. Breakage of epidural catheters was more commonly reported before 1980, when considerable technologic advances in catheter construction were introduced. Crawford recorded the breakage of 12 catheters in 27,000 patients (0.04%) prior to this date.[31] At the Royal Hospital for Women in Sydney, we estimate the current incidence of breakage to be about 1 in 60,000 for nylon catheters, with a much higher incidence for radiopaque[32] and Teflon-coated catheters,[33] which tend to be more brittle. Little information is available on the cause of catheter breakage, with the literature containing mostly isolated case reports and many theories. These include damage caused by withdrawing the catheter through the needle, the use of defective catheters, or "trapping" of the catheter tip by knotting, kinking, or nipping between vertebral laminae or spines.[34, 35]

The caution "Do not withdraw catheter through needle" is clearly printed on almost all epidural kits. This is probably an overemphasis, as the current needles have a blunt, rounded upper edge to their orifice, replacing the previous sharp chisel-like bevel, and catheters used today have a high degree of tolerance incorporated into their construction. It does not appear to be hazardous to withdraw an undamaged catheter through a needle, provided that it moves freely with minimal traction applied. In the laboratory it is virtually impossible to break a "trapped" catheter by withdrawing it through a needle until it has been subjected to considerable force and stretched by more than 30% of its length.[32] However, as unforeseen catheter damage may have occurred during insertion, it is advisable to remove catheter and needle together as one unit in difficult cases.

Another mechanism of breakage has recently been demonstrated in the laboratory during attempts to replicate the situation in two patients who retained fragments of catheter in their backs.[36] Both cases involved difficult catheter insertion in which it appeared that the epidural needle had been advanced and rotated with the catheter already protruding several centimeters from the tip. Heavy contact between the needle and bone almost certainly followed. Animal experiments have shown that this contact may either sever the end of the catheter, leaving it embedded in the bone with the tip pointing outward (Fig. 36–3*A* to *C*), or weaken the catheter sufficiently to allow breakage on removal.

Following breakage of a catheter, the fragment and the epidural needle should be retained and submitted to expert examination. The patient should be fully informed of the situation, reassured, and offered the considered opinion that the vast majority of catheter fragments produce no long-term effects, and that there should be no attempts at retrieval unless worrying symptoms persist.[37] In any case, locating fragments may be impossible even using the most modern imaging techniques and the assistance of experienced neuroradiologists.

Four rules that should be observed to protect the integrity of the catheters and the dura are listed in Table 36–1.

Spinal microcatheters with sizes between 28 and 32 gauge are prone to breakage unless removed from the subarachnoid space with extreme care.[38] They tend to become stretched on removal and fragment just below the skin. Once again, removal is recommended only if troublesome symptoms persist, as may occur if the fragment lies between the subarachnoid space and the subcutaneous tissues.

Table 36–1 PRECAUTIONS TAKEN TO AVOID CATHETER DAMAGE AND INADVERTENT DURAL PUNCTURE

1. If an epidural catheter meets resistance and cannot be advanced to a sufficient length through an epidural needle, then that needle should not be advanced, angulated, or rotated.
2. The manufacturers recommend that a catheter should never be withdrawn through an epidural needle.
3. A long epidural needle (shaft length 11 cm or greater) is rarely required unless the patient has gross obesity.
4. Never use excessive force on needle insertion.

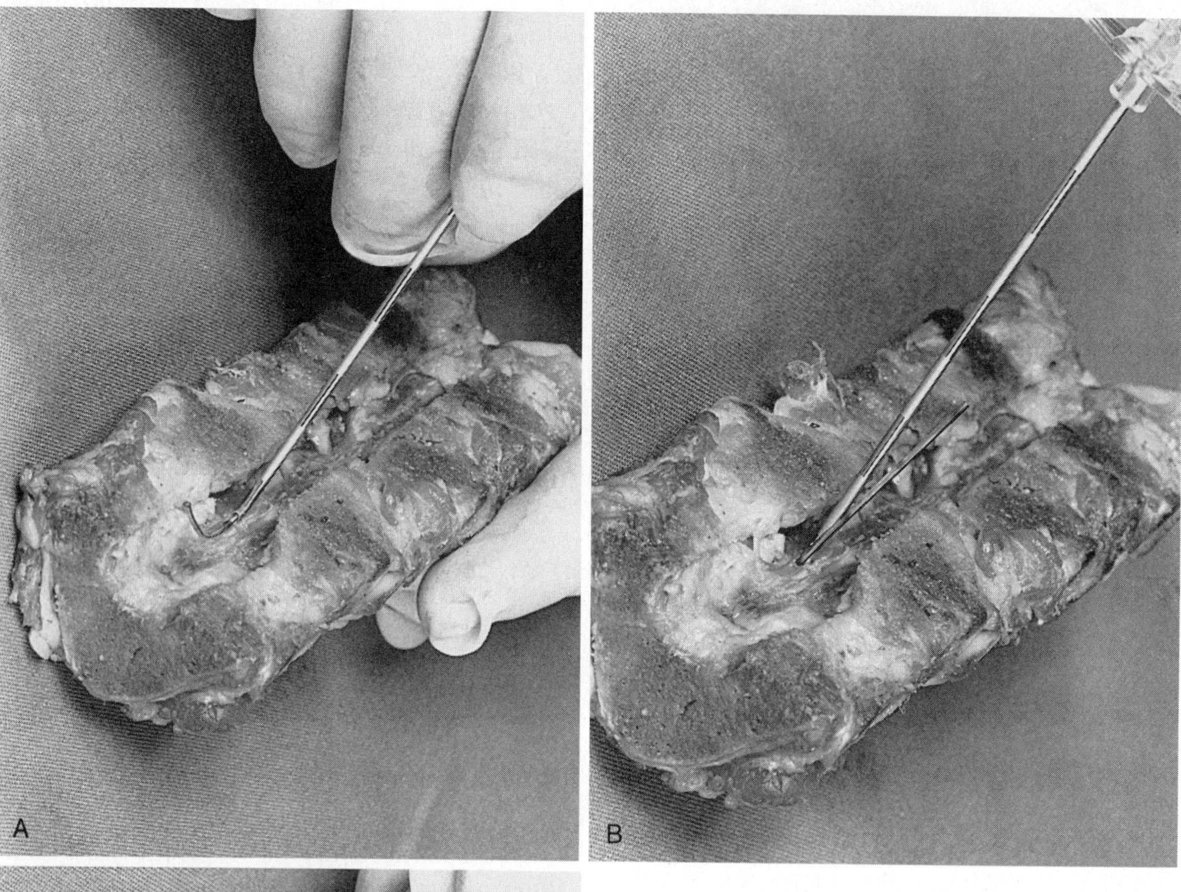

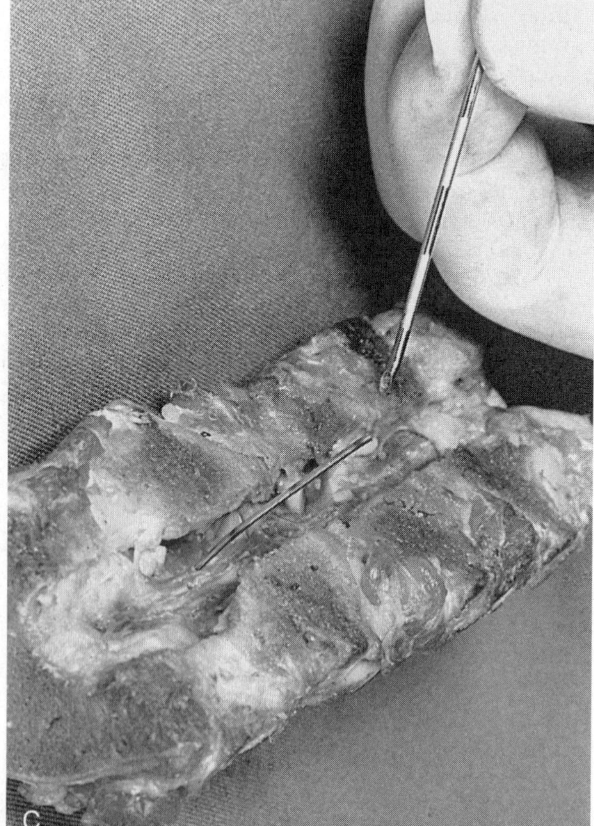

Figure 36–3 Exposed porcine spine showing the point of a Tuohy epidural needle impinging on bone in the anterior wall of the vertebral canal. Approximately 3 cm of catheter has been inserted through the needle. *B*, As the point of the Tuohy needle is advanced into the bone of the vertebral body, the tip of the exposed length of catheter springs back toward the needle. *C*, With further pressure on the Tuohy needle, the catheter is transected, and the proximal 3-cm fragment remains embedded in the bone as the needle is withdrawn.

EARLY COMPLICATIONS FOLLOWING INJECTION THROUGH CORRECTLY PLACED NEEDLES AND CATHETERS

Cardiovascular Complications

Hypotension. This is the commonest complication of all three types of regional anesthesia, with the possible exception of shivering.

Mild hypotension is a side effect of the sympathetic blockade accompanying epidural block. Hypotension may be regarded as a complication when the baseline systolic pressure has fallen by 20% to 30%, and treatment should be immediately commenced with intravenous fluids. Ephedrine, administered as 5- to 6-mg intravenous boluses or as a 0.01% infusion, is probably the vasopressor drug of choice,[39] except in certain groups of cardiac patients who may tolerate the accompanying tachycardia poorly, and phenylephrine may then be preferred.[40] Currently, hypotensive episodes develop in less than 5% of parturients receiving analgesia in labor,[2] probably as a result of the abandonment of large bolus doses of local anesthetic and the avoidance of aortocaval compression. There appears to be little benefit from the use of intravenous fluid preloading prior to analgesia in labor.[41]

When the more extensive and denser blocks for cesarean section are initiated, hypotension is a more common finding, although the incidence is highly variable depending on the volume of fluid preloading, the possible use of a prophylactic vasopressor, and once again, the maternal position. An incidence of 20% would be expected with a T4 block, lateral tilt, and a 1-L crystalloid preload.[42]

Occasionally in the laboring patient, low or even zero diastolic pressures are reported by anxious nursing staff following induction of epidural block. The reason for this unusual finding, which may be noted on manual or automatic pressure recording, is a compensatory vasoconstriction of the brachial artery under the cuff, in response to the onset of vasodilatation in the legs and pelvis. The vasoconstriction may impede the recognition of the diastolic pressure.

With single-dose local anesthetic SAB the degree of sympathetic blockade tends to be greater and the onset of hypotension more rapid than after epidural block. The fall in blood pressure reflects the early onset of the spinal block prior to the physiologic compensatory mechanisms coming into play. Russell reported that hypotension after induction of spinal anesthesia occurred in up to 80% of parturients, despite fluid preloading, and that vasopressor prophylaxis with ephedrine was essential.[43] Others wait for the onset of hypotension (90 mm Hg) or symptoms such as nausea, vomiting, or lightheadedness before administering a vasopressor.[44]

Continuous SAB is reported to offer greater hemodynamic stability than single-dose spinal block, as the local anesthetic may be given more slowly, producing results similar to those obtained with continuous epidural block.[45] The use of subarachnoid opioids has also been associated with unexpected bouts of hypotension in labor, with sufentanil in particular being to blame.[46, 47] This effect of the opioids may be due to weak intrinsic local anesthetic properties or may occur via action on opioid receptors located on preganglionic sympathetic nerve fibers.[25]

Using the CSE technique, smaller doses of subarachnoid local anesthetic may be employed for cesarean section than with pure SAB, as the epidural catheter provides backup in case of an inadequate block. The incidence and severity of hypotension should be decreased,[24] although there is concern regarding hypotension and rapid extension of the spinal block following epidural injections through the catheter.[24]

Comparing CSE and epidural block for labor analgesia, Norris and colleagues found that the incidence and severity of hypotension was the same with both techniques (<5%) when subarachnoid opioid or epidural opioid and local anesthetic were given.[25]

Bradycardia. Significant cardiac slowing may occur during epidural or spinal block, but it is commoner with the latter, and sick sinus syndrome, complete heart block, and asystole may follow on rare occasions.[48] Bradycardia appears to result from two factors: first, blockade of preganglionic cardiac accelerator fibers (T1–T5) with high levels of block, and second, a significant decrease in venous return and right atrial pressure, with reduced afferent activity of right atrial stretch receptors. The onset of action of suxamethonium in a patient with sympathetic blockade is frequently accompanied by intense bradycardia, and occasionally cardiac arrest.

The bradycardia described here usually responds to intravenous atropine, but if it is accompanied by significant hypotension the administration of ephedrine may be required or, on very rare occasions, epinephrine.

Nausea and Vomiting

These unpleasant symptoms are frequently associated with hypotension, and they are subsequently far more common after subarachnoid than after epidural local anesthetic injection. The incidence of nausea following SAB for cesarean delivery has been reported in the range of 14% to 45%.[49] Treatment of the hypotension usually relieves the nausea, and an antiemetic is rarely required. Intrathecal opioids are also associated with more frequent nausea and vomiting than are noted for epidural opioids.[25]

Other Opioid Side Effects

Apart from the problem of nausea and vomiting as just discussed, neuraxial opioids have several other side effects. Included among these is maternal respiratory depression, the foremost; the use of intrathecal morphine, sufentanil, or meperidine probably gives rise to the most concern, with close monitoring required. Pruritus is an annoying accompaniment to the use of neuraxial opioids. It is a common complaint, although symptoms often are not severe, and only a small proportion of patients seek treatment.

Neuraxial opioids may play a part in the development of fetal bradycardia in labor, particularly just after introduction of the block, when larger doses are administered. Urinary retention during and after labor may also present difficulties.

Extensive Block

Even with the most meticulous technique and correct needle or catheter placement, all three types of regional block may occasionally result in extensive blocks.

The dose of local anesthetic required to produce a given level and density of block is a product of the volume and concentration of the agent used.[50] Greater volumes of local anesthetic may increase the extent of sensory blockade, but the relationship is not a linear one and is unpredictable.[51] Volumes as high as 40 mL of 0.5% bupivacaine have been injected incrementally prior to cesarean section without maternal complications.[52] However, on rare occasions extensive spread of motor and sensory block may occur 10 to 20 minutes after the injection of smaller, more typical doses of local anesthetic. These "high" epidural blocks, previously described as "massive" by Bromage,[53] may be associated with numbness and weakness of the hands, and with respiratory difficulty as the intercostal muscles are blocked. The uncoordinated respiratory movements may be impeded by splinting of the diaphragm with the term pregnancy, and not surprisingly, considerable panic is usually evident, often with a feeling of impending death. Hypotension may develop, but not to any marked degree. The patient remains conscious, because the epidural space terminates above at the foramen magnum and the local anesthetic agent does not bathe the brain stem directly as with a high subarachnoid block.

Bromage considered the extensive level of epidural block to be due to a relative overdose of local anesthetic in the epidural space, with inferior vena caval obstruction and distended epidural veins reducing the capacity of the epidural space.[53] Recent magnetic resonance imaging (MRI) studies have demonstrated considerable engorgement of the anterior internal vertebral veins in supine third-trimester patients,[54] and epidurograms in a patient following a high epidural block showed lateral channeling of contrast, with increased cephalic spread (Fig. 36–4).[55] It appears that in about 10% of parturients excessive anterior epidural venous engorgement develops, en-

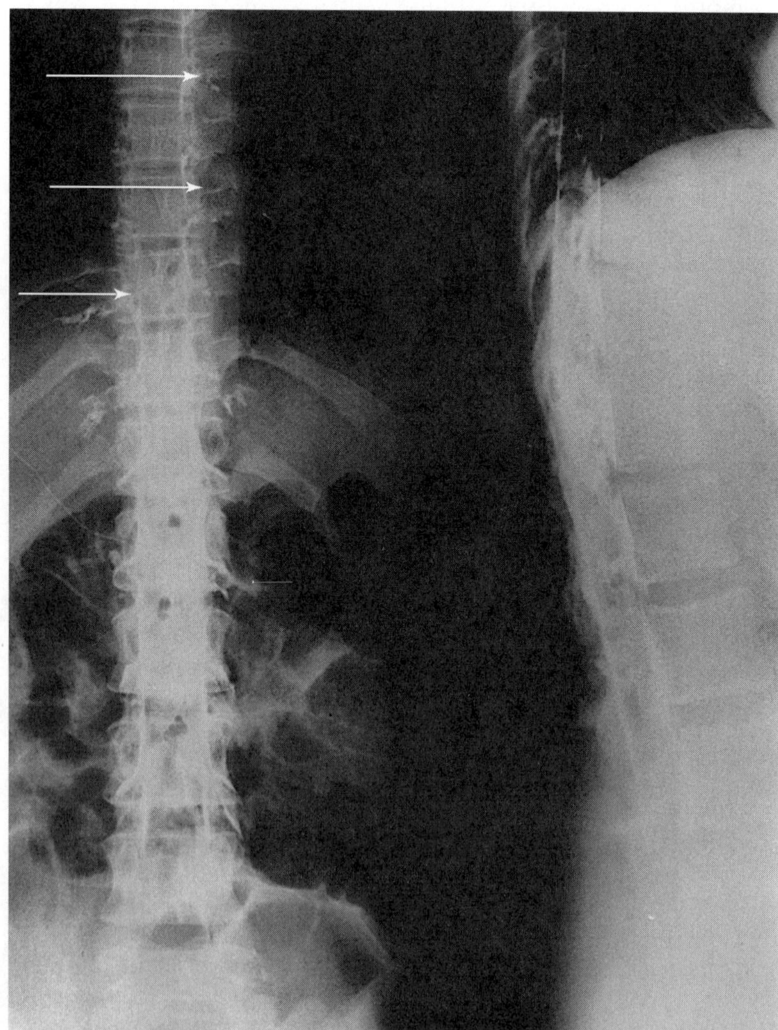

Figure 36–4 Anteroposterior *(left)* and lateral *(right)* views on an epidurogram showing high spread of epidural contrast, reaching the T2 level on the left, with lateral channeling of contrast *(arrows)*. The block extended cephalad to involve the trigeminal nerves.

couraging the lateral and cephalic spread of epidural solutions.[16] This usually goes unrecognized clinically, but it may produce symptoms of high epidural block in approximately 1% to 2% of patients, particularly those undergoing cesarean section. Treatment of a high epidural block consists largely of reassuring the mother of the adequacy of her breathing, while administering oxygen by face mask and having equipment for intubation close at hand, although it is rarely required, as the level of block usually recedes rapidly after 15 to 30 minutes.

It is most unusual for total spinal blockade or even a high spinal block to develop after intentional spinal anesthesia in obstetrics,[56] unless a considerable overdose has been injected or there has been a previous unsuccessful attempt at epidural anesthesia.[14] In the case of failed epidural block there may be a leak of epidural local anesthetic through the dural hole into the CSF, or simply an increased CSF pressure in the epidural space transmitted across the dura with displacement of CSF.[14] Alternatively, CSF may leak out through the dural puncture site, reducing the CSF volume in the subarachnoid space and resulting in a higher than expected block.[57]

There would appear to be no published cases of high blocks following the correct application of the CSE technique,[24] although there is an anecdotal report of total spinal anesthesia developing after a top-up dose administered through the epidural catheter (D. Birnbach, personal communication, March 1998). Restriction of the volume of the epidural dose to 1.5 to 2 mL per unblocked segment is an important factor.[24] However, caution is always required when epidural injection is adjacent to a dural hole, as indicated in three recent reports. In the first, dural puncture with a 26-gauge needle prior to epidural mepivacaine (in nonpregnant subjects) increased the caudal spread of analgesia,[58] while in sheep experiments, prior dural puncture greatly increased the level of morphine in the CSF at the cisterna magna following lumbar epidural injection of morphine.[59] Finally, epidural bupivacaine given to a group of women in labor resulted in significantly higher levels of sensory block when preceded by an intrathecal dose of sufentanil, 10 μg.[60]

Shivering

Shivering is a very common and irritating complication of epidural block, being reported in 20% to 61% of post-block parturients.[61] These involuntary movements frequently disrupt the tranquility in labor that follows the onset of analgesia, and add to the discomfort and concerns of the patient awaiting a cesarean delivery. Pulse, blood pressure, and electrocardiographic (ECG) monitoring as well as oximetry may be impossible with severe shaking, and very occasionally, a differential diagnosis of rigors accompanying the onset of septicemia may be overlooked.

The etiology of shivering remains elusive, despite many ingenious theories, mostly involving a differential inhibition of spinal cord afferent thermoreceptors.[62, 63] However, this cannot be the sole cause, as my colleagues and I have noted severe shaking in one patient with a very limited unilateral block, which on investigation with contrast injection and fluoroscopic screening was shown to result from a misplaced catheter in the ipsilateral paravertebral space.

The onset of symptoms may be within 2 to 3 minutes of epidural local anesthetic injection, although a 10-minute delay is more common. The incidence is greatest when epinephrine-containing solutions are used, and least when plain solutions are warmed to body temperature prior to administration, or when opioids such as fentanyl[61] or sufentanil are added.[64] The application of warming blankets or radiant heat usually diminishes the shaking, as do intravenous opioids or a small dose of midazolam.

Horner's Syndrome

Horner's syndrome is not uncommonly observed in laboring patients following lumbar epidural or caudal block in two distinct situations. More often it appears as an isolated, unexplained finding in the course of a normal block, and only rarely as a component of an excessively high block, particularly after subdural injection. The full clinical picture of ptosis, miosis, enophthalmos, and anhidrosis, which is usually unilateral but may be bilateral, is present in 1% to 4% of epidural block patients,[65] but is frequently overlooked. Pain in the affected eye,[66] a "red eye" from dilated conjunctival vessels, or a unilateral blocked nose may draw attention to the other signs. The syndrome has been reported as early as the 12th week of pregnancy during blockade for cervical cerclage,[67] and has even followed the injection of a 2-mL test dose at the L3 to L4 vertebral level.[68] Symptoms tend to abate without sequelae within 1 to 2 hours and are unlikely to recur with subsequent epidural top-up dosing.

If close inspection is undertaken, isolated pupillary constriction with or without ptosis may be detected after 85% of caudal blocks[69] and after 75% of lumbar epidural blocks.[68] The underlying mechanism is interruption of the sympathetic nerve supply to the pupil, levator palpebrae muscles, conjunctiva, and face. Preganglionic sympathetic fibers emerge predominantly from the upper three thoracic spinal segments, but may also involve the T4 and T5 segments.[67] They then ascend and synapse in the cervical ganglia before reaching the head and neck tissues. The sympathetic fibers are of smaller diameter and are blocked at lower concentrations of local anesthetic than motor or sensory nerves. This may account for those cases of Horner's syndrome in which the upper extent of sensory block was at or below the T7 level.

Allergy

Although it is not unusual for obstetric patients to state that they are "allergic to local anesthetics," true allergy is extremely rare, and may often be excluded by careful history taking. Fisher and his colleagues surveyed 208 patients who were referred to their Anaesthetic Allergy Clinic over a 20-year period, and found only 4 patients who developed anaphylaxis and another 4 who developed delayed allergic reactions following intradermal testing with local anesthetics.[70] They recommend progressive challenge intradermal testing of patients with a history of allergy, and state that it is possible to provide safe local anesthesia for all patients, with satisfactory alternative drugs being available for the rare truly allergic individual.[70]

Local Anesthetic Toxicity

Obstetric epidural block may occasionally be complicated by toxic effects following local anesthetic administration, as a result of the use of an excessive dose or more commonly, following injection into an epidural vein (see later discussion). In labor, the risk of toxicity from a correctly sited epidural local anesthetic is extremely slight, as only low doses of bupivacaine or ropivacaine, in the range of 25 to 50 mg every 2 hours, are usually given. The larger doses required for cesarean section, particularly after a long period of epidural analgesia in labor, are more likely to be associated with toxic episodes, although these are infrequently seen at present probably due to the withdrawal of 0.75% bupivacaine[71] and the avoidance of ropivacaine concentrations greater than 7.5 mg/mL.

Toxicity following systemic absorption usually presents with central nervous system (CNS) symptoms, most often convulsions, the onset of which may be delayed for 20 minutes or more after the last dose.[71] The cardiovascular system is generally more resistant than the CNS to the toxic effects of local anesthetics.[72] The addition of epinephrine to most local anesthetic solutions reduces their epidural absorption, to a greater extent with lidocaine than bupivacaine.[71]

Effects on the Course of Labor

Heated discussion still abounds concerning the effects of regional block, particularly epidural analgesia, on the progress of labor and the incidence of assisted delivery, whether vaginally or by cesarean section.[73] A very comprehensive survey by Miller, which includes 169 references,[74] indicates that no definitive conclusion can be drawn on this highly controversial subject. Miller suggests that it is time to stop asking "Does epidural analgesia affect labor?" and accept that it does in certain circumstances, but that it is only one of many factors to be considered, including the degree of maternal discomfort, the size of the pelvic outlet and the baby, and variations in obstetric management.[74]

Miller found little evidence in support of the time-honored belief that epidural block should be withheld during the latent phase of the first stage of labor, or until a particular degree of cervical dilatation is present.[74] While there is conflicting evidence regarding the duration of the first stage of labor and the rate of cervical dilatation with epidural block, it is accepted that the second stage may be prolonged, although even this is probably of little consequence to the baby.[74] This prolongation may be limited with the use of more dilute local anesthetic solutions.[75]

The use of low and outlet instrumental deliveries seems to be increased after epidural block even when dilute local anesthetics are used, but the incidence of cesarean section appears unaffected, although the evidence is contradictory.[74] Miller concludes by stating that although anesthetic techniques can and do affect uterine activity and the course of fetal descent and delivery, judicious cooperative management by both anesthetists and obstetricians can improve maternal comfort without increasing the risk to mother or baby.[74]

Effects on the Fetus and Neonate

Discussion of any possible adverse effects of regional anesthesia on the fetus and neonate is beyond the scope of this chapter, other than to say that provided the maternal circulation is well supported, both analgesia in labor and surgical anesthesia for cesarean delivery are beneficial to the baby.[76] However, of some concern to both obstetricians and midwives is the development of changes in the fetal heart rate within 10 to 15 minutes of epidural injection of local anesthetic or opioid. Fetal bradycardia with or without decreased beat-to-beat variability may be seen in up to 30% of parturients,[77, 78] particularly, it seems, in those individuals suffering severe pain and distress prior to the block. These heart rate changes are transitory, lasting only 3 to 4 minutes, and should be carefully monitored with the patient in the lateral position breathing oxygen, but they should not give rise to great concern, as long as they are not repeated.

EARLY COMPLICATIONS FOLLOWING INJECTION THROUGH INCORRECTLY PLACED NEEDLES OR CATHETERS

Failed or Inadequate Blocks

A complication of any form of regional anesthesia is that the technique may fail completely or provide only a patchy, inadequate block.

The commonest cause of failed or inadequate epidural blocks (up to about 6%) following correct needle positioning appears to be transforaminal escape of the catheter tip,[79] often as a result of insertion of too great a length of catheter, with 3 to 5 cm being considered sufficient.[80] In about 3% of parturients, persistent unilateral or asymmetric block may result from the presence of a dorsal midline or lateral septum, or similar structure, obstructing the uniform spread of epidural solutions.[79] Other causes of unsatisfactory blocks include spinal deformity, such as scoliosis and catheter malposition or malfunction, as may be seen when catheter eyes are blocked by blood clot or foreign material.[16]

The majority of instances of unsatisfactory blockade may be overcome by withdrawal of the catheter by 1 to 2 cm and injection of further doses of local anesthetic, leaving a residual group of 2% to 3% of patients who require the catheter to be reinserted. However, catheter replacement rates of over 12% have been reported.[81]

Litigation arising from unexpected pain during awake cesarean section is on the increase, and patients should be warned of the possibility of some discomfort during the procedure. Paech and associates have recorded that 1 in 200 of their apparently satisfactory blocks failed because of pain during cesarean section, with general anesthesia being required.[2]

The figures reported for the incidence of failed SAB in obstetrics vary enormously according to the source, from almost 15% in one series[82] down to 0.67% in another,[83] with both groups using a needle-through-needle CSE technique. The problems with the subarachnoid component seem to be related to several factors including the length of spinal needle protruding through the epidural needle, with at least 13 mm being considered optimal,[82] as well as possible movement of the spinal needle out of the subarachnoid space during syringe attachment and injection,[24] although an adjustable interlocking device may overcome this. Furthermore, as the onset of SAB is usually so rapid, any delay in insertion or fixation of the epidural catheter may allow the spinal block to become fixed in a unilateral or low distribution, depending on the patient's posture, although augmentation by the epidural route should enable satisfactory block to be produced.

A report by Lyons has concluded that the use of CSE has reduced the need for rescue general anesthesia to only 1 in 900 cesarean sections.[84]

Accidental Subarachnoid Block

The classic picture of an accidental total spinal (subarachnoid) block, with severe hypotension and early collapse of the patient accompanied by apnea and unconsciousness, following unrecognized dural puncture by an epidural needle or catheter, is difficult to mistake for any other situation, especially if CSF can be aspirated through the catheter. Only a small volume of misplaced local anesthetic (2.5–3 mL of 0.5% bupivacaine or 2% chloroprocaine) may be sufficient to induce a total spinal block.[85, 86] The incidence of this complication is probably on the order of 1 in 10,000 cases[87] and decreasing with the current trend of using smaller volumes of more dilute solutions of local anesthetics (often combined with opioids) and incremental rather than bolus dosing for epidural analgesia.

Weaker local anesthetic solutions usually produce a different and slower sequence of events when injected into the subarachnoid space, and the diagnosis may be difficult, especially if CSF cannot be aspirated, as frequently happens, at least initially. Evans' study of deliberate total spinal anesthesia for general surgery using 1% lidocaine includes descriptions of the likely clinical progression of these blocks.[88] Less extensive blocks that extend above the T1 vertebral level but remain extracranial (high spinals) are far commoner than total spinal blocks but rarely produce marked symptoms. Occasionally, severe dyspnea may develop, but only in about 3 in 10,000 cases.[2]

Treatment of total spinal block involves turning the patient to the supine position with left uterine displacement and ventilation of the lungs with 100% oxygen prior to intubation, which can usually be accomplished without the need for a muscle relaxant. Ventilation may be required for a period of 1 to 2 hours, until consciousness returns together with coordinated movement of the arms. The blood pressure should be restored with rapid fluid infusion together with vasopressors, which may include epinephrine in extreme cases. There would appear to be some value in aspirating 20 to 30 mL of "contaminated" CSF through an epidural catheter when possible, as soon as the diagnosis of subarachnoid injection is made. A large proportion of the subarachnoid local anesthetic or opioid may be recovered, and the extent of the anticipated block may be considerably reduced.[89]

Accidental Subdural Block

The classic picture of an accidental total subdural (extra-arachnoid) block is rarely seen these days. The features include a gradual onset of an extensive sensory block and a moderate degree of hypotension 20 to 40 minutes following an apparently straightforward epidural injection, with further progression to apnea and unconsciousness following intracranial spread of local anesthetic.[90] Many less extensive cases of subdural block occur, but almost certainly go unrecognized, as a result of the current practice of using smaller incremental doses of less concentrated local anesthetics than previously recommended.

A low subdural block may present as merely a higher than expected sensory level, which is usually but not always bilateral. Increased motor block in the legs is noted in about 30% of cases. Higher blocks may involve sensory and sometimes motor block in the arms, together with dyspnea, facial and corneal anesthesia, as well as pupillary changes, most commonly mydriasis. Subdural blocks are most frequently encountered in obstetric practice, with an estimated incidence of 1 in 2000 attempted blocks, and the two frequent predisposing factors are prior dural puncture and rotation of the block needle within the epidural space.[90] Treatment of a total subdural block is the same as described earlier for subarachnoid block, while lower levels of block require constant reassurance of the patient together with careful observation of respiratory movements and arterial oxygen saturation. Subdural opioids produce fairly long-lasting analgesia in low dosage, with few side effects.[91, 92]

A recent case report that bore all the features of an accidental subdural block serves to highlight one of the risks of the CSE technique.[93, 94] The first epidural dose of local anesthetic/opioid following an awake cesarean section was given in the recovery area, prior to the patient's being returned to her room, where 40 minutes later she developed respiratory difficulty and subsequent cardiac arrest. The use of a test dose to exclude subdural catheter placement is impractical, so that the patient should be closely monitored after the first catheter dose, whenever it is given.

Accidental Intravascular Injection

The incidence of convulsions caused by local anesthetic toxicity was recently reported as approximately 1 in 8000 patients following lumbar epidural block, and 1 in 80 to 330 patients following caudal block in a general hospital.[95]

Injection of a local anesthetic into an epidural vein may lead to signs of CNS toxicity within 15 to 30 seconds, depending on the dose and speed of injection. The clinical picture is one of initial CNS stimulation, followed by depression, and is a graded response with signs and symptoms of escalating severity (Table 36–2). A relatively small dose (5–10 mL of 1% lidocaine) may cause ringing in the ears, a metallic taste in the mouth, tongue numbness, drowsiness with decreased awareness, muscular twitching, paresthesias, restlessness, and apprehension. With a larger dose, delirium and dysarthria may ensue and progress to grand mal convulsions and unconsciousness, sometimes with apnea. Hypoxia and hypercarbia may develop if the convulsions are not treated rapidly and efficiently, leading to metabolic and respiratory acidosis. Cardiovascular system toxicity indicates a more severe situation, with depression of cardiac conductivity and contractility often accompanied by hypotension, bradycardia, arrhythmias, and even cardiac arrest. Some of the manifestations of cardiac toxicity may be due directly to brain stem toxicity.[96]

Ropivacaine is less arrhythmogenic than bupivacaine in dogs,[97] and intermediate in terms of cardiotoxicity in sheep between lidocaine (the least toxic) and bupivacaine (the most toxic).[98] Ropivacaine administered by intravenous infusion in human volunteers was again found to be less toxic than bupivacaine.[99] Minor cardiovascular toxicity and mild CNS symptoms occurred at lower dosage and lower plasma concentration with bupivacaine when compared with ropivacaine. The treatment of marked toxicity is based on maintenance of the airway and oxygenation. Seizure activity may be controlled with diazepam or thiopentone, while ephedrine may be given for cardiovascular depression. Cardiopulmonary resuscitation may be required in severe cases, with bretylium (where available) given for the treatment of ventricular tachycardia.[100]

Following intravenous injection, the presence of added epinephrine in the local anesthetic usually leads to the early development of palpitations, which are often the first symptom, accompanied by hypertension, which may be severe enough to precipitate a cerebrovascular accident.

Toxicity may be prevented by the use of appropriate test doses and fractionation of the total dose of local anesthetic, combined with slow epidural injection, with particular caution applied with caudal blocks in parturients.

Table 36-2 NEUROTOXICITY OF LIDOCAINE

Blood Level (μg/mL)	Symptoms
3	Lightheadedness
4	Tongue numbness
6	Visual disturbances
8	Generalized twitching
12	Convulsions
15	Profound coma
20	Respiratory arrest
25	Cardiovascular system depression

Multicompartment Injection

So far in this chapter, complicated blocks have been described as occurring only in isolation, but occasionally they arise in combination as a multicompartment injection.[101] Whereas a combined spinal-epidural anesthetic is a planned and usually well-controlled multicompartment block, the unexpected accidental spread of an epidural solution into the subarachnoid, subdural, or intravascular space may produce major complications. The conduit allowing epidural solutions to flow into two or more compartments is in most cases the epidural catheter with three lateral eyes, which may be incorrectly inserted to lie with its eyes in two or, very rarely, three of the adjacent compartments (primary multicompartment injection), or it may migrate into such a position at a later time (secondary multicompartment injection).[102] As the eyes are spaced 4 mm apart in most lateral eye catheters, being 8, 12, and 16 mm from the tip, and the mean thickness of the dura is approximately 0.5 mm, the possibility of multicompartment positioning is very real (Fig. 36–5). Differential flow through the individual catheter eyes appears to be mostly dependent on the pressure applied to the plunger of the injection syringe.[103]

Multicompartment blocks are also possible with single-terminal-eye catheters and we have recorded an epidural/intravascular injection through a single eye.[104] Subdural and epidural blocks appear to be the commonest type of multicompartment block, although they frequently pass unrecognized. Catheters with "closer eyes" situated 2, 3, and 4 mm from a closed tip have recently been introduced and may overcome the problem of multicompartment injection.[105]

POSTPARTUM COMPLICATIONS

The possibility of long-term complications following regional anesthesia for childbirth is one of the main concerns of parturients, particularly with regard to neurologic damage and backache. The lay press and some childbirth educators have, over the years, instilled undue fear and trepidation among the pregnant population, out of all proportion to the extremely low reported complication rates.

Postpartum Backache

Short-Term Backache. Mild backache is a common complaint for the first 24 to 48 hours following epi-

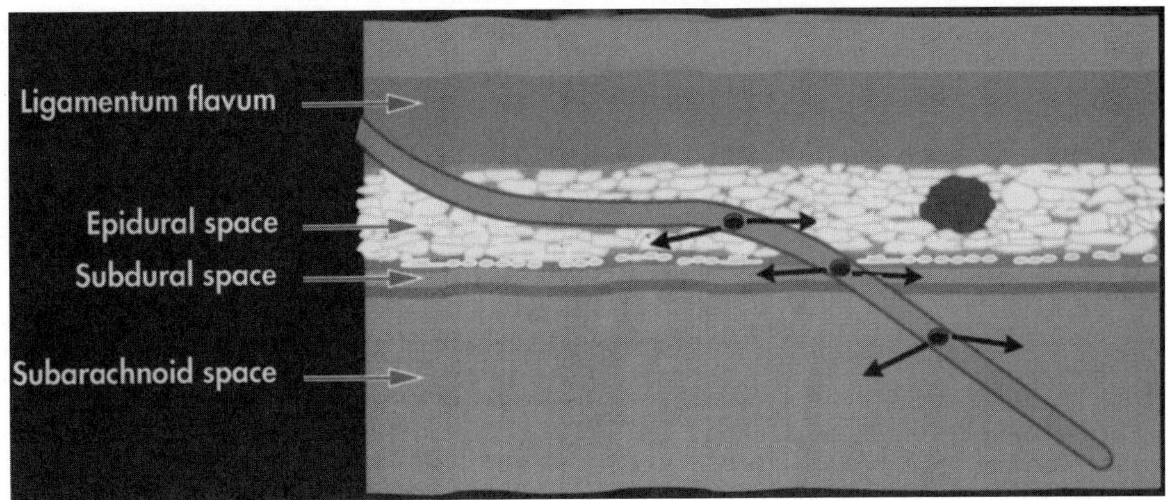

❖ **Figure 36–5** Diagram to illustrate possible multicompartment catheter positioning, with each catheter eye in a different space.

dural block in obstetric practice, and to a lesser extent following SAB. The pain is localized to the injection site, rarely requires treatment, and usually subsides rapidly. Mild to moderate backache is also a common complaint following childbirth in the absence of regional block. This pain is more generalized and often includes a component arising from the sacroiliac joints. In one series of unblocked patients, 40% reported backache after spontaneous vaginal deliveries and 25% after instrumental deliveries.[106] It should be straightforward to distinguish between postblock backache and that caused by childbirth itself.

Long-Term Backache. Very occasionally, localized backache persists for several months or longer, often accompanied by the presence of a small tender lump at the injection site. Crawford reported this finding with an incidence of approximately 1 in 2000 epidural blocks, and considered that it is due to the formation of a hematoma in the supraspinous ligaments that is slow to resolve.[107] This uncommon type of chronic backache is probably the only one that can be attributed directly to the insertion of a needle and catheter into the back. For most other cases of backache, no correlation with a regional anesthetic procedure can be demonstrated,[108] as was noted in one of the studies from the Birmingham Maternity Hospital, where the incidence of backache after elective cesarean section using epidural anesthesia was not significantly higher than that after general anesthesia.[109] Even difficult and repeated attempts at block insertion do not appear to predispose to later back pain.[110]

One theory linking regional block and backache suggested that the muscular relaxation developing in labor with more concentrated local anesthetic solutions allowed parturients to adopt unusual and stressful postures with subsequent symptoms.[109] There has been no prospective randomized study to support this theory,[111] and the use of more dilute solutions has rendered it almost obsolete.

It must be remembered that at least 50% of pregnant women complain of backache at some time in pregnancy,[112] with the most likely causes being an increased lumbar lordosis and sacroiliac joint strain that predispose to muscle and ligament derangement and subsequent pain, in addition to possible prolapse of a lumbar vertebral disk. The gravid uterus may contribute to the development of backache in two ways: by direct compression of nerves or by inducing vascular insufficiency following obstruction of aortic blood flow.[112] In one study, two thirds of patients with antenatal backache reported that their symptoms persisted into the postnatal period.[113]

Three published reports from London,[111] Boston,[114] and Montreal[115] provide clear evidence that epidural blocks in labor do not increase the incidence of long-term backache after childbirth. The results of these studies should be sufficient to allay the fears of women approaching labor, who may be concerned about earlier reports of postnatal backache based largely on the findings of anecdotal case reports and poorly controlled retrospective studies.[108]

NEUROLOGIC COMPLICATIONS OF CHILDBIRTH

Obstetric Causes. It is important to realize that the process of childbirth and the assistance of the obstetrician together account for far more neurologic complications than the administration of a regional block. Postpartum nerve damage was reported as early as 1838,[108] 50 years before the introduction of local anesthesia. At the turn of the century, "maternal obstetric paralysis" could be expected in 2% to 3% of parturients, with footdrop and femoral neuropathy being common findings.[2, 116, 117] Improvements in obstetric techniques over the years, with an increase in cesarean deliveries and a reduction in the practice of high forceps application and difficult fetal head rotations, have substantially reduced both the incidence and severity of neurologic complications, although transient sensory neurologic dysfunction can still be detected in 21% of postpartum women.[118] Fairly recent figures suggest that significant transient paresthesias or motor dysfunction occurs in 1 in 500 unblocked parturients,[119] with prolonged or permanent deficits in 1 in 2500.[120] Similar figures may be derived from groups of parturients who underwent regional block.[120]

Bromage described three different mechanisms, namely neural compression, arterial compression, and venous congestion, for producing postpartum neurologic dysfunction in the absence of regional block.[121]

Neural Compression

The fetal head during its descent through the maternal pelvis may compress the lumbosacral trunk or various individual nerves, with an estimated incidence of 1 in 3000.[121] This intrapelvic entrapment neuropathy is commonly associated with cephalopelvic disproportion, although 15% of cases follow spontaneous vaginal deliveries.[122]

Lumbosacral Trunk (L4–L5 Level). This is probably the commonest neural structure to suffer compression, either by the fetal head at the level of the pelvic brim or by traumatic application of middle or high forceps (Fig. 36–6). The clinical picture may include footdrop and weakness of hip adductors and quadriceps, with sensory loss over the lateral foot and calf. Damage to the sacral nerve roots may cause disturbance of bladder function.

Femoral Nerve (L2–L4 Level). This nerve may be injured in a similar manner to the lumbosacral trunk, although more frequently it is compressed by surgical retractors at cesarean section, leading to quadriceps weakness and loss of anterior thigh and medial calf sensation. The obturator and lateral cutaneous nerves may also be damaged by compression in the pelvis.

Arterial Compression

The fetal head may obstruct the arterial blood supply to the lower part of the spinal cord, resulting in ischemic damage, with an approximate incidence of 1 in 15,000.[121]

Venous Congestion

Arteriovenous malformations of spinal cord blood vessels may occur in up to 10% of individuals,[122] and if subjected to pressure from the fetal head, they may become congested. Cord ischemia and postpartum neurologic deficit may follow in approximately 1 in 20,000 cases.

Incidental Causes. Coincidental neurologic dysfunction, due, for example, to multiple sclerosis, polyneuritis, or prolapse of an intervertebral disk (1 in 10,000 deliveries),[123] may present for the first time after childbirth, and compressive peripheral neuropathies are not uncommon.

Compressive Peripheral Neuropathies. Many peripheral nerves are vulnerable to compression in labor, particularly with the use of the lithotomy position for delivery, and damage to the femoral, sciatic, obturator, common peroneal, saphenous, and lateral femoral cutaneous nerves has been reported.[124] The lithotomy position is not essential for damage to occur and two cases of sciatic nerve palsy following cesarean section have recently occurred.[125] Damage to the lateral femoral cutaneous nerve is probably the commonest lower limb mononeuropathy, with persistent numbness developing in the anterolateral aspect of the thigh, usually in the postpartum period. This condition, known as meralgia paresthetica, results from entrapment of

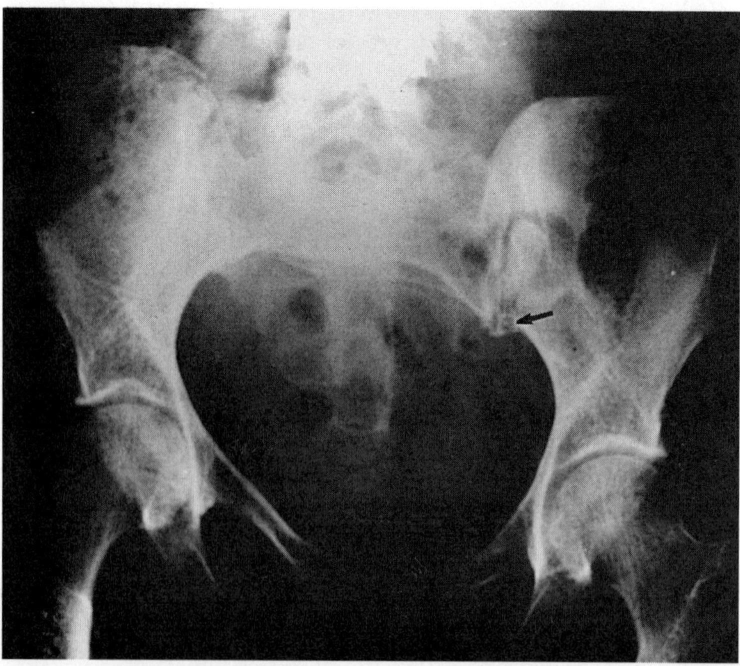

Figure 36–6 Anteroposterior radiograph of the pelvis showing distortion of the pelvic inlet and left sacroiliac joint *(arrow)* following old traumatic fractures. Application of obstetric forceps produced damage to the overlaying left lumbosacral plexus, with immediate pain in the leg and later footdrop and sensory loss.

the nerve as it passes around the anterior superior iliac spine or through the inguinal ligament,[126] and often seems to be related to excessive fluid retention. If a regional block has been undertaken prior to any of these neuropathies appearing, it is almost invariably blamed for the damage, at least in the first instance. The block itself may not be entirely blameless, as the patient may be immobilized and nerve compression and accompanying weakness or numbness may pass without notice in the presence of regional blockade.

When the figures for all these types of obstetric neurologic dysfunction are combined, an overall incidence of 1 in 2000 deliveries may be derived.[108] This value is about six times the incidence of neurologic impairment related to regional anesthesia.

Neurologic Complications of Regional Anesthesia

Minor neurologic dysfunction is frequent in the postnatal period, but as already indicated, regional anesthesia is not usually the cause. Major neurologic complications are extremely unusual in parturients if acknowledged guidelines are followed and an impeccable technique is employed, particularly with regard to maintenance of the circulation in the presence of excessively high blocks. In very rare cases, unrecognized congenital[127] or acquired spinal cord anomalies[128] may contribute to a poor neurologic outcome.

Prolonged Neural Blockade. Delayed recovery from regional anesthesia for obstetrics is occasionally seen, especially after epidural block. This was more frequent when high concentrations of bupivacaine and tetracaine were in widespread usage,[124] with patchy motor and sensory blocks lasting 10 to 48 hours being described.[129] Epidural block may also be prolonged for several hours following injection of more dilute local anesthetic solutions in parturients who have an existing neuropathy, which may or may not have been detected clinically. Prolonged bilateral blocks have been seen in diabetic patients and multiple sclerosis sufferers. Prolonged unilateral blocks have been noted in occasional patients with recurrent prolapsed intervertebral disks and previous sciatica, as well as in poliomyelitis victims several decades after their acute attack. Despite these explanations for prolongation of block duration, close observation of all patients is required until resolution of symptoms, as a more serious condition such as epidural abscess or hematoma may be overlooked.

Bladder Dysfunction. Regional anesthesia may increase the incidence of urinary retention during and after childbirth by causing bladder atonia from blockade of the sacral nerve roots. In addition, intrathecal opioids may reduce tone in the detrusor muscle. Attention to the bladder is mandatory in labor, particularly in the presence of regional block, and the parturient should be encouraged to void at regular intervals, or undergo catheterization. An overfilled and distended bladder may delay descent of the presenting part in labor and result in an atonic bladder postpartum. Long-term bladder dysfunction is unlikely to result from uncomplicated regional anesthesia,[108] but urinary incontinence may herald the onset of a cauda equina lesion.

Major Neurologic Complications of Regional Anesthesia

Nerve Root Lesions

Direct trauma by needles or catheters to nerve roots in the epidural or subarachnoid spaces is a rare occurrence, but may give rise to defects with a specific distribution. The development of paresthesias on block insertion has already been discussed on p. 504.

Although a momentary complaint of pain or paresthesias in one leg is very common on epidural catheter insertion with most types of catheter, the incidence of catheter-induced traumatic neuropathy is extremely low at 1 in 11,000 patients,[2] and the defect is usually transitory. However, use of more rigid catheters in one center over a 12-month period was associated with seven cases of prolonged neurologic dysfunction.[3] All the patients developed hyperesthesia to touch in 1 or 2 adjacent dermatomes in the same distribution as for the catheter-induced paresthesias. Four of the 7 patients also developed pain in the affected areas. Although complete relief of symptoms usually occurred within a few days or weeks, 2 patients had incomplete resolution. Catheters with soft flexible tips rarely produce paresthesias on insertion, which serves as a reminder that nerves are delicate structures that require gentle handling if damage is not to result.

Epidural needles may occasionally be inserted into the subarachnoid space and come into contact with intrathecal nerve roots, producing severe pain. The large, fairly blunt tips of epidural needles appear less likely to actually pierce the nerve roots than their smaller, sharper spinal counterparts. Any nerve dysfunction usually abates within 3 months of epidural needle trauma.

A gentle atraumatic technique is even more important when inserting subarachnoid needles and catheters, as the intrathecal nerve roots are more delicate and unprotected. Permanent nerve damage from direct needling of a spinal nerve occurs in approximately 1 in 80,000 surgical patients,[6] and probably less often in young healthy parturients. There is little evidence in the literature to relate the pain suffered at the time of needle insertion into a nerve or its surrounding tissues to subsequent nerve damage. Although permanent nerve dysfunction has followed cases of "traumatic" needle insertion with repeated attempts at the block producing severe pain, it has also followed straightforward pain-free "atraumatic" insertions.[6] However, it is recommended that the tip of the needle be withdrawn out of the subarachnoid space and redirected at a different angle of approach following one episode of marked nerve root pain, with abandonment of the technique after two or three attempts. Ignoring this advice has led to at least one case of severe, permanent neurapraxia in a parturient.

Lesser degrees of trauma to the nerve roots may result in symptoms for weeks or months. Intraneural injections, as well as producing the most excruciating lancinating pain at the time, can produce neuritis with paresthesias and loss of function that may be permanent.

It is worrying that unexplained neurologic deficits after CSE technique are appearing in the literature[8, 9] and as anecdotal reports, so soon after its widespread introduction. The possibility of dysfunction caused by nerve root trauma in these cases should always be excluded. With all regional techniques it is worth remembering that gentleness, precision, and careful manual control are essential for technical success and the avoidance of trauma and its consequences.[130]

Cauda Equina Syndrome and Paraplegia

These major neurologic problems are extremely rare, but most parturients are acutely aware of them, and considerable anxiety may be generated throughout pregnancy and early labor. Dysfunction of the spinal cord and cauda equina syndrome are usually due to compression by space-occupying lesions or caused by ischemia or neurotoxicity. Compression of the cord may present as paraplegia, while the cauda equina syndrome consists of residual numbness (the block "never wears off"), sphincter disturbance, perineal sensory loss, and varying degrees of lower limb paralysis. Urinary retention may be the first complaint, followed by fecal incontinence, and then other neurologic deficits. Symptoms may persist for weeks or months, or become permanent. The incidence of major complications following spinal or epidural anesthesia in a general hospital population in Finland was recently reported as approximately 0.5 in 10,000 blocks.[6] One would expect an obstetric population to have a far lower incidence, and Scott and Hibbard detected only three major spinal complications in their study of 505,000 obstetric epidural blocks.[131] The space-occupying lesions of importance are hematomas and abscesses.

Spinal Hematoma. Hematomas arising in the epidural, subdural, or subarachnoid spaces are remarkably rare and are usually spontaneous and unrelated to regional anesthesia.[132] They have been reported in pregnancy[133] and in the puerperium.[134] Trauma to blood vessels, in particular the epidural veins, occurs fairly commonly on epidural needle insertion, and possibly also on catheter removal. In the presence of a bleeding disorder, an expanding hematoma may develop over subsequent hours or days leading to cord or cauda equina compression, with ischemia and ultimately neuronal death. Spinal subdural hematoma may follow puncture of the dura, and has been reported following CSE.[135] Surveys of the world literature reveal the rarity of the condition, with only 25 cases of spinal hematoma following epidural or spinal puncture reported.[132] However, the consequences of a hematoma can be so devastating that regional anesthesia is contraindicated in the presence of coagulation abnormalities, which may be suspected in situations such as moderate or severe cases of pregnancy-induced hypertension, intrauterine fetal death, or placental abruption. The usually accepted indication of adequate coagulation is a platelet count of 75 to 100 $\times$ 10^9/L, although with a rapidly falling platelet count even this level may be considered inadequate. There appears to be minimal risk of hematoma from regional block in parturients on low-dose therapy with aspirin[136, 137] or heparin.[138] Individual obstetric departments should have their own protocols in place for managing parturients who are receiving low-molecular-weight heparin (LMWH) therapy.

A spinal hematoma should be suspected if an unusually prolonged block is accompanied by backache and urinary retention. Urgent investigation with MRI (Fig. 36–7) should be undertaken in suspicious cases, followed by surgical decompression if indicated.

Spinal Abscess. As with spinal hematoma, it is important to recognize that abscesses do occur spontaneously in the absence of regional block, and a spontaneous epidural abscess has been reported in the puerperium.[139] Infection in the spinal canal is another extremely rare complication of regional block, with a lower incidence than that of spinal hematoma. Abscess formation is usually secondary to infection elsewhere in the body, although it may result from contaminated needles, catheters, or injectate.[140] The important diagnostic features are severe back pain, overlying local tenderness, fever, and leukocytosis usually appearing within 2 to 3 days of the block, but occasionally delayed for several months. If the infection goes untreated, nerve root pain, weakness, and paralysis may follow.[140]

A catheter for a regional block should not be inserted through an area of skin sepsis, and prolonged catheterization should probably be avoided in the presence of known systemic sepsis, bacteremia, or viremia.[108] However, single-shot subarachnoid block or short-term epidural catheterization has been used satisfactorily in many parturients with chorioamnionitis, including some with bacteremia.[141] Other risk factors for abscess formation include diabetes, steroid administration, and immunocompromised status. Suspicion of the presence of an abscess should lead to urgent MRI examination, and surgical drainage if necessary. Two recent case reports have recorded epidural abscesses following CSE, one of which was treated conservatively.[142, 143] The reasons for a possible increased incidence of spinal infections with CSE are discussed later when meningitis is considered.

Meningitis

Septic Meningitis. Septic meningitis may be bacterial or viral in origin. Bacterial meningitis after spinal[144] or epidural anesthesia[145] has been extremely rare in the past, but a spate of recent reports have described this problem in five parturients following CSE.[146–150] The causative organisms are usually nosocomial, and infection is considered to result in most, but not all, cases from a breach in sterile technique. There appear to be three factors that might predispose CSE patients to an increased risk of meningitis or abscess formation.

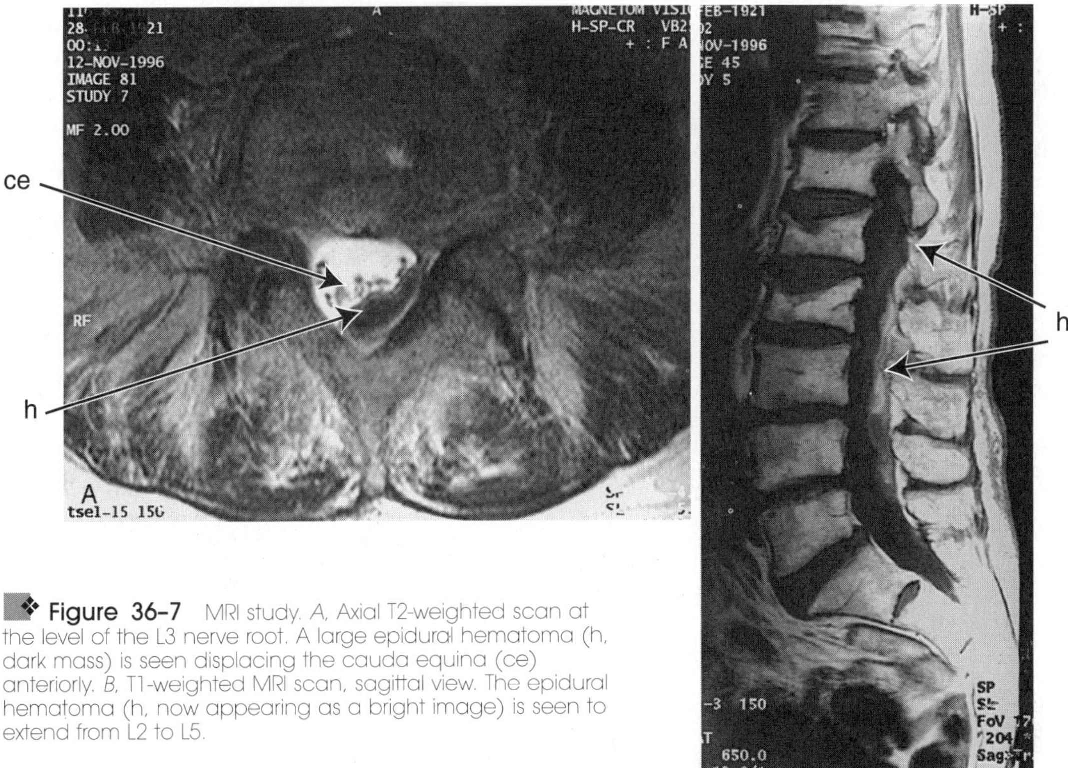

Figure 36–7 MRI study. *A*, Axial T2-weighted scan at the level of the L3 nerve root. A large epidural hematoma (h, dark mass) is seen displacing the cauda equina (ce) anteriorly. *B*, T1-weighted MRI scan, sagittal view. The epidural hematoma (h, now appearing as a bright image) is seen to extend from L2 to L5.

First, once the dura is perforated a protective barrier to the CNS is lost,[24] and at the same time, the epidural catheter allows access to the outside environment. Second, it is now common practice to mix agents for intrathecal use at the bedside, with increased risk of bacterial contamination, rather than using them as prepackaged and sterilized solutions. Third, it has been recognized that, in the past, the antimicrobial effects of spinal local anesthetics may have helped to prevent infections.[151] The current vogue of using intrathecal opioids, which do not have this property, as sole agents may contribute to the apparently increased infection rate. The symptoms of meningitis include headache, neck stiffness, photophobia, and fever. Aggressive treatment with antibiotics is usually instituted.

Viral meningitis may potentially follow regional block in parturients with primary herpes simplex infection,[152] or result from reactivation of herpes zoster infection.

Aseptic Meningitis. Aseptic meningitis mimicks bacterial meningitis and is currently a rare complication of both subarachnoid and epidural block, although a recent case was reported following CSE.[146] Most cases are attributed to disinfectant or detergent contamination of syringes and other equipment, either reusable or disposable.[145]

Arachnoiditis. Arachnoiditis is a rare inflammatory disorder involving all the membranes enveloping the spinal cord and cauda equina, which become thickened, fibrotic, and constrictive of the trapped nervous tissue. The exact cause of this condition is undetermined, although chemical damage, vasoconstrictors, and hemorrhage followed by clot organization have all been incriminated.[153] In 1980, the local anesthetic 2-chloroprocaine with sodium metabisulfite as a preservative was blamed for several cases of arachnoiditis with prolonged sensory and motor loss following inadvertent intrathecal injection of relatively large volumes intended for the epidural space.[49] 2-Chloroprocaine is now supplied free of preservative.

Neurotoxicity

Accidental injection of the wrong solution into the spinal canal can have diastrous consequences, with the epidural space showing a greater resistance to permanent neurologic sequelae than the subarachnoid space.[154] There have been a number of recent reports of potential neurotoxicity following intrathecal hyperbaric 5% lidocaine. In its milder form this toxicity is manifested as "transient radicular irritation" with severe pain in the lower back and/or buttocks, with or without radiation to one or both legs after spinal anesthesia.[155] Two cases have been reported in pregnant patients at 14 to 15 weeks' gestation subsequent to cervical cerclage, with complete recovery within 3 days.[156] The more severe and devastating form of neurotoxicity resulted in the cauda equina syndrome in several patients (none pregnant) following use of the hyperbaric lidocaine in continuous spinal anesthesia administered through microcatheters.[157, 158]

Ischemia

Ischemic damage of the spinal cord and cauda equina may result from prolonged and profound hypotension,

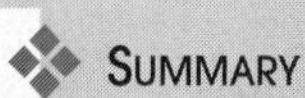

SUMMARY

Key Points

- Combined spinal-epidural anesthesia in the parturient is a relatively new technique, but there are a growing number of reports of complications. The reader must decide which, if any, of these complications are of significant concern and how to minimize these complications.
- The use of regional anesthesia in the anticoagulated parturient remains controversial, particularly related to low-molecular-weight heparin. The possibility of a spinal hematoma should always be considered in the patient with motor block following recovery from neuraxial anesthesia.
- Rapid diagnosis and treatment are necessary to prevent permanent impairment in the patient with a neurologic compromise following regional anesthesia. MRI is usually used for diagnosis of maternal obstetric palsy.

Key Reference

Reynolds F: Maternal sequelae of childbirth. Br J Anaesth 1995; 75:515.

Case Stem

A resident reports that he has had difficulty in removing an epidural catheter that was hard to place several hours previously. Following steady traction, the catheter was removed, but with the terminal 5 cm missing. Discuss the potential causes of this complication, how it can be prevented, and how you would manage this complication.

particularly if there is underlying vascular disease,[159] including that associated with pregnancy induced hypertension. Even though hypotension is usually corrected rapidly in pregnancy to maintain the fetal circulation, cases of anterior spinal artery syndrome with neurologic deficit have been reported.[11, 160, 161] The role of epinephrine added to the local anesthetic is uncertain. The features of spinal cord ischemia include localized back pain and loss of temperature sensation with burning pain in the feet prior to the onset of paraplegia and incontinence.

Auditory and Ocular Effects

Deafness and visual defects are rare but recognized complications of regional anesthesia in obstetrics. Transient hearing loss has been noted after spinal anesthesia for many years, and is presumed to be due to a loss in CSF pressure being transmitted to the perilymph in the cochlea.[162] Conversely, a sudden increase in CSF pressure following an epidural bolus dose may explain the occasional short-lived period (10 minutes) of deafness during epidural anesthesia.

Temporary blindness from a retinal hemorrhage has followed an epidural block in labor. Again, an increase in CSF pressure is believed to have been responsible.[162]

Conclusion. Despite this long and sometimes daunting list of possible complications of regional block in obstetrics, it should not be forgotten that, when these techniques are diligently performed, they are extremely safe and have eased the pain and suffering of countless women and benefited their babies over several decades.

References

1. Rolbin SH, Hew E, Ogilvie G: A comparison of two types of epidural catheter. Can J Anaesth 1987; 34:459.
2. Paech MJ, Godkin R, Webster S: Complications of obstetric epidural analgesia and anaesthesia: a prospective analysis of 10,995 cases. Int J Obstet Anesth 1998; 7:5.
3. Yoshii WY, Rottman RL, Rosenblatt RM, et al: Epidural catheter-induced traumatic radiculopathy in obstetrics: one center's experience. Reg Anesth 1994; 19:132.
4. Hiller A, Rosenberg PH: Transient neurological symptoms after spinal anesthesia with 4% mepivacaine and 0.5% bupivacaine. Br J Anaesth 1997; 79:301.
5. Hopkinson JM, Samaan AK, Russell IF, et al: A comparative multicentre trial of spinal needles for Caesarean section. Anaesthesia 1997; 52:998.
6. Aromaa U, Lahdensuu M, Cozanitis DA: Severe complications associated with epidural and spinal anesthesias in Finland 1987–1993: a study based on patient insurance claims. Acta Anaesthesiol Scand 1997; 41:445.
7. Turner MA, Reifenberg NA: Combined spinal epidural anaesthesia: the single space double-barrel technique. Int J Obstet Anesth 1995; 4:158.
8. Paech MJ: Unexplained neurological deficit after uneventful combined spinal and epidural anesthesia for Cesarean delivery. Reg Anesth 1997; 22:479.
9. Kubina P, Gupta A, Oscarsson A, et al: Two cases of cauda equina syndrome following spinal-epidural anesthesia. Reg Anesth 1997; 22:447.
10. Verniquet AJW: Vessel puncture with epidural catheters: experience in obstetric patients. Anaesthesia 1980; 35:660.
11. Scott DB, Hibbard BM: Serious nonfatal complications associated with extradural block in obstetric practice. Br J Anaesth 1990; 64:537.
12. Reynolds F: Auditing complications of regional analgesia in obstetrics [editorial]. Int J Obstet Anesth 1998; 7:1.
13. Collier CB: Collapse after epidural injection following inadvertent dural perforation. Anesthesiology 1982; 57:427.
14. Beck GN, Griffiths AG: Failed extradural anaesthesia for caesarean section: complication of subsequent spinal block. Anaesthesia 1992; 47:690.
15. Leach A, Smith GB: Subarachnoid spread of epidural local anaesthetic following dural puncture. Anaesthesia 1988; 43:671.
16. Collier CB: Complicated epidural blocks. *In* Collier CB: An Atlas of Epidurograms: Epidural Blocks Investigated. Sydney: Harwood Academic Press; 1998:42–44.
17. Franksson C, Gorth T: Headache after spinal anesthesia and a technique for lessening its frequency. Acta Chir Scand 1946; 94:443.
18. Stride PC, Cooper GM: Dural taps revisited: a 20-year survey from Birmingham Maternity Hospital. Anaesthesia 1993; 48:247.
19. Crawford JS: Experiences with epidural blood patch. Anaesthesia 1980; 35:513.
20. Carbaat PAT, van Crevel H: Lumbar puncture headache: controlled studyon the preventive effect of 24 hours' bed rest. Lancet 1981; 2:1133.
21. Ostman PL: Complications associated with regional anesthesia

in the obstetric patient. *In* Norris MC (ed): Obstetric Anesthesia. Philadelphia: JB Lippincott; 1993:763–799.
22. Brownridge P: The management of headache following dural puncture in obstetric patients. Anaesth Intens Care 1983; 11:4.
23. O'Kell RW, Sprigge JS: Unintentional dural puncture: a survey of recognition and management. Anaesthesia 1987; 42:1110.
24. Rawal N, Van Zundert A, Holmstrom B: Combined spinal-epidural technique. Reg Anesth 1997; 22:406.
25. Norris MC, Grieco WM, Borkowski M, et al: Complications of labor analgesia: epidural versus combined spinal epidural techniques. Anesth Analg 1994; 79:529.
26. Crawford JS: Headache after lumbar puncture. Lancet 1981; 2:418.
27. Reynolds F: Dural puncture and headache: avoid the first but treat the second. BMJ 1993; 306:874.
28. Chadwick HS: An analysis of obstetric anesthesia cases from the American Society of Anesthesiologists closed claims project database. Int J Obstet Anesth 1996; 5:258.
29. Bevacqua BK, Haas T, Brand F: A clinical measure of the posterior epidural space depth. Reg Anesth 1996; 21:456.
30. Szeinfeld M, Ihmeidan IH, Moser MM, et al: Epidural blood patch: evaluation of the volume and spread of blood injected into the epidural space. Anesthesiology 1986; 64:820.
31. Crawford JS: Some maternal complications of epidural analgesia for labour. Anaesthesia 1985; 40:1219.
32. Hutchison GL: The severance of epidural catheters. Anaesthesia 1987; 42:182.
33. Belatti RG, Fromme GA, Danielson DR: Relative resistance to shearing of commercially available epidural catheters versus available epidural needles [abstract]. Anesthesiology 1985; 63:A189.
34. Moerman N, Porcelijn T, Deen L: A broken epidural catheter: case report. Reg Anaesth 1980; 3:17.
35. Tio TO, MacMurdo SD, McKenzie R: Mishap with an epidural catheter. Anesthesiology 1979; 50:260.
36. Collier CB: Epidural catheter breakage: A possible mechanism. Int J Obstet Anesth (in press).
37. Bromage PR: Complications and contraindications. *In* Bromage PR (ed): Epidural Analgesia. Philadelphia: WB Saunders; 1978:654–715.
38. Hurley RJ, Lambert DH: Continuous spinal anesthesia with a microcatheter technique: preliminary experience. Anesth Analg 1990; 70:97.
39. Shnider SM, de Lorimier AA, Holl JW, et al: Vasopressors in obstetrics. I. Correction of fetal acidosis with ephedrine during spinal hypotension. Am J Obstet Gynecol 1968; 102:911.
40. Moran D, Perillo M, La Parta R, et al: Phenylephrine in the prevention of hypotension following spinal anesthesia for cesarean delivery. J Clin Anesth 1991; 3:301.
41. Zamora JE, Rosaeg OP, Lindsay MP, et al: Haemodynamic consequences and uterine contractions following 0.5 or 1.0 litre crystalloid infusion before obstetric epidural analgesia. Can J Anaesth 1996; 43:347.
42. Hallworth D, Jellicoe JA, Wilkes RG: Hypotension during epidural anaesthesia for Caesarean section. Anaesthesia 1982; 379:53.
43. Russell IF: Regional anaesthesia for Caesarean section: current approaches. *In* Bogod DG (ed): Clinical Anaesthesiology, Vol 9; No. 4: Obstetric Anaesthesia. London: Baillière Tindall; 1995:633–648.
44. Norris MC: Spinal anesthesia for cesarean section. *In* Norris MC (ed): Obstetric Anesthesia. Philadelphia: JB Lippincott; 1993:419–446.
45. Kestin IG, Madden AP, Mulvein JT, et al: Comparison of incremental spinal anaesthesia using a 32-gauge catheter with extradural anaesthesia for elective caesarean section. Br J Anaesth 1991; 66:232.
46. Honet JE, Arkoosh VA, Norris MC, et al: Comparison among intrathecal fentanyl, meperidine and sufentanil for labor analgesia. Anesth Analg 1992; 75:734.
47. Cohen SE, Cherry CM, Holbrook RH: Intrathecal sufentanil for labor analgesia—sensory changes, side effects and fetal heart rate changes. Anesth Analg 1993; 77:1155.
48. Juhani TP, Hannele H: Complications during spinal anesthesia for cesarean delivery: a clinical report of one year's experience. Reg Anesth 1993; 18:128–131.
49. Parnass SM, Schmidt KJ: Adverse effects of spinal and epidural anaesthesia. Drug Saf 1990; 5:179.
50. Bromage PR: Mechanism of action of extradural analgesia. Br J Anaesth 1975; 47(suppl 2):199.
51. Grundy EM, Ramamurthy S, Patel KP, et al: Extradural anesthesia revisited: statistical study. Br J Anaesth 1978; 50:805.
52. Crawford JS: Experiences with lumbar extradural for caesarean section. Br J Anaesth 1980; 52:821.
53. Bromage PR: Mechanism of action. *In* Bromage PR (ed): Epidural Analgesia. Philadelphia: WB Saunders; 1978:119–159.
54. Hirabayashi Y, Shimuzu R, Fukuda H, et al: Soft tissue anatomy within the vertebral canal in pregnant women. Br J Anaesth 1996; 77:153.
55. Collier CB: Bilateral trigeminal nerve palsy during an extensive lumbar epidural block. Int J Obstet Anesth 1997; 6:185.
56. Russell IF: Total spinal anaesthesia: the effect of spinal infusions. *In* Reynolds F (ed): Epidural and Spinal Blockade in Obstetrics. London: Baillière Tindall; 1990:107–120.
57. Wagner DL: Total spinal anesthesia during cesarean section hours after previous unintentional dural puncture. Anesthesiology 1994; 81:260.
58. Suzuki N, Koganemaru M, Onizuka S, et al: Dural puncture with a 26-gauge spinal needle affects epidural anesthesia. Reg Anesth 1995; 20(suppl 2):118.
59. Swenson JD, Wisniewski M, McJames S, et al: The effect of prior dural puncture on cisternal cerebrospinal fluid morphine concentrations in sheep after administration of lumbar epidural morphine. Anesth Analg 1996; 83:523.
60. Leighton BL, Arkoosh VA, Huffnagle S, et al: The dermatomal spread of epidural bupivacaine with and without prior intrathecal sufentanil. Anesth Analg 1996; 83:526.
61. Shehabi Y, Gatt S, Buckman T, et al: Effect of adrenaline, fentanyl and warming of injectate on shivering following extradural analgesia in labour. Anaesth Intens Care 1990; 18:31.
62. Holdcroft A, Hall GM, Cooper GM: Redistribution of body heat during anaesthesia: a comparison of halothane, fentanyl and epidural anaesthesia. Anaesthesia 1979; 34:758.
63. Walmsley AJ, Giesecke AH, Lipton JM: Contribution of extradural temperature to shivering during extradural anaesthesia. Br J Anaesth 1986; 58:1130.
64. Sevarino FB, Johnson MD, Lema MJ, et al: The effect of epidural sufentanil on shivering and body temperature in the parturient. Anesth Analg 1989; 68:520.
65. Clayton KC: The incidence of Horner's syndrome during lumbar extradural for elective Caesarean section and provision of analgesia during labour. Anaesthesia 1983; 38:583.
66. Abdelatti MO: Horner's syndrome due to epidural anaesthesia presenting with a painful eye. Anaesthesia 1993; 48:1019.
67. Zoellner PA, Bode ET: Horner's syndrome after epidural block in early pregnancy. Reg Anesth 1991; 16:242.
68. Carrie LES, Mohan J: Horner's syndrome following obstetric extradural block. Br J Anaesth 1976; 48:611.
69. Mohan J, Potter JM: Pupillary constriction and ptosis following caudal epidural analgesia. Anaesthesia 1975; 30:769.
70. Fisher MMcD, Bowey CJ: Alleged allergy to local anaesthetics. Anaesth Intens Care 1997; 25:611.
71. Laishley RS: Local anaesthetic toxicity. *In* Reynolds F (ed): Epidural and Spinal Blockade in Obstetrics. London: Baillière Tindall; 1990:81–94.
72. Reynolds F: Local anaesthetic drugs. Clin Anaesthesiol 1984; 2:577–603.
73. Camann W: Regional analgesia and labor outcome [editorial]. Int J Obstet Anesth 1997; 6:1.
74. Miller AC: The effects of epidural analgesia on uterine activity and labour. Int J Obstet Anesth 1997; 6:2.
75. Paech MJ: Patient controlled epidural analgesia during labour: choice of solution. Int J Obstet Anesth 1993; 2:65.

76. Reynolds F: Effects on the baby of conduction blockade in obstetrics. *In* Reynolds F (ed): Epidural and Spinal Blockade in Obstetrics. London: Baillière Tindall; 1990:207–218.
77. Cohen SE, Tan S, Albright GA, et al: Epidural fentanyl/bupivacaine mixtures for obstetric analgesia. Anesthesiology 1987; 67:403.
78. Viscomi CM, Hood DD, Melone PJ, et al: Fetal heart rate variability after epidural fentanyl during labor. Anesth Analg 1987; 71:679.
79. Collier CB: Why obstetric epidurals fail: a study of epidurograms. Int J Obstet Anesth 1996; 5:19.
80. Beilin Y, Bernstein HH, Zucker-Pinchoff B: The optimal distance that a multiorifice epidural catheter should be threaded into the epidural space. Anesth Analg 1995; 81:301.
81. Eappen S, Segal S, Blinn A, et al: Replacement rate and etiologic factors associated with inadequate block during epidural analgesia in parturients. Reg Anesth 1995; 20(suppl 2):69.
82. Joshi G, McCaroll S: Evaluation of combined spinal-epidural anesthesia using two different techniques. Reg Anesth 1994; 19:169.
83. Westbrook JL, Donald F, Carrie LES: An evaluation of a combined spinal epidural needle set utilizing a 26-gauge, pencil point spinal needle for caesarean section. Anaesthesia 1992; 47:990.
84. Lyons G: Epidural is an outmoded form of regional anaesthesia for elective caesarean section. Int J Obstet Anesth 1995; 4:34.
85. Kim YI, Mazza NM, Marx GF: Massive spinal block with hemicranial palsy after a "test dose" for extradural analgesia. Anesthesiology 1975; 43:370.
86. Stonham J, Moss P: The optimal test dose for epidural anesthesia. Anesthesiology 1983; 58:389.
87. Youngstrom P, Boyd D, Rhoton F: Statistical process control (SPC) in obstetric anesthesia service: six years experience [abstract]. Anesthesiology 1992; 77:A1020.
88. Evans TI: Total spinal anaesthesia. Anaesth Intens Care 1974; 2:158.
89. Southorn P, Vasdev GMS, Chantigian RC, et al: Reducing the potential morbidity of an unintentional spinal anaesthetic by aspirating cerebrospinal fluid. Br J Anaesth 1996; 76:467.
90. Collier CB: Accidental subdural block: four more cases and a radiographic review. Anaesth Intens Care 1992; 20:215.
91. Miller DC, Choi WW, Chestnut DH: Subdural injection of local anesthetics and morphine: a complication of attempted epidural anesthesia. South Med J 1989; 82:87.
92. Collier CB, Gatt SP, Lockley SM: A continuous subdural block. Br J Anaesth 1993; 70:462.
93. Myint Y, Bailey PW, Milne BR: Cardiorespiratory arrest following combined spinal epidural anaesthesia for Caesarean section. Anaesthesia 1993; 48:684.
94. Collier CB: Cardiorespiratory arrest following combined spinal epidural anaesthesia. Anaesthesia 1994; 49:259.
95. Brown DL, Ransom DM, Hall JA, et al: Regional anesthesia and local anesthetic-induced systemic toxicity: seizure frequency and accompanying cardiovascular changes. Anesth Analg 1995; 81:321.
96. Heavner JE: Cardiac dysrhythmias induced by infusion of local anesthetics into the lateral cerebral ventricle of cats. Anesth Analg 1986; 65:133.
97. Feldman HS, Arthur GR, Covino BG: Comparative systemic toxicity of convulsant and supraconvulsant doses of intravenous ropivacaine, bupivacaine and lidocaine in the conscious dog. Anesth Analg 1989; 69:794.
98. Nancarrow C, Rutten AJ, Runciman WG, et al: Myocardial and cerebral drug concentrations and the mechanisms of death after fatal intravenous doses of lidocaine, bupivacaine and ropivacaine in the sheep. Anesth Analg 1989; 69:276.
99. Scott DB, Lee A, Fagan D, Bowler GMR, et al: Acute toxicity of ropivacaine compared with that of bupivacaine. Anesth Analg 1989; 69:563.
100. Kasten GW, Martin ST: Successful cardiovascular resuscitation after massive intravenous bupivacaine overdosage in anesthetized dogs. Anesth Analg 1985; 64:491.
101. Beck H, Brassow F, Doehn M, et al: Epidural catheters of the multi-orifice type: dangers and complications. Acta Anaesthiol Scand 1986; 30:549.
102. Gregoretti S: Uneventful extradural analgesia after unrecognized perforation. Can Anaesth Soc J 1978; 25:509.
103. Power I, Thorburn J: Differential flow from multihole epidural catheters. Anaesthesia 1988; 43:876.
104. Collier CB, Gatt SP: Epidural catheters for obstetrics: terminal holes or lateral eyes? Reg Anesth 1994; 19:378.
105. Collier CB, Gatt SP: A new epidural catheter: closer eyes for safety? Anaesthesia 1993; 48:803.
106. Grove LH: Backache, headache and bladder dysfunction after delivery. Br J Anaesth 1973; 45:1147.
107. Crawford JS: Lumbar epidural block in labour: a clinical analysis. Br J Anaesth 1972; 44:66.
108. Russell R, Reynolds F: Long-term effects of epidural analgesia. *In* Bogod DG (ed): Clinical Anaesthesiology, Vol 9; No. 4: Obstetric Anaesthesia. London: Baillière Tindall; 1995:607–622.
109. MacArthur C, Lewis M, Knox EG, et al. Epidural analgesia and long-term backache after childbirth. BMJ 1990; 301:9.
110. Clark VA, McQueen MA: Factors influencing backache following epidural analgesia in labour. Int J Obstet Anesth 1993; 2:193.
111. Russell R, Groves P, Taub N, et al: Assessing long term backache after childbirth. BMJ 1993; 306:1299.
112. Fast A, Shapiro D, Ducommun E, et al: Low back pain in pregnancy. Spine 1987; 12:368.
113. Berg G, Hammar M, Moller-Nielsen J, et al: Low back pain during pregnancy. Obstet Gynecol 1988; 71:71.
114. Breen TW, Ransil BJ, Groves PA, et al: Factors associated with back pain after childbirth. Anesthesiology 1994; 81:29.
115. Macarthur AJ, Macarthur C, Weeks S. Epidural anesthesia and postpartum back pain [abstract]. Anesthesiology 1993; 79:A973.
116. Hill EC: Maternal obstetric paralysis. Am J Obstet Gynecol 1962; 83:1452.
117. Cole JT: Maternal obstetric paralysis. Am J Obstet Gynecol 1946; 52:372.
118. O'Donnell D, Rottman R, Kotelko D, et al: Incidence of postpartum neurologic dysfunction [abstract]. Anesthesiology 1994; 81:A1127.
119. Ong BY, Cohen MM, Esmail A, et al: Paresthesias and motor dysfunction after labour and delivery. Anesth Analg 1986; 66:18.
120. Holdcroft A, Gibberd FB, Hargrove RL, et al: Neurological complications associated with pregnancy. Br J Anaesth 1995; 75:522.
121. Bromage PR: Neurological complications of regional anesthesia for obstetrics. *In* Shnider SM, Levinson G (eds): Anesthesia for Obstetrics, 3rd ed. Baltimore: Williams & Wilkins; 1993:433–453.
122. Reynolds F: Maternal sequelae of childbirth. Br J Anaesth 1995; 75:515.
123. Ashkan K, Casey ATH, Powell M, et al: Back pain during pregnancy and after childbirth: an unusual cause not to miss. J R Soc Med 1998; 91:88.
124. Datta S: Relief of labor pain by regional analgesia/anesthesia. *In* Datta S (ed): The Obstetric Anesthesia Handbook, 2nd ed. St. Louis: CV Mosby; 1992:115–150.
125. Silva M, Mallinson C, Reynolds F: Case reports: sciatic nerve palsy following childbirth. Anaesthesia 1996; 51:1144.
126. Van Diver T, Camman W: Meralgia paresthetica in the parturient. Int J Obstet Anesth 1995; 4:109.
127. Katz N, Hurley R: Epidural anesthesia complicated by fluid collection within the spinal cord. Anesth Analg 1993; 77:1064.
128. Roscoe MWA, Barrington TW: Acute spinal subdural hematoma: a case report and review of the literature. Spine 1984; 9:672.
129. Bromage PR: An evaluation of bupivacaine in epidural analgesia for obstetrics. Can Anaesth Soc J 1969; 16:46.
130. Wildsmith JAW, Lee JA: Neurological sequelae of spinal anaesthesia. Br J Anaesth 1989; 63:505.
131. Scott DB, Hibbard BM: Serious non-fatal complications associated with extradural block in obstetric practice. Br J Anaesth 1990; 64:537.

132. Bidzinski J: Spontaneous spinal epidural hematoma during pregnancy: case report. J Neurosurg 1966; 24:1017.
133. Crawford JS: Pathology in the extradural space. Br J Anaesth 1975; 47:412.
134. Sage DA: Epidurals, spinals and bleeding disorders in pregnancy: a review. Anaesth Intensive Care 1990; 18:319.
135. Bougher RJ, Ramage D: Spinal subdural haematoma following combined spinal-epidural anaesthesia. Anaesth Intens Care 1995; 23:373.
136. Nelson-Piercy C, De Swiet M: The place of low dose aspirin in pregnancy. Int J Obstet Anesth 1994; 3:3.
137. Sibai B, Caritis SN, Thom E, et al: Low-dose aspirin in nulliparous women: safety of continuous epidural block and correlation between bleeding time and maternal-neonatal bleeding complications. Am J Obstet Gynecol 1995; 172:1553.
138. Letsky EA: Haemostasis and epidural anaesthesia. Int J Obstet Anesth 1991; 1:51.
139. Malc CG, Martin R: Puerperal epidural abscess. Lancet 1973; 1:608.
140. Ngan Kee WD, Joner MR, Thomas P, et al: Extradural abscess complicating extradural anaesthesia for caesarean section. Br J Anaesth 1992; 69:647.
141. Bader AM, Gilbertson L, Kirz L, et al. Regional anesthesia in women with chorioamnionitis. Reg Anesth 1992; 17:84.
142. Schroter J, Wa Djamba D, Hoffman V, et al: Epidural abscess after combined spinal-epidural block. Can J Anaesth 1997; 44:300.
143. Dysart RH, Balakrishnan V: Conservative management of extradural abscess complicating spinal-extradural anaesthesia for Caesarean section. Br J Anaesth 1997; 78:591.
144. Berga S, Trierwiler MW: Bacterial meningitis following epidural anesthesia for vaginal delivery: a case report. Obstet Gynecol 1989; 74(3 pt 2):437.
145. Roberts SP, Petts HV: Meningitis after obstetric spinal anaesthesia. Anaesthesia 1990; 45:376.
146. Harding SA, Collis RE, Morgan BM: Meningitis after combined spinal-extradural anaesthesia in obstetrics. Br J Anaesth 1994; 73:545.
147. Cascio M, Heath G: Meningitis following a combined spinal-epidural technique in a labouring term parturient. Can J Anaesth 1996; 43:399.
148. Aldebert S, Sleth JC: Meningite bacterienne apres anesthesie rachidienne et peridurale combinee en obstetrique. Ann Fr Reanim 1996; 15:687.
149. Bouhemad B, Dounas M, Mercier FJ, et al: Bacterial meningitis following combined spinal-epidural analgesia for labour. Anaesthesia 1998; 53:292.
150. Stallard N, Barry P: Another complication of the combined extradural-subarachnoid technique. Br J Anaesth 1995; 75:370.
151. Ready LB, Helfer D: Bacterial meningitis in parturients after epidural anaesthesia. Anesthesiology 1989; 71:988.
152. Lee JJ, Parry H: Bacterial meningitis following spinal anaesthesia for caesarean section. Br J Anaesth 1991; 66:383.
153. Covino BG, Marx GF, Finster M, et al: Prolonged sensory/motor deficits following inadvertent spinal anesthesia. Anesth Analg 1980; 59:399.
154. Craig DB, Habib GG: Flaccid paraparesis following obstetrical epidural anesthesia: the possible role of benzyl alcohol. Anesth Analg 1977; 56:219.
155. Pinczower GR, Chadwick HS, Woodland R, et al: Bilateral leg pain following lidocaine spinal anaesthesia. Can J Anaesth 1995; 42:217.
156. Newman LM, Iyer NR, Tuman KJ: Transient radicular irritation after hyperbaric lidocaine spinal anesthesia in parturients. Int J Obstet Anesth 1997; 6:132.
157. Rigler ML, Drasner K, Krejcie TC, et al: Cauda equina syndrome after continuous spinal anesthesia. Anesth Analgesia 1991; 72:275.
158. Schell RM, Brauer FS, Cole DJ, et al: Persistent sacral nerve root deficits after continuous spinal anesthesia. Can J Anaesth 1991; 38:908.
159. Usubiaga JE: Neurological complications following epidural anesthesia. Int Anesthesiol Clin 1975; 13:1.
160. Ackerman WE, Juneja MM, Knapp RK: Maternal paraparesis after epidural anesthesia and cesarean section. South Med J 1990; 83:695.
161. Eastwood DW: Anterior spinal artery syndrome after epidural anesthesia in a pregnant diabetic patient with scleroderma. Anesth Analg 1991; 73:90.
162. Day CJE, Shutt LE: Auditory, ocular and facial complications of central neural block: a review of possible mechanisms. Reg Anesth 1996; 21:197.

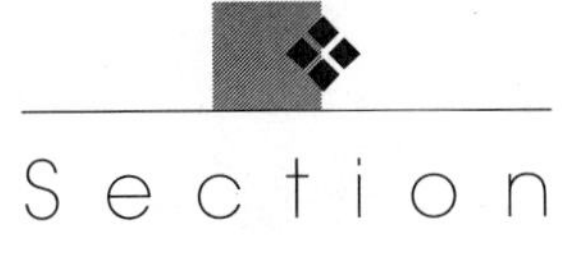

Section

V

Systemic Disease in the Pregnant Patient

37

The Obese Parturient

❖ MAKOTO TANAKA, MD
❖ SEIJI WATANABE, MD, PHD

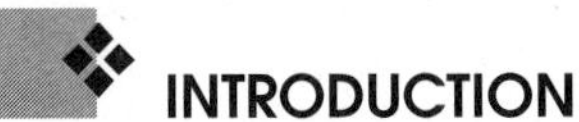

INTRODUCTION

Obesity is perhaps the most common nutritional disorder seen in industrialized countries. Among the various definitions, body mass index (BMI = weight [kg]/height [m]^2) has been most commonly employed to define the extent of obesity (Fig. 37–1).[1] The normal value of BMI is 25, while BMIs between 26 and 29 are classified as overweight. Obesity usually refers to BMI greater than 27.8 for men and 27.3 for women, representing approximately 120% of desirable weight, and morbid obesity is defined as body weight more than twice the ideal weight, or BMI more than 35.[2, 3] Obviously, the proportion of obese individuals depends on geographic location. In the United States, one third of the population is estimated to be overweight, and there have been increases in the incidence of obesity in all sex, race, and age groups in the past decade (Table 37–1).[2, 4] Of note, even though BMI is a simple, useful method to quantify the extent of obesity, the physiologic and pathophysiologic nature of obesity cannot be accurately predicted by this formula. For instance, android obesity (characterized primarily by a truncal distribution of fat) is associated with a high incidence of cardiovascular disorders, whereas in gynecoid obesity (fat distributed to thighs and buttocks), the association incidence of cardiovascular disorders is low.[5] In addition, many individuals whose BMIs are greater than 28 may have no apparent respiratory, cardiovascular, or metabolic pathology. This implies that the clinical relevance of obesity should not rely only on a number derived from the simple calculation, but must be determined based on the coexisting pathophysiologic functions found in each case.

Despite this, the likelihood of abnormal anatomic findings, physiologic functions, and pharmacologic responses is high in the obese population. The incidence of cardiovascular disorders, such as hypertension and coronary artery disease, impaired pulmonary function, adult-onset (insulin-resistant) diabetes mellitus, and gastrointestinal abnormalities, which could all complicate anesthetic management and postoperative care, are reported to be increased in obese patients.[6, 7] As a result, morbidly obese patients present with a greater than twofold increase in surgical mortality.[6, 8] In addition, not only increased maternal prepregnancy weight, but also increased gestational weight gain has to be noted, since gestational weight gain is associated with increased risks of a difficult airway, abnormal labor patterns, certain fetal abnormalities, and emergent cesarean section.[9–11]

PATHOPHYSIOLOGY OF OBESITY

Respiratory

Although the basal metabolic rate usually remains within the normal range, obese individuals have increased oxygen consumption ($\dot{V}O_2$) and carbon dioxide production ($\dot{V}CO_2$) in proportion to the extent of the obesity.[12–14] This is considered to be secondary to the metabolic activity of adipose tissue, as well as the increased energy expenditure due to locomotive and respiratory efforts. Obese patients, therefore, require high minute ventilation to meet the energy requirement and maintain normocarbia against the reduced chest wall compliance, secondary to the fat-loaded truncal structure (restrictive lung disease). Compliance of the lung parenchyma, however, is usually normal unless underlying lung pathology is present.[6] Increases in $\dot{V}O_2$ and $\dot{V}CO_2$ in the obese individual are even more pronounced during exercise, such as during labor and delivery.[12, 14]

More importantly, obese patients have dramatic reduction of residual volume and functional residual capacity compared with lean patients.[15] Even in the upright position, tidal respiration may fall within the closing capacity during the expiratory phase, resulting in ventilation/perfusion mismatching or intrapulmonary right-to-left shunt. This is accentuated in the supine or Trendelenburg position when the functional residual capacity is further reduced, which is the major cause of arterial hypoxemia encountered in the operating suites in this population. Although many healthy obese subjects can maintain adequate minute ventilation and present with normal pulmonary function tests (including the forced vital capacity, forced

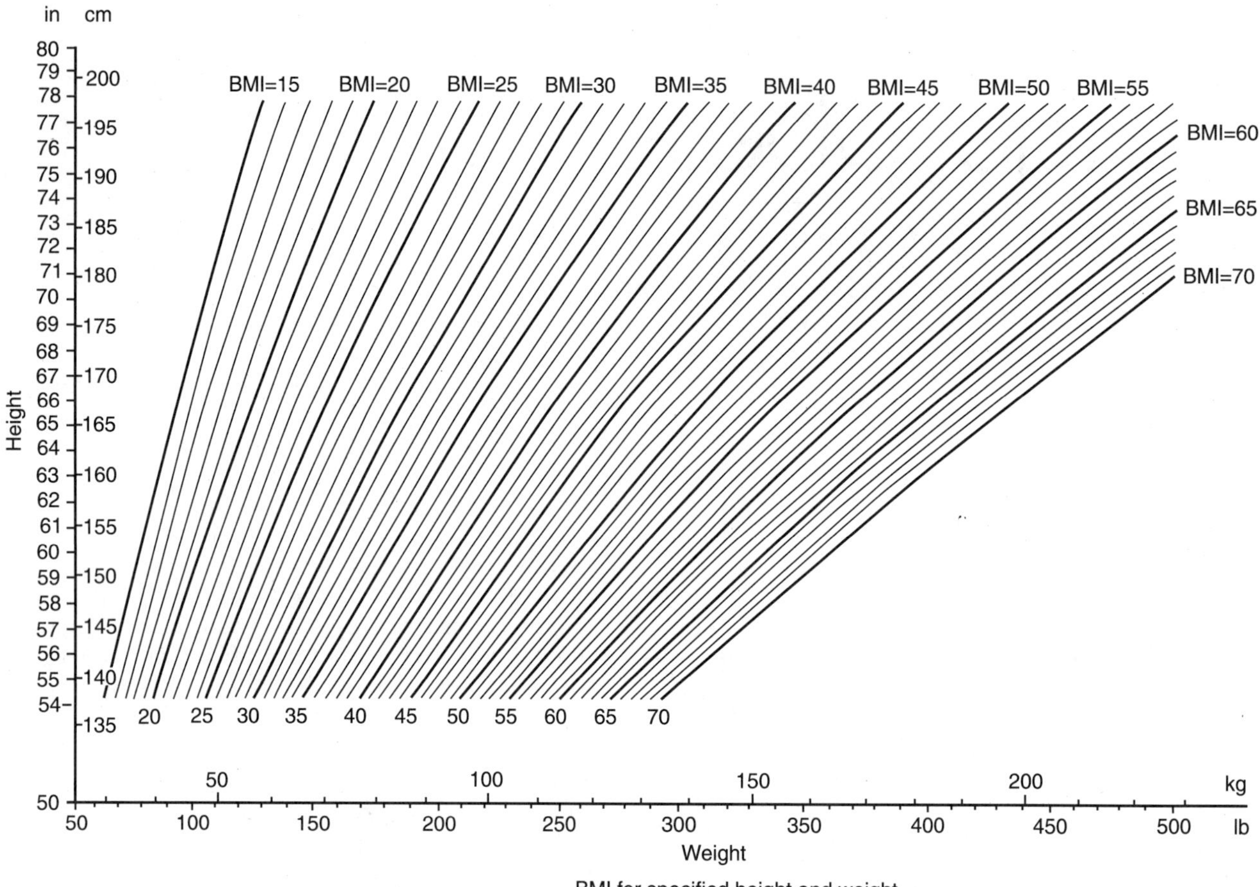

Figure 37–1 Body mass index (BMI) (body weight in kilogram/height in meters²) for specified height and weight. (From Frankel HM: Determination of body mass index. JAMA 1986; 255:1292.)

expiratory volume in 1 second, peak expiratory flow rate, and normal respiratory response to carbon dioxide), some extreme cases may present conditions known as obesity hypoventilation syndrome (pickwickian syndrome).[16] This syndrome, which occurs in approximately 8% of the obese population, is characterized by alveolar hypoventilation, daytime somnolence, and morbid obesity.[17] Chronic arterial hypoxemia and resultant polycythemia are present. Hypercarbia is considered secondary to decreased sensitivity of the brain stem respiratory center to carbon dioxide. Chronic hypoxemia and hypercarbia may cause pulmonary hypertension, and ultimately cor pulmonale and right ventricular failure. The soft tissue mass of the oropharynx is increased, predisposing these patients to develop intermittent obstruction of the upper airway when pharyngeal musculature is relaxed during sleep.[18] As a result, these patients are deprived of sleep, and daytime hypersomnolence ensues. Other common complications associated with the pickwickian syndrome are pulmonary embolism and pneumonia.

Airway

Obesity-related changes in the upper airway include limited flexion of the cervical spine and atlanto-axial joint, limited mouth opening, and narrowed view of the pharyngeal opening. These alterations are due, at least in part, to the cervical, upper thoracic, breast, and mental adipose tissue located subcutaneously. Frequently, an enlarged tongue as well as fleshy pharyngeal and supralaryngeal soft tissue may prevent adequate visualization of the cords and thus make laryngoscopy extremely difficult. In addition, obese pregnant women have a much higher incidence of failed intubation (0.35%) as compared with obese nonpregnant surgical patients (0.04%), indicating that obesity and pregnancy can additively increase the incidence of failed intubation.[9] Furthermore, pregnancy at term, especially when associated with a weight gain of more than 15 kg, is associated with a four times greater incidence of suboptimal laryngoscopic view when compared with nonpregnant women at the corresponding age.[10]

Cardiovascular

Circulating blood volume, plasma volume, and cardiac output are known to increase in proportion to weight in obese subjects.[19, 20] Increased blood viscosity because of polycythemia may also be present in morbidly obese patients and those with obesity hypoventilation syn-

Table 37–1 AGE-ADJUSTED AND AGE-SPECIFIC PREVALENCE OF OVERWEIGHT, US POPULATION 20 THROUGH 74 YEARS OF AGE*

POPULATION GROUP	PREVALENCE OF OVERWEIGHT BY STUDY, %			
	NHES I (1960–1962)†	**NHANES I (1971–1974)**	**NHANES II (1976–1980)**	**NHANES III Phase 1 (1988–1991)**
Age 20–74 y	24.3	25.0	25.4	33.3
Race/sex				
White				
Men	23.0	23.8	24.2	32.0
Women	23.6	24.0	24.4	33.5
Black				
Men	22.1	23.9	26.2	31.8
Women	41.6	43.1	44.5	49.2
Sex/age, y				
Men				
20–74	22.8	23.7	24.1	31.7
20–29	18.4	15.7	15.1	20.2
30–39	21.8	28.4	24.4	27.4
40–49	25.5	30.2	32.4	37.0
50–59	28.8	27.1	28.2	42.1
60–74	23.0	21.6	26.8	40.9
Women				
20–74	25.7	26.0	26.5	34.9
20–29	10.1	12.6	14.7	20.2
30–39	21.9	22.9	23.8	34.3
40–49	26.8	29.7	29.0	37.6
50–59	35.0	35.5	36.5	52.0
60–74	45.6	39.0	37.3	41.3

NHES, National Health Examination Survey; NHANES, National Health and Nutrition Examination Survey.
*Pregnant women excluded.
†A total of 0.9 kg was subtracted from measured weight to adjust for weight of clothing.
From Kuczmarski RJ, Flegal KM, Campbell SM, Johnson CL: Increasing prevalence of overweight amongst US adults: The National Health and Nutritional Examination surveys, 1960–1991. JAMA 1994; 272:205–211.

drome. The increase in cardiac output is in part due to blood flow through the adipose tissue, which accounts for 2 to 3 mL/min/100 g tissue at rest and parallels that of $\dot{V}O_2$. An abrupt rise in cardiac output occurs in obese versus lean patients during exercise,[21] and such changes can be augmented during labor, producing a profound increase in oxygen consumption. Also of concern, the incidence of coronary artery disease is doubled in obese as compared with nonobese subjects.[6, 7] Furthermore, typical symptoms of angina may not be present in diabetic patients. The heart rate at rest is usually unaltered in obese patients, indicating that the increase in stroke volume accounts for the increase in cardiac output.[20]

Hypertension is a frequent coexisting disorder in obese patients. Among the morbidly obese, 50% of patients present with mild and 5% to 10% with severe hypertension.[22] Elevated blood pressure and increased circulating blood volume indicate that both afterload and preload are elevated, even at rest. As a result of these pressure and volume changes, left ventricular end-diastolic pressure is increased, cardiac diameter is increased on the chest radiograph, and left ventricular hypertrophy ensues.[21] Labor- and delivery-induced changes in blood pressure in obese parturients may necessitate continuous infusion of a vasodilatory drug. It is, however, clinically challenging to obtain satisfactory blood pressure control because of the contraction-induced abrupt surges in blood pressure due to both preload and afterload augmentations. This is illustrated by the fact that undiagnosed rupture of a cerebral aneurysm or arteriovenous malformation frequently occurs during labor.[23]

Obese parturients are also vulnerable to pulmonary hypertension.[24] Pulmonary artery occlusion pressure becomes elevated during labor and delivery, which may be accentuated by hypoxic pulmonary vasoconstriction in the morbidly obese parturient who may have preexisting pulmonary pathology.

Endocrine and Metabolic System

Glucose tolerance is frequently impaired in the obese patient as a result of developing resistance to insulin.[25] Hypertrophy of the islets of Langerhans of the pancreas is found, and hyperinsulinemia ensues, reflecting a marked increase in the incidence of adult-onset diabetes mellitus in morbidly obese patients. During pregnancy, a relative insulin deficiency may further impair glucose tolerance.[26] These patients may also present with high serum triglyceride and cholesterol levels, which may possibly be the cause of the increased prevalence of ischemic heart disease.

Gastrointestinal System

There is a proportional increase in the intra-abdominal pressure in obese patients, resulting in a high prevalence of hiatal hernia in this population. Classically, gastric volume is increased and the pH of the gastric fluid is decreased by obesity.[27] Indeed, nearly 90% of fasted morbidly obese patients present with gastric volume greater than 25 mL and the pH less than 2.5, a condition associated with a high risk for developing aspiration pneumonitis should gastric fluid reach the airway. It has, therefore, been a routine practice to administer preoperative antacid with or without gastric prokinetic drugs to obese patients. However, a recent clinical investigation questioned these classic findings and demonstrated a decreased incidence of high-volume, low-pH gastric content for nonmedicated, nondiabetic, fasting obese patients (BMI >30) free of gastroesophageal pathology as compared with nonobese surgical patients (BMI <30).[28] The new study differs from the classic one in that a greater proportion of the obese patients in the classic study received narcotic premedication compared with lean patients.

The findings of Vaughan et al.[27] that almost 90% of obese nonpregnant patients had high-volume, low-pH gastric content is similar to that seen in healthy pregnant patients.[29] Whether the combination of obesity and pregnancy produces even greater risk for aspiration remains to be determined.[30] There is no doubt that pregnancy is associated with an increased incidence of symptomatic hiatal hernia and decreased sphincter tone of the lower esophagus.[31, 32] As the effects of obesity may be superimposed on gastric fluid volume, pH, or lower esophageal sphincter tone during pregnancy, emphasis should be on the benefits of antacid and gastric prokinetic drugs to decrease the likelihood of aspiration pneumonitis in this population.

PROBLEMS ASSOCIATED WITH PREGNANCY

Obese pregnant patients have more difficulties than those who are not obese. These difficulties include an increased incidence of prepregnant medical problems,[33–36] increased incidence of abnormal labor,[11, 32, 37] increased likelihood of cesarean delivery,[11, 35–37] and increased likelihood of fetal abnormality.[11, 33, 35, 37]

Of all medical illness, pregnancy induces perhaps the most striking effect on the incidence of chronic hypertension in the obese woman (Fig. 37–2). Compared with nonobese patients, a 14-fold increase in the incidence of chronic hypertension has been observed, whereas the increase in the incidence of pregnancy-induced hypertension remains minimal.[33–36] The diabetogenic state of pregnancy also puts the obese parturient at risk for developing insulin-dependent diabetes, whereas nonpregnant obese patients are already in an insulin-resistant state.[35–38] Indeed, the pregnancy-induced increase in the incidence of diabetes is twofold to eightfold. More importantly, anesthesia- and surgery-related maternal death is increased in the obese as compared with nonobese parturient.[39–41]

Some studies also suggest that obese patients have an increased likelihood of abnormal labor, including meconium-stained amniotic fluid and late decelerations during labor.[11, 32, 37] Failure to progress, prolonged second stage of labor, and failed response to elective induction of labor have also been reported to occur more frequently in obese parturients.[33] Dystocia is more frequently diagnosed in the obese than nonobese parturient, all of which probably contribute to

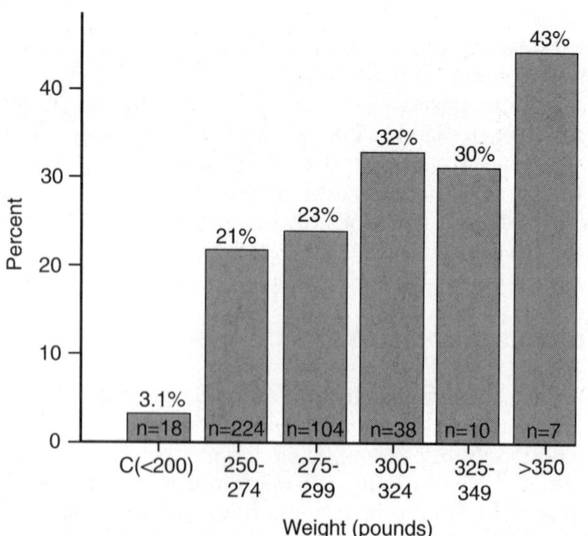

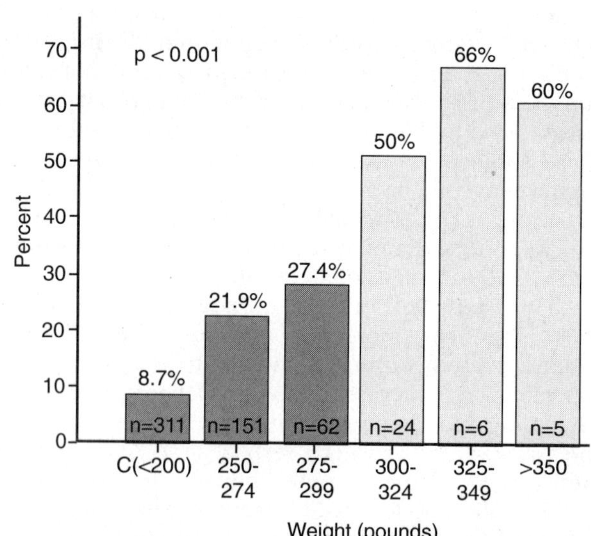

❖ Figure 37–2 Incidence of chronic hypertension in obese parturients stratified in increasing increments of 25 pounds. (From Johnson SR, Kolberg BH, Varner MW, Railsback LD: Maternal obesity and pregnancy. Surg Gynecol Obstet 1987; 164:431–437.)

the increased risk of cesarean section. Other factors associated with the increased likelihood of cesarean delivery in the obese parturient may be abnormal presentations, including shoulder dystocia, fetal macrosomia, and multiple gestation. These are all reported to be higher in obese women.[33, 35, 38] Although macrosomia may be associated with a high incidence of cesarean section, Johnson et al.[33] reported that the increased incidence of cesarean section in obese parturients was independent of the presence of hypertension, diabetes, and macrosomic infants. It has been speculated that intrapelvic fat tissue and perineal and vaginal wall adipose deposits may cause anatomic distortion of the birth canal, producing prolonged labor and the frequent diagnosis of dystocia in this population.[37]

Maternal obesity, increased gestational weight gain, and diabetes are all independent risk factors for developing macrosomia.[11, 35, 37] On the other hand, decreased incidences of preterm delivery and low birthweight are known to occur in the obese patients.[11, 33, 38] Most significant, a higher incidence of neonatal admission to the intensive care unit is seen, and infants of obese patients have a 10-fold increase in perinatal mortality.[36, 42]

PHARMACOKINETIC AND PHARMACODYNAMIC ALTERATIONS IN THE OBESE

Physiologic and pathophysiologic alterations that affect pharmacokinetic and pharmacodynamic considerations include increases in circulating blood volume, cardiac output, organ size, and amount of adipose tissue. Most importantly, the increase in fat tissue alters the pharmacokinetic properties of lipophilic drugs, as opposed to hydrophilic drugs, whose pharmacokinetic property is relatively less affected.[43, 44] A classic belief is that the recovery of obese patients is prolonged following administration of volatile anesthetic agents (which also have high affinity to adipose tissue), but this is not observed after short procedures such as cesarean section.[45, 46]

Lipid-soluble drugs tend to have an increased volume of distribution. Albumin and total protein concentrations are unaffected by obesity, whereas the increased triglyceride, cholesterol, free fatty acid, and α_1-acid glycoprotein may influence the plasma protein binding and the free fraction of the active drug. Increased kidney size and renal blood flow (glomerular filtration rate) facilitate renal clearance. Increased splanchnic blood flow and hypertrophy of the hepatic parenchymal cells may also affect hepatic clearance of drugs through the liver. Obesity, however, is not associated with changes in the phase I metabolism of the liver (oxidation, reduction, and hydrolysis), whereas elimination through the phase II metabolism (conjugation pathway) seems to be faster.

Thiopental and benzodiazepines are highly lipophilic and hence have larger volumes of distribution.[47, 48] Their longer elimination half-life, despite the unchanged clearance values, indicate that these lipid-soluble drugs are more selectively distributed in the fat tissue. These findings imply that obese patients may require larger induction doses of lipid-soluble drugs for general anesthesia, even though decreased anesthetic requirements during pregnancy should also be considered.

Propofol is also a lipophilic agent possessing a fast-onset, short-duration property. Even though the pharmacokinetic data of propofol in obese patients are limited, the initial volume of distribution of propofol does not seem to be modified in obese patients as compared with nonobese subjects.[49] Total body clearance and volume of distribution at steady state were also correlated to body weight. Pharmacokinetic data of propofol also do not seem to be altered during pregnancy, suggesting that propofol accumulation does not occur and that the dosing schemes expressed in milligrams per kilogram body weight (mg/kg) need not be altered in morbidly obese parturients. Ketamine is the induction agent of choice for those with a history of bronchial asthma as well as for those presenting with hypotension.[50] However, the ideal dose of ketamine for obese pregnant patients has not been determined.

Fentanyl, when given on a mg/kg basis, has comparable pharmacokinetic properties in obese as compared with nonobese patients.[51] On the other hand, sufentanil is associated with a larger volume of distribution and unchanged plasma clearance, producing a prolonged elimination half-life.[52] Alfentanil is associated with longer elimination half-life in the obese than nonobese patient, secondary to decreased drug clearance. Volume of distribution at steady state, however, is unaltered.[53]

Fat tissue serves as a reservoir for volatile anesthetic agents, and there is a fear of an increased risk of biotransformation of volatile agents in obese patients. Increased serum inorganic fluoride concentrations have been reported after halothane anesthesia in obese patients compared with nonobese patients.[54] Peak plasma fluoride concentration after administration of enflurane was three times greater than after isoflurane.[55] However, no prospective study has demonstrated an increased incidence of renal toxicity after brief exposure to enflurane in obese patients. Similarly, although halothane hepatitis is epidemiologically associated more frequently with obesity, no evidence suggests increased hepatocellular damage as detected enzymatically after halothane anesthesia in the obese patient.[54] Similarly, sevoflurane biotransformation and plasma inorganic fluoride concentrations seem not to be increased in obese patients, and postoperative hepatic or renal tests do not appear to be different.[56] From these viewpoints, isoflurane may be the volatile agent of choice for obese parturients. For brief procedures like cesarean section, however, the choice of volatile anesthetic agent does not appear to be clinically important.

Plasma cholinesterase activity increases in proportion to BMI,[57] whereas a 25% to 30% reduction of cholinesterase activity is known to occur starting in the first trimester, and continuing during the remainder of pregnancy and postpartum period.[58, 59] Whether the combination of these pathophysiologic states yields greater or less pseudocholinesterase activity, and thus whether the dosing regimen of succinylcholine should be increased or decreased, remains undetermined. Some anesthesiologists are reluctant to administer a relatively large dose of succinylcholine (2 mg/kg) at the time of general anesthesia induction for fear of prolonged paralysis in the event of a failed intubation. In obese as well as pregnant patients, vecuronium produces muscle relaxation that lasts longer than in lean, nonpregnant patients.[60] On the other hand, metabolism and recovery of atracurium-induced muscle relaxation is not affected by obesity. To date, atracurium has not been reported to cause adverse responses in pregnant women, which would be indicative of altered pharmacokinetic parameters. However, if a very high dose is administered as a bolus, it can precipitate histamine release and hypotension. In theory, atracurium may be the muscle relaxant of choice for maintenance of short procedures such as cesarean section. Regardless of the choice of muscle relaxant, use of a nerve stimulator will help objectively assess the onset and duration of neuromuscular blockade.

PREOPERATIVE EVALUATION

In addition to the routine preoperative evaluation for parturients, including prepregnant medical disorders and pregnancy-associated problems, careful and detailed assessment of the airway should be performed in the obese parturient. Any history of previous anesthetics and surgeries should be obtained in detail. If an adverse reaction was noted in association with a previous anesthetic, a strategy should be thoroughly discussed, well in advance of induction of anesthesia. Anesthesiologists should anticipate the worst possible events that may arise at the time of induction of general or regional anesthesia and must be fully equipped to deal with them. It is also essential that the patients be informed of possible upcoming plans. Another important aspect of the preoperative visit is to administer in a timely fashion medications that are mandatory to optimize the patient's condition for surgery and anesthesia. Prophylaxis for aspiration of gastric contents should be done aggressively in all obese pregnant patients. Cardiovascular medication is usually continued up to the time of surgery.

Respiratory System and Airway

Information on the history of preexisting respiratory disorders, treatment, and current status should be obtained. Careful physical examination is mandatory and a chest radiograph is advisable for morbidly obese patients. In addition, a determination of arterial blood gas tensions can provide important information regarding both ventilation and oxygenation. Oxygen saturation measured by a pulse oximeter in both the sitting and the supine position may help assess the degree of compromise of pulmonary function due to obesity. A decrease in oxygen saturation from the recumbent to the supine position suggests airway closing at tidal respiration and gives a guideline for postoperative oxygen therapy. In symptom-free, healthy obese parturients, oxygen saturation by pulse oximeter is routinely determined at our institution under room air in both recumbent and supine positions. More detailed pulmonary investigations are reserved for those with more severe respiratory diseases.

Airway examination in relation to endotracheal intubation is by far the most important part of the preoperative visit. Obesity and pregnancy may additively worsen the condition for laryngoscopy and intubation.[9] A history of sleep obstruction is an ominous sign suggestive of poor laryngoscopic view. An increased fat pad on the back of the neck and shoulder and the fatty anterior chest tissue all make extension and flexion of the neck considerably limited. In addition, achieving optimal positioning for laryngoscopy may be difficult in the obese parturient. Increased chest diameter, enlarged breasts, and decreased chin-to-chest distance all increase the likelihood of difficult laryngoscopy. Furthermore, the laryngoscopic view may be narrowed owing to the enlarged tongue and fleshy pharyngeal and supralaryngeal soft tissue. A recent study demonstrated that more than 15 kg weight gain during pregnancy is associated with threefold increase in the incidence of suboptimal laryngoscopic view, as compared with the view in nonpregnant women at the corresponding age.[10] Through a complete preoperative evaluation of the airway, a possible difficult laryngoscopy/failed intubation can often be predicted, and a step-by-step strategy for airway management can be planned.

Cardiovascular System

Prepregnancy cardiovascular disorders should be thoroughly examined as should pregnancy-induced changes such as pregnancy-induced hypertension. Especially in morbidly obese parturients, possible signs of left or right ventricular failure, pulmonary hypertension, and ischemic heart disease should be sought from the history, electrocardiogram, and chest radiograph. In patients with a long history of diabetes, typical symptoms indicative of angina pectoris may be absent due to "silent ischemia." In healthy obese parturients without evidence of cardiovascular disease, however, an electrocardiogram and chest radiograph may not be routinely obtained in our institution. Caution should be exercised when blood pressure is measured noninvasively in obese parturients. The sphygmomanometric cuff should be of an appropriate size, otherwise systolic and diastolic blood pressure may be overestimated. Occasionally, if noninvasive blood pressure recording is not possible because of patient size, an arterial line will become necessary.

Gastrointestinal and Endocrine System

Obese parturients should be questioned regarding symptoms of esophageal reflux, and medication for these symptoms should be continued up to the time of anesthesia and surgery. Previous laboratory test results, including fasting blood glucose levels and liver function, should be closely examined. History and treatment of diabetes should be obtained. If abnormal liver function is present, HELLP (hemolysis, elevated liver enzymes, low platelets) syndrome should be ruled out.

Miscellaneous

When analgesia using a central neuraxial block is considered for the obese parturient, the needle insertion site should be examined and bony landmarks identified. Anesthesiologists should anticipate the possible need for a longer epidural or spinal needle in the morbidly obese parturient, but often a standard needle will suffice.[61] Establishment of peripheral venous access may also be difficult in the obese parturient. In such cases, a large-bore, single-lumen central venous catheter can be inserted. Because these patients may have increased blood loss, a large-bore catheter is more advantageous than a small-bore multilumen catheter. Administration of medication in the obese parturient is recommended by either the oral or the intravenous route, but not via the intramuscular route, since attempts to give an intramuscular injection may result in intrafat or subcutaneous injection, with variable drug absorption.

PREMEDICATION

Prophylaxis against aspiration pneumonitis is considered the most important aspect of premedication in the morbidly obese parturient. Routine medications in this regard include H_2-blockers (famotidine 20 mg PO or IV, ranitidine 50 mg IV) and a prokinetic drug (metoclopramide 10 mg IV).[62, 63] H_2-blockers have long durations of pharmacologic action and thus should be given as early as possible. In case of an emergency not allowing sufficient time for an intravenous H_2-blocker to exert its effect, 30 mL of 0.3 M sodium citrate solution given orally will rapidly increase the pH of the stomach.[64] It should be noted, however, that its pH-increasing effect dissipates rapidly and its duration of action varies tremendously among individuals. Therefore, it should be given within 10 minutes prior to induction of general anesthesia. Also, repeated administration through the orogastric tube before extubation should be considered in high-risk obese parturients.[29] Anxiolytic drugs are usually not required and, if possible, should be avoided because they may be associated with mild respiratory depression and may also cause suppression of the upper airway protective reflexes.

ANESTHETIC MANAGEMENT

General principles for delivering anesthesia for obese parturients are as follows:

1. Based on previous epidemiologic evidence (Fig. 37–3),[39, 41, 65] regional anesthesia should be chosen unless general anesthesia is the last resort to save the mother or fetus.
2. If possible, at least two experienced anesthesiologists should attend morbidly obese parturients undergoing labor and delivery or cesarean section.

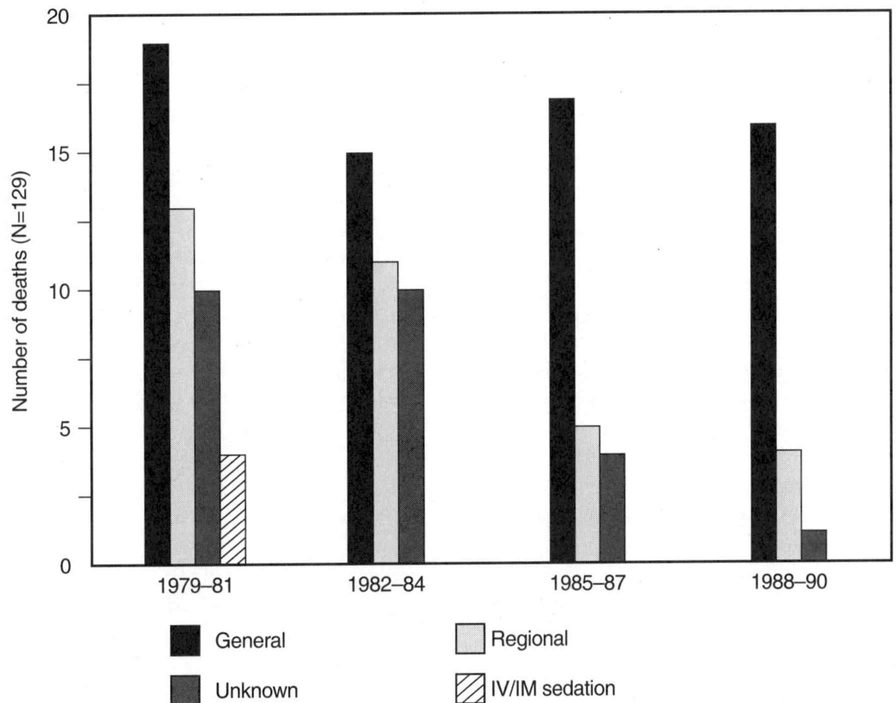

❖ **Figure 37–3** Anesthesia-related maternal deaths by types of anesthesia, United States, 1979 through 1990. (From Hawkins JL, Koonin LM, Palmer SK, Gibbs CP: Anesthesia-related deaths during obstetric delivery in the United States, 1979–1990. Anesthesiology 1997; 86:277–284.)

3. As in all parturients, general anesthesia, if absolutely indicated, should be delivered via endotracheal tube rather than mask, and ventilation should be controlled.
4. Attempts should be made to minimize the risk of aspiration of the gastric contents.
5. Sedation should be minimized or ideally avoided unless respiration is closely monitored by experienced anesthesiologists.

The operating room, monitors, anesthesia machine, difficult airway equipment, and drugs expected for emergency cesarean section and airway management should always be available in close proximity to the labor and delivery rooms. An appropriately sized labor bed and operating table may be required for obese parturients. A sufficient number of personnel is mandatory to transport oversized patients, especially when they are unable to move themselves because of contraction pain and motor weakness from neural blockade. Preparation for airway management should include short-handled laryngoscope, assorted blades (such as Macintosh and Miller) of different sizes, endotracheal tubes of three different sizes with a stylet in each tube, oropharyngeal airways, laryngeal masks, and equipment for transtracheal intubation, jet ventilation, and fiberoptic intubation. A suction device (preferably Yankauer type), should be readily available. This type of suction device can be handled by a single hand, the direction of the tip is easily controlled, and the lumen is not easily obstructed.

Anesthesia for Labor and Delivery

Despite anticipated technical difficulties, administration of epidural analgesia for labor and delivery provides numerous theoretic advantages for obese parturients. Pain relief during contractions reduces the oxygen consumption and attenuates the hypertensive response. Increases in cardiac output are also lessened. Limited data suggest that the administration of epidural anesthesia per se does not increase the likelihood of cesarean section in obese patients.[66] Compared with single-shot intrathecal opioids, drugs can be administered repeatedly through the epidural catheter. Unlike systemic opioids, neonatal depression is usually not associated with epidural analgesia. Hence, anesthesiologists should not be reluctant to perform epidural anesthesia simply because of the anticipated technical difficulties in obese parturients. In light of an increased incidence of cesarean section in the obese parturient,[11, 35, 36] placing a functional epidural catheter in advance is a definite advantage. In addition, epidural analgesia can be extended for postoperative analgesia, when adequate pain relief and optimal care are thought to decrease maternal morbidity in obese patients.

Identification of midline can be problematic in some morbidly obese parturients. The fat pad over the thoracic region of the back is usually thinner than that over the lumbar region. If the thoracic spinous process can be identified, a lumbar midline can be assumed between the thoracic midline and the coccygeal bone. It may be easier to have obese patients sitting up rather than lying on the side, to identify the midline. In theory, an increase in the depth from the skin to the epidural space causes greater angle deviation along which the needle is to be advanced. As a result, the likelihood of introducing the epidural catheter in the lateral part of the epidural space would be increased. Indeed, a higher incidence of failed epidural anesthesia, unilateral block, and more attempts to identify the epidural space have all been reported in morbidly obese patients.[3, 61] A longer than usual length of the catheter should be left in the epidural space, because the epidural catheter position relative to the epidural space is more likely to change due to the excessive fatty subcutaneous tissue. If the epidural is placed with the patient in the sitting position, the patient should be assisted to the lateral position before the catheter is secured. Given the fact that more obese patients will eventually proceed to cesarean section, epidural anesthesia should be checked frequently for its efficacy, and a malfunctioning catheter should be replaced immediately.

Intrathecal opioids (fentanyl, sufentanil) and intravenous opioids (meperidine, butorphanol) can also be effective for labor pain relief. Pudendal block during stage II labor is found to be technically difficult, especially in morbidly obese patients. Inhalational analgesia should not be used because loss of consciousness may precipitate upper airway obstruction in morbidly obese patients who are likely to represent a difficult intubation. In summary, our fundamental approach to obese patients requiring analgesia for labor and delivery is similar to that for nonobese parturients, but a functional epidural or spinal catheter would be imperative to make further anesthetic management of cesarean section and postoperative care safer and smoother.

Regional Anesthesia for Cesarean Section

Among parturients presenting for labor and delivery, cesarean section and morbid obesity are independent risk factors for increased morbidity and mortality.[39–41] A higher percentage of morbidly obese parturients will require cesarean delivery, as compared with nonobese parturients. Given that a considerable proportion of maternal mortality is associated with general anesthesia during cesarean section (see Fig. 37–3),[65] it is rational that indications for general anesthesia should be confined to cases in which general anesthesia is indispensable to save the mother or fetus. General anesthetic should not be delivered to save the fetus at the cost of endangering the mother.

Compared with single-shot spinal anesthesia, epidural anesthesia offers several advantages: first, ability to titrate the dose to achieve the desired level of analgesia; second, ability to extend the block for prolonged surgery; third, a decreased incidence and perhaps slower speed of developing hypotension; and fourth, utilization for postoperative analgesia. There are limited data showing that obese patients undergoing abdominal surgery require smaller doses for induction of epidural anesthesia.[61, 67] In the obese parturient, the administration of local anesthetic should be closely titrated using small incremental doses. Epidural anesthesia alone is usually well tolerated in the obese parturients,[68] and sedating obese patients during cesarean section requires extreme vigilance. Any sedative drug may impair the airway protective reflex. In addition, relaxation of pharyngeal musculature, and narrower than usual oropharyngeal and supraglottic spaces, may increase the likelihood of upper airway obstruction in sedated obese parturients. Given the potential for difficult bag-and-mask ventilation and failed intubation in these parturients, excessive sedation places these patients at a risk for aspiration pneumonitis and life-threatening complications. The level of anesthesia must be carefully tested before the surgeon is allowed to begin. Should epidural anesthesia alone prove inadequate to provide surgical anesthesia, the anesthesiologist should consider replacing the epidural or initiating a continuous spinal technique, as is discussed in Chapter 12.

Extending labor epidural analgesia for cesarean section requires additional local anesthetic of higher concentration than the dilute solutions used to provide labor analgesia. The level of anesthesia required for cesarean section is at least T4-5. The dose of epidural or intrathecal local anesthetic needed to produce a denser and higher block, where some analgesia preexists from an epidural infusion, remains undetermined. Following an injection of a test dose, many anesthesiologists administer incremental doses of 2% lidocaine with epinephrine until the desired effect is attained. Bupivacaine 0.5% and chloroprocaine 3% can also be utilized.

Previous reports have demonstrated conflicting results regarding the dose requirement of spinal anesthesia for obese patients. Some studies have demonstrated a negative correlation between the degree of obesity and the dose requirement for intrathecally administered local anesthetic (i.e., the higher the BMI, the higher the spread of sensory analgesia produced by spinal anesthesia).[69] Other studies, however, have failed to demonstrate any significant correlation.[70] Greene[71] has suggested that the dose requirement is unaltered, but that the spread is affected by obesity. Larger buttocks, engorged epidural veins resulting in a reduced subarachnoid space, exaggerated curvature of the lumbar spinal column, and hormonal changes may all contribute to the change seen in obese patients. Caution should therefore be exercised for consequences of an extensive high block when single-shot spinal anesthesia is selected in obese parturients. A longer period of time is often necessary for obese parturients before the incision can be made, because the subarachnoid blockade may extend in the cephalad direction more slowly and insidiously. In general, however, obese patients tolerate a T4 blockade well in terms of ventilation and oxygenation. Although high thoracic spinal anesthesia may produce a more profound motor blockade than epidural anesthesia, spinal anesthesia produces either no change in arterial gas tensions or only a slight worsening of oxygenation in obese parturients.[72] Rather, cardiovascular compromise may be of greater concern in obese parturients undergoing spinal anesthesia because of a higher incidence of systemic hypotension. Higher and variable extension of autonomic blockade is known to occur in obese patients.[73] In addition, panniculus retraction may exaggerate cardiovascular compromise.[74] Another concern that is associated with single-shot spinal anesthesia is the potential for prolonged surgery in the obese parturient. Continuous spinal anesthesia would alleviate many of the concerns associated with single-shot spinal anesthesia, and the desired level of surgical analgesia could be obtained in a more titratable manner. Post–dural puncture headache is reported to occur less frequently in morbidly obese parturients than in nonobese parturients.[75]

General Anesthesia for Cesarean Section

Whenever general anesthesia is anticipated in obese patients, prophylaxis against regurgitation and aspiration of gastric contents should be initiated in a timely fashion. Thorough preoperative assessment of the airway is mandatory. Anesthetic equipment and medications should be prepared for the worst possible scenario. It is imperative that the airway be secured using an endotracheal tube whenever general anesthetic is delivered to obese parturients. However, the standard techniques of endotracheal intubation may not be successful, because anatomic deviation of the upper airway may be exaggerated by the combination of obesity and pregnancy. Indeed, Buckley et al.[61] estimated that 13% of obese patients pose difficulties in tracheal intubation, whereas the incidence reached 30% among obese parturients. Furthermore, as expected, the degree of obesity is positively correlated with the incidence of difficult intubation.[76]

If the Mallampati classification (Fig. 37–4) suggests a likely difficult intubation (i.e., class IV), awake oral intubation is recommended in obese parturients.[77] Direct laryngoscopy can be performed following topical anesthesia using 4% lidocaine over the base of the tongue, epiglottis, larynx, and posterior pharyngeal wall. If the entire or most of the glottis is visualized, subsequent endotracheal intubation is usually easier than expected. Then, an induction dose of intravenous agent and succinylcholine is administered with cricoid pressure (rapid sequence induction) after denitrogenation is achieved by tidal respiration of 100% oxygen for 3 minutes, or four maximal inspirations of 100% oxygen.[78–80] No previous data have clearly demonstrated that one technique for denitrogenation is considerably better than another. It is reasonable that the urgency of cesarean section should dictate one of those techniques. If, on the other hand, it is impossible to visualize the larynx, awake intubation should be accomplished either by direct laryngoscopy or via fiberoptic guidance. Nasal instrumentation and intubation are not recommended because of mucosal edema during pregnancy and the risk of epistaxis. Multiple attempts at direct laryngoscopy may cause further mu-

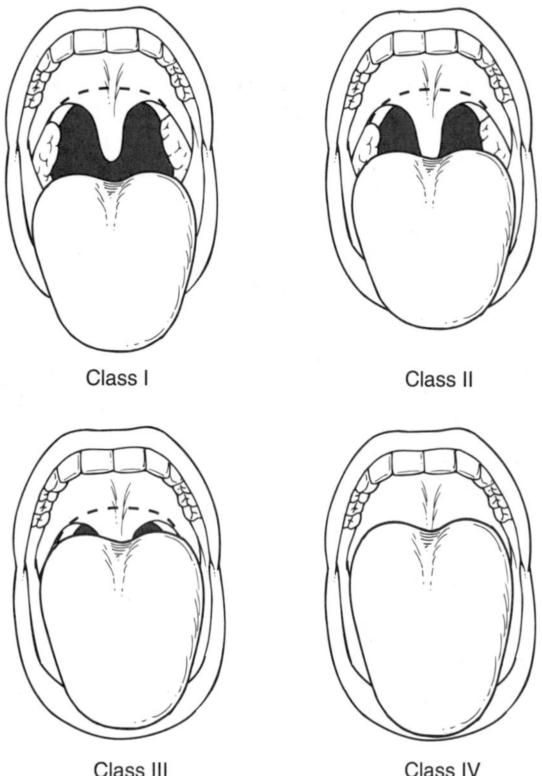

❖ **Figure 37–4** Classification of the upper airway in terms of the size of the tongue and the pharyngeal structures when the mouth is widely opened. Class I, the glottis (including anterior and posterior commissures) could be fully exposed; class II, the glottis could be partly exposed (anterior commissure not visualized); class III, the glottis could not be exposed (corniculate cartilages only could be visualized); class IV, the glottis, including corniculate cartilages, could not be exposed. (Modified from Mallampati SR, Gatt SP, Gugino LD, et al: A clinical sign to predict difficult tracheal intubation: a prospective study. Can Anaesth Soc J 1985; 32:429–434.)

cosal swelling and bleeding, rendering subsequent maneuvers and visualization extremely difficult.

Failure to quickly intubate the trachea after a rapid sequence induction usually necessitates bag-and-mask ventilation with extra personnel applying cricoid pressure continuously, since desaturation occurs rapidly in obese parturients.[81] If the mother and fetus are stable and the situation allows sufficient time to reattempt intubation, awakening the patient may be a reasonable alternative. Otherwise, if there is a good mask airway, cesarean section should be performed while patients are ventilated via anesthetic mask, bearing in mind that the risk of aspiration continues during the entire course of surgical procedure. Cricoid pressure, therefore, should be maintained throughout. If mask-ventilation is found to be difficult, laryngeal mask airway may be a valuable aid.

Tracheal intubation should be confirmed by capnography in addition to auscultation. However, breath sounds may be distant in morbidly obese patients. Once tracheal intubation is confirmed, general anesthesia should be maintained by intermittent positive pressure ventilation rather than spontaneous respiration. Most anesthesiologists use supplemental nitrous oxide as far as the mother can maintain adequate oxygenation. In morbidly obese patients, however, higher inspired concentration of oxygen may be required than in nonobese patients.[82] Larger-than-normal tidal volume and application of positive end expiratory pressure (PEEP) have been suggested to raise PaO_2 and lower alveolar-arterial oxygen tension difference in extremely obese patients.[83] However, increasing PEEP may progressively decrease cardiac output and oxygen availability in this population.[84] Whether application of PEEP increases or decreases oxygen delivery to the fetus remains to be determined in obese parturients. A volatile agent, irrespective of the choice, relaxes uterine smooth muscle in a dose-dependent manner[85] and may increase postpartum hemorrhage in theory. In addition, volatile agents and muscle relaxants decrease functional residual capacity, which is further compromised in the supine position in obese patients. To decrease the general anesthetic requirement, therefore, most anesthesiologists administer supplemental narcotics, such as fentanyl 3 to 5 μg/kg, once the umbilical cord is clamped. Such practice also helps alleviate pain in the immediate postoperative period. At the end of surgery, the neuromuscular blockade should be antagonized completely, confirmed by responses to peripheral nerve stimulation. One should bear in mind that the effect of muscle relaxant during surgery may be overestimated, whereas the reversal effect may be underestimated because of the thickened subcutaneous soft tissue in obese patients. Routine criteria for tracheal extubation should also be strictly followed.

POSTOPERATIVE CONSIDERATIONS

Increased postoperative morbidity is associated with morbidly obese patients after cesarean delivery, but not after vaginal delivery. Among morbidly obese patients undergoing cesarean section, prolonged surgery and intraoperative blood loss are particularly associated with the increase in postoperative morbidity.[32] As expected, obese parturients are more likely to develop postoperative pulmonary complications, such as hypoxemia, atelectasis, and pneumonia.[86, 87] Even in healthy obese patients, postoperative hypoxemia occurs universally after cesarean section under general anesthesia. A vertical abdominal incision as opposed to a horizontal incision is more likely to cause postoperative hypoxemia.[88] Patients should be placed in a semirecumbent position as soon after surgery as possible. In addition to aggressive physiotherapy, supplemental oxygen should be continued, possibly for several days, in morbidly obese parturients, until hypoxemia is no longer of concern.

Previous literature indicates that obese patients are at an increased risk for developing deep vein thrombosis and pulmonary thromboembolism.[89] On the other hand, pregnancy-induced anemia and the resultant decrease in blood viscosity may decrease such complications. However, a recent governmental report from Japan documented that the majority of pulmonary thromboembolism occurred in obese parturients, and that 76% of such complications occurred after cesarean section, suggesting that obesity still remains a major risk factor for developing thromboembolism during pregnancy.[90] The clinical efficacy of low-dose heparin, compression stockings, and regional anesthesia as compared with general anesthesia for prevention of thromboembolic episodes remains to be proved in obese parturients.

In theory, early postoperative mobilization in obese parturients is essential to decrease the likelihood of developing pulmonary complications and thromboembolic episodes. Sufficient dose of analgesic medication should be administered for postoperative analgesia, since adequate pain control is essential to decrease postoperative maternal morbidity. For those who underwent cesarean section under single-shot spinal or general anesthesia, intravenous patient-controlled analgesia (PCA) using morphine or fentanyl is most often utilized in our institution. However, an anecdotal report suggests that PCA could be hazardous in patients with a history of sleep apnea,[91] whereas others have demonstrated that PCA can be used safely for postoperative analgesia in morbidly obese patients.[92] For those who received epidural anesthesia intraoperatively, continuous epidural analgesia or epidural PCA with local anesthetic plus fentanyl usually provides excellent pain relief. Alternatively, epidural morphine may be given intermittently because the analgesic action of epidural morphine is much longer than that of epidural fentanyl.[93] However, respiratory depression of delayed onset may occur following administration of epidural morphine.[94] Therefore, monitoring respiratory variables is mandatory to avoid or detect respiratory depression at the earliest possible time, because respiratory reserve is already marginal in morbidly obese patients. Routine use of pulse oximeter and frequent determinations of respiratory rate and the level of consciousness may facilitate early detection of clinically significant respiratory depression.

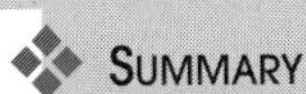

SUMMARY

Key Points

- The obese parturient is at greater risk for medical diseases that can complicate pregnancy, labor, and delivery. These include cardiovascular disease, diabetes, and pulmonary and gastrointestinal abnormalities.
- In the obese parturient with a difficult airway, every effort should be made to initiate an early regional anesthetic via a catheter technique.
- The cesarean section rate is dramatically higher in the morbidly obese parturient. There is an increased incidence of abnormal labor, and dystocia is a common cause of emergency cesarean section.
- Anxiolytic drugs and opioids must be used with great caution in the morbidly obese parturient, as they may be associated with respiratory depression and a supression of the upper airway protective reflexes. Owing to variable drug absorption, intramuscular injections are not advisable in these patients.

Key References

Hamilton CL, Riley ET, Cohen SE: Changes in the position of epidural catheters associated with patient movement. Anesthesiology 1997; 6:778–784.

Hood DD, Dewan DM: Anesthetic and obstetric outcome in morbidly obese parturients. Anesthesiology 1993; 79:1210–1218.

Case Stem

A morbidly obese parturient (BMI 42) who has been in labor for 6 hours is now to undergo an emergent cesarean section for dystocia and "nonreassuring" fetal heart rate tracing. She does not have an epidural catheter in place. Discuss the anesthetic implications of her obesity and your anesthetic plans for the cesarean section.

References

1. Frankel HM: Determination of body mass index. JAMA 1986; 255:1292.
2. Kuczmarski RJ, Flegal KM, Campbell SM, Johnson CL: Increasing prevalence of overweight amongst US adults: The National Health and Nutritional Examination surveys 1960–1991. JAMA 1994; 272:205.
3. Abraham S, Johnson CL: Prevalence of severe obesity in adults in the United States. Am J Clin Nutr 1980; 33:364.
4. Van Itallie TB: Health implications of overweight and obesity in the United States. Ann Intern Med 1985; 103:983.
5. Bray GA, Gray DS: Obesity: Part 1. Pathogenesis. West J Med 1988; 149:429.
6. Bray GA: Complications of obesity. Ann Intern Med 1985; 103:1052.
7. Manson JE, Colditz GA, Stampfer MJ, et al: A prospective study of obesity and risk of coronary heart disease in women. N Engl J Med 1990; 322:882.
8. Drenick EJ, Bale GS, Seltzer F, Johnson DG: Excessive mortality and causes of death in morbidly obese men. JAMA 1980; 243:443.
9. Samsoon GL, Young JRB: Difficult tracheal intubation: A retrospective study. Anaesthesia 1987; 42:487.
10. Shankar KB, Krishna S, Moseley HSL: Airway changes during pregnancy. Anesthesiology 1997; 87:A895.
11. Johnson JWC, Longmate JA, Frentzen B: Excessive maternal weight and pregnancy outcome. Am J Obstet Gynecol 1992; 167:353.
12. Farebrother MJB: Respiratory function and cardiorespiratory response to exercise in obesity. Br J Dis Chest 1979; 73:211.
13. Luce JM: Respiratory complications of obesity. Chest 1980; 78:626.
14. Dempsey JA, Reddan W, Rankin J, Balke B: Alveolar-arterial gas exchange during muscular work in obesity. J Appl Physiol 1966; 21:1807.
15. Vaughan RW: Pulmonary and cardiovascular derangements in the obese patient. *In* Brown BR (ed): Anesthesia and the Obese Patient. Contemporary Anesthesia Practice Series. Philadelphia: FA Davis; 1982:19.
16. Burwell CS, Robin ED, Whaley ED, et al: External obesity associated with alveolar hypoventilation: A Pickwickian syndrome. Am Med 1956; 21:811.
17. Lourenco RV: Diaphragm activity in obesity. J Clin Invest 1969; 48:1609.
18. Wittels EH, Thompson S: Obstructive sleep apnea and obesity. Otolaryngol Clin North Am 1990; 23:751.

19. Reisin E, Frolich ED: Obesity: Cardiovascular and respiratory pathophysiological alterations. Arch Intern Med 1981; 141:431.
20. Alexander JK, Dennis DW, Smith WG, et al: Blood volume, cardiac output, and distribution of systemic blood flow in extreme obesity. Cardiovasc Res Center Bull 1962; 1:39.
21. Alexander JK: The cardiomyopathy of obesity. Prog Cardiovasc Dis 1985; 27:325.
22. Buckley FP: Anesthesia and obesity and gastrointestinal disorders. *In* Barash PG, Cullen BF, Stoelting RK (eds): Clinical Anesthesia, 3rd ed. Philadelphia: Lippincott-Raven; 1997:975.
23. Dias MS, Sekhar LM: Intracranial hemorrhage from aneurysms and arteriovenous malformation during pregnancy and the puerperium. Neurosurgery 1990; 27:855.
24. Paul DR, Hoyt JL, Boutros AR: Cardiovascular and respiratory changes in response to change of posture in the very obese. Anesthesiology 1976; 45:73.
25. Kissebah AH, Vydelingum N, Murray R, et al: Relation of body fat distribution to metabolic complications of obesity. J Clin Endocrinol Metab 1982; 54:254.
26. Farmer G, Hamilton-Nicol DR, Southerland HW, et al: The ranges of insulin response and glucose tolerance in lean, normal, and obese women during pregnancy. Am J Obstet Gynecol 1992; 167:772.
27. Vaughan RW, Bauer S, Wise L: Volume and pH of gastric juice in obese patients. Anesthesiology 1975; 43:686.
28. Harter RL, Kelly WB, Kramer MG, et al: A comparison of the volume and pH of gastric contents of obese and lean surgical patients. Anesth Analg 1998; 86:147.
29. Dewan DM, Floyd HM, Thistlewood JM, et al: Sodium citrate pretreatment in elective cesarean section patients. Anesth Analg 1985; 64:34.
30. O'Brien TF: Lower esophageal sphincter pressure (LESP) and esophageal function in obese humans. J Clin Gastroenterol 1980; 2:145.
31. Van Thiel DH, Gavaler JS, Joshi SN, et al: Heartburn of pregnancy. Gastroenterology 1972; 72:666.
32. Ulmsten U, Sundstrom G: Esophageal manometry in pregnant and nonpregnant women. Am J Obstet Gynecol 1978; 132:260.
33. Johnson SR, Kolberg BH, Varner MW, Railsback LD: Maternal obesity and pregnancy. Surg Gynecol Obstet 1987; 164:431.
34. Tracy TA, Miller GL: Obstetric problems of the massively obese. Obstet Gynecol 1969; 33:204.
35. Gross T, Sokol RJ, King KC: Obesity and pregnancy: Risk and outcome. Obstet Gynecol 1980; 56:446.
36. Perlow JH, Morgan MA, Montgomery D, et al: Perinatal outcome in pregnancy complicated by massive obesity. Am J Obstet Gynecol 1992; 167:958.
37. Garbaciak JA, Richter M, Miller S, Barton JJ: Maternal weight and pregnancy complications. Am J Obstet Gynecol 1985; 152:238.
38. Kliegman RM, Gross T: Perinatal problems of the obese mother and her infant. Obstet Gynecol 1985; 66:299.
39. Endler GC, Mariona FG, Sokol RJ, Stevenson LB: Anesthesia-related maternal mortality in Michigan, 1972 to 1984. Am J Obstet Gynecol 1988; 159:187.
40. Sachs BP, Oriol NE, Ostheimer GW, et al: Anesthetic-related maternal mortality, 1954 to 1985. J Clin Anesth 1989; 1:333.
41. May WJ, Greiss FC: Maternal mortality in North Carolina: A forty-year experience. Am J Obstet Gynecol 1989; 161:555.
42. Rahaman J, Narayansingh GV, Roopnarinesingh S: Fetal outcome among obese parturients. Int J Gynecol Obstet 1990; 31:227.
43. Abernethy DR, Greenblatt DJ: Pharmacokinetics of drugs in obesity. Clin Pharmacokinet 1981; 7:108.
44. Blouin RA, Kolpek JH, Mann HJ: Influence of obesity on drug disposition. Clin Pharm 1987; 6:706.
45. Ladegaard-Pedersen HJ: Recovery from general anesthesia in obese patients. Anesthesiology 1981; 55:720.
46. Cork RC, Vaughan RW, Bentley JB: General anesthesia for morbidly obese patients: An examination of postoperative outcomes. Anesthesiology 1981; 54:310.
47. Jung D, Mayersohn M, Perrier D, et al: Thiopental disposition in lean and obese patients undergoing surgery. Anesthesiology 1982; 56:269.
48. Abernethy DR, Greenblatt DJ, Divoll M, et al: The influence of obesity on the pharmacokinetics of oral alprazolam and triazolam. Clin Pharmacokinet 1984; 9:177.
49. Servin F, Farinotti R, Haberer JP, Desmonts JM: Propofol infusion for maintenance of anesthesia in morbidly obese patients receiving nitrous oxide: A clinical and pharmacokinetic study. Anesthesiology 1993; 78:657.
50. White PF, Way WL, Trevor AJ: Ketamine: Its pharmacology and therapeutic uses. Anesthesiology 1982; 56:119.
51. Bentley JB, Borel JD, Gillespie TJ, et al: Fentanyl pharmacokinetics in obese and nonobese patients. Anesthesiology 1981; 55:A177.
52. Schwartz AE, Matteo RS, Ornstein E, et al: Pharmacokinetics of sufentanil in obese patients. Anesth Analg 1991; 73:790.
53. Bentley JB, Finley JH, Humphrey LR, et al: Obesity and alfentanil pharmacokinetics. Anesth Analg 1983; 62:251.
54. Bentley JB, Vaughan RW, Gandolfi J, et al: Halothane biotransformation in obese and nonobese patients. Anesthesiology 1982; 57:94.
55. Strube PJ, Hulands GH, Halsey MJ: Serum fluoride levels in morbidly obese patients: Enflurane compared with isoflurane anaesthesia. Anaesthesia 1987; 42:685.
56. Frink EJ, Malan TP, Brown RA, et al: Plasma inorganic fluoride levels with sevoflurane anesthesia in morbidly obese and nonobese patients. Anesth Analg 1993; 76:1333.
57. Bentley JB, Borel JD, Vaughan RW, Gandolfi AJ: Weight, pseudocholinesterase activity, and succinylcholine requirement. Anesthesiology 1982; 57:48.
58. Evans RT, Wroe JM: Plasma cholinesterase changes during pregnancy: Their interpretation as a cause of suxamethonium-induced apnoea. Anaesthesia 1980; 35:651.
59. Leighton BL, Cheek TG, Gross JB, et al: Succinylcholine pharmacodynamics in peripartum patients. Anesthesiology 1986; 64:202.
60. Weinstein JA, Matteo RS, Ornstein E, et al: Pharmacodynamics of vecuronium and atracurium in the obese surgical patient. Anesth Analg 1988; 67:1149.
61. Buckley FP, Robinson NB, Simonowitz DA, Dellinger EP: Anaesthesia in the morbidly obese: A comparison of anaesthetic and analgesic regimens for upper abdominal surgery. Anaesthesia 1983; 38:840.
62. Lam AM, Grace DM, Phil D, et al: Prophylactic intravenous cimetidine reduces the risk of acid aspiration in morbidly obese patients. Anesthesiology 1986; 65:684.
63. Manchikanti L, Roush JR, Colliver JA: Effect of preanesthetic ranitidine and metoclopramide on gastric contents in morbidly obese patients. Anesth Analg 1986; 65:195.
64. O'Sullivan GM, Bullingham RE: Noninvasive assessment by radiotelemetry of antacid effect during labor. Anesth Analg 1985; 64:95.
65. Hawkins JL, Koonin LM, Palmer SK, Gibbs CP: Anesthesia-related deaths during obstetric delivery in the United States, 1979–1990. Anesthesiology 1997; 86:277.
66. Hood DD, Dewan DM: Anesthesia and obstetric outcome in morbidly obese parturients. Anesthesiology 1993; 79:1210.
67. Hodgkinson R, Husain FJ: Obesity and the cephalad spread of analgesia following epidural administration of bupivacaine for cesarean section. Anesth Analg 1980; 59:89.
68. Maitra AM, Palmer SK, Bachhuber SR, Abram SE: Continuous epidural analgesia for cesarean section in a patient with morbid obesity. Anesth Analg 1979; 58:348.
69. McCulloch WJD, Littlewood DG: Influence of obesity on spinal analgesia with isobaric 0.5% bupivacaine. Br J Anaesth 1986; 58:610.
70. Norris MC: Height, weight, and the spread of subarachnoid hyperbaric bupivacaine in the term parturient. Anesth Analg 1988; 67:555.
71. Greene NM: Distribution of local anesthetic solutions within the subarachnoid space. Anesth Analg 1985; 64:715.
72. Blass NH: Regional anesthesia in the morbidly obese. Reg Anesth 1979; 4:20.
73. Chamberlain DP, Chamberlain BDL: Changes in the skin temperature of the trunk and their relationship to sympathetic blockade during spinal anesthesia. Anesthesiology 1986; 65:139.
74. Hodgkinson R, Husain FJ: Caesarean section associated with gross obesity. Br J Anaesth 1980; 52:919.

75. Faure E, Moreno R, Thisted R: Incidence of post-dural puncture headache in morbidly obese parturients. Reg Anesth 1994; 19:361.
76. Lee JJ, Larson RH, Buckley JJ, Roberts RB: Airway maintenance in the morbidly obese. Anesthesiol Rev 1980; 7:33.
77. Mallampati SR, Gatt SP, Gugino LD, et al: A clinical sign to predict difficult tracheal intubation: A prospective study. Can Anaesth Soc J 1985; 32:429.
78. Norris MC, Dewan DM: Preoxygenation for cesarean section: A comparison of two techniques. Anesthesiology 1985; 62:827.
79. Gambee AM, Hertzka RE, Fisher DM: Preoxygenation techniques: Comparison of three minutes and four breaths. Anesth Analg 1987; 66:468.
80. Goldberg ME, Norris MC, Larijani GE, et al: Preoxygenation in the morbidly obese: A comparison of two techniques. Anesth Analg 1989; 68:520.
81. Archer GW, Marx GF: Arterial oxygen tension during apnoea in parturient women. Br J Anaesth 1974; 46:358.
82. Vaughan RW, Wise L: Intraoperative arterial oxygenation in obese patients. Ann Surg 1976; 184:35.
83. Eriksen J, Andersen J, Rasmussen JP, Sorensen B: Effects of ventilation with large tidal volumes or positive end-expiratory pressure on cardiorespiratory function in anesthetized obese patients. Acta Anaesthesiol Scand 1978; 22:241.
84. Santesson J: Oxygen transport in venous admixture in the extremely obese: Influence of anaesthesia in artificial ventilation with and without positive end-expiratory pressure. Acta Anaesthesiol Scand 1976; 20:387.
85. Munson ES, Embro WJ: Enflurane, isoflurane, and halothane and isolated human uterine muscle. Anesthesiology 1977; 46:11.
86. Vaughan RW, Engelhardt RC, Wise L: Postoperative hypoxemia in obese patients. Ann Surg 1974; 180:877.
87. Mircea N, Constantinescu C, Jianu E, Busu G: Risk of pulmonary complications in surgical patients. Resuscitation 1982; 10:33.
88. Vaughan RW, Engelhardt RC, Wise L: Postoperative alveolar-arterial tension difference: Its relation to the operative incision in obese patients. Anesth Analg 1975; 54:433.
89. Postlethwait RW, Johnson WD: Complications following surgery for duodenal ulcer in obese patients. Arch Surg 1972; 105:438.
90. Maternal and child health statistics of Japan. Maternal and Child Health Division, Children and Families Bureau, and Statistics and Information Department, Minister's Secretariat, Ministry of Health and Welfare, Japan; 1997.
91. VanDercar DH, Martinez AP, De Lisser EA: Sleep apnea syndromes: A potential contraindication for patient-controlled analgesia. Anesthesiology 1991; 74:623.
92. Levin A, Klein SL, Brolin RE, Pitchford DE: Patient-controlled analgesia for morbidly obese patients: An effective modality if used correctly. Anesthesiology 1992; 76:857.
93. Rosen MA, Hughes SC, Shnider SM, et al: Epidural morphine for the relief of postoperative pain after cesarean delivery. Anesth Analg 1983; 62:666.
94. Bromage PR, Camporesi EM, Durant PA, Nielsen CH: Rostral spread of epidural morphine. Anesthesiology 1982; 56:431.

38

Hypertensive Disorders and Renal Disease in Pregnancy and Labor

❖ STEPHEN P. GATT, OAM, KM, MD, LRCP, MRCS, MRACMA, FFARACS, FANZCA, FFICANZCA

ETIOLOGY, RISK FACTORS, AND PATHOGENESIS

The overall risk of developing preeclampsia is 2.5% to 7.0% of all pregnancies.[1–3]

The 1990s have seen a marked increase in the understanding of the chances of developing preeclampsia.[1, 4, 5] Demographic studies have led to the development of a chart of risk factors by the American College of Obstetrics and Gynecology (Table 38–1).[6] This includes genetic and familial factors (e.g., angiotensin T-235, homozygous and heterozygous), chronic renal disease and hypertension, anticardiolipin syndrome, multiple pregnancy, elderly gravidity, primiparity and diabetes, all of which increase risk, but not low socioeconomic status and young maternal age.[6]

It is recognized that the risk increases from between 2.5% and 7.0% to 28% if the pregnant woman's mother had preeclampsia and to 42% if siblings have preeclampsia. Exposure to the father's seminal fluid seems to confer some protection, so the use of condoms and other barrier methods seems to increase the risk by 2.37 times, whereas frequent exposure to paternal seminal fluid as in oral intercourse or prolonged cohabitation with the father reduces risk.[7] Some protection is also provided by previous autologous blood transfusion.

Less progress has been made with elucidation of etiology, but there is an increasing appreciation of the role of a number of enzymes and receptors ($aV\beta_1$, $aV\beta_3$, vascular endothelial growth factor 1 [GF-1], vascular endothelial cadherin, and platelet endothelium cell adhesive molecule-1), of the thromboxane-to-prostacyclin ratio, of selective prostaglandin H synthetase-2 blockers (NS-398), and of nitrous oxide–mediated and tumor necrosis factor–mediated mechanisms.[5]

It has been shown that women with elevated car-

Table 38–1 FACTORS IMPLICATED IN INCREASED RISK OF DEVELOPING PREECLAMPSIA

RISK RATIO	FACTOR
20:1	Homozygous angiotensin T-235
	Chronic renal disease
10:1	Antiphospholipid syndrome
	Chronic hypertension
5:1	Family history of preeclampsia
4:1	Twin gestation
	Heterozygous angiotensin T-235
3:1	Nulliparity
	Maternal age over 40
2:1	Diabetes
1.5:1	African-American race
nil	Low socioeconomic group
	Maternal age less than 18

Modified from American College of Obstetricians and Gynecologists: Technical Bulletin. Int J Gynecol Obstet 1996; 53:175–183.

Table 38–2 MATERNAL MORTALITY IN PREGNANCY IN THE UNITED STATES, 1980–1985

Cause	Rate (%)
Embolism	17.0
Indirect causes	15.6
Hypertension in pregnancy	12.3
Ectopic pregnancy complications	10.0
Hemorrhage	9.1
Stroke	8.4
Anesthesia	7.0
Complications of termination	5.2
Cardiomyopathy	4.2
Infection	3.5
Other	7.7

Adapted from the US Maternal Mortality Surveillance, 1980–1985. MMWR CDC Surveillance Summary, 1988.

diac output in early pregnancy, as measured by Doppler ultrasonography, are more likely to develop preeclampsia.[8]

MORTALITY STATISTICS

Several interesting new trends in the mortality statistics emerge. For example, the Centers for Disease Control and Prevention in the United States reports that hypertensive disorders of pregnancy have been relegated from the first to the third most common cause of death in the United States (Table 38–2).

There is also a relative increase in adult respiratory distress syndrome and pulmonary edema as causes of death from preeclampsia and a decline in mortality from convulsions. This may be a somewhat artificial statistic resulting from better intensive care management whereby these women are surviving the initial insult (e.g., intracerebral hemorrhage), only to succumb some days later to pulmonary complications.[9] Intracerebral catastrophe (all causes) remains responsible for over 50% of deaths with eclampsia and intracranial hemorrhage accounting for 30% to 40%, cerebral edema for 19%, and hypertensive encephalopathy for a small percentage.[10] Pulmonary edema is responsible for between 30% and 38%, renal failure for up to 10%, and coagulopathy and hemorrhage including abruptio placentae for up to 9%. Airway obstruction, usually from upper airway edema, is uncommon but accounts for up to 6% of deaths. Other causes of mortality include cardiac dysrhythmias and hepatic rupture (Table 38–3).

DEFINITION OF HYPERTENSION IN PREGNANCY

Hypertension in pregnancy is said to exist when systolic arterial systemic pressure (SAP) is 140 mm Hg or greater, or diastolic systemic arterial pressure (DAP) is 90 mm Hg or greater (Korotkoff V-K5, point of disappearance), or both.[11] It should be noted that an SAP of greater than 140 and a DAP of greater than 90 is (1) two standard deviations outside the SAP mean

Table 38–3 CAUSES OF DEATH IN PREECLAMPSIA

Adult respiratory distress syndrome and pulmonary edema
Intracranial hemorrhage, edema, and infarction
Coagulopathy and disseminated intravascular coagulation
Eclampsia and hypertensive encephalopathy
Abruptio placentae and massive blood loss
Cardiac dysrhythmias
Hepatic rupture
Respiratory obstruction and upper airway edema

of the normal pregnant population[12] and (2) associated with a clinically significant increase in perinatal mortality.

Alternatively, hypertension in pregnancy is said to exist if there is a rise in SAP of 25 mm Hg or greater, or a rise in DAP of 15 mm Hg or greater, or both, from SAP before conception or in the first trimester.

Measurements should be made with the patient seated, using a cuff of appropriate size, and a mercury sphygmomanometer.[13, 14]

CLASSIFICATION OF HYPERTENSION IN PREGNANCY

The 1999 Australian Society for the Study of Hypertension in Pregnancy (ASSHP) classification is shown in Table 38–4. It should be noted that preeclampsia is subdivided into mild and severe (but not moderate) and that the hemolysis–elevated liver enzymes–low platelet (HELLP) syndrome is included in the "severe" category (and is not characterized as a separate subtype).[15]

Table 38–4 AUSTRALIAN SOCIETY FOR THE STUDY OF HYPERTENSION IN PREGNANCY CLASSIFICATION OF HYPERTENSIVE DISEASE IN PREGNANCY, 1999

Preeclampsia
Mild
Severe (including HELLP and eclampsia)
Chronic hypertension
Essential hypertension
Secondary hypertension
Chronic hypertension with superimposed preeclampsia
Gestational hypertension (including transient hypertension)

Modified from Brown MA, Gallery EDM, Gatt SP, et al: Consensus Statement: Management of hypertension in pregnancy, consensus statement of the Australasian Society for the Study of Hypertension in Pregnancy, Executive Summary. Med J Aust 1993; 158:700–702.

DEFINITION OF PREECLAMPSIA

Preeclampsia is defined as hypertension occurring after 20 weeks' gestation or in the early postpartum period and returning to normal within 3 months after delivery *and* the onset after 20 weeks' gestation and at least one of the following:

- Proteinuria of >300 mg/24 hr or spot urine protein:creatinine ratio >30 mg/mmol
- Oliguria or serum:plasma creatinine ratio >0.09 mmol/L
- Headaches with hyperreflexia or eclampsia or clonus or visual disturbances
- Elevated liver enzymes, plasma glutathione S-transferase alpha 1-1 or serum alanine aminotransferase or right upper abdominal quadrant pain[16]
- Thrombocytopenia or raised lactate dehydrogenase or hemolysis or disseminated intravascular coagulation
- Intrauterine growth retardation

CLASSIFICATION OF PREECLAMPSIA

The features that differentiate severe from mild preeclampsia are an SAP of 160 mm Hg or greater, a DAP of 110 mm Hg or greater, proteinuria of 5 g/24 hrs or dipstick measurement of 3+ to 4+, oliguria of 500 mL/24 hr or less, headache or visual disturbances, epigastric or right upper quadrant abdominal pain, pulmonary edema or cyanosis and thrombocytopenia, disseminated intravascular coagulation or the HELLP syndrome.[17, 18]

The differentiating features are shown in Table 38–5.

ANESTHETIC ASSESSMENT OF SEVERITY IN TREATED DISEASE

Because most women with severe preeclampsia present to the anesthetist after receiving treatment, some other measure needs to be used to assess risk and to determine the extent of organ damage. Examples include treated DAP, proteinuria, oliguria, neurologic or abdominal symptoms or signs, elevated serum uric acid and antiphospholipid antibodies, and significant thrombocytopenia.[19] Of particular practicality to the anesthetist as a measure of severity in the treated parturient is the degree of proteinuria.[15, 20]

Pre-existing Renal Disease

Pre-existing renal disease or hypertension is best diagnosed and controlled prior to planned pregnancy.[21] Women with serum creatinine levels of less than 0.12 mmol/L should be warned of the considerably increased risk of renal function deterioration and perinatal morbidity and mortality.[20, 22]

The Treated Patient with Severe Preeclampsia

A treated DAP of more than 100 mm Hg and proteinuria of more than 2+ on dipstick measurement (and/or neurologic or abdominal signs) is a useful starting definition of severe preeclampsia for an anesthetist encountering the treated preeclamptic patient for the first time. There should be no doubt that the patient falls into the severe subset if the clinical findings include proteinuria of 5 g/24 hr or greater, cerebral or visual disturbances, oliguria, or epigastric or right upper quadrant abdominal pain or coagulopathy.[23]

Significant proteinuria (more than 2+) and hypoproteinemia, severe thrombocytopenia, elevated serum uric acid, serum iron, β-thromboglobulin concentration or antiphospholipid antibodies, hemoconcentration, coagulopathy, platelet count of less than 75,000/mm^3, raised hematocrit and hemoglobin, and neurologic or hepatic symptoms imply increased severity with end organ damage and, therefore, substantially increased risk.[19, 20, 22, 24–26]

Patients with severe preeclampsia superimposed on chronic hypertension or associated with insulin-dependent diabetes are also at increased risk.[1, 20, 21, 25, 27]

PRE-PREGNANCY MEDICAL TREATMENT OF HYPERTENSION

The main groups of drugs used in the management of hypertension pre-existing before the index pregnancy are the β_1 selective (e.g., metoprolol) and nonselective (e.g., propranolol) beta-blockers; the alpha-blockers (e.g., prazosin); the combined alpha- and beta-blockers

Table 38–5 FACTORS THAT DIFFERENTIATE MILD FROM SEVERE PREECLAMPSIA*

	MILD	SEVERE
Systolic arterial pressure	<160 mm Hg	≥160 mm Hg
Diastolic arterial pressure	<110 mm Hg	≥110 mm Hg
Urinary protein	<5 g/24 hr dipstick + or 2+	≥5 g/24 hrs dipstick 3+ or 4+
Urine output	>500 mL/24 hr	≤500 mL/24 hr
Headache	no	yes
Visual disturbances	no	yes
Epigastric pain	no	yes
Right upper quadrant abdominal pain	no	yes
Pulmonary edema	no	yes
Cyanosis	no	yes
HELLP	no	yes
Platelet count	>100,000/mm^3	<100,000/mm^3

*Not all features need be present in the same patient.

Table 38–6 AGENTS USED FOR THE TREATMENT OF HYPERTENSION

CLASS OF DRUG	SUBCLASS	DRUG
β-Blockers	β_1-Selective	Atenolol, metoprolol, timolol
	Nonselective	Propranolol, oxprenolol, pindolol
α-Blockers		Prazosin
α- and β-Blockers		Labetalol, carvedilol
Centrally acting antihypertensives		Methyldopa, clonidine
Vasodilators		Hydralazine, minoxidil
Thiazide diuretics		Bendrofluazide, chlorothiazide, chlorthalidone, hydrochlorothiazide
Thiazide-like diuretics		Indapamide
Potassium-sparing diuretic combinations		Amiloride/hydrochlorothiazide
		Triamterene/hydrochlorothiazide
ACE inhibitors		Captopril, enalapril, fosinopril, lisinopril, perindopril, quinapril, ramipril, trandolapril
Ca^{++} channel blockers	Dihydropyridines	Amlodipine, felodipine, nifedipine
	Nondihydropyridines	Verapamil, diltiazem
Angiotensin II receptor antagonists		Irbesartan, candesartan

Modified from World Health Organization: International Society of Hypertension Guidelines for the Management of Hypertension. J Hypertens 1999; 17:151–183.

(e.g., labetalol); the thiazide (e.g., hydrochlorothiazide), thiazide-like (e.g., indapamide), and potassium-sparing (e.g., triamterene/hydrochlorothiazide) diuretics; other diuretics (e.g., frusemide); the centrally acting antihypertensives (e.g., methyldopa, clonidine); the vasodilators (e.g., hydralazine); the angiotensin converting enzyme inhibitors (e.g., captopril); the dihydropyridine (e.g., nifedipine) and non-dihydropyridine (e.g., verapamil) calcium channel blockers; and the angiotensin II receptor antagonists (e.g., irbesartan).[28–31] The agents used for the treatment of hypertension are summarized in Table 38–6 and the thiazide and thiazide-like diuretics are classified in Table 38–7.[28, 32]

Suitability of These Agents in Pregnancy

Angiotensin converting enzyme (ACE) inhibitors are best avoided antepartum because they have been associated with neonatal renal failure and fetal wastage.[30, 31, 33, 34]

Table 38–7 THIAZIDE AND THIAZIDE-LIKE DIURETICS

CLASS OF THIAZIDE	AGENT
Thiazide	Bendrofluazide
	Chlorothiazide
	Chlorthalidone
	Hydrochlorothiazide
Thiazide-like	Indapamide
Potassium-sparing combinations	Triamterene + hydrochlorothiazide
	Amiloride + hydrochlorothiazide

Modified from Drug and Therapeutics Information Service. National Prescribing Service (NPS) News 1999; 6:3.

Atenolol is best avoided because it may produce intrauterine growth retardation.

Diuretics can cause further contraction of the intravascular volume and more hemoconcentration. The nonsteroidal anti-inflammatory agents, excluding low-dose aspirin, can further reduce renal blood flow.

Labetalol, oxprenolol, hydralazine, methyldopa, nifedipine, prazosin, and clonidine are all efficacious and safe.[35–38]

The calcium channel blockers are also efficacious for control of antepartum hypertension, but hypotension and respiratory embarrassment have been reported when they are used in combination with magnesium sulfate.[29]

PRINCIPLES OF TREATMENT OF PREECLAMPSIA

Drug Treatment. There is no evidence that drug control of hypertension in preeclampsia confers any major benefits to the fetus and it is aimed mainly at protecting the mother from the complications of extreme hypertension. The most commonly used medications are summarized in Table 38–8 and are subdivided into those used:

1. For home management of preeclampsia and on admission to the hospital when SAP is greater than 160 but less than 170 mm/Hg or DAP is greater than 90 but less than 110 mm/Hg or both (e.g., methyldopa, oxprenolol, labetalol, clonidine, hydralazine, nifedipine)[13, 29]
2. To control an acute hypertensive episodes when SAP is 170 mm Hg or greater or DAP is 110 mm Hg or greater, or both (e.g., hydralazine, labetalol, diazoxide, or, in more

Table 38-8 MAIN GROUPS OF ANTIHYPERTENSIVE AGENTS SHOWING THEIR RELATIVE USE IN PREGNANCY IN 1999

ANTIHYPERTENSIVE AGENT		MANAGEMENT OF: Hypertension in Pregnancy	MANAGEMENT OF: Acute Hypertensive Emergency
Diuretic	Thiazide	0	0
	Frusemide	0	+ + +
β-Blocker	Atenolol, metoprolol	+ +	+ +
	Esmolol	0	+ + +
β/α-Blocker	Labetalol	+ + +	+ +
Adrenergic blocker	Methyldopa	+ + + +	+ +
	Clonidine	+ /0	0
α-Blocker	Phenoxybenzamine	0	0
Postsynaptic α-blocker	Prazosin	+ +	0
Sympathetic postganglionic transmission blocker	Reserpine	+	0
Ganglion blocker	Trimetaphan	0	+ +
Vasodilator	Hydralazine	+	+ + + +
	Diazoxide	+ /0	+ + +
	Nitroprusside	0	+ + + +
	Minoxidil	0	0
	Magnesium	0/ +	0/ +
	Nitroglycerin	0	+ + +
Serotonin II antagonist	Ketanserin	+ /0	0
Sedative	Barbiturate	+	0
Calcium channel blocker	Nifedipine	+ +	+ +
Angiotensin-converting enzyme inhibitor	Captopril	+ /0	0

Column 1 shows drugs used to manage mild preeclampsia on an outpatient basis or if it is mild, and column 2 those drugs used to treat acute hypertensive emergencies and crises.

0, drug not used for this indication; +, drug used only rarely for this indication; + + + +, drug very commonly used for this indication.

severe crises, Na nitroprusside, glyceryl trinitrate, or trimetaphan).[39, 40]

Delivery of the Fetus. Since delivery of the fetus usually produces a marked improvement in maternal condition and a resolution of symptoms, delivery must be timed carefully so as not to allow the preeclampsia to deteriorate beyond fetal salvageability and secure a viable, healthy fetus.[41]

In the main, the primary reason for delivery is either fetal distress or intrauterine growth restriction, but there are some maternal absolute and relative indications for delivery (Table 38–9).[29, 41]

Bedrest. Bedrest is probably of minimal benefit but is still encouraged in some centers.[42]

Aspirin. It was originally thought that low-dose aspirin (60–80 mg) would prevent or modify the severity of preeclampsia, but this was not supported by the large multicenter CLASP study. This study suggests that regional anesthesia is not contraindicated in the presence of low-dose aspirin.[43–45]

Calcium. Calcium supplementation may reduce the likelihood of developing preeclampsia.[46–49]

Fish Oils and Salt Restriction. These do not seem to confer any benefit.[50]

Volume Expansion. Volume expansion can be beneficial if central venous pressure or pulmonary capillary wedge pressure are low; if the woman is oliguric or has deteriorating renal function; prior to placement of epidural, spinal subarachnoid, or combined spinal-epidural block; or before initiating vasodilator therapy.[51–53]

RENAL FUNCTION AND RENAL DISEASE

The most important renal diseases in women of childbearing age are the following:

- Reflux nephropathy
- Glomerulonephritis and glomerular sclerosis
- Hypertensive renal disease: 2% of women in this age group have hypertension, mostly essential.[21]
- Polycystic kidney

In some of these patients, the fetal intrauterine growth restriction is out of proportion to the chronic hypertension.[21, 54] In others, renal function can deteriorate considerably in pregnancy.

Initial testing should include urine dipstick testing for protein, serum creatinine, and uric acid; urine protein: creatinine ratio and urine culture (if urinary tract infection is suspected); 24-hour urine catecholamines (if pheochromocytoma is suspected); and urine sediment microscopy for red blood cells, white blood cells, and casts (if glomerulonephritis is suspected).[19]

Table 38-9 ABSOLUTE AND RELATIVE MATERNAL AND FETAL INDICATIONS FOR DELIVERY OF THE FETUS IN SEVERE PREECLAMPSIA

ABSOLUTE	RELATIVE
Maternal	
Convulsion	Severe hypertension
Cerebral irritability	Right upper quadrant abdominal pain
Heart failure	Heavy proteinuria
Oliguria with urine output <20 mL/hr	
Uncontrollable hypertension	
Rising serum creatinine (>50%)	
Thrombocytopenia	
Disseminated intravascular coagulation	
Clinical placental abruption	
Fetal	
Fetal distress	Intrauterine growth retardation

Modified from Gallery EDM: Hypertension in pregnancy. Practical management recommendations. Drugs 1995; 49:4:561.

PREECLAMPSIA: ANESTHETIC RISK ASSESSMENT

More than 2+ urinary protein, poorly controlled blood pressure, thrombocytopenia of less than 75,000, elevated serum uric acid, and depletion of central vascular volume all augur poorly for the anesthetist. Anesthetic risk is higher when preeclampsia is superimposed on chronic hypertension or associated with insulin-dependent diabetes.[1, 20, 21, 25, 27]

Principles of Pre-anesthetic Preparation

In the absence of urgency for delivery, maternal resuscitation should take precedence over any other activity. There are four main components to this predelivery resuscitation: assessment, choice of anesthetic, optimization of physical condition, and monitoring.

Assessment. Assess degree of recent bleeding (e.g., placental abruption), laryngeal or upper airway edema,[55] severity of thrombocytopenia and other coagulopathy,[24, 45, 56] medications being used (including aspirin),[45] and fetal condition.

Optimization of Physical Condition. Provide control of hypertension, seizure prophylaxis, relief of oliguria, and rehydration.

Choice of Anesthetic. Obtain blood cross-match. For general anesthesia, choose the best attenuator of pressor responses to intubation and laryngoscopy and agents most appropriate for a woman with potential renal or hepatic impairment. Provide preoxygenation and aspiration prophylaxis by observing fasting regimens and by administering clear antacid, H_2-blockers, proton pump inhibitors, and metoclopramide. Avoid supine hypotensive (aortocaval compression) syndrome. For epidural anesthesia, assess the appropriateness of epidural anesthetic in the presence of coagulopathy.[56] This is usually decided on the basis of degree of thrombocytopenia, sometimes coupled with thromboelastography, bleeding time, or both. For spinal and combined spinal-epidural anesthesia, prehydration may minimize the likelihood of hypotension. During active bleeding or if thrombocytopenia is severe, these techniques may be contraindicated.[57]

Monitoring. Noninvasive monitoring should include systemic arterial pressure (NIBP), Doppler or other noninvasive (e.g., differential CO_2 Fick partial rebreathing technique) cardiac output, and the cardiotocogram. Invasive monitoring should include intra-arterial, central venous, and pulmonary artery pressures.[51, 52, 58–64] The last is indicated when the patient is a severely oliguric or anuric pre-eclamptic who does not respond to fluid loading, a severe hypertensive who does not respond to aggressive antihypertensive medication, or in pulmonary edema resistant to standard cardiac failure therapy (Table 38–10).[51, 52, 58–60]

Table 38–10 Preoperative Resuscitation of the Woman with Severe Preeclampsia

Control hypertension
Gradually rehydrate
Re-establish adequate urine output
Secure seizure prophylaxis
Decide which attenuator of pressor responses to intubation and laryngoscopy to use
Institute hemodynamic monitoring
Look for evidence of laryngeal or upper airway edema
Assess degree of recent bleeding (if any)
Assess fetal condition
Choose the best anesthetic
Decide whether neuraxial block is safe
(Remember thrombocytopenia, disseminated intravascular coagulation, renal or liver damage)
Decide whether general anesthesia is safe

From Gatt S: Clinical management of established pre-eclampsia/gestational hypertension: Perspectives of the midwife, neonatologist and anesthetist. *In* Brown M (ed): Baillière's Clinical Obstetrics and Gynaecology, Pregnancy and Hypertension Edition, Baillère's Best Practice and Research. London: Baillère Tindall, 1999; 13:1:95–105.

REGIONAL OR GENERAL ANESTHESIA FOR PREECLAMPSIA

There is mounting evidence that spinal and combined spinal-epidural anesthesia are as safe as epidural anesthesia for the patient with severe preeclampsia.[65, 66] Epidural anesthesia would seem to be superior to general anesthesia for cesarean section, and, in labor and delivery, epidural analgesia also has the added advantage of improved blood pressure control, increased renal and uteroplacental blood flow, and decreased potential for seizures. Nevertheless, in some patients, a regional block is contraindicated by virtue of concurrent coagulopathy or active bleeding.

The risks of general anesthesia in severe preeclampsia include the following:

- Hemodynamic instability at induction and intubation and again at extubation (Fig. 38–1)
- Hypertension and tachycardia leading to raised intracranial pressure[21]

The risks associated with regional anesthesia in this scenario include the following:

- A significant epidural hematoma with spinal cord compression in the thrombocytopenic woman
- The need for pressor agents to correct maternal systemic arterial pressure falls in a population that is occasionally exquisitely sensitive to catecholamines
- Precipitate falls in arterial pressure in the hypovolemic, hemoconcentrated woman with concomitant reduction in uteroplacental and renal blood flow

Nevertheless, there are advantages to both groups of techniques. For both, delivery of the placenta and

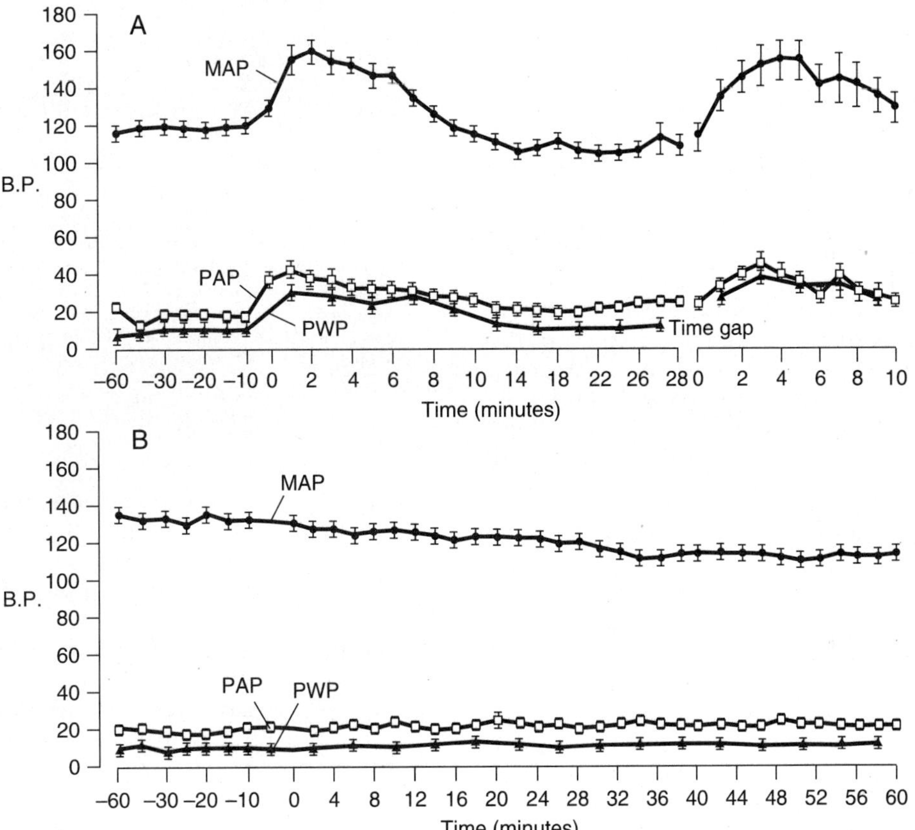

Figure 38–1 Mean arterial systemic pressure (MAP) *(closed circles)*, pulmonary artery pressure (PAP) *(open circles)*, and pulmonary capillary wedge pressure (PCWP) *(triangles)* in patients with preeclampsia undergoing cesarean section under thiopentone-N_2O anesthesia (n=8) *(A)* and epidural anesthesia (n=9) *(B)*. (From Hodgkinson R, Husain FJ, Hayashi RH: Systemic and pulmonary blood pressure during cesarean section in parturients with gestational hypertension. Can Anesth Soc J 1980; 27:389–394.)

infant usually results in cessation of the disease process and a return to pre-pregnancy well-being. Regional techniques may reverse some of the pathophysiologic processes and improve control of systemic vascular pressure and systemic vascular resistance during labor (and in the puerperium), thereby improving uteroplacental blood flow, vasodilating the renal vasculature, and reducing the likelihood of seizures. Also, regional techniques afford good postoperative pain relief (e.g., using 0.1% ropivacaine or bupivacaine with fentanyl or sufentanil). General anesthesia can secure rapid delivery by cesarean section without exposure to the likelihood of epidural bleed.[21]

A number of precautions can be taken to reduce these risks. For example, pressor responses to laryngoscopy and endotracheal intubation can be reduced by esmolol, magnesium, remifentanil, fentanyl, alfentanil, lignocaine, labetalol, thiopentone (thiopental), or propofol.[4, 57] Alternatively, we can pretreat with labetalol, diazoxide, nifedipine, or hydralazine prior to induction. Occasionally, nitroprusside, trimetaphan, or nitroglycerin may be necessary in the untreated or poorly managed patient with severe preeclampsia. Although none can guarantee complete abolition of the systemic arterial pressure rises and the tachycardia, some seem superior to others (e.g., magnesium is superior to alfentanil and lignocaine).[57, 67] Sometimes, these beneficial effects are not achieved without cost. Additional doses of thiopentone can cause hypotension at induction, magnesium will potentiate both the nondepolarizing and the depolarizing muscle relaxants, and opioids can cause respiratory depression in the neonate.

The risk of epidural hematoma following regional anesthesia can be reduced by having guidelines for safe epidural placement.[23, 68] It is best to avoid regional techniques at certain levels of thrombocytopenia because the risk of epidural bleeding rises beyond these lower limits.[24, 69] Patients with HELLP syndrome have markedly decreased platelet counts.[18, 69] All other factors (e.g., degree of anticipated airway difficulty) being equal, the limits vary slightly from one institution to the next (e.g., platelet counts of $<100x10^9$L, $<85x10^9$L, $<80x10^9$L, $<75x10^9$L, or $>50x10^9$/L but $<100x10^9$/L and normal bleeding time, or $>100x10^9$/L but prolonged clotting/coagulation tests, or $>60x10^9$/L but $<100x10^9$/L and normal thromboelastography).[24] Such decision-making should be influenced by the risk-to-benefit ratio of a particular technique in the individual patient. Usually, the nadir of the platelet count occurs at a mean of 29 hours postpartum and returns toward normal within 95 hours postpartum.[70]

Table 38-11 Stratagem for the Prevention of Convulsions in Those Who Have Either Developed Severe Preeclampsia or Experienced a Prior Convulsive (Eclamptic) Episode

- Rigid control of blood pressure including epidural sympathetic blockage
- Magnesium sulphate
- Phenytoin (less commonly)
- Both phenytoin and magnesium (rarely)

From Gatt S: Clinical management of established pre-eclampsia/gestational hypertension: Perspectives of the midwife, neonatologist and anesthetist. *In* Brown M (ed): Baillière's Clinical Obstetrics and Gynecology, Pregnancy and Hypertension Edition, Baillère's Best Practice and Research. London: Baillère Tindall, 1999; 13:1:95–105.

Table 38-12 Hemodynamic Changes in Late Pregnancy*

Value	Change (%)
Cardiac output	up 43
Heart rate	up 17
Systemic vascular resistance	down 21
Pulmonary vascular resistance	down 34
Colloid osmotic pressure (COP)	down 14
COP-Pulmonary capillary wedge pressure gradient	down 28
Mean arterial pressure	NA
Pulmonary capillary wedge pressure (PCWP)	NA
Central venous pressure	NA
Pulmonary artery pressure	NA
Left ventricular stroke work index (LVSWI)	NA
LVSWI/PCWP	NA

NA, unaltered or not affected to an appreciable degree in normal pregnancy.

*Comparison of hemodynamic parameters in normal (not preeclamptic) pregnancies compared at 11–13 weeks postpartum (non-pregnant value) with values at 36–38 weeks' gestation.

Modified from Clark SL, Cotton DB, et al: Central hemodynamic assessment of normal pregnancy. Am J Obstet Gynecol 1989; 161(6): 1439–1442.

Table 38-13 Classical Clinical Picture of Severe, Untreated Preeclampsia

Value	Change
Left ventricular function	Marked elevation
Cardiac output	Moderate elevation
Systemic vascular resistance	Marked elevation
Colloid osmotic pressure	Usually decreased
Mean arterial pressure	Marked elevation
Central venous pressure	Modest decrease
Plasma volume	Modest decrease
Blood viscosity	Small elevation
Red blood cell deformability	Mild increase
Pulmonary vascular resistance	Unaffected
Urine output	Moderate decrease

From Gatt S: Clinical management of established pre-eclampsia/gestational hypertension: Perspectives of the midwife, neonatologist and anesthetist. *In* Brown M (ed): Baillière's Clinical Obstetrics and Gynecology, Pregnancy and Hypertension Edition, Baillère's Best Practice and Research. London: Baillère Tindall, 1999; 13:1:95–105.

MANAGEMENT AND PROPHYLAXIS OF CONVULSIONS

Convulsions should be treated promptly using intravenous thiopentone or diazepam. It is also important to maintain a patent airway, to administer oxygen by face mask, and to apply left lateral pelvic tilt.

The chances of recurrence can be reduced by strict control of hypertension and by prophylactic administration of magnesium sulfate (and, very occasionally, phenytoin) as suggested by the International (n= 1680) and Australian Multicentre Collaborative Eclampsia trials.[71] Women receiving magnesium had a 52% lower risk of recurrence of seizures than those receiving diazepam and a 67% lower risk than those given phenytoin (Table 38–11). Magnesium may be superior to diazepam or phenytoin for the treatment of eclampsia.[71, 72]

DIAGNOSIS AND DIFFERENTIAL DIAGNOSIS

The physiologic changes produced by normal pregnancy are shown in Table 38–12. The most notable are the 43% increase in cardiac output and the 21% decrease in systemic arterial vascular resistance.[8, 73] The superimposed features of severe preeclampsia are shown in Table 38–13 and Figures 38–2, 38–3, and 38–4.[8, 52, 63, 73–75] To these one must add the changes imposed by regional anesthesia (Fig. 38–5) and the atypical picture seen in some preeclamptic patients.[8, 21, 52, 63, 73–75] For example, although the systemic arterial vascular resistance index is often more than 2200 dynes/sec/cm^{-5}/M^2, it is normal (1500–2200) in many patients and low (<1500) in a few. Likewise, although the cardiac index is normal (>3L/min/M^2) or high (>5)in most severe preeclamptics, in a small minority it is low (<3). The large hemodynamic alterations that occur intrapartum and immediately postpartum can make the clinical picture and hemodynamic measurements difficult to interpret.

The differential diagnosis of preeclampsia includes acute cocaine intoxication, essential hypertension, renal disease, idiopathic thrombocytopenic purpura, gallbladder disease, systemic lupus, acute fatty liver of pregnancy, pheochromocytoma, cardiomyopathy, dissecting aortic aneurysm, glomerulonephritis, and ruptured bile duct.

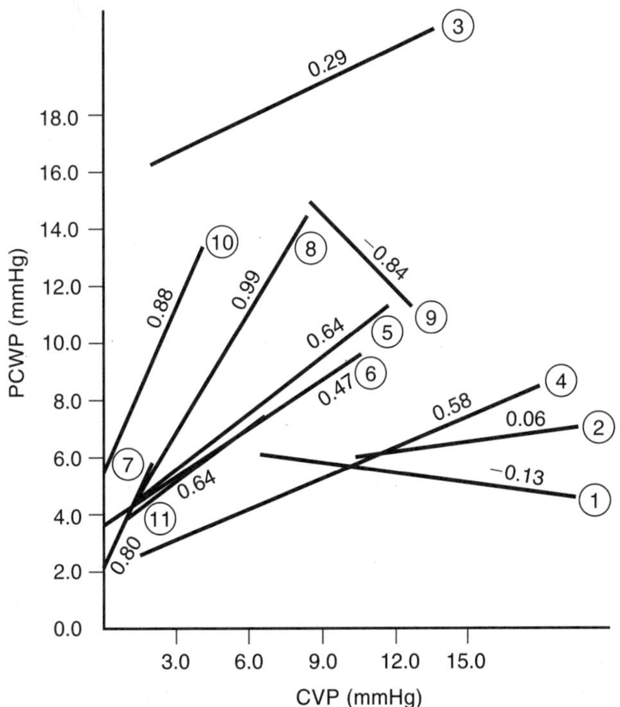

Figure 38–2 Correlation between central venous pressure (CVP) and pulmonary capillary wedge pressure in severe preeclampsia. The correlation is poor and is worst when CVP is less than 6 cm H_2O. (From Newsome LR, Bramwell RS, Curling PE: Hemodynamics in severe preeclamptics. Anesth Analg 1986; 65:33.)

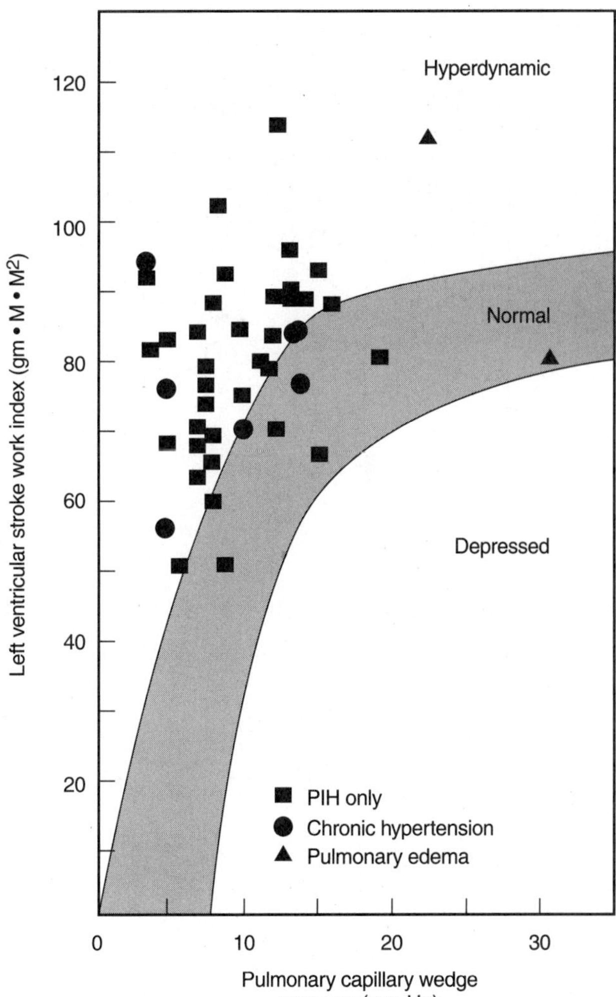

Figure 38–3 Left ventricular curves in women with severe untreated preeclampsia, chronic hypertension, and pulmonary edema. (From Cotton DB, Lee W, Huhta JC, et al: Hemodynamic profile of severe pregnancy-induced hypertension. Am J Obstet Gynecol 1988; 158:523–529.)

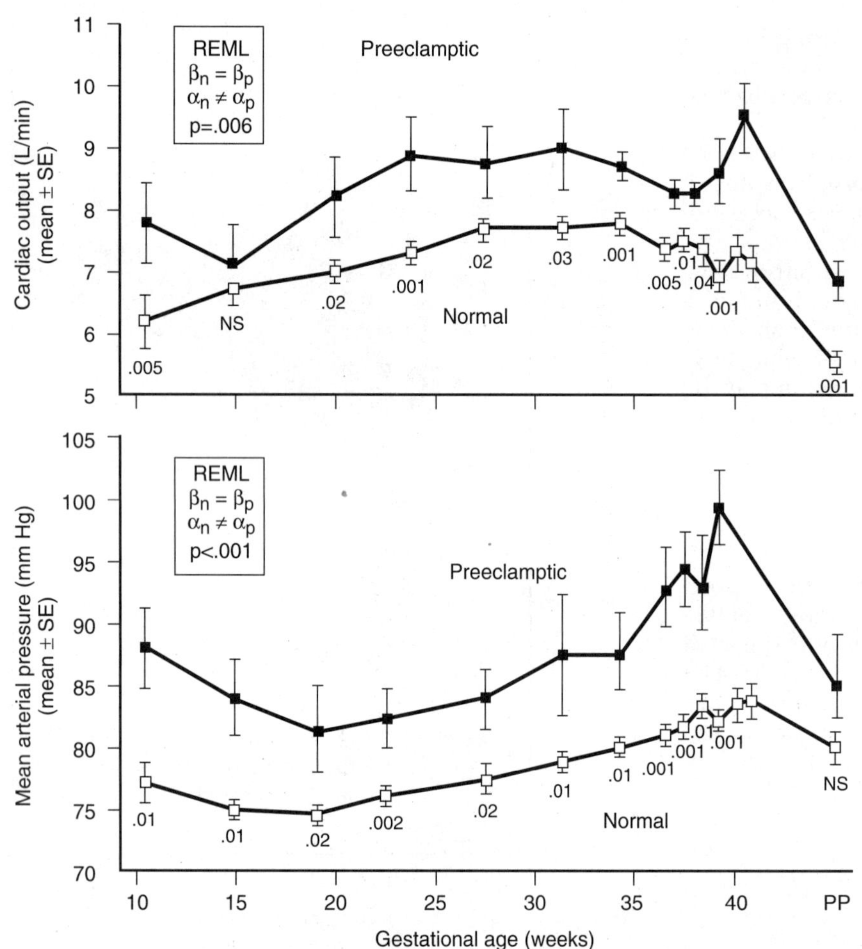

❖ **Figure 38-4** The cardiac output *(upper panel)* and mean systemic arterial pressure *(lower panel)* in normal *(open squares)* and preeclamptic *(closed squares)* pregnancies at different stages of pregnancy and in the postpartum period. (From Easterling TR, Benedetti TJ: Maternal hemodynamics in normal and preeclamptic pregnancies: A longitudinal study. Obstet Gynecol 1990; 76:1061–1069.)

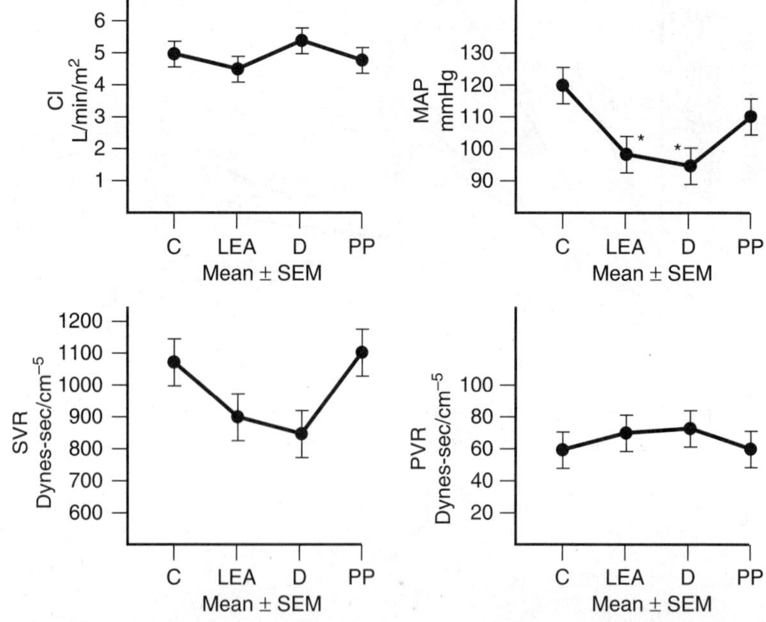

❖ **Figure 38-5** Cardiac index (CI), mean systemic arterial pressure (MAP), systemic vascular resistance (SVR), and pulmonary vascular resistance (PVR) in severely preeclamptic patients at control (C), after lumbar epidural anesthesia (LEA), at delivery (D), and 2 hours post partum (PP). (From Newsome LR, Bramwell RS, Curling PE: Hemodynamics in severe preeclamptics. Anesth Analg 1986; 65:33.)

❖ SUMMARY

Key Points

- Preeclampsia is a multisystem disorder that continues to produce maternal morbidity and mortality.
- Magnesium sulfate remains the agent most often utilized to prevent seizures in the preeclamptic patient. If convulsions occur, they should be immediately treated with intravenous benzodiazepines or thiopental.
- Few preeclamptic patients require invasive monitoring with pulmonary artery catheterization. Indications for invasive monitoring include severe oliguria, pulmonary edema, and severe hypertension unresponsive to aggressive pharmacologic management.
- Epidural anesthesia provides numerous maternal and fetal benefits to the preeclamptic patient by reducing mean arterial pressure and systemic vascular resistance. Thrombocytopenia and disseminated intravascular coagulation may accompany preeclampsia and if present may have an impact on the use of regional analgesia and anesthesia.

Key Reference

Brown MA, Gallery EDM, Gatt S, et al: Consensus Statement: Management of Hypertension in Pregnancy. Australasian Society for the Study of Hypertension in Pregnancy. New Era Printing Pty Ltd., 1993.

Case Stem

A 38-year-old primigravida presents at 31 weeks' gestation complaining of headache and blurred vision. The patient has a blood pressure of 170/105 and has hyperreflexia, clonus, and edema of hands, neck, and lower extremities. Discuss the management, monitoring, and delivery options for this patient.

CONCLUSION

Preeclampsia is a common disease, the management of which is usually straightforward and simple. In some patients, it can be difficult and challenging.

References

1. Gatt S: Anæsthesia and intensive care management of the patient with pre-eclampsia and eclampsia. *In* Davadass A, Wong A (eds). Anaesthesia in the New Millennium. Kuala Lumpur: New Voyager, 1999:155–164.
2. O'Brien WF: Predicting pre-eclampsia. Obstet Gynecol 1990; 75:445–452.
3. Gatt S: Pre-eclampsia *In* Birnbach DJ (ed): Ostheimer's Manual of Obstetric Anesthesia, 3rd ed. Philadelphia: WB Saunders, 1999.
4. Gatt S: Clinical management of established pre-eclampsia/gestational hypertension: Perspectives of the midwife, neonatologist and anæsthetist. *In* Brown M (ed): Baillière's Clinical Obstetrics and Gynæcology, Pregnancy and Hypertension Edition. Baillère's Best Practice and Research. London: Baillère Tindall, 1999; 13:1:95–105.
5. Dekker GA, Sibai BM: Etiology and pathogenesis of preeclampsia: Current concepts. Am J Obstet Gynecol 1998; 178:1359–1375.
6. American College of Obstetricians & Gynecologists: Technical bulletin. Int J Gynecol Obstets 1996; 53:175–183.
7. Klonoff-Cohen HS, Savitz DA, Celafo RC, McCAnn MF: An epidemiologic study of contraception and preeclampsia. JAMA 1989; 262:3143–3147.
8. Easterling TR, Benedetti TJ, et al: Maternal hemodynamics in normal and preeclamptic pregnancies: A longitudinal study. Obstet Gynecol 1990; 76:1061.
9. Moodley J: Treatment of eclampsia. Br J Obstet Gynaecol 1990; 97(1):99–101.
10. Ramanathan J, Angel JJ, Bush AJ, et al: Changes in maternal middle cerebral artery blood flow velocity associated with general anesthesia in severe preeclampsia. Anesth Analg 1999; 88:357–361.
11. de Swiet M, Shennan A: Blood pressure measurement in pregnancy. Br J Obstet Gynecol 1996; 103:862–863.
12. Stone P, Cook D, Hutton J, et al: Measurements of blood pressure, oedema and proteinuria in a pregnant population of New Zealand. Aust N Z J Obstet Gynecol 1995; 35:32–37.
13. Brown MA, Gallery EDM, Gatt S, et al: Consensus Statement: Management of Hypertension in Pregnancy. Australasian Society for the Study of Hypertension in Pregnancy. Sydney, Australia: New Era Printing Pty Ltd. 1993; 15–46.
14. Brown MA, Robinson A, Buddle ML: Accuracy of automated blood pressure recorders in pregnancy. Aust N Z J Obstet Gynecol 1998; 38:262–265.
15. Brown M, Buddle M: What's in a name? Problems with the classification of hypertension in pregnancy. J Hypertension 1997; 15:1049–1054.
16. Knapen MFCM, Mulder TPJ, Bisseling JGA, et al: Plasma glutathione S-transferase alpha 1-1: A more sensitive marker for hepatocellular damage than serum alanine aminotransferase in hypertensive disorders of pregnancy. Am J Obstet Gynecol 1998; 178:161–165.
17. Bernheim J: Hypertension in pregnancy. Nephron 1997; 76:3:254–263.
18. Crosby ET: Obstetrical anaesthesia for patients with the syndrome of haemolysis, elevated liver enzymes and low platelets. Can J Anaesth 1991; 38(2):227.
19. Magann EF, Martin JN: The laboratory evaluation of hypertensive gravidas. Obstet Gynecol Surv 1995; 50(2):138–145.
20. Ferrazini S, Caruso A, de Carolis, et al: Proteinuria and outcome of 444 pregnancies complicated by hypertension. Am J Obstet Gynecol 1990; 162:366–371.
21. Williams K: Hypertension in pregnancy. Can Family Physician 1995; 41:626–632.
22. Gabert HA, Miller JM: Renal disease in pregnancy. Obstet Gynecol Surv 1985; 40:449.
23. Chadwick HS, Easterling T: Anesthetic concerns in the patient with pre-eclampsia. Semin Perinatol 1991; 15(5):397–409.
24. Schindler M, Gatt S, Isert P, et al: Thrombocytopenia and platelet functional defects in pre-eclampsia: Implications for regional anaesthesia. Anaesth Intens Care 1990; 18:169.
25. Chesley LC: Diagnosis of preeclampsia. Obstet Gynecol 1985; 65:423.
26. Redman CW, Bonnar J, et al: Early platelet consumption in preeclampsia. Br Med J 1978; 1:467.
27. Malinow AM: Preeclampsia and eclampsia: Anesthetic management. *In* American Society of Anethesiologists 1996 Annual Refresher Course Lectures. Philadelphia: Lippincott-Raven, 1996; 511:1–7.
28. World Health Organization: International Society of Hypertension guidelines for the management of hypertension. J Hypertens 1999; 17:151–183.
29. Gallery ED: Hypertension in pregnancy: Practical management recommendations. Drugs 1995; 49(4):555–562.
30. Mastrobattista JM: Angiotensin converting enzyme inhibitors in pregnancy. Semin Perinatol 1997; 21:2:124–134.

31. Lewis R, Sibai BM: The use of calcium-channel blockers in pregnancy. New Horizons 1996; 4(1):115–122.
32. Drug and Therapeutics Information Service. National Prescribing Service (NPS) News 1999; 6:3.
33. Constantine G, Beevers DG, Reynolds AL, Luesley DM: Nifedipine as a second line antihypertensive drug in pregnancy. Br J Obstet Gynecol 1987; 94:1136–1142.
34. Burrows RF, Burrows EA: Assessing the teratogenic potential of angiotensin-converting enzyme inhibitors in pregnancy. Aust N Z J Obstet Gynecol 1998; 38:306–309.
35. Mabie WC, Gonzales AR, Sibai BM, Amon E: A comparative trial of labetalol and hydralazine in the acute management of severe hypertension complicating pregnancy. Obstet Gynecol 1987; 70:328–333.
36. Walters BNJ, Redman CWG: Treatment of severe pregnancy-associated hypertension with the calcium antagonist nifedipine. Br J Obstet Gynecol 1981; 21:11–15.
37. Gallery EDM, Ross M, Györy AZ: Antihypertensive treatment in pregnancy: Analysis of different responses to oxprenolol and methyldopa. Br Med J 1985; 291:563–566.
38. Lindow SW, Davies N, Davey DA, Smith JA: The effect of sublingual nifedipine on uteroplacental blood flow in hypertensive pregnancy. Br J Obstet Gynecol 1988; 95:1276–1281.
39. Gatt SP: Gestational proteinuric hypertension. Curr Opin Anesthesiol 1992; 5:354–359.
40. Gatt S: Intravenous nitroglycerine (GTN/NTG) for uterine relaxation. *In* Hochstein E (ed): Clinical Guidelines of the Royal Hospital for Women. Sydney: Wyeth Australia Publications, 1998; 80–81.
41. Pritchard JA, Cunningham FG, et al: The Parkland Memorial Hospital Protocol for the treatment of eclampsia: Evaluation of 245 cases. Am J Obstet Gynecol 1984; 148:951.
42. Duley L: Strict bed rest for proteinuric hypertension in pregnancy. *In* Enkin M, Keirse M, Renfrew M, et al (eds): Pregnancy and Childbirth Module of the Cochrane Database of Systematic Reviews. London. BMJ Publishing, 1995.
43. Redman CW, Roberts JM: Management of pre-eclampsia. Lancet 1993; 341:1451–1454.
44. CLASP: A randomised trial of low dose aspirin for the prevention and treatment of pre-eclampsia among 9364 pregnant women. Lancet 1994; 343:619–629.
45. Macdonald R: Aspirin and extradural blocks. Br J Anaesth 1991; 66:1.
46. Crowther CA, Hillier JE, Pridmore B, et al: Calcium supplementation in nulliparous women for the prevention of pregnancy-induced hypertension, pre-eclampsia and preterm birth: An Australian randomised trial. Aust N Z Obstet Gynecol 1999; 39:12–18.
47. Levine RJ, Hauth JC, Curet LB, et al: Trial of calcium to prevent pre-eclampsia. N Engl J Med 1997; 337:69–76.
48. Lopez-Jarmillo P: Prevention of pre-eclampsia with calcium supplementation and its relation with the L-arginine: Nitric oxide pathway. Brazilian J Med Biol Res 1996; 29:6:731–741.
49. Van den Elzen HJ, Wladimiroff JW, et al: Calcium metabolism, calcium supplementation and hypertensive disorders of pregnancy. Eur J Obstet Gynecol Reprod Biol 1995; 59(1):5–16.
50. Seclier NH, Olsen SE: Fish-oil and pre-eclampsia. Br J Obstet Gynecol 1990; 97:1077–1079.
51. Clark SL, Cotton DB: Clinical indications for pulmonary artery catheterisation in the patient with severe preeclampsia. Am J Obstet Gynecol 1988; 158:453.
52. Wasserstrum N, Cotton DB, et al: Hemodynamic monitoring in severe pregnancy-induced hypertension. Cl Perinatol 1986; 13:781.
53. Sibai BM: Treatment of hypertension in pregnant women. N Engl J Med 1996; 335(4):257–265.
54. Haelterman E, Breart G, Paris-Llado J, et al: Effect of uncomplicated chronic hypertension on the risk of small-for-gestational-age-birth. Am J Epidemiol 1997; 145:689–695.
55. Mallampati RS, Gatt SP, Gugino LD, et al: Clinical sign to predict difficult tracheal intubation: A prospective study. Can Anaes Soc J 1985; 32:429.
56. Barker P, Callander CC: Coagulation screening before epidural analgesia in pre-eclampsia. Anaesthesia 1991; 46:67.
57. Allen RW, James MF, et al: Attenuation of the pressor response to tracheal intubation in hypertensive proteinuric pregnant patients by lignocaine, alfentanil and magnesium sulphate. Br J Anæsth 1991; 66:216.
58. Pritchard JA, Cunningham FG, et al: The Parkland Memorial Hospital Protocol for the treatment of eclampsia: Evaluation of 245 cases. Am J Obstet Gynecol 1984; 148:951.
59. Sise MJ, Hollingworth P, et al: Complications of the flow-directed pulmonary artery catheter. Crit Care Med 1981; 9:315.
60. Elliott CG, Zimmerman GA, et al: Complications of pulmonary artery catheterisation in the care of critically ill patients. Chest 1979; 76:647.
61. Groenendijk R, Trembos MJ, et al: Hemodynamic measurements in pre-eclampsia: Preliminary observations. Am J Obstet Gynecol 1984; 150:232.
62. Gallery ED, Delprado W, et al: Antihypertensive effect of plasma volume expansion in pregnancy-associated hypertension. Aust N Z Med J 1981; 11:20.
63. Cotton DB, Gonik B, et al: Cardiovascular alterations in severe pregnancy induced hypertension: Relationship of central venous pressure to pulmonary capillary wedge pressure. Am J Obstet Gynecol 1985; 151:762.
64. Clark SL, Horenstein JM, et al: Experiences with the pulmonary artery catheter in obstetrics and gynecology. Am J Obstet Gynecol 1985; 152:374.
65. Hood D, Curry R: Spinal versus epidural anesthesia for cesarean section in severely preeclamptic patients. Anaesth 1999; 9(5):1276–1283.
66. Howell P: Spinal anesthesia in severe preeclampsia: Time for reappraisal, or time for caution? Int J Obstet Gynecol 1998; 7:217–219.
67. Liu P, Gatt SP, Gugino LD, et al: Evaluation of esmolol in controlling increases in heart rate and blood pressure during intubation after thiopental and succinylcholine induction. Can Anaesth Soc J 1986; 33:556–562.
68. Barker P, Callander CC: Coagulation screening before epidural analgesia in pre-eclampsia. Anaesth 1991; 46:67.
69. De Boer K, Büller HR, et al: Coagulation studies in the syndrome of hemolysis, elevated liver enzymes and low platelets. Br J Obstet Gynaecol 1991; 98:42.
70. Neiger R, Contag SA, et al: The resolution of preeclampsia-related thrombocytopenia. Obstet Gynecol 1991; 77:5:692.
71. Eclampsia Trial Collaborative Group: Which anticonvulsant for women with eclampsia? Evidence from the collaborative eclampsia trial. Lancet 1995; 345:1455–1463.
72. Lucas MJ, Leveno KJ, et al: A comparison of magnesium sulfate with phenytoin for the prevention of eclampsia. N Engl J Med 1995; 333:4:201–251.
73. Clark SL, Cotton DB, et al: Central hemodynamic assessment of normal pregnancy. Am J Obstet Gynecol 1989; 161(6):1439–1442.
74. Newsome LR, Bramwell RS, Curling PE: Hemodynamics in severe preeclamptics. Anesth Analg 1986; 65:33.
75. Cotton DB, Lee W, Huhta JC, et al: Hemodynamic profile of severe pregnancy induced hypertension. Am J Obstet Gynecol 1988; 158:523–529.

39

Cardiovascular Disease in the Pregnant Patient

❖ JOSE CARVALHO, MD

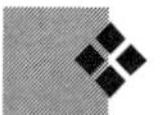

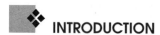

INTRODUCTION

Cardiac disease producing morbidity and mortality in the pregnant patient is seen across the globe. The report on Confidential Enquiries Into Maternal Deaths in the United Kingdom for the years 1991 through 1993[1] reported a significant increase in maternal mortality related to cardiac disease as compared with the previous two triennia. In the city of São Paulo, Brazil, where maternal mortality in the period of 1993 through 1995 was 50.2 per 100,000 live births, 11.3% of these deaths were related to cardiac disease.[2] Different reasons can be used to explain the prevalence of cardiac disease in the pregnant population and the poor outcome in some of the cases, in both developed and developing countries. Many of these maternal deaths are preventable if appropriate prenatal care is provided, and if a coordinated multidisciplinary approach is taken. In addition, it is of paramount importance that the potential risks of cardiac disease in pregnancy not be underestimated by the physicians caring for these patients. As for many other subsets of high-risk pregnant patients, the parturient with cardiac disease often requires specially trained obstetricians, cardiologists, and anesthesiologists to care for their special needs.

The distribution of cardiac disease in the pregnant population varies according to geographic region. At the University of São Paulo, in Brazil, in a series of 1000 pregnant cardiac patients,[3] the most common cardiac disease was rheumatic heart disease (56.3%), followed by cardiomyopathy (15.4%) and congenital heart disease (14.4%). This distribution differs somewhat from the classically described distribution,[4] in which the incidence of cardiomiopathy is less frequent than congenital heart disease. This difference can be attributed to the high incidence of Chagas' disease in Brazil, which is responsible for more than 10% of all cardiac patients. However, as in many other countries, the most common cardiac disease presenting to the anesthesiologist in Brazil is mitral stenosis, either as a sole dysfunction or in combination with other valvular dysfunctions.

PHYSIOLOGIC CHANGES OF PREGNANCY AND THE CARDIAC PATIENT

It is not difficult to understand why pregnancy may worsen underlying disease in a cardiac patient. As described in Chapter 2, pregnancy increases both cardiac work and myocardial oxygen consumption. During the course of normal pregnancy, blood volume increases 40 to 50% and is accompanied by increases of 18% in heart rate and 50% in cardiac output. Additional hemodynamic changes occur during labor and are especially acute during each uterine contraction. An increase of up to 45% in cardiac output is seen during the late second stage of labor.[5–7] Such cardiovascular changes seem to be largely based on sympathetically mediated increases in heart rate, as well as in stroke volume during contractions. Cardiac output may further increase 10 to 20% in the immediate postpartum period as a consequence of postpartum volume shifts, which are due to release of vena cava obstruction by the pregnant uterus and decrease in vascular capacitance associated with the delivery of the fetus and placenta and subsequent uterine contractions. Systemic vascular resistance is suddenly elevated as a result of uterine contractions after placental extraction. Such dramatic preload and afterload changes are readily accommodated by increases in cardiac output in the patient with a normal heart. However, the patient with a relatively fixed cardiac output may be unable to accommodate such hemodynamic fluctua-

tions, and hydrostatic pulmonary edema or congestive heart failure may develop.[8]

There are three periods during the evolution of pregnancy in which cardiac patients are at a greater risk for decompensation. The first is between the 20th and 24th week of gestation, when most of the hemodynamic changes of pregnancy have occurred; many patients with severe cardiac disease may require hospitalization during that phase. The second period of increased risk is during labor and delivery, when contractions, pain, anxiety, and intravascular volume shifts place a larger burden on the cardiovascular system. The third period is immediately post partum, a time that is critical for most cardiac patients as both cardiac output and systemic vascular resistance suddenly increase, leading to extra myocardial work.

For all of these reasons, the anesthetic management of pregnant cardiac patients should provide analgesia and optimal conditions for delivery, and also attempt to provide hemodynamic and cardiovascular stability during the intrapartum period and in the immediate postpartum period.

The cardiovascular changes associated with pregnancy will totally return to non-pregnant status within 6 months post partum, but most of this regression will occur during the first 2 weeks. Therefore, unnecessary surgical and anesthetic procedures in this high-risk group of patients, including postpartum tubal ligation, should be postponed, if possible, until 2 weeks post partum.

PLANNING THE ANESTHETIC MANAGEMENT OF THE CARDIAC PREGNANT PATIENT

The considerations that should guide the anesthetic management of these patients include the pathophysiology and severity of the cardiac disease as well as the cardiovascular adaptations that have occurred during the course of pregnancy.

Pathophysiology

Patients with different cardiac diseases adapt to pregnancy through different mechanisms. The changes in the equilibrium between pulmonary and systemic circulation induced by the stress of labor and delivery and various anesthetic techniques will be tolerated differently in different disease states. Each particular case deserves a comprehensive evaluation of how **heart rate and rhythm, preload, afterload**, and **myocardial contractility** will affect a certain patient. Taking these different variables into account, it is possible to anticipate the desirable hemodynamic profile for most cardiac dysfunctions and to indivualize and optimize the patient's care by administering the anesthetic agents and techniques that will achieve the desired hemodynamic goals (Table 39–1).

Severity of Heart Disease

Based on the New York Heart Association (NYHA) classification,[9] patients can be allocated into functional classes I to IV, which are defined as follows:

Class I: no limitation of physical activity

Class II: symptoms with ordinary physical activity

Class III: symptoms with less than ordinary physical activities

Class IV: symptoms at rest

Severity of heart disease based on this functional classification, while occasionally helpful, should not be an absolute indication or contraindication for a particular anesthetic technique. For example, some class I patients may have a relative contraindication to regional anesthesia (e.g., pulmonary hypertension, aortic and pulmonic stenosis), whereas regional anesthesia techniques may be ideal in other class I parturients, in whom they may even be therapeutic (e.g., mitral stenosis with pulmonary edema). The severity of heart disease should never be considered without a

Table 39–1 EXPECTED IDEAL HEMODYNAMIC FEATURES FOR THE ANESTHETIC TECHNIQUES USED IN THE MANAGEMENT OF CARDIAC PREGNANT PATIENTS

DISEASE	HEART RATE	PRELOAD	AFTERLOAD	CONTRACTILITY
Mitral stenosis	M-SD	M-SD	M-SD	M
Mitral insufficiency	M-SI	M-SD	M-SD	M-SI
Aortic stenosis	M	M-SI	M-SI	M
Aortic insufficiency	M-SI	M-SD	M-SD	M-SI
Pulmonic stenosis	M	M-SI	M-SI	M
Pulmonary hypertension	M	M-SI	M-SI	M
Dilated cardiomyopathy	M	M-SD	M-SD	SI
Hypertrophic cardiomyopathy	M-SD	M-SI	M	M-SD
Left-to-right shunt	M	M-SI	M-SI	M
Right-to-left shunt	M	M-SI	M-SI	M
Ischemic heart disease	M-SD	M-SD	M-SD	M-SD

M, maintain; SD, slight decrease; SI, slight increase.

Adapted and modified from Ramanathan S: Cardiac disease. In Ramanathan S (ed): Obstetric Anesthesia. Philadelphia: Lea & Febiger, 1988: 191.

comprehensive evaluation of the underlying pathophysiology.

Cardiovascular Adaptation to Pregnancy

Detailed clinical observation of cardiac patients during the period of their prenatal care will provide useful information regarding the factors involved in the improvement or in the impairment of their cardiovascular status. Although some patients will benefit from the decrease in systemic vascular resistance associated with pregnancy (e.g., aortic and mitral insufficiency), others will not tolerate increases in blood volume or in heart rate (e.g., mitral stenosis). The response of a particular parturient with cardiac disease to her pregnancy will help the obstetrician and anesthesiologist anticipate the response to various anesthetic techniques. The response of the pregnant patient with cardiac disease to the various drugs used in the control of intercurrent dysrhythmias or other cardiac dysfunctions will also be helpful in anticipating and treating perioperative complications. It is therefore essential for the anesthesiologist to have as complete a history as possible, including both currently and previously prescribed drugs and their effects on that particular patient. If possible, the patient should be examined and oriented before pregnancy is planned. A comprehensive baseline physical examination will be valuable in evaluating symptoms and signs that might be underestimated during pregnancy.[10] Additionally, some patients, such as those using oral anticoagulants, may require a change in their medication.[11]

Adequate Documentation

Adequate workup is absolutely necessary for the understanding of the contribution of preload, afterload, cardiac rhythm, and myocardial contractility to the hemodynamic status of each pregnant patient with cardiac disease. Supplemental tests are fundamental and should include a chest radiograph and electrocardiogram. In addition, when available, echocardiography performed in both the first and third trimesters of gestation is ideal. Echocardiography has been extensively used in the evaluation of pregnant cardiac patients and has been shown to be a very valuable tool in their clinical and anesthetic management. An echocardiographic profile of normal pregnant patients[12] is summarized in Table 39–2. Echocardiographic findings should be complemented by those of electrocardiogram and radiograph. In certain patients (such as those with mitral stenosis), pulmonary congestion is a common feature, often associated with echocardiographic findings suggestive of pulmonary hypertension. It is of utmost importance to differentiate between venous hypertension and arteriolar hypertension in these patients. Sometimes the presence of an increased right ventricular systolic pressure can mislead the anesthesiologist to expect the presence of arteriolar hypertension. In this commonly occurring situation, the electrocardiogram is essential to make the correct differential diagnosis. If there are no signs of right axis deviation and right ventricular hypertrophy is seen, regardless of echocardiographic results, it is unlikely that the patient is suffering from pulmonary arteriolar hypertension. It should be stressed, however, that interpretation of the electrocardiogram in the pregnant patient must take into account the changes induced by normal pregnancy. These include the following:

1. P wave, PR interval, and QTc interval remain stable.
2. QRS axis and T axis are deviated to the left.
3. T wave can be negative in lead III and occasionally in aVF.
4. ST segment depression of 0.5 to 1 mm is acceptable.

Choice of Adequate Anesthetic Technique for the Cardiac Patient Undergoing Cesarean Section

Based on the desirable hemodynamic profile for each cardiac disease and on the hemodynamic implications of different anesthetic drugs and techniques, a guideline for the selection of the anesthetic technique is suggested in Table 39–3. These guidelines should be

Table 39–2 DOPPLER ECHOCARDIOGRAPHIC VARIABLES IN NORMAL PREGNANT PATIENTS IN THE 24TH TO 28TH WEEK OF GESTATION (P1) AND IN THE 32ND TO 36TH WEEK OF GESTATION (P2)

	P1 (MEAN ± SD)	P2 (MEAN ± SD)
Mitral valve area (cm)	3.69 (0.48)	4.31 (0.67)
Left atrium (cm)	2.95 (0.29)	3.25 (0.22)
Left ventricle (cm)	4.93 (0.37)	5.06 (0.44)
Cardiac output (L/min)	4.06 (0.54)	5.39 (1.01)
Systolic volume (mL)	72.39 (27.25)	93.83 (29.16)
Final systolic volume (mL)	29.70 (8.13)	34.26 (10.25)
Final diastolic volume (mL)	116.39 (25.73)	130.35 (35.27)
Ejection fraction (%)	0.74 (0.04)	0.76 (0.04)
Aorta (cm)	2.85 (0.19)	3.06 (0.21)

From Faccioli R: Área da valva mitral estenótica em gestantes portadoras de doença reumática: Correlação com o prognóstico perinatal. Tese de Doutoramento-Faculdade de Medicina da Universidade de São Paulo, 1990.

Table 39–3 SUGGESTED ANESTHETIC TECHNIQUE FOR VARIOUS CARDIAC DISEASES

DISEASE	TECHNIQUE
Mitral stenosis	Regional
Mitral insufficiency	Regional
Aortic stenosis	General
Aortic insufficiency	Regional
Pulmonic stenosis	General
Pulmonary hypertension	General
Dilated cardiomyopathy	Regional?
Hypertrophic cardiomyopathy	General
Left-to-right shunt	General
Right-to-left shunt	General
Ischemic heart disease	Regional?

used as a general approach and each patient should be considered individually.

REGIONAL ANESTHESIA AND ANALGESIA FOR THE PREGNANT CARDIAC PATIENT

There is clear evidence in the literature that regional anesthesia is the most effective way of blocking the stress response during labor and delivery and during cesarean section. Although this is beneficial to all patients, it becomes all the more important in the cardiac patient. The cardiovascular changes induced by regional anesthesia may not always be beneficial to the parturient with cardiac disease and therefore should be considered for each patient, depending on the underlying pathophysiology. Spinal or epidural blocks may have an effect on conductance vessels, resulting in a decrease in systemic vascular resistance (afterload). However, they exert a very important action on capacitance vessels, resulting in a significant pooling of blood and a decrease in venous return (preload). Systemic vascular resistance can be further decreased following initiation of an epidural block if epinephrine is added to the local anesthetic solution. Heart rate is dependent on the reduction of either systemic vascular resistance or venous return, and the concomitant use of epinephrine in association with the local anesthetic solution.

For most patients, regional anesthesia represents a cushion to the hemodynamic fluctuations that occur during labor and delivery. In certain cases, neuraxial blockade may be very beneficial in the postpartum period as well.

The potential benefits of regional anesthesia for pregnant cardiac patients is especially seen in the management of the patient with mitral stenosis. Clark et al.[8] reported the results of invasive monitoring with pulmonary artery catheters in a series of eight patients with mitral stenosis, in the first clinical report of this nature. Patients were NYHA functional class III or IV and all delivered vaginally. It is interesting to note that a mean increase in pulmonary capillary wedge pressure of 10 mm Hg was observed in the immediate postpartum period. Although three of these patients received epidural anesthesia during the active phase of labor, no significant improvement in hemodynamic parameters occurred. However, Hemmings et al.[13] reported on a NYHA class II parturient who was invasively monitored and in whom epidural anesthesia had clearly beneficial effects. Three observations were especially relevant in this case:

- Epidural anesthesia was beneficial in the first stage of labor. When contractions became painful, pulmonary artery pressure (PAP), pulmonary vascular resistance, and systemic vascular resistance increased and cardiac output decreased. After induction of epidural anesthesia with 0.25% bupivacaine, pulmonary vascular resistance, systemic vascular resistance, and PAP decreased while cardiac output increased toward baseline values.
- Dramatic increases in PAP and decreases in cardiac output were observed during bearing-down efforts in the second stage. The patient's urge to bear down was decreased by the epidural, with correction of the hemodynamic profile.
- There was no increase in pulmonary capillary wedge pressure in the immediate postpartum period. The authors related this to the conservative fluid management and to a continued sympathetic blockade to the T-6 dermatomal level.

Mostafa[14] reported on the management of a parturient with severe mitral stenosis and pulmonary edema undergoing emergency cesarean section under a spinal anesthetic, which was performed after unsuccessful epidural anesthesia attempts. This case report illustrates how the understanding of the pathophysiology can lead to successful clinical management. It also illustrates that the functional class of the patient by itself should not lead to the election of general anesthesia as the anesthetic technique of choice. Under such circumstances, general anesthesia, despite the beneficial effects of increasing intra-alveolar pressure during intermittent positive pressure ventilation, could lead to hypertension, tachycardia, dysrhythmias, and increases in pulmonary artery pressure, associated with intubation, extubation, and light anesthesia. General anesthesia would also be unable to accommodate for the excessive venous return during contractions or after delivery.

Patients with mild to severe mitral stenosis, mitral insufficiency, aortic insufficiency, and many cases of dilated cardiomyopathy and ischemic heart disease are candidates for a safely conducted regional technique, both for vaginal delivery and for cesarean section (Table 39–4). Although epidural anesthesia is still a widely used anesthetic technique for the cardiac patient, the use of combined spinal-epidural has gained acceptance worldwide and at this institution it is the technique of choice. Additionally, spinal and spinal-epidural techniques may greatly benefit patients with conduction disturbances or severe myocardial compromise (e.g., parturients with Chagas' cardiomyopathy) in whom large doses of local anesthetics are not well tolerated.

Table 39–4 REGIONAL TECHNIQUES AND SUGGESTED ANESTHETIC MANAGEMENT FOR PREGNANT CARDIAC PATIENTS WITH NO CONTRAINDICATION FOR REGIONAL ANESTHESIA

Vaginal Delivery

- Fluid restriction; Start analgesia early; Left uterine displacement; Monitoring: HR, NIBP, ECG, Spo_2
- Epidural analgesia:
  - Epidural incremental bolus: 10 mL (12.5 mg) of 0.125% bupivacaine plus sufentanil or fentanyl
  - Epidural continuous infusion: 0.0625% bupivacaine plus sufentanil 0.2 μg/mL or fentanyl 2 μg/mL, 8–12 mL/h (titrate to effect)
- Combined spinal-epidural analgesia:
  - Subarachnoid bolus injection: sufentanil 5 μg plus or minus 2.5 mg of bupivacaine;
  - Epidural continuous infusion: 0.05% bupivacaine plus fentanyl or sufentanil, as above

Cesarean Delivery

- Fluid restriction; Oxygen by mask; Lateral uterine displacement
- Maintain systolic blood pressure close to control values with prophylactic vasopressors, e.g., ephedrine (except in mitral stenosis = metaraminol or phenylephrine)
- Monitoring: Pulse, NIPB, ECG, SpO_2
- Oxytocin infusion (10–20 IU) after delivery; avoid ergot derivatives
- Epidural anesthesia
  - 0.5% bupivacaine in incremental doses plus 50 μg fentanyl plus 1–2 mg of morphine;
  - Bring up level very slowly to avoid sudden changes and hemodynamic compromise
- Combined spinal-epidural anesthesia
  - 5–7.5 mg hyperbaric 0.5% bupivacaine plus 25–50 μg of morphine or 7.5–10 mg 0.75% bupivacaine
  - After 15 minutes, incremental doses of 3 mL of plain 0.5% bupivacaine at 5-min intervals
- Continuous spinal anesthesia
  - Epidural catheter threaded into subarachnoid space;
  - 0.5 mL of bupivacaine as first dose, then incremental injections of 0.1–0.2 mL to effect

ECG, electrocardiograph; HR, heart rate; NIBP, noninvasive blood pressure.

For a more comprehensive approach to this group of patients, in whom regional anesthesia may be highly beneficial, a brief description of the general hemodynamic adaptive mechanisms and a proposed anesthetic management are reviewed.

Mitral Stenosis

In normal adults, the mitral valve orifice is 4 to 6 cm^2 and the valvular diastolic gradient is 5 mm Hg or less. If an obstruction to the left atrial outflow is present, a higher intra-atrial pressure is required to send the blood to the left ventricle. When the orifice is reduced to 1 cm^2, 25 mm Hg of pressure gradient is required to maintain cardiac output. The increase in heart rate observed during pregnancy reduces the filling time of the left ventricle and results in elevations in left atrial pressure, which might produce a rise in pulmonary capillary pressure and pulmonary edema.[15] Atrial fibrillation is associated with an increased risk of maternal morbidity and mortality and requires aggressive treatment. β-Adrenergic blockers and digitalis are often used to control heart rate during pregnancy in these patients, with excellent maternal results, without adverse effects on the fetus and neonate.[16] As a complication of long-lasting severe mitral stenosis, pulmonary hypertension may result[17]; however, this is not usually seen in the age range of the pregnant woman. Left ventricular function should be normal in parturients with mitral stenosis. Any abnormality of ventricular dimensions or function indicates the possibility of a different concomitant disturbance. Right ventricular function is also normal, except when in the presence of pulmonary hypertension. Pregnancy raises both preload and heart rate; both factors raise transvalvular gradient, thus impairing cardiac function. Pulmonary congestion and hypertension in the pulmonary venous bed usually occurs; however, this state should be differentiated from a hyper-resistance status in the pulmonary arteriolar bed, as they have different anesthetic implications. As discussed earlier in this chapter, the echocardiogram, chest radiograph, and electrocardiogram should be used to improve the likelihood of making the correct diagnosis. Should pulmonary arterial hypertension occur, major regional anesthesia may be contraindicated.

When considering a pregnant woman with any valvular dysfunction, a complete evaluation of the patient is necessary. In a series of 67 cardiac patients with mitral stenosis undergoing cesarean section at the University of São Paulo, in 1987 through 1991, only 28% of the patients presented with mitral stenosis as the sole dysfunction. Although 75% of the patients presented mitral stenosis either alone or associated with valvular abnormalities that did not contraindicate regional anesthesia, in 25% of the patients the mitral stenosis was associated with other valvular dysfunctions that necessitated general anesthesia.

Basic rules for the anesthetic management of mitral stenosis include the following:

1. Heart rate
   - Avoid tachycardia
   - Provide labor analgesia early to reduce pain and stress
   - Do not use epinephrine associated with the local anesthetic
   - If hypotension occurs, use metaraminol or phenylephrine
   - Treat all acute dysrhythmias
2. Preload
   - Avoid increases in preload
   - Sympathetic blockade will provide a reduction of venous return, especially during contractions and after delivery
3. Afterload
   - Avoid marked decreases
   - Do not use epinephrine-containing local anesthetics
4. Myocardial contractility
   - Avoid myocardial depressants
   - Attempt to maintain myocardial contractility

Mitral Insufficiency

In the presence of mitral regurgitation, the resistance to left ventricular emptying is reduced, thus producing a greater outflow to the left atrium. To maintain cardiac output, the left ventricle must increase myocardial contractility. With the progression of the mitral insufficiency, left atrial enlargement, increased pulmonary capillary pressure, and right-sided heart failure may develop. If left ventricular function deteriorates, the left ventricle will dilate and its compliance will increase. Although cardiac function can deteriorate, the usual evolution of mitral insufficiency is benign and pregnancy is well tolerated.

Aortic Insufficiency

In aortic insufficiency, the regurgitant flow during diastole can be of the same magnitude as the forward stroke volume; the major hemodynamic compensation is an increase in left ventricular end-diastolic volume, which allows the left ventricle to send a larger stroke volume and maintain ejection fraction. As compared with mitral insufficiency, in aortic insufficiency the left ventricular enlargement occurs in the early phases. As the disease progresses, left ventricular dysfunction occurs, ejection fraction is reduced, the left atrium is enlarged, and pulmonary congestion may occur.

Although there are marked differences in their pathophysiology and hemodynamic adaptations to pregnancy, the anesthetic considerations for mitral and aortic regurgitation are quite similar and will be discussed jointly.

Anesthetic Management of Mitral and Aortic Regurgitation

- Heart rate: avoid bradycardia, as heart rate helps maintain cardiac output in mitral regurgitation and reduces the degree of blood regurgitated during diastole in aortic insufficiency; vena cava decompression will avoid marked decreases in venous return with consequent bradycardia; if mitral stenosis is not present, epinephrine can be used in association with local anesthetics.
- Preload: This should be decreased, to reduce left ventricular over-distention; sympathetic blockade will provide reduction in venous return, especially during contractions and after delivery.
- Afterload: This should also be decreased, to reduce the regurgitant flow; early labor analgesia will avoid pain and stress associated with marked increases in peripheral resistance; epinephrine associated with the local anesthetic is useful if mitral stenosis is not present; if hypotension occurs, use ephedrine.
- Myocardial contractility: This should be maintained by avoiding myocardial depressants; inhalation agents should be used with great caution, as these patients are extremely sensitive to them.

Mitral Valve Prolapse

Mitral valve prolapse is a very frequent finding in young women[18] and is usually very well tolerated during pregnancy.[19] Most patients are asymptomatic; however, some may develop palpitations and fatigue. The diagnosis is usually made by echocardiography, whereas these patients exhibit a normal electrocardiographic pattern. However, in some cases, a variety of arrhythmias may occur, and there is also a high incidence of mitral valve prolapse in patients with Wolff-Parkinson-White syndrome.[18]

Anesthetic management does not require special planning. Epinephrine-containing local anesthetic solutions are usually avoided. Specific arrhythmias should be treated accordingly.

Dilated Cardiomyopathy

In dilated cardiomyopathy, the cardiac chambers, especially those on the left side, are enlarged. The primary functional disturbance is the loss of ventricular contractile power, with a reduction in the ejection fraction. As the disease progresses, end-diastolic volume increases and cardiac output decreases. Two major causes of this condition are peripartum cardiomyopathy and Chagas' disease. Chagas' disease is a chronic cardiomyopathy well known not only for cardiac enlargement and thromboembolic phenomena but also for intracardiac conduction disturbance.[20] Peripartum cardiomyopathy is a rare but severe form of heart failure usually occurring in the third trimester of pregnancy or the first several months of the postpartum period.[21–25] It is usually insidious but can rapidly progress to severe cardiac failure, low cardiac output, and elevated filling pressures. Women who develop an episode of postpartum cardiomyopathy are unlikely to return to normal cardiac function.[24–26]

Anesthetic Management of the Parturient with Dilated Cardiomyopathy

- Heart rate: Avoid bradycardia, as it will raise left ventricle end-diastolic volume and compromise ejection fraction; be careful with intubation, succinylcholine, and halothane.
- Preload: This should be reduced; increases in venous return associated with contractions and delivery may precipitate pulmonary edema; sympathetic blockade will reduce venous return and thus improve myocardial function.
- Afterload: This should also be reduced; if peripheral resistance rises, left ventricular failure might occur; early labor analgesia is suggested; if general anesthesia is required, avoid light anesthesia.
- Myocardial contractility: This should be maintained or increased; large doses of local anesthetic can impair myocardial function; if a conduction disturbance is present (e.g., Chagas' disease) large doses of local anesthetics should also be avoided: epidural blockade can be used for labor and delivery, but spinal or combined spinal-epidural anesthesia are generally the techniques of choice for cesarean section; avoid inhalation agents if possible.

If myocardial function is severely compromised, with a marked reduction in the ejection fraction, these patients may benefit from a combination of epidural and general anesthesia. Epidural anesthesia, with a low dose and dilute concentration of local anesthetics, will provide protection against sudden increases in venous return and peripheral resistance, without further compromising left ventricular function.

The Pregnant Patient with a Transplanted Heart

There have been several reports of women who have undergone cardiac transplantation and subsequently given birth.[27–29] The transplanted heart has no afferent or efferent autonomic or somatic innervation.[30–32] Baseline heart rate tends to be higher, because vagal innervation is not present. Additionally, drugs acting by means of the vagus nerve are ineffective. If sympathomimetic agents are required, the direct-acting agents should be used. These agents should, however, be used with caution; as a consequence of heart denervation, an up-regulation of the cardiac adrenergic receptors is observed, with increased sensitivity. If epidural anesthesia is to be used, epinephrine should be avoided.[33] Regional and general anesthesia have been successfully used in these patients.[34]

RESTRICTIONS TO REGIONAL ANESTHESIA IN THE PREGNANT CARDIAC PATIENT

Most parturients presenting with mitral stenosis, mitral insufficiency, aortic insufficiency, and dilated cardiomyopathy can be optimally managed with regional anesthesia. Parturients with other cardiac lesions, however, may have contraindications to neuraxial techniques. Each patient, therefore, must be extensively evaluated before the anesthetic technique is chosen. The use of regional techniques in the parturient with cardiac disease has dramatically increased, thanks in part to the introduction of new drugs and techniques, which have provided practitioners with new options. The most important restrictions to regional anesthesia in the cardiac patient are anticoagulation, pulmonic stenosis, aortic stenosis, left-to-right and right-to-left shunts with significant hemodynamic implications, primary and secondary pulmonary hypertension, and hypertrophic cardiomyopathy (see Table 39–3).

Anticoagulation

Anticoagulation is very common among pregnant patients with cardiac disease. Indications for anticoagulation include mechanical prostheses, chronic atrial fibrillation, previous stroke, presence of thrombi detected by the echocardiography, dilated cardiomyopathies, and cyanotic cardiopathies. Active anticoagulation is an absolute contraindication to spinal or epidural techniques, owing to the increased risk of bleeding, leading to the possible development of an epidural hematoma. If interruption of heparin therapy is possible, it should be done prior to labor and delivery and can then be safely reintroduced in the immediate postpartum period, as documented by Rao et al.[35] If the heparin is discontinued for 12 hours and the coagulation profile is within normal limits, regional anesthesia can be used. If interruption of anticoagulation is not possible, pain relief with a neuraxial technique is not advisable, either for labor or cesarean section. Should the situation (such as premature labor) occur in which a laboring parturient is still taking oral anticoagulants, which are usually associated with a prolonged half-life, regional anesthesia is also contraindicated. The use of low molecular weight heparin for these patients has recently gained acceptance among cardiologists and obstetricians. If these drugs are being used, regional anesthesia can be used 12 hours after a prophylactic dose of low molecular weight heparin. If anticoagulation is to be instituted after regional anesthesia, an interval of 4 hours after needle puncture or catheter removal should be allowed before the actual administration of the drug.[36]

Primary and Secondary Pulmonary Hypertension

A striking example of a case in which neuraxial techniques are usually contraindicated is the parturient with primary pulmonary hypertension. Maternal mortality among women presenting with primary pulmonary hypertension ranges between 40 and 60% during the third trimester and postpartum period.[37] Hemodynamic features include PAP in excess of 30/15 mm Hg or a mean PAP greater than 25 mm Hg, right ventricular hypertrophy, and, eventually, heart failure with a low, fixed cardiac output. Two principles must be considered in the management of patients with primary pulmonary hypertension: (1) the primary goal is to minimize increases in pulmonary vascular resistance secondary to hypercarbia, hypoxia, acidosis, stress, and pain; (2) major hemodynamic changes should be avoided, especially marked decreases in systemic vascular resistance and venous return.

There are many case reports in the literature describing the anesthetic management of patients with primary pulmonary hypertension, with different opinions as to the optimal anesthetic technique. These include combination of intrathecal morphine and pudendal block[38]; combination of segmental epidural block with pudendal block[39]; double catheter epidural technique[40]; and continuous epidural infusion of local anesthetics and opiates.[41] At present, combined spinal-epidural with the administration of intrathecal opiates followed by low-dose, low-concentration epidural infusions of local anesthetics combined with opiates have proven, in our experience, to be effective and safe for use in the laboring parturient with pulmonary hypertension, either primary or secondary.

If cesarean section is indicated, regional anesthesia represents a real risk to these patients. Although major regional blockade, under invasive central monitoring and with careful titration of local anesthetics, has been used in a few reported cases,[42] general anesthesia provides a much more stable hemodynamic condition and should be considered for these patients.

Two subgroups of secondary pulmonary hypertension should be considered. When the disease is secondary to acquired valvular heart disease (usually mitral dysfunction), pulmonary hypertension develops later and has a more benign course. In fact, in this situation, there is usually no pulmonary arteriolar hypertension with underlying anatomic modifications of the vessels and consequently no right chamber impairment. These patients are usually in a state of pulmonary congestion, with venous hypertension, and greatly benefit from the use of regional anesthesia, as it reduces venous return. In other cases, however, evidence of pulmonary arteriolar hyperresistance exists, and in such circumstances general anesthesia should be considered.

If pulmonary hypertension is secondary to congenital heart disease (as in Eisenmenger's syndrome), arteriolar hypertension with underlying anatomic modifications is certainly present. Preload and afterload reduction associated with major regional anesthesia may be dangerous in these patients, owing to an increased right-to-left shunt and a compromise of both oxygenation and myocardial function. Patients undergoing labor and delivery should be managed as those presenting with primary pulmonary hypertension, with a very dilute local anesthetic epidural infusion or a combined spinal-epidural technique, as previously described. Patients undergoing cesarean section should receive general anesthesia.

Pulmonic and Aortic Stenosis

Lesions of the pulmonic and aortic valves are discussed together, as they pose similar problems to the anesthesiologist. Early in the disease course of these patients, the right or left ventricle is hypertrophic, the compliance is low, the systolic volume is somewhat fixed, and the venous return must be optimized to maintain cardiac output.

The choice of anesthetic technique in parturients with these lesions has been a matter of some controversy.[43] At the University of São Paulo, we are very selective in the use of regional anesthesia in these patients, depending on the severity of the disease.

Echocardiography has proven to be a useful tool to assess the severity of the disease in these patients. Both valvular area and transvalvular gradients are important in defining the severity of the case (Table 39–5).

Patients with mild aortic or pulmonic stenosis have few hemodynamic implications and can receive regional anesthesia both for labor and delivery and for cesarean section. Patients with moderate to severe aortic or pulmonic stenosis are optimally managed during labor and delivery with parenteral opioids or very dilute epidural infusions, as described for primary pulmonary hypertension. If cesarean section becomes necessary, general anesthesia is preferred.

Hypertrophic Cardiomyopathy

Hypertrophic cardiomyopathy is in many ways similar to aortic and pulmonic stenosis as regards the anesthetic management. The basic cardiac dysfunction is a dynamic obstruction to left ventricular outflow due to increased contractility of the left ventricle. In these cases, the left ventricle is hypertrophic and its compliance is low. Decreases in preload and afterload are not tolerated in these patients. During labor and delivery, these patients should be managed as those presenting with pulmonary hypertension. If general anesthesia is required for cesarean section, low-concentration vola-

Table 39-5 ECHOCARDIOGRAPHY IN AORTIC AND PULMONIC STENOSIS

SEVERITY OF DISEASE	AORTIC GRADIENT (mm Hg)	AORTIC VALVULAR AREA (cm)	PULMONIC GRADIENT (mm Hg)
Severe	>80	<0.7	>80
Significant	50–80	0.7–0.9	—
Moderate	30–50	1.0–1.2	40–80
Mild	<30	1.3–1.5	<40

tile agents are beneficial in association with a high-dose opiate technique, to reduce myocardial contractility. Isoflurane, however, may not be the best agent to use in these situations, since it may increase cardiac rate and reduce peripheral resistance.

Left-to-Right Shunts

Ventricular septal defect, atrial septal defect, and patent ductus arteriosus are associated with left-to-right shunts. Small communications are not associated with marked hemodynamic changes and these patients can be managed with regional techniques. If larger defects are present, however, there may be a marked increase in pulmonary blood flow and thus pulmonary hypertension may develop. In the presence of pulmonary hypertension (Eisenmenger's syndrome), a right-to-left shunt or bi-directional shunt is an associated finding. In such situations, regional analgesia for labor and delivery may be conducted as for primary pulmonary hypertension. Cesarean section, however, is usually performed under general anesthesia.

Pregnancy in women with Eisenmenger's syndrome is associated with high mortality rates. Avila et al.[44] studied 12 women who opted to continue with their pregnancy despite physician recommendation for therapeutic abortion. Mean systolic and diastolic pulmonary artery pressures were 112.7 mm Hg and 61.7 mm Hg, respectively. There were three spontaneous abortions, one premature labor at 23 weeks of gestation, and two maternal deaths during the 23rd and 27th weeks of gestation. Seven patients reached the end of pregnancy. One of these patients, however, died on the 30th day post partum. All patients underwent cesarean section under an opiate-based general anesthetic technique. Some authors suggest prophylactic anticoagulation during the perioperative period; although this is a standard procedure at the University of São Paulo, it is unclear whether this improves maternal outcome.

Right-to-Left Shunt

Tetralogy of Fallot is representative of a right-to-left shunt. The tetralogy consists of infundibular pulmonary artery stenosis, right ventricular hypertrophy, overriding aorta, and a ventricular septal defect. These patients do not tolerate decreases in preload or afterload, which will further increase their right-to-left shunt. Anesthetic management is similar to that used in pulmonary hypertension if patients have not been surgically treated. For those who have been surgically treated, the shunt should no longer be present, and regional anesthesia techniques are usually acceptable. A detailed evaluation of right ventricular outflow is suggested in these patients. Fortunately, although pulmonic stenosis is usually present, it tends to be of minor importance and does not appear to limit the use of regional techniques.[45]

Myocardial Infarction

Although very uncommon, myocardial infarction in pregnancy is associated with a high maternal mortality rate of 30 to 40%.[46] The prognosis is better if the myocardial infarction occurs in the first or second trimester than in the third trimester. If possible, all obstetric and anesthetic procedures should be postponed for at least 2 weeks after the acute event. Vaginal delivery seems to be associated with a lower incidence of complications,[46] as compared with cesarean section. Regional anesthesia can be beneficial in reducing stress response and avoiding extra cardiac work.[47] The stress response to endotracheal intubation in cases in which general anesthesia is required can be a serious challenge to these patients. Continuous electrocardiographic tracing in lead V5 should be carefully followed for signs of ischemia, which should be immediately treated with nitrates. If myocardial function is adequate, regional anesthesia can be used. If myocardial function is severely compromised as a consequence of the myocardial infarction, however, restrictions to regional anesthesia apply, and if cesarean section is required, general anesthesia is often used.

In the group of patients in whom the cardiac lesions contraindicate the use of a **dense** regional anesthetic block for surgery, it is still often possible to provide safe and effective analgesia for labor and delivery by a continuous epidural infusion of **dilute** local anesthetic plus opioid or by a combined spinal-epidural technique (see Table 39–4). If cesarean section is indicated, however, general anesthesia, unless otherwise contraindicated, is considered to be the first-choice technique.

GENERAL ANESTHESIA FOR THE PREGNANT CARDIAC PATIENT

Opiates constitute the basis of general anesthesia in the cardiac patient, usually providing a rather stable hemodynamic status. Induction agents that allow maximal hemodynamic stability include etomidate and midazolam. Low-concentration inhalational agents must be carefully titrated, as they can seriously compromise myocardial function in some patients. Isoflurane is suitable for situations in which myocardial dysfunction is present, especially if a reduction of peripheral resistance and tachycardia are acceptable (mitral insufficiency and aortic insufficiency). It is, however, contraindicated in situations in which tachycardia or decreases in peripheral resistance would not be tolerated, such as in Eisenmenger's syndrome, mitral and aortic stenosis, and hypertrophic cardiomyopathy. Nitrous oxide can be used following delivery unless pulmonary hypertension is present, in which case its use is controversial. Succinylcholine, especially in cases in which repeated doses are necessary to facilitate endotracheal intubation, must be used carefully because of the bradycardia that is occasionally associated with its use. General anesthesia will not provide the same degree of perioperative hemodynamic stability as regional anesthesia, and one should therefore be prepared to overcome this via the use of vasoactive drugs to control either preload (nitroglycerin) or afterload (sodium nitroprusside), as appropriate.

If general anesthesia becomes necessary, a high-

Table 39–6 GENERAL ANESTHESIA FOR THE PREGNANT CARDIAC PATIENT

- Prepare and monitor the patient
- Maintain IV rate, but avoid overhydration
- Right wedge to maintain left uterine displacement
- Preoxygenation for 3 minutes
- Fentanyl 15 μg/kg + etomidate 0.2 mg/kg
- Succinylcholine 0.5–1 mg/kg
- Sellick's maneuver + tracheal intubation
- Start surgery as soon as endotracheal tube position is verified
- Maintenance:
  - Etomidate 0.05–0.1 mg/kg as required
  - Succinylcholine infusion or nondepolarizing agent as required
  - 50% N_2O if appropriate
  - Supplementary fentanyl 5 μg/kg as required
- Oxytocin infusion (10 IU) after delivery; avoid ergot derivatives

LR, Lactated Ringer's solution.

dose opiate technique is suggested (Table 39–6), although variations of this technique can be adapted to specific cases. Physiologic changes of pregnancy, including increased volume of distribution, higher levels of endorphins, and progesterone-induced stimulation of the respiratory center, are probably responsible for the successful response of this group of patients to the high-dose opiate techniques. Neonatal respiratory depression is not frequent but is certainly possible, and therefore preparation for neonatal resuscitation must be made. To minimize the risk of neonatal depression, the induction-to-delivery time must be as short as possible, thus reducing placental transfer of maternally administered anesthetic agents. Portela et al.[48] have reported the use of 10 μg/kg of fentanyl during general anesthesia for cesarean section and detected neonatal plasma levels lower than 3.0 ng/mL, which is the level known to produce respiratory depression in adults.[49] In that series, neonatal Apgar scores varied from 6 to 9 in the first minute and from 8 to 10 in the fifth minute; all neonates had an Apgar score of 10 in the 10th minute of life.

General anesthesia plays a very important role in the management of pregnant cardiac patients. Despite the well established preference for regional anesthesia in obstetrics, even in the presence of cardiac disease, a certain number of these patients will require general anesthesia. At our institution, general anesthesia for cesarean section is used six times more frequently in the group of cardiac patients than in the general obstetric population.

In a series of 54 cardiac patients undergoing cesarean section at the University of São Paulo in 1987 through 1989, the most frequent indications for general anesthesia were those already highlighted in this chapter; in some patients, however, insufficient documentation of the patient was the primary reason for avoiding regional anesthesia. In this series, no major complications occurred in the group of patients receiving regional anesthesia for cesarean section (34 patients) as compared with six complications in the group undergoing general anesthesia (20 patients). These results may be explained, in part, by the more critical clinical conditions of the patients who underwent general anesthesia. However, it is clear that in some cases, the anesthetic management itself may have contributed to the complication. Overhydration and the use of inhalational agents were found to be the most important causes of cardiac impairment in the perioperative period. Hypervolemia is a frequent intraoperative and postoperative complication associated with pulmonary edema. All efforts should be made to avoid excessive hydration, which may further increase the naturally occurring volume shifts during labor and delivery. In patients who are likely to develop pulmonary congestion and pulmonary edema, diuretics are often introduced intraoperatively or immediately after delivery to reduce the risk of fluid overload.

Preparing the Patient for Surgery

Monitoring. The severity of the disease and the underlying pathophysiology will dictate the standard of monitoring. NYHA functional class I and II patients can usually be managed with continuous noninvasive blood pressure, electrocardiogram, pulse oximeter, and urinary catheter monitoring. NYHA functional class III and IV patients are usually managed with an intra-arterial line, electrocardiogram, central venous pressure, pulse oximeter, and urinary catheter monitoring. The use of a pulmonary artery catheter is helpful when left ventricular function is severely compromised. Although the risk associated with its use is probably no greater in the pregnant patient than in the non-pregnant patient, the Swan-Ganz catheter has been associated with significant morbidity and mortality.[50–52]

Antibiotics. All patients with valvular or congenital defects, whether surgically corrected or not, should receive prophylactic antibiotics. The recommended prophylactic regimen includes ampicilin 2.0 g IV 1 hour before surgery and gentamicin 1.5 mg/kg IM 1 hour before surgery. These drugs should be repeated after 6 hours. If an obstetric infection such as chorioamnionitis is suspected, therapeutic doses of antibiotics should be administered.

CONCLUSION

Successful management of the pregnant patient with underlying cardiac disease depends on the cooperative work of the cardiologist, the obstetrician, and the anesthesiologist. Thorough prenatal care will provide the best clinical conditions and sufficient information on the underlying pathophysiology and its adaptation to pregnancy. A comprehensive understanding of the exact contribution of preload, afterload, heart rate, and myocardial contractility to each particular patient is essential for appropriate indication of the anesthetic technique. Regional anesthesia should be used whenever appropriate, as its hemodynamic effects help accommodate the dramatic hemodynamic fluctuations occurring during labor, delivery, and the immediate postpartum period. The vast majority of patients can receive regional analgesia for labor and delivery. General anesthesia, however, will be necessary for cesarean delivery in certain cases. Should general anesthesia be indicated, a high-dose opiate-based anesthesia technique is often chosen, as it provides good cardiovascular stability. Although neonatal respiratory depression may occur when general anesthesia is utilized, it should nonetheless be used when indicated by maternal condition. General anesthesia does not offer the same degree of protection against the profound hemodynamic fluctuations as regional anesthesia. Fluid overload and the use of myocardial depressants are the most common causes of cardiac dysfunction in these patients. Invasive monitoring is not usually necessary unless the disease is severe and is not easily applicable to the pregnant patient. The anesthesiologist should rely on a comprehensive preoperative evaluation of the case and careful planning of the anesthetic technique following consultation with cardiologist, obstetrician, and intensivist, to provide the best standard of care.

❖ SUMMARY

Key Points

- Cardiac patients will often have worsening of their symptoms between 20 and 24 weeks of gestation and may even require hospitalization during that period.
- Most parturients presenting with mitral stenosis, mitral insufficiency, aortic insufficiency, or dilated cardiomyopathy can be optimally managed with regional anesthesia.
- Aortic stenosis and pulmonary hypertension are not necessarily absolute contraindications to regional anesthesia; however, slow induction of neuraxial block is necessary and single-shot techniques should not be attempted in these patients.
- The successful management of the pregnant patient with underlying cardiac disease depends on the cooperative interaction between cardiologist, obstetrician, and anesthesiologist.

Key Reference

Brighouse D, Whitfield A, Holdcroft A: Anaesthesia for caesarean section in patients with aortic stenosis: The case for regional anaesthesia and the case for general anaesthesia. Anaesthesia 1998; 53:107–112.

Case Stem

A 34-year-old primiparous Asian parturient with a history of rheumatic heart disease and mitral stenosis is admitted in active labor complaining of dyspnea. The patient had an echocardiogram prior to this pregnancy, at which time the valve orifice was 1 cm^2 and moderate pulmonary hypertension was reported. Discuss the obstetric management as well as the anesthetic options you would consider.

References

1. Report on confidential enquiries into maternal deaths in the United Kingdom 1991–1993. London, HMSO, 1996.
2. Boyacyan K, Marcus PAF, Veja CEP, et al: Maternal mortality in São Paulo City from 1993 to 1995. Rev Bras Ginecol Obstet 1998; 20:13–18.
3. Ávila WS, Grinberg M: Gestação em portadoras de afecções cardiovasculares. Experiência com 1000 casos. Arq Bras Cardiol 1993; 60:5–11.
4. Mangano DT: Anesthesia for the pregnant cardiac patient. In Shnider SM, Levinson G (eds): Anesthesia for Obstetrics. Baltimore: Williams & Wilkins, 1987.
5. Ueland K, Hansen JM: Maternal cardiovascular dynamics II. Posture and uterine contractions. Am J Obstet Gynecol 1969; 103:1–7.
6. Ueland K, Hansen JM: Maternal cardiovascular dynamics. III. Labor and delivery under local and caudal analgesia. Am J Obstet Gynecol 1969; 103:8–18.
7. Ueland K, Novy M, Peterson E, Metcalf J: Maternal cardiovascular dynamics. IV. The influence of gestational age on the maternal cardiovascular response to posture and exercise. Am J Obstet Gynecol 1969; 104:156–164.
8. Clark SL, Phelan JP, Aldahl D, Horenstein J: Labor and delivery in the presence of mitral stenosis: Central hemodynamic observations. Am J Obstet Gynecol 1985; 152:984–988.
9. Criteria Committee of the New York Heart Association: Nomenclature and Criteria for Diagnosis of Diseases of the Heart and Great Vessels. New York: New York Heart Association, 1979.
10. Marcus FI, Ewy GA, O'Rourke RA, et al: The effect of pregnancy on the murmurs of mitral and aortic regurgitation. Circulation 1970; 41:795–805.
11. Shaul WL, Hall JG: Multiple congenital anomalies associated with oral anticoagulants. Am J Obstet Gynecol 1977; 27:191–198.
12. Faccioli R: Area da valva mitral estenótica em gestantes portadoras de doenca reumática: Correlação com o prognóstico perinatal. Tese de Doutoramento. Faculdade de Medicina da Universidade de São Paulo, 1990.
13. Hemmings GT, Whalley DG, O'Connor PJ, et al: Invasive monitoring and anaesthetic management of a parturient with mitral stenosis. Can J Anaesth 1987; 34:182–185.
14. Mostafa SM: Spinal anaesthesia for caesarean section management of a parturient with severe cardiovascular disease. Br J Anaesth 1984; 56:1275–1277.
15. Braunwald E: Valvular heart disease. In Braunwald E (ed): Heart Disease, 4th ed. Philadelphia: W. B. Saunders; 1992: 1011.
16. Al Kasab SM, Sabag T, Al Zeibag M: Beta-adrenergic blockade in the management of pregnant women with mitral stenosis. Am J Obstet Gynecol 1990; 165:37–40.
17. Rapaport E: Natural risk of aortic and mitral valve disease. Am J Cardiol 1975; 35:221–227.
18. Hanson EW, Neerhut RK, Lynch C: Mitral valve prolapse. Anesthesiology 1995; 85:178–195.
19. Shapiro EP, Trimble EL, Robinson JC, et al: Safety of labor and delivery in women with mitral valve prolapse. Am J Cardiol 1985; 56:806–807.
20. Moraes TABPP: Pregnancy in patients with Chagas' disease. Rev Soc Cardiol Estado de São Paulo 1994; 6:547–551.
21. George LM, Gatt SP, Lowe S: Peripartum cardiomyopathy: Four case histories and a commnetary on anaesthetic management. Anaesth Intensive Care 1997; 25:292–296.
22. Brown CS, Bertolet BD: Peripartum cardiomyopathy: A comprehensive review. Am J Obstet Gynecol 1998; 178:409–414.
23. Sanderson JE, Adesanaya CO, Anjorin FI, Parry EH: Maternal cardiomyopathy of pregnancy: Heart failure due to volume overload? Am Heart J 1979; 97:613–621.
24. Lampert MB, Weinert L, Hibbard J: Contractile reserve in patients with peripartum cardiomyopathy and recovered left ventricular function. Am J Obstet Gynecol 1997; 176:189–195.
25. Witlin AG, Mabie WC, Sibai BM: Peripartum cardiomyopathy: A longitudinal echocardiographic study. Am J Obstet Gynecol 1997; 177:1129–1132.
26. Witlin AG, Mabie WC, Sibai BM: Peripartum cardiomyopathy:

An ominous diagnosis. Am J Obstet Gynecol 1997; 176:182–189.

27. Kim KM, Sukhani R, Slogoff S, Tomich PG: Central hemodynamic changes associated with pregnancy in a long-term cardiac transplant recipient. Am J Obstet Gynecol 1996; 174:1651–1653.
28. Eskandar M, Gader S, Ong BY: Two successsful vaginal deliveries in a heart transplant recipient. Obstet Gynecol 1996; 88:880.
29. Scott JR, Wagoner LE, Olsen SL, et al: Pregnancy in heart transplant recipients: Management and outcome. Obstet Gynecol 1993; 82:324–327.
30. Leachman RD, Cokkinas DV, Cabrera R: Response of the transplanted, denervated heart to cardiovascular drugs. Am J Cardiol 1971; 27:272–276.
31. Yusef S, Theodoropoulos S, Mathias CJ, et al: Increased sensitivity of the denervated transplanted human heart to isoprenaline both before and after adrenergic blockade. Circulation 1987; 75:696–704.
32. Kossoy LR, Herbert CM, Wentz AC: Management of heart transplant recipients: Guidelines for the obstetrician-gynecologist. Am J Obstet Gynecol 1988; 159:490–499.
33. Camann WR, Goldman GA, Johnson MD, et al: Cesarean delivery in a patient with a transplanted heart. Anesthesiology 1989; 71:618–620.
34. Hosenpud JD, Bennett LE, Keck BM, et al: The registry of the international society for heart and lung transplantation: Fourteenth official report. J Heart Lung Transplant 1997; 16:691–712.
35. Rao TLK, El-Etr AA: Anticoagulation following placement of epidural and subarachnoid catheters. Anesthesiology 1981; 55:618–620.
36. American Society of Regional Anesthesia: Neuraxial Anesthesia and Anticoagulation. American Society of Regional Anesthesia Consensus Statement, May, 1998.
37. Nelson DM, Main E, Crafford W, Ahumada GG: Peripartum heart failure due to primary pulmonary hypertension. Obstet Gynecol 1983; 62:58S–63S.
38. Abboud T, Raya J, Noueihed R, Daniel J: Intrathecal morphine for relief of labor pain in a parturient with severe pulmonary hypertension. Anesthesiology 1983; 59:477–479.
39. Sorensen MB, Korshin JD, Fernandes A, Secher O: The use of epidural analgesia for delivery in a patient with pulmonary hypertension. Acta Anesthesiol Scand 1982; 26:180–182.
40. Slomka F, Salmeron S, Zetlaoui P, et al: Primary pulmonary hypertension and pregnancy: Anesthetic management for delivery. Anesthesiology 1988; 69:959–961.
41. Robinson DE, Leicht CH: Epidural analgesia with low-dose bupivacaine and fentanyl for labor and delivery in a parturient with severe pulmonary hypertension. Anesthesiology 1988; 68:285–288.
42. Spinnato JA, Kraynack BJ, Cooper MW: Eisenmenger's syndrome in pregnancy: Epidural anesthesia for elective cesarean section. N Engl J Med 1981; 304:1215–1217.
43. Brighouse D, Whitfield A, Holdcroft A: Anaesthesia for caesarean section in patients with aortic stenosis: The case for regional anaesthesia and the case for general anaesthesia. Anaesthesia 1998; 53:107–112.
44. Avila WS, Grinberg M, Snitcowsky R, et al: Maternal and fetal outcome in pregnant women with Eisenmenger's syndrome. Eur Heart J 1995; 16:460–464.
45. Carvalho JCA, Mathias RS, Siaulys MM, et al: Anesthesia for cesarean section in patients with surgically corrected tetralogy of Fallot. Braz J Anesthesiol Int Issue 1993; 4:32–34.
46. Hankins GDV, Wendel GD, Leveno KJ, Stoneham J: Myocardial infarction during pregnancy: A review. Obstet Gynecol 1985; 65:139–145.
47. Hands ME, Johnson MD, Saltzman DH, Rutherford JD: The cardiac, obstetric, and anesthetic management of pregnancy complicated by acute myocardial infarction. J Clin Anesth 1990; 2:258–268.
48. Portela AAV, Reis GFF, Melo GA, Cyreno NU: General anesthesia for cesarean section with fentanyl: Maternal and fetal plasma concentrations. Braz J Anesthesiol Int Issue 1990; 3:35–37.
49. Stoeckel H, Schuttler J, Magnussen H, Hengstmann JH: Plasma fentanyl concentration and the ocurrence of respiratory depression in volunteers. Br J Anaesth 1982; 54:1087–1095.
50. Devitt JW, Noble WH, Byrick BJ: A Swan-Ganz catheter related complication in a patient with Eisenmenger's syndrome. Anesthesiology 1982; 57:335–337.
51. Robinson S: Pulmonary artery catheters in Eisenmenger's syndrome: Many risks, few benefits. Anesthesiology 1983; 58:588–589.
52. Schwalbe SS, Deshmukh SM, Marx GF: Use of pulmonary artery catheterization in parturients with Eisenmenger's syndrome. Anesth Analg 1990; 71:442–443.

40

Pulmonary Disease in the Pregnant Patient

DAN BENHAMOU, MD
FRÉDERIC J. MERCIER, MD
MARIE-LOUISE FELTEN, MD

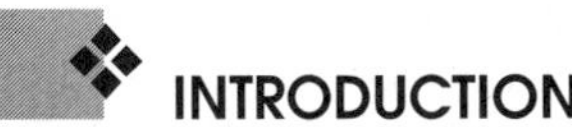

INTRODUCTION

Major alterations occur in the respiratory system during pregnancy which serve to meet the increased oxygen demand by the growing fetus. These changes have been reviewed in detail by Lapinsky and colleagues[1] and are described in Chapter 2 of this text and are not detailed here. Hyperventilation and increased cardiac output arise to meet the increased metabolic rate and limit the physiologic reserve of the cardiorespiratory system, thus explaining why any preexisting cardiac or respiratory disease may easily decompensate during pregnancy. Moreover, because of the associated increase in blood volume, pulmonary edema may occur even in the absence of any preexisting disease. This occurs as a consequence of several triggering factors including aspiration of gastric contents, preeclampsia, or sepsis. This chapter reviews the current knowledge on the clinical course of acute respiratory failure occurring in pregnant patients as well as the influence of labor and delivery on respiratory function. Finally the influence of pregnancy on chronic respiratory illness is detailed, with special emphasis on asthma.

ACUTE RESPIRATORY FAILURE IN PREGNANCY

Definition and General Problems

According to a recent consensus conference,[2] acute lung injury (ALI) is defined as a disease of acute onset with a Pa_{O_2}/F_{IO_2} of 300 mm Hg or less (regardless of positive end-expiratory pressure [PEEP]) and with bilateral infiltrates seen on the frontal chest radiograph. Acute respiratory distress syndrome (ARDS) is defined by the same criteria except that Pa_{O_2}/F_{IO_2} should be less than 200 mm Hg (regardless of the level of PEEP). Although the mechanisms and causes are similar for both situations, the severity of hypoxemia in ARDS may require more aggressive therapy, which by itself may produce undesired consequences. High levels of PEEP may reduce cardiac output and subsequently decrease oxygen delivery to the mother. Moreover, hypoxemia and decreased oxygen delivery may have deleterious consequences on the fetus and may require cesarean delivery to relieve fetal hypoxia, decrease oxygen consumption, and facilitate maternal care.[3] Maternal sedation that may be required to facilitate mechanical ventilation may also sedate the fetus and render difficult the analysis of fetal heart rate tracings. Recent data also suggest that the prone position may, in severe lung disease, improve oxygenation dramatically, thereby allowing decreased airway pressure and reduced F_{IO_2}.[4] The enlarged uterus, however, impedes ventral positioning and venous return, thereby leading to more difficult therapy. By contrast, when ARDS occurs after delivery therapeutic rules are similar to those used in nonpregnant patients.[5] There are no data comparing outcomes with ARDS in pregnant and nonpregnant women. This would, however, be useful because pregnancy-induced cardiopulmonary changes have been said to potentiate respiratory deterioration and to increase the risk of death. For example, it has been postulated that the prominent role of aspiration of gastric contents as a cause of death in pregnant women is related to pregnancy-related cardiopulmonary changes.[6] Moreover, it is unclear if imbalance of the immune system occurs during pregnancy and predisposes to increased severity of septic complications.[7]

Causes of Acute Lung Disease in Pregnancy

Most conditions leading to acute respiratory failure in pregnancy are pregnancy related. Moreover, they do not usually occur in isolation and are very often associated with a complicated pregnancy or parturition, which often requires an urgent cesarean delivery. In the largest series of ARDS in pregnancy reported to date, the syndrome occurred in 1 in 2900 deliveries and primarily in the third trimester.[8] The most common causes were infection (50%), preeclampsia-eclampsia (25%), and hemorrhage (12.5%). Two thirds of the infants were delivered before or soon after the maternal diagnosis, and maternal mortality was 44%. In the *Report on Confidential Enquiry into Maternal Deaths in the United Kingdom*,[9] a special chapter on ARDS as the main cause of death was included, in order to highlight this acute disease as a risk of death. Hemorrhage, pneumonia, and aspiration were the most frequent causes of ARDS. Sepsis and preeclampsia, while potential causes of ARDS, were less common.

Pulmonary Aspiration. Aspiration of gastric contents has long been the main cause of anesthetic-related maternal mortality. After recognition that rapid-sequence induction and tracheal intubation during general anesthesia may protect the airway from aspiration, a decline in aspiration-related deaths occurred, but an increase in difficult intubation–related deaths was also seen. In total, the overall number of anesthetic deaths has decreased, thus suggesting an increased quality of anesthetic care. In the most recent Triennial Report of 1994 to 1996, no deaths related to aspiration were seen.[10] In addition, Warner and colleagues[11] reported that no aspiration occurred in 456 cesarean deliveries, while the pulmonary aspiration syndrome occurred in 1 in 895 cases of emergency nonobstetric surgery. Unfortunately, aspiration-related deaths recurred in the Triennial Report of 1991 to 1993. Chestnut,[12] in an astute editorial, warned against the risk of considering aspiration a disappearing condition and reemphasized that well-accepted precautions (i.e., fasting guidelines, antacid prophylaxis, rapid-sequence induction, tracheal intubation, and cricoid pressure), although perhaps of equivocal efficacy in individual cases, should be used in every case to maintain present commendable results.

Even when maternal mortality does not occur, aspiration may be of significant concern, because it can cause severe lung disease. Sibai and colleagues[13] have reported that gastric aspiration is the most frequent respiratory complication causing ARDS during pregnancy and immediately post partum. More recent reports, however, have not shown that aspiration is a leading cause of maternal admission to an intensive care unit. For example, Kilpatrick and Matthay[14] described only one patient who aspirated among 8 cases of acute lung injury in pregnant women, and in a recent series of causes of acute respiratory failure, none was related to aspiration. Thus, the declining role of aspiration is likely related to the widespread use of prophylactic maneuvers during induction of general anesthesia.

Preeclampsia and Eclampsia. Today, in many countries pulmonary edema has become a rare complication of preeclampsia-eclampsia, but this has not always been the case, but it still occurs in countries where parturients do not receive the benefits of modern health care. In 1954, Donnelly and Lock reported on 533 patients who died from pregnancy induced hypertension and in their report, pulmonary edema was considered the cause of death in 25% of the cases.[13] In the largest recent series, 37 cases have been reported by Sibai and colleagues,[13] who reported an overall incidence of pulmonary edema of 2.9% in preeclamptic patients. Unfortunately, this incidence was reduced to only 1.7% when considering patients with no superimposed disease. In their series of 37 cases, four deaths occurred, but pulmonary edema was not the main cause of death in any of these patients. Rather, in most cases, pulmonary edema was only one feature of multiple organ failure, with coagulopathy occurring in 50% of patients and acute renal failure in 27% of patients. The onset of pulmonary edema occurred before delivery in only one third of their patients and almost all these patients (10 of 11) had preexisting chronic hypertension. It is unknown from the data presented by these authors how severe the ventilation-perfusion mismatch was, because their report included no information on oxygenation or mechanical ventilation. Unfortunately, the results of the hemodynamic investigations performed in 18 of 37 patients were also not reported, so that we are left with only speculations as regards the mechanism of pulmonary edema. The authors do emphasize that most cases of pulmonary edema occurred 2 to 3 days after delivery and might have been a consequence of large volume expansion at the time of delivery and of delayed postpartum mobilization of extracellular fluids. Diuretics such as furosemide may help prevent the occurrence of pulmonary edema, as well as treat any significant increase in arterial blood pressure. Recent data[15] also suggest that low-dose dopamine may have a diuretic action in postpartum preeclamptic women with oliguria.

Sepsis. Sepsis may also lead to pulmonary edema and to ARDS in pregnant patients, just as it can in nonpregnant patients. Sepsis syndrome, with or without hypotension, can manifest with signs both of systemic inflammation and of organ dysfunction, including the lung.[2] Pyelonephritis is the most common cause of sepsis, and about 2% of pregnant patients with sepsis syndrome develop some degree of respiratory insufficiency.[16] The incidence of ARDS in this situation is unclear because strict criteria were not provided. It has been noted that less severe urinary tract infections may also lead to pulmonary edema, especially when systemic tocolysis is used.[17] In other words, a majority of patients in preterm labor destined to develop pulmonary edema while being treated with systemic tocolytic agents may have an underlying infection. A similar negative role of tocolytics has also been described in other maternal infections. In 49 patients with appendicitis during pregnancy,[18] pulmonary edema developed in 18% of them. None of these patients was suspected to have suffered from aspiration during anesthesia.

β_2-Adrenergic Agonists. Maternal injection of β_2-agonists can also lead to pulmonary edema. Pisani and Rosenow[19] in a literature review of 58 cases found that the incidence of pulmonary edema in pregnant women who receive tocolytic agents may be as high as 5%. Mechanical ventilation was required in 4 (7%) patients with pulmonary edema, and mortality occurred in the 2 patients (3.5%) who developed features resembling ARDS. Otherwise, rapid clinical response, usually occurring in less than 12 hours, was the rule and the maternal outcome was excellent. Of note, in 15 of 58 patients symptoms developed after discontinuation of therapy, and a mean duration of tocolysis of 54 hours was observed before pulmonary edema occurred. As stated previously, this pulmonary edema is most likely caused primarily by hemodynamic disturbances, because increased pulmonary capillary permeability has not been demonstrated in humans.[20] Fluid overload occurs as a consequence of antidiuretic hormone and renin release by β-adrenergic agonists, which leads to water and salt retention.[21] Large volumes of fluid are also often administered, in part to compensate for the vasodilator effect of these agents. Altered heart function and increased heart rate may also contribute.[20] In the Triennial Report of 1991 to 1993,[22] simple guidelines are proposed: infusion through a controlled device is preferable, and a maximum concentration of 6 μg/kg/min of ritodrine should be used, such that the total daily dose should not exceed 120 mg. Frequent observations of respiratory symptoms and of heart rate are mandatory, while particular caution should be exercised in patients with cardiac disease, multiple pregnancy, infection, and diabetes.

Less frequently, other causes of sepsis can also produce pulmonary edema or ARDS. Chorioamnionitis, staphylococcal septicemia,[23] and surgical emergencies other than appendicitis have anecdotally been reported as precipitating pulmonary edema. When lung infection becomes diffuse and severe enough to meet the ALI/ARDS definition, the consensus is now to consider other causes of ALI/ARDS.[2] In a series of 71 pregnant women admitted with community-acquired pneumonia, chronic underlying maternal disease was identified in 31 of 71 women (44%) with asthma being the most common cause.[24] The etiology, however, was established in only 19 of 71 women.

***Streptococcus pneumoniae* and Varicella.** Pneumonia in pregnancy is caused by *S. pneumoniae* or varicella infection in 5 out of 71 (7%) women. Varicella pneumonia is the most common infectious childhood disease occurring in adults. Although varicella infection occurs in as few as 1 to 5 per 10,000 pregnant patients, it requires special attention for several reasons. Pulmonary involvement is more common in pregnancy than in the adult normal population (up to 50% of cases) and if the problem goes untreated, mortality may be as high as 45%.[25] Smoking and any previous respiratory disease both contribute to an increased severity. The time profile for pulmonary infiltrates correlates well with that of the skin rash and of pharyngeal lesions. Delivery of the infant, if possible, should be avoided in the days immediately before or after the onset of skin rash. Acyclovir in high doses (15–45 mg/kg/day) decreases symptoms, and mortality is significantly decreased if treatment is started early (within the first 72 hours of dyspnea). Acyclovir poses no threat to the fetus, and the newborn should be treated with varicella immunoglobulin. With adapted and early treatment, mortality from varicella pneumonia has decreased but remains at 15% to 20%.

Tuberculosis. Although tuberculosis was not seen in the series reported by Richey and coinvestigators,[24] testing with intradermal tuberculin is recommended in symptomatic immigrant, indigent pregnant women as well as in those in whom immunodepression (most frequently as a consequence of human immunodeficiency virus infection) is detected. Data on antibiotics necessary to treat tuberculosis in pregnancy are rare. Generally because of the severity of the disease itself, treatment cannot be delayed.

Pulmonary Embolism. Acute pulmonary embolism remains a major cause of death in pregnant women.[26] The real incidence of deep vein thrombosis (DVT) and of pulmonary embolism is not well known because diagnosis is difficult. In one study using venography,[27] monthly rates of DVT of 0.01 per 1000 patients during pregnancy and of 0.6 per 1000 patients in the postpartum period have been reported. In those studies in which the diagnosis was made only on clinical grounds, much higher incidences have been reported. Many also believe that the rate of DVT is greater in the postpartum period. However, in recent series, DVT did not appear to be more frequent in the postpartum period, probably because early mobilization is now common.[28] DVT is more often seen in the left leg because of compression by the iliac artery and by the uterus.[28] Physiologic changes of pregnancy, including an increase in coagulation factors and the changes in venous system compliance, increase the likelihood of DVT.[1] Several risk factors are also well known: age greater than 35 years, cesarean delivery, bed rest during pregnancy, and obesity all join to increase the risk of DVT.[26] More importantly, a previous history of DVT during pregnancy increases the risk, particularly when hereditary thrombophilia is recognized. Not all congenital deficits are linked with a major risk,[29] and a hereditary deficit of antithrombin carries a much higher risk than a factor V Leiden mutation.[30] Unfractionated heparin has long been considered the main drug for treatment and prophylaxis; however, several recent studies have demonstrated the effectiveness and safety profile of low-molecular-weight heparins (LMWHs).[31] The clinical diagnosis of DVT or of pulmonary embolism is often difficult, and invasive tests may be necessary if the appropriate patients are to receive anticoagulants. When acute severe pulmonary embolism is suspected, unfractionated heparin should be started intravenously and may be replaced by LMWH after several days of effective anticoagulation. Treatment should be continued during the entire pregnancy and maintained for 4 to 6 weeks post partum. The total duration of treatment should not be less than 3 months.[26] Prophylaxis against thromboembolism after cesarean section is based mostly on anecdotal recommendations, because there are very few studies in this area. Uncomplicated cesarean delivery in healthy parturients should not be followed by prophylactic treatment. By contrast, moderate- or high-risk situations may benefit from unfractionated heparin or LMWH.[32]

Acute Respiratory Failure During Labor and Delivery

Dyspnea. Dyspnea or more severe respiratory failure is very uncommon during delivery. Labor pain increases ventilation, and effective pain relief by epidural analgesia decreases oxygen consumption and alveolar ventilation. Expulsive efforts have been suggested to induce fatigue of the diaphragm[33] as evidenced by electromyography analysis (reduced high/low frequency ratio) and by a decrease of maximal inspiratory pressure immediately after delivery (from 103 to 72 cm H_2O). However, several limitations of this study (in particular the nonspecific value of reduced spectral electromyographic analysis and the changes in lung volume after delivery) preclude definitive conclusions. An increase in alveolar pressure may also lead to Hamman's syndrome, that is, pneumomediastinum and subcutaneous emphysema related to rupture of marginal alveoli.[34] Pain occurring immediately after air escape from the alveoli may be intense, and the differential diagnosis includes angina pectoris, myocardial infarction, dissecting aneurysm of the aorta, and pulmonary embolism. Pneumothorax may also occur, however, with a very low incidence.

Anesthesia-Related Respiratory Failure. Other causes of respiratory failure during labor may be related to anesthesia, such as opioid-induced respiratory depression. This may occur after either systemic opioid administration[35] or epidural analgesia[36] or, more recently described, after the use of intrathecal lipophilic opioids.[37] Respiratory paralysis during epidural anesthesia as a consequence of inadvertent total spinal block is also possible.

Amniotic Fluid Embolism. Perhaps the most common cause of acute life-threatening respiratory failure during labor is amniotic fluid embolism. As discussed in Chapter 31, this relatively rare event carries a high risk of mortality[38] and often includes acute respiratory failure, circulatory shock, and coagulopathy. Although many risk factors have been discussed, this catastrophic event remains impossible to predict. This is also reflected by our complete lack of understanding of its pathophysiology. Pulmonary vasospasm and obstruction as well as left ventricular failure contribute to cardiorespiratory complications.[39] It is hoped that since early diagnosis and treatment are more frequent because of the increased presence of anesthesiologists in labor and delivery, favorable outcomes will be seen more frequently.[40]

Postpartum Respiratory Complications

Respiratory problems may also occur in the postpartum period. Some of these are frequent and often unrecognized. Pleural effusions, for example, occur in as many as 67% of patients in the first 24 hours after vaginal delivery. Most of these effusions are quite small and not indicative of cardiopulmonary abnormality.[41] Increased blood volume during pregnancy and Valvasa maneuvers typical of second-stage labor may explain the occurrence of these effusions. They almost never require any intervention.

Cesarean delivery itself may lead to decreased lung volume, but in the vast majority of patients this resolves without any consequence. Cesarean delivery, as any other abdominal surgical procedure, may produce reflex diaphragmatic dysfunction and/or increased tension of abdominal muscles. These changes are already observed during the surgery, because epidural anesthesia also causes a restrictive syndrome.[42]

Other respiratory complications may be more serious and lead to ALI and/or ARDS. Their causes are similar to those previously discussed. Management of ARDS, regardless of cause, is much easier after delivery of the infant.

EXACERBATION OF CHRONIC RESPIRATORY DISEASE DURING PREGNANCY

Asthma

Definition and Epidemiology. Recent research has underlined the central role of airway inflammation and the variability of its consequences. Asthma is "a chronic inflammatory disorder of the airways in which many cells play a role . . . . In susceptible individuals this inflammation causes symptoms which are usually associated with widespread but variable airflow obstruction that is often reversible, . . . and causes an associated increase in airway responsiveness to a variety of stimuli."[43] Asthma is the most common chronic pulmonary disease of pregnancy. The prevalence of asthma in the general population has been reported to be increasing in the United States, Europe, New Zealand, and Australia.[43] In fact, recent information suggests that up to 7% of pregnancies are complicated by asthma.[44]

Effect of Pregnancy on Asthma. As with many other chronic diseases, pregnancy has an unpredictable effect on asthma. It has been reported that asthma becomes worse in one third of pregnant women and less severe in one third and remains unchanged in the other third.[45, 46] This contrasts with the marked twofold reduction in sensitivity to methacholine reported during the second and third trimesters of pregnancy.[47] Statistically, patients with severe asthma are at greater risk for deterioration during pregnancy, particularly between 17 and 36 weeks' gestation.[46] Adequate treatment also plays a major role in the course of asthma. Interestingly, acute asthma is uncommon during the last month of pregnancy, and more specifically asthma is often quiescent during labor and delivery.[46, 48] Although symptoms were reported in 10% of 366 asthmatic women during labor and delivery, only 2 parturients (0.5%) required systemic medication (aminophylline) and no complications occurred.[46] In one study, acute exacerbations of asthma were shown to be much more frequent after cesarean section (18-fold higher relative risk) than after vaginal delivery.[49] However, despite a 28% cesarean section rate, asthma caused no emergencies in a series of 198 deliveries.[50] In most patients, asthma reverts to its prepregnancy status during the 3 months post partum.[46] Sixty percent of women follow the same pattern during subsequent pregnancies. The asthma rarely worsens, but it may be better if treatment has been reevaluated and adjusted earlier.[50]

Effect of Asthma on Pregnancy. As a result of maternal hypoxia, uncontrolled asthma may result in adverse outcomes, including increased rate of cesarean section,[49, 50] low birthweight, prematurity, or even perinatal morbidity and mortality. In addition, some studies have reported increased incidence for hyperemesis gravidarum, antepartum and postpartum hemorrhage, placenta previa, neonatal hypoxia, and neonatal hyperbilirubinemia.[46] Schatz[46] suggests that the goals of gestational asthma therapy should include optimization of pulmonary function (i.e., forced expiratory volume in 1 second [FEV_1]) in addition to achievement of symptomatic control. Stenius-Aarniala and associates[50] reported normal neonatal outcomes and a low increased risk for mild hypertension. These good results were recently confirmed by very large case-controlled studies.[44, 46] The only clinically significant concern in one study was an increased risk for antepartum and postpartum hemorrhage, which was independent of medication usage.[44] Thus, the overall message to the pregnant woman with asthma should be reassurance, provided that her asthma remains carefully controlled by adequate treatment.[51]

Asthma Management During Pregnancy

The course of asthma during pregnancy remains largely unpredictable for each individual. As a consequence, women with asthma need to be followed more closely during pregnancy, and their medications should be adjusted as required. Many indirect and direct data support the concept that the better controlled the asthma, the better the outcome in terms of intrauterine growth, term birth, and perinatal well-being.[46] Accordingly, the main goals for asthma therapy, defined in 1993 by the Working Group on Asthma and Pregnancy, are full control of symptoms (including nocturnal symptoms), maintenance of (near) normal pulmonary function, and prevention of acute asthmatic episodes.[45, 48] To achieve these goals, the Working Group recommended a four-component program of pulmonary monitoring, control of asthma triggers, pharmacologic management, and patient education.[45]

Pulmonary Monitoring. Objective measurements of lung volumes and flow rates are considered essential for assessing and monitoring severity of asthma in order to make appropriate therapeutic recommendations.[45, 48] Although changes in some lung volumes occur during pregnancy, FEV_1 and the peak expiratory flow rate (PEFR) normally remain unchanged. Predicted values of PEFR are in the range of 380 to 550 L/min, but the use of a "personal best" PEFR as a reference is more informative. Pregnant women with moderate to severe asthma should make PEFR measurements twice daily (in the morning on rising and 12 hours later), and these records should be brought to each antenatal visit.

Control of Asthma Triggers. The avoidance and control of asthma triggers is too often neglected, although it is a major factor in reducing the risk of exacerbations and medication requirements. Many triggers should be considered and this is best done by an asthma specialist. For example, the removal of furred or feathered pets from the patient's bedroom or household may be required, mattresses and pillows should be encased, and air conditioning may be useful. Patients who are sensitive to sulfites from food additives or drugs such as aspirin should avoid exposure to them. Exposure to tobacco smoke and β-blockers should be eliminated.

Pharmacologic Management. A step-care pharmacologic management of chronic asthma is recommended. Only pregnant patients with *mild* and *intermittent* asthma may use only inhaled β_2-agonists on an as-needed basis. These patients have episodes of wheezing, coughing, and difficult breathing less than twice a week, have nocturnal cough and wheezing less than twice a month, and are free of any symptoms between episodes.[45] The safety of inhaled β_2-agonists is well documented during pregnancy.[45, 52]

DAILY ANTI-INFLAMMATORY THERAPY. Daily anti-inflammatory therapy is recommended for all patients with more than mild and intermittent asthma. The Working Group suggested either cromolyn sodium or inhaled corticosteroids. Cromolyn sodium is safe in pregnancy[52] and virtually devoid of side effects.[45] If cromolyn sodium was effective prior to pregnancy, it should be continued throughout the pregnancy. Inhaled corticosteroids are now considered as first-line therapy in the treatment of nonpregnant adults with persistent asthma.[53] Moreover, two recent studies have documented dramatic beneficial effects during pregnancy. In a prospective nonrandomized study, only 4% of the 257 patients treated with inhaled beclomethasone or budesonide, from the beginning of pregnancy, had an acute attack of asthma compared with 17% of the 177 patients not initially treated with inhaled corticosteroids.[54] In a second study, 65 patients hospitalized for acute asthma were randomized, on discharge, to receive either albuterol with an oral steroid taper only, or the same regimen plus inhaled beclomethasone. The addition of inhaled beclomethasone produced a nearly three-fold decrease in the readmission rate (12% vs. 33%).[55] Full benefit of inhaled corticosteroids may require 2 to 4 weeks' treatment[45] (unless a tapering course of oral steroid is used). Systemic effects are minimal with the relatively low doses (100–400 μg) that are needed to control moderate asthma.[45] Despite previous concerns, the safety of inhaled corticosteroids during pregnancy is now well established;[46, 52] however, as in nonpregnant patients, the use of a spacer is recommended.

SUSTAINED-RELEASE THEOPHYLLINE. Sustained-release theophylline has been advocated as once-daily therapy for patients with primarily nocturnal symptoms.[45] However, the recent availability of long-acting inhaled β_2-agonists has challenged this specific indication. Theophylline, however, may be considered as a third-line agent.[49] Nonetheless, it has been suggested that the addition of theophylline to β_2-agonists may not confer additional benefits.[55] In addition, theophylline clearance may vary during pregnancy, and thus close monitoring with reduction in dose may be required. Theophylline freely crosses the placenta and newborns exposed in utero may exhibit transient jitteriness, vomiting, and tachycardia when serum theophylline levels are just above the upper recommended range for the mother (12 mg/mL).[45] Although theophylline has a wide and long-standing use in pregnancy,[46] recent evidence suggests a possible (weak) association with congenital malformations.[52] An ongoing multicenter, double blind, randomized clinical trial will undoubtedly help to define the role, if any, of theophylline in asthma during pregnancy.[56]

ORAL CORTICOSTEROIDS. Oral corticosteroids are indicated as a short tapering course when progressive deterioration of asthma develops despite the combination of bronchodilators and inhaled corticosteroids even at increased doses.[45] Gradual reductions in PEFR (more than 20–30% during worst exacerbations) and/or development of nocturnal symptoms usually characterize such a deterioration. Chronic therapy (>2 weeks) should be reserved for patients with severe asthma (<5% of asthma patients[49]) and administered under the supervision of a specialist.[45] Oral corticosteroids may be associated theoretically with many side effects. However, these effects are dose- and duration-dependent and in a population of 824 pregnant women with asthma subjected to multivariate analysis, only a low increase in preeclampsia was related to oral corticosteroids.[46] Of note, a placental enzyme metabolizes nearly 90% of the prednisone[49] to prednisolone, which does not significantly cross the placenta.

ANTICHOLINERGICS. Anticholinergic agents have no clear established role in day-to-day management of the pregnant patient with asthma. However, ipratropium (which lacks atropine's side effects) has been shown to be effective for adjunctive therapy in acute exacerbations of asthma.[45]

Patient Education. Patient education is essential to avoid undertreatment related to maternal fears over possible harm to the fetus.[51] The pregnant woman should be reminded that she is breathing for two.[48] General practitioners' information is essential as well.[51]

Asthma Management During Labor and Delivery

It is of the utmost importance to continue asthma medications throughout labor and the peripartum period. It should also be remembered that β-blockers, prostaglandin $F_{2\alpha}$, and ergot alkaloids (methylergonovine and ergonovine) are relatively contraindicated in the parturient with asthma because they may precipitate bronchospasm.[45] Oxytocin, however, may be safely used for induction of labor. The bronchodilating effect of prostaglandin E_2 has been extensively documented,[45, 46, 57] but paradoxical bronchoconstriction with its use has been reported. Prostaglandin E_2, however, remains the safest analogue as second-line treatment to control uterine atony and bleeding in patients with asthma when oxytocin is not sufficient.[45]

Preanesthetic Assessment. The preanesthetic assessment of a pregnant woman with asthma should optimally be performed several weeks before delivery, during an antenatal visit. Mainly on the basis of history and recordings of PEFR (if performed by the patient), the anesthesiologist can determine the severity of the asthma and if it is optimally controlled. If the asthma is not adequately controlled, the several weeks available before delivery will be very useful, particularly in allowing sufficient time to gain full benefit from inhaled corticosteroids. If the asthma proves to be severe and not treated optimally, the patient should be referred without delay to an asthma specialist.[45]

Anesthesia Management. Adequate labor analgesia is useful to decrease oxygen consumption and maternal hyperventilation and stress, the last two being common triggers of acute asthmatic attacks. Compared with alternative methods of labor management, neuraxial techniques provide reliable and profound analgesia[58] and offer patients with asthma considerable benefit.[45] In addition, ongoing epidural analgesia provides the opportunity to enhance the block quickly and safely, in the event that anesthesia is required for an obstetric intervention such as cesarean section. For this purpose, proper placement and functioning of the catheter in the epidural space should be assessed as early as possible. Because this crucial information on epidural catheter placement is delayed until intrathecal analgesia has vanished during sequential combined spinal-epidural (CSE) analgesia, this technique may be suboptimal in the specific setting of these high-risk patients.[59] Because of its numerous benefits, epidural analgesia for labor should be recommended to the patient and the obstetrician when the asthma is severe, even if the woman does not ask for it. The use of a dilute concentration of a local anesthetic in combination with fentanyl or sufentanil[60] minimizes the risk of motor blockade, which is particularly undesirable in parturients with asthma. In the very rare situation when epidural analgesia is contraindicated, alternative methods such as systemic opioids and/or inhalation analgesia may be used. However, the risk of respiratory depression and/or hypoxia makes these alternatives inappropriate for the patient with uncontrolled severe asthma. In this setting, pudendal blocks may be useful for second-stage analgesia.

Cesarean Section. As detailed previously, the risk of an acute attack of asthma is probably much higher during birth by cesarean section.[49] It has been shown that a high dose of methylprednisolone (2 mg/kg/day) increases the sensitivity to β-adrenergic agonists within 48 hours in dogs.[61] A short taper (2–4 days) is thus indicated in patients with moderate asthma not chronically treated with inhaled corticosteroids, as methylprednisolone is virtually devoid of side effects when used for such a short period.[62] Elective cesarean section should be delayed if asthma is unstable to allow better control before surgery.

Regional anesthesia is the preferred technique in patients with asthma undergoing cesarean section. Indeed, compared with general anesthesia plus endotracheal intubation (which is mandatory during cesarean section because of the high risk of aspiration), regional anesthesia is associated with much less bronchospasm.[63] However, the high sensory level required during cesarean delivery may have adverse effects on the parturient with asthma. First, the associated blockade of the accessory muscles of respiration may be deleterious in patients with unstable asthma. However, only peak expiratory pressure (which largely depends on abdominal musculature) was noticeably decreased during cesarean delivery performed under lumbar epidural anesthesia and, interestingly, this decrease was milder when 0.5% bupivacaine instead of 2% lidocaine with epinephrine (1:200,000) was used.[64] Single-shot spinal anesthesia, which produces a faster onset of a more dense motor block than that with epidural anesthesia, may not be tolerated as well as a slow, controlled epidural injection in parturients with severe and unstable asthma. In addition, the upper level of anesthesia during single-shot spinal anesthesia cannot be as precisely titrated as it can with epidural or CSE anesthesia. It has also been suggested that blockade of pulmonary and adrenal medulla sympathetic innervation might precipitate bronchospasm during cesarean delivery in asthmatic parturients. Yet, two studies on high thoracic epidural anesthesia have provided very reassuring results.[65, 66] The first study, performed in humans with documented bronchial hyperreactivity, showed that the acetylcholine threshold concentration (used for provocative tests) was increased threefold after epidural anesthesia when compared with baseline. However, the same threefold increase in acetylcholine threshold was also obtained after intravenous injection of local anesthetic, suggesting that the epidural route provided no specific benefit.[65] This corresponds to the well-documented preventive effect of intravenous lidocaine on reflex bronchoconstriction.[62, 67] Conversely, another recent study reported an increased pulmonary responsiveness to methacholine in guinea pigs after spinal anesthesia,[68] a result in agreement with bronchial hyperreactivity observed in humans with spinal cord transection above the T6 vertebral level.[69] Thus, even in patients with moderate asthma, catheter techniques may be a better alternative than single-shot spinal anesthesia. A lower spinal block extended with epidural injections (using the CSE technique) may combine the efficacy of the spinal technique with the flexibility and safety of an epidural block and thus may be an attractive choice in patients with asthma.

General anesthesia is sometimes mandatory for cesarean delivery because of dire fetal distress and/or absolute contraindications to neuraxial blockade.

Anesthetic Agents. Although endotracheal intubation during induction of general anesthesia increases the risk of bronchospasm considerably,[63] it must be performed even in pregnant patients with asthma to protect them against the catastrophic consequences of aspiration of gastric contents. As a means of aspiration prophylaxis in the healthy parturient, we advocate the use of histamine type 2 (H_2) receptor antagonists. These drugs, however, should theoretically be avoided in patients with asthma.[62] Classically, ketamine is considered as a very appropriate induction agent for patients with reactive airway disease who require rapid-sequence induction of anesthesia.[62] In addition, a clinically appropriate dose of ketamine has been shown to enhance the bronchodilating properties of epinephrine.[70] Propofol also has pronounced antiasthma action.[71, 72] However, Brown and Wagner[73] have recently demonstrated in sheep that ketamine was more potent than propofol at preventing neurally induced bronchoconstriction. On the other hand, ketamine in doses larger than 1.0 to 1.5 mg/kg may increase uterine tone and decrease uteroplacental perfusion. Practically considered, both ketamine and propofol appear to be reasonable options to induce general anesthesia in patients with moderate to severe asthma. Succinylcholine remains the neuromuscular blocking agent of choice for induction of patients with asthma undergoing cesarean section, because it provides the most rapid onset of muscle relaxation. Atropine or glycopyrrolate (which may also prevent neostigmine-induced airway constriction) can reverse adverse muscarinic activation. Nondepolarizing muscle relaxants that induce histamine release (e.g., atracurium) or prejunctional muscarinic type 2 receptor activity (e.g., pancuronium) are best avoided in parturients with asthma.[62] A study in dogs showed that pancuronium and atracurium enhanced pulmonary resistance induced by vagus nerve stimulation.[74] However, Cadwell and colleagues found no adverse respiratory effects with atracurium when used in asthmatic patients.[75]

Anesthesia Maintenance. Maintenance of anesthesia with volatile halogenated anesthetics is recommended because of their well-established ability to produce bronchodilation.[62] High concentrations of halothane and isoflurane appear equally effective[62] but halothane was found more potent when a low dose (0.6 minimum alveolar concention [MAC]) was being used in dogs.[76] However, when it is available, isoflurane is a much better choice than halothane. The arrhythmic threshold of epinephrine is much lower in the presence of halothane as compared with isoflurane (or sevoflurane or desflurane).[77, 78] Because β_2-agonists are very useful in preventing or treating acute asthma during general anesthesia, the use of a volatile anesthetic less likely to precipitate arrhythmias is a cautious preventive measure.

SEVOFLURANE. Recent data suggest that sevoflurane is a better bronchodilator than isoflurane[79] and therefore sevoflurane appears to be a suitable alternative to isoflurane during cesarean section.[80] The clinical effects of narcotics in asthmatic patients are poorly documented but these agents can be used provided that they do not induce histamine release (as does high-dose morphine) and that a sufficient depth of anesthesia is achieved with the induction agent alone.[62]

ISOFLURANE. Isoflurane does not add to the bronchodilating effect of a β_2-adrenergic agonist after tracheal intubation.[81] Conversely, it can be argued that 2 puffs of the β_2-adrenergic agonist albuterol does not add to the bronchodilating effect of 0.6 MAC isoflurane alone used for longer than 10 minutes.[82] Nonetheless, the subanesthetic concentration of isoflurane remaining at emergence from general anesthesia does not reduce the bronchial hyperreactivity in asthmatic patients.[83] Thus, an inhaled β_2-agonist should be administered in asthmatic patients who are not receiving chronic β_2-therapy, to prevent bronchoconstriction during the risky periods of induction and emergence. Intravenous lidocaine also attenuates reflex bronchoconstriction, whereas aerosol may provoke initial bronchoconstriction.[62] In addition, a combination of intravenous lidocaine and an inhaled β_2-agonist performs better than each alone.[67] However, we believe that administration of lidocaine should be delayed until the emergence period. Indeed, during this period, intravenous lidocaine is particularly useful because neither volatile nor intravenous anesthetics can lessen the stimulus of the endotracheal tube (which cannot be removed early, in order to prevent inhalation of gastric contents).

Bronchospasm. The initial management of intraoperative bronchospasm is similar to that recommended in nonpregnant patients. Kinking or obstruction of the endotracheal tube, pulmonary edema, pulmonary embolism, aspiration of gastric contents, pneumothorax, or anaphylaxis must be quickly eliminated as the cause. The treatment of asthmatic bronchospasm relies mainly on β_2-agonists given by aerosol by the intravenous route if necessary. Intravenous lidocaine, deepening of the anesthesia with nonarrhythmogenic volatile anesthetics, and the administration of intravenous ketamine or propofol may be useful additive measures. Intravenous corticosteroids are a second-line measure because they do not act rapidly. One particular problem linked to cesarean delivery is that most bronchodilators (namely, β_2-agonists and volatile anesthetics) are also potent tocolytics. In this regard, ketamine might be advantageous for use following delivery, as it increases uterine tone.

The use of prostaglandin F_2 is contraindicated, and even prostaglandin E_2 in the setting of bronchospasm is highly controversial. Thus, surgical (artery ligation) or radiologic (embolization) control of bleeding should be quickly implemented if large doses of oxytocin prove insufficient to reverse uterine atony and stop hemorrhage.

Other Chronic Lung Diseases

Very little new information is available on other chronic lung diseases and pregnancy. Chronic obstructive lung disease (asthma excluded) occurs rarely in young women. However, when FEV_1 is less than 1 L, caution should be exercised and rest is recommended in the late part of pregnancy. Restrictive lung disease (e.g., following lung resection or kyphoscoliosis) is usually well tolerated, and patients with severe disease should have minimal exertion or frequent bed rest

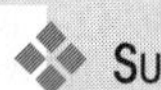

SUMMARY

Key Points

- If cesarean section is necessary in the pregnant patient with respiratory disease, regional anesthesia should be used, if possible, as it will allow avoidance of endotracheal intubation. Use of a catheter technique further reduces the likelihood of the need for intubation.
- Asthma is the most common chronic respiratory disease in pregnant women and should be controlled carefully to avoid deleterious outcomes, such as cesarean section, low birthweight, and hemorrhage.
- Pulmonary edema may occur as a consequence of aspiration of gastric contents, preeclampsia, sepsis, or exacerbation of underlying cardiac disease, or following administration of tocolytic agents.

Key Reference

Lapinsky SE, Kruczinski K, Slutsky AS: Critical care in the pregnant patient. Am J Respir Crit Care Med 1995; 152:427–455.

Case Stem

A nulliparous woman with poorly controlled asthma (peak flow rate = 280 L/min) caused, in part, by low compliance with her medications (β-agonist and inhaled steroid) is admitted to labor and delivery for premature labor at 35 weeks' gestation. Discuss the anesthetic and obstetric management.

during the third trimester of pregnancy. Patients with cystic fibrosis now survive long enough to become pregnant. They are, however, thought to have low fertility.[84] When they become pregnant, good tolerance and stable pulmonary function is usually observed even for women with severe disease. Maternal weight and nutritional status and fetal well-being should be closely monitored. In all these situations, epidural analgesia is thought to be useful because it decreases maternal ventilatory stress during labor. Dermatomal spread should, however, be carefully controlled to avoid block of the thoracic muscles.

References

1. Lapinsky SE, Kruczinski K, Slutsky AS: Critical care in the pregnant patient. Am J Respir Crit Care Med 1995; 152:427–455.
2. Bernard GR, Artigas A, Brigham KL, et al: Report of the American-European consensus conference on ARDS: definitions, mechanisms, relevant outcomes and clinical trial coordination. Intens Care Med 1994; 20:225–232.
3. Daily WH, Katz AR, Tonnesen A, et al: Beneficial effect of delivery in a patient with adult respiratory distress syndrome. Anesthesiology 1990; 72:383–386.
4. Tobin A, Kelly W: Prone ventilation—it's time. Anaesth Intens Care 1999; 27:194–201.
5. Guinard N, Beloucif S, Gatecel C, et al: Interest of a therapeutic optimization strategy in severe ARDS. Chest 1997; 111:1000–1007.
6. MacLennan FM: Maternal mortality from Mendelson's syndrome: an explanation? Lancet 1986; March 15:587–589.
7. Reid TMS: Striking a balance in maternal immune response to infection. Lancet 1998; 351:1670–1671.
8. Mabie WC, Barton JR, Sibai BM: Adult respiratory distress syndrome in pregnancy. Am J Obstet Gynecol 1992; 167(4 pt 1):950–957.
9. Adult respiratory distress syndrome (ARDS). *In* Report on Confidential Enquiries into Maternal Deaths in the United Kingdom, 1988–1990. London: Her Majesty's Stationery Office; 1994: 97–99.
10. Deaths associated with anaesthesia. Why mothers die. *In* Report on Confidential Enquiries into Maternal Deaths in the United Kingdom, 1994–1996. London: Her Majesty's Stationery Office; 1998:92–102.
11. Warner MA, Warner ME, Weber JG: Clinical significance of pulmonary aspiration during the perioperative period. Anesthesiology 1993; 78:56–62.
12. Chestnut DH: Anesthesia and maternal mortality. Anesthesiology 1997; 86:273–276.
13. Sibai BM, Mabie BC, Harvey CJ, et al: Pulmonary edema in severe preeclampsia-eclampsia: analysis of thirty-seven consecutive cases. Am J Obstet Gynecol 1987; 156:1174–1179.
14. Kilpatrick SJ, Matthay MA: Obstetric patients requiring critical care: a five-year review. Chest 1992; 101:1407–1412.
15. Mantel GD: Low dose dopamine in postpartum pre-eclamptic women with oliguria: a double blind, placebo, controlled, randomised trial. Br J Obstet Gynaecol 1997; 104:1180–1183.
16. Cunningham F, Lucas M, Hankins G: Pulmonary injury complicating antepartum pyelonephritis. Am J Obstet Gynecol 1987; 156:797–807.
17. Hatjis CG, Swain M: Systemic tocolysis for premature labor is associated with an increased incidence of pulmonary edema in the presence of maternal infection. Am J Obstet Gynecol 1988; 159:723–726.
18. De Veciana M, Towers CV, Major CA, et al: Pulmonary injury associated with appendicitis in pregnancy: who is at risk? Am J Obstet Gynecol 1994; 171:1008–1013.
19. Pisani RJ, Rosenow EC III: Pulmonary edema associated with tocolytic therapy. Ann Intern Med 1989; 110:714–718.
20. Clesham GF, Scott J, Oakley CM, et al: β-Adrenergic agonists and pulmonary œdema in preterm labour. BMJ 1994; 308:260–262.
21. Armson BA, Samuels P, Miller F, et al: Evaluation of maternal fluid dynamics during tocolytic therapy with ritodrine hydrochloride and magnesium sulfate. Am J Obstet Gynecol 1992; 167:758–765.
22. Deaths associated with the use of ritodrine. *In* Report on Confidential Enquiries into Maternal Deaths in the United Kingdom, 1991–1993. London: Her Majesty's Stationery Office; 1996:105–107.
23. Greenberg LR, Moore TR: Staphylococcal septicemia and adult respiratory distress syndrome in pregnancy treated with extracorporeal carbon dioxide removal. Obstet Gynecol 1995; 86(4 pt 2):657–660.
24. Richey SD, Roberts SW, Ramin KD, et al: Pneumonia complicating pregnancy. Obstet Gynecol 1994; 84(4 pt 1):525–528.
25. Davis TA, Angel J: Varicella pneumonia in pregnancy. Int J Obstet Anesth 1997; 6:274–278.
26. Toglia MR, Weg JG: Venous thromboembolism during pregnancy. N Engl J Med 1996; 335:108–114.
27. Bergqvist A, Bergqvist D, Hallbook T, et al: Deep vein thrombosis during pregnancy: a prospective study. Acta Obstet Gynaecol Scand 1983; 62:443–448.
28. Ginsberg JS, Brill-Edwards P, Burrows RF, et al: Venous thrombosis during pregnancy: leg and trimester of presentation. Thromb Haemost 1992; 67:519–520.
29. Friederich PW, Sanson B-J, Simioni P, et al: Frequency of pregnancy-related venous thromboembolism in anticoagulant factor-deficient women: implications for prophylaxis. Ann Intern Med 1996; 125:955–960.
30. McColl MD, Ramsay JE, Tait RC, et al: Risk factors for pregnancy associated venous thromboembolism. Thromb Haemost 1997; 78:1183–1188.
31. Hunt BJ, Doughty H-A, Majumdar G, et al: Thromboprophylaxis with low molecular weight heparin (Fragmin) in high risk pregnancies. Thromb Haemost 1997; 77:39–43.
32. Prophylaxis against thromboembolism in caesarean section. Why mothers die. *In* Report on Confidential Enquiries into Maternal Deaths in the United Kingdom, 1994–1996. London: Her Majesty's Stationery Office; 1998:105–107.
33. Gandevia SC: Does the diaphragm fatigue during parturition? Lancet 1993; 341:347.
34. Gaspar LS: Hamman's syndrome: pneumomediastinum and subcutaneous emphysema occurring in labour. Int J Obstet Anesth 1997; 6:55–58.
35. Reed PN, Colquhoun AD, Hanning CD: Maternal oxygenation during normal labour. Br J Anaesth 1989; 62:316–318.
36. Porter JS, Bonello E, Reynolds F: The effect of epidural opioids on maternal oxygenation during labour and delivery. Anaesthesia 1996; 51:899–903.
37. Lu JK, Manullang TR, Staples MH, et al: Maternal respiratory arrests, severe hypotension, and fetal distress after administration of intrathecal, sufentanil, and bupivacaine after intravenous fentanyl. Anesthesiology 1997; 87:170–172.
38. Clark SL, Hankins GDV, Dudley DA, et al: Amniotic fluid embolism: analysis of the National Registry. Am J Obstet Gynecol 1995; 172(4 pt 1):1158–1169.
39. Hankins GDV, Snyder RR, Clark SL, et al: Acute hemodynamiuc and respiratory effects of amniotic fluid embolism in the pregnant goat model. Am J Obstet Gynecol 1993; 168:1113–1130.
40. Petroff S, Thill B, Levacher S, et al: Embolie amniotique avec évolution favorable. Ann Fr Anesth Reanim 1994; 13:135–137.
41. Hughson WG, Friedman PJ, Feigin DS, et al: Postpartum pleural effusion: a common radiologic finding. Ann Intern Med 1982; 97:856–858.
42. Harrop-Griffiths AW, Ravalia A, Browne DA, et al: Regional anaesthesia and cough effectiveness: a study in patients undergoing Caesarean section. Anaesthesia 1991; 46:11–13.
43. National Heart, Lung and Blood Institute, and National Institutes of Health: International Consensus Report on the Diagnosis and Treatment of Asthma. NIH Publication No. 92–3091. Bethesda, MD: National Institutes of Health; March 1992. Also in Eur Respir J 1992; 5:601–641.
44. Alexander S, Dodds L, Armson BA: Perinatal outcomes in

women with asthma during pregnancy. Obstet Gynecol 1998; 92:435–440.
45. National Heart, Lung and Blood Institute: Report of the Working Group on Asthma and Pregnancy: Management of Asthma During Pregnancy. NIH Publication No. 93–3279. Bethesda, MD: National Institutes of Health; September 1993.
46. Schatz M: Interrelationships between asthma and pregnancy: a literature review. J Allergy Clin Immunol 1999; 103:S330–S336.
47. Juniper EF, Daniel EE, Roberts RS, et al: Improvement in airway responsiveness and asthma severity during pregnancy: a prospective study. Am Rev Respir Dis 1989; 140:924–931.
48. Luskin AT: An overview of the recommendations of the Working Group on Asthma and Pregnancy. J Allergy Immunol 1999; 103:S350–S353.
49. Mabie WC: Asthma in pregnancy. Clin Obstet Gynecol 1996; 39:56–69.
50. Stenius-Aarniala B, Piirilä P, Teramo K: Asthma and pregnancy: a prospective study of 198 pregnancies. Thorax 1988; 43:12–18.
51. Moore-Gillon J: Asthma in pregnancy. Br J Obstet Gynaecol 1994; 101:658–660.
52. Rosa F: Databases in the assessment of the effects of drugs during pregnancy. J Allergy Clin Immunol 1999; 103:S360–S361.
53. Boushey HA: Effects of inhaled corticosteroids on the consequences of asthma. J Allergy Clin Immunol 1998; 102:S5–S16.
54. Stenius-Aarniala BS, Hedman J, Teramo KA: Acute asthma during pregnancy. Thorax 1996; 51:411–414.
55. Wendel PJ, Ramin SM, Barnett-Hamm C, et al: Asthma treatment in pregnancy: a randomized controlled study. Am J Obstet Gynecol 1996; 175:150–154.
56. Dombrowski M, Thom E, McNellis D: Maternal-Fetal Medicine Units (MFMU) studies of inhaled corticosteroids during pregnancy. J Allergy Clin Immunol 1999; 103(suppl): S356–S359.
57. Gauvreau GM, Watson RM, O'Byrne PM: Protective effects of inhaled PGE_2 on allergen-induced airway responses and airway inflammation. Am J Respir Crit Care Med 1999; 159:31–36.
58. Ranta P, Spalding M, Kangas-Saarela T, et al: Maternal expectations and experiences of labour pain—options of 1091 Finnish parturients. Acta Anaesthesiol Scand 1995; 39:60–66.
59. Mercier FJ, Bouaziz H, Benhamou D: Transition from intrathecal analgesia to epidural anesthesia for emergency cesarean section using a combined spinal epidural technique [letter]. Anesth Analg 1996; 83:434.
60. Chestnut DH, Owen CL, Bates JN, et al: Continuous infusion epidural analgesia during labor: a randomized, double-blind comparison of 0.0625% bupivacaine/0.0002% fentanyl versus 0.125% bupivacaine. Anesthesiology 1988; 68:754–759.
61. Sauder RA, Lenox WC, Tobias JD, et al: Methylprednisolone increases sensitivity to beta-adrenergic agonists within 48 hours in Basenji greyhounds. Anesthesiology 1993; 79:1278–1283.
62. Hirshman CA: Perioperative management of the asthmatic patient. Can J Anaesth 1991; 38:R26–R32.
63. Olsson GL: Bronchospasm during anesthesia: a computer-aided incidence study of 136,929 patients. Acta Anesthesiol Scand 1987; 31:244–252.
64. Yun E, Topulos GP, Body SC, et al: Pulmonary function changes during epidural anesthesia for cesarean delivery. Anesth Analg 1996; 82:750–753.
65. Groeben H, Schwalen A, Irsfeld S, et al: High thoracic epidural anesthesia does not alter airway resistance and attenuates the response to an inhalational provocation test in patient with bronchial hyperreactivity. Anesthesiology 1994; 81:868–874.
66. Yuan HB, Tang GJ, Kou YR, et al: Effects of high thoracic epidural anaesthesia on the peripheral airway reactivity in dogs. Acta Anaesthesiol Scand 1998; 42:85–90.
67. Groeben H, Silvanus MT, Beste M, et al: Combined intravenous lidocaine and inhaled salbutamol protect against bronchial hyperreactivity more effectively than lidocaine or salbutamol alone. Anesthesiology 1998; 89:826–828.
68. Capellozzi M, Arantes FM, Paiva PS, et al: Spinal anesthesia increases pulmonary responsiveness to methacholine in guinea pigs. Anesth Analg 1998; 87:874–878.
69. Dicpinigaitis PV, Almenoff PL: Effect of pulmonary sympathetic blockade on bronchial responsiveness. Anesthesiology 1995; 82:794–795.
70. Hirota K, Hashimoto Y, Skai T, et al: In vivo spasmolytic effect of ketamine and adrenaline on histamine-induced airway constriction: direct visualisation method with a superfine fiberoptic bronchoscope. Acta Anaesthesiol Scand 1998; 42:184–188.
71. Pizov R, Brown RH, Weiss YS, et al: Wheezing during induction of general anesthesia in patients with and without asthma: a randomized, blinded trial. Anesthesiology 1995; 82:1111–1116.
72. Eames WO, Rooke GA, Wu RS, et al: Comparison of the effects of etomidate, propofol, and thiopental on respiratory resistance after tracheal intubation. Anesthesiology 1996; 84:1307–1311.
73. Brown RH, Wagner EM: Mechanisms of bronchoprotection by anesthetic induction agents: propofol versus ketamine. Anesthesiology 1999; 90:822–828.
74. Vettermann J, Beck KC, Lindahl SG, et al: Actions of enflurane, isoflurane, vecuronium, atracurium, and pancuronium on pulmonary resistance in dogs. Anesthesiology 1988; 69:688–695.
75. Cadwell JE, Lau M, Fisher DM: Atracurium versus vecuronium in asthmatic patients: a blinded, randomized comparison of adverse events. Anesthesiology 1995; 83:986–991.
76. Brown RH, Zerhouni EA, Hirshman CA: Comparison of low concentrations of halothane and isoflurane as bronchodilators. Anesthesiology 1993; 78:1097–1101.
77. Johnston RR, Eger EI II, Wilson C: A comparative interaction of epinephrine with enflurane, isoflurane, and halothane in man. Anesth Analg 1976; 55:709–712.
78. Hikasa Y, Okabe C, Takase K, et al: Ventricular arrhythmogenic dose of adrenaline during sevoflurane, isoflurane, and halothane anaesthesia either with or without ketamine or thiopentone in cats. Res Vet Sci 1996; 60:134–137.
79. Rooke GA, Choi JH, Bishop MJ: The effect of isoflurane, halothane, sevoflurane, and thiopental/nitrous oxide on respiratory system resistance after tracheal intubation. Anesthesiology 1997; 86:1294–1299.
80. Gambling DR, Sharma SK, White PF, et al: Use of sevoflurane during elective cesarean birth: a comparison with isoflurane and spinal anesthesia. Anesth Analg 1995; 81:90–95.
81. Wu RS, Wu KC, Wong TK, et al: Isoflurane anesthesia does not add to the bronchodilating effect of a $beta_2$-adenergic agonist after tracheal intubation. Anesth Analg 1996; 83:238–241.
82. Choi JH, Rooke GA, Wu SC, et al: Reduction in post-intubation respiratory resistance by isoflurane and albuterol. Can J Anaesth 1997; 44:717–722.
83. Mercier FJ, Benhamou D, Denjean A: Lack of bronchodilator effect after administration of subanaesthetic concentration of isoflurane in mild asthmatic subjects challenged with methacholine. Br J Anaesth 1995; 74:301–305.
84. ACOG Technical bulletin: Pulmonary disease in pregnancy. Int J Gynecol Obstet 1996; 54:187–196.

41

Anesthetic Management of Diabetic Parturients

SANJAY DATTA, MD, FFARCS (ENG)

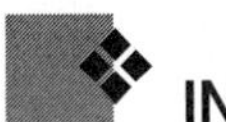

INTRODUCTION

Diabetes still remains the most common medical problem during pregnancy. The incidence of insulin-dependent diabetes mellitus (IDDM) at the present time is close to 0.5% of all pregnancies. Since the introduction of insulin and the knowledge of strict control of IDDM pregnant patients, the maternal and neonatal prognoses have improved considerably. Currently, the perinatal mortality rate among this group closely matches that of the general population.[2] Significant maternal morbidity, however, still exists. Such morbidity is related to hypoglycemia, diabetic ketoacidosis, hypertension, exacerbation of nephropathy, and retinopathy; whereas neonatal morbidity is related to respiratory distress syndrome (RDS) and congenital anomalies. Close communications between perinatologists and anesthesiologists are important in achieving optimal maternal and neonatal outcomes. This chapter deals with the pathophysiology of this disease in pregnancy, maternal and fetal effects, and obstetric and anesthetic management. A concise discussion of immediate neonatal resuscitation is also presented.

PATHOPHYSIOLOGY

Diabetes is generally classified into two groups: type I, or IDDM, and type II. Type I is characterized by insulin dependence, juvenile onset, and a tendency to ketosis. Type II is characterized by the lack of insulin dependence, and by adult onset, ketosis resistance, and obesity. The vast majority of the pregnant patients in these groups fall into the IDDM category. IDDM is a chronic autoimmune disease caused by the destruction of pancreatic B cells. The disease has a genetic predisposition, and it has been suggested that the relevant genes are located on chromosome 6 in association with the major histocompatibility complex.[1] The incidence of diabetes in the offspring of IDDM parturients varies between 1% and 3%. The risk is greater (6.1%) if the father has IDDM, whereas it is highest (20%) if both parents have IDDM.

MATERNAL EFFECTS

As far back as 1949, Priscilla White[3] from the Joslin Clinic classified diabetic parturients on the basis of duration of the disease as well as association of microvascular and macrovascular complications. During that time, White's classification was correlated to both maternal and neonatal mortality and morbidity rates. In other words, the higher the class, the greater the incidence of mortality and morbidity. However, at the present time, White's classification (Table 41–1) is used mainly for discussing epidemiologic data, and for clinical trials. On the other hand, Pedersen's classification may be more relevant clinically. According to this, four maternal complications—diabetic ketoacidosis, preeclampsia, pyelonephritis, and maternal neglect—are associated with poor pregnancy outcome. Tight metabolic control can improve these outcomes, except in patients with preeclampsia.

Uteroplacental Insufficiency

In the anesthesia team's monitoring of diabetic parturients, decreased placental perfusion is one of the most important pathophysiologic changes. A further decrease in placental perfusion from the anesthetics and other techniques can significantly affect the fetus.

Placental pathology is very significant in severe uncontrolled diabetes; however, abnormalities can be seen in mild diabetes, in addition to well-controlled diabetes. Nylund and colleagues[4] observed uteropla-

Table 41–1 Modified White's Classification of Diabetes Pregnancy

1. **Gestational Diabetes Mellitus**
   Gestational diabetes mellitus non–insulin-requiring (GDMNI): Abnormal carbohydrate tolerance during pregnancy, only not requiring insulin.
   Gestational diabetes mellitus insulin requiring (GDMI): Abnormal carbohydrate tolerance during pregnancy, only requiring insulin
2. *Class A:* Abnormal carbohydrate tolerance in the nonpregnant state identified prior to the present pregnancy that does not require insulin either prior to or during the pregnancy
   Class B: Onset of insulin-requiring diabetes after 20 years of age, with duration of less than 10 years
   Class C: Onset of insulin-requiring diabetes between ages 10 and 20 years with duration of less than 20 years, or duration of 10 to 20 years regardless of age at onset
   Class D: Onset of insulin-requiring diabetes prior to age 10 years, or duration greater than 20 years, regardless of age at onset, or onset of insulin-requiring diabetes with chronic hypertension, or insulin-requiring diabetes with benign retinopathy
   Class F: Insulin-requiring diabetes with diabetic nephropathy (proteinuria of greater than 500 mg in a 24-h urine collection)
   Class R: Insulin-requiring diabetes with proliferative retinopathy
   Class T: Insulin-requiring diabetes with renal transplantation
   Class H: Insulin-requiring diabetes with coronary artery disease

From White P: Pregnancy and diabetes: medical aspects. Med Clin North Am 1965; 49:1015–1019.

cental blood flow using intravenous indium-113 in 26 diabetic parturients and compared them with 41 healthy pregnant individuals. The uteroplacental blood flow index was decreased 35% to 45% in diabetes. The blood flow index was further decreased in the presence of increased blood glucose. The authors did not observe any difference in the blood flow index between the gestational diabetic patients and the parturients with preexisting diabetes. Radioactive compound studies are no longer used in pregnant patients, with Doppler ultrasonography having become the technique of choice for the determination of uteroplacental blood flow. Using Doppler ultrasonography, Reece and associates[5] observed the fetal umbilical artery blood flow in 56 diabetic parturients. A total of 14 of these patients exhibited associated vascular complications.[5] Systolic/diastolic (S/D) ratios were higher in diabetic patients with vasculopathy compared to those of healthy parturients. The S/D ratio was greater than 30 in about 50% of patients with vasculopathy. An S/D ratio higher than 40 was associated with a worse neonatal outcome. Doppler indices significantly increased in the presence of vasculopathy, with associated hypertension and deteriorating renal insufficiency. Intrauterine growth retardation and neonatal metabolic complications were associated with decreased blood flow in the umbilical artery. Although the exact etiology of decreased uteroplacental blood flow in these patients is unknown, Bjork and Persson[6] found enlarged villi, with associated reduction of intervillous space.

Fetal Oxygenation

Hemoglobin A_{1c} (HbA_{1c}) is glycosylated hemoglobin whose concentration is proportional to the level of blood glucose for the 6 weeks prior to the former's estimation. Maternal glycemic control is important in IDDM parturients; estimation of HbA_{1c} concentration has been found to be a good indicator for this purpose. HbA_{1c} also has an important physiologic implication for fetal oxygenation. Madsen and Ditzel[7] observed decreased oxygen saturation and P_{50} values with increased HbA_{1c} (Figs. 41–1 and 41–2). Hence, in parturients with uncontrolled diabetes, fetal oxygenation will be decreased.

Diabetic Ketoacidosis (DKA)

Diabetic ketoacidosis is one of the major causes of fetal mortality and morbidity: fetal loss can be as high as 50% if this disorder is not properly treated.[8] The different etiologies of DKA include (1) changes in the insulin requirement in the presence of infection; (2) the omission of insulin doses; (3) pump malfunction if the subcutaneous pump is used for continuous infusion; (4) tocolytic therapy with a β-mimetic drug; and (5) the use of a glucocorticoid to promote maturation of fetal lungs. Usually, DKA occurs in the presence of a relative or absolute deficiency of insulin or an absolute increase in the major counter-regulatory hormone, glucagon. One or both of these conditions increase hepatic glycogenolysis and decrease peripheral glucose utilization, ultimately causing severe hyperglycemia. Beta-stimulation, produced either by an exogenous β-mimetic drug or endogenous epinephrine resulting from stress due to infection, decreases insulin-induced glucose transport in the peripheral tissues. Hyperglycemia initiates osmotic diuresis, causing dehydration. Potassium and sodium concentrations are decreased because of osmotic diuresis. Increased concentrations of β-oxidative enzymes in the liver metabolize free fatty acids to ketone bodies. β-Hydroxybutyrate and acetoacetate decrease maternal pH and stimulate the respiratory center. Intracellular potassium is replaced by hydrogen ions, and thus total body potassium is depleted. The loss of maternal plasma volume decreases cardiac output and blood pressure and ultimately will produce cardiovascular collapse and shock.

Interestingly, diabetic parturients can develop ketoacidosis with blood glucose levels as low as 200 mg/dL.

The clinical features of DKA include (1) anorexia, (2) nausea, (3) vomiting, (4) polyuria, (5) polydipsia, (6) tachycardia, and (7) abdominal pain or muscle cramps. In severe cases, other features include (1) Kussmaul hyperventilation, (2) hypotension and oliguria due to severe hypovolemia, (3) lethargy due to

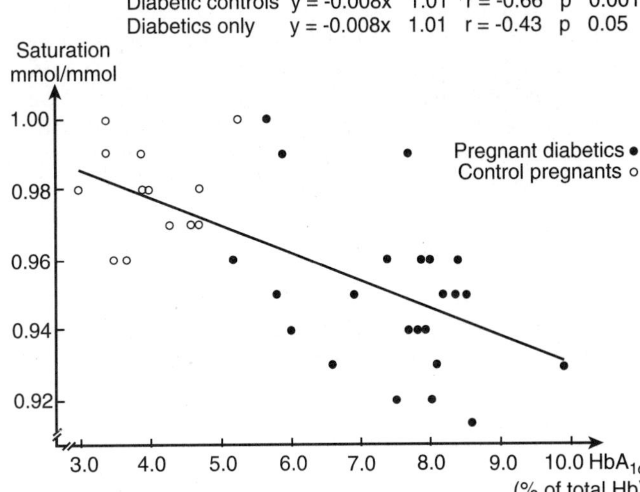

❖ **Figure 41-1** Correlation between HB A_{1c} and arterial oxygen saturation in diabetic women. (From Madsen H, Ditzel J: Changes in red blood cell oxygen transport in diabetic pregnancy. Am J Obstet Gynecol 1982; 143:421–424.)

coma, (4) normal or cold body temperature, and (5) fruity odor.

The presence of ketones, maternal arterial pH of less than 7.30, and anion gap confirm the diagnosis.

Maternal Infections

The rate of infections is higher in IDDM parturients than that in normal pregnant patients, a finding that may be related to inadequate metabolic control. The infections are usually genitourinary, respiratory, endometrial, or wound related. Infection from *Candida* occurs more often in diabetic parturients.

Preeclampsia

Preeclampsia is more common in IDDM parturients (13.6% versus 5%). The incidences increase according to the severity of the diabetes. Also increased is the perinatal mortality rate. The mortality increases from 3.3 per 1000 live births in normotensive diabetic parturients to 60 per 1000 live births in IDDM parturients with preeclampsia. Preeclampsia is also difficult to diagnose in this patient population, especially in the presence of diabetic nephropathy with associated hypertension. There is an imbalance between the normal thromboxane/prostacyclin ratio in preeclamptic patients. This imbalance is also observed in IDDM parturients, which might be one of the reasons for higher incidences of preeclampsia in this group. Although the prophylactic use of minidose aspirin did not prove to be useful in preeclamptic parturients, it may be indicated in diabetic parturients with associated nephropathy and hypertension.

Diabetic Nephropathy

A total of 5% of diabetic pregnant patients have associated pathologic nephropathy. Interestingly, hypertension is observed in patients with diabetic nephropathy in 30% of cases during the first trimester and in as much as 75% by the time of delivery. The preterm delivery rate is much higher, and 50% to 60% undergo cesarean section. Many of the patients with long-standing nephropathy have hypoalbuminemia, low colloid oncotic pressure (COP), and associated severe edema

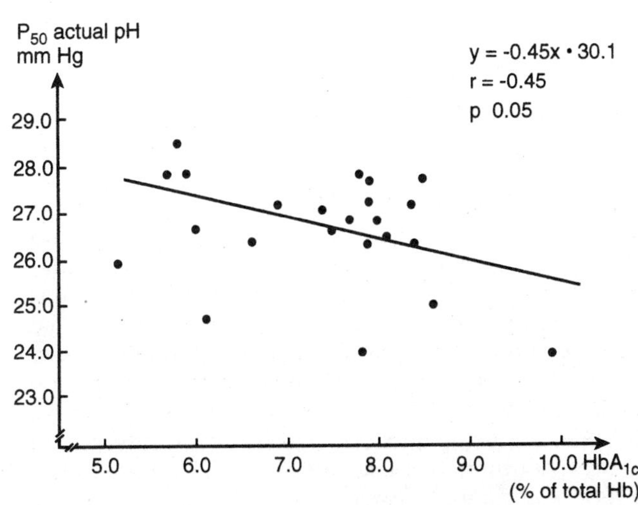

❖ **Figure 41-2** Correlation between Hb A_{1c} and P_{50} at actual pH in diabetic women. (From Madsen H, Ditzel J: Changes in red blood cell oxygen transport in diabetic pregnancy. Am J Obstet Gynecol 1982; 143:421–424.)

and, rarely, pulmonary edema. Perinatal outcome may be poor in IDDM parturients with nephropathy, if the urinary protein excretion exceeds 3 g/24 h and creatinine concentration increases above 1.5 mg/dL, a high mean arterial pressure (>107 mm Hg) will worsen the situation.[9] Long-term prognosis is also poor in these cases.

Diabetic Retinopathy

Proliferative retinopathy most probably gets worse during pregnancy.[10] Valsalva maneuvers should be prevented to avoid the possibility of retinal hemorrhage.

Diabetic Neuropathy

Diabetic autonomic neuropathy can get worse and cause postural hypotension; gastrostasis is common in diabetic parturients. Hirsch and Shamoon[11] observed the response of counter-regulatory hormones to hypoglycemia in IDDM pregnant patients and compared it with that of healthy parturients. Normal increases in plasma growth hormone (GH), norepinephrine, and cortisol were observed; however, there was a decreased or absent response in plasma epinephrine and glucagon in diabetic patients in response to hypoglycemia.[11]

Jones and colleagues[12] observed the counter-regulatory hormone responses to insulin-induced hypoglycemia in eight adult patients with IDDM and six age-matched normal subjects in three sets of conditions: (1) awake during the day; (2) asleep at night; and (3) awake at night.[12] The authors measured plasma free insulin, epinephrine, norepinephrine, cortisol, and GH during the study period. The sleep state was monitored by polysomnography. The plasma epinephrine and norepinephrine concentrations were decreased during sleep, and cortisol levels did not change in diabetic subjects during hypoglycemia. The authors concluded that sleep might impair counter-regulatory hormone responses to hypoglycemia in diabetic subjects during sleep. Autonomic dysfunction as well as the impairment of the response of counter-regulatory hormones to hypoglycemia may be important during both regional and general anesthesia for these patients.

Effect on the Cardiovascular System

Cardiac function may be impaired in diabetic parturients. Airaksinen and colleagues[13] observed by using echocardiography the adaptation of the heart to an increase in blood volume during pregnancy in diabetic subjects. Mean duration of diabetes was 14 years, and 6 of these 17 subjects had associated microvascular complications. Slightly smaller left ventricle size was observed in diabetic parturients compared to normal patients. The pregnancy-related increase in left ventricular size, stroke volume, and heart rate was impaired in IDDM patients. The decreased responses in stroke volume and heart rate were associated with decreased cardiac output in diabetic parturients. The exact mechanism is not known; however, the possible factors that have been suggested are (1) preclinical diabetic cardiomyopathy and (2) subclinical autonomic neuropathy. Anesthetic implications may be important in such a situation.

Diabetic Stiff Joint Syndrome

Stiff joint syndrome is a symptom complex, associated with (1) juvenile-onset diabetes, (2) nonfamilial short stature, and (3) joint contractures.[14] These patients may be complicated by limited atlanto-occipital extension; hence, difficult intubation. An awake intubation or, if necessary, fiberoptic intubation may be necessary. A positive "prayer sign" may be present in parturients with diabetic stiff joint syndrome. A positive prayer sign is defined by the patient's inability to approximate the palmar surfaces of the interphalangeal joints despite maximal effort, secondary to connective tissue changes of these joints.

Diabetic scleredema is synonymous with stiff joint syndrome.[15] In this condition, there are certain changes in the epidural spaces as well as the spinal cord blood supply: (1) the epidural space becomes rigid because of pathologic changes in the connective tissues and ligaments, possibly making the epidural space less compliant; and (2) diminished arterial supply of the spinal cord. Because of the noncompliant epidural space and decreased vascular supply of the spinal cord, the use of an excessive volume of local anesthetic and associated hypotension in the patient should be avoided.

Gestational Diabetes

In the original White classification, gestational diabetes was not included. The importance of the clinical implications of gestational diabetes has become obvious. Among diabetic pregnant patients, the incidence of gestational diabetes mellitus (GDM) is most frequent. GDM is diagnosed in about 90,000 women in the United States each year.[16] GDM is defined as carbohydrate intolerance of varying severity when it is diagnosed first during pregnancy. GDM can be further subdivided to (1) diet control, not requiring insulin, and (2) GDM requiring insulin. The majority of these patients do have normal carbohydrate tolerance before pregnancy, and the tolerance returns to normal after delivery. There is a significant controversy regarding the clinical implications of GDM so far as the maternal and neonatal outcomes are concerned. The Toronto Gestational Diabetes Project was interested in observing the clinical importance of the carbohydrate intolerance with the onset or first diagnosis during pregnancy.[17] They recorded the results from the screening test and the full oral glucose tolerance test (OGTT) of more than 3800 individuals aged 24 years or older. Patients with OGTT values above threshold were treated; for the rest of the patients the caregivers were blinded for the OGTT values and the authors observed a direct relationship between OGTT results and adverse pregnancy outcome, including preeclampsia, neonatal macrosomia, and cesarean section. A significant independent impact of OGTT results was found, when other significant risk factors were considered. GDM was associated with increased rates of macrosomia. The authors maintained that aggressive management of maternal glycemia as early as possible can decrease the incidences of macrosomia.

FETAL EFFECTS

Strict maternal glucose control, improved prenatal fetal monitoring, and better neonatal intensive care management have improved neonatal outcome. However, congenital anomalies and "unexplained" fetal death still remain the major problem. Several important factors influence fetal morbidity and mortality: (1) chronic hypoxia with polycythemia, (2) increased platelet aggregation, and (3) hypertrophic cardiomyopathy. The fetus of the IDDM mothers may have chronic hypoxia; associated hyperglycemia will make the situation worse, as this can decrease the umbilical artery oxygen dramatically. Fetal hypertrophic cardiomyopathy may also be the reason for sudden intrauterine fetal death.

Incidence of congenital anomalies are much higher in the infants of diabetic mothers—about two to four times higher compared to normal parturients.[18] A total of 40% of the perinatal deaths in diabetic patients are due to severe congential anomalies. The major factors that are responsible for the congenital anomalies include (1) uncontrolled or poorly controlled diabetes preconception,[19] (2) duration of diabetes for more than 10 years, and (3) genetic susceptibility. The different congenital anomalies include (1) neural tube anomalies, (2) caudal regression syndrome, (3) cardiac abnormalities causing ventricular septal defects, transposition of the great vessels, and coarctation of the aorta, (4) renal anomalies, and (5) gastrointestinal anomalies.

Extremes of fetal growth have been noted in the diabetic population. Macrosomia and also marked intrauterine growth retardation (IUGR) have been observed (Fig. 41–3). Macrosomia may be related to maternal hyperglycemia causing fetal hyperglycemia and hyperinsulinemia. Hence, this might be present more often in poorly controlled or uncontrolled diabetic parturients. However, even with rigid maternal glycemic control, the incidences of macrosomia vary between 8% and 43%. This high incidence might be related to the following:[20] (1) difficult glycemic control, especially in patients with long-standing IDDM; (2) maternal weight; and (3) genetic factors. In an interesting study, Menon and colleagues[21] observed that a significant amount of antibody-bound insulin was transferred across the placenta from the IDDM mother to the fetus. The amount of transfer was related to the concentrations of maternal anti-insulin antibody. The authors concluded that the correlation between macrosomia and the cord blood animal insulin levels indicated that the transferred insulin may have biologic activity. They further suggested that the formation of antibody to insulin in the mother may be a determinant of fetal outcome independent of maternal blood glucose levels. At the other extreme, in diabetic parturients with associated vascular involvements and superimposed preeclampsia, the incidence of IUGR is high. This also increases the risk of fetal morbidity and mortality.

OBSTETRIC CONSIDERATIONS

Screening for GDM

The method of screening is controversial. Some authors suggest routine biochemical screening for all parturients, whereas others maintain the usefulness of screening, depending on the historical risk factors. There is evidence that universal biochemical screening, combined with aggressive therapy, may reduce the incidence of macrosomia and ultimate operative delivery.[22]

Antenatal Fetal Monitoring

Although sudden fetal demise can happen in this group; the incidences have decreased significantly because of diligent fetal monitoring. A weekly nonstress test (NST), and then an oxytocin challenge test (OCT), are done routinely from 32 weeks onward. These are performed twice a week from 36 weeks until delivery.[23] A biophysical profile as well as Doppler analysis of blood flow in the umbilical artery have become popular at the present time for the determination of fetal well-being.

Lung Maturity Test

Incidences of RDS are high among infants of IDDM mothers. In this group, infant lung maturity is delayed compared to that of infants of nondiabetic women, and the incidences of RDS are significantly higher in the presence of a normal lecithin/sphingomyelin (L/S) ratio in infants of normal subjects. Hence, a lung maturity test is routinely done in these subjects if the delivery is contemplated before 39 weeks of gestation. The estimation of saturated phosphatidylcholine (SPC) is done to predict lung maturity. An L/S ratio of 3.5 and an SPC count of 1000 μg/dL are found to be optimal, and the patient with such values is extremely unlikely to develop RDS.

Route and Timing of Delivery

There are concerns for both the route and the gestational weeks of delivery. The problem with early delivery was higher incidences of RDS, whereas late delivery may be associated with sudden intrauterine fetal death (IUFD). Close monitoring of the fetus has decreased the numbers of IUFD. The incidences of macrosomia—hence abdominal delivery—are much higher in this patient population. Bernstein and Catalano[24] observed risk factors of cesarean section in pregnant IDDM patients. In this study, infant birthweight was not different between the vaginal delivery and cesarean section groups (3374 ± 559 g versus 3520 ± 456 g).

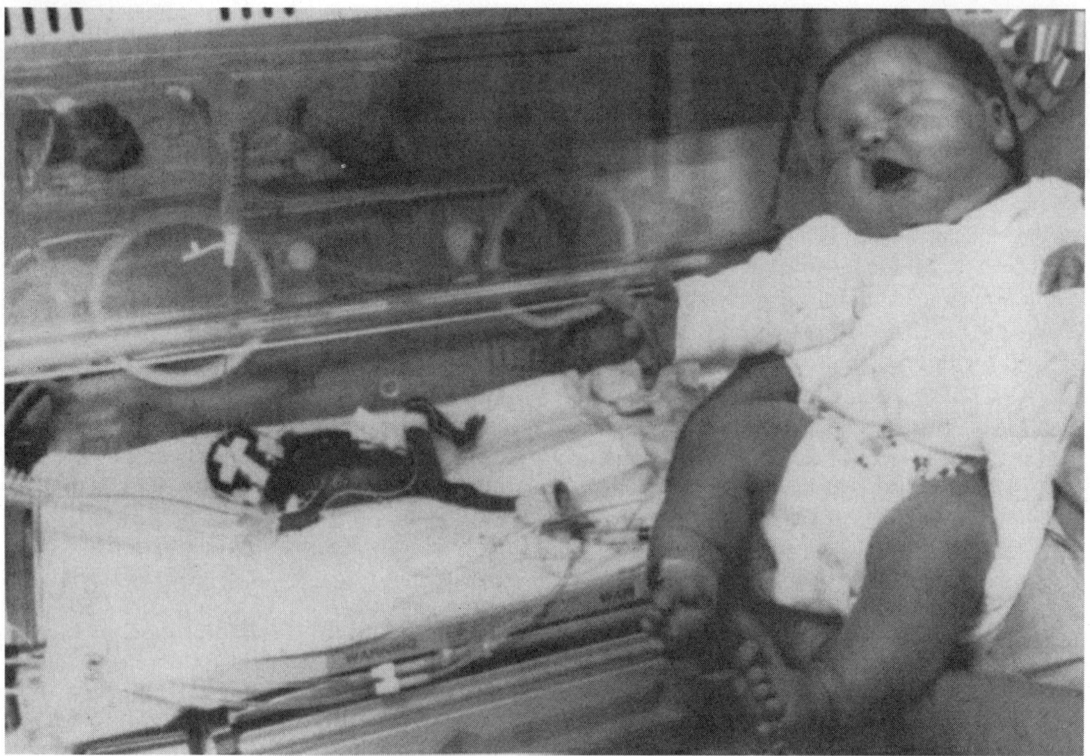

❖ **Figure 41–3** Two extremes of growth abnormalities in infants of diabetic mothers. The small, growth-retarded infant on the left weighs 470 g and is the offspring of a woman with nephropathy and hypertension, delivered at 28 weeks of gestation. The neonate on the right is the 5100-g baby of a woman with suboptimally controlled class C diabetes. (From Landon MB: Diabetes mellitus and other endocrine diseases. *In* Gabbe SG, Niebyl JR, Simpson JL (eds): Obstetrics: Normal and Problem Pregnancies, 3rd ed. New York: Churchill Livingstone; 1996:1043.)

However, the factors that were significant for the cesarean section were (1) nulliparity, (2) maternal pregravid body mass index, (3) fetal position at delivery, and (4) all estimates of neonatal body fat. Interestingly, the authors concluded that increased newborn fat was associated independently with the rate of cesarean section. Elective deliveries are usually planned between 38 and 40 weeks after performing a fetal lung maturity test (SPC) if necessary. Ultrasound examination is done for the estimation of fetal weight. Pelvic delivery is usually planned if fetal weight is less than 4000 g. If fetal weight is above this level, cesarean section is usually indicated.

Treatment of Diabetic Ketoacidosis

Because maternal hypovolemia is a major problem, volume replacement with two intravenous lines is important: one for rapid fluid infusion, and the other one for insulin therapy. Initial treatment should include fluid replacement with normal saline (15 to 20 mL/kg/h), approximately 1 L/h for the first 2 hours of resuscitation. Accurate monitoring of urine output is important and at the same time provides volume replacement. From the third hour of resuscitation, the fluid rate can be decreased to 7.5 mL/kg/h according to the clinical situation and urine output. With the decline of blood glucose of 250 mg/dL, the intravenous solution should be replaced with 5% dextrose in water. Insulin replacement should be started early and via the intravenous route. A bolus dose of 10 units may be administered first, followed by a continuous infusion of 5 to 10 units/h.[25] Patients with DKA are usually insulin resistant; hence, if hyperglycemia and anion gap are not improved by 2 hours the infusion rate may have to be doubled to overcome the resistance. Treatment with bicarbonate is indicated only in the presence of severe metabolic acidosis with a maternal pH of less than 7.10. Because of excessive potassium loss, frequent measurement of extracellular potassium is important, and potassium replacement may be necessary. Intravenous fluid should be continued until there is a resolution of nausea, and the patients are able to drink an adequate amount of fluid by mouth. In most instances, fetal heart rate (FHR) monitoring will suggest a nonreassuring pattern, with loss of beat-to-beat variability. The FHR gradually improves with proper maternal volume replacement as well as the treatment of the maternal metabolic disorder.[25]

Insulin Therapy

The goal of therapy is to maintain proper plasma glucose concentrations during the antepartum, intrapartum, and postpartum periods. The insulin requirement may vary,[27] depending on the different stages of pregnancy (Fig. 41–4*A*). The majority of patients will achieve adequate control with mixed therapy, a combination of regular and intermediate-acting insulin. In a few institutions, continuous subcutaneous insulin infusion (CSII) via pump has been used, with some success. The disadvantages of this regimen are (1) cost of supplies, (2) pump malfunction, and (3) uncertainty about whether this method offers significant advantages.[28] Oral hypoglycemic agents are not useful in IDDM pregnant patients.

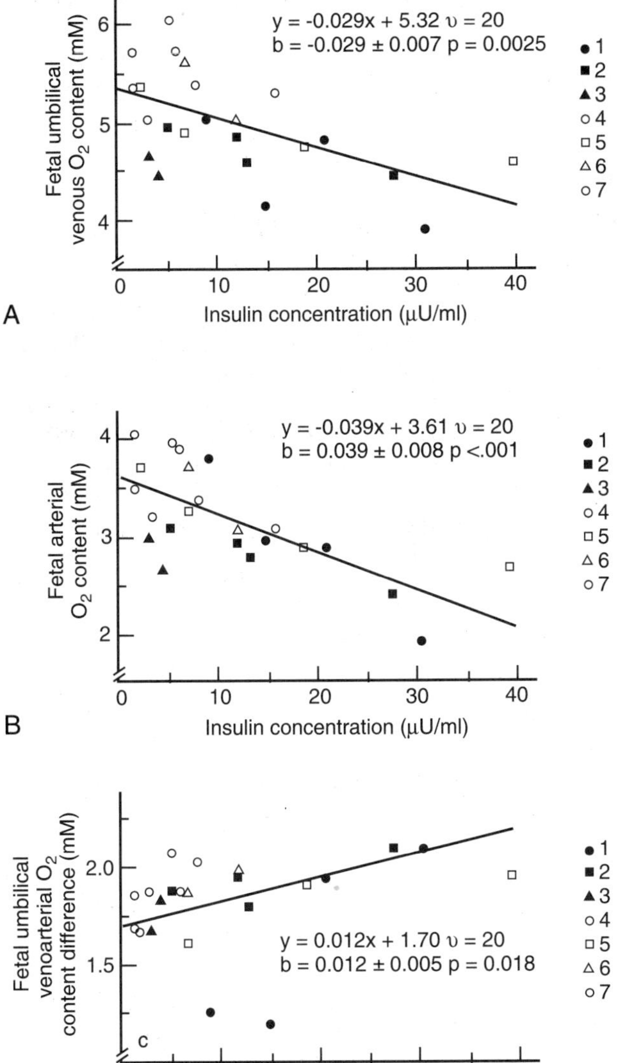

Figure 41–4 The association between fetal plasma insulin concentration and fetal umbilical venous oxygen content (*A*), fetal arterial oxygen content (*B*), and fetal umbilical venoarterial oxygen content difference (*C*). Shown is the regression line, as determined by analysis of covariance. Also shown are the regression equations and the slopes with their standard errors and P values. Data from seven animals are represented by the symbols shown in the figure. (From Milley JR, Rosenberg AA, Philipps AF, et al: The effect of insulin on ovine fetal oxygen extraction. Am J Obstet Gynecol 1984; 149:673.)

Management for Labor and Delivery

A tight control of maternal blood glucose is important during labor. Both hypoglycemia and hyperglycemia can affect the fetus. Glucose crosses the placenta by passive diffusion. Oakley and colleagues[29] observed a difference of blood glucose of 20 mg/dL or less between mother and fetus at the physiologic range of maternal glucose. The authors also observed a plateauing of fetal blood glucose (150 to 200 mg/dL)—even the maternal blood glucose level rose more than 300 mg/dL. In my institution, different results were observed. We found a direct correlation between maternal and fetal blood glucose levels, and there was no upper limit of placental transfer of glucose. Umbilical blood glucose was found to be higher than 300 mg/dL following acute maternal volume expansion with 5% of dextrose solution. Maternal hyperglycemia produces fetal hyperglycemia and hyperinsulinemia and ultimately neonatal hypoglycemia. Lactate concentrations in the fetus were found to be increased in the presence of high glucose and fructose concentrations in the mother.[30] In an animal model, Shelley[31] observed an increased accumulation of lactate in fetal lambs during hyperglycemia and hypoxia. In an interesting study, Robillard and colleagues[32] compared fetal blood gases, pH, and plasma lactate concentrations at different stages of hyperglycemia in well-oxygenated sheep fetuses. Plasma lactate concentration increased, with an associated decrease of fetal pH (7.38 to 7.32); however, the fetal blood gases were stable in the fetus when the fetal plasma glucose concentration was above 150 mg/dL. On the other hand, a severe metabolic acidosis and concomitant decreases in blood gases and pH (from 7.38 to 7.18) occurred when the fetal plasma glucose level was more than 300 mg/dL. In a primate study, we observed severe fetal metabolic acidosis in the presence of maternal hyperglycemia and acute hypoxia.[33] For labor and delivery one third to one half of the pregnancy dose of insulin can be given in the morning, as the insulin requirement goes down significantly following delivery. West and Lowy[34] used low-dose intravenous insulin together with dextrose during labor. A normal dose of insulin was given to the patient the day before the induction of labor and delivery; food was withheld after 10 p.m. The following morning the patient received 1 liter of 5% dextrose solution every 6 hours, together with 1 to 2 units/h of Actrapid insulin. Maternal blood glucose levels were observed frequently, and the insulin infusion was adjusted to maintain the maternal blood glucose concentrations between 90 and 125 mg/dL. None of the neonates were hypoglycemic. In my institution maternal fasting blood glucose (FBG) remains an important marker. If the FBG is less than 120 mg/dL, intermediate-acting insulin is administered in one third of the daily dose given during pregnancy, and capillary blood glucose levels are measured every 1 to 2 hours during labor. If capillary blood glucose levels exceed 120 mg/dL, an intravenous infusion of 0.5 to 2 units of regular insulin per hour is added. However, if the baseline FBG is higher than 120 mg/dL, an intravenous infusion of insulin is used at the onset. In the case of cesarean delivery, usually no insulin is given if the surgery is scheduled in the early morning. If the abdominal delivery is planned later in the day, one third of the regular dose is given in the presence of normal FBG. Blood glucose is routinely checked in the postanesthesia care unit (PACU), and the dose of insulin is adjusted accordingly. Lev-Ran[35] noted a significant drop in the insulin requirement for 1 or 2 days in 11 of 12 patients undergoing cesarean section.

The exact mechanism of the immunogenicity of the animal insulin in the human is unknown; however, the differences in the composition of amino acids between the bovine, porcine, and human insulin could be one of the mechanisms. Hence, technology has been focused on reshaping the amino acid structure of human insulin to make it more advantageous with regard to subcutaneous use as well as to the other important pharmacologic profiles. Insulin Lispro has been approved for clinical use in the United States.[36] This new insulin has a few distinct clinical advantages. However, it has not been used in parturients, as not enough data are available at the present regarding its teratogenic effect. Future studies may ultimately lead to its use in IDDM pregnant patients.

Anesthetic Management

Decreased uteroplacental perfusion is the most important pathologic change that can take place in diabetic parturients. The fetus of a mother with uncontrolled IDDM will be hypoxic because of (1) increased maternal HbA_{1c}, (2) hyperglycemia and hyperinsulinemia, and (3) significantly decreased uteroplacental perfusion. Hence, hypotension because of regional anesthesia or vena caval compression should be prevented. For labor and delivery, moderate pain relief can be obtained by intramuscular or intravenous narcotics in the early part of labor. Lumbar epidural or combined spinal epidural anesthesia[37] (if the airway is normal) will provide excellent pain relief both for labor and delivery. A continuous infusion of a low concentration of local anesthetic mixed with fentanyl can be used for continuous epidural infusion without adverse fetal effect.[38] Pearson[39] observed that the fetus commenced the second stage in a less acidotic state when mothers were given epidural anesthesia than when mothers received no anesthesia. Acidosis was metabolic in origin and was related to high lactate concentration. Shnider and colleagues[40] observed decreased maternal catecholamine concentrations associated with excellent pain relief following the use of epidural anesthesia. A decreased catecholamine will indirectly increase placental perfusion, provided that maternal blood pressure is maintained. The other advantage of epidural analgesia is the prevention of maternal hyperventilation. Maternal alkalosis causes fetal acidosis. Valsalva maneuvers may be contraindicated in parturients with diabetic retinopathy, because it might predispose to vitreous hemorrhage.[10] Dense perineal anesthesia prevents the urge to push. For forceps delivery, dense anesthesia may be necessary; 3% 2-chloroprocaine or 2% plain lidocaine produces excellent results. Close attention to maternal blood pressure is important. If the mother is already receiving intravenous insulin mixed with 5% dextrose, a second intravenous line may be beneficial for volume expansion with nondextrose solution. Continuous fetal heart rate monitoring is absolutely essential throughout labor. In the absence of epidural anesthesia, spinal anesthesia may be indicated for forceps delivery. A small amount of 1.5% hyperbaric lidocaine or 0.75% bupivacaine may be used. Maternal hypotension should be treated promptly with aggressive volume replacement and the use of vasopressors.

Cesarean Sections

Several important pathophysiologic changes that take place in these patients should be considered. These are (1) uteroplacental insufficiency, (2) associated fetal hypoxia, (3) diabetic neuropathy, (4) preclinical cardiomyopathy, and (5) diabetic scleredema. Because of these pathophysiologic changes, parturients will be more prone to hypotension. In some situations, hypotension (severely diabetic patient, according to White's classification) may be difficult to treat.

Datta and Brown[41] compared spinal and general anesthesia for cesarean section in healthy pregnant and diabetic mothers (Table 41–2). The infants of diabetic mothers who had received spinal anesthesia were more acidotic than the infants of the mothers who received general anesthesia. Acidosis was related

Table 41–2 Maternal-Neonatal Acid-Base Values

	No Hypotension	Hypotension
1977 Study* (Spinal Anesthesia for Cesarean Section)		
Umbilical Artery		
pH	7.24±0.02†	7.16±0.01§
Po_2 (mm Hg)	19±2	16±2
Pco_2 (mm Hg)	65±3	71±4
Base deficit (mEq/L)	4.35±0.88	8.25±1.74§
1981 Study¶ (Epidural Anesthesia for Cesarean Section)		
Umbilical Artery		
pH	7.26±0.02†	7.16±0.01§
Po_2 (mm Hg)	25±2.5	18±1.3§
Pco_2 (mm Hg)	52±2	65±3§
Base deficit (mEq/L)	5±1.2	10±0.6§

*Data from Datta S, Brown WU Jr: Acid-base status in diabetic mothers and their infants following general or spinal anesthesia for cesarean section. Anesthesiology 1977; 47:272–276.

†Mean±SE.

§$P < 0.05$.

¶Data from Datta S, Brown WU Jr, Ostheimer GW, et al: Epidural anesthesia for cesarean section in diabetic parturients: maternal and neonatal acid-base status and bupivacaine concentration. Anesth Analg 1981; 60:574–580.

to maternal diabetes and hypotension. Subsequent study from the same group observed the neonatal acid-base values following the use of epidural anesthesia for cesarean section.[42] The incidence of neonatal acidosis (umbilical artery pH 7.20 or less) was 60%. Fetal acidosis was associated with the severity of maternal diabetes and hypotension. The umbilical artery pH was always greater than 7.20 in the absence of maternal hypotension. In both studies, 5% dextrose solution was used for acute volume expansion.

The mechanisms of fetal acidosis following regional anesthesia for cesarean section are complex; however, several factors may be involved. The human placenta produces lactate in vitro, especially during hypoxia,[43] and in the presence of increased glycogen deposition, as it occurs in diabetes. The placenta of the ewe can also produce lactic acid.[44] In sheep, lactate metabolism accounts for 25% of fetal oxygen consumption, whereas glucose metabolism accounts for 50%. A glycogen-rich placenta in the diabetic parturient can contribute lactate in fetal blood during conditions of relative hypoxia, which may happen during decreased placental blood flow following maternal hypotension. In human pregnancy, elevated fetal blood glucose may be associated with acidosis at birth. Swanstrom and Bratteby[45] observed a significant correlation between umbilical cord blood glucose concentrations and base deficit with the neonate's low 1-minute Apgar score. Kenepp and colleagues[46] observed lower umbilical artery pH values in the presence of higher umbilical artery glucose produced by maternal volume expansion with dextrose solution. Fetal lactic acidosis may occur in the presence of maternal hyperglycemia, followed by fetal hyperglycemia and associated maternal hypotension. Kitzmiller and colleagues[33] observed the effect of maternal hypoxia, following the administration of intravenous normal saline or dextrose solution, on maternal and fetal acid-base values in Rhesus monkeys. The hyperglycemic fetus had (1) a greater reduction in arterial oxygen tension and content than that of normoglycemic control subjects, despite similar values for maternal arterial oxygen partial pressure in each group, and (2) severe metabolic acidosis, compared with a modest reduction of arterial pH in normoglycemic fetuses. However, hyperglycemic monkey fetuses exposed to moderate maternal hypoxia did not have greater increases in blood lactate levels compared to normoglycemic fetuses. Beside fetal hypoxia and acidosis, the other ill effect of fetal hyperglycemia is higher incidences of neonatal hypoglycemia. Soler and Malins[47] observed an incidence of more than 40% of neonatal hypoglycemia in the presence of maternal blood glucose of more than 130 mg/dL. In an interesting study using sheep models, Carson and colleagues[48] observed that chronic infusion of insulin directly into the sheep fetus increased fetal glucose utilization, using oxygen, and subsequently decreased fetal arterial oxygen content (Fig. 41–4*B* and *C*). The authors speculated that in uncontrolled diabetes, associated fetal hyperglycemia and hyperinsulinemia will be associated with fetal hypoxia and acidosis. Datta and colleagues[49] reevaluated the acid-base status of 20 rigidly controlled IDDM parturients; 10 had received spinal anesthesia and 10 had undergone general anesthesia. With Ringer's lactate (dextrose-free) solution, volume expansion and aggressive treatment of any drop in maternal blood pressure was achieved using ephedrine as the vasopressor. No significant differences were observed in acid-base values between diabetic and nondiabetic mothers, as well as in infants between the groups (Table 41–3). The authors concluded that in the presence of well-controlled maternal blood glucose acute volume expansion with Ringer's lactate and aggressive management of a drop in maternal blood pressure, spinal anesthesia will be associated with a good neonatal outcome.

Spinal Versus Epidural Anesthesia for Cesarean Section

Spinal anesthesia is the preferred method for cesarean section at the present time unless contraindicated. Because of the rapidity of onset, the incidence of hypotension is higher following subarachnoid block. The incidences of hypotension may be significant in parturients with severe diabetes, as the occurrences of cardiomyopathy and autonomic dysfunction are higher in these patients. With the known existence of aforementioned problems, epidural anesthesia may be a better option. A large volume of local anesthetic should not be injected during a short time period in patients with stiff joint syndrome; a case of temporary anterior spinal artery syndrome was reported following the use of 35 mL of 3% 2-chloroprocaine via epidural catheter for cesarean section. Possible mechanisms, as suggested by the author, were (1) less compliant epidural space, (2) diminished arterial supply to the spinal cord due to the increased epidural space pressure, and (3) preexisting microvascular disease in the spinal cord.

Combined spinal epidural technique can also be used in such a situation.[50]

General anesthesia in diabetic parturients may be associated with a few important problems: (1) gastroparesis, (2) limited atlanto-occipital joint extension in patients with diabetic stiff joint syndrome, and (3) impaired counter-regulatory hormone responses to hypoglycemia during sleep.

Table 41–3 1982 Study (Spinal Anesthesia for Cesarean Section)

	No Hypotension	Hypotension
Umbilical artery		
pH	7.27±0.01*	7.30±0.01
Po_2 (mm Hg)	20±2	22±2
Pco_2 (mm Hg)	56±2	50±2.5
Base deficit (mEq/L)	4±1	3±0.7

*Mean±SE.

Data from Datta S, Kitzmiller JL, Naulty JS, et al: Acid-base status of diabetic mothers and their infants following spinal anesthesia for cesarean section. Anesth Analg 1982; 61:662–665.

As erythromycin possesses a gastric emptying effect similar to that of the hormone motilin, Janssens and colleagues[51] observed the effect of erythromycin in gastric emptying in 10 patients with IDDM and gastroparesis. Erythromycin significantly shortened the gastric emptying times for both liquids and solids. Metoclopramide should be used routinely preoperatively to enhance gastric emptying as well as to increase the tone of the gastroesophageal sphincter. Diabetic parturients with a positive "prayer sign" should be thoroughly examined for the proper extension of the atlanto-occipital joint. Vohra and associates[52] observed the cardiovascular responses to tracheal intubation in 10 diabetic patients with proven abnormal autonomic function and compared them with 10 healthy patients. There was a greater increase in heart rates, mean arterial pressure, and vascular resistance in the diabetic group. The authors speculated that the exaggerated pressure response to tracheal stimulation in diabetic subjects may be related to autonomic dysfunction. Although no clinical study exists on this hypothesis, one should speculate that the IDDM parturients may be in a better condition to undergo cesarean section under regional than under general anesthesia. Under regional anesthesia, patients will be able to vocalize signs of hypoglycemia; cardiovascular responses to hypoglycemia may be blunted when patients are under general anesthesia. For postoperative pain relief, intrathecal morphine may be used following regional anesthesia, whereas patient-controlled analgesia should be used for parturients who are to undergo cesarean section under general anesthesia. In the PACU, routine blood glucose estimation must be performed and insulin doses should be adjusted accordingly.

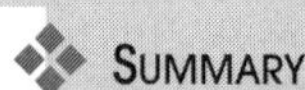

SUMMARY

Key Points

- Because the incidence of respiratory distress syndrome (RDS) is very high among the neonates of IDDM parturients, the establishment of lung maturity is important.
- The incidence of superimposed preeclampsia is high in class F diabetics. It may be difficult to distinguish between hypertensive diabetic nephropathy and preeclampsia.
- The cesarean section rate is much higher in diabetic women. Epidural analgesia is an ideal technique for labor and delivery analgesia and can also be used for cesarean section.
- Pregnancy produces a progressive increase in peripheral resistance to insulin. Since insulin requirements decrease significantly in the postpartum period, the insulin regimen may need to be adjusted at that time.

Key Reference

Ramanathan S, Khoo P, Arismendy J: Perioperative maternal and neonatal acid-base status and glucose metabolism in patients with insulin-dependent diabetes mellitus. Anesth Analg 1991; 73:105–111.

Case Stem

A 32-year-old primigravida with class F-R diabetes is admitted for induction of labor at 38 weeks of gestation. Discuss the anesthetic management.

NEONATAL CONSIDERATIONS

Because of high incidences of RDS, hypoglycemia, major congenital anomalies, macrosomia, and severe IUGR, the neonatologist should be present at the time of both vaginal and abdominal delivery.

With the advent of modern ventilatory support, including high-frequency ventilation and surfactant therapy, the survival rate of infants with RDS has increased significantly. Rarely, severe polycythemia can produce thrombosis, especially in the renal veins. Hyperbilirubinemia and hypocalcemia also occur more frequently in these infants. Mothers should be delivered in hospitals with access to a neonatal intensive care unit.

References

1. Garner P: Type I diabetes mellitus and pregnancy. Lancet 1995; 46:157–161.
2. Beard RW, Lowy C: The British survey of diabetic pregnancies. Br J Obstet Gynaecol 1982; 89:783–785.
3. White P: Pregnancy and diabetes: medical aspects. Med Clin North Am 1965; 49:1015–1019.
4. Nylund L, Lunell NO, Lewander R, et al: Uteroplacental blood flow in diabetic pregnancy: measurements with indium 113m and a computer-linked gamma camera. Am J Obstet Gynecol 1976; 144:298–302.
5. Reece EA, Hagay Z, Assimakopoulos E, et al: Diabetes mellitus in pregnancy and assessment of umbilical artery wave forms using pulsed Doppler ultrasonography. J Ultrasound Med 1994; 13:73–80.
6. Bjork O, Persson B: Placental changes in relation to the degree of metabolic control in diabetes mellitus. Placenta 1983; 3:367–378.
7. Madsen H, Ditzel J: Changes in red blood cell oxygen transport in diabetic pregnancy. Am J Obstet Gynecol 1982; 143:421–424.
8. Drury MI, Greene AT, Stronge JM: Pregnancy complicated by clinical diabetes mellitus: a study of 600 pregnancies. Obstet Gynecol 1977; 49:51–60.
9. Hare JW: Diabetic complications of diabetic pregnancies. Semin Perinatol 1994; 18:451–458.
10. Klein BEK, Moss SE, Klein R: Effect of pregnancy on progression of diabetic retinopathy. Diabetes Care 1990; 13:34–40.
11. Hirsch BR, Shamoon H: Defective epinephrine and growth hormone responses in Type I diabetes are stimulus specific. Diabetes 1987; 36:20–26.
12. Jones TW, Porter P, Sherwin RS, et al: Decreased epinephrine responses to hypoglycemia during sleep. N Engl J Med 1998; 338:1657–1662.
13. Airaksinen KEJ, Ikaheimo MJ, Slmea PI: Impaired cardiac adjustment to pregnancy in type I diabetes. Diabetes Care 1986; 9:376–381.
14. Hogan K, Rusy D, Springman SR: Difficult laryngoscopy and diabetes mellitus. Anesth Analg 1988; 67:1162–1164.
15. Eastwood DW: Anterior spinal artery syndrome after epidural anesthesia in a pregnant diabetic patient with scleroderma. Anesth Analg 1991; 73:90–91.
16. Fagen C, King JD, Erick M: Nutrition management in women with gestational diabetes mellitus: a review by ADA's diabetes

care and education dietetic practice group. J Am Diet Assoc 1995; 95:460–467.

17. Naylor CD, Sermer M, Chen E, Sykora K: Cesarean delivery in relation to birth weight and gestational glucose tolerance: pathophysiology or practice style? JAMA 1996; 275:1165–1170.
18. Rowenn B, Miodovnik M, Combs CA, et al: Glycemic thresholds for spontaneous abortion and congenital malformations in insulin-dependent diabetes mellitus. Obstet Gynecol 1994; 84:515–520.
19. Reece EA, Hobbins JC: Diabetic embryopathy: pathogenesis, prenatal diagnosis and prevention. Obstet Gynecol Surv 1986; 41:325–335.
20. Campanaro J, Okun N, Stenstrom R, Garner PR: Macrosomia: the relative importance of diabetes as a predisposing factor. Am J Obstet Gynecol 1991; 164:136–137.
21. Menon RK, Cohen RM, Sperling MA, et al: Transplacental passage of insulin in pregnant women with insulin dependent diabetes mellitus: its role in fetal macrosomia. N Engl J Med 1990; 323:309–315.
22. Coustan DR, Imarah J: Prophylactic insulin treatment of gestational diabetes reduces the incidence of macrosomia, operative delivery, and birth trauma. Am J Obstet Gynecol 1984; 150:836–840.
23. Miller JM, Horger EO: Antepartum heart rate testing in diabetic pregnancy. J Reprod Med 1985; 30:515–520.
24. Bernstein IM, Catalano PM: Examination of factors contributing to the risk of cesarean delivery in women with gestational diabetes. Obstet Gynecol 1994; 83:462–465.
25. Luzi L, Barrett EJ, Groop LC, et al: Metabolic effects of low-dose insulin therapy on glucose metabolism in diabetic ketoacidosis. Diabetes 1988; 37:1470–1477.
26. Rigg LA, Petie RH: Fetal biochemical and biophysical assessment. *In* Reece EA, Coustan DR (eds): Diabetes Mellitus in Pregnancy: Principles and Practice. New York: Churchill Livingstone; 1988:375.
27. Tyson JE, Felig P: Medical aspects of diabetes in pregnancy and the diabetogenic effects of oral contraceptives. Med Clin North Am 1971; 55:947.
28. Coustan DR, Reece EA, Sherwin RS, et al: A randomized clinical trial of the insulin pump vs. intensive conventional therapy in diabetic pregnancies. JAMA 1986; 255:531–536.
29. Oakley NW, Beard RW, Turner RC: Effect of sustained maternal hyperglycemia in normal and diabetic pregnancies. Br Med J 1972; 1:466–469.
30. Ames AC, Cobbolds MJ: Lactic acidosis complicating treatment of ketosis in labour. Br Med J 1975; 4:511–513.
31. Shelley HJ: The use of chronically catheterized foetal lambs for the foetal metabolism in combine. *In* Gross RS, Dawes KW, Nathanielsz PW (eds): Foetal and Neonatal Physiology. London: Cambridge University Press; 1973:360–381.
32. Robillard JE, Session C, Kennedy RL, Smith FG Jr: Metabolic effects of constant hypertonic glucose infusion in well-oxygenated fetuses. Am J Obstet Gynecol 1978; 130:199–203.
33. Kitzmiller JL, Phillipe M, VanOeyen P, et al: Hyperglycemia, hypoxia and fetal acidosis in rhesus monkeys. [Abstracts of scientific papers.] St. Louis: Society for Gynecologic Investigation; 1981:98.
34. West TET, Lowy C: Control of blood glucose during labour in diabetic women with combined glucose and low dose insulin infusion. Br Med J 1977; 1:1252–1254.
35. Lev-Ran A: Sharp temporary drop in insulin requirement after cesarean section in diabetic patients. Am J Obstet Gynecol 1974; 120:905–908.
36. Holleman F, Hoekstra JBL: Insulin Lispro. N Engl J Med 1997; 183:176–183.
37. Campbell DC, Camann WR, Datta S: The addition of bupivacaine to intrathecal sufentanil for labor analgesia. Anesth Analg 1995; 81:305–309.
38. Bader A, Fragneto R, Terui K, et al: Maternal and neonatal fentanyl and bupivacaine levels after epidural infusion during labor. Anesth Analg 1995; 81:829–832.
39. Pearson JF: The effect of continuous lumbar epidural block on maternal and fetal acid-base balance during labor and at delivery. *In* Doughty A (ed): Proceedings of the Symposium on Epidural Analgesia in Obstetrics. London: Lewis; 1972:16–30.
40. Shnider SM, Abboud T, Artal R, et al: Maternal endogenous catecholamines decrease during labor after lumbar epidural anesthesia. Am J Obstet Gynecol 1983; 147:13–15.
41. Datta S, Brown WU Jr: Acid-base status in diabetic mothers and their infants following general or spinal anesthesia for cesarean section. Anesthesiology 1977; 47:272–276.
42. Datta S, Brown WU Jr, Ostheimer GW, et al: Epidural anesthesia for cesarean section in diabetic parturients: maternal and neonatal acid-base status and bupivacaine concentration. Anesth Analg 1981; 60:574–580.
43. Gabbe SG, Demer SLM, Greep RO, Villee AC: The effects of hypoxia on placental glycogen metabolism. Am J Obstet Gynecol 1972; 114:540–545.
44. Shelley JH, Bassett JM, Milner RDG: Control of carbohydrate metabolism in the fetus and newborn. Br Med Bull 1975; 31:37–43.
45. Swanstrom S, Bratteby LE: Metabolic effects of obstetric regional analgesia and of asphyxia in the newborn infant during the first two hours after birth. Acta Paediatr Scand 1981; 70:791–800.
46. Kenepp NB, Shelley WC, Kuman S, et al: Effects on newborn of hydration with glucose in patients undergoing cesarean section with regional anaesthesia. Lancet 1980; 1:645–646.
47. Soler NG, Malins JM: Diabetic pregnancy: management of diabetes on the day of delivery. Diabetologia 1978; 15:441–446.
48. Carson BS, Philipps AF, Simmon MA, et al: Effects of a sustained insulin infusion upon glucose uptake and oxygenation of the ovine fetus. Pediatr Res 1980; 13:147–152.
49. Datta S, Kitzmiller JL, Naulty JS, et al: Acid-base status of diabetic mothers and their infants following spinal anesthesia for cesarean section. Anesth Analg 1982; 61:662–665.
50. Rawal N, Schollin J, Wesstrom G: Epidural versus combined spinal epidural block for cesarean section. Acta Anaesthesiol Scand 1988; 32:61–66.
51. Janssens J, Peeters RL, Vantrappen G, et al: Improvement of gastric emptying in diabetic gastroparesis by erythromycin: preliminary studies. N Engl J Med 1990; 322:1028–1031.
52. Vohra A, Kumar S, Charlton AJ, et al: Effect of diabetes mellitus on the cardiovascular responses to induction of anaesthesia and tracheal intubation. Br J Anaesth 1993; 71:258–261.

42

Hematologic Disease

MICHAEL LOTTAN, MD
ROY MASHIACH, MD
MICHAEL NAMESTNIKOV, MD

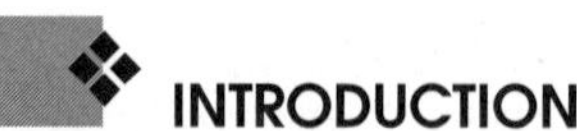

INTRODUCTION

The physiologic adaptations to pregnancy involve profound changes, many of which begin soon after conception and continue throughout gestation. Most of these remarkable changes occur in response to physiologic stimuli provided by the fetus and the placenta. Some of these changes may mimic several hematologic disorders and thus make the assessment of these disorders during pregnancy more difficult. An understanding of the physiologic changes of pregnancy provides the basis for better understanding of pathologic processes, as they relate to the hematologic system.

BLOOD VOLUME

Pregnancy-induced hypervolemia serves to meet the demands of the enlarged uterus with its hypertrophied vascular system, to protect the mother and the fetus against the deleterious effects of impaired venous return in the supine and erect positions, and to safeguard the mother against the adverse effects of blood loss associated with parturition. The maternal blood volume increases markedly during pregnancy. It starts to increase during the first trimester, expands most rapidly during the second trimester, and then rises at a much slower rate during the third trimester. This increased blood volume (40% to 45%) results from an increase in both plasma (50%) and erythrocytes (33%). Moderate erythroid hyperplasia is present in the bone marrow, and the reticulocyte count is slightly elevated during normal pregnancy. This is due, in part, to a threefold increase in maternal plasma erythropoietin levels.[1] The increase in the volume of erythrocytes is accomplished via accelerated production. Despite augmented erythropoiesis, the concentration of hemoglobin, erythrocytes, and hematocrit decrease slightly during normal pregnancy because of increased plasma volume. Consequently, whole blood viscosity decreases.[2] The hemoglobin concentration at term averages 12.5 g/dL. In most women, a hemoglobin of less than 11.0 g/dL during late pregnancy should be considered abnormal, and is usually due to iron deficiency, rather than to the hypervolemia of pregnancy.

The iron requirements of normal pregnancy total about 1000 mg. About 300 mg are actively transferred to the fetus and placenta, about 200 mg are lost by excretion, and 500 mg are utilized by the body to increase the volume of circulating erythrocytes. The amount of iron absorbed from the diet, together with that mobilized from stores (300 mg), is usually insufficient to meet the demands imposed by pregnancy. Therefore, during normal pregnancy, especially during its second half, serum iron and ferritin concentrations decline, and transferrin levels increase.

During normal vaginal delivery of a single fetus, the average blood loss is about 500 to 600 mL. The average blood loss associated with cesarean delivery or with vaginal delivery of twins varies between 800 and 1000 mL.[3]

BLOOD LEUKOCYTES

The blood leukocyte count (mainly polymorphonuclear) varies considerably, ranging from 5000 to 12,000/mL during normal pregnancy. The increase in the polymorphonuclear leukocytes appears to be estrogen-stimulated.[4, 5] During labor, the leukocyte count may become markedly elevated, averaging 14,000 to 16,000/mL, but can reach as high as 25,000/mL. The cause for this marked increase is not known, but probably represents the reappearance in the circulation of leukocytes previously shunted out of the active circulation.[6] The leukocyte count returns to nonpregnant values within 6 days post partum.[7, 8]

The changes in white blood count are associated with an increase in their metabolic activity. There is an increased activity of leukocyte alkaline phosphatase, hexose monophosphates, myeloperoxidase, and glucose oxidation. These are needed for improved phagocytosis and intracellular destruction of bacteria and fungi, which are increased during pregnancy.[9, 10] Lymphocyte function is suppressed, and cell-mediated immunity is depressed. Human chorionic gonadotropin and/or prolactin can be the cause of suppressed function of lymphocytes. However, the lymphocyte count does not change significantly during pregnancy.[11] The depression of cell-mediated immunity during pregnancy is associated with decreased resistance to viral infections, such as herpes, influenza, poliomyelitis, rubella, and hepatitis.[12, 13]

BLOOD PLATELETS

Platelet concentrations may decrease moderately with the progression of pregnancy,[14] as a consequence of increased platelet consumption throughout normal pregnancy.[15] The mean platelet volume is mildly elevated, and platelet distribution width significantly increases as pregnancy advances.[14] In addition, platelet half-life is shorter in the pregnant state compared with the nonpregnant state.[12]

Platelets produced in the bone marrow from megakaryocytes have a life span of 9 to 12 days, with most being engulfed in the reticuloendothelial system. A decline in platelet count is occasionally observed in the third trimester. This decline is usually attributed to hemodilution and/or low-grade chronic intravascular coagulation within the uteroplacental circulation.

COAGULATION

The levels of plasma fibrinogen during normal pregnancy can increase by about 50%, to as much as 600 mg/dL in the third trimester, compared with nonpregnant women (200 to 400 mg/dL). This contributes greatly to the increase in the erythrocyte sedimentation rate.[16] Factors VII, VIII, IX, and X all are increased appreciably during normal pregnancy. Factor II is increased only slightly, whereas factors XI and XIII are decreased.[17]

Antithrombin III levels remain within the normal range throughout pregnancy. Both protein C and protein S decrease during pregnancy. Inherited hypercoagulability states such as protein C, protein S, and antithrombin III deficiencies account for 15% to 20% of thromboembolic episodes during pregnancy. D-dimer levels increase with gestational age.[18, 19]

The level of plasminogen in plasma increases considerably. This increase may be secondary to the increase in the estrogen levels. Despite this change, the fibrinolysis is distinctly prolonged, compared with that of the normal nonpregnant state, and thromboelastography demonstrates a hypercoagulable state.

The hypercoagulable state associated with pregnancy is helpful because of the potential need for higher amounts of clotting factors. This situation allows a reduction of the bleeding that usually occurs during delivery and thus allows the new mother to quickly achieve a satisfactory coagulation status.

ANEMIA

The effect of anemia on pregnancy is important, as maternal and perinatal outcome can change markedly. Anemia is defined as a hemoglobin concentration of less than 12 g/dL in nonpregnant women and less than 10 g/dL (1%) during pregnancy.[6] The hemoglobin concentration is usually lowest in midpregnancy. The Centers for Disease Control and Prevention (CDC) has defined anemia as less than 11.0 g/dL in the first and third trimesters and less than 10.5 g/dL in the second trimester. This modest fall in hemoglobin is caused by plasma volume expansion, which exceeds the increase in the hemoglobin mass and red cell volume. This effect has been called "physiological anemia." The disproportion between the rates at which plasma and erythrocytes are added to maternal circulation reaches its peak during the second trimester.[6] The frequency of anemia varies considerably during pregnancy, depending primarily on whether supplemental iron is taken. In women who received iron supplementation, hemoglobin levels at term averaged 12.7 g/dL, compared with 11.2 g/dL in women who did not.[20]

Iron Deficiency

The most common cause of anemia during pregnancy is iron deficiency. During single-fetus pregnancy, maternal iron consumption is about 1000 mg. A total of 300 mg is invested in the fetus and placenta, and 500 mg in maternal hemoglobin, and 200 mg are shed through the gut, urine, and skin. Unless the difference between the amount of stored iron available to the mother and the iron requirements of normal pregnancy cited is compensated for by absorption of iron from the gastrointestinal tract, iron deficiency anemia develops. With rapid expansion of blood volume, iron shortage increases. Iron deficiency anemia during pregnancy is the consequence primarily of expansion of plasma volume without equal expansion of the hemoglobin mass.

The classic morphologic evidence of iron deficiency anemia is erythrocyte hypochromia and microcytosis. Serum iron binding capacity is elevated, serum ferritin levels decrease, and normoblastic hyperplasia of the bone marrow is found. Evaluation includes measurements of hemoglobin, hematocrit, red blood cell indices, smear of peripheral blood, and iron and ferritin levels.

Treatment of elemental iron deficiency can be accomplished by oral supplementation. The response may be detected by an elevated reticulocyte count. To replenish iron stores, oral therapy should be continued for 3 months or more. Transfusions of iron, red blood cells, or whole blood are seldom indicated, unless hypovolemia from blood loss exists and an operative procedure must be performed.

PREGNANCY COMPLICATED BY HEMOGLOBINOPATHY

Hemoglobinopathies are abnormalities resulting from alternation in the structure or production of hemoglobin. The etiology of thalassemia syndromes involves diminished production of normal hemoglobin, while the etiology of sickle cell anemia is substitution of one or more amino acids in the globin chain.

Sickle Cell Anemia

The defect associated with hemoglobin S (HbS) occurs when the neutrally charged amino acid valine is replaced by the negatively charged glutamic acid. The defect associated with hemoglobin C (HbC) occurs when lysine is replaced by glutamic acid. These structural changes are inherited in an autosomal recessive manner. In the 1950s and 1960s, sickle hemoglobinopathies were thought to be a contraindication to pregnancy. Since the 1970s, mainly because of sickle cell centers offering aggressive surveillance and treatment, a dramatic decrease in morbidity and mortality has been achieved. Now, normal pregnancy can usually be completed for many women with sickle hemoglobinopathies.

The sickle hemoglobinopathies are classified as major or minor, depending on the severity of clinical symptoms. The minor hemoglobinopathies are associated with urinary tract infections and anemia during pregnancy. Hemoglobin SS (HbSS), hemoglobin SC (HbSC), and hemoglobin S-beta thalassemia (HbS-beta thal.) represent the vast majority of the clinically significant hemoglobinopathies and are called "sickle cell disease." The disease is more common in people of African ancestry and in people of the Mediterranean, Middle Eastern, and East Indian origin.[21] Hemoglobin S, when in the deoxyhemoglobin state, tends to bind and create strands of polymerized hemoglobin within the erythrocyte, thus changing to a sickle shape. When reoxygenated, the cell returns to its regular form. Repeated polymerization-aggregation cycles lead to membrane rigidity and shorter half-life for the erythrocyte (17 days, as compared to 120 in the normal population), thus resulting in a chronic anemia of 6.5 to 9.5 g/dL.[21] The odd-shaped erythrocyte, with its rigid membrane, tends to occlude small vessels, thus increasing intracellular hypoxia, acidosis, and 2,3-diphosphoglycerate (2,3-DPG) production, leading to further sickling and tissue hypoxia. This vicious cycle leads to necrosis or infarction of various organs, which manifests as painful events and end-organ failure. The clinical manifestations of this disease can occur at any time during pregnancy. Virtually all the signs and symptoms are secondary to hemolysis, vaso-occlusive crises, and increased susceptibility to infections.[21] Vaso-occlusive crises manifest as pain in long bones, abdomen, chest, or back. There may be low-grade fever and leukocytosis. Many precipitating factors, as illustrated in Table 42–1, have been implicated. These events are more frequent in the second half of pregnancy.

Although rare in clinical obstetrics, aplastic crises manifesting as weakness and pallor without icterus are the most common hematologic crises occurring during pregnancy.[22] These crises are usually associated with infection, and although ordinarily mild, if they go untreated they can result in cardiac failure. The crises usually resolve with aggressive transfusion therapy and treatment of the precipitating factors (e.g., treating infection, restoring adequate oxygenation, and correcting metabolic acidosis). The liberal use of parenteral analgesic, usually an opiate derivative, is indicated during such crises. Recently, the administration of high-dose methylprednisolone was demonstrated to decrease the duration and severity of the crises in children and adolescents, although such use has never been tested in parturients.

Pregnancy can cause exacerbation of sickle cell disease. The increased incidence of clinical manifestations during pregnancy is probably the result of increased metabolic demands, the hypercoagulable state, and the increased vascular stasis common to all pregnant patients. Vaso-occlusive crises are more common in the second half of pregnancy, when vascular stasis and oxygen demands increase. An altered immune system makes sickle cell patients prone to pyelonephritis and cholelithiasis, both of which are more common than in the normal gravid population.

Pregnancy outcome in women with sickle cell disease is often determined by the severity of the anemia. Diagnosis is dependent on the presence of HbS. With the major syndromes, manifestations occur in early childhood; thus, it is unusual for patients to become pregnant with an undiagnosed disease. All patients with sickle hemoglobinopathies are encouraged to take 1 mg of folate supplementation per day; iron supplementation is withheld unless there is evidence of iron deficiency. The goal of this treatment is to maintain the hemoglobin percentage at rates higher than 20% and thus increase the overall oxygen-carrying capacity. This treatment lowers the incidence of vaso-occlusive crises during pregnancy but is associated with the known risks of transfusion therapy. Intrapartum management should contain supportive measures that ensure adequate hydration, oxygenation, reduction of stress, and avoidance of hypotension or hypertension. Early ambulation, adequate hydration, and aggressive management of infection are also essential in the postpartum period. Oral analgesics should be administered generously.

Table 42–1 PRECIPITATING FACTORS FOR SICKLE CRISES

Dehydration
Hypotension
Hypothermia and shivering
Increase in hemoglobin S > 50%

Thalassemia

The term "thalassemia" is used to designate a number of hereditary disorders in which there is a failure or reduction of structurally normal hemoglobin. Women who have β-thalassemia major and survive childhood are usually infertile. Women with β-thalassemia minor tend to have an average hemoglobin level of 8 to 10 g/dL late in the second trimester, with an increase to 9 to 11 g/dL near term. They rarely require treatment.[23]

THROMBOCYTOPENIA

Thrombocytopenia is second only to anemia as a hematologic complication of pregnancy. Usually, the plate-

Table 42-2 CAUSES OF THROMBOCYTOPENIA IN THE PREGNANT PATIENT

Idiopathic	Septicemia
Acquired	Systemic lupus erythematosus
Preeclampsia/eclampsia	Megaloblastic anemia
HELLP syndrome	Viral infections
Severe obstetric hemorrhage	Aplastic anemia
Transfusion	Radiation exposure
Placental abruption	Medications

let count falls slightly, owing to hemodilution and to increased turnover. However, the platelet count should not fall below 100,000 in normal pregnancy. Thrombocytopenia in pregnancy may be idiopathic, but it is more often associated with various disorders or medications, as illustrated in Tables 42–2 and 42–3.

Until the 1980s, all patients with unexplained thrombocytopenia carried a diagnosis of immune thrombocytopenic purpura (ITP). Traditional immunologic tests cannot distinguish between ITP, thrombocytopenia of preeclampsia, and gestational thrombocytopenia.[24] The difference between these disorders is important, however, since each has distinct maternal and neonatal implications.

Gestational Thrombocytopenia

The incidence of low platelet counts (<150,000/L) in normal pregnancy was reported as 7.6%, and counts of less than 100,000/L were reported in 0.9% of normal pregnancies. It appears that isolated mild maternal thrombocytopenia detected during the second half of pregnancy is not associated with adverse consequences to the mother or the fetus. The clinician must exercise care to exclude the presence of occult preeclampsia or hemolysis, elevated liver enzymes, and low platelets (HELLP). The possibility of undiagnosed ITP or thrombotic thrombocytopenic purpura (TTP) must also be considered.[25, 26]

Immune Thrombocytopenic Purpura

The entity previously called "idiopathic thrombocytopenic purpura" is usually a condition caused by production of antiplatelet antibodies. Acute idiopathic thrombocytopenic purpura most often follows a viral infection. Most of the cases resolve spontaneously, and about 10% become chronic. ITP is primarily a disease of young women and rarely resolves spontaneously.[27] Despite the fact that 1 to 3 per 1000 pregnancies are affected, ITP requires much attention because of the potential for profound neonatal thrombocytopenia in infants born to mothers with this condition. No predisposing factor for fetal thrombocytopenia has been found. A neonatal morbidity rate of 278 per 1000 was reported for infants born to mothers with true ITP. The neonatal morbidity includes intraventricular hemorrhage, hemopericardium, gastrointestinal bleeding, and extensive cutaneous manifestation of bleeding.[28]

Pregnancy has not been determined to be a cause of ITP or to change its severity. Most cases are discovered during pregnancy because the disease is usually subclinical and manifested only in blood count, which is often taken for the first time during routine pregnancy care.

Orally administered corticosteroids are the initial treatment, followed by intravenous therapy if necessary. Approximately 80% of pregnant women will respond to this therapy. Others may respond to high-dose immunoglobulin or splenectomy, usually performed during the second trimester.[27]

Obtaining fetal blood for thrombocytopenia assessment by percutaneous cordocentesis or intrapartum scalp sampling is difficult and cannot always predict neonatal bleeding disorders.[28]

Obstetric management of parturients with a stable platelet count above 50,000 is not different from that of normal parturients.[28] Contraindications to the use of regional anesthesia and a higher risk associated with general anesthesia do, however, exist if platelet count falls below this level. When attempting to determine the advisability of initiating regional anesthesia in these women, anesthesiologists should look at previous platelet counts to determine whether platelet count is stable. Clinical examination is also of great importance.

The fetus may be severely thrombocytopenic; thus, trauma resulting from vaginal delivery should be avoided when severe fetal thrombocytopenia is suspected. Abdominal delivery, however, which may be best for the neonate, may be more risky to the mother.

Thrombocytopenia Related to Severe Preeclampsia, HELLP Syndrome, and Other Microangiopathies

As discussed in Chapter 38, hypertensive disorders account for a substantial portion of the cases of pregnancy-related thrombocytopenia. Thrombocytopenia will develop in 15% to 18% of patients suffering from preeclampsia and 30% of those with eclampsia.[29] Because of the high maternal and fetal mortality and morbidity, every woman presenting with undiagnosed thrombocytopenia in the second or third trimester should be considered to have preeclampsia unless clinical and laboratory evaluations suggest otherwise. The pathogenesis of thrombocytopenia with preeclampsia-eclampsia is obscure. There is some evidence in favor of accelerated destruction of platelets owing to microangiopathy as well as to abnormal activation of

Table 42-3 MEDICATIONS KNOWN TO INDUCE PLATELET DYSFUNCTION

- Aspirin
- Nonsteroidal anti-inflammatory drugs (NSAIDs)
- Adenyl cyclase stimulators, including prostaglandin and prostacyclin
- Antibiotics
- Heparin
- Phosphodiesterase inhibitors (theophylline)

the coagulation system. Treatment, which is generally achieved via the expedient removal of all gestational products from the uterus, should not be delayed. Although some patients with mild thrombocytopenia can be managed expectantly by obstetricians in the community, if the condition worsens, the patient should be cared for, whenever possible, at a tertiary care center with perinatology, obstetric anesthesiology, and neonatology specialists all readily available. Platelet counts of less than 100,000 may correlate with evidence of hepatic and renal dysfunction, and disseminated intravascular coagulation (DIC) due to intravascular hemolysis (HELLP syndrome). Dexamethasone and platelet replacement can be used, depending on the platelet count and mode of delivery. The resolution of thrombocytopenia usually begins 72 to 96 hours post partum.[24, 27]

Thrombotic Thrombocytopenic Purpura

This disease is characterized by microangiopathic hemolytic anemia and severe thrombocytopenia. Pregnancy does not predispose to this condition, but this condition should be considered in the differential diagnosis when one evaluates a pregnant woman with severe thrombocytopenia. Thrombotic thrombocytopenic purpura has been characterized by the pentad of thrombocytopenia, fever, neurologic abnormality, renal impairment, and hemolytic anemia.[24] However, only 40% of patients present with all five components. About 75% of these parturients have a triad of microangiopathic hemolytic anemia, thrombocytopenia, and neurologic changes.[24] The pathologic substrate of this disease is thrombotic occlusion of arterioles and capillaries. This occlusion may cause multiple organ involvement without specific clinical manifestations. The clinical presentation depends on which organs are involved. The exact pathophysiology of TTP remains unclear, but diffuse endothelial damage and impaired fibrinolytic activity are hallmarks of this disorder, similar to severe preeclampsia.

Microangiopathic hemolytic anemia with thrombocytopenia can lead to postpartum renal failure. This complication usually develops on the first or second day after delivery. However, it has been described to occur as long as 26 days after delivery. Maternal mortality from this may exceed 50 percent in the postpartum period.[30]

COAGULATION DISORDERS

Major changes occur in the clotting system during pregnancy. Hemorrhage and thrombosis, two major hazards of the pregnant woman, are consequences of a malfunction of the clotting system. Hemostasis in pregnancy, as in the nonpregnant state, depends on a complex interaction between vasculature, platelets, coagulation factors, and fibrinolysis.

On occasion, the anesthesiologist is confronted with a patient suffering from a coagulation disorder. Diagnosis is often made during labor and before delivery. Routine laboratory screening tests (thrombin, prothrombin, partial thromboplastin, platelet count) usually reveal a need for further studies to identify the abnormality. On occasion, the discovery of a coagulation disorder during surgery or delivery leads to instability and creates anxiety for obstetricians and anesthesiologists. Hence, understanding of the coagulation mechanism, laboratory evaluation, and treatment of common coagulation disorders are essential.

DIC can result from a variety of clinical conditions and can range from life-threatening fulminant disease to a mild presentation. A high index of suspicion and an understanding of the etiology are crucial for the treatment of obstetric patients, because a number of obstetric and hematologic complications are associated with such coagulopathies.

Disseminated intravascular coagulation is essentially consumption of coagulation factors (procoagulant proteins) and platelets, resulting from a triggering event. The clotting, in turn, activates the fibrinolytic proteins through the vascular system, a normal physiologic response. In this pathologic, diseased state, these processes lose the normal balance that provides homeostasis in the circulation. Thrombosis or bleeding may predominate. Initiation of the complement cascade and kinin contributes to extreme vascular permeability, and vasodilatation that is augmented by fibrin deposition within the microvasculature (Shwartzman reaction) may cause end-organ damage and necrosis. Factors such as endothelial cell damage (disruption), endotoxin release by bacteria, and fetal-placental thromboplastic material can be triggers for this abnormal coagulation. Through either the extrinsic or the intrinsic pathway, factor X activates factor V, which provides the conversion of prothrombin to thrombin.[31]

Thrombin induces the cleavage of fibrinogen to fibrin, to create a stable clot. Thrombin at the same time induces the cleavage of plasminogen to form plasmin, which checks and balances the system since plasmin results in the degradation of the clot and prevents its further propagation. Fibrin degradation products (FDP), created from fibrinolysis, directly inhibit the conversion of fibrinogen to fibrin by thrombin as well as platelet-mediated coagulation.[31]

Antithrombin III, the principal physiologic inhibitor of coagulation in the normal state, binds irreversibly to several clotting factors, most importantly to factor X, crucial for both the extrinsic and the intrinsic pathways. It also slowly inactivates thrombin. In DIC, fibrin is deposited in the microvasculature and coats circulating platelets. Thrombocytopenia results from both the irreversible entrapments of platelets by fibrin deposits and the increased clearance of fibrin-coated platelets by the reticuloendothelial system.[31]

Pregnancy represents a hypercoagulability state accompanied by increased levels of many clotting factors and increased levels of fibrinogen and FDP. Hence, some authors consider it a state of low-grade self-limited DIC, or at least consider that pregnant women have an increased susceptibility for DIC.[31]

The preeclampsia/eclampsia syndrome is the most common cause of DIC in parturients. Many of these women have a chronic, subclinical coagulopathy, but only rarely do these patients experience massive hemorrhage.

Women suffering from preeclampsia/eclampsia may have increased fibrin deposits in their glomerular, hepatic, and placental microvasculature. Increased levels of FDP and decreased activity of antithrombin III are seen in the same patients. It is not known what etiologic factor triggers DIC in this syndrome, or why coagulopathy is rarely clinically apparent and thrombocytopenia may be the only detected hematologic abnormality in an otherwise asymptomatic patient.[32]

Placental abruption is another common cause of acute DIC in obstetric patients. Here, coagulopathy results from the local, extravascular consumption of clotting factors and from systemic activation of fibrin synthesis and degradation by release of thromboplastin into maternal circulation. The common findings in these patients include increased FDP, hypofibrinogenemia, and thrombocytopenia. The clinical severity of the hemostatic abnormality usually correlates with the degree of placental separation. The disturbance is self-limited, and patients tend to normalize as the release of thromboplastin ceases with delivery. These patients are, however, at increased risk for postpartum hemorrhage.[31]

Intrauterine fetal death can be associated with DIC, probably owing to the release of fetal and/or placental thromboplastin into the maternal circulation. The onset of DIC is gradual and related to the amount of time the dead fetus was retained. If the dead fetus was retained more than 4 weeks, a thorough investigation of the coagulation status is necessary.[31] However, as chronic abruption may be an important cause of intrauterine fetal demise (IUFD), the tests of clotting parameters are necessary in every IUFD patient.

Amniotic fluid embolism is a fulminant life-threatening crisis that is likely to result in hemodynamic collapse. Amniotic fluid has a procoagulant effect, stimulating the conversion of fibrinogen to fibrin and platelet activation. Maternal mortality is very high, usually within hours of the initial cardiopulmonary insult. A thorough description of this topic can be found in Chapter 31.

Another important cause of DIC in the pregnant woman is gram-negative infection. Circulatory collapse may be caused by endotoxins via an enhanced release of kinins, histamine, serotonin, and prostaglandins. Fibrinogen production increases initially because it is an acute phase reactant, but later, with development of uncontrolled consumption, hypofibrinogenemia results. Thrombocytopenia can also be severe.[33]

Monitoring and Diagnosis of Coagulation Abnormalities

A history of bleeding is very important in the preoperative evaluation of the parturient.[34] Points requiring attention include bleeding lasting for more than 24 hours or rebleeding following dental extractions, recurrent epistaxis, or excessive bleeding requiring transfusion following a simple surgical procedure. Any patient with a history of thrombosis or thrombocytopenia should be evaluated for hereditary or acquired deficiencies of protein C or S, because these may increase the thrombotic problems in pregnancy.[35] Antithrombin III, protein S, and protein C are the natural inhibitors of the coagulation system. Deficiency in any of them is referred to as thrombophilia. Increased frequency of genetic thrombophilia was found in women with complications of pregnancy including severe preeclampsia, placental abruption, and intrauterine growth retardation.[36] Patients should be examined for any signs of bleeding, mainly bruising, bleeding from mucous membranes, or bleeding from venipuncture points or inserted intravenous lines.

Attention should also be paid to the type of bleeding. Bleeding due to platelet shortage or dysfunction is usually at mucocutaneous surfaces. Deep bleeding (e.g., into joints or muscles) is usually related to a deficiency of coagulation factors.[37]

Low platelet counts may be erroneous and should be checked manually, because falsely low counts may be related to pseudothrombocytopenia caused by platelet clumping. Useful information about platelet consumption and production can be obtained from the mean platelet volume (MPV). Younger platelets are larger and an increase in the MPV is indicative of activation of marrow production. Significant increases in MPV have been reported in patients with preeclampsia and in pregnant patients with incidental thrombocytopenia.[38] It is important to remember that an adequate number of platelets do not necessarily imply adequate function. Evaluation of platelet function is difficult to obtain because it depends on a large variety of factors, including concentration of sodium citrate anticoagulant, storage time, temperature, and pH of the blood sample—as well as factors such as age, sex, race, and hematocrit. Even a profound platelet abnormality cannot be used to predict the risk of hemorrhage in individual patients. Although at one time the bleeding time (BT) was considered to be the best in vivo test of platelet function, its use has fallen from favor. In their extensive review of the BT, Rodgers and Levin[39] concluded that bleeding time is not a specific in vivo indicator of platelet function. There is no evidence that BT is a predictor of the risk of hemorrhage in individual patients. Prothrombin time (PT) measures the extrinsic and final common pathway. Thromboplastin (brain lipoprotein) and calcium are added to the sample of citrated platelet-poor plasma, and the time to fibrin formation is evaluated. PT is prolonged when factors V, VII, and X are reduced to less than 50% of normal values, prothrombin to less than 30%, or fibrinogen to less than 1 g/L. Because factor VII is vitamin K dependent, PT is generally used to monitor warfarin therapy. PT is most sensitive to factor VII deficiency and least sensitive to fibrinogen and prothrombin deficiencies.[38] For standardization of this test, all thromboplastins are allocated to an International Standardized Index (ISI). Following PT measurement, the ratio of the patient's PT to control PT is calculated. This result is taken to the power of the ISI and then becomes the International Normalized Ratio (INR), which is a more objective presentation of the PT.[40]

Blood Coagulation Tests During Pregnancy

The levels of several blood coagulation factors are increased during pregnancy. Plasma fibrinogen levels rise from a nonpregnant average of 300 mg/dL to 450 mg/dL during pregnancy. The increase is most likely owing to the increase in the erythrocyte sedimentation rate.[41] Other clotting factors that increase markedly during pregnancy are factors VII, VIII, IX, and X. Factor II levels increase slightly, whereas the levels of factors XI and XIII decrease.[42]

PT and partial thromboplastin time (PTT) shorten slightly as pregnancy progresses and the clotting time of whole blood does not change significantly during pregnancy. D-dimer levels increase during pregnancy. The evidence concerning the levels of protein S and C (measured by antigenic activity or levels of free protein) are conflicting. Although there is a decrease in free protein S levels during the second trimester, levels of total protein S remain unchanged.[42] Other investigators have found no change.[43]

During normal pregnancy, the levels of plasminogen in plasma increase, probably owing to high levels of estrogen. Even so, fibrinolytic activity is prolonged during pregnancy. Thromboelastography (TEG), which observes all clotting factors, is fast becoming a popular method of predicting coagulation problems (Figs. 42–1 and 42–2). Harter first reported the use of TEG in 1948.[44] Long popular in Europe, TEG has only recently attracted interest in the United States,

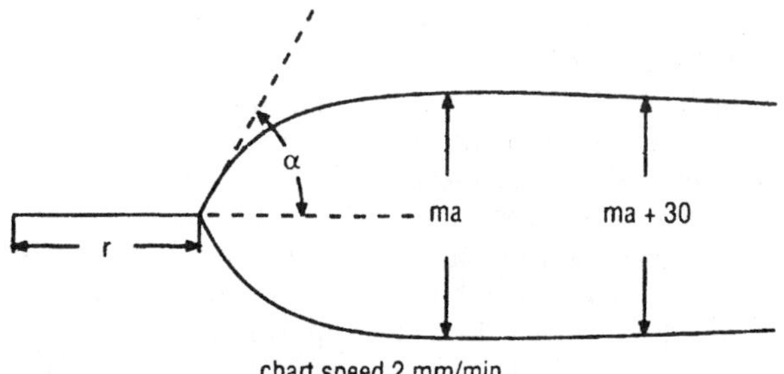

Variable	Measures	Abnormality	
r reaction time	thromboplastin generation via the intrinsic pathway	↑r	Factor deficiency Heparin Severe thrombocytopenia
α angle of divergence	rate of clot formation	↓α	Hypofibrinogenemia Thrombocytopenia Thrombocytopathy
ma maximum amplitude	maximum clot strength/elasticity	↓ma	Thrombocytopenia Thrombocytopathy Hypofibrinogenemia Factor XIII deficiency
ma + 30	clot retraction after 30 minutes	↓ma + 30	Fibrinolysis

❖ **Figure 42–2** Typical thromboelastogram (TEG) pattern and variables measured and normal values. r = 21–30 mm; α = 30–41°; ma = 45–54 mm; ma+30 = minimal reduction. (Modified from Faust RJ: Functional platelet disorders. *In* Faust RJ (ed): Anesthesiology Review, 2nd ed. 1994, p 481.)

following its use in liver transplantation and cardiopulmonary bypass. TEG enables global assessment of hemostatic function based on a single small specimen (0.36 mL) of blood. The machine is easy to use and allows patient assessment of all aspects of clotting within 20 to 30 minutes. Information about subsequent clot stability and fibrinolysis becomes available over the next 60 minutes. Along with rapid evaluation and diagnosis of coagulation status, TEG enables assessment of the response to therapeutic interventions.[45]

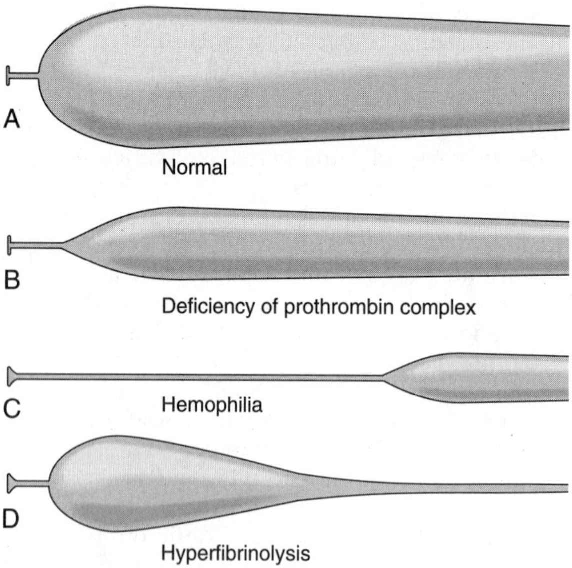

❖ **Figure 42–1** Typical thromboelastogram patterns: examples include a normal pattern and some abnormal tracings.

PREGNANCY AND CONGENITAL DISORDERS OF HEMOSTASIS

Abnormalities of the coagulation process are relatively rare. A history of a successful previous delivery is not necessarily an indicator of the lack of abnormality. A family history of bleeding disorders should raise the possibility of a congenital coagulopathy. Although most of these disorders are inherited with autosomal or sex-linked distribution, penetrance may be variable. Since coagulation factors are present at levels several times greater than those needed for normal clotting, even a 50% decrease may not be clinically evident. Almost all coagulation factors can be deficient,[46] but in women only a few clotting factor deficiencies are of clinical importance.[47] Therefore, when a factor deficiency is known before surgery or vaginal delivery, replacement of that specific factor can be considered.

Von Willebrand's Disease

Von Willebrand's disease is the most prevalent coagulation disorder in women of childbearing years, with an incidence in the general population of 1:10,000.[48] It is a family of disorders, inherited mainly as an autosomal dominant trait. The pathologic basis of the disease is a marked decrease in or absence of the Von Willebrand portion of the factor VIII complex, which plays a major role in platelet aggregation and helps prevent the removal of factor VIII:C from the circulation.[49] Thus, patients with von Willebrand's disease show a pattern of bleeding similar to that found in disorders of platelet function (i.e., mucosal and gingival bleeding, menorrhagia, intestinal hemorrhage, or epistaxis). Serious blood loss may occur immediately after trauma, including vaginal delivery or surgery.[50] Criteria for the laboratory diagnosis of von Willebrand's disease are reviewed in Table 42–4.

For the pregnant woman with von Willebrand's disease, the factor VIII level should be checked periodically during the antenatal course and pretreatment reserved for patients with levels below 25% of normal. Bleeding associated with von Willebrand's disease is best treated with infusion of cryoprecipitate.[31] This therapy is also useful in factor VIII deficiency and hypofibrinogenemia. Usually, 6 to 10 units are given. However, until a specific diagnosis for hemorrhage is made, fresh frozen plasma should be administered in addition to cryoprecipitate. In the absence of clinical deterioration, coagulation profiles should be rechecked at least every 6 to 8 hours.

DDAVP (1-diamino-8-D-arginine vasopressin) can be administered instead of cryoprecipitate for cases known to be responsive, including type I, and in some patients with type IIa. Treatment is usually begun when the patient is in labor. Treatment is repeated every 12 hours; however, the infusion often becomes less effective.

Despite the fact that serious bleeding is rare when factor levels are above 25% of normal and BT is less than 15 minutes, when cesarean section is needed for obstetric reasons treatment is indicated if the level is 40% of normal or less. Cryoprecipitate treatment should begin 24 hours preoperatively to allow new factor VIII synthesis in addition to the elevation obtained from the cryoprecipitate. In the case of acute bleeding or when emergent cesarean section is performed, the initial therapeutic dose should be increased by approximately 50%, and a second dose should be given approximately 12 hours later. After vaginal delivery or cesarean section, the level should be checked daily and therapy given if the level falls below 25% of normal or if bleeding with no obstetric cause occurs.[51]

Table 42–4 LABORATORY FINDINGS IN VON WILLEBRAND'S DISEASE

Slight to moderate reduction in aPTT
Active factor VIII level (15%–30% of normal)
Prolonged bleeding time
Abnormal platelet adhesiveness
Lack of ristocetin-induced platelet aggregation
Factor VIII coagulating activity-to-factor VIII antigen ratio of 1.[48]

In women with von Willebrand's disease, a major anesthetic risk is bleeding into the epidural space during regional blockade and subsequent hematoma formation, with its risk of permanent neurologic damage. Therefore, neuraxial block for delivery or cesarean section in these women should be performed only after full evaluation of the patient's hemostatic status. Any significant abnormality found should be corrected by administration of cryoprecipitate. Since depletion of coagulation factors can occur during labor or in the postpartum period, a coagulation investigation should be performed every 3 or 4 hours while the epidural is sited, and any diagnosed abnormality must be treated promptly.[52]

If general anesthesia is indicated, care must be taken to perform laryngoscopy and intubation of the trachea carefully and gently. Airway bruising can result in production of expanding hematomas that can cause severe respiratory compromise intraoperatively or postoperative respiratory complications.

Since the disease is autosomal dominant, the baby must be assumed to have a coagulopathy. Some authors recommend elective cesarean section to prevent neonatal complications, although fetal disability because of bleeding during labor is rare.[52] Periventricular hemorrhage in a 32-week fetus that inherited type IIa von Willebrand's disease has been reported. Scalp electrodes should be avoided, if possible, and circumcision postponed until the diagnosis is confirmed. Prenatal diagnosis using percutaneous umbilical blood sampling is possible.[53]

Hemophilia

Hemophilia is usually inherited as an X-linked recessive disorder and therefore commonly affects males. Pregnant patients, however, can be carriers of the disease. An affected woman would have to be the offspring of the uncommon match between an affected male and a carrier female. Although some cases of carriers suffering from bleeding tendency have been reported,[54] anesthesia implications are rare, and therefore the disease will be only briefly mentioned in this chapter.

Early knowledge of fetal gender is crucial when one treats a patient who is a hemophilia carrier. The risk of hemophilia in a male fetus is 50%. Fetal blood, obtained through cordocentesis, can be checked for factor VIII:C and VIII:RAg ratios.

A few affected homozygous women have been reported to deliver,[55] and postpartum hemorrhage can be treated by cryoprecipitate, fresh frozen plasma, and factor VIII:C concentrate. Replacement is indicated when factor VIII:C levels are reduced to half or when cesarean section is planned. It is recommended to keep the level at 80% of normal during the surgery.

Deficiencies in Other Clotting Factors

Factor VII deficiency is a rare autosomal recessive disorder. With about 50 cases reported,[56] an unusual feature of this disorder is the large variation in response to surgery that does not appear to correlate with laboratory abnormalities.[57] These patients may be prone to thromboembolic disorders. Factor XI deficiency (plasma thromboplastin antecedent deficiency), an incompletely recessive autosomal disorder, is found with increased frequency in the Ashkenazi Jewish population. Most affected pregnancies do not have bleeding problems, despite the lower levels of factor XI found in gestation. Fresh frozen plasma is the treatment of choice.

Factor XII (Hageman factor) deficiency is rare and has usually minimal clinical significance. Ironically, this deficiency leads to a higher thrombotic tendency.

Congenital Regulatory Protein Disorders

Genetic disorders, which impair the level or function of regulator proteins, increase the tendency for thrombosis. These disorders were given the name thrombophilias because they are associated with recurrent thromboembolism. Examples include antithrombin III deficiency, protein S deficiency, protein C deficiency, and activated protein C resistance (APC-R). The risk of thromboembolism appears to be about 3% per year for otherwise asymptomatic patients.[58] In pregnancy, the risk is cited to be higher.[59]

Antithrombin III Deficiency

Congenital antithrombin III deficiency is a group of disorders characterized by a deficiency in antithrombin III function or concentration. The classic disorder, named type 1, is an autosomal disorder affecting 1 in 5000 persons. The prevalence of the overall disorder is about 1 in 2000, and heterozygotes have 25% to 60% of the normal level.[60] Only the heterozygous state is seen in the pregnant woman, since the homozygous state is lethal. The first presentation of this disease is usually as deep vein thrombosis by the second or third decade of life. Precipitating factors include trauma, surgery, and oral contraceptives containing more than 50 μg of estradiol. During pregnancy, 50% to 70% of pregnant women with antithrombin III deficiency develop deep vein thrombosis, with 75% occurring before labor. Prophylactic heparin can be beneficial in preventing thrombosis.

It is recommended that a dose of anticoagulation that prolongs the patient's PTT to 5 to 10 seconds beyond the patient's baseline be used.[61] Prophylaxis should be initiated as soon as pregnancy is confirmed. Gravid patients may be relatively resistant to heparin and require 30,000 to 45,000 IU per day. Fresh frozen plasma is a good source of antithrombin III and can be used with heparin. Heated antithrombin III is preferable, and it can be given intravenously. In the postpartum period, warfarin should be substituted for the heparin.

Protein C deficiency is inherited in an autosomal dominant pattern, with incomplete penetrance. The frequency is about 1 in 200 to 1 in 300. Protein C levels below 65% of normal are associated with deep and superficial thrombosis. Pulmonary embolism is not rare in patients with protein C deficiency. However, many patients with protein levels of 50% of normal are asymptomatic. The first manifestation of the disorder is often during pregnancy. Deep vein thrombosis has been observed in 25% of 93 affected pregnancies.[62]

Protein S is a cofactor of protein C, and the deficiency is inherited as an autosomal dominant trait. The clinical manifestation is similar to protein C deficiency. Several authors recommend heparin treatment throughout gestation.[59]

Activated protein C resistance is a thrombophilia characterized by resistance of plasma to the anticoagulant effect of activated protein C and appears to be more common than the other disorders.

TRANSFUSION THERAPY

Although the vast majority of parturients do not require transfusion therapy, when blood transfusion becomes necessary, a massive quantity may be required. It is critical that physicians correctly estimate the amount of blood loss in pregnant patients. Acute blood loss of 15% of the normal blood volume does not require transfusion. A 15% to 30% loss may require transfusion; however, most of these patients can be stabilized with the use of crystalloids. An acute blood loss of 10% to 40% usually results in a reduction of systolic pressure, tachypnea, and tachycardia. A loss of more than 40% is often life-threatening and will require transfusion.[63]

The primary indication for transfusion of erythrocytes in a parturient is to maintain or restore the blood's oxygen-carrying capacity. At this time, the erythrocyte is still the only material that efficiently carries oxygen. To prevent a shortage of fresh cross-matched blood, fresh whole blood is not usually administered; component therapy is the mainstay of blood therapy. Table 42–5 reviews the indications for administration of packed erythrocytes in the peripartum period.

Platelets are usually given only if the platelet count is less than 20,000 or less than 50,000 in a patient scheduled for surgery. Cryoprecipitate should be given to patients who are bleeding and are to undergo surgery only if they have a demonstrated factor deficiency or uremia. Some clotting factors are not found in cryoprecipitate, thus necessitating fresh frozen plasma administration. Fresh frozen plasma administration may

Table 42–5 Indications for Administration of Packed Red Blood Cells in the Peripartum Period

Hemoglobin level below 8 g/dL with hemodynamic instability
Hematocrit < 24%
The patient is symptomatic (syncope, dizziness, or other hypovolemic-related symptoms)
Evidence of massive blood loss
Signs of acute hypoxia

be indicated in the symptomatic patient with a PTT or PT 1.5 times greater than normal. Other relative indications include parturients who require reversal of warfarin treatment or parturients with HELLP syndrome in whom blood exchange treatment is employed.

The risks of transfusion are mainly transmission of infection and adverse immunologic response. The principal infectious complication is hepatitis, which occurs in approximately 1% of patients who receive blood. The incidence of non-A non-B hepatitis is approximately 1 in 3000 transfusions. Other forms of hepatitis are rare. The risk of transmission of HIV is less than 1:500,000. Because of improved techniques for selecting and testing blood donors, the overall incidence of viral transmission is rare.[64]

Adverse immunologic responses to blood transfusion can be divided into minor and major reactions. The minor reactions do not necessarily require discontinuation of the transfusion, and include low-grade fever and minor allergic reactions. The usual approach in these cases is the administration of diphenhydramine and careful observation. Major reactions are due to hemolysis, usually from administration of incompatible blood. These are rare and should be treated with immediate discontinuation of infusion as well as prompt rechecking of the blood being transfused and cross-matching it with the patient's blood.

❖ SUMMARY

Key Points

- When attempting to determine the advisability of initiating regional anesthesia in parturients with thrombocytopenia, previous platelet counts should be reviewed for a trend. Clinical examination is also of great importance. There is no evidence that a bleeding time predicts which patient will be at risk for bleeding in the epidural space.
- Frank coagulopathy is an absolute contraindication to neuraxial anesthesia—isolated laboratory findings without clinical evidence of coagulopathy are not. Regional anesthesia has been safely used in parturients with hemoglobinopathies.
- Obtaining fetal blood for thrombocytopenia assessment by percutaneous cordocentesis or intrapartum scalp sampling is difficult and is not always predictive of neonatal bleeding disorders.
- Pregnancy can cause exacerbation of sickle cell disease. There are several steps that should be routinely performed in order to help prevent crisis in these parturients. They include prevention of dehydration, hypotension, and hypothermia.

Key Reference

Sage DJ: Epidurals, spinals and bleeding disorders in pregnancy: a review. Anaesth Intensive Care 1990; 18:319–326.

Case Stem

A primiparous full-term parturient with a current platelet count of 78,000 is requesting labor analgesia. Can neuraxial analgesia be administered and are there any laboratory or clinical tests that need to be done before initiation of the block?

References

1. Shulman NR: The physiologic basis for therapy of classic hemophilia and related disorders. Ann Intern Med 1967; 67:856–882.
2. Good W, MacDonald HN, Hancock KW, Wood JE: Haematological changes in pregnancy following ovulation-induction therapy. Obstet Gynaecol Br Commonw 1973; 80:486–490.
3. Ueland K: Maternal cardiovascular dynamics. VII. Intrapartum blood volume changes. Am J Obstet Gynecol 1976; 126:671–677.
4. Cruickshank JM, Morris R, Butt W, et al: The relationship of total and differential leukocyte counts with urinary estrogen and plasma cortisol levels. J Obstet Gynaecol Br Commonw 1970; 79:450.
5. Jacobs AA, Selvaraj RJ, Strauss RR, et al: Role of the phagocyte in host-parasite interactions: stimulation of bactericidal activity of myeloperoxidase-containing leucocyte fraction by estrogens. Am J Obstet Gynecol 1973; 117:671.
6. Jones E, Curzen E, Gaugas GM: Suppressive activity of pregnancy on mixed lymphocyte reaction. J Obstet Gynaecol Br Commonw 1973; 80:603.
7. Cruickshank JM: The effect of parity on leucocyte count in pregnant and nonpregnant woman. Br J Haematol 1970; 18:531.
8. Good W, MacDonald HN, Hancock KW, et al: Haematological changes in pregnancy following ovulation induction therapy. J Obstet Gynaecol Br Commonw 1973; 80:486.
9. Brain E, Marston RH, Gordon J: Immunological response in pregnancy. Br Med J 1972; 4:488.
10. St. Hill CA, Finn R, Denie V: Depression of cellular immunity in pregnancy due to serum factor. Br Med J 1973; 3:513.
11. Pearlman M, Faro S: Obstetric septic shock: a pathophysiologic basis for management. Clin Obstet Gynecol 1990; 33:482.
12. Purtilo DT, Hallgren HM, Yunis EJ: Depressed maternal response to phytohaemagglutinin in human pregnancy. Lancet 1972; 1:769.
13. Rigby FB, Nolan TE: Inherited disorders of coagulation in pregnancy. Clin Obstet Gynecol 1995; 1938; 3:497–5.
14. Taylor DJ, Phillips P, Lind T: Puerperal haematological indices. Br J Obstet Gynaecol 1981; 88:601–606.
15. Fay RA, Hughes AO, Farron NT: Platelets in pregnancy: hyperdestruction in pregnancy. Obstet Gynecol 1983; 61:238–240.
16. Orlikowski CE, Rocke DA: Coagulation monitoring in the obstetric patient. Int Anesthesiol Clin 1994; 32:174–191.
17. Coopland A, Alkjaersig N, Fletcher AP: Reduction in plasma factor 13 (fibrin stabilizing factor) concentration during pregnancy. J Lab Clin Med 1969; 73:144–153.
18. Bremme K, Ostlund E, Almqvist I, et al: Enhanced thrombin generation and fibrinolytic activity in normal pregnancy and the puerperium. Obstet Gynecol 1992; 80:132–137.
19. Gatti L, Tenconi PM, Guarneri D, et al: Hemostatic parameters and platelet activation by flow-cytometry in normal pregnancy: a longitudinal study. Int J Clin Lab Res 1994; 24:217–219.
20. Lund CJ: Studies on the iron deficiency anemia of pregnancy including plasma volume, total hemoglobin, erythrocyte protoporphyrin in treated and untreated normal and anemic patients. Am J Obstet Gynecol 1951; 62:947.
21. Rust OA, Perry KG: Pregnancy complicated by sickle hemoglobinopathy. Clin Obstet Gynecol 1995; 38:472–484.
22. Martin JN, Morrison JF: Sickle cell crisis. *In* Clark SL, Cotton DB, et al (eds): Critical Care Obstetrics, 2nd ed. Cambridge, MA: Blackwell Scientific Publications; 1991:212.

23. Niehius AW: Thalassemia major: molecular and clinical aspects. Ann Intern Med 1979; 91:883–897.
24. Samuels P, Bussel JB, Braitman LE, et al: Estimation of the risk of thrombocytopenia in the offspring of pregnant women with presumed immune thrombocytopenic purpura. N Engl J Med 1990; 323:229.
25. Tygart SG, McRoyan DK, Spinnato JA, et al: Longitudinal studies of platelet indices during normal pregnancy. Am J Obstet Gynecol 1986; 154:883–887.
26. Stubbs TM, Lasarchick J, Van Dorester JP, et al: Evidence of accelerated platelet production and consumption in nonthrombocytopenic preeclampsia. Am J Obstet Gynecol 1986; 155:263–265.
27. Glantz JC, Roberts DJ: Pregnancy complicated by thrombocytopenia secondary to human immunodeficiency virus infection. Obstet Gynecol 1994; 83(5 Pt 2):825–827.
28. Samuels P, Bussel JB, Braitman LE, et al: Estimation of the risk of thrombocytopenia in the offspring of pregnant women with presumed immune thrombocytopenic purpura. N Engl J Med 1990; 323:229.
29. Rakoczi I, Tallian F, Bagdany S, Gati I: Platelet life-span in normal pregnancy and pre-eclampsia as determined by a non-radioisotope technique. Thromb Res 1979; 15(3–4):553–556.
30. Robson JS, Martin AM, Ruckley V, Macdonald MK: Irreversible post-partum renal failure: a new syndrome. Q J Med 1968; 37:147, 423–435.
31. Weiner C: The obstetrics patient and disseminated intravascular coagulation. Clin Perinatol 1986; 13:705.
32. Leduce L, Wheeler JM, Kirshon B, et al: Coagulation profile in severe preeclampsia. Obstet Gynecol 1992; 79:14.
33. Pearlman M, Faro S: Obstetric septic shock: a pathophysiologic basis for management. Clin Obstet Gynecol 1990; 33:482.
34. Laposata M, Teruya J: Reappraisal of preoperative coagulation testing [editorial Laposata]. Am J Clin Pathol 1990; 94:795–796.
35. Crowley JP: Coagulopathy and bleeding in the parturient patient. RI Med J 1989; 72:135–143.
36. Kupferminc MJ, Eldor A, Steinman N, Lessing JB: Increased frequency of genetic thrombophilias in women with complications of pregnancy. N Engl J Med 1999; 7:340:9–13.
37. George JN, Shattil SJ: The clinical importance of acquired abnormalities of platelet function. N Engl J Med 1991; 324:27–39.
38. Fay RA, Hughes AO, Farron NT: Platelets in pregnancy: hyperdestruction in pregnancy. Obstet Gynecol 1983; 61:238–240.
39. Rodgers RPC, Levin J: A clinical reappraisal of the bleeding time. Semin Thromb Hemost 1990; 16:1–20.
40. Orlikowski CE, Rocke DA: Coagulation monitoring in the obstetric patient. Intern Anaesth Clin 1994; 32:174–191.
41. Ozanne P, Linderkamp O, Miller FC, Meiselman HJ: Erythrocyte aggregation during normal pregnancy. Am J Obstet Gynecol 1983; 147:576–583.
42. Cunningham FG, MacDonald PC, Gant NF, et al (eds): Hematological disorders. *In* Williams Obstetrics, 20th ed. Appleton & Lange 1997; 51:1197.
43. Faught W, Garner P, Jones G, Ivey B: Changes in protein C and protein S levels in normal pregnancy. Am J Obstet Gynecol 1995; 172(1 Pt 1):147–150.
44. Franz RC, Coetzee WJC: The thromboelastographic diagnosis of hemostasic defects. Surg Annu 1981; 13:75–107.
45. Mallet SV, Cox DJA: Thromboelastography. Br J Anaesth 1992; 69:307–313.
46. Greenwood RJ, Rabin SC: Hemophilia-like postpartum bleeding. Obstet Gynecol 1967; 30:362.
47. Saidi P, Siegelman M, Mitchel VB: Effect of factor XII deficiency on pregnancy and parturition. Thromb Haemost 1979; 41:523.
48. Bloom AL: The Von Willebrand syndrome. Semin Hematol 1980; 17:215.
49. Evans PC: Obstetric and gynecologic patients with von Willebrand's disease. Obstet Gynecol 1971; 38:37.
50. Lipton RA, Ayromlooi J, Colle BS: Severe von Willebrand's disease during labor and delivery. JAMA 1982; 248:1355.
51. Perkins HA: Correction of hemostatic defect in von Willebrand disease. Blood 1966; 30:375.
52. Cohen S, Goldiner PL: Epidural analgesia for labor and delivery in a patient with von Willebrand's disease. Reg Anesth 1989; 14:95–97.
53. Mullaart RA, Van Dongen P, Gabreëls FJ, van Oostrom C: Fetal periventricular hemorrhage in von Willebrand's disease: short review and first case presentation. Am J Perinatol 1991; 8:190–192.
54. Veltcamp JJ, Van Tilberg NH: Autosomal haemophilia. Br J Haematol 1974; 26:141–152.
55. Kasper CK, Boylem AL, Ewing NP, et al: Hematologic management of hemophilia a for surgery. JAMA 1985; 253:1279–1283.
56. Marder VJ, Shulman NR: Clinical aspects of congenital factor VII deficiency. Am J Med 1964; 37:182.
57. Jonnaess H: Cold-promoted activation of factor VII. Gynecol Invest 1973; 4:61.
58. Pabinger I, Kyrle PA, Heistinger M, et al: The risk of thromboembolism in asymptomatic patients with protein C and protein S deficiency: a prospective cohort study. Thromb Haemost 1994; 71:441–445.
59. De Stefano V, Leone G, Mastrangelo S, et al: Thrombosis during pregnancy and surgery in patients with congenital deficiency of antithrombin III, protein C, protein S [letter]. Thromb Haemost 1994; 71:799–800.
60. Rodgers RP, Levin J: A critical reappraisal of the bleeding time. Semin Thromb Hemost 1990; 16:1–20.
61. Hellgren M, Tengborn L: Pregnancy in women with antithrombin III deficiency: experience of treatment with heparin and antithrombin. Gynecol Obstet Invest 1982; 14:127.
62. Conard J, Horellou MH, Van Dreden P, et al: Thrombosis and pregnancy in congenital deficiencies in AT III, protein C or protein S: study of 78 women. Thromb Haemost 1990; 63:319–320.
63. Babineau TJ, Dzik WH, Borlase BC, et al: Reevaluation of current transfusion practices in patients in surgical intensive care units. Am J Surg 1992; 164:22–25.
64. Gillon R: Resuscitation policies—action required [editorial]. J Med Ethics 1992; 18:115–116.

43

Autoimmune Disease

❖ PETER STONE, MD, MBChB, DDU, FRCOG, FRNZCOG

❖ GRAHAM SHARPE, MBChB, FANZCA

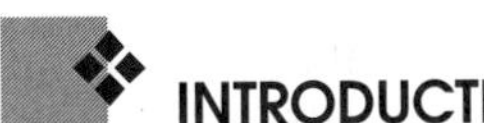

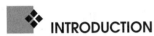

INTRODUCTION

Successful pregnancy requires maternal immune and vascular adaptations that can tolerate and promote the growth of the fetal allograft. A number of changes occur in the maternal immune system in pregnancy, but whether these reflect immune suppression or immune adaptation to the fetoplacental unit is unclear because the exact nature of the immunologic basis of normal pregnancy remains to be elucidated. This chapter briefly reviews immune changes in pregnancy, discusses a number of autoimmune conditions that have implications for maternal or fetal welfare, describes the effects of pregnancy on these autoimmune conditions, and discusses special anesthetic considerations relating to these conditions.

Autoimmune disease occurs when immune activation against self constituents occurs. The mechanisms by which the autoimmune condition causes clinical disease and adverse outcomes in pregnancy vary and are not always indicated directly by the activity of autoantibodies. In the antiphospholipid syndrome and systemic lupus erythematosus (SLE) the autoimmune mechanisms remain unclear.

Management of the clinical disease states requires an understanding not only of the primary immune abnormality if this is known but also of the end-organ derangements, which are more clearly related to pregnancy outcomes.

Autoimmune conditions discussed in this chapter include the antiphospholipid syndrome, systemic lupus erythematosus, rheumatoid arthritis, and other less common rheumatologic conditions such as polyarteritis nodosa, ankylosing spondylitis, and scleroderma.

IMMUNE CHANGES IN PREGNANCY

Most immune function in pregnancy is normal, although increased susceptibility to certain infections has been attributed to decreased cellular immune responses to some antigens. There is an increase in the total white blood cell count, mostly caused by increases in polymorphonuclear leukocytes. The increase persists for 6 to 8 weeks post partum. The erythrocyte sedimentation rate (ESR) is also raised and cannot be used as a marker of infection or immune activity.

Cell Mediated Immunity. Thymus-dependent, or T, cells bearing the CD4 antigens can be divided into TH1 and TH2 clones based on their cytokine production. TH1 mediates cell-mediated immune responses and produces a number of cytokines harmful to the maintenance of pregnancy, for example, by stimulating natural killer cell activity. In pregnancy, TH1 cytokine responses are decreased. The clinical implications of decreased TH1 activity are seen in an improvement in the majority of patients with rheumatoid arthritis, which is a TH1 cell–mediated autoimmune disease. Similarly, the majority of multiple sclerosis patients experience remission or improvement in pregnancy.

The TH1 profile is associated with infectious disease resistance. The response to infection with organisms causing tuberculosis, leprosy, and leishmaniasis is critically related to a TH1 rather than a TH2 profile. Pregnant women normally have a TH2 cytokine profile, which down-regulates the TH1 profile,[1] which is protective against infection in the nonpregnant state. This explains why certain infections such as malaria are particularly dangerous for the pregnant woman.

Humoral Immunity. Antibody production is normal in pregnancy. There are no changes in circulating B cells, plasma cells, or levels of immunoglobulin classes G, M, and A. Animal and indirect human evidence supports the predominance of a TH2 cytokine profile over TH1. This means that there is increased production of the immunosuppressive cytokines (IL-4 and IL-10). Th2 cells are the principal stimulators of humoral immunity. This would explain the exacerbation of TH2-mediated immune responses that is seen in pregnant patients with SLE.

The Fetoplacental Unit. Normal trophoblast does not express the classic HLA antigens and produces complement regulatory proteins. Both factors may enhance the ability of the trophoblast to be tolerated by the maternal immune system. Pregnancy proteins and hormones such as early pregnancy factor, human chorionic gonadotropin, α-fetoprotein, corticosteroids, and sex steroids all may be involved in reducing the maternal immune response, at least in part by stimulating TH2 cells and causing downregulation of TH1 cytokines.[2]

Summary. Further clarification of the immune nature of pregnancy is required before the relationships between autoimmunity, effector mechanisms, and disease activity can be determined. In practice, the implications of autoimmune disease are best assessed by clinical symptoms and signs. Disease severity is currently judged by end-organ response; this includes the fetoplacental unit, which can be considered a target organ in autoimmune conditions.

ANTIPHOSPHOLIPID SYNDROME

The group of clinical and laboratory criteria making up the antiphospholipid syndrome (APS), or Hughes syndrome, is one of the most important causes of hypercoagulability, an acquired autoimmune thrombophilia. APS may be associated with conditions affecting many organ systems. The causes of hypercoagulability are shown in Table 43–1 and include both pregnancy and inherited and acquired conditions that can adversely affect a pregnant patient. Thus the importance of excluding all these potential causes when a pregnant woman suffers a thrombotic event should be emphasized.

Antiphospholipids are a heterogeneous group of antibodies directed against negatively charged phospholipids in cell membranes. Although the presence of antiphospholipids constitutes an acquired autoimmune condition, a number of childhood diseases in which a coagulopathy exists have been associated with antiphospholipids.

Adverse maternal and fetal or neonatal outcomes were one of the original features of APS in women with no other recognizable signs of autoimmune disease. These patients are said to have primary APS, whereas those with SLE or other connective tissue disorders have secondary APS.

The hallmark of APS is a coagulopathy, but the overlap of the clinical and laboratory constituents between the primary and secondary forms implies that clinical manifestations could involve multiple organ systems, and this is indeed the case. The author has seen myocardial infarction in a young woman in association with arterial vasculopathy secondary to APS.

The fluctuating nature of the presence of antiphospholipid antibodies has been reported both in pregnant and nonpregnant subjects despite ongoing clinical manifestations.[3] This fact suggests that antiphospholipid antibodies are secondary markers of a process currently not fully understood. Indeed, serum β_2-glycoprotein I deposition has been found in placentas from patients with higher antiphospholipid antibody titers than in normal subjects, although this was not related to histologic changes in the villi.[4]

Diagnosis

The clinical features suggestive of APS are listed in Table 43–2. The diagnosis is based on the history and clinical suspicion, supported by laboratory features.

Table 43–1 CAUSES OF HYPERCOAGULABILITY

Primary (Genetic) Causes	Secondary (Acquired) Causes
Protein C and S deficiencies	Pregnancy and postpartum states
Antithrombin III deficiency	Bed rest, trauma, after surgery
	Diabetes mellitus
Factor V Leiden mutation	Hyperlipidemia
Homocysteinemia	Combined oral contraceptives
Abnormal fibrinolysis	
Familial antiphospholipid syndrome	Malignancy
	Vasculitides
	Antiphospholipid syndrome

Table 43–2 CLINICAL CRITERIA SUGGESTIVE OF THE ANTIPHOSPHOLIPID SYNDROME

Pregnancy Abnormalities
Recurrent spontaneous miscarriage
Unexplained fetal death
Atypical preeclampsia
Deteriorating outcomes in consecutive pregnancies

Thrombosis
Venous
Arterial including cerebrovascular (stroke)

Autoimmune Thrombocytopenia

Other Manifestations by System
Skin
- Livedo reticularis

Vascular
- Cutaneous ischemia and infarcts
- Splinter hemorrhages
- Leg ulcers, superficial thrombophlebitis

Cardiac
- Angina and myocardial infarction
- Valvular vegetations, intracardiac thrombus
- Postpartum cardiomyopathy

Pulmonary
- Pulmonary hypertension

Gastrointestinal
- Budd-Chiari syndrome, liver infarction

Renal
- Renovascular (and occlusion), accelerated hypertension, glomerular thrombosis

Ophthalmologic
- Retinal artery or vein occlusion, retinopathy, ischemic optic neuropathy

Endocrine
- Adrenal failure

Musculoskeletal
- Avascular necrosis of bone

Neurologic
- Chorea
- Seizures

Interpretation of laboratory results requires some understanding of the pathogenesis of the condition and awareness of other conditions in pregnancy that may influence hematologic and biochemical tests. It is also necessary for the laboratory to use accepted methodology to ensure consistent accuracy of test results.

The three antiphospholipids for which accepted assays are available include

- Biologic false-positive Venereal Disease Research Laboratory (VDRL) test for syphilis
- Anticardiolipin antibody (standard sera from the Antiphospholipid Standardization Laboratory, Louisville, KY)
- Lupus anticoagulant (a misnomer, because in vivo it reflects hypercoagulability), determined by phospholipid-dependent tests (including the activated partial thromboplastin time [APTT], dilute Russell viper venom time, and kaolin clotting time)

Clearly, in the presence of antiphospholipids these tests cannot be used to assess coagulation or monitor treatment.

Thrombocytopenia may also occur in APS and may be difficult to distinguish from other causes, such as disseminated intravascular coagulation as seen in preeclampsia, or in the presence of a placental abruption, both of which occur much more frequently in women with APS.

Apart from benign gestation thrombocytopenia, a low platelet count in pregnancy can occur in association with thrombosis in APS, but it also occurs in thrombotic thrombocytopenic purpura, as part of atypical preeclampsia or in the HELLP syndrome (*h*emolysis, *e*levated *l*iver enzymes, *l*ow *p*latelets), or it may be drug induced (including heparin). Generally platelet counts greater than 100,000/mm^3 do not require specific evaluation, although the trend derived from taking serial measurements is important.[5]

There is also evidence that warfarin monitoring using the International Normalized Ratio (INR) is invalid in patients with the lupus anticoagulant.[6] The tests listed in Table 43–3 have generally been used to confirm the diagnosis of APS. Other antiphospholipids have not shown an association with the clinical syndrome of APS. Lupus anticoagulant (LA) and anticardiolipin (ACL) antibodies may represent the same group or family of autoantibodies. The significance of IgA anticardiolipin is uncertain. Although many other antiphospholipid antibodies exist—usually in the presence of LA or ACL—their clinical importance is unknown.

Table 43–3 DIAGNOSTIC TESTS FOR THE ANTIPHOSPHOLIPID SYNDROME

Lupus Anticoagulant
Activated partial thromboplastin time
Kaolin clotting time
Dilute Russell viper venom time
Anticardiolipin
IgM MPL units medium or high positive
IgG GPL units medium or high positive
15–20 IgG binding units

GPL, immunoglobulin G anticardiolipin; MPL, immunoglobulin M anticardiolipin.

Antiphospholipids do not bind directly to phospholipids in the cell membrane but bind to a complex including the protein cofactor β_2-glycoprotein 1. It would appear that this cofactor is necessary for antiphospholipids to cause adverse pregnancy outcomes, although the clinical relevance of this protein is uncertain because assays of ACL currently use β_2-glycoprotein–containing sera.[7, 8]

While an awareness of the varied manifestations of APS is important for the assessment of clinical signs and management, the majority of these features are uncommon. The most specific clinical features are pregnancy abnormalities or loss, thrombosis, and autoimmune thrombocytopenia.[9, 10] In addition to unexplained fetal death, recurrent spontaneous miscarriage ($\geq$3 consecutive miscarriages and no more than 1 live birth), early or atypical preeclampsia, and increasingly adverse pregnancy outcomes warrant investigation for APS. Repeated intrauterine growth failure and progressively smaller or early deliveries may suggest an underlying acquired autoimmune condition, and APS should be excluded.

Thrombosis may be arterial or venous or involve the small vessel circulation in the skin, digits, and organs such as the kidney. The most common arterial thrombo-occlusive event is cerebral infarction,[11] and in patients with chorea, cerebral infarcts identified by computed tomography or magnetic resonance imaging occur in 35% of cases.[12] The main discerning feature of cerebral ischemia or infarction in patients with no other manifestations of APS was an IgG anticardiolipin greater than 40 GPL. Seizures occurring in these patients were associated with focal brain infarction.[13] The prevalence of thrombocytopenia in APS is in the range of 23%, and it is not associated with any other particular features of the syndrome.[14]

A less frequent complication of APS is cardiac involvement. This may take a number of forms including cardiomyopathy associated with postpartum exacerbation of APS.[15, 16] Unlike the Libman-Sacks vegetations on heart valves in acute SLE, which are generally asymptomatic, valve involvement in APS and chronic SLE causes thickening, nodularity, poor coaptation, and regurgitation.[17] The valve lesions in APS may involve all valves with intravalvular fibrin deposits, but little inflammation.[18] In addition to functional regurgitant lesions, patients with primary APS have a high risk of acute myocardial infarction, pulmonary hypertension, and pleural effusion compared with case-matched controls.[19]

Obstetric Risks and Management

Adverse pregnancy outcomes with APS relate to increased pregnancy loss, preeclampsia, fetal growth failure, preterm delivery, and the impact of medications, in addition to implications of the other clinical manifestations of APS. These maternal and fetal risk factors are discussed in the following text.

Maternal Risks

Thrombosis. The risk of developing thrombosis or stroke during pregnancy is unclear but appears to be higher if there is a positive lupus anticoagulant titer, high titers of anticardiolipin, and history of a previous thrombotic episode. In a prospective study of patients with SLE and lupus anticoagulant, 50% of the patients had a thrombotic episode.[20] A retrospective cohort study also found a high risk of thrombosis in APS occurring in 30% of cases.[21] Two prospective series have reported a 5% to 12% risk of thrombosis during pregnancy.[22, 23]

Women in pregnancy and those with high titers of anticardiolipin[24] or lupus anticoagulant have improved outcomes after treatment with antithrombotic therapy.[23] In Lima and coworkers' study, there were no thrombotic events in those patients receiving a low-molecular-weight heparin (LMWH) regimen.[23] Although the initial studies that showed improved pregnancy outcomes in APS used prednisone and aspirin,[25] it is now apparent that prednisone is associated with the complications of corticosteroids, and aspirin or heparin in combination with aspirin currently appears to offer the best outcome with fewer adverse side effects.[26] Heparin-aspirin combination therapy has been shown to lead to a higher live birth rate than aspirin alone.[27]

There appears to be considerable advantage to using LMWH, and this treatment has been used throughout pregnancy, labor, delivery, and the puerperium[28] without any adverse effects, particularly hemorrhage. The risk of osteopenia from long-term heparin use is unclear, since it has been shown that in normal pregnancy, lumbar spine bone density decreases are similar to those in women treated with heparin.[29]

Preeclampsia. A high rate of preeclampsia, often of early onset or complicated by the HELLP variant of preeclampsia, has been a consistent feature of many series of patients with APS.[22, 23] Preeclampsia rates of 16% to 50% have been described compared with the rate in a normal population of 3%.[30]

The severity of the preeclampsia may often necessitate early delivery. This often leads to cesarean section owing to a combination of factors including maternal and fetal condition, fetal presentation, the state of the cervix, and the likelihood of successful induction of labor and vaginal delivery. Close surveillance before, during, and after delivery is important especially in cases of early delivery for preeclampsia, as such patients are at increased risk for developing the complications of preeclampsia and the organ involvement seen in APS.

Fetal Risks. Fetal risks include early pregnancy loss, unexplained intrauterine death, poor fetal growth, and the complications associated with preterm delivery performed for maternal and fetal reasons. As discussed previously, treatment is associated with improved fetal outcomes but close monitoring of pregnancy is necessary because even with treatment, up to 30% of fetuses fail to reach their expected growth potentials.[22, 31]

In patients with APS requiring treatment, that is, those with high titers of lupus anticoagulant or IgG anticardiolipin, preterm delivery is common with up to 30% of patients being delivered before 32 weeks' gestation.[22]

Treatment

Management in Pregnancy

A number of treatment regimens have been promoted as improving outcomes in pregnancy, and new strategies such as intravenous immunoglobulin or prepregnancy hydroxychloroquine are being investigated.[32] Currently, aspirin in a dosage up to 150 mg/day and aspirin in combination with thromboprophylactic doses of heparin up to 20,000 U/day are the most widely used treatments.

Not all patients with antiphospholipid antibody require treatment,[33] but usually those who have sought obstetric specialist surveillance have a history of pregnancy loss and significant antiphospholipid antibody levels and require treatment.

Low-dose aspirin (60–150 mg) is unlikely to be associated with any serious complications as demonstrated by the CLASP trial.[34] Unfractionated heparin has been given subcutaneously, 5000 to 25,000 U, in once- or twice-daily doses. Evidence of the superiority of LMWH in general use,[35] and the limited evidence in pregnancy, support its use. Generally, a dose equivalent to fosfestrol sodium, 5000 U daily, is given, and in patients with previous proven thromboembolic events or active antiphospholipid activity, twice this dose has been given without maternal complications. It would appear that monitoring of factor Xa levels is not required, nor is it necessary to monitor antiphospholipid titers as an indicator of response to treatment.

In the puerperium, LMWH therapy may be continued or, alternatively, warfarin may be substituted. There are no contraindications to breast-feeding while the mother is on warfarin therapy. In documented thrombotic episodes, long-term anticoagulation needs to be considered, as this may reduce the risk of subsequent thrombosis.

Labor Management

Anesthetic Considerations. Anesthesia for the patient with APS must take into account the following:

- The presence or absence of end-organ dysfunction
- Any treatment the patient is receiving, especially anticoagulants
- The anticipated route of delivery

Organ Dysfunction

Respiratory. Although pulmonary hypertension is a rare complication of APS, its presence imposes a marked increase in risk for the parturient. Increases in pulmonary vascular resistance, such as that caused by pain, stress, or hypoxia must be avoided. Similarly, rapid decreases in systemic vascular resistance must be prevented.

Epidural anesthesia or analgesia is not necessarily contraindicated in patients with pulmonary hypertension but must be initiated and established slowly with appropriate monitoring. The use of anticoagulants in these patients may preclude the use of regional anesthesia.

CARDIAC. Myocardial infarction is also a rare complication of APS. If possible, delaying delivery until at least 2 weeks postinfarction has been advised.[36] The choice of vaginal or cesarean delivery appears to be based on anecdotal reports, but vaginal delivery has been recommended as the preferred option.[37]

Regional anesthesia can reduce the stress response to delivery or surgery but must be instituted carefully with appropriate monitoring. Anticoagulation may preclude its use.

General anesthesia may be required for cesarean section. The technique chosen must avoid the stress response to intubation as much as possible. β-blockers and opiates may be indicated, but their use may have implications for the fetus; pediatric staff should be informed by the anesthetist if such drugs are to be administered to the mother.

ANTICOAGULATION. The use of anticoagulant therapy in the parturient with APS has implications for the use of regional anesthesia. Concerns have been expressed regarding the use of regional anesthesia in patients receiving LMWH, with case reports of spinal hematoma. The U.S. Food and Drug Administration has alerted clinicians to these concerns.[38] Similar alerts also exist in other countries.

A review article advises a 10- to 12-hour wait before placing an epidural catheter in a patient receiving LMWH and a further 2-hour wait before an additional dosage of LMWH.[39] Similar time periods are also advised before catheter removal. Close observation of the patient's neurologic status is, of course, mandatory.

It should be noted that the concurrent use of aspirin therapy poses an additional risk for spinal hematoma following regional anesthesia in patients receiving LMWH treatment.

Although the use of regional anesthesia in APS patients, particularly those with associated preeclampsia or hypertension, appears a very attractive option, the anesthetist must take into account any concurrent anticoagulant therapy and then proceed with caution. In cases in which anesthesia is required for emergency delivery, especially for cesarean section, and the time limits advised cannot be adhered to, general anesthesia may be the more prudent option.[39] The anesthetist also needs to take into account other factors such as recent oral intake and airway status assessment. The final decision then becomes one of risk-benefit analysis.

A recent review reminded clinicians of the importance of other thromboprophylactic measures and advocated the use of epidurals in ambulatory parturients ("walking epidurals") to further lessen the chance of thrombotic episodes during labor.[40]

SYSTEMIC LUPUS ERYTHEMATOSUS

The effects of systemic lupus erythematosus (SLE) on pregnancy and on the fetus and neonate may be considerable. There is some overlap with APS, in part because antiphospholipid antibodies may be common to both conditions. However, some important differences are specific to SLE. These include specific organ involvement, risk of congenital heart block, and neonatal lupus erythematosus. Recurrent pregnancy loss may precede overt clinical lupus.

In patients with SLE, antiphospholipid antibodies are generally absent or of low titer. When antiphospholipid antibodies are present in SLE (secondary APS), the pregnancy outcome is much worse.

Pathogenic Mechanisms. The vasculitis of SLE is inflammatory in contrast to that of primary APS. This distinction and the differentiation of SLE from primary APS is of importance, because SLE is treated with immunosuppressive therapy including glucocorticoids, whereas primary APS is managed with heparin and aspirin.

Maternal Risks

SLE FLARE IN PREGNANCY. There is controversy whether pregnancy is associated with exacerbations in SLE, but flare of SLE has been found to occur in less than 25% of cases.[41] Flares tend to be mild and are generally easily treated with glucocorticoids.[42] Contrary to many reports, a recent prospective study has found that flares were more common during the pregnancy than in the puerperium.[43] Patients with SLE who are stable on hydroxychloroquine before pregnancy should continue this treatment while pregnant, since cessation may precipitate a flare. Markers of SLE may occur in pregnant women who do not have SLE, such as proteinuria, thrombocytopenia secondary to anemia, and classic pathway hypocomplementemia.

It may be difficult to distinguish SLE with active renal involvement from preeclampsia. Patients with SLE are at increased risk for developing preeclampsia. The factors listed in Table 43–4 may help in differentiating between the two conditions. Reliable indicators of SLE include rising antinuclear antibodies (ANA), alternative pathway hypocomplementemia, and clinical signs such as arthritis, skin rash, muscle aches, and lymphadenopathy.

HYPERTENSIVE DISEASE AND PREECLAMPSIA. Gestational hypertension and preeclampsia are more likely to occur in patients with SLE. Lupus nephritis and the use of corticosteroids are particular risk factors for developing pregnancy induced hypertension and preeclampsia.

RENAL DISEASE. Renal involvement is common in patients with SLE and presents with proteinuria. Diffuse proliferative glomerulonephritis is the most severe

Table 43-4 Laboratory Tests Helpful in Distinguishing Preeclampsia From SLE Nephritis

Test	PET	SLE
Hematology		
Blood film (abnormal in HELLP)	Yes	No
Microangiopathic hemolytic anemia	Yes	No
Autoimmune hemolytic anemia (Coombs-positive, anti-red cell antibodies)	No	Yes
Thrombocytopenia	Yes	Yes
White blood cell count	Raised	Low
Biochemistry		
Serum creatinine	Raised if severe	Markedly increased
Serum hepatic transaminases (ALT)	Raised	Normal
Urinalysis		
Hematuria	If fulminating	Present
Cellular casts	No	Present
Serology/Antibodies		
Elevated anti-DS DNA	Normal	Elevated
Decreased complement	Variable	Decreased

ALT, alanine aminotransferase.

renal lesion in SLE. It presents with hypertension, proteinuria (nephrotic syndrome), hematuria, pyuria, casts, and hypocomplementemia. Treatment is with glucocorticoids, cytotoxic agents such as cyclophosphamide, and aggressive antihypertensive medication.

Exacerbations of SLE and superadded preeclampsia may lead to deteriorating maternal and fetal welfare and require preterm delivery, usually by cesarean section because of the state of the mother and the fetus and the difficulties establishing labor before term.

Fetal Risks

Fetal Loss. Patients with SLE appear to have increased risks of miscarriage and second and third trimester pregnancy loss. This is particularly so when antiphospholipid antibodies and lupus nephritis are present.

Preterm Delivery. It is difficult to distinguish iatrogenic from spontaneous preterm delivery in SLE, but it is thought that preterm delivery is more likely with a flare. A recent prospective review has confirmed the high rate of preterm birth, but prematurity was generally unrelated to disease flare.[43]

Some connective tissue disorders, for example, Ehlers-Danlos syndrome, are associated with preterm rupture of the fetal membranes,[44] but this effect is less clear for SLE.

Fetal Growth Failure. The association of preeclampsia and APS with SLE explains the frequent occurrence of poor fetal growth seen in up to one third of cases. Poor fetal growth, evidence on antenatal ultrasound of deterioration in amniotic fluid volume, and abnormal fetal Doppler velocimetry are all indications for early delivery, often by cesarean section.

Neonatal Lupus Erythematosus. A full discussion of this condition is beyond the scope of this chapter. Neonatal lupus has dermatologic hematologic, and cardiac manifestations. The majority of cases are associated with maternal anti-Ro/SSA or anti-La/SSB antibodies. Presence of these antibodies should alert clinicians to the possibility of neonatal lupus. Conversely, in a fetus with persistent brachycardia consistent with a congenital heart block, SLE in the mother should be excluded.

Treatment

Management in Pregnancy. Apart from prepregnancy and regular pregnancy review by an obstetrician or a rheumatologist, specific drug therapy is used to control symptoms or treat an exacerbation. Glucocorticoids are safe for the human fetus but increase the chance of gestational diabetes and hypertension. The use of glucocorticoids and heparin in patients with severe SLE has been associated with osteoporotic fractures of the vertebral column. Other immunosuppressive agents have been used. Azathioprine is not a teratogen in humans, but cyclophosphamide used for lupus nephritis may be teratogenic. Antimalarial agents have been associated with ocular toxic effects and ototoxicity, but the risks seem small and there is a trend to treat women before pregnancy with hydroxychloroquine to reduce antiphospholipid activity.[32]

Labor and Delivery Management. Special considerations include steroid boluses for patients on glucocorticoids, thromboprophylaxis for those with anticardiolipin and lupus anticoagulant antiphospholipid antibodies, and continuous fetal heart rate monitoring in labor.

Postnatal care includes close observation for SLE exacerbation, recommencing prepregnancy maintenance therapy, and careful examination of the baby for signs of SLE-associated problems.

Anesthetic Considerations. Anesthetic considerations for pregnant patients with SLE are similar to pregnant women with APS. Pericardial effusion can complicate SLE. End-organ damage to the kidney may result in renal failure. Pulmonary involvement may cause restrictive lung disease. These possibilities should all be accounted for in assessing the pregnant patient with SLE.

Preanesthesia evaluation, including serum creatinine and electrolytes, chest x-ray, and echocardiography, should be done, if indicated. The choice of anesthetic agents may be affected by laboratory findings.

Concurrent administration of anticoagulant agents has implications for the use of regional anesthesia similar to APS. Patients with SLE may also be receiving steroid therapy, and additional doses must be allowed for.

The choice of anesthesia may be governed by some or all of the above-mentioned factors, but in most cases regional anesthesia is to be preferred.

RHEUMATOID ARTHRITIS

This common systemic inflammatory arthritis has been found to frequently improve during pregnancy. This is consistent with the effects of pregnancy on cell-mediated immunity. Decreased immune complexes have been found in patients undergoing remission of rheumatoid arthritis (RA) in pregnancy. Occasionally, the first manifestations of RA become apparent during pregnancy.

Of particular importance for obstetric and anesthetic management is involvement of the temporomandibular joints and the larynx in the inflammatory process. Problems with the synovial joints of the hips are a late manifestation of the disease and are rarely of concern for delivery.

Effects on the Pregnancy. There appears to be little evidence for adverse obstetric outcomes in patients with RA. In contrast to most of the other autoimmune rheumatologic conditions, there is no increase in fetal loss or preterm delivery with RA.

Effect of Pregnancy on Rheumatoid Arthritis. The majority of patients with RA with active disease at conception show remission of symptoms, generally during the early weeks of pregnancy. However, the disease frequently flares as soon as 2 to 3 weeks after delivery.

Treatment

Management in Pregnancy. Simple analgesia with paracetamol or aspirin is often adequate and is safe for the fetus. Of the other agents used, sulfasalazine appears to have few adverse effects. Nonsteroidal anti-inflammatory drugs (NSAIDs), particularly the cyclooxygenase type I inhibitors such as indomethacin, may be associated with impairment of fetal renal function which may persist postnatally. These drugs may also cause premature closure of the ductus arteriosus in the fetus and neonate. Antimalarial drugs may have effects on fetal ocular development and the ear, as discussed previously in the section on SLE.

Although prednisone and hydrocortisone do not cross the human placenta in any great amount because of placental hydrolysis, these drugs are associated with maternal complications including hypertension and gestational diabetes in addition to the longer-term effects of osteoporosis.

Labor and Delivery Management

ANESTHETIC CONSIDERATIONS. In the pregnant patient with RA, the known potential for airway management problems associated with the pregnancy may be worsened by the disease status, especially involvement of the temporomandibular joints. These patients should be considered at risk for difficult intubation and appropriate precautions instituted. In extreme situations, awake intubation using a fiberoptic bronchoscope may be the safest option.

It must be remembered that cervical spine manipulation in patients with RA may in itself be life-threatening.[45] When possible, preanesthetic evaluation should include appropriate radiologic investigation of the neck[45] as well as clinical evaluation of the airway.[46] Furthermore, it should be noted that the cricoarytenoid joints may have rheumatoid involvement, adding to the potential for airway management difficulties.[47]

The pregnant patient with RA may also have cardiac or respiratory involvement. Pericarditis may be present and an associated pericardial effusion may compromise cardiac output necessitating extreme caution when instituting regional anesthesia. Restrictive lung disease associated with RA may have implications for anesthetic management including postoperative care. Allowing for the possible dangers of x-rays in pregnant patients, there must nevertheless be a low threshold for radiologic examination of the chest, with particular emphasis on checking for the presence of pleural and pericardial effusions.

As with SLE, concurrent use of steroid therapy should be taken into consideration when planning anesthetic care. Many of these patients take aspirin, which does not appear to be a contraindication for regional anesthesia.

Although RA does not in itself contraindicate the use of regional anesthesia, careful evaluation of the patient's spinal anatomy and peripheral neurologic status should be assessed before instituting epidural anesthesia. In most instances, regional anesthesia techniques are to be preferred, in light of the potential airway problems. If general anesthesia is required, consideration should be given to awake intubation using local anesthesia. It has been recommended that transtracheal injection be avoided in these patients.[48]

ANKYLOSING SPONDYLITIS

Effects on the Pregnancy. The evidence available suggests that the disease has no adverse effect on pregnancy outcomes. Ostensen and Husby[49] found no differences in the various serologic parameters used to monitor disease activity. It appears that only in situations of severe disease requiring aggressive drug therapy is pregnancy outcome unfavorable, and this may be as much a result of the medications as the effect of the disease itself on the fetus.[50]

Effect of Pregnancy on Ankylosing Spondylitis. In contrast to rheumatoid arthritis, ankylosing spondylitis may show a more variable course in pregnancy with the majority of patients either having no change in disease activity or having an exacerbation. In one prospective review, remission occurred in only 20% of patients.[49] It was noted in that study that anterior uveitis occurred during pregnancy or in the first 6 months after delivery in 20% of patients, but there were no cases of cardiac or pulmonary disease.[49]

SCLERODERMA

This is a rare condition of unknown etiology leading to multiorgan involvement in connective tissue fibrosis. It is commoner in females. Its importance lies in the apparent risk of serious maternal and fetal sequelae documented in the few reports of pregnancies in patients with the condition.[51] Of concern are the risks of developing serious cardiopulmonary and renal problems, especially early in the course of the disease. Involvement of the esophagus in scleroderma is well recognized, and life-threatening hemorrhage from Mallory-Weiss tears has been documented.[52]

Most of the maternal mortality in scleroderma has been associated with renal disease and hypertension or with pulmonary fibrosis with superimposed infection. The hypertension associated with renal involvement in scleroderma appears to be effectively managed with angiotensin-converting enzyme inhibitors such as captopril. Although these drugs are generally contraindicated in pregnancy because of negative fetal effects, including renal toxicity, anuria-oligohydramnios, and hypocalvaria, they may on occasion be needed in this condition.[53]

Anesthetic Considerations. These include difficulties with intravascular access owing to the thickened skin, flexion contractures, and vasoconstriction. Pulmonary hypertension, heart failure, and cardiac conduction defects, in addition to hypertension, may complicate anesthesia at delivery.

Intubation may be difficult, and fiberoptic techniques may be necessary. Even if regional anesthesia is planned, contingencies should be in place in the event that intubation proves necessary.[54]

Postpartum Care. Renal, respiratory, or multiorgan failure may occur postpartum, and intensive monitoring of the mother's condition is necessary following delivery.

POLYARTERITIS NODOSA

This is an unusual vasculitis involving the small and medium-sized arteries that leads to a destructive necrotizing inflammation of the vessel walls. The weakened areas of the vessels may form small aneurysms. If an aneurysm ruptures, a subcutaneous nodule may form, hence the name of the condition. Polyarteritis tends to occur in males and in the fifth decade of life, but it may occur in females in the reproductive age group and, as such, deserves mention.

The most commonly affected organs are the heart, the kidneys, the gut, and muscle, with skin involvement being one of the clinical manifestations of the disease.

Effects on the Pregnancy. The few reports that are available suggest a very poor prognosis with a significant maternal mortality.[55] This may relate to the level of disease activity and the association of other complications such as preeclampsia, which accords with the authors' experience. There have been case reports of good outcomes related to quiescence of the disease.[56]

In the authors' experience, the main adverse effects of polyarteritis nodosa on pregnancy appear to have been severe, early-onset hypertensive complications leading to the need for preterm delivery. There are case reports of maternal death related to coronary periarteritis and thrombosis with multiorgan failure.

Effect of Pregnancy on Polyarteritis Nodosa. There are reports of polyarteritis nodosa appearing to have its onset during pregnancy or in the immediate postpartum period.[55] These patients seem to have a poorer prognosis than those with preexisting disease who are in a stable condition at the onset of the pregnancy.

Labor and Delivery Management. Preparation for delivery includes an assessment of maternal and fetal welfare to plan the most appropriate route to deliver the baby. Maternal assessment includes an electrocardiogram and renal and liver function tests. Fetal assessment includes an estimate of size, amniotic fluid volume, umbilical arterial Doppler velocimetry, and cardiotocography, examining the response of the baby to changes in its intrauterine environment, such as fetal movements and behavioral state patterns.

Patients with active disease are generally treated with corticosteroids as first-line therapy, and consideration should be given to increasing the dosages during the time of delivery. Thromboprophylaxis given post partum, especially after a complicated delivery, may protect against small vessel occlusion but there are few data on the efficacy of this approach in this rare condition.

THYROID DISEASE

In this section, the implications of autoimmune thyroid disease on the mother and fetus are briefly summarized along with a review of anesthetic considerations.

Graves' disease and autoimmune thyroiditis, also called Hashimoto's disease, constitute the two groups of autoimmune thyroid conditions. Whereas thyroid-stimulating hormone (TSH) does not cross the placenta, and triiodothyronine (T_3) and thyroxine (T_4)

do so only in small amounts, antithyroid drugs as well as thyroid antibodies readily cross the placenta.

Thyroid Function in Pregnancy. A number of factors alter the assessment of thyroid function in pregnancy. Thyroid-binding globulin increases owing to estrogen causing increased hepatic synthesis. This leads to increased output of T_4 from the thyroid gland to maintain normal circulating levels, but the TSH does not increase. Human chorionic gonadotropin, a glycoprotein with an α chain similar to TSH, has a weak intrinsic thyroid-stimulating effect. The increased iodine requirement in pregnancy, which is caused by the increased renal excretion of iodine, is generally compensated for except in iodine-deficient geographic regions.

Graves' disease often improves in the second trimester of pregnancy. The reason for this is not clear, although levels of maternal thyrotropin receptor antibodies (TRAb) do fall.[57] The condition may exacerbate in the postnatal period.

The fetal hypothalamic-pituitary-thyroid axis is functional by 12 weeks' gestation. Thyrotropin-releasing hormone crosses the placenta, but neither TSH nor T_4 does to any significant amount. Iodine is transferred actively to the fetus and importantly, maternal thyroid antibodies also cross the placenta even if the mother has been rendered euthyroid by treatment. During pregnancy, the fetus should be observed for growth failure, tachycardia, and the development of a goiter, which may occur in the presence of TRAb even if the mother is euthyroid. This is one of the reasons why all women with autoimmune thyroid disease should be screened for TRAb in early pregnancy.

In hypothyroidism, it has been found that if treated women do become pregnant, there may be increased requirements for T_4 necessitating an adjustment to the dosage of thyroxine.[58] Thyroiditis may occur post partum. The serum marker for postpartum thyroiditis is the presence of thyroid microsomal antibodies. Almost 50% of patients with these antibodies develop postpartum thyroiditis. There appears to be a relationship between the presence of these thyroid antibodies and the development of postnatal depression, but it is unresolved whether there is benefit to be gained from screening for these microsomal antibodies in every pregnancy.

Most of the drugs used to treat thyrotoxicosis may be used in pregnancy. Both carbimazole and propylthiouracil are used, although the latter is found in lower amounts than carbimazole in breast milk. There is no evidence that it is of value to use blocking-replacement regimens such as carbimazole and thyroxine.

β-Blocking agents are needed only to control cardiovascular complications of thyrotoxicosis and in thyroid crisis.

Anesthetic Considerations. The two main considerations are management of the airway and metabolic derangements, which are discussed in Chapters 32 and 53, respectively.

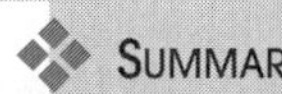

SUMMARY

Key Points

- Most immune function is pregnancy is normal, although increased susceptibility to certain infections in pregnancy has been attributed to decreased cellular immune responses.
- Autoimmune diseases may produce abnormalities in the pulmonary and cardiac systems and may have an impact on both regional and general anesthesia.
- Parturients with high titers of anticardiolipin or lupus anticoagulant have improved outcomes if treated with antithrombotic therapy.
- Glucocorticoids, used to treat several autoimmune diseases, are safe for the human fetus, but increase the risk of gestational diabetes and hypertension.

Key Reference

Horlocker TT, Heit JA: Low molecular weight heparin: Biochemistry, pharmacology, perioperative prophylaxis regimens, and guidelines for regional anesthetic management. Anesth Analg 1997; 85:874–875.

Case Stem

A 38-year-old gravida 5 para 0 is sent to you for a pre-delivery anesthetic consultation at 26 weeks of gestation. She suffers from severe SLE and has severe renal involvement and hypertension. Her obstetric history is positive for numerous second trimester miscarriages. Her medications include glucocorticoids, antihypertensives, and thromboprophylaxis. What will you advise her regarding anesthesia analgesia?

References

1. Buyon JP, Nelson JL, Lockshin MD: The effects of pregnancy on autoimmune diseases. Clin Immunol Immunopathol 1996; 78:99–104.
2. Formby B: Immunological response in pregnancy: its role in endocrine disorders of pregnancy and influence on the course of maternal autoimmune diseases. Endocr Metab Clin North Am 1995; 24:187–205.
3. Topping S, Quenby S, Farquharson RGF, et al: Marked variation in antiphospholipid antibodies during pregnancy: relationship to pregnancy outcome. J Obstet Gynaecol 1998; 18:515–516.
4. La Rosa L, Meroni PL, Tincani A, et al: β_2-Glycoprotein I and placental anticoagulant protein I in placentae from patients with antiphospholipid syndrome. J Rheumatol 1994; 21:1684–1693.
5. Burrows RF, Kelton JG: Incidentally detected thrombocytopenia in healthy mothers and their infants. N Engl J Med 1998; 319:142.
6. Moll S, Ortel TL: The INR is invalid in monitoring warfarin anticoagulant therapy in patients with lupus anticoagulants [abstract]. Lupus 1996; S552.
7. Cabiedes J, Cabral AR, Alarcon-Segovia D: Clinical manifestations of the antiphospholipid syndrome in patients with systemic lupus erythematosus associate more strongly with anti-beta 2-glycoprotein-1 than with antiphospholipid antibodies. J Rheumatol 1995; 22:1899–1906.

8. McNally T, Mackie IJ, Machin SJ, et al: Increased levels of beta 2 glycoprotein-1 antigen and beta 2 glycoprotein-1 binding antibodies are associated with a history of thromboembolic complications in patients with SLE and primary antiphospholipid syndrome. Br J Rheumatol 1995; 34:1031–1036.
9. Lockshin MD: Antiphospholipid antibody: babies, blood clots, biology. JAMA 1997; 277:1549–1551.
10. Harris EN: Syndrome of the Black Swan. Br J Rheumatol 1986; 26:324–326.
11. Brey RL, Levine SR: Treatment of neurologic complications of antiphospholipid antibody syndrome. Lupus 1996; 5:473–476.
12. Cervera R, Asherson RA, Font J, et al: Chorea in the antiphospholipid syndrome: clinical, radiologic and immunologic characteristics of 50 patients from our clinics and the recent literature. Medicine 1997; 76:203–212.
13. Levine SR, Brey RL: Neurological aspects of antiphospholipid antibody syndrome. Lupus 1996; S:347–353.
14. Cuadrado MJ, Mujic F, Mundz E, et al: Thrombocytopenia in the antiphospholipid syndrome. Ann Rheum Dis 1997; 56:194–196.
15. Kochenour NK, Branch DW, Roten S, et al: A new postpartum syndrome associated with antiphospholipid antibodies. Obstet Gynecol 1987; 69:460–468.
16. Airoldi ML, Eid O, Tosetto C, et al: Post partum dilated cardiomyopathy in antiphospholipid positive women. Lupus 1996; 5:247–250.
17. Shahian DM, Labib SB, Schneebaum AB: Etiology and management of chronic valve disease in antiphospholipid antibody syndrome and systemic lupus erythematosus. J Card Surg 1995; 10:133–139.
18. Garcia-Torres R, Amigo MC, de la Rosa A, et al: Valvular heart disease in primary antiphospholipid syndrome (PAPS): clinical and morphological findings. Lupus 1996; 5:56–61.
19. Badui E, Solorio S, Martinez E, et al: The heart in the primary antiphospholipid syndrome. Arch Med Res 1995; 26:115–120.
20. Glueck HI, Kant KS, Weiss MA, et al: Thrombosis in systemic lupus erythematous: relation to the presence of circulating anticoagulant. Arch Intern Med 1985; 145:1389–1395.
21. Krnic-Barrie S, O'Connor CR, Looney SW, et al: A retrospective review of 61 patients with antiphospholipid syndrome: analysis of factors influencing recurrent thrombosis. Arch Intern Med 1997; 157:2101–2108.
22. Branch DW, Silver RM, Blackwell JL, et al: Outcome of treated pregnancies in women with antiphospholipid syndrome: an update of the Utah experience. Obstet Gynecol 1992; 80:614–620.
23. Lima F, Khamashta MA, Buchanan NM, et al: A study of sixty pregnancies in patients with the antiphospholipid syndrome. Clin Exp Rheumatol 1996; 14:131–136.
24. Silver RM, Porter TF, Van Leeuween I, et al: Anticardiolipin antibodies: clinical consequences of "low titres." Obstet Gynecol 1996; 87:494–500.
25. Lubbe WF, Butler WS, Palmer SJ, et al: Fetal surveillance after prednisone suppression of maternal lupus anticoagulant. Lancet 1983; 1:1361–1363.
26. Cowchock FS, Reece EA, Balaban D, et al: Repeated fetal losses associated with antiphospholipid antibodies: a collaborative randomised trial comparing prednisone to low dose heparin treatment. Am J Obstet Gynecol 1992; 166:1318–1327.
27. Rai R, Cohen H, Dave M, et al: Randomised controlled trial of aspirin plus heparin in pregnant women with recurrent miscarriage associated with antiphospholipid antibodies. BMJ 1997; 314:253–257.
28. Dulitzki M, Pauzner R, Langevitz P, et al: Low molecular weight heparin during pregnancy and delivery: preliminary experience with 41 pregnancies. Obstet Gynecol 1996; 87:380–383.
29. Shefras J, Farquharson RG: Bone density studies in pregnant women receiving heparin. Eur J Obstet Gynecol Reprod Biol 1996; 65:171–174.
30. Stone P, Cook D, Hutton J, et al: Measurement of blood pressure, oedema and proteinuria in a pregnant population of New Zealand. Aust N Z J Obstet Gynaecol 1995; 35:32–37.
31. Kutteh WH: Antiphospholipid antibody associated recurrent pregnancy loss: treatment with heparin and low dose aspirin is superior to low dose aspirin alone. Am J Obstet Gynecol 1996; 174:1584–1589.
32. Petri M: Pathogenesis and treatment of the antiphospholipid antibody syndrome. Med Clin North Am 1997; 81:151–177.
33. Cowchock S, Reece EA: Do low-risk women with antiphospholipid antibodies need to be treated? Am J Obstet Gynecol 1997; 176:1099–1100.
34. CLASP [Collaborative Low-Dose Aspirin in Pregnancy Trial]: A randomised trial of low dose aspirin for the prevention and treatment of pre-eclampsia among 9364 pregnant women. Lancet 1994; 343:619–629.
35. Pineo GF, Hull RD: Low molecular weight heparin: prophylaxis and treatment of venous thromboembolism. Annu Rev Med 1997; 48:79–91.
36. Carvalho JCA, Van Zundert A, Ostheimer GW: Cardiac disease. *In* Pain Relief and Anesthesia in Obstetrics. New York: Churchill Livingstone; 1996:547–557.
37. Hankins GDV, Wendall GD, Leveno KJ, et al: Myocardial infarction in pregnancy: a review. Obstet Gynecol 1985; 65:139–146.
38. Federal Drug Administration: Health advisory for certain anticoagulant drugs. FDA Talk Paper 1997; 15 December: T97-63.
39. Horlocker TT, Heit JA: Low molecular weight heparin: biochemistry, pharmacology, perioperative prophylaxis regimens and guidelines for regional anaesthetic management. Anaesth Analg 1997; 85:874–885.
40. Ringrose DK: Anaesthesia and the antiphospholipid syndrome: a review of 20 obstetric patients. Int J Obstet Anaesth 1997; 6:107–111.
41. Boumpas DT, Fessler BJ, Austin HA, et al: Systemic lupus erythematosus: emerging concepts. Ann Intern Med 1995; 123:42–53.
42. Lockshin MD: Pregnancy does not cause systemic lupus erythematosus to worsen. Arthritis Rheum 1989; 32:665–670.
43. Le Thi Huong D, Wechsler B, Vauthier-Brouzes D, et al: Outcome of planned pregnancies in systemic erythematosus: a prospective study on 62 pregnancies. Br J Rheumatol 1997; 36:772–777.
44. Parry S, Strauss JF: Premature rupture of the fetal membranes. N Engl J Med 1998; 338:663–670.
45. McArthur A, Kleiman S: Rheumatoid cervical disease—a challenge to the anesthetist. Can J Anesth 1993; 40:154–159.
46. Popitz MD: Anaesthetic implications of chronic disease of the cervical spine. Anesth Analg 1997; 4:672–683.
47. Funk D, Raymon F: Rheumatoid arthritis of the cricoarytenoid joints: an airway hazard. Anaesth Analg 1975; 54:742–745.
48. Longmire S: Autoimmune diseases. *In* Gambling DR, Douglas MJ (eds): Obstetric Anaesthesia and Uncommon Disorders. Philadelphia: WB Saunders; 1998; 381–404.
49. Ostensen M, Husby G: A prospective clinical study of the effect of pregnancy on rheumatoid arthritis and ankylosing spondylitis. Arthritis Rheum 1983; 26:1155–1159.
50. Ostensen M, Romberg O, Husby G: Ankylosing spondylitis and motherhood. Arthritis Rheum 1982; 25:140–143.
51. Steen VD: Scleroderma and pregnancy. Rheum Dis Clin North Am 1997; 23:133–147.
52. Chin KAJ, Kaseba CM, Weaver JB: Mallory-Weiss syndrome complicating pregnancy in a patient with scleroderma: diagnosis and management. Br J Obstet Gynaecol 1995; 102:498–500.
53. D'Angelo R, Miller R: Pregnancy complicated by severe preeclampsia and thrombocytopenia in a patient with scleroderma. Anesth Analg 1997; 85:839–841.
54. Younker D, Harrison B: Scleroderma and pregnancy: anaesthetic considerations. Br J Anaesth 1985; 57:1136–1139.
55. Pitkin R: Polyarteritis nodosa. Clin Obstet Gynecol 1983; 6:579–586.
56. Reed NR, Smith MT: Periarteritis nodosa in pregnancy: report of a case and review of the literature. Obstet Gynecol 1980; 55:381–384.
57. Hall R: Pregnancy and autoimmune endocrine disease. Clin Endocrinol Metab 1995; 9:137–155.
58. Larsen PR: Monitoring thyroxine treatment during pregnancy. Thyroid 1992; 2:153–154.

44

Hepatic Disease

❖ CHONG JIN LONG, MD

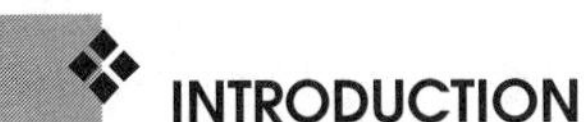

INTRODUCTION

The liver is the largest parenchymal organ in the human body and is perfused by approximately 25% of the cardiac output through a dual circulation from the portal vein and the hepatic artery. It has vital roles in general metabolism, plasma protein production, and drug detoxification. In normal pregnancy, hepatic function is not significantly impaired,[1] and although the development of vascular spiders and palmar erythema might be erroneously attributed to liver disease, it is most likely due to physiologic increases of circulating estrogens. This is confirmed by the finding that these lesions disappear with delivery.

A wide variety of liver disorders occur in pregnancy. The incidence is 1 in 500 to 1 in 5000 pregnancies.[2, 3] Liver disease is therefore an uncommon problem in pregnancy. Liver disease can occur in many forms in the pregnant patient, and the severity may range from mild dysfunction to fulminant hepatic failure. Since liver function can be affected by pregnancy, it may be difficult to distinguish these changes from early or mild liver disease.

Liver disease occurring in pregnancy can be categorized into three groups. The first group includes diseases caused by pregnancy. Among these are acute fatty liver of pregnancy, hypercholestasis of pregnancy, and disorders associated with preeclampsia, for example, the HELLP syndrome (hemolysis, elevated liver enzymes, and low platelets). The second group includes liver diseases that are coincident with pregnancy, such as drug-induced liver disease and acute viral hepatitis. Viral infections such as hepatitis are usually benign but they can be exacerbated by pregnancy. However, some forms of viral hepatitis can lead to fulminant hepatic failure. The last group comprises patients who have preexisting liver disease. These diseases include chronic viral hepatitis, autoimmune chronic active hepatitis, Wilson's disease, and Budd-Chiari syndrome. This last group is small because patients with previous liver disease are subfertile. The incidence of these cases may increase in the future as medical therapies enable such patients to become pregnant.

Liver diseases severe enough to cause jaundice in pregnancy are uncommon. Jaundice occurs in about 1 in 1500 pregnancies, an incidence of approximately 0.067%.[3] Forty percent of cases in which jaundice occurs during pregnancy are due to an acute viral hepatitis and about 20% are due to intrahepatic cholestasis.[4]

NORMAL CHANGES IN THE LIVER DURING PREGNANCY

In normal pregnancy with adequate nutrition, the metabolic changes seem to be without significant effect on liver metabolism and function. The liver in pregnancy also shows no undue susceptibility to drugs and toxins. Abnormal liver function tests suggest liver disease or a hepatic complication of an incidental medical problem of pregnancy. In the nonpregnant individual, hepatic blood flow represents 25% to 35% of the cardiac output. Although cardiac output in pregnancy increases by about 40% at term, absolute blood flow to the liver remains the same, thus leading to a smaller proportion of the increased cardiac output passing through the liver. Hence in percentage terms with respect to cardiac output, there is a relative decrease.

Clearance of drugs with high hepatic extraction ratios is significantly unaltered.[5] Metabolism of some compounds may be decreased during pregnancy. For example, caffeine clearance was decreased by 50% during pregnancy in monkeys in the third trimester. Hepatic excretion of sulfobromophthalein is impaired during the latter half of pregnancy. This may infer that the clearance of compounds by microsomal oxidizing enzymes is impaired during the latter half of pregnancy.

Biochemical changes do occur. There is a mild increase in total and direct serum bilirubin in about 20% of pregnant women, which reflects mild physiologic cholestasis related to the increasing circulating estrogens.[6]

There appear to be minimal histologic changes in the liver despite the biochemical changes seen during pregnancy. However, minor subcellular alterations, including some involving bile canaliculi, have been reported in pregnancy. The changes include occasional binucleate cells, increased glycogen content, and slight periportal lymphocytic infiltration. Electron microscopy reveals proliferation of smooth endoplasmic reticulum and enlarged mitochondria.

LABORATORY TESTS IN PREGNANCY

Abnormal biochemical tests occur in 1 in 10 of all normal pregnancies. While most of the so-called liver enzymes are normal, certain less specific blood chemistries may progressively rise or fall throughout pregnancy. Levels of enzymes that are raised during pregnancy include serum cholesterol, triglyceride, plasminogen, some clotting factors, and the erythrocyte sedimentation rate. Biochemical tests show a rise in serum alkaline phosphatase. Serum total cholesterol is raised, serum albumin is reduced, and globulin rises prior to delivery. Serum transaminases may be abnormal prior to delivery and in the postpartum period. The normal pregnant state is mildly cholestatic, as evidenced by the slower excretion of bile.[7]

Serum cholesterol and triglyceride levels begin to rise in the fourth month of pregnancy and peak at term. Cholesterol levels may increase by 50% to levels of about 6 to 8 mmol/L, and serum triglyceride levels may increase up to 180 mg/dL. There is also a small rise in the aspartate aminotransferase (AST) and alkaline phosphatase (ALP) during the third trimester. The AST may be as high as 35 IU/L and ALP may increase to about 135 IU/L.

LIVER DISEASE UNIQUE TO PREGNANCY

The diseases that are unique to pregnancy are acute fatty liver of pregnancy, intrahepatic cholestasis of pregnancy, liver disease related to preeclampsia and HELLP syndrome, and hyperemesis gravidarum (Table 44–1).

Acute Fatty Liver of Pregnancy (AFLP). There is no universally acceptable definition of this disease. The earliest description of acute fatty liver of pregnancy is attributed to a case reported by Stander and Cadden in 1934,[8] but the earliest description is probably that by Sheehan in 1940.[9] The incidence is estimated to be very low—1 in 10,000 to 1 million pregnancies.[10, 11] The etiology is unknown. Some have suggested it may be related to abnormalities in fatty acid metabolism.

Table 44–1 LIVER DISEASE IN PREGNANCY

Disorder	Clinical Features	Anesthetic Implications
Acute fatty liver of pregnancy	Presents acutely in the last trimester Elevated bilirubin and ALP Defect in coagulation, e.g., DIC Preeclampsia occurs frequently Associated with high mortality Hypoglycemia Metabolic acidosis	Monitor blood glucose, liver function, and coagulation Control blood pressure Early termination of pregnancy Epidural anesthesia for labor and operative delivery if no coagulopathy Intensive care management required Problems resolve after delivery
Intrahepatic cholestasis of pregnancy	Presents in latter half of pregnancy with pruritus and jaundice Usually innocuous but fetal loss can occur	Optimize medical management Possible postpartum hemorrhage
Hyperemesis gravidarum	Severe vomiting Liver enzymes mildly elevated Dehydration can occur	Increased risk of fetal death Correct fluid and electrolyte imbalances
Viral hepatitis	Most common cause of jaundice in pregnancy Many forms; hepatitis A-E, G and herpes simplex Presents as nonspecific viral infection with jaundice Hepatitis E and herpes simplex hepatitis potentially deadly AST and ALP very high	Anesthesia and surgery are risky Avoid drugs that damage liver Optimize fluid balances and correct coagulation defects Isoflurane and desflurane a better choice than halothane
Wilson's disease	Uncommon; problem of copper metabolism leading to liver damage Copper deposits in various organs; treatment is with penicillamine, trientine, or zinc Zinc sulfate the preferred drug in pregnancy	Assess and monitor liver function and coagulation, and assess for bleeding varices Therapy should continue during pregnancy For general anesthesia use drugs that are appropriate for liver dysfunction
Budd-Chiari syndrome	Hepatic vein occlusion Leg edema, portal hypertension, and ascites are presenting features Associated with resistance to protein C	Monitor liver function and coagulation Look for lupus anticoagulant and if present, treatment is heparin Bleeding varices may occur
Primary biliary cirrhosis	Variable presentation Can present as liver cirrhosis or pruritus Antimitochondrial antibodies and liver biopsy are diagnostic	Monitor liver function and coagulation Use vitamin K and blood when indicated

ALP, alkaline phosphatase; AST, aspartate aminotransferase; DIC, disseminated intravascular coagulation.

However, there is no unifying, easily identifiable defect that is reliably specific to AFLP. There are reports that it can recur with subsequent pregnancies.[12] Diagnosis can be confirmed by liver biopsy that reveals microvesicular fatty deposit in the hepatocytes. AFLP is a potentially fatal disease. It can lead to maternal as well as perinatal mortality. The only treatment is to terminate the pregnancy. The symptoms disappear once the baby is delivered. Occasionally liver transplantation is necessary because of hepatic failure. Previously, both maternal and perinatal mortality were as high as 85%, but in recent years rates have fallen to less than 10% to 20% with early diagnosis and aggressive treatment. AFLP typically presents during the third trimester with a mildly jaundiced patient who has features of impending hepatic failure. The features include symptomatic malaise, headache, and anorexia with pain at the right hypochondrium. Moderately elevated transaminases with mild elevation of bilirubin are evident. As the disease progresses, the features of hepatic failure and encephalopathy ensue. Coagulopathy with an elevated prothrombin time and activated partial thromboplastin time is typically seen. Disseminated intravascular coagulation (DIC) can also be present. However, thrombocytopenia by itself is not a feature of AFLP. After the onset of jaundice the patient frequently goes into early spontaneous labor, and the delivery may be associated with excessive bleeding. Gastrointestinal hemorrhage has also been reported. Hypoglycemia and renal failure can complicate this disease, with the patient going into progressive liver failure; 20% to 40% of these patients also have signs of preeclampsia, that is, hypertension and proteinuria.[14]

The clinical diagnosis is based on a high index of suspicion. Although the confirmatory diagnostic test is liver biopsy, this is often not possible because of coagulopathy. Laboratory tests of liver function invariably reveal a cholestatic pattern with serum transaminases below 500 U/L and the serum bilirubin usually less than 10 mg/dL. Total white cell counts may be elevated to about 20,000 to 30,000/μL. Diagnostic imaging techniques to assist diagnosis are often inconclusive, but there are reports that features of fatty liver on computed tomography (CT) scan can be helpful. The liver has a lower density compared with the spleen on the CT scan.[15] Fatty liver can also be seen in other disorders, such as liver disease associated with the HELLP syndrome. AFLP may be coincident with preeclampsia as well. Reye's syndrome liver exhibits histologic features similar to AFLP, and this may possibly suggest that they have a common etiology.

It is important to note that jaundice and hyperbilirubinemia may continue to increase for several days postpartum before AFLP begins to resolve. Management of the patient with AFLP is supportive. Hemorrhagic episodes should be treated with vitamin K, blood, fresh-frozen plasma, and platelets whenever necessary. Proper assessment should be performed prior to administration of anesthesia. General anesthesia and narcotics should be used with caution. Regional anesthesia is often contraindicated secondary to coagulopathy. Drugs that are hepatotoxic should be avoided.

Intrahepatic Cholestasis of Pregnancy. This disorder, which is also known as pruritus gravidarum, recurrent intrahepatic cholestasis of pregnancy, and obstetric hepatosis, occurs in pregnant women as well as those who are on oral contraceptives. It typically resolves with the termination of pregnancy or cessation of oral contraceptives. Although the etiology is unknown, it is possibly related to the high estrogen and progesterone levels of pregnancy. It occurs more frequently in some ethnic groups including Scandinavians and Araucanian Indians from Chile, and there is a definite possibility that it may be transmitted by an autosomal dominant gene. The mother usually presents in the third trimester with jaundice, and the course of the disease is variable, with a high incidence of poor fetal outcome. Intrahepatic cholestasis of pregnancy accounts for 20% of all cases of jaundice during pregnancy and is second only to hepatitis in terms of frequency of jaundice. Increased concentrations of bile salts are known to cause umbilical vasoconstriction. Intermittent pruritus with periods of intense itch is another feature. The pruritus usually precedes jaundice by about a week. Bilirubin and alkaline phosphatase levels are elevated, but serum transaminases are only mildly increased (<250 U/L). Unlike AFLP, intrahepatic cholestasis does not progress to hepatic failure or a coagulation defect. An increase in fetal prematurity and death are common complications of this syndrome but the cause is not established. Treatment consists of administration of cholestyramine. Occasionally, intense pruritus calls for the administration of phenobarbitone, which has relieved some patients of their pruritus. Some patients may become vitamin K–deficient because of the cholestasis, so vitamin K should be given to these patients. Careful monitoring of the fetus is important as well, and early delivery is indicated if the fetus shows signs of jeopardy.

Ursodeoxycholate has recently shown efficacy in this condition. It appears to stimulate the biliary excretion of sulfated progesterone metabolites.[16, 17] *S*-adenosylmethionine may also be useful but, as with the evidence for ursodeoxycholate treatment, the data come from anecdotal and poorly controlled trials.

Anesthetic management is usually not different from that for normal parturients.

Preeclampsia and HELLP Syndrome. Preeclampsia and eclampsia is a syndrome that occurs in the third trimester in 5% to 7% of pregnancies and is characterized by hypertension (>140/90 mm Hg; or a >30 mm Hg rise in the systolic pressure or a >15 mm Hg rise in diastolic pressure), edema, and proteinuria with or without convulsion. Liver dysfunction is usually not a feature of early disease. However, in severe preeclampsia liver dysfunction may be as high as 50%. Other possible complications are DIC and hyperuricemia.

Very occasionally, preeclampsia is accompanied by the HELLP syndrome, that is, *h*emolysis, *e*levated *l*iver enzymes, and *l*ow *p*latelet count. This occurs in approximately 0.2% to 0.6% of pregnancies. On CT scan, hepatic subcapsular hemorrhage may be seen. Patients may thus present with abdominal pain. HELLP syndrome may not have the other features of preeclampsia.

The definitive treatment of preeclampsia and HELLP syndrome is delivery of the fetus. Hepatic subcapsular hemorrhages with preeclampsia may lead to hepatic rupture and catastrophic outcome. Hepatic rupture is characterized by sudden or rapidly progressive right upper abdominal pain with the development of shock. Treatment is rapid surgical intervention.

Anesthetic care of these patients involves aggressive resuscitation, control of hemodynamics, and administration of general anesthesia for laparotomy and cesarean delivery. Availability of blood and blood products is vital to successful resuscitation. Correction of coagulopathy and control of blood pressure are essential before planned cesarean delivery.

Hyperemesis Gravidarum. Hyperemesis gravidarum can be defined as intractable nausea and vomiting during pregnancy. It can be so severe that the patients may require hospital admission. Unfortunately, patients with this disease attract little attention and often receive little sympathy from their physicians. There are very few large studies on this disease. Nausea and vomiting are common early in pregnancy, occurring in as many as 60% to 90% of pregnant women. They are so common that conventional wisdom holds that nausea and vomiting are usual and almost invariable signs of pregnancy. Hyperemesis gravidarum, however, is not so common. Its incidence varies from 0.3% to 1% of all pregnancies.

Factors that predispose to an increased risk for this disease are maternal age less than 35 years, obesity, twin gestation, and nulliparity. It is generally a disorder of the first trimester with onset between the 4th and 10th weeks of gestation. In most cases, the nausea and vomiting resolve by 20 weeks' gestation. Patients with hyperemesis gravidarum may present with dehydration, ketosis, and altered electrolyte levels, including low sodium and potassium. Often, an increase in hematocrit occurs, indicating contracted fluid volume. There may also be elevated levels of AST and alanine aminotransferase (ALT) and/or serum bilirubin.

If liver function tests are abnormal, acute hepatitis, either viral or drug induced, must be included in the differential diagnosis. Severe renal dysfunction and hypercalcemia can also occur in pregnancy and present with recurrent intractable vomiting. Hyperemesis gravidarum may also be associated with hyperthyroidism. The thyroid dysfunction is transient and is concurrent with the hyperemesis gravidarum. The incidence of hyperthyroidism may be as high as 60%. There seems to be a correlation between the severity of the nausea and vomiting and the elevation of thyroxine and depression of thyroid-stimulating hormone (TSH). The possible etiologies of hyperemesis gravidarum include psychologic, hyperthyroidism and hyperparathyroidism, hormonal changes, and autonomic dysfunction during pregnancy. Treatment is symptomatic, with hospitalization for intactable vomiting, dehydration, or malnutrition often necessary. Intravenous rehydration is first-line therapy. Treatment with antiemetics such as prochlorperazine, promethazine, or metoclopramide is often required.

COINCIDENT LIVER DISEASE IN PREGNANCY

Acquired liver diseases can be caused by infections, toxins, drugs, and alcohol abuse or sometimes by unknown causes. The most common cause is viral infection.

Viral Hepatitis. Acute viral hepatitis is the leading cause of jaundice during pregnancy. Usually it is a mild illness, but it can become catastrophically fulminant. In particular, hepatitis E and herpes simplex virus infections can result in maternal and/or fetal death. The approach to the management of acute viral hepatitis is to provide supportive care and to prevent further liver damage, cross-infection to health care workers, and vertical transmission to the neonate. Vertical transmission may lead to neonatal hepatitis. Clinical symptoms of acute viral hepatitis range from vague constitutional symptoms to overt jaundice. Physical examination often reveals tender hepatomegaly. The hepatic transaminases, for example, AST and alanine-leucine transaminases, are in the 1000 IU/L range during acute infection. Although viral hepatitis has not been found to influence the course of pregnancy, it is associated with preterm delivery.

Hepatitis A. Hepatitis A virus (HAV) was formerly known as infective hepatitis. It is the most common acute viral infection of the liver in the developing world, whereas hepatitis B infection is more common in developed countries. HAV is transmitted through the oral-fecal route and can also be transmitted vertically. The incubation period is 15 to 50 days, and the diagnosis is confirmed by serologic testing. Acute HAV infection is marked by the presence of immunoglobulin M class (IgM) anti-HAV antibody. IgG antibody to HAV antigen indicates a previous exposure. Unlike hepatitis B, a carrier state does not occur. The symptomatic period lasts about 6 weeks. The condition is usually self-limiting. Management is usually supportive. Immunization with a recombinant antigen vaccine reliably protects against infection when there is high risk of exposure.

Hepatitis B. Hepatitis B infection was formerly known as serum hepatitis. The hepatitis B virus (HBV) is a partially double-stranded DNA virus that replicates in part through an RNA intermediate. The viral genome is one of the smallest known at the present time. The incubation period is from 30 to 180 days. HBV is transmitted parenterally or through contact with body fluids.[18] The infection presents as a mild clinical hepatitis or as an incidental finding. Unlike hepatitis A, HBV may progress to a chronic carrier state. Infection during infancy often progresses to a chronic hepatitis, whereas acute infection in the adult tends to be self-limiting. Diagnosis is made by serologic testing, that is, by the detection of antibody to the hepatitis B core antigen (HBcAg). There are at least eight distinct serotypes.

During acute HBV infection, multiple arms of the immune system are activated and probably act in concert to effect viral clearance. Together with the development of "transaminitis" during acute HBV infection, antibodies specific for HBV proteins develop. The earliest antibody to appear is IgM directed against HBcAg. IgM is produced by virtually all infected patients, and both IgM and IgG HBc antibody may persist for years after the infection. Anti–hepatitis B early antigen (anti-HBeAg) is not universally produced but, at least in some patients, this may be associated with termination of viral replication. The development of hepatitis B surface antigen (HBsAg) marks the resolution of the acute phase of the illness. Anti-HB is neutralizing, and the presence of it is sufficient to protect from viral infection.

In 1% to 10% of patients infected with HBV, the viral infection is not cleared and is followed by chronic liver disease. The viral or host factors that permit this development have not been defined. It is well known that age at acquisition determines the likelihood of chronic infection, with neonatal infection representing the highest risk period, but whether this is due to a relative immune hyporesponsiveness in neonates or high levels of maternal viremia are unknown. Certain HLA haplotypes (B8, SC01, DR3) are associated with relative vaccine hyporesponsiveness. The common hallmark of chronic infection is the failure to produce anti-HBs with the persistence of HBsAg in the blood. In contrast to individuals who have only an acute infection and also those who respond to vaccination, those with chronic infection and non–vaccine responders have a more vigorous cellular-mediated response in the peripheral blood.

Unfortunately, there is no cure for HBV infection. The only treatment approach is to prevent infection based on immunization. Immunoglobulin (HBIG) together with vaccine is indicated in persons exposed to the disease. HBIG alone protects against disease transmission to neonates in about 70% of cases, while HBIG with vaccination affords protection in 90% to 95% of cases.

Hepatitis C. The hepatitis C virus (HCV) was first discovered in 1989 by Choo and colleagues[19] and accounts for approximately 20% of cases of acute hepatitis, 70% of chronic hepatitis, and 30% of end-stage liver disease.[20] HCV is a single-stranded, enveloped RNA virus. The incubation period is 30 to 160 days and is symptomatic and icteric in only one third of the patients. Rarely, HCV goes on to a fulminant form. The prevalence in some parts of the world is relatively high. The mean period from onset of acute hepatitis to the development of anti-HCV is 12 weeks; therefore, during an acute episode of hepatitis, the anti-HCV may be negative. In this setting, an HCV-RNA polymerase chain reaction (PCR) test can be helpful to clinch the diagnosis. In a report from Mumbai, India, 15.9% of volunteer blood donors tested seropositive for HCV.[21] Like hepatitis B, HCV transmission is by parenteral, salivary, and sexual routes. Unlike hepatitis B, the antigen is not detected by normal laboratory tests. The antibody to HCV is tested using the enzyme-linked immunosorbent assay (ELISA). The present laboratory test, ELISA-3, can have a very high incidence of false-positive results. Therefore a positive test is reconfirmed by a more specific test, that is, by a recombinant immunoblot assay (RIBA). The incidence of HCV is higher in those who have had multiple blood transfusions and hemodialysis. The risk of progression to chronic hepatitis is about 80% of those infected with the virus. Many infected patients become carriers. Chronic infection can lead to cirrhosis in 20% of the individuals, and 10% eventually develop hepatocellular carcinoma. At present, there is no vaccine available. Antisera can afford partial protection, and chronic hepatitis with HCV has been treated with interferon. Vertical transmission occurs, and risk appears to be higher in HIV-positive mothers. An important issue is that HCV may be transmitted via breast-feeding. HCV has been detected in low concentrations in breast milk samples in some studies.

Hepatitis D. The hepatitis D virus (HDV) was discovered in 1977 by Rizzetto and colleagues in Italy.[22] The delta particle was first found in liver biopsy material from hepatitis B antigen–positive individuals. HDV is an incomplete virus. It infects the patient either in concurrence with hepatitis B or as a result of superinfection. In coinfection, the serum shows both HDV markers and IgM anti-HBc antibodies. In acute infection, patients do not have anti-HBc IgM in the serum. By and large, superinfection is associated with a worse natural history than coinfection. It can lead to chronic active hepatitis. Spread is through the parenteral route. At higher risk are parenteral drug abusers and hemophiliacs who have received plasma products. HDV has a worldwide distribution, but the populations of some geographic locations appear to be particularly at risk. These areas include southern Italy, Venezuela, Colombia, and the western part of Asia. It can also be very fulminant.[23] The significance of this viral infection is still relatively undefined.

However, a combined acute HBV/HDV infection may take a more fulminant course when compared with an acute infection by HBV alone. Because HDV cannot exist on its own, immunization against HBV may prevent superinfection with HDV. The postdelivery administration of HBIG and hepatitis B vaccine to a neonate whose mother has active HBV/HDV infection should effectively prevent 95% of the vertical transmission of HDV.

Hepatitis E. The hepatitis E virus (HEV) is clinically similar to HAV in that it is transmitted via oral-fecal spread and is also a single-stranded, nonenveloped RNA virus. The clinical course of the disease resembles acute HAV infection. However, for as yet unknown reasons, the mortality in pregnant women is very high (>20%). Hepatitis E infection has been reported to be endemic in Asia, Africa, and Mexico. Often it is endemic in areas where there is an unhealthy combination of an undernourished population and low standards of hygiene.[24] Pathologic changes in the liver during acute HEV infection are somewhat variable. Some cases have a cholestatic picture, while others demonstrate a more typical hepatitic pattern. The peak of viremia and "transaminitis" is just prior to the appearance of antibody. The first antibody to be detected is IgM, which declines during the convalescent phase. None of the available animal models develop the fulminant hepatitis that is seen in pregnant women. The mechanism of fulminant liver disease remains obscure. Death rates are high in pregnant women. For this reason, it was advocated that pregnant women with HEV infection or exposure be given intravenous serum immunoglobulin (IVIG). A recent study in India found that IVIG does not confer any significant protection in exposed women because of the weak anti-HEV titer in the immunoglobulin.

The incubation period of HEV is 3 to 9 weeks, the average being 6 weeks. Very often young adults are victims. It is usually a self-limiting disease, with patients usually making a full recovery. In nonpregnant patients, the risk of fulminant hepatitis is about 0.5%, compared with a 20% risk in pregnant women in the third trimester. No treatment is prescribed for this disease other than supportive care.

Hepatitis G. The hepatitis G virus (HGV) is a hepatotropic virus that is associated with blood-transfusion, non-A to E hepatitis.[25] It often occurs with other hepatitic infection. Vertical transmission has been reported to occur.[26] Not much is known about HGV's effects on the liver except that it probably does not have much effect on its own. Its hepatic action is probably similar to that of cytomegalovirus and herpesviruses in that it manifests under certain immune deficiency conditions.

Herpes Simplex Virus Hepatitis. Although the hepatitis caused by herpes simplex virus (HSV) is most commonly found in immunosuppressed patients, some cases have been reported during pregnancy. HSV usually presents in the third trimester. Pregnant patients usually have features of a systemic illness, including fever with a diffuse vesicular skin rash. Leukopenia is also common. Coagulopathy occurs in 90% of these patients. The patient tends to be anicteric. Without therapy, the mortality rate is 43%. A high index of suspicion is important because treatment with acyclovir may be successful. Prompt delivery of the fetus may improve the outcome.

Anesthetic Considerations in Acute Viral Hepatitis. Anesthesia and surgery are particularly hazardous in patients with acute viral hepatitis. The risk of mortality is high.[27] Inhalational anesthetic agents that are hepatotoxic and interventions that lead to decreased hepatic blood flow should be used sparingly, if at all.

Drug-Induced Hepatitis. Liver manifestations of drug-induced hepatitis can be divided into two main groups: drugs that predominantly affect the hepatocyte and those that cause cholestasis. Some agents produce a combination of both. Drugs that cause liver dysfunction by affecting the liver independent of the pregnancy include antiemetic agents (e.g., chlorpromazine), methyldopa, isoniazid, acetaminophen, and ranitidine. The only treatment is to withdraw the drug and to avoid subsequent exposure. Steroids may improve symptoms. Halothane is known to have the potential to cause liver dysfunction and should be avoided in cases in which drug-induced hepatitis exists.

PREEXISTING LIVER DISEASE

Preexisting chronic liver disease requires careful monitoring of the patient (for worsening of the disease) and the fetus. Normally, the woman who has preexisting liver disease is able to carry the fetus safely to term.

Autoimmune Chronic Active Hepatitis. Autoimmune hepatitis is a heterogeneous group of diseases with presentations ranging from subclinical to severe, fulminant hepatitis. Classically, it is associated with the presence of nonspecific antibodies; anti–smooth muscle antibodies and antinuclear antibodies are positive in many of these patients. Often the condition is diagnosed because of an abnormal laboratory investigation. Flareup of chronic active liver disease has been reported during pregnancy, but it is not known whether the cause is pregnancy itself or whether it is due to chance because autoimmune hepatitis is known to have sporadic spontaneous flareups. Drugs, such as azathioprine and prednisolone, that are used to treat the autoimmune diseases can be continued during pregnancy. The incidence of stillbirths and premature labor is high in patients with autoimmune hepatitis.

Chronic Viral Hepatitis. There is little evidence that pregnancy influences the clinical outcome of either chronic active or chronic persistent viral hepatitis. Rarely, a worsening of chronic HBV and HCV has been reported. The possibility of vertical transmission of the infection should be remembered. Standard guidelines and precautions should be observed in the handling of blood and tissue fluids.

Primary Biliary Cirrhosis. This disease may be an incidental finding or it may present as lethargy, pruritus, and right-sided abdominal pain. It may be associated with Raynaud's syndrome. These patients tend to have jaundice, pruritus, and possibly, portal hypertension. The biochemical features are those of cholestasis with raised antimitochondrial antibodies. Pregnancy leads to an increase in the biochemical parameters of cholestasis in women with primary biliary cirrhosis.

Ascites and variceal hemorrhage often occur in end-stage disease. After delivery, prepregnant values return. It is postulated that the disease is a result of an immune attack on the bile ducts. Since the disease commonly occurs in older women, very few pregnant women are expected to have this condition. The life expectancy after diagnosis is about 10 years. Treatment is often to relieve the pruritus using oral cholestyramine, 4 to 16 g daily, but there is no definitive treatment except for orthoptic liver transplantation when the patient develops end-stage liver failure.

Liver Cirrhosis. Many cirrhotic women tend to be able to sustain a normal pregnancy without worsening of their condition. These women are less fertile when compared to those without cirrhosis. This is attributed to an altered metabolism of sex steroids. They tend to have a higher rate of premature infants and stillbirths. Hepatic failures have been reported. Esophageal varices may develop in these women if not already present before pregnancy. It is not known whether they tend to bleed more often than nonpregnant patients with cirrhosis. A history of variceal bleeding in one gestation is not necessarily predictive of hemorrhage in a subsequent pregnancy.

The maternal death rate in cirrhotic patients is reported to range from 10.3% to 18%.[28] The most common cause of death is gastrointestinal hemorrhage. About half of pregnant women with cirrhosis have transient esophageal varices. The progressive increase in circulating blood volume, elevation in portal pressure, and added pressure from the gravid uterus on the inferior vena cava divert blood to the azygos system, leading to gastroesophageal varices.

Bleeding varices can be treated by endoscopic banding or sclerotherapy. Vasopressin is contraindicated because of its effect on the uterus. Transjugular intrahepatic portosystemic shunting is a possible interventional tool; however, there are at present no reports of its use in pregnancy. Treatment of hepatic encephalopathy is with lactulose or oral neomycin. Anesthetic management should be directed at avoiding further liver damage, and provision should be made to prepare for massive hemorrhage from portal hypertension or coagulopathy. Preoperative assessment should include a thorough liver and renal function assessment. Intravascular volume should be optimized during anesthesia and surgery to avoid further reduction of liver and renal blood flow.

Wilson's Disease. This is a rare disorder of copper metabolism with autosomal recessive inheritance. It is also known as hepatolenticular degeneration. The incidence is 1 in 30,000 and half of these patients present in adulthood. The condition occurs because the hepatic lysosomes lack the normal mechanism to excrete copper into the bile for subsequent elimination. Very often it leads to copper toxicity and death before the age of 30 years. The accumulation of copper leads to organ toxicity of the liver, brain, and other organs. Fifty percent of the patients present with cirrhosis or chronic hepatitis; the others present with neurologic or psychiatric disturbances. Occasionally, patients present with hemolytic anemia or repeated spontaneous abortion. Confirmation of the diagnosis is made by detection of low blood ceruloplasmin levels or a liver biopsy with characteristic copper deposit patterns. Patients with Wilson's disease are treated with penicillamine, trientine, or zinc. Penicillamine and trientine chelate copper, while zinc blocks copper absorption from the intestinal tract. Therapy should be maintained during pregnancy[29] because these drugs have been shown to be quite safe. Withdrawal of penicillamine has been associated with worsening of the disease. Very often vitamin B_6 is given to counter the antipyridoxine effect of penicillamine. Zinc is also another therapy often used in pregnancy because of its lack of toxicity. It is also reported to be better tolerated than penicillamine.[30] Penicillamine has been reported to produce a myasthenia-like syndrome and can prolong the action of neuromuscular agents. Penicillamine may also cause bone marrow suppression that predisposes the patient to sepsis because of depression of the immune system.

High copper levels may affect the fetal liver. The pregnant patient should continue with the therapy, as a relapse may cause the patient to develop fulminant hepatitis and/or hemolysis.

Regional anesthesia is preferred unless it is contraindicated as a result of the presence of coagulopathy, or neurologic or psychiatric disorders. When general anesthesia is chosen, care must be made to avoid drugs with hepatotoxic properties.

Budd-Chiari Syndrome. The Budd-Chiari syndrome is characterized by large hepatic vein occlusion that can lead to hepatocellular damage. The prevalence is about 2.4 per million, and the etiology is unknown. It is associated with polycythemia rubra vera and coagulopathy. The main clinical features are hepatomegaly, leg edema, ascites, and venous dilatation over the trunk. Deaths occur as a result of liver failure, variceal bleeding, and hepatocellular carcinoma.[31] Pregnancies have been reported in this condition, but the obstetric outcome is poor.[32] It has been postulated that certain hypercoagulable conditions, such as resistance to activated protein C, together with pregnancy can precipitate this condition. Some cases of Budd-Chiari syndrome have been reported to occur 1 to 3 weeks postpartum. A careful search for hemolytic anemia, lupus anticoagulant, and other hypercoagulable states should be made in addition to performing a coagulation screen.

ANESTHETIC IMPLICATIONS OF LIVER DISEASE IN PREGNANCY

General Considerations. The patient with liver disease presents to the anesthesiologist for the management of labor pain, operative delivery, and intensive care unit therapy. When a patient presents with jaundice, the anesthesiologist should enlist the help of a hepatologist to make an accurate diagnosis.

Anesthetic assessment should be directed toward optimizing treatment of the liver condition and monitoring the maternal and fetal condition. Some conditions require more aggressive management than others. Acute fatty liver of pregnancy and HELLP syndrome are examples of conditions that need a more aggressive approach to achieve a good outcome.

Liver function should be evaluated prior to anesthesia and surgery. Liver function tests and coagulation screen are essential and should include prothrombin time, activated partial thromboplastin time, platelet count, and the international normalized ratio (INR). A platelet count of more than 100,000/μL is considered safe for performing an epidural block, although many anesthesiologists routinely perform neuraxial blockade in patients with platelet counts greater than 75,000, and occasionally when it is less than 75,000/μL.

Liver blood flow should be preserved as far as possible and hepatotoxic drugs should be avoided. Surgery can lead to a decrease in liver blood flow. The stress of surgery gives rise to increased catecholamine levels and hepatic vasoconstriction. While general anesthesia has been implicated in causing hepatic dysfunction and decreases in hepatic blood flow, a coagulation defect may necessitate the use of general anesthesia for operative delivery. A regional analgesia/anesthesia technique is not contraindicated if a coagulation defect is absent. In fact, elective forceps delivery and epidural anesthesia have been successfully used in a patient with portal hypertension and esophageal varices.[33] Regional anesthesia in the absence of hypotension improves liver perfusion.

The effect of sodium thiopental on liver blood flow is not well established, as some studies demonstrate no effect while others have shown a decrease.[34] In contrast, propofol has been shown to have no effect on liver blood flow. Halothane, enflurane, and methoxyflurane can cause hepatic dysfunction. Isoflurane and desflurane have no deleterious effect on hepatic blood flow and there is minimal rise in serum transferase concentration. However, using more sensitive analysis (glutathione transferase alpha) investigators have reported that isoflurane and desflurane may cause mild derangement in hepatocellular integrity[35] and that sevoflurane may also produce some degree of hepatocellular disturbance.[36]

Intensity of anesthetic management depends on the severity of the disease. Patients with mild liver disease can be managed the same way as normal pregnant patients. In more severe forms of liver disease it is necessary to ensure that the patient is not developing hepatic encephalopathy or coagulopathy. In the patient with chronic liver disease, the metabolism and protein binding of drugs become issues. Cardiovascular changes (e.g., reduction of systemic vascular resistance) can be caused by the presence of an arteriovenous shunt and increased cardiac output. Tense ascites may impair venous return and aggravate supine hypotension. Central venous monitoring should be considered for cesarean section when cardiomyopathy and ascites are present.[37] Presence of portal hypertension should be assessed. Impaired liver function leads to decreased production of clotting factors I, II, V, VII, and X. Vitamin K corrects coagulopathy if malabsorption is the cause of decreased liver synthesis; it does not correct coagulopathy if parenchymal disease is the cause. Hypoxemia can be present and may be caused by portal-pulmonary venous shunting and pulmonary atelectasis caused by the splinting of the diaphragm secondary to the gravid uterus and tense ascites.

Metabolic changes that may occur in the parturient with hepatic disease include hypoglycemia, hyponatremia, hypokalemia, and acid-base disturbances. Hypoglycemia should be corrected prior to administration of general anesthesia. Hepatic encephalopathy may occur and is produced by the unmetabolized ammonium products, increased γ-aminobutyric acid levels and, possibly, increased influx of false transmitters into the brain. These patients may be at risk for aspiration if their level of consciousness is impaired. Prophylactic administration of a histamine H_2 receptor antagonist is warranted to reduce gastric complications.

In acute fatty liver of pregnancy, cesarean delivery treats the condition as well as provides a better perina-

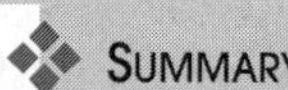

Summary

Key Points

- The new onset of hepatic disease is serious but uncommon in pregnancy.
- Intrahepatic cholestasis of pregnancy is a benign disease in the mother but may be associated with fetal difficulties.
- Acute fatty liver of pregnancy may be life-threatening and may actually represent a severe subset of preeclampsia.
- Pregnancy does not change the long-term survival following hepatic transplantation.
- Patients with hepatic disease may be coagulopathic, and therefore a coagulation profile should be obtained prior to initiation of a regional anesthetic.

Key Reference

Reily CA: Hepatic disease in pregnancy. Am J Med 1994; 96 (Suppl):18S–22S.

Case Stem

A 28-year-old primigravida presents at 36 weeks' gestation with severe right-sided abdominal pain. She states that she has had anorexia and malaise for 1 week. Physical examination reveals jaundice and mild peripheral edema. Laboratory findings include elevated serum transaminase and alkaline phosphatase levels. Discuss the obstetric and anesthetic implications.

tal outcome. Correction of hydration and coagulation is necessary prior to the administration of anesthesia. Vitamin K and fresh-frozen plasma should be used to correct coagulopathies. Intra-arterial blood pressure monitoring is helpful. Regional anesthesia is not absolutely contraindicated if the coagulation defects are corrected. Epidural or continuous spinal anesthesia is preferred, as the accompanying hemodynamic changes are not as abrupt as that produced by single-shot spinal anesthesia. Regional anesthesia has the added benefit of preserving hepatic blood flow. Good intravenous access with a large-gauge venous cannula (to treat possible excessive bleeding) is desirable. Grouping and matching of blood should be arranged prior to operative delivery. If general anesthesia is chosen, an intravenous induction should be conducted using propofol, as it does not cause a decrease in liver blood flow and its pharmacokinetics are not affected in cirrhosis.[38]

Postoperative pain management is an important issue because it is necessary to prevent a decrease in liver blood flow that can occur from the high catecholamine levels associated with uncontrolled pain. Pain relief can be provided using a patient-controlled analgesia device or epidural narcotics. Morphine excretion may be impaired in severe liver dysfunction. Intramuscular injections should be avoided if the patient has impaired coagulation. When neuraxial anesthesia is performed for surgery, the addition of epidural or intrathecal morphine can provide excellent postoperative pain relief.

CONCLUSION

Severe liver disease in pregnancy is uncommon. Reports describing the anesthetic management of these patients have demonstrated that good outcome is possible.[39] Attention should be paid to proper assessment, optimizing medical therapy, and avoiding factors that may further harm the liver.[40]

References

1. Strunin L, Eagle CJ: Hepatic disease. *In* Benumof JL (ed): Anesthesia and Uncommon Diseases, 4th ed. Philadelphia: WB Saunders; 1997: 147–173.
2. Gabraith RM: Liver and pancreas. *In* Gleicher N (ed): Principles and Practice of Medical Therapy in Pregnancy, 2nd ed. Stamford, CT: Appleton & Lange; 1995: 957–959.
3. Rustgi VK: Liver disease in pregnancy. Med Clin North Am 1989; 73:1041–1046.
4. Haemmmerli UR: Acta Med Scand Suppl 1966; 197:444.
5. Steven MM: Pregnancy and liver disease. Gut 1981; 592–614.
6. Knopp RH, Bergelin RO, Wahl PW, et al: Clinical chemistry alterations in pregnancy and oral contraceptive use. Obstet Gynecol 1985; 66:682–690.
7. Sherlock S: The liver in pregnancy. *In* Philipp E, Barnes J, Newton M (eds): Scientific Foundations of Obstetrics and Gynaecology. Stoneham, MA: William Heinemann Medical Books; 1986: 499–504.
8. Stander HJ, Cadden JF: Acute yellow atrophy of the liver in pregnancy. Am J Obstet Gynecol 1934; 28:61.
9. Sheehan HL: The pathology of acute yellow atrophy and delayed chloroform poisoning. J Obstet Gynaecol Br Empire 1940; 47:49.
10. Fagan E: Disorders of the liver, biliary system and pancreas. *In* de Swiet M (ed): Medical Disorders in Obstetric Practice, 3rd ed. Cambridge, MA: Blackwell Sci; 1992: 321–356.
11. Varmer M, Ronderknecht NK: Acute fatty metamorphosis of pregnancy: a maternal mortality and literature review. J Reprod Med 1980; 24:177.
12. Visconti M, Manes G, Giannattasio F, Uomo G: Recurrence of acute fatty liver of pregnancy. J Clin Gastroenterol 1995; 21:243–245.
13. Latham P: Liver diseases. *In* Gleicher N (ed): Principles and Practice of Medical Therapy in Pregnancy. Stamford, CT: Appleton & Lange; 1991: 960–968.
14. Pockros PJ, Peters RL, Reynolds TB: Idiopathic fatty liver of pregnancy: findings in ten cases. Medicine 1984; 63:1–11.
15. Bova JG, Schenker S: Acute fatty liver of pregnancy. N Engl J Med 1985; 313:1608.
16. Meng LJ, Reyes H, Palma J, et al: Effects of ursodeoxycholic acid on conjugated bile acids and progesterone metabolites in serum and urine of patients with intrahepatic cholestasis of pregnancy. J Hepatol 1997; 27:1029–1040.
17. Palma J, Reyes H, Ribalta J, et al: Ursodeoxycholic acid in the treatment of cholestasis of pregnancy: a randomized, double-blind study controlled with placebo. J Hepatol 1997; 27:1022–1028.
18. Towers CV: Hepatitis in pregnancy. *In* Mishell DR (ed): The 1997 Yearbook of Obstetrics and Gynecology. St. Louis: Mosby–Year Book; 1997: xvii–xxiv.
19. Choo QL, Kuo G, Weiner AJ, et al: Isolation of a cDNA clone derived from a blood borne non-A, non-B hepatitis. Science 1989; 244:362–364.
20. Hoofnagle JH: Hepatitis C: the clinical spectrum of disease. Hepatology 1997; 26(suppl):15S–20S.
21. Gosavi MS, Shah SK, Shah SR, et al: Prevalence of hepatitis C virus (HCV) infection in Mumbai. Indian J Med Sci 1997; 51:378–385.
22. Rizzetto M, Canese MG, Arico S, et al: Immunofluorescence detection of a new antigen/antibody system (delta/antidelta) associated with hepatitis B virus in liver and serum of HbsAg carriers. Gut 1997; 18:997–1003.
23. Buitrago B, Popper H, Hadler SC, et al: Specific histologic features of Santa Marta hepatitis: a severe form of hepatitis delta-virus infection in northern South America. Hepatology 1986; 6:1285–1291.
24. De Cock KM, Bradley DW, Sanford WD, et al: Epidemic non-A, non-B hepatitis in patients from Pakistan. Ann Intern Med 1987; 106:277.
25. Magriples U: Hepatitis in pregnancy. Semin Perinatol 1998; 22:112–117.
26. Inaba N, Okajima Y, Kang XS, et al: Maternal-infant transmission of hepatitis G virus. Am J Obstet Gynecol 1997; 177:1537–1538.
27. Powell-Jackson P, Greenway B, Williams R: Adverse effects of exploratory laparotomy in patients with unsuspected liver disease. Br J Surg 1982; 69:449.
28. Pajor A, Lehoczky D: Pregnancy in liver cirrhosis: assessment of maternal and fetal risks in eleven patients and review of the management. Gynecol Obstet Invest 1994; 38:45–50.
29. Anderson LA, Hakojarvi SL, Boudreaux SK: Zinc acetate treatment in Wilson's disease. Ann Pharmacother 1998; 32:78–87.
30. Brewer GJ: Practical recommendations and new therapies for Wilson's disease. Drugs 1995; 50:240–249.
31. Czlonkowska A, Gajda J, Rodo M: Effects of long-term treatment in Wilson's disease with D-penicillamine and zinc sulphate. J Neurol 1996; 243:269–273.
32. Reid R: Liver disease. *In* Chestnut D (ed): Obstetric Anaesthesia: Principles and Practice. St. Louis: Mosby–Year Book; 1994:883–889.
33. Heriot JA, Steven M, Sattin RS: Elective forceps delivery and extradural anaesthesia in a primigravida with portal hypertension and oesophageal varices. Br J Anaesth 1996; 76:325–327.
34. Okuda H, Yamagata H, Obata H, et al: Epidemiological and clinical features of Budd-Chiari syndrome in Japan. J Hepatol 1995; 22:1–9.
35. Fickert P, Ramshack H, Kenner L, et al: Acute Budd-Chiari

syndrome with fulminant hepatic failure in a pregnant woman with Factor V Leiden mutation. Gastroenterology 1996; 111:1670–1673.
36. Gelman S: General anaesthesia and hepatic circulation. Can J Physiol Pharmacol 1987; 65:1762.
37. Servin F, Cockshott ID, Farinotti R, et al: Pharmacokinetics of propofol infusion with cirrhosis. Br J Anaesth 1990; 65:177–183.
38. Taivainen T, Tiainen P, Meretoja OA, et al: Comparison of sevoflurane and halothane on the quality of anaesthesia, serum glutathione transferase alpha and fluoride in paediatric patients. Br J Anaesth 1994; 73:590–595.
39. Antognini JF, Andrews S: Anaesthesia for Caesarean section in a patient with acute fatty liver of pregnancy. Can J Anaesth 1991; 38:7904–7907.
40. Corke PJ: Anaesthesia for Caesarean section in a patient with acute fatty liver of pregnancy. Anaesth Intensive Care 1995; 23:215–218.

45

Musculoskeletal Disorders

❖ DAVID C. CAMPBELL, MD, MSc, FRCPC

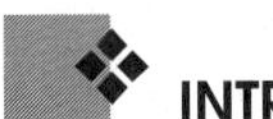

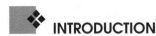

INTRODUCTION

Parturients commonly report musculoskeletal complaints that are usually benign and resolve within the postpartum period. For some, however, particularly those with preexisting musculoskeletal disease, the symptoms may be debilitating and present a significant anesthetic challenge. The purpose of this chapter is to review musculoskeletal disorders and discuss the anesthetic management of the affected parturient.

LOW BACK PAIN

Antenatal Low Back Pain

Low back pain (LBP) is common in the general population, with an incidence of 60% to 80%.[1–4] Antenatal LBP is a frequent complaint during pregnancy, reported by more than 80% of parturients.[5–11] Predisposing factors include prepregnancy LBP, LBP in a previous pregnancy, young age, increased body mass index, lower socioeconomic class, and possibly macrosomia.[6–10] The etiology of LBP of pregnancy results from both mechanical and hormonal factors. Mechanical factors involve (1) direct pressure of the gravid uterus on lumbosacral nerve roots; (2) inefficient and insufficient support from abdominal muscles; and (3) enlarging gravid uterus necessitating a progressive lumbar lordosis with a change in the center of gravity.[1] The primary hormonal factor involves relaxin, which is released from the corpus luteum. The 10-fold increase in relaxin levels during pregnancy contributes to the laxity, mobility, and ultimate instability of the sacrococcygeal, sacroiliac, and pubic joints.[12] Between 10% and 21% of pregnant women experience severe, incapacitating LBP that is often associated with radiating leg pain[7, 10, 13, 14] and has been reported to be responsible for up to 7.5 weeks of sick leave in the antenatal period.[7] Of note, acute herniated lumbar intervertebral disk disease is uncommon, with a reported incidence of only 1 in 10,000 parturients.[15, 16] Acute lumbar intervertebral disk herniation can be differentiated from benign LBP of pregnancy by the presentation of neurologic symptoms other than radiating leg pain.

Anesthetic Management

There is no evidence that the mode of delivery (vaginal versus cesarean) will affect the natural progression of antenatal LBP. An instrumented (vacuum or low outlet forcep) vaginal delivery may decrease maternal stress and reduce the aggravation of LBP during the second stage of labor.[17] Delaying maternal expulsive efforts until the fetal head presents on the perineum may also reduce maternal stress and aggravation of LBP.

There is no evidence that regional analgesia or anesthesia is contraindicated in pregnant women with LBP, sciatica, or acute lumbar intervertebral disk herniation. The use of lumbar-epidural analgesia (LEA) may potentially result in several beneficial effects during labor and delivery, which may also avoid the aggravation of LBP. First, the provision of effective analgesia results in a restoration of maternal composure and control. This may avoid any uncontrollable abrupt positioning changes commonly observed with parturients attempting to cope with the intense pain of labor that may aggravate LBP. Second, the use of dilute local anesthetic solutions of bupivacaine or ropivacaine combined with an opioid (e.g., fentanyl 1–2 μg/mL) produce minimal motor block, thereby permitting the early detection of the onset of new or intensifying neurologic deficits. The use of ropivacaine (0.8%) combined with fentanyl (2 μg/mL) commonly permits ambulation, and initial experience suggests that it might be optimal in these circumstances.[18] A dilute solution of bupivacaine plus opioid can serve the same purpose. Third, the intense somatic (pressure) sensations associated with the transition and second stage of labor can be obviated with the use of an epidural bolus dose of fentanyl (1 μg/kg) or higher concentrations of local anesthetic (e.g., 2% lidocaine), or both.

This permits the expectant mother to remain comfortable and composed until the fetal head presents on the perineum. Fourth, the use of high-concentration local anesthetics (e.g., 2% lidocaine) facilitates the surgical anesthesia necessary for the placement of low-outlet forceps.

Although delayed onset and ineffective epidural anesthesia have occasionally been observed in parturients presenting with antenatal LBP, sciatica, and herniated lumbar intervertebral disk disease,[19] this is not common and does not imply that LEA should be avoided in these parturients. Herniated intervertebral disks that occur in the lumbar region may produce scarring or adhesions within the epidural space. This may result in a lack of sufficient cephalad spread above the lesion or produce unilateral spread of epidural analgesic solutions resulting in ineffective analgesia.[20] Should regional analgesia be desired, intrathecal analgesia provides effective analgesia and avoids the complications of inadequate spread due to scarring or adhesions within the epidural space. The combination of intrathecal sufentanil (5–10 μg) and bupivacaine (2.5 mg) with or without epinephrine (200 μg) provides rapid, profound ambulatory analgesia during the first and second stages of labor for 2 to 4 hours.[21–23] This intrathecal analgesic solution can be administered either through a spinal needle, as a single shot, or as part of the combined spinal-epidural technique. Should an inadvertent dural puncture occur, the epidural catheter might be placed in the intrathecal space and utilized to facilitate analgesia. As with an epidural catheter, an intrathecal catheter can facilitate the conversion from analgesia to anesthesia, should surgical intervention become necessary.

Alternatively, intravenous narcotics may be utilized when LEA is not available, contraindicated, technically impossible, or ineffective. Intravenous fentanyl produces analgesia with fewer maternal and neonatal adverse effects than meperidine.[24–25] Intravenous fentanyl is administered at our institution as an initial loading dose of 2 to 3 μg/kg, and analgesia is maintained using a patient-controlled intravenous analgesia (50 μg with a lock-out period of 5–10 minutes) with frequent adjustments in dosage, particularly during the transition period.

In conclusion, regional analgesia or anesthesia is not contraindicated in parturients presenting with antenatal LBP. All pregnant women with moderate to severe LBP should ideally be assessed by an anesthesiologist during the antenatal period. During this assessment, evidence can be sought for any neurologic compromise. Such deficiencies should be documented and consultation sought with either a neurologist or a neurosurgeon. Following identification of any neurologic deficit and with appropriate consultation, regional analgesia should be offered after a thorough risk-and-benefit discussion with the parturient. Ideally, all pregnant women, particularly those with LBP, should also be counseled in the antenatal period with regard to the various labor analgesic options and concurrently informed of anesthetic options (regional and general) for surgical delivery. Prenatal education affords the parturient an opportunity to make informed choices regarding labor analgesia as well as to become aware of potential concerns and limitations of various options.

Postpartum Low Back Pain

Postpartum LBP is a common complaint in the immediate postpartum period, reported by as many as 87% of parturients.[7, 11, 26, 27] The location of the postpartum LBP is consistently in the lumbosacral areas. In women with no history of antenatal LBP, the incidence significantly decreases within the first week of delivery to 30% to 40%,[11, 26] and by 6 weeks the incidence further reduces to 20%.[26] A recent prospective survey 12 months following delivery reported an incidence of LBP of 12% in women with no history of antenatal LBP.[28] Two surveys, one from the United States[27] and the other from Sweden,[7] suggest that the prevalence of all women with LBP remains approximately 50% at 12 to 18 months postpartum. This is not surprising considering the incidence of antenatal LBP of 50%, particularly when combined with the physical exertion and musculoskeletal trauma associated with delivery, which is unlikely to improve antenatal LBP.

The risk factors identified for persistent postpartum LBP include a history of antenatal LBP, young maternal age, primiparity, obesity, short stature, and physically strenuous work.[7, 8, 27, 29] The suggested association between epidural labor analgesia and LBP from several retrospective reports[29–32] has been the cause of great debate. Several recent prospective studies dispute this association and clearly demonstrate that the incidence of LBP is not related to epidural labor analgesia.[26–28, 33] However, difficult epidural needle placement necessitating multiple attempts to identify the epidural space may cause direct trauma to the periosteum. This will result in point tenderness over the epidural insertion site, which may persist for several weeks postpartum.

Anesthetic Management

With the high incidence of postpartum LBP (50–80%) and the concurrent increasing availability of epidural labor analgesia, it is understandable that anesthesiologists will be consulted more frequently to assess this complaint. It is extremely important to take the time to assess those patients for whom a formal consultation has been forwarded. During the assessment, a thorough chart review and history should be taken to identify any potential precipitating factors of LBP, including a history of antepartum LBP, difficult epidural placement, and prolonged second-stage labor. Physical examination should concentrate on identifying any evidence of herniated lumbar intervertebral disk disease, sciatica, or neurologic sequelae. In the majority of patients, no identifiable etiology will be ascertained and therefore it is extremely important to inform patients of the prevalence of this complaint. Expectant mothers must be informed of the importance of appropriate back care and that further assessment and consultation with practitioners of physiotherapy or other appropriate therapy may be invaluable. Finally, reassurance must be offered that the postpartum LBP is unlikely related to the epidural labor analgesia technique and will likely resolve with time.

SCOLIOSIS

One of the most common nontraumatic musculoskeletal disorders of childhood and adolescence is structural scoliosis. Consequently, as they mature to the childbearing age, many women with scoliosis eventually present as parturients. Structural scoliosis represents a complex alteration in the anteroposterior spinal alignment associated with lateral curvature, rotation of the vertebrae, and deformity of the rib cage.[34] With the prevention of poliomyelitis and the introduction of school screening programs, the majority of affected children are identified early with curvatures less than 20 degrees.[35, 36] Of the children screened, it appears that less than 1% will eventually require active treatment. Owing to this early detection and intervention, the presentation of parturients with uncorrected moderate to severe scoliotic curves is uncommon. Therefore, most parturients with scoliosis would be expected to have obstetric outcomes similar to those of the general population. However, the implications for the pregnant woman with uncorrected moderate to severe scoliosis are reviewed in this chapter so that the reader can better optimize anesthetic care during labor and delivery.

The most common form of scoliosis is adolescent idiopathic scoliosis; however, several other conditions are associated with scoliosis as outlined in Table 45–1.[37] Adolescent idiopathic scoliosis (AIS) is defined as a lateral curvature of the spine that begins at or near the onset of puberty for which no cause has been identified.[38] A minimum curvature of 10 degrees as measured by the Cobb method is required to make the diagnosis of AIS.[39] The majority of AIS cases present as a thoracic curvature, of which 96% are right-sided convexity with involvement of an average of six vertebrae from T5-T6 to T11-T12. The curvatures of AIS may also present as a lumbar (76% left convexity from T11-T12 to L3-L4); thoracolumbar (80% right convexity from T6-T7 to L1-L2); or double (90% right thoracic and left lumbar convexity from T5-T6 to L4).[40] In the area of the apex of the curvature, the spinous processes and vertebrae rotate away from the convexity and the disks and vertebral bodies become wedge-shaped. In patients with curvatures greater than 40 degrees, distortion of the vertebral bodies on the concave side produces a narrower vertebral canal as well as shorter, thinner pedicles and laminae.[41]

Table 45–1 CLASSIFICATION OF CONDITIONS ASSOCIATED WITH SCOLIOSIS

Congenital
Congenital rib fusions
Spinal vertebrae deformity (e.g., hemivertebrae)
Abnormal spinal cord development (e.g., spina bifida)
Neuromuscular
Neurologic disorders
Lower motor neuron (e.g., polio)
Upper motor neuron (e.g., cerebral palsy)
Myopathic disorders
Progressive (e.g., muscular dystrophy; myotonic dystrophy)
Static (e.g., amyotonia)
Friedreich's ataxia
Connective tissue disorders
Marfan's syndrome
Rheumatoid arthritis
Neurofibromatosis
Osteochondrodystrophies
Osteogenesis imperfecta
Infection
Tuberculosis
Post-traumatic
Vertebral (e.g., fracture, surgical)
Extravertebral (e.g., burns)

Surveys of AIS undertaken in North America, Brazil, Great Britain, Norway, Sweden, Italy, Greece, South Africa, China, and Japan consistently report a prevalence of 2% to 3% with Cobb angles greater than 10 degrees.[40, 42–45] However, the prevalence significantly decreases as the Cobb angle increases to greater than 20 degrees. The overall female-to-male prevalence is 3.6:1, although with small curvatures (<20 degrees) the prevalence is approximately equal.[40, 46] The incidence of severe scoliosis, which is much more common in females, is uncommon in parturients and ranges from 1:1500 to 1:12,000.[47, 48]

Pathologically, severe uncorrected scoliosis involving thoracic curvatures adversely affects the cardiopulmonary system. Due to a common embryologic development, the incidence of mitral valve prolapse is approximately 25% in AIS.[49] Thoracic curvatures can interfere with the development of the lungs, ultimately affecting pulmonary function, commonly with a restrictive pattern.[50] Restriction of chest wall movement and resistance to airflow increase the work of breathing. Therefore, it is not uncommon for patients with curvatures greater than 100 degrees to present with dyspnea following mild exertion even in the nonpregnant state.[51] An inverse relationship has been demonstrated between vital capacity, forced expiratory volume in one second (FEV_1) and increasing severity of the curvature. However, significant (<80% predicted) reductions in vital capacity, functional residual capacity, and FEV_1 generally do not occur until the uncorrected curvature is severe (>120 degrees).[52] Such alterations lead to alveolar hypoventilation, producing an increased alveolar-to-arterial oxygen gradient with reduced arterial oxygen tension (PaO_2) and normal arterial carbon dioxide tension ($PaCO_2$). Deformity of the thoracic cage may also impair the development of the pulmonary vasculature. These abnormalities of pulmonary development and alveolar hypoventilation are sufficient to produce pulmonary hypertension and ultimately right ventricular hypertrophy.[37] Sleep apnea, night-time hypoxemia, and daytime hypercapnia are common in those with severe (>100 degrees) scoliosis.[53] In the most severe cases, the natural progression may include early death from cardiopulmonary failure.[54, 55]

The physiologic changes of pregnancy may significantly worsen the condition of women with severe uncorrected thoracic scoliosis or kyphoscoliosis. Scoliotic curve progression during pregnancy remains the same as in the nonpregnant state. Stable curvatures that are less than 25 degrees reportedly do not progress throughout pregnancy.[56–58] Pregnancy appears to increase back pain in women with uncorrected scoliosis but not in those with surgical correction.[56] Of particular importance, mortality and morbidity, although attributed to the severity of the curvature, are more likely related to the women's preexisting cardiopulmonary status.[59–61] Several of the physiologic changes of normal pregnancy may have a significant impact on the cardiopulmonary system of women with severe thoracic scoliosis. The normal increase in minute ventilation becomes dependent on an increased respiratory rate rather than on the usual increase in tidal volume due to the noncompliant chest wall. This significantly increases the work of breathing, particularly in the third trimester as the gravid uterus further encroaches on the nondistensible chest wall. The reduction in functional residual capacity to 20% of prepregnancy levels reduces available oxygen storage. During labor, minute ventilation may increase 150% and to a further 300% in the second stage and oxygen consumption increases by 30% to 40% and up to 70% in second stage in unmedicated women. This situation may be unattainable for the severely scoliotic parturient and may lead to respiratory failure.[59] Should pulmonary function testing reveal prepregnant lung volumes of greater than 50%, the pregnancy will likely progress normally.[57, 59] Women with severe thoracic scoliosis are likely to have pulmonary hypertension and right ventricular hypertrophy, and the normal increase in blood volume (30–40%) and cardiac output (40–50%) by the third trimester may precipitate right ventricular failure. In parturients with pulmonary hypertension, significant decompensation typically occurs either at the time of delivery or in the early postpartum period.

Obstetric Management of Uncorrected Scoliosis

The majority of parturients with scoliosis tolerate pregnancy, labor, and delivery well and should be expected to have obstetric outcomes similar to those of the general population.[57, 59] Maternal morbidity and mortality appear to be related to severe curvatures in which significant preexisting cardiopulmonary insufficiency has developed. Preterm labor is reportedly more common with severe curvatures, likely reflecting embarrassment of the cardiopulmonary system.[59, 62] In the majority of parturients with scoliosis, there is little to no involvement of the pelvis and therefore normal vaginal delivery should be anticipated. Cesarean delivery may be indicated in the presence of a mechanical deformity of the pelvis, particularly if fetal malpresentation occurs. Of importance, cesarean delivery may also be necessary in uncorrected severe scoliosis resulting in maternal compromise and cephalopelvic disproportion.[60, 61, 63] Although uncommon, anesthesiologists must be aware of the potential for surgical difficulty during the cesarean delivery. The orientation of the uterus in the small abdominal cavity may make the lower uterine segment inaccessible and necessitate a classic cesarean delivery.[61, 63]

Anesthetic Management of Uncorrected Scoliosis

The majority of parturients with scoliosis have no cardiopulmonary impairment. Therefore, the anesthetic management remains similar to that used for the healthy parturient population. Rotary deviation of the vertebrae is relatively uncommon with curvatures less than 20 degrees. However, even mild curvatures with slight torsion of the lower lumbar spinous processes may slightly increase the risk of inadvertent dural puncture.

For the woman with significant uncorrected scoliosis, specific anesthetic evaluation should occur early in the pregnancy and ideally reassessments should take place every few months until the third trimester. For optimal management, a multidisciplinary approach involving anesthesiology, obstetrics, pulmonology, cardiology, intensive care, and nursing departments should be initiated from the onset. During the third trimester, women should optimally be assessed at least every 2 weeks, or more frequently if necessary. Specific attention should be paid to eliciting evidence of dyspnea and changes in exercise tolerance. Cardiology consultation should be sought to assess cardiac status, with particular emphasis on the detection of pulmonary hypertension, right ventricular malfunction, and evidence of congenital cardiac disease, particularly mitral valve prolapse, which may require antibiotic prophylaxis. Pulmonary consultation should be undertaken early in the pregnancy with particular emphasis directed to pulmonary function testing to determine lung volumes and evidence of adequacy of gas exchange with arterial blood gas tests.

Should vaginal delivery be planned, an indwelling arterial catheter will provide the means to facilitate blood work as well provide beat-to-beat blood pressure assessments. Because of the concerns of respiratory compromise during labor, pulmonary status should be monitored by continuous pulse oximetry as well as intermittent arterial blood gas evaluations. Supplemental oxygen should be delivered by face mask. As previously outlined, the pain of labor significantly increases minute ventilation, maternal oxygen consumption, and cardiac output, all of which may be poorly tolerated in a parturient with preexisting cardiopulmonary insufficiency. Consequently, it is a good practice to initiate neuraxial analgesia as soon as labor is established or when the obstetric plan is made to commit the woman to delivery. Effective epidural or spinal labor analgesia will significantly reduce minute ventilation, maternal oxygen consumption, and cardiac output associated with the pain of labor. This is of particular importance in parturients with little cardiopulmonary reserve, for example those who exhibit antepartum dyspnea at rest.

In parturients with lumbar scoliosis, significant distortion of the lumbar skeletal anatomy and usual landmarks may make location of the epidural space a significant challenge. Of importance, in relation to the spinous process that deviates toward the concavity of the curvature, the middle of the epidural space is deviated toward the convexity of the curvature. Consequently, the epidural needle should be directed toward the convexity of the curvature, particularly if attempting to identify the epidural space at the L3-L4 or L4-L5 interspaces. Previous radiographic evidence may provide useful information regarding the extent of the distortion of the lumbar skeletal anatomy. A lower placement at L5-S1 may prove less difficult, as distortion of the anatomy is usually less dramatic at this level. The risk of an inadvertent dural puncture due to the significantly distorted anatomy in this small subset of patients is certainly a real possibility. In light of the technical difficulties, the occurrence of inadvertent dural puncture even in experienced hands is high. If inadvertent dural puncture occurs, 3 cm of the 20-gauge, or 21-gauge, multiple orifice epidural catheter may be placed into the subarachnoid space.[64] Intrathecal labor analgesia may then be provided initially with 5 to 10 μg of sufentanil and 2.5 mg of bupivacaine.[21–23] This should provide analgesia in both stage I and stage II of labor and last for approximately 3 hours. Should additional labor analgesia be requested, then a reduction in doses of both sufentanil and bupivacaine is warranted. Further analgesia can then be administered by intermittent intrathecal injections of 5 to 10 μg of sufentanil and 1.25 mg bupivacaine.[65] Surgical anesthesia using small (0.5 mL) injections of hyperbaric 0.75% bupivacaine may also be administered through the intrathecal catheter should an instrumented or surgical delivery become necessary. Of note, intrathecal microcatheters (27- or 29-gauge) are no longer available in the United States or Canada and therefore the only available intrathecal catheter acceptable for continuous intrathecal analgesia and anesthesia in North America is the standard 20-gauge or 21-gauge epidural catheter.

For a planned cesarean delivery, consultation and cooperation with the obstetrician are imperative. Many of these parturients are unable to lie supine and will likely require the semisitting position during surgery. This potential problem should be discussed with the obstetrician preoperatively. Depending on the woman's respiratory status, prior to the initiation of anesthesia an arterial line should be placed to facilitate blood work as well as to allow a continuous assessment of the blood pressure. The placement of central venous monitoring should be determined based on the woman's cardiac status. In cases of significant cardiac compromise, a pulmonary artery catheter offers many advantages. Continuous pulse oximetry will permit continuous assessment of maternal oxygenation. The anesthetic plan should be focused on attempting to avoid manipulation of the woman's airway as well as avoiding a worsening of the cardiopulmonary status due to the effects of positive pressure ventilation. However, awareness that the parturient may not tolerate even a slight reduction in ventilatory function must be acknowledged and equipment must be readily available to induce general anesthesia, if necessary. Lumbar epidural anesthesia facilitates the slow titration of regional anesthesia, and its use has been reported in a parturient with severe uncorrected idiopathic kyphoscoliosis and a vital capacity of less than 800 mL.[66] Should an inadvertent dural puncture occur, then the epidural catheter can be placed intrathecally. Intrathecal anesthesia can then be slowly titrated via the catheter. Once a level of T10 is achieved in the sitting position, attempts can be made to place the woman in a more recumbent position. The anesthetic level can then be slowly titrated to achieve a T4-T6 block. The importance of uterine displacement can not be overemphasized. Constant vigilance of the parturient's pulmonary status and vitals signs is imperative. Constant reassurance as the level of the block is raised is also of paramount importance. The significant acute alterations in volume status immediately postpartum, as well as those that occur with the regression of the regional block, require aggressive monitoring and treatment. This is of particular importance if the parturient has underlying pulmonary hypertension and a noncompliant right ventricle.

Pregnant women with significant antenatal cardiopulmonary embarrassment as a result of scoliosis should be monitored in an intensive care setting for at least 24 to 48 hours following delivery. The control of postoperative pain without producing hypoxemia due to a reduction in respiratory drive will reduce oxygen consumption. Postoperative analgesia for 24 hours can be provided with preservative-free morphine. Breakthrough pain is effectively managed with 30 mg of intravenous ketorolac rather than systemic opioids. Ketorolac provides effective postoperative analgesia, particularly in settings in which systemic narcotization should be avoided. Oral or rectal nonsteroidal anti-inflammatory medications are important adjuvants to the intrathecal/epidural opioids to optimally control post–cesarean delivery pain in these women.

Scoliosis Corrective Surgery

The treatment options for AIS were historically based primarily on the degree of curvature. The ultimate goal of surgical instrumentation is to improve cardiopulmonary status and prevent progression of the deformity. Curvatures less than 20 degrees are considered benign and do not require treatment.[67] A large Canadian prospective series observed curve progression in 78.8% of patients with initial curvatures between 20 to 39 degrees.[68] It is suggested that these children be followed closely and receive orthotic treatment. If significant progression is observed, surgery is indicated. The majority of AIS cases involving thoracic curvatures greater than 45 degrees are treated surgically. Currently, decisions to surgically intervene are based on skeletal maturity and balance, not simply on an arbitrary Cobb angle.[69] Owing to early detection and surgical intervention in childhood or adolescence, it is now becoming uncommon for pregnant women to present with severe uncorrected scoliosis and associated cardiopulmonary compromise. Consequently, parturients with previous surgical correction are much more common today. The impact of surgical intervention is reviewed here.

Surgical correction has involved several approaches, including Harrington rod instrumentation,[70] Luque instrumentation,[71] Wisconsin instrumentation,[72] and Cotrel-Dubousset instrumentation.[73] A review of these various surgical techniques of the past decade describes the extent of the instrumentation and provides an excellent reference to elucidate the potential impact on regional anesthesia.[74] Many recent advances have taken place in the surgical treatment of scoliosis and currently one of the most popular approaches involves an anterior release with posterior segmental instrumentation and spinal fusion.[69] These techniques now attempt to preserve the spinous processes and instrument no further caudad than the L3 level. Although modern surgical techniques have changed, many women who are currently of childbearing age have undergone previous, more aggressive surgical techniques that were popular in the past. Consequently, many of today's parturients underwent instrumentation that extended down to or below L4 as an adolescent. This may have a significant impact on attempts to successfully achieve regional anesthesia.

Anesthetic Management in Patients with Previous Corrective Surgery

The anesthetic assessment should focus on the same concerns outlined previously for parturients with uncorrected scoliosis. Of note, due to the high incidence of mitral valve prolapse, the antenatal examination should specifically attempt to identify this abnormality. Several considerations should be given to parturients who have previously undergone corrective spinal surgery. First, technical difficulties attempting to identify the epidural space at the usual L3-L4 or L4-L5 level are likely to be encountered because of bone grafting during the instrumentation surgery.[75] Success depends on the extent of the fusion. In several reports, the epidural space was identified in all parturients with Harrington rod manipulation except those with a fusion that extended to L3 or below.[76–78] Second, the usual tactile landmarks utilized to identify the intraspinous spaces are often obliterated due to the removal of the spinous processes during the fusion procedures, thus making placement more difficult. Although the incisional scar usually extends below L4, scoliosis instrumentation rarely involves the L5-S1 interspace[79] and should provide a location of high success for locating the epidural space. Lumbar radiographs and operative reports can provide important information regarding the extent of the surgical manipulation in the lumbar area. Third, successful identification of the epidural space and catheter placement does not guarantee effective analgesia or anesthesia.[76] Analgesic solutions injected through the epidural catheter may not spread sufficiently in a cephalad direction because of obliteration of the epidural space at the level of surgical correction.[75, 80] Consequently, this loss of epidural space continuity may result in ineffective labor analgesia or surgical anesthesia, even with an appropriately sited epidural catheter.[76]

The analgesic plan for the management of labor pain and the anesthetic plan for the provision of surgical anesthesia should be outlined well in advance of labor and delivery. If a vaginal delivery is planned, the concerns regarding the efficacy of LEA and possible alternatives should be discussed. Of note, it remains worthwhile to attempt LEA if the patient is willing and accepting of the higher risk of an inadvertent dural puncture and the risk of a post–dural puncture headache. Previous radiographic evidence may provide useful information regarding the extent of the distortion of the lumbar skeletal anatomy. Should accidental dural puncture occur, the epidural catheter should be placed intrathecally and used to provide either spinal analgesia or anesthesia. An intentional dural puncture with an 18-gauge or 17-gauge epidural needle will facilitate the intrathecal placement of the 20-gauge or 21-gauge epidural catheter as a means to deliver continuous spinal analgesia or anesthesia. Spinal catheters, whether placed intentionally or as a result of unintentional dural puncture, provide a means to deliver effective labor analgesia. More importantly, a correctly placed intrathecal catheter may provide an opportunity to facilitate surgical anesthesia while concurrently avoiding the risks of manipulating the airway.[81] Recently, patient-controlled intravenous analgesia fentanyl has gained popularity, and it provides a safe, viable alternative for regional analgesia in a parturient in whom regional analgesia is either contraindicated or technically impossible.[82] The protocol used at my institution includes a 2 to 3 μg/kg intravenous bolus of fentanyl followed by patient-controlled intravenous analgesia 50 μg every 10 minutes with no hourly limit and no restrictions on usage in the second stage. As the labor progresses, a reduction is made in the lockout interval and, if necessary, increases in the fentanyl dose (75–100 μg). Although naloxone must be readily available for neonatal resuscitation at the time of delivery, it is required only rarely.[83]

The presence of previous spinal instrumentation is not an indication for an elective cesarean delivery. The indications for operative delivery should not differ from those of the general population. However, cesarean delivery may be indicated if deterioration in maternal cardiopulmonary status occurs or an existing distortion of the maternal pelvis precludes fetal descent and delivery. Of note, the need for operative delivery is reportedly higher in parturients with a history of corrective spinal surgery than in the general population.[84] Again, a review of the previous radiographs may provide useful information regarding the extent of the surgical instrumentation of the lumbar skeletal anatomy. Whenever possible, even in these high-risk women, it is preferable to avoid general anesthesia and to provide regional anesthesia in the form of spinal anesthesia for elective, urgent, and very urgent cesarean delivery. The management of an epidural or intrathecal catheter has been discussed. A report of a successful spinal anesthetic for cesarean delivery after the initial epidural anesthetic technique failed to provide adequate anesthesia in a woman with prior surgical correction of scoliosis, using a midline approach with a 22-gauge atraumatic spinal needle at the L4-L5 interspace, has been made.[80] Another report described a successful spinal anesthetic for cesarean delivery using a 25-gauge atraumatic spinal needle at the L5-S1 interspace with a midline approach after multiple unsuccessful attempts to identify cerebrospinal fluid (CSF) at the L3-L4 interspace using both a midline and a paramedian approach.[85] A reasonable way to proceed would be to first attempt a midline approach with a 25-gauge atraumatic spinal needle at the L4-L5 or L5-S1 interspaces. If difficulty is encountered, particularly passing bone, then attempts with a 22-gauge atraumatic spinal needle can be made. Patience and perseverance on the part of the patient, obstetrician, and anesthesiologist are often necessary. Once clear, free-flowing CSF is identified, a mixture of 10.5 mg (1.4 mL) of 0.75% bupivacaine in aqueous 8.25% dextrose, 10 μg (0.2 mL) of fentanyl, and 200 μg (0.4 mL) of preservative-free morphine[86] can be administered via the spinal needle. This combination provides both effective intraoperative anesthesia and effective postoperative analgesia.

In summary, parturients presenting with either corrected or uncorrected scoliosis represent unique challenges to anesthesiologists. Early consultation with an anesthesiologist and a multidisciplinary approach will ensure that the parturient is well informed and that labor and delivery management is optimized.

SPONDYLOLISTHESIS

Spondylolisthesis is a ventral displacement of one vertebra upon another. This disorder was first described by an obstetrician who observed a bony prominence ventral to the sacrum that occasionally interfered with vaginal delivery.[87] Spondylolisthesis, which occurs in 6% of the general population,[88] has been classified into five distinct types[89]:

- Type I (dysplastic): congenital defects involving the superior sacral or inferior L5 facets with gradual ventral displacement of L5
- Type II (isthmic): fractures at the pars interarticularis
- Type III (degenerative): usually involving the L4-L5 joints
- Type IV (traumatic): other than involving the pars interarticularis
- Type V (pathologic)

Types I and II are more common in children and adolescents and involve L5-S1.[90] Degenerative spondylolisthesis (type III) is most common in females and most frequently involves L4-L5.[91] Spondylolisthesis is graded according to the amount of ventral displacement: grade I (0–25%), grade II (26–50%), grade III (51–75%), and grade IV (76–100%).[92]

Most women with spondylolisthesis are completely asymptomatic, but some have varying degrees of LBP.[91] Neurologic deficits are uncommon, except in severe spondylolisthesis.[93] Surgical decompression and fusion are indicated for ventral displacements of 30% or greater, incapacitating symptoms, or neurologic deficits. Pregnancy appears to be an important factor in the etiology of degenerative[94] but not isthmic[95] spondylolisthesis and will aggravate LBP in most parturients. Pregnant women with spondylolisthesis should be expected to have obstetric outcomes similar to the general population, and this condition does not preclude vaginal delivery.[96]

The anesthetic management previously outlined for LBP and previous lumbar surgery should be applied to parturients presenting with spondylolisthesis. Antenatal consultation is important to delineate symptoms, review radiographs, and develop and discuss management strategies with these women.

ACHONDROPLASTIC DWARFISM

Achondroplastic dwarfism is the most common form of disproportionate dwarfism, with a prevalence rate in North America of 0.5 to 1.5 per 10,000 births.[97, 98] Approximately 80% of cases are the result of a spontaneous mutation; however, the remaining 20% show an autosomal dominant inheritance pattern.[99–101] Short stature results from abnormal endochondral bone formation due to defective cartilage production, primarily at epiphyseal growth plates.[102] Patients have shortened limbs, thus rarely achieving a height greater than 130 cm, but have normal truncal length.[103] Characteristic craniofacial features include megalocephaly, frontal bossing, depressed nasal bridge, maxillary hypoplasia, large mandible, and large tongue.[99, 102] Patients often have kyphosis or kyphoscoliosis that may lead to pulmonary embarrassment owing to the exaggerated detrimental effect on functional residual capacity and closing capacity of the intra-abdominal gravid uterus.[104, 105] Respiratory compromise is of particular concern during the last 2 months of gestation because of the increased size of the extrapelvic uterus.[106] Spinal and subsequent neurologic abnormalities including lumbar hyperlordosis, thoracolumbar spinal canal stenosis, narrowed subarachnoid and epidural spaces with a normal-sized spinal cord, malformed vertebral bodies, and intervertebral disk disease are also common.[107–112] Foramen magnum stenosis has also been identified, particularly in parturients with neurologic symptoms.[113, 114] Of note, nonachondroplastic dwarfs also have a high incidence of atlantoaxial instability.[100, 115]

Anesthetic Management

Owing to the progressive pathophysiologic disorders associated with achondroplasia, these women ideally should be assessed early in the pregnancy and followed closely for evidence of cardiopulmonary compromise. Concurrently, an anesthetic plan can be developed and incorporated in the multidisciplinary approach to the parturient's management. The incidence of cephalopelvic disproportion and malpresentation necessitating the need for cesarean delivery is extremely high in dwarfism.[105, 106] Consequently, management should ultimately center on a plan for an elective cesarean delivery, once fetal lung maturity has been confirmed at term gestation, in an attempt to avoid emergency surgery.

The choice of either regional or general anesthesia in the patient with achondroplastic dwarfism has been a source of debate. Proponents of general anesthesia[116–118] cite the risk of potential injury to the spinal cord[100, 106, 118, 119] with regional anesthesia as justification for the use of general anesthesia. However, general anesthesia is also of concern, due to difficulties with airway manipulation[100] and the documentation of at least one failed intubation.[120] Proponents of regional anesthesia cite the growing number of case reports of successful use of continuous spinal[121] or epidural[122–127] anesthesia with no resultant adverse neurologic consequences. Single-shot spinal anesthesia, however, is best avoided because of the unpredictability of the cephalad spread of the block, which may occur because of the atypical spinal anatomy and short stature. No matter which modality is chosen, difficult-airway equipment such as an intubating light wand, fiberoptic bronchoscope, laryngeal mask airway, and cricothyrotomy or tracheotomy set should be immediately available. If airway manipulation becomes necessary, a small (5.5–6.0-mm) cuffed oral endotracheal tube should be chosen.[97]

A prudent anesthetic approach in the patient with achondroplastic dwarfism is to provide regional anesthesia via continuous lumbar epidural anesthesia for cesarean delivery, initiated in the sitting position. This should be undertaken in an operating room setting and only after the parturient has received a minimum of 20 mL/kg of a balanced salt solution. If the parturient has cardiopulmonary disease, radial artery pressure monitoring should be established prior to the initiation of anesthesia. Due to the prevalence of kyphoscoliosis, location of the epidural space may be difficult and care must be taken to avoid an inadvertent dural puncture. Once the epidural space is identified, the multiorifice epidural catheter is placed approximately 3 cm within the epidural space. An assessment for inadvertent intravascular or intrathecal placement should be carefully undertaken. Passive observation for blood or CSF should be followed by active, gentle aspiration for blood or CSF.[128–130] Owing to the lack of predictability of single-shot spinal anesthesia, a very small mass of local anesthetic should be administered.[122, 123] It is advisable to wait approximately 5 minutes between each injection and to assess the effect of each bolus prior to subsequent injections. Once a bilateral level of T8 has been achieved, the parturient may then be placed in the supine position with particular attention paid to ensure adequate left uterine displacement. Once hemodynamic stability has been established, subsequent incremental doses of the anesthetic solution can be administered to achieve the desired level of T4. Of note, as little as 10 to 12 mL of the anesthetic solution may be required to achieve cephalad levels of T4 for cesarean delivery.[122, 123, 127, 131]

If unintentional dural puncture occurs during epidural catheter placement, the epidural catheter should be placed intrathecally. As with epidural administration, incremental doses of medication can be administered to reach the desired effect. Small (<0.5 mL) incremental boluses of hyperbaric 0.75% bupivacaine can be used to achieve the desired level of surgical anesthesia in a controlled fashion. Each incremental dose must be accompanied by constant vigilance to assess the clinical effect.

For postoperative analgesia, epidural preservative-free morphine can be administered in a single dose of no greater than 3 mg.[125] The use of nonsteroidal anti-inflammatory agents and patient-controlled intravenous analgesia using 1 mg morphine boluses with a 5-minute lock-out period has recently been reported to provide effective postoperative analgesia.[122] It is important to carefully monitor these women for potential neurologic deficits postoperatively.

As with many high-risk conditions, the importance of an obstetric anesthesiology consultation early in the pregnancy and communication with the obstetric and neonatal care teams is vital to the successful perinatal management of women presenting with achondroplastic dwarfism.

OSTEOGENESIS IMPERFECTA

Osteogenesis imperfecta is a rare group of disorders of collagen synthesis, characterized by excessive fragility of bones with increased propensity to fracture.[132–134] The disorder results from a genetic mutation that affects type 1 collagen, the primary protein of bone.[133] The mutations can cause decreased collagen synthesis, production of defective collagen, or both.[135] This disorder was recognized several centuries ago[136] and subsequently observed to have not only a familial pattern but also nonskeletal manifestations, which typically include ligamentous laxity and blue sclerae.

Originally, osteogenesis imperfecta was classified into two categories, depending on the age at onset of fractures, either congenita (birth or infancy) or tarda (childhood). Currently, the disorder is classified into four types, incorporating biochemical, genetic, and morphologic characteristics.[137, 138] The prevalence of all types of osteogenesis imperfecta is reported to be 1 to 2 in 10,000.[133] Type 1 is the most common and inherited as an autosomal dominant trait that usually presents in childhood. It is the mildest form of the disorder, resulting from an abnormally low production of normal type 1 collagen. Bone deformity is not as severe as the other types, as it results from fractures rather than abnormal bone development. Affected women have normal fertility, and the least severe and most common represent the majority of parturients.[137] The other types, 2 through 4, represent severe forms and result from the production of abnormal collagen. Type

4 is the most common of the severe forms and typically results in dwarfism and kyphoscoliosis. There is a high incidence of intrauterine or neonatal death associated with types 2 and 3.[139]

Osteogenesis imperfecta may involve various systems that affect anesthesia. Musculoskeletal abnormalities include fractures from minor trauma, dwarfism, kyphoscoliosis, pectus excavatum, and other chest wall abnormalities leading to restrictive pulmonary dysfunction. Other abnormalities include conductive hearing loss, shortened cervical spine with limited mobility, odontoid hypoplasia, micrognathia, and brittle teeth. Hyperthyroidism has been observed in at least 50% of patients with osteogenesis imperfecta.[140] This may contribute to the excessive diaphoresis and elevations in temperature that are likely related to accelerated cellular metabolism or dysfunction in temperature regulation. Elevations in temperature are not associated with malignant hyperthermia and can be treated symptomatically. Capillary fragility has been observed in a few patients, but the majority had normal bleeding times.[141] One study found abnormalities of several laboratory platelet function studies, but all patients were clinically asymptomatic and all usual laboratory coagulation test results (platelet count, bleeding time, partial thromboplastin time, prothrombin time) were normal.[142] The clinical significance of these inconsistent laboratory observations with regard to the development of an epidural hematoma is suspect. It is also important to note that none of the patients studied in these series were parturients, who are normally in a hypercoagulable state. With the revelation that the bleeding time could neither accurately assess platelet function nor be used to predict risk of excessive bleeding, this test is not regularly used.[143, 144] The decision to undertake regional anesthesia should be determined following an assessment of a parturient's coagulation status, including a clinical history and examination and routine coagulation tests (platelet count, activated partial thromboplastin time, and INR). Some authors have also suggested the use of thromboelastography to evaluate risk of bleeding.[145, 146] Excessive uterine bleeding due to abnormalities of connective tissue in the uterus has been reported in women with osteogenesis imperfecta.[147, 148]

The majority of women who survive to childbearing age have type 1 osteogenesis imperfecta and will achieve full-term pregnancies.[149] Type 1 has an inheritance pattern of autosomal dominance and therefore the fetus of a woman with this type has a 50% chance of also having the disorder. Consequently, care must be taken with the handling of both the parturient and the neonate. Because of the risk of postpartum hemorrhage, the parturient should have large-bore intravenous access established and blood products readily available prior to delivery. Monitoring during the peripartum period should include the usual monitors. However, automatic noninvasive blood pressure devices should be avoided or used with great caution, as overinflation of the cuff may result in fracture of the humerus.[150] Placement of a radial arterial line avoids the risk of inadvertent aggressive manual blood pressure assessments and provides beat-to-beat blood pressure data as well as a single site for blood sampling.

Cesarean delivery is common in these women due to cephalopelvic disproportion or previous pelvic fracture.[147] The mode of delivery remains somewhat controversial, although if ultrasonographic evidence suggests that the fetus is affected, then an atraumatic cesarean delivery may be warranted.[149] In situations in which the fetus appears unaffected, elective cesarean delivery may still be advantageous, since it can avoid the risks of (1) maternal fractures during maternal expulsive efforts at the time of vaginal delivery, (2) a potential instrumental (forceps or vacuum) delivery, and (3) the potential "rough" handling of the parturient during an urgent or emergent surgical delivery. For a vaginal delivery, the use of effective, modern, ambulatory, epidural labor analgesia will relieve labor pain.[18] This may avoid accidental self-inflicted maternal injury associated with uncontrolled movements during attempts to cope with labor pain. The avoidance of epidural analgesics that result in dense lower extremity motor blockade may also prevent malpositioning conducive to accidental trauma. The concerns about excessive maternal expulsive efforts can be avoided with the combination of effective epidural labor analgesia followed by dense perineal epidural anesthesia at the time of delivery. This will permit a well-controlled spontaneous vaginal delivery with minimal maternal expulsive efforts. In a review of a series of nine vaginal deliveries between 1953 and 1968, only one complication, a fracture of pubic rami, was reported in a parturient, and she did not receive epidural labor analgesia.[147]

Anesthetic considerations for cesarean delivery will be dependent on the clinical status of the parturient and the severity of the osteogenesis imperfecta. Because of the potential for a difficult intubation, odontoid hypoplasia, and restrictive pulmonary insufficiency, general anesthesia ideally should be avoided for elective cesarean delivery. If general anesthesia is administered, succinylcholine may induce fasciculations that could potentially result in fractures, particularly of the long bones. However, there have been no case reports to date of this complication in pregnant women, most likely due to the decreased propensity of parturients to fasciculate. General anesthesia has been safely administered to a parturient with osteogenesis imperfecta who refused a regional anesthetic.[151] The administration of epidural rather than one-shot spinal anesthesia may be advantageous, as the anesthetic level via a catheter can be slowly titrated to the appropriate level. This is of particular importance considering that many of these parturients will be of short stature. Epidural anesthesia has been successfully used for women undergoing elective cesarean delivery.[152, 153]

TRANSIENT OSTEOPOROSIS OF THE HIP

Transient osteoporosis of the hip is a benign, self-limiting condition of transient localized demineralization and is of unknown etiology. It is characterized by an onset of discomfort during the third trimester that significantly increases in intensity, often sufficient to preclude ambulation.[154, 155] There is no history of trauma or infection, and previous pregnancies may have been unaffected, although it may recur in subsequent pregnancies.[156] Symptoms may affect one or both hips and are relieved by rest and aggravated by weight-bearing.[157] Examination reveals an antalgic gait and significant reduction in the range of motion of the hip due to pain. Magnetic resonance imaging examination is highly sensitive, revealing osteopenia of the femoral head with occasional involvement of the femoral neck and acetabulum.[158] As treatment includes reduced weight-bearing and mobility, parturients require prophylactic anticoagulation, including subcutaneous heparin and anti-embolism stockings. Complications of a stress fracture, osteoarthrosis, or avascular necrosis of the affected hip have been reported; however, the majority of cases resolve completely in the postpartum period.[156, 159, 160]

The majority of severely affected parturients will require elective cesarean section, as the necessary hip position for vaginal birth is too painful to assume.[155, 156, 161–165] Regional anesthesia for cesarean delivery is preferred. Care must be taken when positioning parturients following the induction of anesthesia and during the resolution of the spinal anesthetic to avoid the risk of unrecognized hip fracture. The use of intrathecal morphine (200 μg) combined with nonsteroidal anti-inflammatory drugs will provide effective postoperative analgesia of sufficient but limited duration. This will prevent the comfortable parturient from assuming positions that may increase the risk of hip injury in the postpartum period. Should the parturient be permitted to labor, effective epidural analgesia should be administered. Epidural labor analgesia will likely prevent the parturient from uncontrollably assuming positions during painful labor that may result in hip fracture. The importance of avoiding concentrations of bupivacaine or ropivacaine sufficient to result in anesthesia, rather than labor analgesia, thus removing the "protective pain" associated with certain hip positions, should be emphasized.

❖ SUMMARY

Key Points

- Low back pain is a common complaint in the pregnant woman and is not a contraindication to the use of neuraxial techniques.
- Epidural anesthesia may be technically more difficult in the pregnant woman who has had corrective surgery for scoliosis. In addition, epidural catheters, even when correctly sited, may not provide adequate analgesia/anesthesia following scoliosis surgery. In many of these parturients, spinally placed epidural catheters are a reasonable alternative.
- Epidural anesthesia or intentional intrathecal placement of an epidural catheter can be safely utilized in the pregnant woman with achondroplastic dwarfism. Single-shot spinal anesthesia is best avoided, owing to the lack of predictability of spread.
- The optimal management of the pregnant woman with a musculoskeletal disorder requires early consultation and a multidisciplinary approach.

Key References

Crosby ET, Halpern SH: Obstetric epidural anaesthesia in patients with Harrington instrumentation. Can J Anaesth 1989; 36:693–696.

Berkowitz ID, Raja SN, Bender KS, Kopits SE: Dwarfs: Pathophysiology and anesthetic implications. Anesthesiology 1990; 73:739–759.

Case Stem

A 31-year-old gravida 3 parous 1 woman in active labor at full term requests labor analgesia. Her past history is significant for corrective scoliosis surgery for adolescent idiopathic scoliosis. The orthopedic operative report suggests that the surgical instrumentation extends to the L4 vertebra. Discuss the analgesia options, including risks and benefits, that can be offered to this parturient. In addition, discuss the anesthetic plan for cesarean delivery, should that become necessary.

CONCLUSION

Parturients with preexisting musculoskeletal disorders may pose a special challenge to obstetric anesthesiologists. Knowledge of the interaction between the physiologic changes of pregnancy and these disorders is important for optimal management of parturients with these disorders. The need for early consultation and a multidisciplinary approach to many of these complex problems is essential. The multidisciplinary consultative process also provides an excellent opportunity to outline and reinforce anesthetic concerns to our obstetric colleagues, which will ultimately provide better communication and management of subsequent parturients with musculoskeletal disorders.

Acknowledgment

The assistance and helpful comments provided by Dr. Anne Dzus, Associate Professor, Director of Pediatric Orthopedic Surgery, Department of Surgery, University of Saskatchewan, are very much appreciated.

References

1. Jackson RP, Simmons EH, Stripinis D: Incidence and severity of back pain in adult idiopathic scoliosis. Spine 1983; 8:749–756.
2. Kosttuik JP, Bentivoglio J: The incidence of low-back pain in adult scoliosis. Spine 1981; 6:268–273.
3. Bjure J, Nachemson A: Non-treated scoliosis. Clin Orthop 1973; 93:44–52.
4. Nagi SZ, Riley LE, Newby LG: A social epidemiology of back pain in the general population. J Chron Dis 1973; 26:769–779.
5. Kristiansson P, Svardsudd K, Schoultz BV: Back pain during pregnancy: A prospective study. Spine 1996; 21:702–709.

6. Orvieta R, Achiron A, Ben-Rafael Z, et al: Low-back pain of pregnancy. Acta Obstet Gynecol Scand 1994; 73:209–214.
7. Ostgaard HC, Andersson GBJ: Postpartum low-back pain. Spine 1992; 17:53–55.
8. Ostgaard HC, Andersson GBJ: Previous back pain and risk of developing back pain in a future pregnancy. Spine 1991; 16:432–436.
9. Fast A, Shapiro D, Ducommun JD, et al: Low back pain in pregnancy. Spine 1987; 12:368–371.
10. Mantle MJ, Greenwood RM, Curry HLF: Backache in pregnancy. Rheumatol Rehabil 1977; 16:95–101.
11. Grove LH: Backache, headache and bladder dysfunction after delivery. Br J Anaesth 1973; 45:1147–1149.
12. MacLennan A, Nicolson R, Green RC, Bath M: Serum relaxin and pelvic pain of pregnancy. Lancet 1986; 2:243–245.
13. Fast A, Weiss L, Ducommun EJ, et al: Low-back pain in pregnancy: Abdominal muscles, sit-up performance, and back pain. Spine 1990; 15:28–30.
14. Berg G, Hammar M, Moller-Nielson J, et al: Low back pain during pregnancy. Obstet Gynecol 1988; 71:71–75.
15. Crawford JS: Some maternal complications of epidural analgesia for labour. Anaesthesia 1985; 40:1219–1225.
16. LaBan MM, Perrin JCS, Latimer FR: Pregnancy and the herniated lumbar disc. Arch Phys Med Rehabil 1983; 64:319–321.
17. Artal R, Friedman MJ, McNitt-Gray JL: Orthopedic problems in pregnancy. Physician Sportsmed 1990; 18:93–105.
18. Zwack RM, Campbell DC, Sawatzky K, et al: Ambulatory epidural analgesia in labor: Ropivacaine versus bupivacaine. Anesthesiology 1999; 90:A89.
19. Benzon HT, Braunschweig R, Molloy RE: Delayed onset of epidural anesthesia in patients with back pain. Anesth Analg 1981; 60:874–877.
20. Schachner SM, Abram SE: Use of two epidural catheters to provide analgesia of unblocked segments in a patient with lumbar disc disease. Anesthesiology 1982; 56:150–151.
21. Campbell DC, Banner R, Crone LA, et al: Addition of epinephrine to intrathecal sufentanil for ambulatory labor analgesia. Anesthesiology 1997; 86:525–531.
22. Viscomi CM, Rathmell JP, Pace NL: Duration of intrathecal labor analgesia: Early versus advanced labor. Anesth Analg 1997; 84:1108–1112.
23. Campbell DC, Camann WR, Datta S: The addition of bupivacaine to intrathecal sufentanil for labor analgesia. Anesth Analg 1995; 81:305–309.
24. Rayburn WF, Smith CV, Parriott JE, Woods RE: Randomized comparison of meperidine and fentanyl during labor. Obstet Gynecol 1989; 74:604–606.
25. Rayburn W, Rathke A, Leuschen P, et al: Fentanyl citrate during labor. Am J Obstet Gynecol 1989; 161:202–206.
26. Macarthur A, Macarthur C, Weeks S: Epidural anaesthesia and low back pain after delivery: A prospective cohort study. Br Med J 1995; 311:1336–1339.
27. Breen TW, Ransil BJ, Groves PA, Oriol NE: Factors associated with back pain after childbirth. Anesthesiology 1994; 81:29–34.
28. Macarthur AJ, Macarthur C, Weeks SK: Is epidural anesthesia in labor associated with chronic low back pain? A prospective cohort study. Anesth Analg 1997; 85:1066–1070.
29. Russell R, Groves P, Taub N, et al: Assessing long-term backache after childbirth. Br Med J 1993; 306:1299–1303.
30. MacLeod J, MacIntyre C, McClure JH, Whitfield A: Backache and epidural analgesia. Int J Obstet Anesth 1995; 4:21–25.
31. Macarthur C, Lewis M, Know EG, Crawford JS: Epidural anaesthesia and long-term backache after childbirth. Br Med J 1990; 301:9–12.
32. Massey Dawkins CJ: An analysis of the complications of extradural and caudal block. Anaesthesia 1969; 24:554–563.
33. Russell R, Dundas R, Reynolds F: Long-term backache after childbirth: Prospective search for causative factors. Br Med J 1996; 313:755–756.
34. Roaf R: Rotation movements of the spine with special reference to scoliosis. J Bone Joint Surg 1958; 40B:312–332.
35. Ashworth MA: Symposium on school screening for scoliosis: Scoliosis Research Society and British Scoliosis Society. Spine 1988; 13:1177–1200.
36. Lonstein JE, Bjorklund S, Wanninger MH, Nelson RP: Voluntary school screening for scoliosis in Minnesota. J Bone Joint Surg 1982; 62A:481–488.
37. Kafer ER: Respiratory and cardiovascular functions in scoliosis and the principles of anesthetic management. Anesthesiology 1980; 52:339–351.
38. Weinstein SL: Adolescent Idiopathic Scoliosis: Prevalence, Natural History, Treatment Indications. Iowa City: University of Iowa Printing Service; 1985: 1–12.
39. Kane WJ: Scoliosis prevalence: A call for a statement of terms. Clin Orthop 1977; 126:43–46.
40. Weinstein SL: Adolescent idiopathic scoliosis: Prevalence and natural history. *In* Weinstein SL (ed): The Pediatric Spine: Principles and Practice. New York: Raven Press; 1994: 463–477.
41. Sevastik JA, Aaro S, Normelli H: Scoliosis: Experimental and clinical studies. Clin Orthop 1984; 191:27–34.
42. Lonstein JE: Adolescent idiopathic scoliosis: Screening and diagnosis. Instr Course Lect 1989; 38:105–113.
43. Carter OD, Haynes SG: Prevalence rates for scoliosis in US adults: Results from the first National Health and Nutrition Examination Survey. Int J Epidemiol 1987; 16:537–544.
44. Winter RB: Adolescent idiopathic scoliosis. N Engl J Med 1986; 314:1379–1380.
45. Ascani E, Bartolozzi P, Logroscino CA, et al: Natural history of untreated idiopathic scoliosis after skeletal maturity. Spine 1986; 11:784–789.
46. Chow D: Scoliosis: A surgical perspective. Probl Anesth 1991; 5:40–43.
47. To WW, Wong MW: Kyphoscoliosis complicating pregnancy. Int J Gynaecol Obstet 1996; 55:123–128.
48. Hung CT, Pelosi M, Langer A, Harrigan JT: Blood gas measurements in the kyphoscoliotic gravida and her fetus: Report of a case. Am J Obstet Gynecol 1975; 121:287–288.
49. Hirshfeld SS, Rudner C, Nash CL, et al: The incidence of mitral valve prolapse in adolescent scoliosis and thoracic hypokyphosis. Pediatrics 1982; 70:451–454.
50. Hamilton PP, Byford LJ: Respiratory and cardiovascular functions in musculoskeletal disorders. Probl Anesth 1991; 5:91–106.
51. Keston S, Garfinkel SK, Wright T, Rebuck AS: Impaired exercise capacity in adults with moderate scoliosis. Chest 1991; 99:663–666.
52. Weinstein SL, Zavala DC, Ponseti IV: Idiopathic scoliosis: Long-term follow-up and prognosis in untreated patients. J Bone Joint Surg 1981; 63A:702–712.
53. Mezon BL, West P, Israels J, Kryger M: Sleep breathing abnormalities in scoliosis. Am Rev Respir Dis 1980; 122:617–621.
54. Pehrsson K, Larsson S, Oden A, Nachemson A: Long-term follow-up of patients with untreated scoliosis: A study of mortality, causes of death, and symptoms. Spine 1992; 17:1091–1096.
55. Bunnell WP: The natural history of idiopathic scoliosis. Clin Orthop 1988; 229:20–25.
56. Betz RR, Bunnell WP, Lambrecht-Mulier E, MacEwan GD: Scoliosis and pregnancy. J Bone Joint Surg 1987; 69A:90–96.
57. Berman AT, Cohen DL, Schwentker EP: The effects of pregnancy on idiopathic scoliosis: A preliminary report on eight cases and a review of the literature. Spine 1982; 7:76–77.
58. Blount WP, Mellemcamp DD: The effect of pregnancy on idiopathic scoliosis. J Bone Joint Surg 1980; 62A:1083–1087.
59. Sawicka EH, Spencer GT, Branthwaite MA: Management of respiratory failure complicating pregnancy in severe kyphoscoliosis: A new use for an old technique? Br J Dis Chest 1986; 80:191–196.
60. Siegler D, Zorab PA: Pregnancy in thoracic scoliosis. Br J Dis Chest 1981; 75:367–370.
61. Kopenhager T: A review of 50 pregnant patients with kyphoscoliosis. Br J Obstet Gynecol 1977; 84:585–587.
62. Visscher W, Lonstein JE, Hoffman DA, et al: Reproductive outcomes in scoliosis patients. Spine 1988; 13:1096–1098.
63. Phelan JP, Dainer MJ, Cowherd DW: Pregnancy complicated by thoracolumbar scoliosis. South Med J 1978; 71:76–78.

64. Moran DH, Johnson MD: Continuous spinal anesthesia with combined hyperbaric and isobaric bupivacaine in a patient with scoliosis. Anesth Analg 1990; 70:445–447.
65. Schultz R, Campbell DC, Crone LA, et al: Intrathecal bupivacaine and sufentanil for ambulatory labor analgesia: Effect of dose reductions. Anesthesiology 1998; 88:A18.
66. Carlson DW, Engelman DR, Bart AJ: Epidural anesthesia for cesarean section in kyphoscoliosis. Anesth Analg 1978; 57:125–128.
67. Lonstein JE, Carlson JM: The prediction of curve progression in untreated idiopathic scoliosis during growth. J Bone Joint Surg 1984; 66A:1061–1071.
68. Rogala EJ, Drummond DS, Gurr J: Scoliosis: Incidence and natural history: a prospective epidemiological study. J Bone Joint Surg 1978; 60A:173–176.
69. Bridwell KH: Surgical treatment of adolescent idiopathic scoliosis: The basics and the controversies. Spine 1994; 19:1095–1100.
70. Harrington PR: Treatment of scoliosis: Correction and internal fixation by spine instrumentation. J Bone Joint Surg 1962; 44A:591–610.
71. Luque ER: Segmental spinal instrumentation for correction of scoliosis. Clin Orthop 1982; 163:192–198.
72. Drummond D, Guadagni J, Keene JS, et al: Interspinous process segmental spinal instrumentation. J Pediatr Orthop 1984; 4:397–404.
73. Cotrel Y, Dubousset J, Guillaumat M: New universal instrumentation in spinal surgery. Clin Orthop 1988; 227:10–23.
74. Tolo VT: Surgical treatment of adolescent idiopathic scoliosis. Instr Course Lect 1989; 38:143–156.
75. Feldstein G, Ramanathan S: Obstetrical lumbar epidural anesthesia in patients with previous posterior spinal fusion for kyphoscoliosis. Anesth Analg 1985; 64:83–85.
76. Daley MD, Roblin SH, Hew EM, et al: Epidural anesthesia for obstetrics after spinal surgery. Reg Anesth 1990; 15:280–284.
77. Crosby ET, Halpern SH: Obstetric epidural anaesthesia in patients with Harrington instrumentation. Can J Anaesth 1989; 36:693–696.
78. Hubbard CH: Epidural anesthesia in patients with spinal fusion. Anesth Analg 1985; 64:843.
79. Winter RB: Posterior spinal fusion in scoliosis: Indications, technique and results. Orthop Clin North Am 1979; 10:787–800.
80. Pascoe HF, Jennings GS, Marx GF: Successful spinal anesthesia after inadequate epidural block in a parturient with prior surgical correction of scoliosis. Reg Anesth 1993; 18:191–192.
81. Hawkins JL, Koonin LM, Palmer SK, Gibbs CP: Anesthesia-related deaths during obstetric delivery in the United States, 1979–1990. Anesthesiology 1997; 86:277–284.
82. Muir HA, Breen TW, Campbell DC, Halpern SH: Is intravenous PCA fentanyl an effective method for providing labor analgesia? Anesthesiology 1999; 90:A28.
83. Halpern SH, Breen TW, Campbell DC, Muir HA: Intravenous PCA fentanyl vs epidural PCA fentanyl/bupivacaine: Neonatal effects. Anesthesiology 1999; 90:A19.
84. Cochran T, Irstam L, Nachemson A: Functional changes in patients with adolescent idiopathic scoliosis treated by Harrington rod fusion. Spine 1983; 8:576–584.
85. Kardash K, King BW, Datta S: Spinal anaesthesia for caesarean section after Harrington instrumentation. Can J Anaesth 1993; 40:667–669.
86. Gerancher JC, Floyd H, Eisenach J: Determination of an effective dose of intrathecal morphine for pain relief after cesarean delivery. Anesth Analg 1999; 88:346–351.
87. Herbinaux G: Triate sur divers accouchements laborieux, et sur polypes de la matrice. Brussels: J.L. De Boubers, 1782.
88. Fredrickson BE, Baker D, McHolick WJ, et al: The natural history of spondylolysis and spondylolisthesis. J Bone Joint Surg 1984; 66:699–707.
89. Wilste LL, Newman PH, Macnab I: Classification of spondylolysis and spondylolisthesis. Clin Orthop 1976; 117:23–29.
90. Thompson GH: Back pain in children. Instr Course Lect 1994; 43:221–230.
91. Rosenberg NJ: Degenerative spondylolisthesis: Predisposing factors. J Bone Joint Surg 1975; 57A:467–474.
92. Meyerding HW: Spondylolisthesis. Surg Gynecol Obstet 1932; 54:371–377.
93. Boxall D, Bradford DS, Winter RB, Moe JH: Management of severe spondylolisthesis in children and adolescents. J Bone Joint Surg 1979; 61A:479–495.
94. Sanderson PL, Fraser RD: The influence of pregnancy on the development of degenerative spondylolisthesis. J Bone Joint Surg 1996; 78B:951–954.
95. Saraste H: Spondylolysis and pregnancy: A risk factor. Acta Obstet Gynecol Scand 1986; 65:727–729.
96. Dandy DJ, Shannon MJ: Lumbo-sacral subluxation. J Bone Joint Surg 1971; 53B:578–595.
97. Mayhew JF, Katz J, Miner M, et al: Anaesthesia for the achondroplastic dwarf. Can Anaesth Soc J 1986; 33:216–221.
98. Orioli IM, Castilla EE, Barbosa-Neto JG: The birth prevalence rates for skeletal dysplasias. J Med Genet 1986; 23:328–332.
99. Feingold M, Pashayan H: Genetics and Birth Defects in Clinical Practice. Boston: Little, Brown; 1990: 686–689.
100. Walts LF, Finerman G, Wyatt GM: Anaesthesia for dwarfs and other patients of pathologic short stature. Can Anaesth Soc J 1975; 22:703–709.
101. Murdoch JL, Walker BA, Hall JG, et al: Achondroplasia: A genetic and statistical survey. Ann Hum Genet 1970; 33:227–244.
102. Fairbank TJ: The hereditary chondrodysplasias. *In* Scott RB (ed): Price's Textbook of the Practice of Medicine, 12th ed. London: Oxford University Press; 1978: 981.
103. Berkowitz ID, Raja SN, Bender KS, Kopits SE: Dwarfs: Pathophysiology and anesthetic implications. Anesthesiology 1990; 73:739–759.
104. Stokes DC, Pyeritz RE, Wisa RA, et al: Spirometry and chest wall dimensions in achondroplasia. Chest 1988; 93:364–369.
105. Tyson JE, Barnes AC, McKusick VA, et al: Obstetric and gynecologic considerations of dwarfism. Am J Obstet Gynecol 1970; 108:688–704.
106. Allanson JE, Hall JG: Obstetric and gynecologic problems in women with chondrodystrophies. Obstet Gynecol 1986; 67:74–78.
107. Wynne-Davies R, Walsh WK, Gormley J: Achondroplasia and hypochondroplasia: Clinical variation and spinal stenosis. J Bone Joint Surg 1981; 63A:508–515.
108. Betham D, Winter RB, Lutter L, et al: Spinal disorders of dwarfism. J Bone Joint Surg 1981; 63A:1412–1425.
109. Morgan DF, Young RF: Spinal neurologic complications of achondroplasia. J Neurosurg 1980; 52:463–472.
110. Kopits SE: Orthopedic complications of dwarfism. Clin Orthop 1976; 114:153–179.
111. Nelson MA: Spinal stenosis in achondroplasia. Proc R Soc Med 1972; 65:1028–1029.
112. Bergstrom K, Laurent U, Lundberg PO: Neurologic symptoms in achondroplasia. Acta Neurol Scand 1971; 47:59–70.
113. Wang H, Rosembaum ARE, Reid CS, et al: Pediatric patients with achondroplasia: CT evaluation of the craniocervical junction. Radiology 1987; 164:515–519.
114. Hecht JT, Nelson FW, Butler IJ, et al: Computerized tomography of the foramen magnum: Achondroplastic values compared to normal standards. Am J Med Genet 1985; 29:355–360.
115. Perovic MN, Kopitis SE, Thompson RC: Radiological evaluation of the spinal cord in congenital atlanto-axial dislocation. Radiology 1973; 109:713–716.
116. Mcarthur RDA: Obstetric anaesthesia in an achondroplastic dwarf at a regional hospital. Anaesth Intensive Care 1992; 20:376–378.
117. Kalla GN, Fening E, Obiaya MO: Anaesthetic management of achondroplasia. Br J Anaesth 1986; 58:117–119.
118. Bancroft GH, Lauria JI: Ketamine induction for cesarean section in a patient with acute intermittent porphyria and achondroplastic dwarfism. Anesthesiology 1983; 59:143–144.
119. DiNardo SK: Anesthetic considerations for the achondroplastic dwarf. J Am Assoc Nurse Anesth 1988; 56:42–48.
120. Mather JS: Impossible laryngoscopy in achondroplasia: A case report. Anaesthesia 1966; 21:244–248.

121. Crawford M, Dutton DA: Spinal anaesthesia for caesarean section in an achondroplastic dwarf. Anaesthesia 1992; 47:1007.
122. Morrow MJ, Black IH: Epidural anaesthesia for caesarean section in an achondroplastic dwarf. Br J Anaesth 1998; 81:619–621.
123. Carstoniu J, Yee I, Halpern S: Epidural anaesthesia for caesarean section in an achondroplastic dwarf. Can J Anaesth 1992; 39:708–711.
124. Wardall GJ, Frame WT: Extradural anaesthesia for caesarean section in achondroplasia. Br J Anaesth 1990; 64:367–370.
125. Brimacombe JR, Caunt JA: Anaesthesia in a gravid achondroplastic dwarf. Anaesthesia 1990; 45:132–134.
126. Waugaman WR, Kryc JJ, Andrews MJ: Epidural anesthesia for cesarean section and tubal ligation in an achondroplastic dwarf. J Am Assoc Nurse Anesth 1986; 54:436–437.
127. Cohen SE: Anesthesia for cesarean section in achondroplastic dwarfs. Anesthesiology 1980; 52:264–266.
128. Norris MC, Ferrenbach D, Dalman H, et al: Does epinephrine improve the diagnostic accuracy of aspiration during labor epidural analgesia? Anesth Analg 1999; 88:1073–1076.
129. Norris MC, Fogel ST, Dalman H, et al: Labor epidural analgesia without an intravascular "test dose." Anesthesiology 1998; 88:1495–1501.
130. Mulroy MF, Norris MC, Liu SS: Safety steps for epidural injection of local anesthetics: Review of the literature and recommendations. Anesth Analg 1997; 85:1346–1356.
131. Nguyen TT, Papadakos PJ, Sabnis LU: Epidural anesthesia for extracorporeal shock wave lithotripsy in an achondroplastic dwarf. Reg Anesth 1997; 22:102–104.
132. Cole WG: Etiology and pathogenesis of heritable connective tissue diseases. J Pediatr Orthop 1993; 13:392–403.
133. Byers PH, Steiner RD: Osteogenesis imperfecta. Annu Rev Med 1992; 43:269–282.
134. Gertner JM, Root L: Osteogenesis imperfecta. Orthop Clin North Am 1990; 21:151–162.
135. Byers PH, Wallis GA, Willing MC: Osteogenesis imperfecta: Translation of mutation to phenotype. J Med Genet 1991; 28:433–442.
136. Weil UH: Osteogenesis imperfecta: Historical background. Clin Orthop 1981; 159:6–10.
137. Sillence D: Osteogenesis imperfecta: An expanding panorama of variants. Clin Orthop 1981; 159:11–25.
138. Sillence DO, Senn A, Danks DM: Genetic heterogeneity in osteogenesis imperfecta. J Med Genet 1979; 16:101–116.
139. Cole WG, Dalgleish R: Perinatal lethal osteogenesis imperfecta. J Med Genet 1995; 32:284–289.
140. Libman RH: Anesthetic considerations for the patient with osteogenesis imperfecta. Clin Orthop Rel Res 1981; 159:123–125.
141. Evensen SA, Myhre L, Stormorken H: Haemostatic studies in osteogenesis imperfecta. Scand J Haematol 1984; 33:177–179.
142. Hathaway WE, Solomons CC, Ott JE: Platelet function and pyrophosphates in osteogenesis imperfecta. Blood 1972; 39:500–509.
143. Rodgers RPC, Levin JA: A critical reappraisal of the bleeding time. Semin Thromb Hemost 1990; 16:1–20.
144. Lind SE: The bleeding time does not predict surgical bleeding. Blood 1991; 77:2547–2552.
145. Campbell DC, Sawatzky K, Yip RW: Thromboelastographic evaluation of thrombocytopenic parturients. Anesthesiology 1999; 90:A12.
146. Chandler WL: The thromboelastograph and the thromboelastograph technique. Semin Thromb Hemost 1995; 21:1–6.
147. Key TC, Horger EO: Osteogenesis imperfecta as a complication of pregnancy. Obstet Gynecol 1978; 51:67–71.
148. Young BK, Gorstein F: Maternal osteogenesis imperfecta. Obstet Gynecol 1968; 31:461–470.
149. Carlson JW, Harlass FE: Management of osteogenesis imperfecta in pregnancy. J Reprod Med 1993; 38:228–232.
150. Oliverio RM: Anesthetic management of intramedullary nailing in osteogenesis imperfecta: Report of a case. Anesth Analg 1973; 52:232–236.
151. Cho E, Dayan SS, Marx GF: Anaesthesia in a parturient with osteogenesis imperfecta. Br J Anaesth 1992; 68:422–423.
152. Cunningham AJ, Donnelly M, Comerford J: Osteogenesis imperfecta: Anesthetic management of a patient for cesarean section—a case report. Anesthesiology 1984; 61:91–93.
153. Bullard JR, Alpert CC, James WF: Anesthetic management of a patient with osteogenesis imperfecta undergoing cesarean section. J South Carolina Med Assoc 1977; 73:417–419.
154. Khovidhunkit W, Epstein S: Osteoporosis in pregnancy. Osteoporos Int 1996; 6:345–354.
155. Beaulieu JG, Razzano CD, Levine RB: Transient osteoporosis of the hip in pregnancy: Review of the literature and a case report. Clin Orthop 1987; 122:197–202.
156. Brodell JD, Burns JE, Heiple KG: Transient osteoporosis of the hip of pregnancy: Two cases complicated by pathologic fracture. J Bone Joint Surg 1989; 71A:1252–1257.
157. Shifrin LZ, Reis ND, Zinman H, Besser MI: Idiopathic transient osteoporosis of the hip. J Bone Joint Surg 1987; 69B:769–773.
158. Urbanski SR, de Lange EE, Eschenroeder HC: Magnetic resonance imaging of transient osteoporosis of the hip: A case report. J Bone Joint Surg 1991; 73A:451–455.
159. Fokter SK, Vengust V: Displaced subcapital fracture of the hip in transient osteoporosis of pregnancy: A case report. Int Orthop 1997; 21:201–203.
160. Goldman GA, Friedman S, Hod M, Ovadia J: Idiopathic transient osteoporosis of the hip in pregnancy. Int J Gynaecol Obstet 1994; 46:317–320.
161. Jolliffe DM: Anaesthesia and transient osteoporosis of the hip in pregnancy. Int J Obstet Anaesth 1997; 6:63–66.
162. Guerra JJ, Steinberg ME: Distinguishing transient osteoporosis from avascular necrosis of the hip. J Bone Joint Surg 1995; 77A:616–624.
163. Ben-David Y, Bornstein J, Sorokin Y, et al: Transient osteoporosis of the hip during pregnancy: A case report. J Reprod Med 1991; 36:672–674.
164. Bramlett KW, Killian JT, Nasca RJ, Daniel WW: Transient osteoporosis. Clin Orthop 1987; 222:197–202.
165. Campbell DC, Epp A, Turnell R: Emergent uterine relaxation with intravenous nitroglycerine for a vaginal breech delivery: Clinical report and review. J Soc Obstet Gynaecol Can 1997; 19:415–420.

46

Anesthesia for the Parturient with Neurologic Disease

CATHERINE S. DOWNS, MBBS (Hons 1), FANZCA

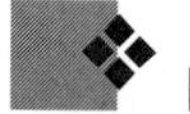

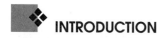

INTRODUCTION

The parturient with neurologic disease provides an interesting challenge to the anesthetist. This chapter outlines the anesthetic, obstetric, and neonatal considerations for several of the more common neurologic diseases that affect women of childbearing age. Up-to-date evidence on the role of regional anesthesia for labor and cesarian section in each condition is summarized. Key features of the anesthetic consultation have been included in table form for easy reference in the antenatal anesthesia clinic.

EPILEPSY

Maternal seizure disorders occur in 0.5% of all parturients.[1, 2] The aim of therapy is to prevent seizures, especially status epilepticus, while minimizing teratogenic effects of anticonvulsant medications. There are several types of seizure disorders (Table 46–1).

Seizure frequency is unchanged during pregnancy in 60 to 85% of patients with a seizure disorder.[3] An increased seizure frequency is seen in approximately one in four epileptics and is often associated with sleep deprivation, poor compliance with therapy, and changing pharmacokinetics.[4] It is also clearly associated with adverse perinatal outcome.[5] Sabers et al.[6] found no change in seizure frequency in 66% of 151 pregnant women, with an increased frequency in 21%.

The new onset of seizures in pregnancy is usually caused by eclampsia but may be due to neoplasm, cerebrovascular disease, or metabolic, toxic, or infective conditions.[7, 8] Of all women with epilepsy, 13% have their first seizure during pregnancy, and 40% of these (5.2% overall) have seizures only during pregnancy.[9] Usually, isolated seizures do not have a deleterious effect on the fetus,[10] although injury to mother or fetus and in utero deaths after seizures have been reported.[1, 11]

Status epilepticus can result in fetal and maternal death, and immediate management must include protection of the airway, uterine displacement, and administration of an anticonvulsant medication such as diazepam, lorazepam or thiopental.[12] These parturients may require general anesthesia with controlled ventilation.

Table 46–1 SEIZURE DISORDERS

Seizure Disorders
Focal (partial) seizures
Generalized seizures
Grand mal
Petit mal
Focal progressing to generalized seizures

Pharmacologic Therapy

A small proportion of women who are planning to get pregnant and are seizure-free can have antiepileptic drugs (AEDs) withdrawn. If this is not possible, then a switch to monotherapy at the lowest effective dose is recommended. AEDs used in pregnancy include carbamazepine, phenytoin, phenobarbital, valproate, primidone, clonazepam, and ethosuxamide. Apart from trimethadione, which is contraindicated during pregnancy,[11] the Consensus Guidelines[13] state that the AED chosen should be the one that stops seizures in a given patient because no single AED has consistently proven to be more or less teratogenic than the others.[4]

Samren et al.,[14] in a study of 192 children, recently found an increased relative risk (RR = 2.3) for major congenital malformations in children exposed to AEDs during gestation compared to nonepileptic control subjects, and that this was significantly higher for both carbamazepine (RR = 4.9) and valproate (RR = 4.9), especially at higher doses. Valproate and carbamazepine are associated with a 1 to 2% incidence of neural tube defects and high-dose folate (5 mg/day) before conception and during pregnancy may be recommended.[15] The two newer second line AEDs, gabapentin and lamotrigine, do not appear to be teratogenic in animal studies.[10]

Serum levels of most AEDs decrease during pregnancy due to changing pharmacokinetics and reduced compliance because of emesis and fear of teratogenicity. Free drug levels should be assessed every month early during pregnancy, weekly during the last month of pregnancy, and at the onset of labor.[11] The doses must then be readjusted during the postpartum period to avoid toxicity.[2]

Obstetric Considerations

The literature regarding the incidence of pregnancy complications experienced by women with epilepsy is not conclusive. Studies exist that show an increase in many complications, including preeclampsia, bleeding, and premature labor, whereas others show no difference compared with the nonepileptic population.[1, 5, 16, 17] Most women with epilepsy can have a normal vaginal delivery although obstetric intervention, such as induction of labor, mechanical rupture of membranes, forceps delivery, and cesarian section, are more common in these patients than in the general population.[2]

A grand-mal seizure during labor occurs in 1 to 2% of women with epilepsy and within 24 hours of delivery in another 1 to 2%.[16] Sabers et al.,[6] in a retrospective review of 151 pregnancies in epileptic mothers, found an incidence of seizures of 2.6% during labor and delivery and 5% in the puerperium. When seizures occur during labor, fetal bradycardia is common. The postictal parturient may then require urgent cesarian section.

Neonatal Considerations

Approximately 95% of infants born to women with epilepsy are healthy[2]; the remaining 5% comprises stillbirth, perinatal mortality, congenital malformations, dysmorphism, and developmental delay.[3] An increased perinatal mortality of 1.2- to 3-fold has been widely reported.[16] Sabers et al.[6] reported a perinatal mortality rate of 1.3%, which was more frequent (but not significantly increased) compared with the background population of 0.5%.

An increase in congenital malformations in the children of epileptic mothers has been observed. Sabers et al.[6] found an incidence of 5.3%, compared with 1.5% in the nonepileptic control subjects. The most common congenital abnormalities are cardiac and orofacial malformations, microcephaly, and neural tube defects.[2] Variables that have been identified as important in this increased risk include AEDs, maternal seizures during pregnancy, and maternal epilepsy itself.[18] Congenital malformations attributable to AEDs include fetal hydantoin syndrome and neural tube defects. Maternal seizures in the first trimester have been associated with an increased risk of malformation, although this may be related to drug treatment rather than seizures.[19] Nulman et al.[20] observed that some congenital abnormalities occurred more commonly in the offspring of nontreated epileptic mothers and concluded that the drugs and the epilepsy have independent effects on the developing fetus, and that some malformations may be genetically linked to epilepsy itself. Neonatal hemorrhage is also a concern if the mother has been on anticonvulsant medications, and vitamin K may be given orally to the parturient (10 mg/day) during the last 2 to 4 weeks of pregnancy[2, 4] and also intramuscularly to the neonate at birth.

Anesthetic Considerations

Anesthetic consultation should take place before the onset of labor, especially if seizures have been poorly controlled. The aims of the anesthetic consultation are outlined in Table 46–2.

Systemic Analgesia

Myoclonus and seizures following pethidine (meperidine) administration are well described and are attrib-

Table 46–2 ANESTHETIC CONSULTATION IN EPILEPSY

1. Determine seizure history during current and previous pregnancies.
2. Ensure recent compliance with AEDs and check or repeat serum levels as necessary.
3. Ensure that AEDs are continued throughout labor. If oral therapy is not tolerated, consider intravenous phenytoin or a benzodiazepine.[108]
4. Consider elective cesarean section in consultation with obstetrician and neurologist if patient has had poor recent control of epilepsy or prior occurrence of severe seizures during times of physical or mental stress.
5. Explain the importance of good analgesia for labor, as respiratory alkalosis may exacerbate seizure disorders.
6. Obtain informed consent for regional anesthesia in case it is required.
7. Consider intravenous access during labor and be prepared to manage a seizure on the labor floor.
8. Remember that epilepsy may be associated with an increase in obstetric complications and interventions and that there is an increased incidence of stillbirth, congenital malformation, and neonatal hemorrhage.

AED, antiepileptic drug.

uted to its metabolite norpethidine, which has a long half-life (14–21 hours). AEDs and phenothiazines have been demonstrated to increase the conversion of pethidine to norpethidine in humans, while phenothiazines themselves may lower the seizure threshold.[21] Thus pethidine and phenothiazines are best avoided in the epileptic parturient. Nitrous oxide has an extremely low epileptogenic potential,[21] and its use in labor appears safe.

Regional Anesthesia

Low blood concentrations of local anesthetics, as occur with routine obstetric epidural blocks, have been shown to be anticonvulsant.[12, 22] Epidural anesthesia has been safely used in the epileptic parturient for labor, delivery and cesarian section and should not be withheld. Spinal anesthesia has also been safely used, although there are case reports of seizures under spinal anesthesia in which intravascular injection was unlikely and patients were not hypotensive or hypoxic.[23] The use of caffeine in the management of post–dural puncture headache has been implicated in causing a postpartum seizure.[24]

General Anesthesia

Anticonvulsants must be continued throughout the fasting period. Methohexital, ketamine, etomidate, and propofol have all been associated with seizure-like activity in predisposed individuals.[12, 25, 26] Prolonged recurrent seizures for greater than 36 hours after propofol exposure have been described in a nonepileptic patient following miscarriage.[27] General anesthesia is frequently induced with thiopental and succinylcholine and maintained with oxygen, nitrous oxide, and isoflurane. Enflurane, though not contraindicated, is best avoided in high concentrations or in conjunction with hypocarbia.[21] If muscle relaxants are used, they should be monitored, with a nerve stimulator, as chronic anticonvulsant therapy may induce resistance. Of the commonly used nondepolarizing agents, atracurium pharmacokinetics are least affected.[28] Although patient-controlled analgesia can be used for postoperative analgesia, it may be prudent to avoid pethidine (meperidine).

MULTIPLE SCLEROSIS

Multiple sclerosis (MS), a demyelinating disease of the central nervous system affects 1 in 1000 people in western countries[29] and is more common in women than men in a ratio of 2:1. Two-thirds of patients have their first symptoms between the ages of 20 and 40 years. Symptoms include visual disturbances, muscle weakness, spasticity, paresthesias, sphincter dysfunction, ataxia, and fatigue. Most patients experience exacerbations and remissions at unpredictable intervals, although some have a chronic progressive form of the disease. Factors implicated as contributing to relapse of MS include stress and emotional upset, infection, trauma, and increased body temperature.[30]

There is no known cure for MS. Pharmacologic management includes immunosuppressive agents such as corticosteroids, azathioprine, methotrexate, and the newer agents interferon beta and copolymer. Other medications to treat the symptoms of MS include baclofen, amantadine, pemoline, and carbamazepine.[31] Most of these drugs have uncertain fetal effects, and to use them during pregnancy, the clinician must carefully weigh risks and benefits. Methotrexate is contraindicated for use during pregnancy.

Obstetric and Neonatal Considerations

Multiple sclerosis does not affect the course of pregnancy or fetal outcome. The relapse rate during pregnancy is similar to that in the non-pregnant population in the first and second trimester and is reduced during the third trimester.[29, 31] Spontaneous labor and vaginal delivery are usually achieved and rates of infant mortality and congenital malformations do not differ from those in the general population.[31]

In the first 6 months postpartum, patients with relapsing-remitting MS have a two to three times increased rate of exacerbation, primarily in the first 3 months.[29, 31] Achiron et al.[32] administered intravenous immunoglobulin to nine patients with a history of MS exacerbation after childbirth; none of the treated patients relapsed during the first 6 months after delivery. No study has clearly demonstrated a negative consequence of pregnancy on the long-term course of MS.[31] Interestingly, Runmarker and Andersen[33] found a significantly decreased risk of entering a progressive course in women who became pregnant after MS onset.

Anesthetic Considerations

The anesthetic consultation should take place early in the third trimester. Important goals are outlined in Table 46–3. Patients treated with greater than 10 to 20 mg per day of prednisone, or its equivalent, should receive steroid coverage during labor and delivery.

Table 46–3 ANESTHETIC CONSULTATION IN MULTIPLE SCLEROSIS

1. Assess the degree of fatigability and neuromuscular weakness, especially respiratory compromise.
2. Determine the need for corticosteroid supplementation.
3. If severe disease, consider the potential for autonomic hyperreflexia and succinylcholine-induced hyperkalemia.
4. Ensure that the patient is aware of the high incidence of postpartum relapse.
5. Discuss the evidence that epidural anesthesia is safe in multiple sclerosis and does not alter relapse rate.
6. Obtain informed consent for epidural anesthesia in case it is required.
7. Consult with obstetrician and neurologist to unify a management plan.

The recommended course is 100 mg hydrocortisone intramuscularly or intravenously on admission and every 8 hours until no further complications are anticipated.[34]

Systemic Analgesia

Parenteral and inhalational analgesics may be used safely in the majority of patients. If MS is severe and respiratory reserve is limited, it may be prudent to avoid respiratory depressants.

Regional Anesthesia

The safety of regional anesthesia in MS has long been controversial. Epidural anesthesia has been used successfully for labor, vaginal delivery, and cesarian section. Confavreux et al.[29] studied 269 pregnancies in women with MS, of whom 42 received epidural analgesia. They concluded that epidural analgesia had no adverse effect on the rate of relapse or on the progression of disability in MS. Bader et al.[35] reviewed epidurals in nine women who delivered vaginally and five who had cesarian section and detected no difference in relapse rates, but all of the women who experienced postpartum relapses had received concentrations of bupivacaine greater than 0.25%. These authors concluded that a higher concentration of drug over a longer period of time may adversely influence the relapse rate. Crawford et al.[36] reported 57 cases of epidural block, 7 of which were in labor, with only 1 postoperative relapse. Salvador et al.[37] reported the safe use of epidural bupivacaine and fentanyl in low doses for vaginal delivery. Jones and Healy[38] stated that epidural anesthesia does not adversely affect the disease process in MS but that there is sufficient evidence to advise moderation in the total dose of local anesthetic used because of the known disturbance in the blood-brain barrier. This disturbance occurs in less than 25% of patients[39] and may result in enhanced cerebrospinal fluid concentrations of local anesthetics as they traverse the blood-brain barrier. Thus the consensus is that epidural analgesia should not be withheld in the presence of MS, but that the use of the lowest effective dose may be prudent.

Fewer reports are available concerning the use of subarachnoid anesthesia in MS. The conservative approach to the use of this technique stems from animal studies on the effect of local anesthetic agents on the spinal cord as well as a small number of case reports of the deterioration of MS after surgery under spinal anesthetic in humans.[40] Tui et al.[41] showed that very high levels of cerebrospinal fluid procaine, nupercaine, and monocaine cause transient reversible histologic changes in cat and rabbit spinal cords. It is possible that the demyelinated nervous tissue in MS may be even more sensitive to these potentially neurotoxic effects of local anesthetics.

Bamford et al.[42] presented data on eight MS patients who received a total of nine spinal and three caudal anesthetics; only one patient experienced aggravation of MS in the month after a spinal anesthetic for childbirth. Stenuit and Marchand[43] described 19 cases of spinal anesthetic in patients with MS in which symptoms were aggravated in only two cases following general surgery. Berger et al.[44] reported a case of intrathecal tetracaine and morphine for penile surgery in a male with MS; this patient had also previously had a prostate resection under spinal anesthesia. No adverse effects were noted. Leigh et al.[45] described a patient with advanced MS and respiratory compromise who underwent sigmoid colectomy under spinal anesthesia with heavy amethocaine and diamorphine. Postoperative analgesia was provided for 4 days with intermittent intrathecal diamorphine. Again, no adverse effects were noted.

Because MS relapse can be associated with emotional or physical stress, or a rise in body temperature, it is difficult to relate isolated case reports of relapse to the anesthetic technique. Clearly, more research is needed in this area. Despite the fact that deleterious effects of spinal local anesthetics have not been proven, epidural administration is usually the preferred technique where possible. The final choice of anesthetic technique, however, must take into account the risks and benefits for the individual patient in the given situation.[46]

General Anesthesia

General anesthesia itself does not increase the relapse rate in MS unless there is an associated postoperative fever, and there is no clear association between anesthetic drugs used and clinical deterioration.[30] Sevoflurane has been safely used for nonobstetric anesthesia in an MS patient.[47] If disease is severe, succinylcholine-induced hyperkalemia, autonomic hyperreflexia, and postoperative respiratory insufficiency should be considered. A correlation between pyrexia and aggravation of the disease makes avoidance of postoperative fever of paramount importance.

MOTOR NEURON DEGENERATION

Amyotrophic Lateral Sclerosis

Amyotrophic lateral sclerosis is a degenerative disease of the central nervous system affecting upper and lower motor neurons with sparing of the sensory apparatus, coordination, and intellect. It affects males more commonly than females, with a peak incidence between the ages of 40 and 50. An uncommon familial form of the disease has its onset in the late teens. There are few reports of amyotrophic lateral sclerosis in pregnancy.[48]

Amyotrophic lateral sclerosis begins with weakness, atrophy, and fasciculations in the limbs and usually progresses over 1 to 2 years to involve most muscles, including bulbar muscles. Spasticity may also occur. Death is usually from respiratory failure within 6 years.

Obstetric and Neonatal Considerations

Although pregnancy places the parturient with amyotrophic lateral sclerosis at increased risk of respiratory complications, it does not adversely affect the course of the disease or increase the incidence of abnormal fetal development. Delivery is usually normal, spontaneous, and associated with an uneventful postpartum course.[48]

Anesthetic Considerations

The parturient should be assessed for the degree of bulbar involvement and respiratory reserve. There is no evidence contraindicating the use of regional anesthesia for labor or cesarian section. Regional anesthesia may be preferable, to avoid the respiratory depression associated with inhalational agents and parenteral analgesia for labor. If general anesthesia is deemed necessary, then aspiration prophylaxis with metoclopramide and an H_2 antagonist is important. Succinylcholine should be avoided because of the risk of hyperkalemia. Enhanced sensitivity to nondepolarizing neuromuscular blockers should be considered and neuromuscular monitoring utilized.[49] Postoperative ventilation may be required.

Spinal Muscular Atrophy

The spinal muscular atrophies (SMAs) are a group of inherited diseases of motor neurons characterized by selective degeneration of the anterior horn cells of the spinal cord. Proximal SMA is the second most common autosomal recessively inherited disorder after cystic fibrosis, with an estimated incidence of 1 in 10,000 children.[50] The onset of muscular weakness and atrophy is in infancy, childhood, or early adulthood and often progresses slowly; thus, women of childbearing age may be affected. In severe disease, skeletal abnormalities such as kyphoscoliosis and contractures as well as restrictive lung disease may occur.[51]

Obstetric and Neonatal Considerations

Pregnancy complications in patients with SMA include recurrent urinary tract infections, worsening pulmonary function, musculoskeletal pain, exacerbation of muscle weakness, and fatigue. Rudnik-Schöneborn et al.[50] reviewed 17 deliveries in 12 women with SMA. An increased incidence of premature labor (35%) and prolonged labor (24%) was noted. Five patients (42%) claimed their pregnancies were responsible for a permanent exacerbation of SMA, and although the long-term course was still mild in most cases, three patients experienced delayed recovery of between 1 and 2 years. Two of the 17 children later developed SMA.

Vaginal delivery is usually possible,[50] although assistance may be required in the second stage.[52] Cesarian section may need to be performed if disease is severe because pelvic deformities and cephalopelvic disproportion may prohibit vaginal delivery.[51,52] Infants born to these patients may show a muscular hypotonia in the neonatal period but are usually otherwise healthy.[53] They have a small chance of developing SMA, which depends on the SMA subtype and mode of inheritance.[51]

Anesthetic Considerations

The anesthesiologist should be involved at an early stage. An assessment of the severity of the disease is important, especially respiratory reserve, muscle weakness, and fatigability. The lumbar spine should be inspected for likely difficulty with regional anesthesia; if severe kyphoscoliosis and pelvic deformity are present, elective cesarian section may be planned.

Systemic Analgesia. If respiratory reserve is limited, it may be prudent to avoid administration of parenteral or inhalational agents that cause respiratory depression.

Regional Anesthesia. Epidural anesthesia has been used safely for vaginal delivery and cesarian section,[52] and there is no evidence that it affects the course of the disease. In patients with SMA who have kyphoscoliosis, regional anesthesia should still be considered where clinically appropriate, although it may be technically difficult to perform and a patchy block may occur. The use of subarachnoid block in patients with SMA has not been reported.

General Anesthesia. General anesthesia may be required for cesarian section. The airway must be assessed carefully, especially in cases of kyphoscoliosis, and succinylcholine should be avoided because of the risk of hyperkalemia. Hypersensitivity to nondepolarizing neuromuscular blockers should also be considered; the combination of these factors may make awake intubation occasionally necessary. If restrictive lung disease is severe, postoperative ventilation may be required.

Landry-Guillain-Barré Syndrome or Acute Idiopathic Polyneuritis

Landry-Guillain-Barré Syndrome (LGBS) is an acute, immune-mediated, demyelinating polyradiculoneuritis of unknown etiology that affects both sexes and occurs in people of all ages. The syndrome affects 0.7 to 1.9 persons per 100,000 population per year, but the incidence may be slightly lower during pregnancy[54] and higher in the first month postpartum.[55] In about half of patients, neurologic symptoms are preceded by viral gastroenteritis, cytomegalovirus or Epstein-Barr virus infection, or respiratory tract infection by 1 to 8 weeks.[56] Surgery, malignancy, vaccination, and pregnancy[54] have also been implicated as antecedent events.[56]

The syndrome usually presents with motor weakness and a raised protein level but normal cell count in the cerebrospinal fluid. Paralysis usually begins in the lower limbs and may ascend to involve the upper limbs, trunk, and cranial nerves. Thus, in severe cases, total flaccid motor paralysis, bulbar palsy, and respiratory failure can occur. Sensory loss is not usually present, although paresthesias (sometimes painful) can occur. Autonomic dysfunction with hemodynamic instability often occurs. Symptoms peak at 2 to 4 weeks.

Treatment is mostly supportive. Endotracheal intubation may be required for airway protection and respiratory support,[57] especially if vital capacity falls below 13 to 15 mL/kg.[58] Hurley et al.[59] reviewed 31 cases of LGBS in pregnancy and reported that respiratory support was required in 35% of pregnant patients but only 16% of non-pregnant patients. Autonomic instability, which manifests as fluctuating blood pressure, sinus tachycardia, and diaphoresis, may necessitate invasive blood pressure monitoring. Thromboembolic prophylaxis should be considered and physiotherapy is important.

Plasmapheresis, if instituted within 7 days of the onset of symptoms, produces significant improvement in severe cases.[60] High-dose intravenous immunoglobulins may be as effective and have fewer side effects than plasma exchange.[60, 61] Both have been used safely in pregnancy.[59, 62, 63] Corticosteroids are no longer recommended.

Recovery usually begins 2 to 4 weeks after progression stops and is virtually complete in 80% of patients by 6 months. The mortality rate of 10% in pregnancy is greater than the general mortality rate in LGBS patients of 2 to 5%.[60] Death is usually due to pulmonary or thromboembolic complications or cardiac arrhythmia.[64]

Obstetric and Neonatal Considerations

Premature labor may occur, especially in patients requiring ventilatory support.[65] Vaginal delivery is preferable, usually with vacuum or forceps assistance during the second stage, since abdominal muscles are often weak. Unnecessary obstetric intervention must be resisted[65] and induction of labor and cesarian section should be performed only for the usual obstetric indications. Several case reports have reported deterioration of LGBS after cesarian section, which has not been seen after vaginal delivery. Bolik et al.[60] advise that termination by cesarian section is not advantageous, especially in cases of severe respiratory insufficiency.

Most infants born to mothers with LGBS are normal. Nelson et al.[66] in a review of the literature in 1985, found fetal survival in 26 of 27 reported cases of LGBS; the one neonatal death was associated with prematurity. Luijckx et al.[62] reported a tetraplegic parturient on respiratory support who vaginally delivered at 38 weeks' gestation. On day 12, the neonate developed LGBS, which was treated with intravenous immunoglobulin. Both mother and child made a good recovery.

Anesthetic Considerations

The parturient with LGBS should be assessed by the anesthetist at an early stage. Regular measurement of vital capacity is important,[58] as borderline respiratory function may be worsened by the progress of pregnancy. If disease is mild near term, or if it has peaked in the first or second trimester and is remitting, then spontaneous vaginal delivery with epidural block, if indicated, should be an achievable goal.[66–68]

If disease is severe near term and positive pressure ventilation is required, premature labor may be more likely to occur and painless contractions have been described.[65] The parturient should be allowed to labor spontaneously and deliver vaginally when possible, although assistance in the second stage will often be required.[62, 65, 68] Invasive blood pressure monitoring should be instituted if autonomic instability is present, and the possibility of autonomic hyperreflexia, as seen in paraplegics, should be considered.

Systemic Analgesia. If there is limited respiratory reserve, it may be prudent to avoid the parenteral or inhalational administration of respiratory depressant analgesics.

Regional Anesthesia. Epidural anesthesia has been used for both labor[66] and cesarian section.[67] McGrady[67] reported a patient who presented at 38 weeks' gestation with severe limb weakness and adequate respiratory function and went into spontaneous labor 2 weeks later. A lumbar epidural with 4 mL of 0.25% bupivacaine initially provided adequate analgesia and four further 4 mL top-ups were required. Eight hours later, a cesarian section was required because of failure to progress and fetal bradycardia, and an additional 7 mL of 0.5% bupivacaine was used. McGrady[67] commented on the small doses of local anesthetic required. Neuraxial anesthesia is well reported in patients with LGBS, since lower limb pain in non-pregnant patients with this disease is often managed with epidural infusions of bupivacaine, fentanyl, and morphine.[69–72] However, some concern over the use of epidurals has been expressed. The onset of LGBS following epidural anesthesia for delivery, surgical procedures, and analgesia has been described.[73, 74] LGBS after surgery without epidural is also well described, and no clear causal relationship between epidurals and LGBS has been established. Gautier et al.[75] reported one case in which a parturient developed LGBS 24 hours after obstetric epidural for delivery. The authors suggested that a relationship between the two is unlikely.

Currently, there is no evidence that epidural anesthesia should be withheld in patients with active LGBS or a history of the disease. If regional anesthesia is chosen, one must ensure good intravenous hydration, especially in the presence of autonomic instability, and establish the block slowly, as small doses may be all that is required.

Although lumbar puncture is performed routinely, there are no reports of subarachnoid anesthesia in patients with LGBS.

General Anesthesia. Avoidance of general anesthesia for cesarian section is important, especially for parturients who retain adequate respiratory function without ventilation.[67] Invasive blood pressure monitoring should be used with careful intravenous hydration.

If autonomic instability is present, the patient may be sensitive to intravenous induction agents. Succinylcholine should be avoided because of the risk of hyperkalemia. Increased sensitivity to nondepolarizing neuromuscular blockers may occur, even after apparent full recovery of muscle strength from previous LGBS.[76] Postoperative ventilation may be required.

SPINAL CORD INJURY

Spinal cord injury (SCI) in women of childbearing age is most commonly due to trauma; other causes include neoplasia, infection, and vascular anomalies. The obstetric anesthetist may be involved in the management of acute spinal cord injury in the pregnant patient or, more commonly, the management of a patient with chronic SCI presenting for delivery.

Acute Spinal Cord Injury

The anesthetic management of the pregnant trauma patient begins with assessment of the airway and breathing, with stabilization of the cervical spine. Circulatory management follows, with attention to lateral uterine displacement. In the third trimester, fetal monitoring should be applied early, as it provides information about both maternal perfusion status and fetal well-being. One must keep in mind that due to the physiologic expansion of blood volume in pregnancy, in the third trimester the loss of 30 to 35% of the circulating blood volume can occur prior to changes in heart rate and blood pressure.[77] In all cases of severe trauma in the third trimester, an obstetrician should be consulted urgently to evaluate the condition of the fetus and to manage premature labor, should it develop. The obstetrician should consider delivery by cesarian section if either the fetus is in distress and the mother is stable, or if it is certain the mother will not survive and the fetus is of a viable gestational age.[78]

The evaluation and management of the pregnant patient after severe trauma is even more challenging if an acute SCI is present. The acute SCI may itself create hemodynamic and respiratory compromise and also obscure signs of injury in the lower body. Loss of thermoregulation below the level of injury occurs, so attention to maintaining normothermia is important.

Hypotension in a patient with acute SCI may be due to neurogenic shock, although other causes, particularly hypovolemia, must be excluded. Bradycardia may also occur if the cardiac accelerator fibers are involved, and certain maneuvers such as intubation or tracheal suctioning may precipitate severe bradycardia or even asystole. Pretreatment with oxygen and atropine before such maneuvers has been advocated.[79] The initial treatment of hypotension is judicious fluid replacement guided by heart rate, urine output, and invasive measurement of arterial and central venous pressures. Pulmonary capillary wedge pressure measurement may also be helpful. Once hypovolemia is excluded, the use of positive inotropes such as dopamine and dobutamine in the lower dose range may be desirable, bearing in mind they may have β-adrenergic effects on uterine smooth muscle.[80] Continuous fetal monitoring should be used if inotropes are required, as they may reduce uterine blood flow.[81]

Respiratory compromise is common following trauma to the spinal cord rostral to C-5 and may be exacerbated by the physiologic changes of pregnancy. Acutely, spirometry and arterial blood gas parameters should be monitored. If intubation is required, an awake technique is often preferable due to the combination of the oropharyngeal edema of pregnancy and cervical spine instability. Chest physiotherapy should be commenced early.

The usual signs of intraperitoneal hemorrhage may be obscured by both the SCI and the gravid uterus. If peritoneal lavage is required in late pregnancy, it should be performed through a high gastric entry point with an open technique.[80] The fetus should be shielded from diagnostic radiation where feasible, although diagnostic studies should not be withheld for this reason.[77]

It has been reported by Bracken et al.[82] that high-dose methylprednisolone given by intravenous infusion within 8 hours (and preferably within 3 hours) of an acute SCI with neurologic deficit, improves neurologic outcome. A loading dose of 30 mg/kg body weight should be infused over several minutes, followed by an infusion of 5.4 mg/kg/hr for 23 hours. Blood sugar levels should be monitored frequently during the infusion, especially if gestational diabetes is present.

Thromboembolic prophylaxis with intermittent pneumatic calf compression, compression stockings, or low molecular weight heparin[77] should be commenced early. A nasogastric tube and indwelling urinary catheter should be inserted, pressure area relief every 2 hours commenced, and a parenteral H_2 receptor antagonist commenced as prophylaxis against stress ulceration of the gastrointestinal tract.

The period of neurogenic shock usually lasts 1 to 3 weeks, but may be as short as a few days or as long as 6 to 8 weeks.[79] According to Gilson et al.,[80] during this period if the level of SCI is above T-10 and complete transection has occurred, surgery can be performed without anesthesia. No case reports of this were found in the literature and one must be aware that the transition phase may be difficult to define and therefore the risk of autonomic hyperreflexia may exist.

Chronic Spinal Cord Injury

The chronic state that develops following spinal cord injury is characterized by muscle atrophy and spasticity with exaggerated reflexes and hypertonicity. The patient is then at risk of developing autonomic hyperreflexia and mass motor response.

Chronic SCI problems that may be exacerbated by pregnancy include urinary tract infections, chronic renal failure, postural and resting hypotension,[83] spasticity, anemia, decubitus ulcers, and deep venous thrombosis. Routine prophylactic anticoagulation is not recommended unless other risk factors for deep venous thrombosis exist.[78]

The parturient with a cervical or high thoracic injury, with intercostal muscle paralysis, may have borderline respiratory function. Diaphragmatic respiration may be impaired by the advancing pregnancy and may produce the need for ventilatory support, especially with the increased demands of labor. These patients require serial measurements of vital capacity[78] and will generally need ventilation if vital capacity falls below 15 mL/kg.[58] Medications used in the treatment of spasticity, such as baclofen, clonidine, and dantrolene, are uncommonly prescribed in pregnancy.[78]

Most women with SCI know their disability well. Medical and nursing staff must listen to the patient, as she is the expert on management of her day-to-day skin care, bowel care, and bladder care. Cooperation between the anesthetist, spinal physician, and obstetrician as well as nursing staff from these three specialty areas is essential.

Autonomic Hyperreflexia

Eighty-five percent of patients with a lesion at T-6 or above develop autonomic hyperreflexia (AH) in response to cutaneous or visceral stimuli below the level of the spinal cord lesion.[84–87] Common precipitants include urinary retention (e.g., blocked catheter), constipation, tight clothing, or decubitus ulceration. Uterine contractions and surgical stimulus may also precipitate AH. This potentially life-threatening complication results from generalized autonomic overactivity and is characterized by hypertension relative to normal baseline blood pressure due to peripheral and splanchnic vasoconstriction. Other features include vagally mediated bradycardia (and other arrhythmias), sweating, headache, increased spasticity and cutaneous vasodilation above the level of the lesion.[87] In severe circumstances, seizures,[88] intracranial hemorrhage,[79, 86, 89, 90] and death may occur.[91]

During labor or cesarean section, continuous monitoring of blood pressure, electrocardiogram, uterine activity, and fetal well-being are recommended for all parturients at risk for AH (see Anesthetic Considerations). AH often occurs at the onset of labor but has been reported in the antepartum, intrapartum, and postpartum periods.[87, 88, 92, 93]

Preeclampsia is an important differential diagnosis. The onset of symptoms before, rather than with, the onset of labor occurs in most cases of preeclampsia.[85] The pattern of cyclic hypertension in which blood pressure rises during uterine contractions and falls between contractions seen in AH may help distinguish it from the persistent hypertension seen with preeclampsia. Augmentation of reflexes above the spinal lesion implies preeclampsia rather than AH.[85] Unlike AH, preeclampsia most often persists into the postpartum period. AH may also be associated with mass motor response, in which muscle spasms occur in distal muscle groups.

Treatment of AH includes removal of any known precipitating stimulus, such as a full bladder. Tight clothing should be loosened and the patient sat upright whenever possible[86, 94] to induce postural changes in blood pressure. Antihypertensive treatment with drugs such as nifedipine, hydralazine, nitroprusside, phentolamine,[87] labetalol, and nitroglycerin[78, 86, 94] can be used, with short-acting agents recommended to avoid hypotension and fetal compromise between contractions. Regional and general anesthesia are also effective (see Anesthetic Considerations).

Obstetric and Neonatal Considerations

Pregnancy rates[95] and incidence of spontaneous abortions, stillbirth, and intrauterine growth retardation are not affected by chronic SCI,[78, 89] but there is controversy as to whether there is a slightly increased risk of premature labor in these women.[78] In cases in which premature labor does occur, it may be precipitated by infection, usually of the urinary tract.[94] The majority of women with chronic SCI, including those with high lesions, are able to perceive labor in some way.[92] It may manifest as pain, pressure, abdominal or leg spasms, difficulty breathing, or symptoms of AH.[85] Despite this, there will always be a subset of patients with no perception of labor and it is reasonable to instruct all parturients with chronic SCI how to palpate for uterine activity to detect contractions at home. The parturients who are most likely not to perceive labor at all are those with a complete SCI at or above T-10[88] but not high enough (above T-6) to expect symptoms of AH with uterine contractions. In such a case, the risk for unattended delivery at home exists and regular external tocodynamometry[80] and weekly cervical examinations during the third trimester may be recommended.[85, 88, 93] Many patients are admitted to a spinal unit[94] after 36 weeks or when cervical changes occur, to prevent delivery at home. With the introduction of home uterine activity monitoring, it is hoped that more patients may remain at home until closer to term.[96]

The labor of the parturient with chronic SCI does not seem to differ significantly from that of the general population, however, low forceps or vacuum may be required in the second stage because of weakness of expulsive efforts or hypertension or both. Induction of labor should be performed only if obstetric indications exist,[78] as it may increase the risk of AH.[89, 90, 96, 97] A local anesthetic jelly should be used for vaginal examinations in unanesthetized patients at risk of AH.[78, 89] Similarly, local anesthetic on the urinary catheter should minimize this problem.[98]

Cesarean section is appropriately restricted to circumstances in which an obstetric indication exists.[99] It may occasionally be required because of complications of the paraplegia, such as bony deformity of the spine or pelvis, or due to intractable AH unresponsive to antihypertensives or regional block in which the time to vaginal delivery seems remote.[78, 98] Ergot-containing drugs should not be used in the third stage.[94]

Anesthetic Considerations

The obstetric anesthesiologist should be consulted at the time of acute SCI if it occurs during pregnancy. In chronic SCI, consultation should take place early in the third trimester. Important goals of the anesthetic consultation are outlined in Table 46–4.

The parturient at risk for AH should have intravenous access established at the onset of labor and be instructed to communicate any symptoms of AH. If the risk of AH is relatively low (lesion below T-7 with no history of AH), regular noninvasive measurement of blood pressure will suffice initially. If symptoms or signs of AH develop or if the risk is high from the outset, an epidural catheter should be inserted and invasive blood pressure monitoring commenced via a radial artery cannula.[98] This gives beat-to-beat arterial pressure changes with a low risk of complications. These high-risk patients should also have continuous electrocardiographic monitoring because rhythm disturbances, including second-degree atrioventricular block and ventricular bigeminy, may occur.[85]

Monitoring of uterine contractions and continuous fetal monitoring[98] by Doppler or fetal scalp electrode is recommended. One must be aware that constraining abdominal belts can precipitate AH.[89] If respiratory compromise is a concern, pulse oximetry should also be used[100] and mechanical support of ventilation should be immediately available.[98]

Table 46–4 Anesthetic Consultation in Chronic Spinal Cord Injury

1. Assess the level of the lesion.
2. Determine the time since injury and the safety of succinylcholine (high risk 3 days to 9 months)
3. Determine the severity of associated problems, including urinary tract infection, spasms, and decubitus ulcers.
4. History of spinal surgery, especially lumbar or cervical.
5. Inquire about symptoms of cardiovascular instability, such as a history of postural dizziness or symptoms of AH (e.g., headache and sweating with full bladder).
6. Assess for respiratory insufficiency or respiratory tract infection; measure and record vital capacity. Consider arterial blood gas analysis and pulmonary function tests as appropriate.
7. Assess the airway and cervical spine mobility.
8. Medications, especially low molecular weight heparin, and allergies, particularly to latex.
9. Measure:
   Complete blood cell count—anemia is common.
   Urea, electrolytes and creatinine—chronic renal failure may occur.
10. Assess previous anesthetic and other records where available.
11. Discuss the role of epidural analgesia in the management of labor pain (lesion below T-10[99]), spasms, and AH (lesion above T-7).
12. Obtain informed consent for regional anesthesia. Include a discussion of potential technical difficulties and possible failure.
13. Inform the patient that peripheral nerve injury may occur with pregnancy, obstetric interventions, and herniated lumbar disc not related to anesthesia care.[109]
14. If the patient is at high risk for AH, particularly discuss:
    Risks and benefits of epidural analgesia commenced before labor.
    Invasive blood pressure, electrocardiographic, pulse oximetry, and fetal monitoring during labor.
15. If risk of respiratory compromise exists, discuss possibility of mechanical ventilation because of the advancing pregnancy and the work of labor.
16. Discuss with obstetrician and spinal physician a plan for delivery.

AH, autonomic hyperreflexia.

Systemic Analgesia. Parturients at low risk of AH and respiratory insufficiency may be given parenteral analgesics as required. If the risk is high, however, regional anesthesia should be instituted early, to reduce the risk of both AH and respiratory depression with systemic analgesics.

Regional Anesthesia. Both subarachnoid block and epidural anesthesia have been used successfully for labor and cesarean section (Table 46–5). By interrupting noxious sensory input, these neuraxial techniques have advantges over antihypertensive medications in the management of AH, as well as preventing mass motor response. Epidural anesthesia is the most common method used in labor, usually by infusion of local anesthetic solution to maintain a constant level of blockade.[99] A correctly sited epidural block can effectively prevent the development of AH for the duration of labor[101] and the early postpartum period,[79, 88, 99] as well as during cesarean section.[102] It has been recommended that an epidural be placed before the onset of labor in those with high lesions or a history of AH[99] and it may be appropriate to leave the catheter in situ for 48 hours post-delivery, when the risk of AH subsides.[103]

Bupivacaine has been the most commonly reported local anesthetic used for labor in these patients. In cases in which low concentrations have failed to control AH, increasing the concentration up to 0.5% will often be effective.[101] Epidural fentanyl alone is not successful in preventing AH.[100] One report of the successful use of epidural pethidine alone (100 mg in 10 mL saline) to prevent AH has been attributed to its local anesthetic properties.[84] Opiates such as pethidine may be added to the infusion of local anesthetic to minimize the dose of local anesthetic required and the loss of sympathetic tone.[100]

An epidural anesthetic may, however, fail to control AH. Failure to block some segments due to a distorted epidural space is the most likely explanation and may be compounded by difficulty in accurately assessing the completeness of the epidural block.[79] In the situation in which epidural anesthesia has failed to control AH in labor,[97] subarachnoid block with a continuous catheter technique is the treatment of choice. During the second stage of labor, however, a pudendal block or even local infiltration for episiotomy, delivery and repair may be helpful.[78, 94]

Subarachnoid block is the anesthesia technique of choice for general surgery in the patient with chronic SCI who is at risk for AH.[87] It has been widely reported

Table 46-5 TECHNICAL ASPECTS OF REGIONAL ANESTHESIA IN PATIENTS WITH SPINAL CORD INJURY

1. If the spine has not yet been stabilized, the patient may be "log-rolled" onto her side, with the aid of neurosurgeons providing head control, to achieve regional anesthesia.
2. Positioning of patient and placement of needle may be difficult in the parturient with chronic SCI if spasms cause lordosis or if fixed distortion of the vertebral column such as kyphoscoliosis is present. Despite this, SAB is usually possible.[104]
3. Previous back surgery, even if instrumentation remains in situ, does not contraindicate regional anesthesia.[110]
4. Decubitus ulcers in the lumbar region must be avoided and may make regional anesthesia impossible.
5. Parturients should be vigorously prehydrated[87] and uterine displacement performed.
6. The room should be warm and the patient kept covered to prevent hypothermia.
7. Significant hypotension is not a common problem with SAB*[104] or epidural if the block is established slowly,[99] probably owing to the already low levels of sympathetic tone.
8. Ephedrine can be used with care to correct hypotension[104]; an anticholinergic should also be readily available.
9. Local anesthetic solutions containing epinephrine have been used,[99] but care should be taken because of the greater sensitivity of the patient with chronic SCI to catecholamines.[79, 96]
10. Accidental intrathecal injection of an epidural test dose of local anesthetic may not be noticed and one must proceed with caution, with the risk of total spinal anesthesia in mind.[104]
11. Assessment of the level of the block may be difficult in high spinal injury, and one should look for flaccid paralysis with loss of spasticity, loss of reflexes such as knee-jerk and abdominal reflexes, and improved control of blood pressure.
12. Good fixation of epidural catheters is important, as tape may become loose if the patient develops autonomic hyperreflexia.[103]

SAB, subarachnoid block; SCI, spinal cord injury.
*<3% of non-pregnant population.

as being more effective than epidural anesthesia in preventing AH.[104, 105] Subarachnoid block is also recommended when emergency cesarean section is required.[80] For elective cesarean section, a combined spinal-epidural technique may be preferable to either technique alone in the patient at risk for AH, providing dense intraoperative block plus postoperative interruption of afferent stimuli by epidural infusion.

General Anesthesia. Regional anesthesia is the technique of choice for cesarean section but is not always possible, for example for technical reasons, such as previous lumbar surgery or large decubitus ulcers,[87] or if the urgency of the situation necessitates general anesthesia. Gastric emptying is delayed in patients with high spinal cord injury[79] even in the non-pregnant state, so antacid prophylaxis is essential. Premedication with oral nifedipine should be considered if the risk of AH is high and an antihypertensive should be prepared for use in addition to general anesthesia, if required. Routine monitoring, including pulse oximetry, capnography, and electrocardiography, should be enhanced by the addition of temperature measurement and invasive blood pressure monitoring. Measurement of central venous pressure may also be helpful, especially in cases in which significant blood loss is anticipated.

There may be a greater sensitivity to intravenous induction agents in these patients, due to the lower blood volume and thus volume of distribution.[79] Therefore, adequate prehydration is essential to minimize hypotension.[104] Judicious use of direct-acting vasoactive drugs may be required to allow sufficient depth of anesthesia to prevent AH.[87] Indirectly acting sympathetic agents should be used with care because of the greater sensitivity of the patient with chronic SCI to catecholamines.[79, 96]

Depolarizing muscle relaxants such as succinylcholine should not be used for a period beginning 72 hours after acute SCI[106, 107] for at least 9 months, owing to the risk of severe hyperkalemia and cardiac arrest. Nondepolarizing neuromuscular blockers may be used to facilitate intubation and mechanical ventilation and to prevent mass motor response of the abdominal muscles,[87] although smaller doses may be required than in non-SCI patients.[79]

Patients with a high lesion (above T-4) causing interruption of cardiac accelerator fibers will have bradycardia and decreased inotropy. They have a high incidence of conduction defects, heart block, and ventricular arrhythmias due to high vagal tone and should have a preoperative electrocardiogram.[87] Profound bradycardia may occur on intubation, and prior administration of atropine should be considered, especially in the early stages of neurogenic shock or if the heart rate is less than 60.

Airway management may be challenging with the combination of airway edema and cervical spine disease, especially if depolarizing muscle relaxants are contraindicated. Techniques such as awake intubation and the use of the newer, rapid-onset nondepolarizing neuromuscular blockers in a modified rapid-sequence induction should be considered. The technique chosen must ultimately be based on the risk and benefit for each individual.

General anesthesia of adequate depth is required to prevent AH, the depth of anesthesia during surgery being more important than the choice of volatile agent.[86, 104] Isoflurane has advantages over other inhalational agents because of its direct depression of peripheral vascular tone with minimal negative inotropy and arrhythmogenic action.[87] Hypotension with deep levels of anesthesia is a risk,[79] and Baker and Cardenas[78] have recommended supplementing general anesthesia with regional anesthesia to limit inhalational agent requirement and also to reduce the risks of neonatal depression and blood loss due to uterine atony.

Patients with high chronic SCI lesions are more

sensitive to hypotension associated with positive pressure ventilation and myocardial depressants and are unable to compensate for blood loss, so losses must be replaced diligently. Pressure areas should be carefully padded and body temperature checked regularly. Techniques such as warming the operating room and using a warming blanket, fluid warmer, and humidifier should be implemented. Tracheal extubation should not be considered unless the patient is warm and cardiovascularly stable with no residual neuromuscular blockade or volatile agent. Respiratory insufficiency may warrant postoperative ventilation.[87] AH may occur in the recovery room or the postoperative period after general anesthesia.[104] This may be reduced by epidural supplementation. Deep venous thrombosis prophylaxis is important in the postoperative period.

CONCLUSION

Most women with neurologic disease have normal fertility and can achieve a vaginal delivery with good neonatal outcome. A tertiary institution with experience in managing complicated parturients is recommended.

Epidural anesthesia has been widely used in parturients with epilepsy, MS, LGBS, and chronic SCI. There is no evidence that it is detrimental to the course of any of the neurologic diseases discussed. Subarachnoid block may have advantages over epidural in chronic SCI parturients at risk of AH but should be used cautiously in the parturient with MS until further evidence supporting its safety is available. General anesthesia is best avoided, but, when it is necessary, the potential for hyperkalemia with succinylcholine and increased sensitivity to nondepolarizing neuromuscular blockers must be considered.

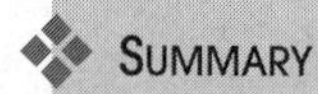

Summary

Key Points

- Most parturients with neurologic disease will be able to vaginally deliver a normal, healthy infant.
- In the parturient with epilepsy, meperidine (pethidine) and phenothiazines should be avoided, as they may be proconvulsant, whereas epidural local anesthetics may have an anticonvulsant effect.
- The parturient with multiple sclerosis must be informed that she has a two- to threefold increase in the risk of exacerbation in the postpartum period. She should be reassured that epidural analgesia has no adverse effect on the rate of relapse or the progression to disability. The use of subarachnoid anesthesia is more controversial.

Key Reference

Confavreux C, Hutchinson M, Hours MM, et al: Rate of pregnancy-related relapse in multiple sclerosis. N Engl J Med 1998; 30:285–291.

Case Stem

A 25-year-old nullipara has had a chronic SCI at the level of T-5 since a motor vehicle accident 18 months previously. She is now at 34 weeks' gestation and is referred for an anesthetic consultation. List the main aims of the anesthetic assessment and describe your anesthetic plan for labor and delivery.

References

1. Sawhney H, et al: Pregnancy with epilepsy: A retrospective analysis. Int J Gynecol Obstet 1996; 54:17–22.
2. Schachter S, Yerby M: Management of epilepsy: Pharmacologic therapy and quality-of-life issues. Postgrad Med 1997; 101:133–153.
3. Yerby M, Devinsky O: Epilepsy and pregnancy [review]. Adv Neurol 1994; 64:45–63.
4. Blume W: Epilepsy: Advances in management. Eur Neurol 1997; 38:198–208.
5. Eller D, Patterson C, Webb G: Maternal and fetal implications of anticonvulsive therapy during pregnancy. Obstet Gynecol Clin North Am 1997; 24:523–534.
6. Sabers A, et al: Pregnancy and epilepsy: A retrospective study of 151 pregnancies. Acta Neurol Scand 1998; 97:164–170.
7. Cheng A, Kwan A: Perioperative management of intra-partum seizure. Anaesth Intensive Care 1997; 25:535–538.
8. Awada A, Watson T, Obeid T: Cavernous angioma presenting as pregnancy-related seizures. Epilepsia 1997; 38:844–846.
9. Fox M, Harms R, Davis D: Selected neurologic complications of pregnancy. Mayo Clin Proc 1990; 65:1595–1618.
10. Crawford P: Epilepsy and pregnancy: Good management reduces the risk. Prof Care Mother Child 1997; 7:17–18.
11. Shuster E: Epilepsy in women. Mayo Clin Proc 1996; 71:991–999.
12. Modica P, Tempelhoff R, White P: Pro- and anticonvulsant effects of anesthetics (part 2). Anesth Analg 1990; 70:433–444.
13. Delgado-Escueta A, Janz D: Consensus guidelines: Preconception counseling, management and care of the pregnant women with epilepsy. Neurology 1992; 42(Suppl 5):149–160.
14. Samren E, et al: Maternal use of antiepileptic drugs and the risk of major congenital malformations: A joint European prospective study of human teratogenesis associated with maternal epilepsy. Epilepsia 1997; 38:981–990.
15. Brodie M, Dichter M: Antiepileptic drugs. N Engl J Med 1996; 334:168–175.
16. Hiilesmaa V: Pregnancy and birth in women with epilepsy. Neurology 1992; 42(Suppl 5):8–11.
17. Svigos J: Epilepsy and pregnancy. Aust N Z J Obstet Gynaecol 1984; 24:182–185.
18. Yerby M: Teratogenic efffects of antiepileptic drugs: What do we advise patients? Epilepsia 1997; 38:957–958.
19. Lindhout D, et al: Antiepileptic drugs and teratogenesis in two consecutive cohorts: Changes in prescription policy paralleled by changes in pattern of malformations. Neurology 1992; 42(Suppl 5):94–110.
20. Nulman I, et al: Findings in children exposed in utero to phenytoin and carbamazepine monotherapy: Independent effects of epilepsy and medications. Am J Med Genet 1997; 68:18–24.
21. Modica P, Tempelhoff R, White P: Pro- and anticonvulsant effects of anesthetics (part 1). Anesth Analg 1990; 70:303–315.
22. Merrell D, Koch M: Epidural anesthesia as an anticonvulsant in the management of hypertensive and eclamptic patients in labour. S Afr Med J 1980; 58:875–877.
23. Sun K: Convulsion following spinal anesthesia [correspondence]. Anaesth Intensive Care 1995; 23:520–521.
24. Bolton V, Leicht C, Scanlon T: Postpartum seizure after

epidural blood patch and intravenous caffeine sodium benzoate. Anesthesiology 1989; 70:146–149.
25. Evans D: Anaesthesia and the epileptic patient: A review. Anaesthesia 1975; 30:34–45.
26. Hansen H, Drenck N: Generalised seizures after etomidate anaesthesia. Anaesthesia 1988; 43:805–806.
27. Harrigan P, Browne S, Quail A: Multiple seizures following re-exposure to propofol. Anaesth Intensive Care 1996; 24:261–264.
28. Ornstein E, et al: The effect of phenytoin on the magnitude and duration of neuromuscular block following atracurium or vecuronium. Anesthesiology 1987; 67:191–196.
29. Confavreux C, et al: Rate of pregnancy-related relapse in multiple sclerosis. N Engl J Med 1998; 339:285–291.
30. Siemkowicz E: Multiple sclerosis and surgery. Anaesthesia 1976; 31:1211–1216.
31. Damek D, Shuster E: Pregnancy and multiple sclerosis. Mayo Clin Proc 1997; 72:977–989.
32. Achiron A, et al: Intravenous immunoglobulin treatment in the prevention of childbirth-associated acute exacerbations in multiple sclerosis: A pilot study. J Neurol 1996; 243:25–28.
33. Runmarker B, Andersen O: Pregnancy is associated with a lower risk of onset and a better risk in multiple sclerosis. Brain 1995; 118:253–261.
34. Davis R, Maslow A: Multiple sclerosis in pregnancy: A review. Obstet Gynecol Survey 1992; 47:290–296.
35. Bader A, et al: Anesthesia for the obstetric patient with multiple sclerosis. J Clin Anesth 1988; 1:21–24.
36. Crawford J, et al: Regional analgesia for patients with chronic neurological disease and similar conditions [letter]. Anaesthesia 1981; 36:821.
37. Salvador M, et al: Multiple sclerosis and obstetric epidural analgesia. Rev Esp Anestesiol Reanim 1997; 44:33–35.
38. Jones R, Healy T: Regional analgesia for patients with chronic neurological disease and similar conditions [letter reply]. Anaesthesia 1981; 36:821–822.
39. Eickhoff K, et al: Protein profile of cerebrospinal fluid in multiple sclerosis with special reference to the function of the blood brain barrier. J Neurol 1977; 214:207–215.
40. Hammes E: Neurological complications associated with spinal anaesthesia (eight cases). Minnesota Med 1943; 36:339–345.
41. Tui C, et al: Local nervous tissue changes following spinal anesthesia in experimental animals. J Pharmacol Exp Ther 1944; 81:209–217.
42. Bamford C, Sibley W, Laguna J: Anesthesia in multiple sclerosis. Can J Neurol Sci 1978; 5:41–44.
43. Stenuit J, Marchand P: Les sequelles de rachi-anesthesie. Acta Neurol Psychiatr Belg 1968; 68:626–635.
44. Berger J, Ontell R: Intrathecal morphine in conjunction with a combined spinal and general anesthetic in a patient with multiple sclerosis. Anesthesiology 1987; 66:400–402.
45. Leigh J, Fearnley S-J, Lupprian K: Intrathecal diamorphine during laparotomy in a patient with advanced multiple sclerosis. Anaesthesia 1990; 43:640–642.
46. Leigh J: Intrathecal diamorphine and multiple sclerosis [reply to comment]. Anaesthesia 1990; 45:1084–1085.
47. Kohno K, et al: Sevoflurane anesthesia in a patient with multiple sclerosis. Masui 1994; 43:1229–1232.
48. Levine M, Michels R: Pregnancy and amyotrophic lateral sclerosis. Ann Neurol 1977; 1:408.
49. Rosenbaum K, Neigh J, Strobel G: Sensitivity to nondepolarizing muscle relaxants in amyotrophic lateral sclerosis: Report of two cases. Anesthesiology 1971; 35:638–641.
50. Rudnik-Schöneborn S, et al: Pregnancy and spinal muscular atrophy. J Neurol 1992; 239:26–30.
51. Carter G, Bonekat H, Milio L: Successful pregnancies in the presence of spinal muscular atrophy: Two case reports. Arch Phys Med Rehabil 1994; 75:229–231.
52. Wilson R, Williams K: Spinal muscular atrophy and pregnancy. Br J Obstet Gynaecol 1992; 99:516–517.
53. Dietz U, Gigon U: Pregnancy and labor in chronic anterior horn lesion [in German]. Z Geburtshilfe Perinatol 1989; 193:155–158.
54. Jiang G-X, et al: Pregnancy and Guillain-Barré syndrome: A nationwide register cohort study. Neuroepidemiology 1996; 15:192–200.
55. Mendizabal J, Bassam B: Guillain-Barré syndrome and cytomegalovirus infection during pregnancy. South Med J 1997; 90:63–64.
56. Laufenburg H, Sirus S: Guillain-Barré syndrome in pregnancy. AFP 1989; 39:147–150.
57. Gracey D, et al: Respiratory failure in Guillain-Barré syndrome: A 6-year experience. Mayo Clin Proc 1982; 57:742–746.
58. Macklem P: Muscular weakness and respiratory function [editorial]. N Engl J Med 1986; 314:775–776.
59. Hurley T, et al: Landry Guillain-Barré Strohl syndrome in pregnancy: Report of three cases treated with plasmapheresis. Obstet Gynecol 1991; 78:482–485.
60. Bolik A, Wissel J, Rolfs A: Guillain-Barré syndrome in pregnancy: Two case reports and a discussion on management. Arch Gynecol Obstet 1995; 256:199–203.
61. Thornton C, Griggs R: Plasma exchange and intravenous immunoglobulin treatment of neuromuscular disease. Ann Neurol 1994; 35:260–268.
62. Luijckx G, et al: Guillain-Barré syndrome in mother and newborn child [letter]. Lancet, 1997; 349:27.
63. Kuller J, et al: Pregnancy complicated by Guillain-Barré syndrome. South Med J 1995; 88:987–989.
64. Winer JB, Hughes RA, Greenwood RJ, et al: Prognosis in Guillain-Barré syndrome. Lancet 1985; 1(8439):1202–1203.
65. Quinlan D, et al: Guillain-Barré syndrome in pregnancy: A case report. S Afr Med J 1988; 73:611–612.
66. Nelson L, McLean W: Management of Landry-Guillain-Barré syndrome in pregnancy. Obstet Gynecol 1985; 65(Suppl):25S–29S.
67. McGrady E: Management of labour and delivery in a patient with Guillain-Barré syndrome. Anaesthesia 1987; 42:899.
68. Sudo N, Weingold A: Obstetric aspects of the Guillain-Barré syndrome. Obstet Gynecol 1975; 45:39–43.
69. Ali M, Hutfluss R: Epidural fentanyl-bupivacaine infusion for management of pain in the Guillain-Barré syndrome. Reg Anesth 1992; 17:171–174.
70. Connelly M, Shagrin J, Warfield C: Epidural opioids for the management of pain in a patient with the Guillain-Barré syndrome. Anesthesiology 1990; 72:381–383.
71. Longobardi J, Comens R, Jacobs A: Epidural morphine as an adjuvant to the treatment of pain in a patient with acute inflammatory polyradiculopathy secondary to Guillain-Barré syndrome. J Foot Surg 1991; 30:267–268.
72. Genis D, et al: Epidural morphine analgesia in Guillain Barré syndrome. J Neurol Neurosurg Psych 1989; 52:999–1001.
73. Rosenberg S, Stacey B: Postoperative Guillain-Barré syndrome, arachnoiditis, and epidural analgesia. Reg Anesth 1996; 21:486–489.
74. Steiner I, et al: Guillain-Barré syndrome after epidural anesthesia: Direct nerve root damage may trigger disease. Neurology 1985; 35:1473–1475.
75. Gautier P, et al: Guillain-Barré syndrome after obstetrical epidural analgesia. Reg Anesth 1989; 14:251–252.
76. Sibert K, Sladen R: Impaired ventilatory capacity after recovery from Guillain-Barré syndrome. J Clin Anesth 1994; 6:133–138.
77. Nunn C, Bass J, Eddy V: Management of the pregnant patient with acute spinal cord injury. Tennessee Med 1996; 89:335–337.
78. Baker E, Cardenas D: Pregnancy in spinal cord injured women. Arch Phys Med Rehabil 1996; 77:501–507.
79. Hambly P, Martin B: Anaesthesia for chronic spinal cord lesions. Anaesthesia 1998; 53:273–289.
80. Gilson G, et al: Acute spinal cord injury and neurogenic shock in pregnancy. Obstet Gynecol Surv 1995; 50:556–560.
81. Rolbin S, Levinson G, Shnider S: Dopamine treatment of spinal hypotension decreases uterine blood flow in the pregnant ewe. Anesthesiology 1979; 51:36–40.
82. Bracken M, et al: A randomized, controlled trial of methylprednisolone or naloxone in the treatment of acute spinal-cord injury. N Engl J Med 1990; 322:1405–1411.
83. Westgren N, et al: Pregnancy and delivery in women with a traumatic spinal cord injury in Sweden, 1980–1991. Obstet Gynecol 1993; 81:926–930.

84. Baraka A: Epidural meperidine for control of autonomic hyperreflexia in a paraplegic parturient. Anesthesiology 1985; 62:688–690.
85. Wanner M, Rageth C, Zach G: Pregnancy and autonomic hyperreflexia in patients with spinal cord lesions. Paraplegia 1987; 25:482–490.
86. Colachis S: Autonomic hyperreflexia with spinal cord injury. J Am Paraplegia Soc 1992; 15:171–186.
87. Amzallag M: Autonomic hyperreflexia. Int Anesthesiol Clin 1993; 31:87–102.
88. Cross L, et al: Pregnancy, labor and delivery post spinal cord injury. Paraplegia 1992; 30:890–902.
89. McGregor J, Meeuwsen J: Autonomic hyperreflexia: A mortal danger for spinal cord-damaged women in labor. Am J Obstet Gynecol 1985; 151:330–333.
90. Verduyn W: Pregnancy and delivery in tetraplegic women. J Spinal Cord Med 1997; 20:371–374.
91. Abouleish E: Hypertension in a paraplegic parturient. Anesthesiology 1980; 53:348–349.
92. Craig D: The adaption to pregnancy of spinal cord injured women. Rehabil Nurs 1990; 15:6–9.
93. Baker E, Cardenas D, Benedetti T: Risks associated with pregnancy in spinal cord-injured women. Obstet Gynecol 1992; 80:425–428.
94. Hughes S, et al: Management of the pregnant woman with spinal cord injuries. Br J Obstet Gynaecol 1991; 98:513–518.
95. Comarr A: Observations on menstruation and pregnancy among female spinal cord injury patients. Paraplegia, 1966; 3:263–272.
96. Verduyn W: Spinal cord injured women, pregnancy and delivery. Paraplegia 1986; 24:231–240.
97. Nath M, Vivian J, Cherny W: Autonomic hyperreflexia in pregnancy and labor: A case report. Am J Obstet Gynecol 1979; 134:390–392.
98. Greenspoon J, Paul R: Paraplegia and quadriplegia: Special considerations during pregnancy and labor and delivery. Am J Obstet Gynecol 1986; 155:738–741.
99. Crosby E, et al: Obstetrical anaesthesia and analgesia in chronic spinal cord-injured women. Can J Anaesth 1992; 39:487–494.
100. Abouleish E, Hanley E, Palmer S: Can epidural fentanyl control autonomic hyperreflexia in a quadriplegic parturient? Anesth Analg 1989; 68:523–526.
101. Stirt J, Marco A, Conklin K: Obstetric anesthesia for a quadriplegic patient with autonomic hyperreflexia. Anesthesiology 1979; 51:560–562.
102. Plotz J, von Hugo R: Autonomic hyperreflexia, pregnancy and delivery in para-tetraplegia. The obstetric anesthesiologic viewpoint on a case. Anaesthesist 1996; 45:1179–1183.
103. Kamani A: Obstetrical anaesthesia and analgesia in chronic spinal cord-injured women [commentry]. Can J Anaesthesia 1992; 39:492–493.
104. Schonwald G, Fish K, Perkash I: Cardiovascular complications during anesthesia in chronic spinal cord injured patients. Anesthesiology 1981; 55:550–558.
105. Broecker B, Hranowsky N, Hackler R: Low spinal anesthesia for the prevention of autonomic dysreflexia in the spinal cord injury patient. J Urology 1979; 122:366.
106. John D, et al: Onset of succinylcholine-induced hyperkalemia following denervation. Anesthesiology 1976; 45:294–299.
107. Gronert G, Theye R: Pathophysiology of hyperkalemia induced by succinylcholine. Anesthesiology 1975; 43:89–99.
108. Rochester J, Kirchner J: Epilepsy in pregnancy. Am Fam Phys 1997; 56:1631–1636.
109. Ong B: Obstetrical anaesthesia and analgesia in chronic spinal cord-injured women. Can J Anaesth 1992; 39:493–494.
110. Crosby E, Halpern S: Obstetric epidural anaesthesia in patients with Harrington instrumentation. Can J Anaesth 1989; 36:693–696.

47

Intracranial Disease During Pregnancy: Anesthetic Management

❖ Peter R. Isert, MBBS, FFARACS, FANZCA

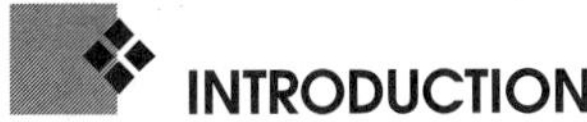

INTRODUCTION

Intracranial disease manifesting during pregnancy is uncommon and neurosurgical intervention during pregnancy is a rare event in most obstetric units. The attending obstetric anesthetist may be required to manage patients with acute or chronic intracranial pathology during labor and delivery or during cesarean section. Occasionally, craniotomy may be indicated during pregnancy. Finally, maternal or fetal disease may require that both craniotomy and safe delivery of the child occur during one anesthetic delivery. A multidisciplinary approach is clearly required for optimal management of these clinical scenarios, and early liaison with obstetric, neurosurgical, and neuroanesthesia colleagues is essential. Striking the right balance between several specialists with often competing priorities is both challenging and rewarding. A detailed and frank discussion with the patient and family is necessary in order to attain true informed consent prior to anesthetic intervention.

Impact of Pregnancy. The physiologic changes of pregnancy that impact on patients with intracranial pathology occur maximally in late pregnancy, during labor and delivery, and immediately postpartum. Of particular relevance are the changes in cardiac output, which increases by 40% by the end of the third trimester[1] and by a further 45% during labor because of pain-induced catecholamine surges and autotransfusion during uterine contractions. These changes return to normal several weeks postpartum. Episodic hypertension is a feature of painful labor, while marked increases in intrathoracic, cerebrovenous, and cerebrospinal fluid (CSF) pressures occur in labor caused by the Valsalva maneuver while pushing and bearing down.[2, 3] It has been suggested that this simultaneous increase in systolic blood pressure (BP) and intracranial pressure (ICP) during painful contractions may in fact prevent bleeding from intracranial arterial anomalies during labor by preventing any transmural pressure gradient from developing.[4] However, the fragile veins of an arteriovenous malformation (AVM) may still distend or bleed because of the dramatically increased cerebral venous pressure.[5] In addition, the release of the Valsalva maneuver at the cessation of painful contractions leads to sudden increased venous return to the heart and elevated BP levels, an acute reduction in ICP,[6] and consequently increased transmural pressure gradients across any partially tamponaded neurovascular lesion. Increase in minute ventilation during pregnancy causes a mild reduction in arterial carbon dioxide (CO_2) tension to approximately 32 mm Hg at term, while hyperventilation during painful labor may result in severe progressive hypocarbia to between 24 mm Hg and 16 mm Hg[7] with subsequent cerebral vasoconstriction. Salt and water retention also increase during pregnancy and may precipitate symptoms of raised ICP in patients with shunted hydrocephalus[8] and together with the increases in estrogen, progesterone, and glucocorticoids occurring during pregnancy may lead to increased growth and edema surrounding certain cerebral tumors.[9, 10] CSF pressure otherwise remains normal until labor, despite lumbar lordosis and uterine compression.[3]

The effects of these gradual and acute changes in cerebral blood flow (CBF), cerebrovenous pressure, BP, and ICP may result in exacerbation of symptoms in patients with known or occult intracranial lesions. The magnitude of these effects during pregnancy, labor, and delivery and in the postpartum period are determined by the patient's cerebral autoregulation, CO_2 responsiveness, and intracranial compliance. The integrity of any abnormal cerebral blood vessels, the presence of any critically ischemic areas of brain, and both the size and nature of the intracranial lesion are also clearly important determinants of patient outcome.

GENERAL PRINCIPLES OF ANESTHESIA MANAGEMENT

Anesthetic management is dictated by the progression of any neurologic symptoms during pregnancy and whether vaginal delivery or cesarean section is planned. Although controversial, pregnant patients with either stable intracranial disease (e.g., shunted hydrocephalus)[8] or stable intracranial lesions (e.g., a small benign tumor,[11] a small asymptomatic aneurysm,[12] or quiescent AVM[13]) may be allowed to reach term before any definitive neurosurgical treatment and to deliver either vaginally or by cesarean section, based on obstetric indications.[14] Early intervention during labor by the anesthetist is important in these patients to optimize pain relief and prevent Valsalva effects.[15]

Regional or general anesthesia may be used for cesarean delivery, if indicated.

In the majority of patients with a cerebral aneurysm,[12, 16] or with unstable intracranial lesions (e.g., a malignant tumor,[10] increasing hydrocephalus caused by a malfunctioning CSF shunt,[8] or intracranial hemorrhage [ICH] caused by a leaking aneurysm, AVM or head injury), if fetal viability is in doubt (<30 weeks' gestation), then craniotomy may be indicated during the pregnancy to prevent further increases in tumor growth,[17] rises in ICP,[8] or fatal rebleeding.[13] This is especially true for aneurysms in contrast to AVMs presenting during pregnancy. The principles of neuroanesthesia management for craniotomy must be modified during pregnancy to ensure safety of both mother and fetus. Perioperative fetal monitoring is essential, and obstetric staff should be immediately available to manage fetal distress or premature labor should it occur in the perioperative period. Less invasive treatment options for neurovascular lesions such as embolization or balloon occlusion should also be considered. Neurosurgically treated patients are considered stable, especially if treatment has been in the second or third trimester and are subsequently managed along standard obstetric guidelines.[12, 16, 18, 19] However, anesthetic management during subsequent labor and delivery must minimize the potential for bleeding or edema in recently operated areas of brain.

Should such neurologically unstable patients present closer to term or if previously stable patients deteriorate during late pregnancy or labor, consideration should be given to early delivery by cesarean section followed immediately by craniotomy and definitive neurosurgical treatment. Delivery before the craniotomy in these patients is important to prevent fetal sequelae from the use of hyperventilation, hypotension, osmotic diuretics, and hypothermia; to minimize neonatal somnolence from anesthetic drugs, especially narcotics given to the mother; and to enable certain, otherwise impractical, positions to be used for the neurosurgery. Principles of neuroanesthesia and neuroresuscitation are vital in preventing further elevations in ICP, intracranial bleeding, and cerebral ischemia in unstable patients, especially if drowsy or moribund,[20] while at the same time optimizing neonatal chances of survival.

LABOR AND DELIVERY

In patients with stable, previously treated, or untreatable intracranial lesions, avoiding the pain of labor and the Valsalva maneuver is of paramount concern and is best achieved by well-functioning continuous epidural blockade. Several case reports and small series suggest that epidural analgesia is safe and effective in selected patients with cerebral tumor,[15, 21, 22] shunted hydrocephalus,[8, 23] recently treated or untreated intracranial aneurysm,[4, 24, 25] and in radically[26] or partially[5] excised AVMs.

Optimal Analgesia. A short second stage to minimize bearing-down efforts and pushing, with perhaps low-forceps delivery is preferable,[13, 15, 22] and early cesarean section should be considered if labor fails to progress or if analgesia is inadequate. Spinal opiates have been suggested as an alternative form of analgesia,[5] but as with paracervical or bilateral lumbar sympathetic nerve blocks, they do not prevent the Valsalva maneuver unless a pudendal or caudal nerve block is used during the second stage. Systemic narcotics and inhaled nitrous oxide are inadequate alternate forms of analgesia compared with an effective epidural block and in addition may cause excessive sedation, hypercarbia, increased cerebral blood volume, and subsequent further increases in ICP during labor, especially if intracranial compliance is already reduced.[27, 28]

Two particular issues concerning the use of epidural block in these patients for either vaginal delivery or cesarean section are, first, the potential for increased ICP caused by the injection of anesthetic drugs into the epidural space, and second, the consequences of inadvertent dural puncture with an epidural needle in the presence of an intracranial lesion.

Increased Intracranial Pressure with Epidurals. ICP is known to increase when boluses of as little as 5 mL are injected into the lumbar epidural space, and the magnitude of this rise in ICP is directly related to both the volume injected and the baseline ICP value[29] and inversely related to the speed of injection.[30] Bolus doses of epidural local anesthetics have in fact been reported to precipitate the onset of new neurologic symptoms and signs in patients with undiagnosed elevated ICP during labor and delivery. One patient with an unrecognized large acoustic neuroma and hydrocephalus developed paresthesias and convulsions following a 4-mL epidural bolus in labor,[31] while another patient with unrecognized recent subarachnoid hemorrhage (SAH) developed headaches and facial twitching following a 20-mL epidural bolus[32] and died 2 days post partum. These symptoms and signs may initially be attributed to inadvertent intravenous administration of local anesthetic solution, further delaying the correct diagnosis. Rapid large-bolus injections, either to initiate or top up epidural analgesia, should be avoided in an attempt to prevent these increases in ICP.[29, 33] Clearly, a continuous epidural infusion is preferable during labor in this regard. However, any amelioration in the increases in ICP by an infusion rather than boluses of local anesthetics may be difficult to demonstrate. Furthermore, epidural infusions are less likely to cause sudden hypotension with subsequent reduced cerebral perfusion pressure leading to further increases in ICP secondary to autoregulatory vasodilation of cerebral arterioles.[34] Sudden hypotension may also cause nausea and vomiting, which may lead to a Valsalva maneuver and raised ICP, or it may mask developing intracranial problems also initially heralded by nausea and vomiting. The use of epidural blocks in patients with the potential to develop increased ICP during labor because of intracranial lesions, benign intracranial hypertension, or preeclampsia continues to be debated.[35, 36]

Inadvertent Dural Puncture. The risk of acute neurologic deterioration occurring as a result of dural puncture in patients with space-occupying lesions and raised ICP is known,[37, 38] but is rarely described in the obstetric population.[39, 40] Furthermore, the expectation of an ensuing postdural puncture headache can delay the diagnosis of an underlying intracranial lesion.[39, 40] Interestingly, the dangers of CSF leakage from lumbar puncture and subsequent downward, often asymmetric, displacement of intracranial contents are caused by the presence of a space-occupying lesion such as a cerebral tumor, hematoma, or AVM rather than by the presence of uniformly distributed increases in ICP, such as in benign intracranial hypertension, in which lumbar punctures are considered therapeutic.[41] The incidence of inadvertent dural puncture during epidural anesthesia is low, especially in experienced hands, and may be further reduced if the parturient is placed in the lateral decubitus rather than the sitting position.[22] Avoiding the dural sac by approaching the epidural space via the caudal approach should also be associated with less increase in ICP associated with epidural bolus and should reduce, but not completely prevent,[35] the risk of inadvertent dural puncture.[22] Although continuous caudal anesthesia has been used successfully in several patients with symptomatically raised ICP in labor,[21, 22] the caudal approach is considered less reliable and requires greater volumes of local anesthetic drug to be effective.[42]

Patients with Raised Intracranial Pressure. Even though epidural analgesia blunts much of the hemodynamic and intracranial sequelae of labor and delivery,[3, 22] extreme caution must be taken in the known presence of raised ICP or vasospasm (e.g., reduced level of consciousness or focal neurologic deficits) during labor. Even in the absence of pain and the Valsalva maneuver, patients with a known large cerebral tumor[43] or known recent SAH[4] who are allowed to labor with an epidural block may exhibit fluctuating consciousness and worsen during delivery. This occurs presumably because of autotransfusion during even painless contractions, small reductions in cerebral perfusion pressure between contractions, or because of increases in ICP associated with intermittent epidural injection. The concomitant use of steroids and judicious small doses of mannitol[21] may "buy time" in this scenario by reducing ICP and improving cerebral perfusion pressure, but early cesarean section under general anesthesia, with or without definitive neurosurgical treatment, may be a better alternative in these patients.

Additional Monitoring. An arterial line for continuous and direct BP monitoring is recommended, especially if antihypertensive drugs are administered during labor, while continuous fetal heart rate monitoring more rapidly detects any developing fetal distress. Ready access to prompt neurosurgical opinion, operating suites that manage both obstetric and neurosurgical procedures and to intensive care facilities are all essential when managing these high-risk parturients.

Summary. Effective epidural analgesia during labor and delivery has many physiologic benefits for the majority of parturients with intracranial lesions, has a proven safety record, and allows the mother to safely remain awake during the delivery of her child. However, there is an increased risk of neurologic deterioration with the use of epidural blocks in patients presenting with, or who develop, symptomatic raised ICP during labor. It is especially in these patients that the risks of the labor and epidural block must be balanced against the anesthetic challenges required for the alternative choice of an elective or urgent cesarean section.

CESAREAN SECTION

The decision to deliver the child of a woman with a stable intracranial lesion by elective cesarean section should be made primarily on obstetric grounds.[13, 14] Cesarean section may become indicated because of failed epidural analgesia in labor, failure to progress, fetal distress, or maternal neurologic deterioration,[12] and as with all urgent cesarian sections, anesthetic management is influenced by the degree of urgency involved.

Regional and general anesthesia have both been described for use during cesarean section in parturients with cerebral tumor[15, 22]; Arnold-Chiari malformation[44]; shunted hydrocephalus[8]; previously treated,[45] untreated,[45–49] or recently bleeding[26] AVMs; recently treated[50] or untreated[51] cerebral aneurysm; and penetrating head injury.[52] Epidural or spinal anesthesia is preferred if time permits in the absence of raised ICP and if the parturient is agreeable, while general anesthesia[45, 48, 52] is an option in extreme urgency, in the presence of raised ICP, in cases in which patient cooperation is in doubt, or because of obstetric considerations. Epidural anesthesia may also be used in combination with general anesthesia for cesarean section in order to minimize perioperative hypertension and improve postoperative analgesia.[49]

Hemodynamic Stability and Invasive Monitoring. Continuous direct BP monitoring is essential because of the extreme importance of ensuring maternal cardiovascular stability. Hypertension increases CBF in areas of brain with impaired autoregulation, for example, surrounding intracranial tumors or neurovascular lesions, potentially increasing ICP, cerebral edema, or ICH. Hypotension may precipitate cerebral ischemia in those areas of the brain where ICP is high or CBF is already reduced as a result of vasospasm or vascular shunting.[53] In the conscious patient, hypotension may also lead to vomiting or retching with resultant increases in ICP, the risk of bleeding from a preexisting aneurysm or AVM, and potential masking of developing intracranial hypertension during the surgery. Correct patient positioning, appropriate fluid loading, and the judicious and early use of small doses of vasopressors are important in this regard. Drugs with the potential for causing maternal hypotension such as local anesthetics, induction agents, and oxytocin should be administered slowly and incrementally, while potentially hypertensive drugs such as ergometrine should be avoided.[51] Adequate postoperative pain relief by continuous epidural infusion of local anesthetics and narcotics, or by patient-controlled analgesia are also clearly important[45, 47] to minimize the hemodynamic and ICP responses to pain.

Regional or General Anesthesia. Regional anesthesia avoids the hypertensive response to laryngoscopy and intubation during the typically light general anesthetic induction used for cesarean section,[54] is associated with less cardiovascular instability compared with general anesthesia during delivery,[55] and avoids the potential for coughing and straining with resultant Valsalva effects during extubation. Observation of any change in mental state and appropriate patient questioning detect any adverse intracranial event much earlier and is clearly only possible during regional anesthesia. In addition, neonatal depression caused by higher doses of anesthetic drugs or narcotics required to obtund dangerous surges in CBF and ICP under general anesthesia is prevented by using a regional technique. Neuroanesthesia principles and techniques of achieving hemodynamic and intracranial stability, especially during induction of general anesthesia, are discussed in further sections of this chapter and should be equally applied to patients with intracranial disease undergoing elective or urgent cesarean section under general anesthesia. This is especially important in acute neurologic deterioration when definite neurosurgical treatment is not undertaken immediately following cesarean section.[20, 45, 56]

Epidural Versus Spinal Anesthesia. As with vaginal delivery, care must be taken to prevent increases in ICP associated with epidural local anesthetic injection by using slow incremental dosing[35] and also the smallest volume required, while the risk of inadvertent dural puncture should be avoided at all costs. Spinal anesthesia has been recommended for cesarean section in this patient group[5, 26] and is unlikely to be associated with increases in ICP because of the very small volume of anesthetic solution required for injection in the subarachnoid space. However, in patients with space-occupying lesions and raised ICP the associated lumbar puncture clearly carries a finite risk of acute neurologic deterioration caused by the acute leakage of CSF, downward displacement of intracranial contents, and in extreme cases, compression of vital midbrain structures and reduction in their blood supply.[37] To what extent the risk is ameliorated by the use of small-caliber pencil-point, bullet-head, spinal needles that let very little, if any, CSF escape through the needle, and actually separate rather than cut dural fibers causing less CSF leakage through the dural hole,[57, 58] is unknown. However, even slow continued seepage of CSF after the spinal needle has been withdrawn may be responsible for some cases of delayed neurologic deterioration,[37] although the presence of an epidural catheter adjacent to the dural hole as is the case in the combined spinal-epidural technique, may be associated with less CSF leakage as reflected by an extraordinarily low incidence of postdural puncture headache.[59]

Whether epidural is preferable to spinal anesthesia in patients with intracranial disease having cesarean section is unclear since CSF leakage through an inadvertent dural puncture with an epidural needle is much greater. Neurologic decompensation caused by inadvertent or deliberate dural puncture can occur even in the absence of papilledema,[37, 38] and symptoms and signs such as worsening headache, increasing drowsiness, or the development of focal neurologic signs seem to be as important in pregnant patients with increasing ICP.[38] A preoperative neurosurgical opinion regarding any recent progression of the intracranial lesion, as well as computed tomography (CT) or magnetic resonance imaging (MRI) looking for radiologic evidence of raised ICP, especially lateral shift of midline structures, loss of basal cisterns, or obliteration of the fourth ventricle,[60] are essential in the anesthetic decision-making process.

Symptomatic Raised Intracranial Pressure. There are no easy decisions in patients with symptomatic raised ICP or unstable intracranial pathology requiring cesarean section because each anesthetic technique has inherent dangers that risk worsening the neurologic outcome. Each case must be dealt with on an individual basis. At least from the medicolegal standpoint, given the sometimes unpredicted and catastrophic consequences of sudden CSF leakage from lumbar puncture, it would seem reasonable to contraindicate the use of regional anesthesia for cesarean section in the presence of obvious symptomatic or radiologic evidence of raised ICP. Priority should by given to minimizing the potential detrimental cardiovascular and intracranial changes occurring during general anesthesia, short-term use of steroids and perhaps small doses of mannitol to reduce ICP, and organizing early definitive neurosurgical treatment.

CRANIOTOMY DURING PREGNANCY

Craniotomy may be indicated before delivery if an intracranial lesion is acutely unstable or likely to worsen during pregnancy and when concerns regarding fetal viability preclude combined cesarean section and craniotomy. General anesthetic techniques have been described in pregnant patients requiring insertion of a CSF shunt for obstructive hydrocephalus,[61] or who undergo craniotomy for cerebral tumor,[62, 63] bleeding AVM,[5, 26, 45, 64, 65] or aneurysm.[25, 50, 66–72] Unlike other patients that neuroanesthetists usually care for, pregnant patients are at increased risk of gastric acid aspiration and generally require antacid prophylaxis and cricoid pressure prior to intubation, require careful positioning to prevent aortocaval compression by the gravid uterus after the first trimester, and must not be exposed to drugs or techniques that might potentially affect the fetus or precipitate premature labor.

Neuroanesthesia Principles

Induction of general anesthesia should aim to prevent further increases in ICP in the presence of a space-occupying lesion or prevent fresh intracerebral hemorrhage from neurovascular lesions. Laryngoscopy and intubation must be performed when the patient is deeply anesthetized and fully paralyzed in order to prevent surges in systemic BP and ICP, or coughing. Hypotension needs to be aggressively treated to prevent reduced cerebral perfusion pressure and cerebral ischemia in areas of brain where ICP is high or where CBF is already low, and in areas of impaired autoregulation. Sudden reductions in ICP and brain bulk must also be avoided in order to prevent expansion of a recent ICH or detamponading of a bleeding neurovascular lesion. Maintenance of anesthesia should provide sufficient brain relaxation to allow the surgeon ready access to cerebral lesions without the need for undue retraction, while manipulation of BP and CBF may be required to facilitate safe obliteration of vascular lesions or to help control bleeding. Hemodynamic stability and prevention of the Valsalva maneuver are also important during emergence, extubation, and in the early postoperative period in order to minimize edema or hemorrhage into adjacent areas of normal brain. Continuous invasive arterial BP monitoring is integral to the perioperative care of the neurosurgical patient.

The effects on the fetus of neuroanesthetic drugs and techniques used to achieve these aims depend on any potential teratogenicity, associated changes in uteroplacental blood flow, or direct effects caused by placental transfer of drugs. Fortunately, many potentially adverse intraoperative techniques such as severe hypocarbia, deliberate hypotension, osmotic diuresis, and induced moderate hypothermia are now no longer routinely used because of recent advances in neurosurgical instrumentation and operative microscopy. In addition, the effects of narcotics and general anesthetic drugs on fetal sleep patterns and uterine muscle tone are of little consequence if delivery is planned for a later date.

Rapid-Sequence Induction? Achieving an intracranially stable induction may be especially challenging given the increased risk of gastric acid aspiration, arterial oxygen desaturation, and difficult intubation associated with the pregnant patient, especially considering the usual hemodynamic instability of a standard rapid-sequence induction using thiopentone and succinylcholine alone. Furthermore, the use of succinlycholine may itself be detrimental in patients with preexisting raised ICP because of increases in CBF and ICP caused by increased afferent stimulation with the onset of muscle fasciculations.[73, 74] Pretreatment by prior administration of a defasciculating dose of nondepolarizing muscle relaxant may or may not prevent this rise in ICP.[75, 76] Other techniques, such as administration of a large dose of nondepolarizer prior to the induction agent[61] or using a shorter-acting nondepolarizer such as rocuronium instead,[77] remain potential but controversial ways of avoiding the use of succinylcholine in these patients.

Slow intravenous induction, administration of a nondepolarizer, gentle mask ventilation with cricoid pressure, and then deepening of anesthesia with either intravenous or inhalational drugs prior to intubation is an alternative technique of avoiding the hemodynamic instability of rapid-sequence induction in patients at increased risk of aspiration,[6, 45, 65, 71, 78] but is potentially hazardous in later pregnancy unless succinylcholine is substituted as the choice of muscle relaxant. Other methods of deepening anesthesia prior to intubation in order to blunt the hypertensive and ICP responses to a standard rapid-sequence induction in pregnant patients include higher doses of intravenous thiopentone,[61, 79] propofol for induction,[80] or supplemental intravenous lidocaine, magnesium, alfentanil,[81–84] droperidol, or fentanyl.[84, 85] Remifentanil may prove especially useful in this regard[86] because of its rapid onset of profound narcosis, while its rapid elimination despite high bolus doses or infusion are of particular benefit if it can reduce neonatal respiratory depression when cesarean section is performed prior to the craniotomy.

Antihypertensive Drugs. The short-term use of vasodilators such as hydralazine, sodium nitroprusside or glyceryl trinitrate, or short-acting intravenous β-blockers (e.g., esmolol) also help obtund hemodynamic responses during rapid-sequence induction.[87] Labetalol appears to be the β-blocker of choice because of its additional α-blocking properties, moderate maternal hypotensive effects without reflux tachycardia, and absence of any fetal bradycardia or hypoglycemia.[88, 89] Esmolol may cross the placenta and cause fetal bradycardia,[90] especially if uteroplacental blood flow is already compromised.[91] However, interestingly, the combination of esmolol and sodium nitroprusside infusions used for induced hypotension during cerebral aneurysm surgery in pregnancy causes only minor alterations in the fetal heart rate (FHR).[69] When used to prevent or treat hypertension and tachycardia during craniotomy,[65] any effect on FHR is only mild and transient because of the high levels of circulatory maternal catecholamines. Although some chronically administered β-blockers during pregnancy can lead to intrauterine growth retardation and inhibition of neonatal sympathetic responses,[92] brief use of short-acting β-blockers for specific indications seems unlikely to affect fetal growth or increase the risk of premature labor by increasing uterine tone.[90] The drugs used to help reduce the hemodynamic response to rapid-sequence induction have been shown to be efficacious primarily in patients with severe preeclampsia or cardiac disease undergoing cesarean section, but are of equal relevance in patients with intracranial lesions undergoing cesarean section, craniotomy during pregnancy, or combined cesarean section and craniotomy. Combination therapy using several familiar drugs probably yields the best results with the least complications.

Experience with the use of antihypertensives and the newer anesthetic drugs, especially during the first trimester of pregnancy is still very limited, and the potential for teratogenicity should always be considered. An up-to-date search for any reports of adverse fetal effects should be sought before these drugs are administered to the mother.

Fetal Monitoring. Although the prone position can be used safely in early pregnancy for posterior fossa craniotomy,[45] most patients are positioned supine, and left lateral tilt to avoid aortocaval compression is vital to ensure maternal cardiovascular stability and fetal perfusion during surgery. Continuous perioperative monitoring of FHR and uterine tone by cardiotocography (CTG) is practical in neurosurgical patients and although its interpretation may be difficult, CTG is essential after the first trimester to attempt to monitor fetal well-being or to detect premature labor which may be masked by the use of postoperative narcotics. Baseline FHR should be assessed preoperatively and experienced personnel should be present or immediately available to interpret any changes detected in FHR patterns or uterine contractility during surgery or in the early postoperative period. Loss of beat-to-beat FHR variability is common during and shortly after general anesthesia and is not necessarily a sign of fetal distress.[71, 93] However, the onset of fetal decelerations or bradycardia usually indicates a dangerous reduction in uteroplacental blood flow and may lead to changes in anesthetic management, such as the cessation of hyperventilation or deliberate hypotension[66, 94] sometimes used to improve neurosurgical conditions.

Hyperventilation. There is a growing appreciation of the unpredictable and potentially adverse cerebral effects of hyperventilation and hypocarbia when used during craniotomy to reduce ICP.[95] Hypocarbia may worsen or precipitate cerebral ischemia by cerebral vasoconstriction, a left shift in the hemoglobin-oxygen dissociation curve, or because of the reduced cardiac output associated with hyperventilation. Maternal hyperventilation also leads to reduced uteroplacental blood flow with resultant fetal hypoxia, acidosis, and distress.[96, 97] In the context of pregnant patients undergoing craniotomy, routine hyperventilation should be avoided and operating conditions optimized instead by using a head-up posture to reduce cerebrovenous pressure, appropriate choice of general anesthetic drugs, or small doses of diuretics if needed. Short-term use of hyperventilation should be reserved to treat severe life-threatening intracranial hypertension prior to definitive decompressive craniotomy but it should be remembered that the normal progressive reduction in arterial CO_2 level during pregnancy may alter the $Pa{CO_2}$ "set point" for any therapeutic effect from hyperventilation.[98] Furthermore, arterial blood gas determination of $Pa{CO_2}$ is recommended because of the unpredictable nature of the arterial–end tidal CO_2 gradient,[95] especially during pregnancy.[99]

Deliberate Hypotension. The routine use of deliberate hypotension during neurosurgery for resection of cerebral aneurysm or AVM has gradually lost popularity because of concerns of inducing cerebral ischemia in areas of impaired autoregulation, vasospasm, or excessive brain retraction and because of the increasing use of temporary clips applied to feeder blood vessels to effectively produce local hypoperfusion.[13, 100] However, hypotension is occasionally required to reduce aneurysmal wall tension during handling of complex or fragile neurovascular lesions and is clearly justified to reduce bleeding and improve visibility if the aneurysm or AVM ruptures. The prevention of hypertensive responses during emergence from craniotomy and extubation is also important to prevent fresh hemorrhage into recently operated areas of brain. The short-term use of β-blockers or hypotensive drugs often required to prevent this hypertension should not adversely affect the fetus if BP remains normal.[65] When necessary, brief periods of deliberate hypotension have been used safely during craniotomy for neurovascular lesions in pregnant patients,[25, 66–69, 72] but may need to be curtailed if FHR changes suggest fetal hypoperfusion.[66, 94] Because of the potential for fetal cyanide toxicity with large doses or prolonged infusion of sodium nitroprusside,[101] the use of deep halothane[25] or isoflurane anesthesia[66, 72] or the concomitant administration of β-blockers or other vasodilators to reduce sodium nitroprusside requirements[102] seems wise. Isoflurane has the additional benefits of reducing cerebral oxygen requirements during periods of hypotension and maintains normal fetal oxygenation and acid-base balance at 1.5 minimum alveolar concentration (MAC)[103] for up to 30 minutes.[104] However, higher concentrations for longer periods reduce uteroplacental blood flow[103, 104] and may also impair cerebral autoregulation and raise ICP.

Normovolemia and Use of Vasoconstrictors. Maternal hypovolemia should be aggressively treated if bleeding from neurovascular lesions occurs (especially if a brief period of controlled hypotension is requested) in order to prevent catastrophic falls in uteroplacental blood flow. The use of a β-agonist such as ephredrine should replace the usual neuroanesthesia vasoconstrictors (such as the α-agonist metaraminol) when treating brief periods of inadvertent hypotension, in order to prevent detrimental effects to placental perfusion.[105, 106] Continuous direct monitoring of BP using an arterial line is essential, and a peripherally placed central venous pressure line is also useful in the cardiovascular management of the pregnant patient undergoing craniotomy. Finally, although the hemodynamic changes associated with pregnancy may protect parturients with cerebral aneurysm from the deleterious effects of vasospasm, the use of colloids, calcium channel blockers, and induced hypertension may still be indicated if a focal neurologic deficit occurs following aneurysm clipping in order to optimize cerebral perfusion pressure and CBF. Nimodopine is probably not teratogenic in humans but may reduce uteroplacental blood flow.[107] Small boluses of selected α-agonists such as phenylephrine do not necessarily adversely affect the fetus when used to treat maternal hypotension, especially if patients are preloaded with intravenous fluids,[108] but the effect of various catecholamine infusions on uteroplacental blood flow when used to augment maternal BP and cardiac output to supranormal levels is unknown. Any effects are dependent on the relative α- or β-actions of the drug which may be dose-dependent, as well as on the cardiac reserve and fluid status of the parturient. β-Agonists such as ephredrine or dopamine[109] or combination therapy using volume loading with colloids and, if required, ephredrine and low-dose phenylephrine infusions, may be more appropriate choices, but the net effect on placental perfusion is difficult to predict. If needed during pregnancy, these drugs should be used with caution and with FHR monitoring.[13]

Osmotic Diuresis. The osmotic diuretic mannitol is sometimes used during craniotomy to help reduce brain bulk or ICP before dural opening, especially in the presence of large cerebral tumors or recent intracerebral or subarachnoid hemorrhage. Injudicious use of mannitol may lead to severe diuresis, electrolyte disturbance, and hypotension and is often unnecessary during routine craniotomy, especially if small amounts of CSF are removed via ventriculostomy or a spinal subarachnoid drain. In large doses, mannitol crosses the placental barrier causing a net flow of water from fetus to mother and fetal dehydration.[110, 111] If mannitol is considered necessary, however, a small bolus dose of 0.25 to 0.5 g/kg is unlikely to be problematic as long as maternal hypovolemia is avoided.[13, 20, 66] Loop diuretics such as furosemide may also be a safer alternative for the fetus. Perioperative use of dexamethasone may also reduce cerebral edema during craniotomy, and steroids have been used safely during pregnancy for many non-neurosurgical conditions without adverse fetal effects.[112] Many commonly used anticonvulsants such as phenytoin are known to be teratogenic,[112] and the prevention and treatment of perioperative convulsions in the pregnant patient remain difficult management issues.[12, 13]

Induced Hypothermia. The growing appreciation of the importance of mild hypothermic cerebral protection has led to the increasing use of induced mild hypothermia during craniotomy, especially for neurovascular procedures in which patients are at increased risk for perioperative cerebral ischemia.[113, 114] Mild hypothermia of 33° to 34°C leads to a substantial reduction in neuroexcitatory amino acid release during ischemia[115] and is more protective than deep anesthesia despite less cerebral metabolic suppression.[116] Mild hypothermia is not associated with cardiac arrhythmias or coagulopathy that is associated with moderate hypothermia of 26° to 28°C. The latter was used much more commonly in the 1960s and 1970s for cerebral protection and improvement of neurosurgical operating conditions. Many case reports and reviews in the anesthetic literature from that era attest to the safety of carefully managed induced moderate hypothermia in pregnant patients with head injury[117] or who had undergone craniotomy for resection of a large tumor, aneurysm, or AVM.[62, 64, 70, 118] Fetal wastage did occur, however, especially in early pregnancy, with bleeding or if metabolic acidosis or hypoxia were not prevented perioperatively,[119] and was considered more likely with deeper levels of hypothermia.[64] Fetal temperature parallels reductions in maternal temperature,[120] and reductions in FHR closely follow the maternal bradycardia caused by progressive hypothermia.[62, 70] Hypothermia increases uterine muscle tone causing reduced uteroplacental blood flow[121] which may adversely affect placental oxygenation of fetal blood.[122] Even though moderate hypothermia reduces fetal oxygen requirements, thereby potentially protecting the fetus from periods of maternal hypotension,[120] premature uterine contractions may still be precipitated.[123] There is little information available concerning any adverse fetal effects of induced mild hypothermia. Maternal temperature of 34°C has been associated with fetal bradycardia, although the FHR mirrored associated reductions in maternal heart rate and there was no loss of FHR variability, implying the absence of fetal distress.[124] The use of induced mild hypothermia in pregnant patients during craniotomy is likely to be safer to both mother and fetus alike but should be used with caution and limited to periods of potential cerebral ischemia only. Uteroplacental blood flow should be otherwise optimized and CTG should be monitored.

Choice of Anesthetic Drugs. A variety of inhalational[5, 25, 26, 50, 63–68, 71, 72] and intravenous[45, 62, 69, 70] anesthetic drugs have been used during craniotomy in pregnant patients. However, even in the absence of currently available data to suggest that any particular anesthetic drugs, except perhaps the benzodiazepines, are either teratogenic or precipitate spontaneous abortion in humans,[125–127] it seems prudent to delay surgery if possible and to avoid drug exposure to the developing fetus, especially during organogenesis and ossification in the first trimester.[128] In nonpregnant patients, propofol is commonly used for induction of anesthesia for intracranial procedures, and propofol infusion is often preferred to isoflurane for maintenance because of its cerebral vasoconstrictor activity and consequent reduction in ICP and brain bulk, maintenance of cerebral autoregulation, rapid emergence, and reduced incidence of postoperative nausea and vomitting.[129] However, propofol rapidly crosses the placenta and continued fetal uptake during an infusion together with slower elimination in the fetus compared with the mother, lead to high concentrations of the drug in the fetus.[130, 131] High propofol concentrations may increase the risk of embryotoxicity, but there remains no published data implicating propofol teratotoxicity in humans.[126] Uteroplacental blood flow, fetal hemodynamics, and acid-base status are not adversely affected by propofol infusion for short periods.[132] Propofol infusion has been used for both maintenance of anesthesia and postoperative sedation in a pregnant patient who underwent craniotomy for AVM at 25 weeks' gestation,[45] as well as in the neurointensive care management of ICH and raised ICP during late pregnancy.[133] Despite the benefits of propofol infusion in optimizing neurosurgical operating conditions and reducing ICP postoperatively, the potential exists for the metabolic acidosis and myocardial failure seen following prolonged high-dose propofol infusion in children[134] to develop in the fetuses of pregnant patients administered prolonged propofol infusion during surgery. Although the dangers of propofol infusions in children appear to have been overstated,[135] there is limited experience or data concerning their use in neonates and the issue must be balanced against the perceived advantages of using a propofol infusion before propofol is administered to a pregnant patient for prolonged periods. Total propofol dosage may be reduced by concomitant use of low-dose isoflurane[45] or nitrous oxide during maintenance, while predominantly isoflurane or narcotic-based techniques are acceptable alternatives for many elective craniotomies.[136]

COMBINED CESAREAN SECTION AND CRANIOTOMY

The conduct of general anesthesia for cesarean section in late pregnancy followed immediately by craniotomy in a patient with acutely unstable or deteriorating intracranial disease is indeed a challenge. Consultation with obstetric and neonatal colleagues is essential to ensure fetal viability if combined surgery is planned before term. Fetal viability is generally considered probable after approximately 30 to 32 weeks' gestation. Anesthesia for combined cesarean section and craniotomy during late pregnancy has been described in patients with a large cerebral tumor[22, 61, 137, 138] or cerebral aneurysm.[78, 139–141] If the etiology of an acute intracranial catastrophe during late pregnancy or labor is uncertain or in the context of severe head injury occurring in late pregnancy, urgent cesarean section may be indicated, followed by a brief period of neuroradiologic investigation and then subsequent craniotomy.[20, 56] Lastly, despite probable fetal viability, craniotomy for treatment of symptomatic cerebral aneurysm has also been performed in late pregnancy without a preceding cesarean section.[50, 66, 72]

Achieving a hemodynamically stable rapid-sequence induction for the cesarean section is crucial, especially in acute neurologic deterioration, in order to prevent dangerous surges in maternal BP or ICP and to avoid the risk of gastric acid aspiration. Because cesarean delivery is performed promptly after induction, the drugs used to obtund the cardiovascular responses to intubation should be chosen to prevent neonatal hemodynamic instability and to minimize neonatal respiratory depression and somnolence.

Advantages. Performing the cesarean section before the craniotomy prevents many of the management problems encountered during craniotomy in pregnant patients and has been recommended for many years.[22, 142] The fetus is not exposed to the detrimental effects of commonly used neuroanesthetic techniques or drugs described in the previous section of this chapter; alternative positions such as prone, park bench, or sitting positions are practical and without risk of aortocaval or fetal compression; and the potential for intraoperative premature labor is avoided. Following delivery, oxytocin is administered to prevent concealed uterine bleeding and craniotomy is then performed using standard neurosurgical and neuroanesthetic techniques. Such immediate definitive neurosurgical treatment avoids the potential for further neurologic deterioration in parturients with raised ICP or unstable intracranial lesions during prolonged labor or following cesarean section.

Neonatal Respiratory Depression. As described previously, many drugs help obtund the hypertensive responses to rapid-sequence induction in a patient with raised ICP or at risk for developing or worsening acute ICH. Shorter-acting narcotics, especially alfentanil,[45, 56, 83] (potentially) remifentanil,[86] or even fentanyl[85] are useful in this regard without necessarily causing undue neonatal respiratory depression. This is especially so if these agents are used in moderate dosage, if concomitant use of an inhalational anesthetic drug is minimized prior to delivery, and in the absence of fetal distress or neonatal asphyxia. Other techniques such as the avoidance of rapid-sequence induction,[78] using higher induction doses of thiopentone, or the use of propofol, adrenergic blockers, or vasodilator infusions have also been used successfully. They are preferred[61, 139–141] for the specific reason of avoiding even the possibility of neonatal respiratory depression caused by narcotics.[81, 84] Combinations of short-acting narcotics plus hypotensive drugs are commonly used in neuroanesthetic induction and may be able to reduce narcotic dosage before delivery of the neonate. Acceptance of the potential for transient neonatal respiratory depression requiring naloxone reversal or a brief period of ventilatory support, in order to prevent maternal intracranial catastrophe at induction, appears reasonable. In addition, the presence of a skilled neonatologist in the operating suite and ongoing neonatal intensive care facilities are required when embarking on these complex cases, whether or not narcotics are used prior to delivery.

Anesthetic Drugs and Techniques. The use of propofol for induction and maintenance of anesthesia would seem an appropriate choice for combined cesarean section and craniotomy. Propofol bolus followed by continuous infusion is associated with less hypertension in the 5 to 10 minutes following rapid-sequence induction for cesarean section,[143, 144] and, as discussed previously, provides stable, rapidly titratable neuroanesthesia, excellent intracranial operating conditions, intact cerebral autoregulation, and rapid emergence even after prolonged anesthesia.[129] Furthermore, propofol infusion used for cesarean section does not cause uterine atony or increase uterine bleeding.[144] Even though neonatal Apgar scores and acid-base status are not adversely affected when compared with inhalational anesthetics,[143, 144] subtle neonatal assessments such as the Neurologic and Adaptive Capacity Score suggest greater neonatal depression when propofol infusion is used in high dosage[145] or when induction-to-delivery times are long.[143] However, the observed differences in neurobehavioral testing are transient, and are unlikely to be of clinical importance[143, 145] or affect maternal bonding, especially in the context of combined cesarean section–craniotomy, in which the mother herself is anesthetized and sedated for at least several hours following delivery of her child. Isoflurane may alternatively be used for maintenance up until delivery or throughout the combined procedure,[61, 137, 139, 141] while the use of narcotic boluses or infusion following delivery helps prevent hemodynamic responses during the subsequent craniotomy.

An alternative approach to general anesthesia for combined cesarean section and craniotomy is the use of either local infiltation[22] or regional blockade[140, 141] for the cesarean section, to allow the mother to witness the birthing experience while avoiding the risks of neonatal depression and then to induce general anesthesia for the craniotomy. Regional anesthesia is associated with less cardiovascular instability during cesarean delivery,[54, 55] while the administration of local anesthesia or narcotics via epidural or spinal catheter may improve postoperative analgesia and reduce perioperative hypertension. During craniotomy, a sufficiently large-diameter spinal catheter may also be used for gradual CSF drainage to reduce ICP just prior to dural opening and to improve neurosurgical access to an intracranial aneurysm.[98, 140] Despite these potential benefits of combined regional and general anesthesia, the technique would seem inappropriate if the cesarean section is urgent or if the patient is confused or uncooperative, or has symptomatic or radiologic evidence of raised ICP, because of the dangers in these patients of epidural injection or inadvertent or deliberate dural puncture.

Postoperative Care. Pregnancy increases the risk of thromboembolism following surgery and because of the traditional avoidance of heparin prophylaxis in neurosurgical patients, other preventive methods such as antithrombosis stockings and calf compressors must be used perioperatively.[61] Postoperative analgesia may also be difficult because of the combined surgery and the requirement to avoid excessive maternal sedation in order to allow early bonding with the neonate and accurate neurologic assessment. Patient-controlled analgesia with small doses of intravenous narcotics and antiemetics may be useful in this regard, depending on the mother's postoperative mental state. Finally, many of the alterations in cardiorespiratory physiology, blood volume, and drug effects associated with pregnancy persist into the early postpartum period and the loss of the gravid uterus and placental shunt alter hemodynamic responses. These may be important con-

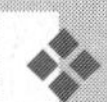
SUMMARY

Key Points

- In patients with stable, previously treated, or untreatable intracranial lesions, avoiding the pain of labor and the Valsalva maneuver is of major concern and can usually be achieved with neuraxial techniques.
- In parturients with intracranial lesions, a short second stage is advisable and can be achieved via a forceps delivery following neuraxial block. Early cesarean section should be considered if labor fails to progress or if analgesia is inadequate.
- Craniotomy may be indicated before delivery if an intracranial lesion is acutely unstable or likely to worsen during pregnancy. Anesthesia for combined cesarean section and craniotomy has been reported.

Key References

Ong B, Littleford J, Segstro R, et al: Spinal anesthesia for caesarean section in a patient with a cervical arteriovenous malformation. Can J Anaesth 1996; 43:1052–1058.

Conklin K, Herr G, Fung D: Anaesthesia for caesarean section and cerebral aneurysm clipping. Can Anaesth Soc J 1984; 31:451–454.

Case Stem

A morbidly obese parturient with a recently diagnosed leaking cerebral aneurysm is to undergo a combined cesarean section and craniotomy. Discuss the neurosurgical, obstetric, and anesthetic implications of this case.

siderations in the postoperative and neurointensive care management of these complex patients.

Conclusion. The anesthetist plays a pivotal role in the proper management of the parturient with stable or unstable intracranial disease. Labor and delivery, cesarean section, or definitive neurosurgical treatment can all occur safely without compromising maternal or fetal well-being. Neuroanesthesia principles and techniques need to be successfully incorporated into obstetric anesthesia practice.

References

1. Ueland K, Novy M, Peterson E, Metcalfe J: Maternal cardiovascular dynamics. IV. The influence of gestational age on the natural cardiovascular response to posture and exercise. Am J Obstet Gynecol 1969; 104:856–864.
2. Hendricks C, Quilligan E: Cardiac output during labour. Am J Obstet Gynecol 1956; 71:953–972.
3. Marx G, Zamaitis M, Orkin L: Cerebrospinal fluid pressures during labour and obstetrical anaesthesia. Anesthesiology 1961; 22:348–354.
4. Young D, Leveno K, Whalley P: Induced delivery prior to surgery for ruptured cerebral aneurysm. Obstet Gynecol 1983; 61:749–752.
5. Visconti C, Wilson J, Bernstein I: Anesthetic management of a parturient with an incompletely resected cerebral arteriovenous malformation. Reg Anesth 1997; 22:192–197.
6. Glosten B: Anesthesia and coexisting maternal disease. II. Diabetes mellitus, obesity, pulmonary and neurologic disease. In Norris M (ed): Obstetric Anesthesia. Philadelphia: J. B. Lippincott; 1993:473–497.
7. Anderson G, Walker J: The effect of labour on the maternal blood gas and acid base status. J Obstet Gynaecol Br Commonw 1970; 77:289–293.
8. Wisoff J, Kratzert J, Handwerker S, et al: Pregnancy in patients with cerebrospinal fluid shunts: report of a series and review of the literature. Neurosurgery 1991; 29:827–831.
9. Roelvink N, Kamphorst W, van Alphen H, Rao B: Pregnancy-related primary brain and spinal tumours. Arch Neurol 1987; 44:209–215.
10. Simon R: Brain tumours in pregnancy. Semin Neurol 1988; 8:214–221.
11. Depret-Mosser S, Jomin M, Monnier J, et al: Tumeurs cérébrales et grossesse. J Gynecol Obstet Biol Reprod 1993; 22:71–80.
12. Stoodley M, Loch Macdonald R, Weir B: Pregnancy and intracranial aneurysms. Neurosurg Clin North Am 1998; 9:549–556.
13. Dias M: Neurovascular emergencies in pregnancy. Clin Obstet Gynecol 1994; 37:337–353.
14. Dias M, Sekhar L: Intracranial haemorrhage from aneurysms and arteriovenous malformations during pregnancy and the puerperium. Neurosurgery 1990; 27:855–865.
15. Finfer S: Management of labour and delivery in patients with intracranial neoplasms. Br J Anaesth 1991; 67:784–787.
16. Reichman O, Karlman R: Berry aneurysm. Surg Clin North Am 1995; 75:115–121.
17. Falconer M, Stafford-Bell M: Visual failure from pituitary and parasellar tumours occurring with favourable outcome in pregnant women. J Neurol Neurosurg Psychiatry 1975; 38:919–930.
18. Weibers D: Subarachnoid haemorrhage in pregnancy. Semin Neurol 1988; 8:226–229.
19. Holcomb W, Petrie R: Cerebrovascular emergency in pregnancy. Clin Obstet Gynecol 1990; 33:467–472.
20. Kofke W, Wuest H, McGinnis L: Cesarean section following ruptured cerebral aneurysm and neuroresuscitation. Anesthesiology 1984; 60:242–245.
21. Kepes E, Andrews I, Rodnay P, et al: Conduct of anesthesia for delivery with grossly raised cerebrospinal fluid pressure. N Y State J Med 1972; 72:1155–1156.
22. Marx G, Scheinberg L, Ramney S: Anesthetic management of the parturient with intracranial tumour. Obstet Gynecol 1964; 24:122–126.
23. Gast M, Grubb R, Strickler R: Maternal hydrocephalus and pregnancy. Obstet Gynecol 1983; 62:29S–31S.
24. Laubstein M, Kotz H, Hehre F: Obstetric and anesthetic management following spontaneous subarachnoid haemorrhage. Obstet Gynecol 1962; 20:661–667.
25. Willoughby J: Sodium nitroprusside, pregnancy and multiple intracranial aneurysms. Anaesth Intensive Care 1984; 12:358–371.
26. Handa F, Tanaka M, Toyooka H: Anesthetic management of parturients with intracranial arteriovenous malformation. Japan J Anesth 1997; 46:1110–1113.
27. Greenberg J, Alavi A, Reivich M, et al: Local cerebral blood volume response to carbon dioxide in man. Circ Res 1978; 43:324–331.
28. Moss E, McDowall D: ICP increases with 50% nitrous oxide in oxygen in severe head injuries during controlled ventilation. Br J Anaesth 1979; 51:757–761.
29. Hilt H, Gramm H-J, Link J: Changes in intracranial pressure associated with extradural anaesthesia. Br J Anaesth 1986; 58:676–680.
30. Usubiaga J, Usubiaga L, Brea L, Goyena R: Epidural and subarachnoid space pressures and relation to postspinal anesthesia headache. Anesth Analg 1967; 46:293–296.
31. Wakeling H, Creagh Barry P: Undiagnosed raised intracranial pressure complicating labour. Int J Obstet Anesth 1995; 4:117–119.
32. McCleod A, Bevan R: Transient seizure: a subtle clue to diagnosis of subarachnoid haemorrhage. Int J Obstet Anesth 1997; 6:122–125.
33. Wildsmith J: Extradural blockade and intracranial pressure. Br J Anaesth 1986; 58:579.
34. Rosner M, Rosner S, Johnson A: Cerebral perfusion pressure: management protocols and clinical results. J Neurosurg 1995; 83:949–962.
35. Abouleish E: Intracranial hypertension and caudal anaesthesia. Br J Anaesth 1987; 59:1478–1479.
36. Selwyn-Crawford J: Extradural blockade and intracranial pressure. Br J Anaesth 1987; 59:1478.
37. Duffy D: Lumbar puncture in the presence of raised intracranial pressure. BMJ 1969; 1:407–409.
38. Richards P, Towu-Aghanste E: Dangers of lumbar puncture. BMJ 1986; 292:605–606.
39. Dutton D: A 'postspinal headache' associated with incidental intracranial pathology. Anaesthesia 1991; 46:1044–1046.
40. Boyd A, Pigstan P: Postpartum headache and cerebral tumour. Anaesthesia 1992; 47:450–451.
41. Katz V, Peterson R, Cefalo R: Pseudotumour cerebri and pregnancy. Am J Perinatol 1989; 6:442–445.
42. Russell P, Coakley C: Re-evaluation of continuous caudal anaesthesia for obstetrics. Surg Gynecol Obstet 1964; 119:531–534.
43. Goroszeniuk T, Howard R, Wright J: The management of labour using continuous lumbar epidural analgesia in a patient with a malignant cerebral tumour. Anaesthesia 1986; 41:1128–1129.
44. Semple D, McClure J, Wallace E: Arnold-Chiari malformation in pregnancy. Anaesthesia 1996; 51:580–582.
45. Hudspith M, Popham P: The anaesthetic management of intracranial haemorrhage from arteriovenous malformation during pregnancy: Three cases. Int J Obstet Anesth 1996; 5:189–193.
46. Sharma S, Herrera E, Sidawi J, Leveno K: The pregnant patient with an intracranial arteriovenous malformation. Reg Anesth 1995; 20:455–458.
47. Laidler J, Jackson I, Redfern N: The management of caesarean section in a patient with an intracranial arteriovenous malformation. Anaesthesia 1989; 44:490–491.
48. Uchide K, Terada S, Akasofu K, Higashi S: Cerebral arteriovenous malformations in a pregnancy with twins: case report. Neurosurgery 1992; 31:780–782.
49. Terao M, Kubota M, Tamakawa S, et al: Anaesthesia for cesarean section in a patient with intracranial AV malformation. Japan J Anesth 1995; 44:1700–1702.

50. Gill E, Mani S, Dessables D: Anesthetic management of cerebral aneurysm clipping during pregnancy: A case report. J Am Assoc Nurse Anesthetists 1993; 61:282–286.
51. Gupta A, Hesselvik F, Eriksson L, Wyon N: Epidural anaesthesia for cesarean section in a patient with a cerebral artery aneurysm. Int J Obstet Anaesth 1993; 2:49–52.
52. Aker J, Parker K: Anesthetic management for emergent cesarean section in a patient with penetrating head injury. Nurse Anesthesia 1993; 4:125–129.
53. Ong B, Littleford J, Segstro R, et al: Spinal anaesthesia for caesarean section in a patient with a cervical arteriovenous malformation. Can J Anaesth 1996; 43:1052–1058.
54. Loughran P, Moore J, Dundee J: Maternal stress response associated with cesarean delivery under general and epidural anesthesia. Br J Obstet Gynaecol 1986; 93:943–949.
55. Milson I, Forssman L, Biber B, et al: Maternal haemodynamic changes during cesarian section: a comparison of epidural and general anaesthesia. Acta Anaesthesiol Scand 1985; 29:161–167.
56. Cheng A, Kwan A: Perioperative management of intra-partum seizure. Anaesth Intensive Care 1997; 25:535–538.
57. Westbrook J, Uncles D, Sitzman B, Carrie L: Comparison of the force required for dural puncture with different spinal needles and subsequent leakage of cerebrospinal fluid. Anesth Analg 1994; 79:769–772.
58. Morrison L, McCrae A, Foo I, et al: An in vitro comparison of fluid leakage after dural puncture with Atraucan, Sprotte, Whitacre and Quincke needles. Reg Anesth 1996; 21:139–143.
59. Brownridge P: Spinal anaesthesia in obstetrics. Br J Anaesth 1991; 67:663–667.
60. Gower D, Baker A, Bell W, Ball R: Contraindications to lumbar puncture as defined by computed cranial tomography. J Neurol Neurosurg Psychiatry 1987; 50:1071–1074.
61. Karula G, Farling P: Anesthetic management of a combined cesarean section and posterior fossa craniotomy. J Neurosurg Anesth 1998; 10:30–33.
62. Strange K, Halldin M: Hypothermia in pregnancy. Anesthesiology 1983; 58:460–461.
63. Molins Gauna N, Gargallo Lopez M, Castells Armenter M, et al: Anaesthesia for brain tumour surgery during pregnancy: report of one case. Rev Esp Anestesiol Reanim 1990; 37:291–293.
64. Matsuki A, Oyama T: Operation under hypothermia in a pregnant woman with an intracranial arteriovenous malformation. Can Anaesth Soc J 1972; 19:184–191.
65. Losasso T, Muzzi D, Cucchiara R: Response of fetal heart rate to maternal administration of esmolol. Anesthesiology 1991; 74:782–784.
66. Newman B, Lam A: Induced hypotension for clipping of a cerebral aneurysm during pregnancy. Anesth Analg 1986; 65:675–678.
67. Danchin Y, Amirov B, Sahar A, Yarkani S: Sodium nitroprusside for aneurysm surgery in pregnancy. Br J Anaesth 1978; 50:849–851.
68. Rigg D, McDonogh A: Use of sodium nitroprusside for deliberate hypotension during pregnancy. Br J Anaesth 1981; 53:985–987.
69. Larson C, Shuer L, Cohen S: Maternally administered esmolol decreases fetal as well as maternal heart rate. J Clin Anesth 1991; 2:427–429.
70. Hess O, Davis C: Electronic evaluation of the fetal and maternal heart rate during hypothermia in a pregnant woman. Am J Obstet Gynecol 1964; 89:801–807.
71. van Buul B, Nijhuis J, Slappendel R, et al: General anesthesia for surgical repair of intracranial aneurysm in pregnancy: effects on fetal heart rate. Am J Perinatol 1993; 10:183–186.
72. Maissin F, Mesz M, Roualdes G, et al: Hypotension a l'isoflurane pour cure d'aneurysme intracraniel en fin de grossesse. Ann Fr Anesth Reanim 1987; 6:453–456.
73. Mori K, Iwabuchi K, Fujita M: The effects of depolarising muscle relaxants on the electroencephalogram and the circulation during halothane anaesthesia in man. Br J Anaesth 1973; 45:605–610.
74. Lanier W, Milde J, Michenfelder J: Cerebral stimulation following succinylcholine in dogs. Anesthesiology 1986; 64:551–559.
75. Stirt J, Grosslight K, Bedford R, Vollmer D: "Defasciculation" with metacurine prevents succinylcholine-induced increases in intracranial pressure. Anesthesiology 1987; 67:50–53.
76. Lanier W, Iaizzo P, Milde J: Cerebral function and muscle afferent activity following intravenous succinylcholine in dogs anesthetized with halothane: The effect of pretreatment with a defasciculating dose of pancuronium. Anesthesiology 1989; 71:87–95.
77. Abouleish E, Abboud T, Lechevalier T, et al: Rocuronium (Org 9426) for caesarian section. Br J Anaesth 1994; 73:336–341.
78. Lennon R, Sundt T, Gronert G: Combined cesarean section and clipping of intracerebral aneurysm. Anesthesiology 1984; 60:240–242.
79. Kosoka Y, Takahashi T, Mark L: Intravenous thiobarbiturate anesthesia for cesarian section. Anesthesiology 1969; 31:489–506.
80. Gin T, O'Meara M, Kan A, et al: Plasma catecholamines and neonatal condition after induction of anaesthesia with propofol or thiopentone at caesarean section. Br J Anaesth 1993; 70:311–316.
81. Allen R, James M, Usy P: Attenuation of the pressure response to tracheal intubation in hypertensive proteinuric pregnant patients by lignocaine, alfentanil and magnesium sulphate. Br J Anaesth 1991; 66:216–233.
82. Redfern N, Bower S, Bullock R, Hull C: Alfentanil for cesarean section complicated by severe aortic stenosis. Br J Anaesth 1987; 59:1309–1312.
83. Dann W, Hutchinson A, Cartwright D: Maternal and neonatal responses to alfentanil administered before induction of anaesthesia for cesarian section. Br J Anaesth 1987; 59:1392–1396.
84. Rout C, Rocke D: Effects of alfentanil and fentanyl on induction of anaesthesia in patients with severe pregnancy-induced hypertension. Br J Anaesth 1990; 65:468–474.
85. Lawes E, Downing J, Duncan P, et al: Fentanyl-droperidol supplementation of rapid sequence induction in the presence of severe pregnancy-induced and pregnancy-aggravated hypertension. Br J Anaesth 1987; 59:1381–1391.
86. Kan R, Hughes S, Rosen M, et al: Intravenous remifentanil: placental transfer, maternal and neonatal effects. Anesthesiology 1998; 88:1467–1474.
87. Ramanathan J: Pathophysiology and anaesthetic implications in preeclampsia. Clin Obstet Gynecol 1992; 35:414–425.
88. Ramanathan J, Sibai B, Mabie W, et al: The use of labetalol for attenuation of the hypertensive response to endotracheal intubation in preeclampsia. Am J Obstet Gynecol 1988; 159:650–654.
89. Jouppila P, Kirkinen P, Koivula A, Ylikorkala O: Labetalol does not alter the placental and fetal blood flow or maternal prostanoids in pre-eclampsia. Br J Obstet Gynaecol 1986; 93:543–547.
90. Eisenach J, Castro M: Maternally administered esmolol produces fetal beta-adrenergic blockade and hypoxemia in sheep. Anesthesiology 1989; 71:718–722.
91. Ducey J, Knape K: Maternal esmolol administration resulting in fetal distress and cesarean section in a term pregnancy. Anesthesiology 1992; 77:829–832.
92. Koaja R, Hiilesmaa V, Holma K, Jarvenpaa J-L: Maternal antihypertensive therapy with beta-blockers associated with poor outcome in very-low birth weight infants. Int J Gynecol Obstet 1992; 38:195–199.
93. Liu P, Warren T, Ostheimer G, et al: Fetal monitoring in parturients undergoing surgery unrelated to pregnancy. Can Anaesth Soc J 1985; 32:525–532.
94. Minielly R, Yuzpe A, Drake C: Subarachnoid haemorrhage secondary to ruptured cerebral aneurysm in pregnancy. Obstet Gynaecol 1979; 53:64–70.
95. Isert P: Control of carbon dioxide levels during neuroanaesthesia: current practice and appraisal of our reliance upon capnography. Anaesth Intensive Care 1994; 22:435–441.
96. Motoyama E, Rivard G, Acheson F, Cook C: Adverse effect of maternal hyperventilation on the fetus. Lancet 1966; 1:286–288.

97. Levinson G, Shnider S, de Lorimier A, Steffenson J: Effects of maternal hyperventilation on uterine blood flow and fetal oxygenation and acid-base status. Anesthesiology 1974; 40:340–347.
98. Eng C, Lam A: Cerebral aneurysms: anaesthesic considerations. In Cottrell J, Smith D (eds): Anaesthesia and Neurosurgery, 3rd ed. St. Louis: CV Mosby; 1994:376–405.
99. Shanker K, Moseley Y, Kumar Y, Vemula V: Arterial to end-tidal carbon dioxide tension difference during caesarean section anaesthesia. Anaesthesia 1986; 41:698–702.
100. Boulard G, Ravussin P, Bissonnette B: Controlled hypertension: pro. J Neurosurg Anesth 1996; 8:244–248.
101. Naulty J, Cefalo R, Lewis P: Fetal toxicity of nitroprusside in the pregnant ewe. Am J Obstet Gynecol 1981; 139:708–711.
102. Willoughby J: Sodium nitroprusside and pregnancy and multiple intracranial aneurysms. Anaesth Intensive Care 1984; 12:351–357.
103. Palahniuk F, Shnider S: Maternal and fetal cardiovascular and acid-base changes during halothane and isoflurane anaesthesia in the pregnant ewe. Anesthesiology 1974; 41:462–472.
104. Bachman C, Biehl D, Sitar D, et al: Isoflurane potency and cardiovascular effects during short exposures in the fetal lamb. Can Anaesth Soc J 1986; 33:41–47.
105. Ralston D, Shnider S, deLorimier A: Effects of equipotent ephedrine, metaraminol, mephentermine and methoxamine on uterine blood flow in the pregnant ewe. Anesthesiology 1974; 40:354–370.
106. Tong C, Eisenach J: The vascular mechanism of ephedrine's beneficial effect on uterine perfusion during pregnancy. Anesthesiology 1992; 76:792–798.
107. Magee L, Schick B, Donnenfeld A, et al: The safety of calcium channel blockers in human pregnancy: a prospective, multicenter cohort study. Am J Obstet Gynecol 1996; 174:823–828.
108. Ramanathan S, Grant G: Vasopressor therapy for hypotension due to epidural anaesthesia for cesarean section. Acta Anaesthesiol Scand 1988; 32:559–565.
109. Clark R, Brunner J: Dopamine for the treatment of spinal hypotension during cesarian section. Anesthesiology 1980; 53:514–517.
110. Bruns P, Linder R, Drose V, Battaglia F: The placental transfer of water from fetus to mother following the intravenous infusion of hypertonic mannitol to the maternal rabbit. Am J Obstet Gynecol 1963; 86:160–166.
111. Battaglia F, Prystowski H, Smisson C, et al: Fetal blood studies. XIII. The effect of the administration of fluids intravenously to mothers upon the concentrations of water and electrolytes in plasma of human fetuses. Pediatrics 1960; 25:2–10.
112. Briggs G, Freeman R, Yaffe S (eds): Drugs in Pregnancy and Lactation: A reference guide to fetal and neonatal risk, 5th ed. Williams & Wilkins; 1998:859–866.
113. Baker K, Young W, Stone J, et al: Deliberate mild intraoperative hypothermia for craniotomy. Anesthesiology 1994; 81:361–367.
114. Plattner O, Kurz A, Sessler D, et al: Efficacy of intraoperative cooling methods. Anesthesiology 1997; 87:1089–1095.
115. Illievich U, Zornow M, Choi K, et al: Effect of hypothermic metabolic suppression on hippocampal glutamate concentrations after transient global cerebral ischaemia. Anesth Analg 1994; 78:905–911.
116. Sano T, Drummond J, Patel P, et al: A comparison of the cerebral protective effects of isoflurane and mild hypothermia in a model of incomplete forebrain ischaemia in the rat. Anesthesiology 1992; 76:221–228.
117. Rowbotham G, Bell K, Akenhead J, Cairn S: A serious head injury in a pregnant woman treated by hypothermia. Lancet 1957; 1:1016–1019.
118. Hehre F: Hypothermia for operations during pregnancy. Anesth Analg 1965; 44:424–428.
119. Boba A: Hypothermia: appraisal of risk in 110 consecutive patients. J Neurosurg 1962; 19:924–933.
120. Vandewater S, Paul W: Observations on the foetus during experimental hypothermia. Can Anaesth Soc J 1960; 7:44–51.
121. Assali N, Westin B: Effects of hypothermia on uterine circulation and on the fetus. Proc Soc Exp Biol Med 1962; 109:485–488.
122. Hawkins J, Paape K, Adkins T, et al: Extracorporeal circulation in the fetal lamb: effects of hypothermia and perfusion rate. J Cardiovasc Surg 1991; 32:295–300.
123. Pomini F, Mercogliano D, Cavalletti D, et al: Cardiopulmonary bypass in pregnancy. Ann Thorac Surg 1966; 61:259–268.
124. Jadhon M, Main E: Fetal bradycardia associated with maternal hypothermia. Obstet Gynecol 1988; 72:496–497.
125. Mozze R, Källén B: Reproductive outcome after anaesthesia and operation during pregnancy: a registry study of 5405 cases. Am J Obstet Gynecol 1989; 161:1178–1185.
126. Hein H, Putman J: Is propofol a proper proposition for reproductive procedures? J Clin Anesth 1997; 9:611–613.
127. Vincent R: Anaesthesia for the pregnant patient. Clin Obstet Gynecol 1994; 37:256–273.
128. Gin T: Pharmacokinetic optimisation of general anaesthesia in pregnancy. Clin Pharmacokinet 1993; 25:59–70.
129. Ravussin P, de Tribolet N, Wilder-Smith O: Total intravenous anaesthesia is best for neurological surgery. J Neurosurg Anesth 1994; 6:285–289.
130. Gin T: Propofol during pregnancy. Acta Anaesthesiol Sin 1994; 32:127–132.
131. Gin T, Yau G, Jong W, et al: Disposition of propofol at caesarean section and in the postpartum period. Br J Anaesth 1991; 67:49–53.
132. Alan E, Ball R, Gillie M, et al: Effects of propofol and thiopental on maternal and fetal cardiovascular and acid-base variables in the pregnant ewe. Anesthesiology 1993; 78:562–576.
133. Bacon R, Razis P: The effect of propofol sedation in pregnancy on neonatal condition. Anaesthesia 1994; 49:1058–1060.
134. Parke T, Stevens J, Rice A, et al: Metabolic acidosis and fetal myocardial failure after propofol infusion in children: five case reports. BMJ 1992; 305:613–616.
135. Pepperman M, Macrae D: A comparison of propofol and other sedative use in paediatric intensive care in the United Kingdom. Paediatr Anaesth 1997; 7:143–153.
136. Todd M, Warner D, Sokoll M, et al: A prospective comparative trial of three anaesthetics for elective supratentorial craniotomy: propofol/fentanyl, isoflurane/nitrous oxide and fentanyl/nitrous oxide. Anesthesiology 1993; 78:1005–1020.
137. Ismail K, Coakham H, Walters F: Intracranial meningioma with progesterone positive receptors presenting in late pregnancy. Eur J Anaesth 1998; 15:106–109.
138. Kuhnigk H, Danhauser-Leistner I: Cesarean section with subsequent craniotomy in the area of the posterior cranial fossa. Anasthesiol Intensivmed Notfallmed Schmerztherap 1994; 29:184–187.
139. D'Haese J, Christiaens F, D'Haens J, Camu F: Combined cesarean section and clipping of a ruptured cerebral aneurysm: a case report. J Neurosurg Anesth 1997; 9:341–345.
140. Conklin K, Herr G, Fung D: Anaesthesia for caesarean section and cerebral aneurysm clipping. Can Anaesth Soc J 1984; 31:451–454.
141. Whitburn R, Laishley R, Jewkes D: Anaesthesia for simultaneous caesarean section and clipping of intracerebral aneurysm. Br J Anaesth 1990; 64:642–645.
142. Scudmore J, Chassar Moir J: Rupture of an intracranial aneurysm during pregnancy. J Obstet Gynaecol Br Commonw 1966; 73:1019–1020.
143. Yau G, Giu T, Ewart M, et al: Propofol for induction and maintenance of anaesthesia at caesarean section. Anaesthesia 1991; 46:20–23.
144. Abboud T, Zhu J, Richardson M, et al: Intravenous propofol vs. thiamylal-isoflurane for caesarean section: comparative maternal and neonatal effects. Acta Anaesthesiol Scand 1995; 39:205–209.
145. Gin T, Yau G, Chan K, et al: Disposition of propofol infusions for cesarean section. Can J Anaesth 1991; 38:31–36.

48

Drug Abuse in Pregnancy

❖ David A. O'Gorman, MD, FFARCSI
❖ David J. Birnbach, MD

DRUG ABUSE IN PREGNANCY

Although it has been suggested that the abuse of some substances may be on the decline in the United States, substance abuse among young women appears to be increasing. Drug abuse with its associated social and medical consequences remains a major problem in our society. A 1994 survey of trends in drug abuse among children and young adults revealed that illicit drug consumption had risen in excess of 30%. Similarly, the increase in use of licit or gateway drugs was also impressive, with 15% of 8th graders and 24% of 10th graders having had five or more consecutive drinks in the 2 weeks preceding the survey. The incidence of cigarette smoking was also high in all groups, with 31% of 12th graders abusing tobacco.[1] Emergency rooms visits for the management of the adverse effects of illicit drugs also increased by more than 68% between 1988 and 1994.[2]

Reports of pregnant patients who are using illicit drugs have been published by authors throughout the world. Data from the 1990 National Institute on Drug Abuse stated that of 60 million women of childbearing age, 50.8% used alcohol, 29% used cigarettes, 6.5% used marijuana, 0.9% used cocaine, and 8.0% used any illicit drug during the previous month.[3] A study by Chasnoff et al.[4] of 36 urban hospitals indicated that illicit drug use during pregnancy varied between 0.4% and 27% of mothers by geographic location. Chasnoff et al. also reported that almost 15% of parturients in their patient population in the United States had a positive urine toxicology screen for cocaine, marijuana, alcohol, or heroin. In addition, multiple drug use is not uncommon in pregnancy. Recent studies reported that women who used cocaine were much more likely to have used a combination of drugs rather than any single drug.[5] Drugs reportedly used by pregnant patients include cocaine, opioids, amphetamines, marijuana, alcohol, and cigarettes.[6]

Substance abuse in pregnancy has emerged as a major public health problem of the 1990s and therefore it is hardly surprising that anesthesiologists are now encountering an increasing number of parturients who use illicit substances.[7] These substances can have a major impact on both the pregnant woman and the developing fetus, and often present clinical challenges to all physicians responsible for their care. In particular, the use of cocaine has increased dramatically in the United States during the past decade and has led to many high-risk situations for both mother and fetus.[8] The clinically challenging situations that arise in the drug-abusing parturient can be due to many factors. The anesthesiologist's first encounter with these patients may include emergency management of clinical situations involving abruptio placentae and fetal or maternal arrhythmias.

Alcohol, nicotine, and most psychoactive drugs cross the placenta easily. Infrequent maternal ingestion may lead to prolonged fetal drug exposure due to slow fetal catabolism, enterohepatic circulation, and amniotic fluid pooling. Multiple drug exposure, variable prenatal care, concomitant infections, withdrawal, trauma, and poor nutrition all contribute to increased morbidity of both mother and child. Of all the many risks associated with maternal drug abuse, the absence of prenatal care has been shown to be of greatest importance. In the drug-abusing pregnant population, as many as 50 to 75% receive little or no prenatal care.[9] Many illicit drugs impair the ability of the developing fetus to use nutrients and thus low birthweight infants are commonly born to cocaine- and heroin-abusing mothers, even after controlling for race and cigarette smoking.[10] Premature labor is also common, with the proportion of births under 34 weeks being four times as high among cocaine users versus nonusers.[11]

Identification of the drug-abusing pregnant patient presents a challenge for all healthcare professionals. All patients, especially those considered to be high risk, should be questioned in a nonjudgmental manner regarding their use of licit and illicit substances. Surveys have found that only 40% of physicians ask their patients about alcohol use and only 20% of physicians inquire about abuse of other substances.[12] Even with direct questioning, denial is a major problem among substance-abusing patients.[13] There is evidence that self-reporting of drug abuse by pregnant patients underestimates actual use as determined by laboratory testing.[14, 15]

COCAINE AND PREGNANCY

Cocaine (benzoylmethylecgonine, $C_{17}H_{21}NO_4$) is an alkaloid derived from the plant *Erythroxylon coca* that is indigenous to Peru, Bolivia, and Ecuador.[16] The alkalinized form of cocaine, which is usually smoked, is known as "crack" and is currently widely used throughout the world.[17] The pharmacologic effects of cocaine are mediated through the norepinephrine, dopamine, and serotonin neurotransmitter systems.[18] Cocaine blocks the presynaptic reuptake of these sympathomimetic transmitters and thus produces an accumulation and prolongation of their effects. Hypertension, tachycardia, and vasoconstriction may be produced from this adrenergic stimulation. Chronic abuse however, may lead to depletion of presynaptic neurotransmitters. Owing to the extremely addictive properties of the drug, the intense need for drug may lead the pregnant woman to engage in other hazardous activities, such as exchanging sex for drugs, endangering both herself and her developing fetus.

Cocaine use has increased dramatically, with more than 5 million Americans abusing this drug on a regular basis.[19] More than 30% of young adults in the United States have tried cocaine, and it is estimated that as many as 8 to 10% of women in the United States use cocaine during pregnancy, many of whom may experience preterm labor.[20] The prevalence of cocaine use in the obstetric population has dramatically increased during the past decade and has resulted in a variety of maternal and perinatal complications.[21] Positive cocaine toxicology results have been reported in pregnant patients from all geographic, socioeconomic, and cultural groups. Because many cocaine-abusing patients deny drug abuse, the exact extent of perinatal cocaine use is unknown.[22] It has been estimated, however, that a large number of high-risk women cared for at many urban hospitals in the United States may be using cocaine.[23] Statistics regarding the number of drug-exposed infants born annually have varied, but in New York City, where these trends have been followed, the current rate is thought to approximate 33 per 1000.[24] Although patients who do not receive prenatal care tend to have the highest incidence of cocaine use, registered private patients in suburban settings have also been found to be cocaine positive.[25] Although comprehensive care of the cocaine-abusing parturient appears to be associated with improved outcomes, prenatal care is critical even if it is not specialized for high-risk patients or linked to drug treatment programs.[10]

The benefits of participation in a traditional, non-gender specific, publicly funded treatment program for cocaine dependency in the indigent population was compared with benefits of a modified program incorporating both gender and pregnancy needs. Statistically and clinically significant improvements in treatment retention were identified after implementation of a pregnancy-specific assistance program.[26] Women in general tend to underutilize the chemical dependency treatment programs, which are often male-oriented models with family exclusion.[27] Pregnant women often have other children, and the fundamental logistic barriers to their accessing treatment include the lack of specific resources for those children.[28]

New approaches currently being investigated in the treatment of cocaine addiction include the synthesis of therapeutic cocaine vaccines. In animal studies, these vaccines were demonstrated to induce a cocaine-specific antibody response. These antibodies bind to circulating cocaine, preventing entry into the central nervous system.[29–31] Although the vaccines have no direct effect on the actual neurobiologic basis of drug craving, it is thought that the lack of gratification from cocaine use may prevent further consumption. However, saturation of the antibody effect by increased cocaine consumption may limit the effectiveness of this form of treatment. This underscores the key factor in all aspects of addiction management, that no modality will succeed without the motivation and commitment of the abuser.

In 1989, a New York City survey of programs revealed that of the few programs that would accept pregnant women, 67% would not accept Medicaid as payment, and only 13% would accept cocaine-addicted Medicaid patients.[32] Medicolegal concerns about detoxification protocols for mother and infant and fear of program liability for negative birth outcomes further limit the resources for pregnant women.[33]

Perinatal cocaine abuse has been linked to significant maternal and neonatal morbidity. As illustrated in Table 48–1, maternal complications linked to

Table 48-1 LIFE-THREATENING MATERNAL COMPLICATIONS OF COCAINE ABUSE

SYSTEM	COMPLICATION
Central Nervous[59]	Seizures
	Cerebrovascular hemorrhage
Pulmonary[36]	Aspiration
	Bronchospasm
	Pneumothorax
Cardiovascular[42]	Myocardial infarction
	Hypertensive crisis
	Arrythmia
	Aortic dissection
Hepatic[41]	Hepatic failure
	Hepatic rupture
Renal[40]	Uremia
Hematologic[39]	Thrombocytopenia
	Disseminated intravascular coagulation
Other[37, 38]	Uterine rupture

cocaine abuse include placental abruption, pneumothorax, uterine rupture, preterm labor and delivery, renal failure, hepatic rupture, cerebral infarction, and cardiac dysrhythmias with infarction and death.[34–43] The morbidity associated with these cardiac sequelae may be increased, since pregnancy results in an increased sensitivity to the cardiovascular effects of cocaine.[44] Figure 48–1 reviews the pathophysiology of cocaine-induced cardiac dysfunction.

Abruptio placentae is a rare and serious complication that may be caused by maternal cocaine use; however, only one study has had large enough numbers to clearly assess the correlation.[45] The risk of cocaine-induced spontaneous abortion is supported by animal studies, but this is difficult to establish clinically, as abortion may occur prior to the knowledge of conception. Cocaine abuse may also be associated with shorter gestational periods and may precipitate labor, reduce fetal oxygen supply, and reduce contraction strength.[46]

Urogenital anomalies are clearly defined among neonates born to cocaine-abusing mothers.[47] Intracranial deficits and congenital heart and limb reduction defects have also been reported in this population, although these findings are difficult to correlate with the lack of control of smoking and other factors. Similarly, maternal hypertension and reduced placental blood flow secondary to cocaine-induced vasoconstriction may account for neonatal cerebral ischemia and hemorrhage reported in brains of exposed infants.[48] In addition to the immediate short-term neonatal concerns of cocaine abuse, evidence suggests that alcohol and drug use is involved in over 75% of child welfare cases and that substance abuse has led to a surge of child abuse and neglect. The number of children in foster care who have been exposed to drugs has doubled in the past decade. A meta-analysis of eight studies to assess the long-term effect of prenatal cocaine exposure on school-aged children showed reliable decrements in cognitive function. These effects were small as demonstrated by Intelligence Quotient findings; however, larger effects on more subtle domains of language were clearly identified. Therefore, although prenatal cocaine use does not necessarily produce devastating brain damage, it may lead to subtle anatomic

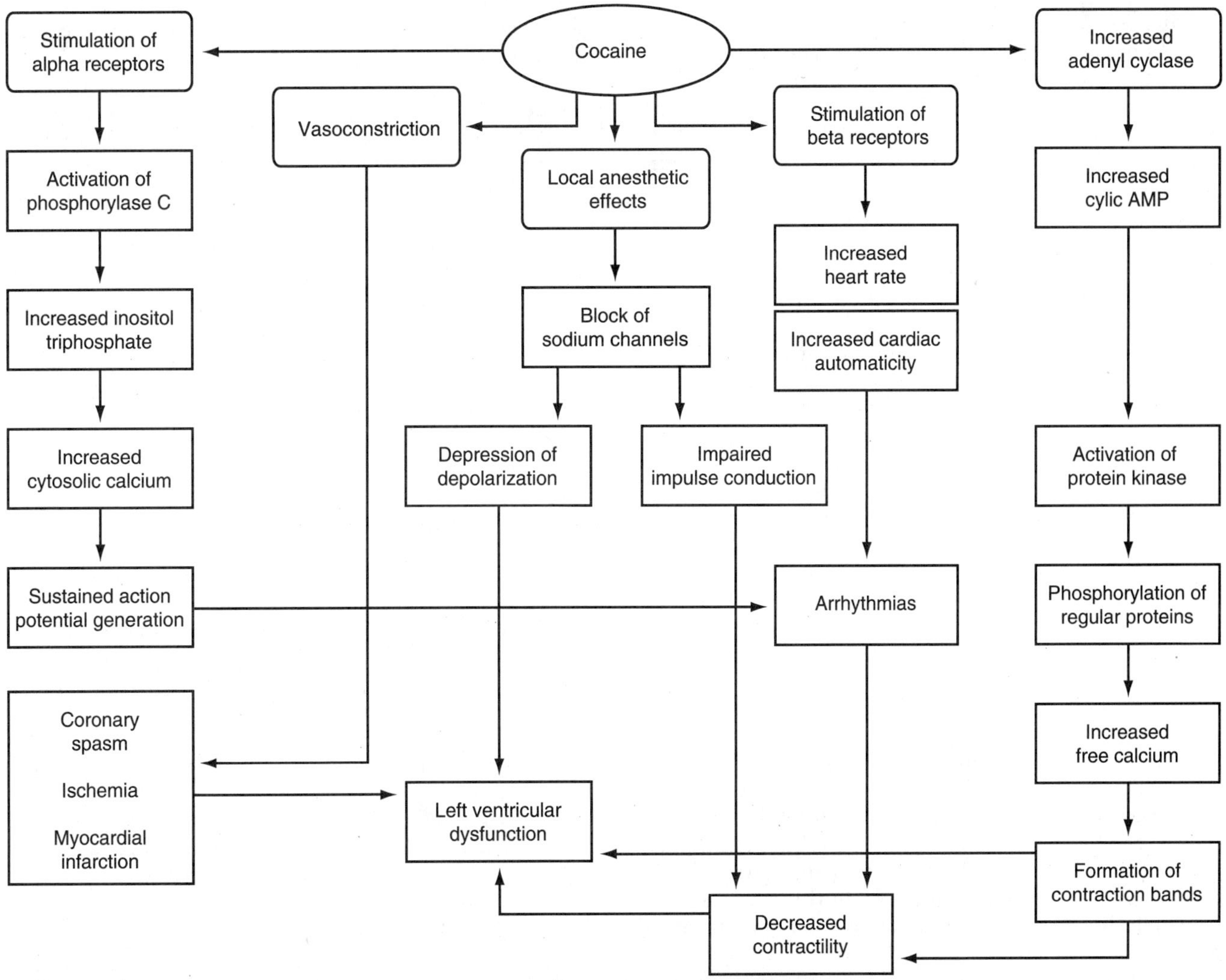

Figure 48–1 Mechanisms of cocaine-induced myocardial depression and dysfunction. (From Chestnut DH (ed): Obstetric Anesthesia. St. Louis: Mosby, 1999.)

Table 48–2 Maternal and Fetal Effects of Maternal Cocaine Abuse

Spontaneous abortion[56]
Preterm labor[47]
Placental abruption[46]
Impaired uteroplacental perfusion[49]
Fetal distress[47]
Congenital malformations[48]
Intrauterine fetal death[47]
Maternal and neonatal myocardial ischemia[45, 54]
Perinatal cerebral infarction[49]

and molecular effects with consequent learning and language difficulties.[49]

Studies in pregnant and non-pregnant animals treated with progesterone to stimulate pregnancy levels have suggested that the metabolism of cocaine is altered by pregnancy and the physiologic effects amplified.[50] Neonatal complications of maternal cocaine abuse include preterm delivery and a multitude of associated problems, congenital abnormalities, myocardial ischemia or myocardial infarction, and intrauterine fetal demise.[51–55]

As illustrated in Table 48–2, cocaine use in pregnancy has been shown to be dangerous to both mother and fetus.[56] Even after confounding variables such as age, race, alcohol abuse, and smoking are taken into account, life-threatening complications are still seen, possibly due to the effects on the placenta. The interaction of cocaine with the human placental serotonin transporter has been investigated, and it has been suggested that the function of the placental serotonin transporter may be severely impaired by maternal use of cocaine during pregnancy.[57] Cocaine is rapidly transferred across the placenta by simple diffusion without metabolic conversion and is thought to have direct effects on the fetal vasculature.[58] The effects of maternal cocaine use are thought to be incremental and cumulative, although it has been reported that the erratic use of cocaine in pregnancy may result in similar perinatal complications to those associated with daily bingeing.[43]

The American College of Obstetrics and Gynecology has recognized that cocaine use is a major public health concern and has published a Committee Opinion that reviews cocaine abuse in pregnancy.[59] It reports that the medical complications found in association with cocaine use include the following: acute myocardial infarction; cardiac arrhythmias, including life-threatening ventricular arrhythmias; rupture of the ascending aorta; stroke; seizures; bowel ischemia; hyperthermia; malnutrition; sexually transmitted disease; and hepatitis. This publication made several recommendations, including the following: all pregnant women should be asked about drug use during their initial prenatal visit and warned about the dangers; women admitting to cocaine use must be counseled regarding the perinatal ramifications of cocaine use and offered treatment; urine testing throughout pregnancy for the patient who admits to cocaine use, and drug screening in certain suspicious situations; and knowledge of state legislation of in utero exposure to drugs, which in some states is a form of neglect or abuse.

One of the most difficult aspects of medical care in the management of the cocaine-abusing parturient is recognition of her cocaine use. A majority of cocaine abusers deny drug use when interviewed by physicians, and physical examination may be misleading because cocaine intoxication is one of several different causes of hypertension in the parturient (Table 48–3). Of particular concern is the difficulty in distinguishing between the effects of cocaine and preeclampsia.[60, 61] Lack of prenatal care and cigarette smoking have been shown to be of predictive value in the recognition of a cocaine abuser.[62] It has been suggested that certain detrimental perinatal effects attributed to cocaine use may actually be due, at least in part, to other factors, including lack of prenatal care, cigarette smoking, and poor nutrition.[63] There is a strong association among crack-cocaine use, high-risk sexual practices, sexually transmitted diseases, and human immunodeficiency virus infection, which may lead to numerous problems for both mother and fetus. As previously mentioned, it has also been suggested that the abuse of cocaine to the exclusion of other drugs is probably so rare that most cocaine users are polydrug abusers.[64]

Current laboratory screening methods for cocaine metabolites include gas chromatography, mass spectrometry, radioimmunoassay, and latex agglutination testing. The disadvantage of many of these laboratory tests is the delay between taking the sample and final analysis report. There may also be difficulty in identifying the cocaine abusing patient, since cocaine metabolites are detected in urine for only 14 to 60 hours after the last use.[65] Thus, only very recent cocaine use will be detected with many screening methods. In some hospitals, it may take several days to receive mass spectrometer toxicology results and therefore these results may be of little benefit to the physician. Although the reliability of urine testing depends on the time of exposure and pharmacokinetics, alternative testing methods are available. An instant latex agglutination test for cocaine metabolites (OnTrak Assay, Roche Diagnostic Systems, Branchburg, NJ) can provide an accurate result within 4 minutes and has been shown to be highly sensitive and specific when used by anesthesiologists.[66] Other studies have evaluated newborn meconium and maternal hair for detection of substance abuse and have found greatly improved detection of cocaine use in pregnancy.[15, 67, 68] Anesthesiologists frequently encounter cocaine-abusing patients in an emergency setting because of the associated higher

Table 48–3 Differential Diagnosis of Hypertension in Pregnancy

Hypoxia/hypercarbia	Pheochromocytoma
Drug withdrawal	Preeclampsia/eclampsia
Essential hypertension	Pain
Drug abuse	Malignant hyperthermia

incidence of cesarean section due to "fetal distress" and abruptio placentae in this population.[22, 69] The choice of anesthetic technique may be dictated by the hemodynamic consequences of drug use. Severe hypertension or, rarely, hypotension may occur as a result of the sympathetic stimulation and myocardial dysfunction, respectively. General endotracheal anesthesia is usually selected for the profoundly hypotensive parturient. In more controlled situations, however, the anesthesiologist should choose the anesthetic technique based on the risks and benefits of regional and general anesthesia individualized to each patient. Epidural or spinal anesthesia may be successfully used to anesthetize the cocaine-abusing patient for cesarean section.[22, 69] It has been demonstrated that the cocaine-abusing patient may require more supplemental intravenous medication than non–drug abusing patients.[22]

This has been explained by changes in both μ and κ opioid receptor densities that have been identified following binge patterns of cocaine administration in central regions with abundant dopaminergic terminals.[70] The binding of opioid receptors by specific receptor-selective ligands have also been reported.[71]

"Life-threatening" events that occurred under anesthesia in the cocaine-abusing parturient have been evaluated, and evidence suggests that severe hypertension and arrhythmias are more common during general anesthesia than during regional anesthesia.[22] Since severe hypertension was most often associated with laryngoscopy, blood pressure should be controlled prior to undertaking intubation. Regardless of the anesthetic technique, patients with a history of chronic cocaine use need to be monitored preoperatively, intraoperatively, and postoperatively for signs of myocardial ischemia.

Cocaine toxicity is often seen many hours after its administration, pointing to a potential role of cocaine metabolites in toxicity.[72] Several drugs that can be used to control blood pressure in the cocaine-abusing patient have been evaluated. β-Blockade, using propranolol, to control blood pressure in the cocaine-abusing patient is contraindicated due to unopposed α-adrenergic stimulation, with possible profound exacerbation of hypertension.[73] In addition, blockade has been reported to enhance cocaine-induced coronary vasoconstriction.[74] An evaluation of hydralazine for the treatment of hypertension in cocaine-positive patients has concluded that hydralazine resulted in profound maternal tachycardia and did not restore uterine blood flow.[75] Hughes et al.[76] studied the effects of hydralazine and labetalol in the treatment of acute cocaine intoxication during parturition and concluded that labetalol may be preferable. Hollander,[77] however, has suggested that labetalol should not be used in cocaine-abusing patients, since the β-antagonistic effects are more potent than the α-antagonistic effects. In addition, in animal studies, labetalol increased both seizure activity and mortality. Although research in this area is ongoing, there is controversy about the efficacy of calcium channel blockers in the treatment and prevention of cocaine toxicity.[77–79]

In the event that general anesthesia becomes necessary, any agent, such as halothane, that sensitizes the myocardium to the effects of catecholamines should be avoided.[80] Although isoflurane has been administered to cocaine-abusing patients without problem, it has been reported that cocaine toxicity during isoflurane anesthesia is associated with a marked increase in systemic vascular resistance and a tendency to produce cardiac arrhythmias.[81] Ketamine should be used with extreme caution in the cocaine-abusing patient, since it may potentiate the cardiac effects of cocaine by further increasing catecholamine levels or produce myocardial depression in cases in which catecholamines have been depleted.[82] There has also been a report of a prolonged block from succinylcholine in a cocaine-abusing patient; therefore, caution should be exercised and neuromuscular blockade assessed prior to initiation of nondepolarizing muscle blockade.[83]

Although offering several advantages over general anesthesia, the use of regional anesthesia in the cocaine-abusing parturient may also be associated with serious complications and life-threatening risks.[22, 84] The patient who has recently used cocaine may be uncooperative or even combative, making placement difficult. The use of regional anesthetic techniques may rarely present an increased risk of epidural hematoma formation due to cocaine-induced thrombocytopenia. Hypotension that is resistant to ephedrine may occur following local anesthetic–induced sympathetic blockade. Titration of low doses of phenylephrine may be required to restore normal blood pressure. These patients may be abusing multiple drugs and these combinations may produce even more profound hemodynamic instability.[22, 84]

Cocaine is a proarrhythmogenic agent producing sinus tachycardia, atrial premature contractions, ventricular tachycardia, ventricular premature contractions, ventricular fibrillation, and asystole.[85] Sodium bicarbonate appears to have an important role in the setting of acute cocaine abuse.[79] This may be due to the metabolic and respiratory acid-base abnormalities, which are often associated with cocaine toxicity.[86] Nitroglycerin has been found to be safe and possibly effective in the treatment of cocaine-associated chest pain.[87] Despite theoretical concerns that lidocaine may enhance cocaine toxicity, lidocaine has been used to treat arrhythmias in cocaine-abusing patients and has not been associated with significant cardiovascular or central nervous system toxicity in these patients.[88] Signs of central nervous system hyperexcitability can be treated with a benzodiazepine.[89]

AMPHETAMINES AND PREGNANCY

Amphetamines are noncatecholamine sympathomimetics that resemble the sympathetic neurotransmitter norepinephrine without hydroxyl groups at the 3′ and 4′ position on the benzene ring. They have a wide distribution and long duration of action, partly due to the ineffectiveness of catechol-*O*-methyltransferase (COMT) and monoamine oxidase (MAO) in their metabolism. The presence of the hydroxyl groups in positions 3 and 4 on the benzene ring and a methylated alpha carbon prevents metabolism of amphetamines by COMT and MAO, respectively.[90] Crystal methamphetamine, also referred to as "ice" or "blue ice," is a more potent form of the drug that may be smoked.

The primary effects of amphetamines are dose-dependent central nervous system stimulation with increased alertness, decreased fatigue, sleeplessness, euphoria, and exhilaration. They may be abused by patients alone or in conjunction with other drugs. Acute administration of amphetamines produces signs and symptoms similar to those of cocaine abuse. Amphetamines enhance the release of presynaptic norepinephrine in the central nervous system, leading to vasoconstriction and tachycardia.[91] Cerebrovascular accidents are common sequelae of amphetamine abuse in the non-pregnant state; however, this has not been reported in the pregnant population.[91–94]

Use of amphetamines during pregnancy can be associated with maternal hypertension, tachycardia, proteinuria, premature labor, and placental hemorrhage. Often, these symptoms may be mistaken for preeclampsia or eclampsia.[95]

Many patients abusing amphetamines receive little or no prenatal care, significantly affecting both maternal and fetal well-being. The anorectic effect of amphetamines may lead to poor maternal nutrition and related growth problems in the fetus.[12]

However, as with many illicit drugs, attributing use in pregnancy to outcome is often complicated by confounding environmental factors. Amphetamine use has been associated with intrauterine growth retardation, intrauterine fetal demise, and abruptio placentae.[96] Associated fetal malformations and adverse outcomes include cleft lip, cardiac defects, low birthweight, growth reduction, reduced head circumference, biliary atresia, prematurity, stillbirth, hyperbilirubinemia, cerebral hemorrhage, body fat reduction, systolic murmurs, and undescended testis.[97–101] A prospective study performed over a 14-year period revealed that only 22% of children born to maternal amphetamine users were with their biological mother since birth. In addition, achievements in mathematics, language, and sports were found to be statistically below those of their classmates. Therefore, maternal amphetamine abuse during pregnancy may influence children at least up to the age of 14 or 15 years, even if the maternal environment is avoided for significant portions of time.[102]

Amphetamine use may precipitate fetal distress, necessitating emergency cesarean section. The associated hemodynamic and central effects of amphetamines have major implications in the administration of anesthesia. Cardiac arrest in amphetamine-abusing patients undergoing cesarean section using both general and regional anesthetic techniques has been reported.[103, 104] Acute ingestion of amphetamines increases the dose requirements for general anesthetic agents, whereas the chronic ingestion of these drugs decreases the minimum alveolar concentration of volatile anesthetic agents.[105] Since it is often difficult to differentiate between chronic and acute amphetamine use, judicious titration of all anesthetic agents is essential. Avoidance of halothane is recommended in the presence of acute amphetamine consumption due to the risk of myocardial sensitization to catecholamines. Although regional anesthesia has been used safely in these patients, severe hypotension may occur following induction, and the response to vasoactive agents may be unpredictable.

The drug 3,4-methylene-dioxymethamphetamine (MDMA) also called "ecstasy" is a three-ring substituted methoxylated analogue of methamphetamine. MDMA shares properties with both amphetamines and hallucinogenic drugs. MDMA has an undeserved reputation for safety and duration of action. Its appeal is based on the effect of induced empathy and closeness toward others.[106] Side effects include sedation, tachycardia, fatigue, and muscle spasms. Serious adverse effects include serious and fatal heat injury, fluid and electrolyte depletion, and central nervous system, cardiac, muscular, renal, and hepatic dysfunction. The main mortality associated with the drug is profound disturbances in thermoregulation (heat stroke).[107]

Several toxicology screening tests for the amphetamine class of drugs of abuse can detect MDMA but at about 50% reduced sensitivity. Treatment of the acute toxic reaction includes rapid cooling, rehydration, and electrolyte and organ homeostasis.[107, 108] Reports of acute and fatal chronic toxicity associated with ingestion are common. Serious morbidity and mortality have occurred from fulminant hyperthermia, cardiac arrhythmia, disseminated intravascular coagulation, rhabdomyolysis, acute renal failure, and hepatic toxicity. MDMA is also a selective serotoninergic neurotoxin, and increased psychomotor drive is a sympathetic nervous system effect. Psychedelic effects include sensory enhancement, distortion, and illusions without overt hallucinations. Rehydration, cooling, management of anxiety, anti-arrhythmic therapy, fluid and electrolyte replacement, and maintenance of urine output are all essential goals of treatment. Dantrolene has been used for MDMA-induced spasms and cramping.[109, 110] Ecstasy consumption produces acute symptomatic hyponatremia with the syndrome of inappropriate antidiuretic hormone secretion.[111]

OPIOID ABUSE IN PREGNANCY

It has been estimated that in the United States, 250,000 women are intravenous drug abusers, 90% of whom are of childbearing age.[112] The abuse of various opioid drugs, including heroin, morphine, meperidine, and methadone, have all been reported in pregnancy. The prevalence of opioid use in pregnancy has been estimated at up to 21% in certain geographic locations.[113] In 1992, approximately 88,000 women in the United States were using heroin regularly, with 650,000 having used it at least once.[114] In 1986, 74,000 people in the United States were enrolled in methadone programs; since then, this number has steadily increased.[115] Recent reports have estimated that 9000 babies are born to opioid-addicted mothers each year and 300,000 infants are exposed to opiates in utero.[9, 116]

Opioid abuse and subsequent addiction in pregnant women results in multiple health problems for both mother and fetus. Maternal medical problems associated with intravenous opioid use include cellulitis, abscess formation, hepatitis, endocarditis, renal disease, and human immunodeficiency virus infection.[117, 118] Poor nutrition, polydrug use, and lack of prenatal care are also associated with this form of drug abuse in pregnancy.

Opioids have both central and peripheral sites of action. Direct depressant effects of opioids on ventilatory centers in the brain stem may lead to hypoventilation or apnea, whereas nausea and vomiting result from direct stimulation of the chemoreceptor trigger zone.[119] Peripheral effects of opioid use in the parturient include decreased uterine and vascular tone. Prolonged abuse leads to tolerance to and physical dependence on opiates, which may lead to symptoms of withdrawal in both mother and neonate upon cessation.

Although opioid dependence usually results from duration of opioid consumption in excess of several weeks, shorter onset of dependence has been reported. Opioid withdrawal is extremely uncomfortable for patients, but is seldom life-threatening in the absence of cardiac disease. Recognition of maternal opioid use and possible withdrawal is essential when treating an opioid-abusing patient. Acute withdrawal syndrome in the mother may be recognized by symptoms and signs of lacrimation, rhinorrhea, restlessness, diarrhea, dehydration, sweating, insomnia, tachycardia, tachypnea, and hypertension.[119] Use of opioid antagonists or agonist-antagonist drugs via parenteral or neuraxial routes may precipitate acute withdrawal and therefore should not be used in these patients.[120]

Withdrawal symptoms usually begin within 4 to 6 hours following the last opioid administration, and peak at 72 hours. Several nonopioid agents can be used to treat the symptoms of withdrawal. These adjuvant agents include clonidine, doxepin, and diphenhydramine.[121] To prevent withdrawal in a known opioid-abusing patient, the patient's daily opioid dose should be calculated and administered as a minimum daily requirement, irrespective of additional considerations such as analgesia for labor.[122]

Opioid overdose must be considered early in the management of parturient presenting with coma, miosis, or respiratory depression to the emergency room. In addition to standard supportive measures in treatment, airway protection is critical to decrease the risk of aspiration and associated problems.

Neonatal opioid withdrawal is present in 42% to 68% of heroin-exposed neonates and 63% to 85% of methadone-exposed neonates.[116] Symptoms of neonatal withdrawal include irritability, poor feeding, hypertonicity, diarrhea, respiratory distress, apnea, and autonomic dysfunction. Symptoms in heroin-exposed neonates present within 24 hours of delivery and 2 to 7 days after birth in methadone-exposed neonates.

Regional anesthetic techniques in this group of patients can provide a comfortable parturition without the need for intravenous opioid administration. The opioid-abusing patient may have developed a pain intolerance due to a decreased level of endogenous opioid peptides and, therefore, may be intolerant of the pain of labor. The same patient may have developed tolerance to opioids and thus have increased intravenous opioid requirements to attain analgesia. To avoid symptoms of withdrawal in the dependent parturient, opioid replacement must be continued throughout prolonged labor or postoperatively following cesarean section. Appropriate conversion of oral methadone to intravenous opioids for maintenance is necessary in the postoperative phase, until oral medications are tolerated. Methadone bioavailability is approximately 50% and is equipotent to parenteral morphine.

The aim of maintenance is to prevent or reduce withdrawal symptoms and craving, to prevent relapse to addictive drugs, and to restore toward normal any physiologic function disrupted by drug abuse. Overall, perinatal care participation among methadone program patients has been reported, but conflict exists between earlier studies that demonstrate an improved fetal growth and outcome for women taking methadone. A retrospective evaluation of women enrolled in methadone maintenance programs revealed that birth outcome was not significantly different between methadone and cocaine abusers. In addition, findings suggested that women receiving methadone maintenance were likely to abuse other illicit drugs.[123]

TOBACCO AND PREGNANCY

Tobacco is still the most commonly abused drug during pregnancy. It has been suggested that 15% of low birthweight cases could be prevented if women did not smoke during pregnancy.[124] In 1990, it was estimated that 29% of American women of childbearing age smoked cigarettes.[115] Thirty percent of women are believed to smoke during pregnancy.[9] Despite the fact that there is no longer any doubt that cigarette smoking has adverse effects on mother and fetus, only 20% of women in the United States quit smoking during pregnancy.[125]

Smoking during pregnancy has been associated with intrauterine growth retardation, spontaneous abortion, premature rupture of membranes, placenta previa, abruptio placentae, and sudden infant death syndrome.[126, 127] The chemical composition of cigarette smoke is more closely related to reduction in fetal growth than the number of cigarettes smoked. The effects of smoking on the fetus could be due to any of the numerous chemical substances in tobacco smoke, but apart from carbon monoxide and nicotine, little is know about the effects of other toxins, which number almost 1000. Nicotine can decrease placental blood flow due to vasoconstriction and contribute to fetal hypoxia.[128] Because of the fetal risks of maternal cigarette smoking, a strong emphasis is placed to encourage quitting in the antenatal period.[129]

The respiratory effects of cigarette smoke include abnormalities in mucus secretion, ciliary transport, and small airway function.[130] Postoperative respiratory morbidity is therefore a risk of general anesthesia in patients who smoke cigarettes. Although 4 to 6 weeks of abstinence is required to allow a decrease in the risk of postoperative respiratory complications, after as little as 48 hours of abstinence, carboxyhemoglobin levels fall and oxygen delivery increases. In addition, a few days of abstinence will improve mucociliary transport. The use of regional anesthesia is particularly beneficial to the cigarette smoker undergoing cesarean section, allowing an alternative to general anesthesia, reducing the risk of bronchospasm during airway manipulation. In addition, regional anesthesia may also avoid postoperative pulmonary complications.

Several treatment modalities have been investigated to aid smoking cessation in pregnancy. In addition to behavioral modification, relaxation techniques and acupuncture, many pharmacologic adjuvants are available that may have significance to the obstetric anesthesiologist. The most commonly encountered agents include buspirone, bupropion (Zyban), and various forms of nicotine replacement therapy. Buspirone was initially advocated as an efficacious agent, but placebo-controlled laboratory and clinical studies have revealed inconsistent and contradictory results.[131]

Bupropion is an atypical antidepressant that has dopaminergic and adrenergic actions.[132] The sustained-release preparation of bupropion became available as a prescription item in 1998 under the trade name Zyban (Glaxo-Wellcome, Research Triangle Park, NC), specifically for smoking cessation. This treatment is available for patients in whom nicotine replacement therapy is not indicated or unsuitable. Patients begin bupropion therapy 1 week prior to cessation at 150–300 mg/day and continue treatment for 7 to 12 weeks. Studies have demonstrated that bupropion consistently doubles quit rates compared with placebo.[133, 134]

The tablet has a bitter taste and produces a sensation of local anesthesia on the oral mucosa. Bupropion works well in the absence and presence of depression, suggesting that its mechanism of action is not due to an antidepressant effect.[135] Adverse reactions are mild and most commonly include dry mouth and insomnia.[136] Earlier studies using high doses of immediate-release preparations suggested that bupropion increased the risks of seizures.[137] More recently with use of therapeutic dosages of sustained-release preparations (up to 300 mg/day), this risk was demonstrated to be no greater than that with any other antidepressant agent. No seizure activity was observed in a study of 2400 volunteers undergoing a smoking cessation trial following use of screening precautions.[134] However, concurrent administration of bupropion with other agents that lower seizure threshold should be undertaken with extreme caution. Side effects with bupropion are rare but include postural hypotension, stroke, tachycardia, syncope, complete atrioventricular block, extrasystoles, hypotension, myocardial infarct, phlebitis, pulmonary embolism, and bronchospasm.[134, 138, 139] Bupropion has a low abuse potential despite a few reported cases of dependence and withdrawal phenomena.[140]

Carcinogenicity studies were performed in mice and rats at doses up to 150 mg/kg and 300 mg/kg, respectively. There was no impairment noted at these doses, which are approximately 2 and 10 times, respectively, the maximum recommended human dose (MRHD) on a mg/m^2 basis. Teratology studies have been performed at doses up to 450 mg/kg of bupropion in rats (approximately 14 times the MRHD on a mg/m^2 basis). No evidence of impaired fertility or fetal morbidity due to bupropion was demonstrated.[141] Although animal reproductive studies are not always predictive of human responses, there are no adequate well-controlled studies in pregnancy. To monitor the fetal outcome of pregnant women exposed to bupropion, Glaxo-Wellcome maintains a Bupropion Pregnancy Register.[142]

Tobacco smoke has been shown to contain nicotine, hydrogen cyanide, and carbon monoxide. Nicotine itself has been shown in clinical studies to cause fetal harm, thus nicotine replacement therapy (NRT) itself may also be implicated in fetal morbidity.[143] Spontaneous abortion has been reported with both NRT and smoking, therefore nicotine cannot be excluded as a contributing factor.[144] All the currently available NRTs appear to be efficacious in the management of smoking cessation, approximately doubling the quit rate compared with placebo. Combination of NRT with bupropion may also increase the quit rate compared with single therapy.

Nicotine from any source can be toxic and addictive. Smoking causes lung cancer, heart disease, and emphysema and may have adverse effects for both mother and fetus. In the presence of pregnancy and concurrent disease, the risk-benefit effect of continued smoking versus use of adjuvant agents needs to be carefully considered. NRT systems should not remain applied during labor and delivery until their effects on both mother and fetus are firmly established. Clearly these drugs should be used during pregnancy only if absolutely essential. Pregnant women should be educated about potential risks and encouraged to attempt cessation using educational and behavioral approaches before pharmacologic methods are used.

SOLVENT ABUSE AND PREGNANCY

Inhalants are a chemically diverse group of centrally acting substances composed of organic solvents and volatile agents. Studies have indicated that between 5 and 15% of young people in the United States have abused inhalants at some point, which may be a measure of their ease of availability and low cost. In 1993 an estimated 889,000 people abused inhalants, of which 68% were children and young adults.[145] Solvents can be taken orally or may be sniffed directly from an open container or "huffed" in a concentrated form from bags or soaked rags. Once inhaled, blood levels rise rapidly, producing an intense central stimulation and disinhibition. The effects of inhalants are similar to those of alcoholic intoxication: distortion of perception of sensory stimuli and depression at higher doses. Headache, nausea, vomiting, loss of coordination, and respiratory compromise are common following inhalation.[146]

Toluene is an industrial solvent widely used as a drying, cleaning, and thinning agent. It is a major component in many household paints, lacquers, adhesives, and cleaning agents. Recreational inhalation of toluene-based solvents has been reported in pregnancy and is associated with an increased incidence of intrauterine growth retardation, preterm labor, and perinatal death.[147, 148]

Toluene abuse may be associated with irreversible encephalopathy, cerebellar degeneration, optic neuropathy, sensorimotor deficits, and diffuse brain atrophy.[149–152] Non-neurotoxic effects of solvent abuse or exposure include renal toxicity, hepatotoxicity, pulmonary hypertension, acute respiratory distress, increased airway resistance, and ventricular fibrillation.[153, 154] Changes in cardiac autonomic function, mainly parasympathetic activity, have been demonstrated with occupational exposure to *n*-hexane, xylene, and toluene.[155]

Solvents cause a unique distal and proximal tubular acidosis with resultant metabolic imbalance and amino acid depletion, respectively. Solvent-induced renal tubular acidosis has been reported in pregnancy, in which three of the five pregnancies revealed growth retardation. In this series, the mothers responded to treatment for their metabolic imbalance after 72 hours of abstinence.[156] In animal studies, perinatal toluene exposure resulted in an ataxic syndrome in the neonatal period.[157]

Studies in mothers with a chronic history of solvent exposure have suggested the existence of a possible fetal solvent syndrome, although the evidence is inconclusive.[158] However, the patients reported on in this series consumed paint thinner and spray paints in addition to alcohol. This combination, coupled with environmental factors, suggest that the syndrome may be multifactorial in origin. Toluene may augment fetal alcohol syndrome by lowering the threshold of dosage at which the syndrome becomes manifest.[159]

Optimal management of these patients requires early recognition of the problem. In a recent review of inhalant abuse in pregnancy, it was suggested that although it is not possible to link a specific birth defect or developmental problem to prenatal exposure to a specific chemical, it is clear that inhalant abuse and its associated lifestyle place mother and child at risk.[158]

ALCOHOL AND PREGNANCY

Evidence suggests that 25% of the 15 million alcoholics in the United States are women.[160] Maternal complications of alcohol abuse include poor nutrition, liver disease such as hepatitis or cirrhosis, coagulopathy, pancreatitis, and cardiomyopathy. In addition, withdrawal from alcohol may present problems for both mother and fetus. Manifestations of alcohol withdrawal result from increased sympathetic discharge and include tachycardia, hypertension, dysrhythmias, cardiac failure, delirium, hallucinations, and seizures.[161] Symptoms can occur as early as 6 to 48 hours and up to 10 days following alcohol consumption.

Alcohol is a well established teratogen and its use in pregnancy is associated with fetal alcohol syndrome.[162] This syndrome is characterized by physical anomalies, growth restriction, and mental handicap. Laboratory studies have consistently demonstrated the toxic effects of ethanol exposure in utero on myelination and neural differentiation.[163, 164] Although the exact incidence of fetal alcohol syndrome varies with inclusion criteria and geographic location, estimates of 9.1 per 1000 live births have been reported.[165] Children with complete fetal alcohol syndrome are usually born to mothers who consume large volumes of alcohol throughout pregnancy. However, since no safe level of alcohol intake has been established, abstinence is considered the safest course in pregnancy.[166]

Regional anesthesia can be utilized safely in an alcoholic patient in the absence of coagulopathy, neuropathy, or infection. Occasionally, psychotic or combative behavior in the acutely intoxicated patient may make the procedure both technically and logistically impossible. Alcohol increases gastric acid secretion and decreases protective airway reflexes; therefore, should general anesthesia become necessary, the risks of aspiration are even further increased. Alcoholic patients with associated hepatic or cardiac disease may exhibit increased sensitivity to the myocardial depressant effects of anesthetic agents, especially in the presence of hypoalbuminemia and cardiac failure. Suggestions that chronic alcohol consumption is associated with increased induction requirements for barbiturates have not been borne out by subsequent pharmacokinetic and pharmacodynamic investigation.[167, 168]

MARIJUANA AND PREGNANCY

Marijuana is the most widely abused illicit drug in the United States. A recent study of trends in drug abuse reported that 56% of women 18 to 25 years of age acknowledged marijuana use. It is estimated that the use of marijuana during pregnancy ranges from 9.5% to 27%. Marijuana exerts its effects through delta-9-tetrahydrocannabinol (THC), which readily crosses the placenta and accumulates in the fetus. Despite its widespread abuse, there is little evidence of the detrimental effects of marijuana on fetal outcome. Multiple studies have suggested that perinatal use of marijuana leads to delayed maturation of the nervous system.[116, 169] Neonates exposed to marijuana in utero have demonstrated increased plasma norepinephrine levels at birth, which may account for early neurobehavioral disturbances.[170] Outcome studies have shown cognitive dysfunction among 9- to 12-year olds exposed to marijuana in the perinatal period.[171] Controversy exists over whether in utero exposure to marijuana is responsible for low birthweight.[172, 173] It has been clearly demonstrated that women who abuse marijuana during pregnancy are more likely to use other substances, thus confounding outcome studies and further contributing to neonatal morbidity.[174]

The maternal effects of acute marijuana use include increased sympathetic discharge, tachycardia, conjunctival congestion, and anxiety. Chronic marijuana use may lead to lethargy, irritability, and respiratory problems such as chronic bronchitis or frequent upper respiratory tract infections.[3] Anesthetic requirements may be increased in patients with a history of acute marijuana use, as a result of increased catecholamine discharge. Respiratory problems associated with chronic marijuana use make regional anesthesia an attractive alternative to general anesthesia. Depletion of catecholamines associated with chronic marijuana use may lead to decreased anesthetic requirements.

CONCLUSION

Despite ongoing educational and rehabilitative measures at both local and national levels, drug abuse during pregnancy remains a significant problem in our society. The obstetric complications of substance abuse present many serious problems that must be recognized and dealt with urgently. It is vital for the physician caring for the substance-abusing patient to identify and treat the patient appropriately, given the effects of these substances on both mother and fetus. Recognition of such a patient is the initial step in care, as signs and symptoms of substance abuse may be confused with other pregnancy-related disease states. This requires a high index of suspicion, combined with nonjudgmental questioning and screening of every patient. Improved techniques in drug detection have enabled more accurate diagnosis of drug use in both mother and child. The long-term effects of substance abuse are exacerbated by several environmental factors that have ramifications beyond the duration of labor and anesthesia.[175] Optimal management of the drug-abusing parturient requires a continuum of care with input from the family practitioner, social worker, psychiatrist, obstetrician, anesthesiologist, and pediatrician. Close communication within this multidisciplinary network is essential to ensure maximal care of this vulnerable patient population.

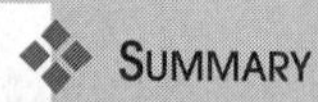

Summary

Key Points

- The majority of drug-abusing parturients deny their drug abuse.
- Drug abuse should be considered in the differential diagnosis for parturients who are unregistered or who present with placental abruption, profound hypertension, or arrhythmias.
- Cocaine abuse represents a relative contraindication to administration of a β-blocking drug, as unopposed α-stimulation may occur.

Key Reference

Kain ZN, Rimar S, Brash PG: Cocaine abuse in the parturient and effects on the fetus and neonate. Anesth Analg 1993; 77:835–845.

Case Stem

An unregistered 28-year-old gravida 3 para 2 woman is admitted at 30 weeks' gestation with a diagnosis of abruptio placentae. Despite a blood loss of 1 L, her blood pressure is 160/110. The patient is unregistered but denies drug abuse. The obstetrician wishes to proceed with an urgent cesarean section for presumed fetal jeopardy. Discuss the obstetric and anesthetic implications.

References

1. Johnston LD, O'Malley PM, Bachman JC: National Survey: Results on Drug Use 1975–94, Vol. 1. Rockville, MD, U.S. Department of Health and Human Services, NIDA, 1995.
2. Treaster JB: Hospital data shows increase in drug abuse. The New York Times July 9, 1992. Page B1.
3. Wheeler SF: Substance abuse during pregnancy. Prim Care 1993; 20:191–207.
4. Chasnoff IJ, Landress HJ, Barrett ME: The prevalence of illicit drug or alcohol use during pregnancy and discrepancies in mandatory reporting in Pinellas County, Florida. N Engl J Med 1990; 322:1202–1206.
5. Bendersky M, Alessandri S, Gilbert P, Lewis M: Characteristics of pregnant substance abusers in two cities in the northeast. Am J Drug Alcohol Abuse 1996; 22:349–362.
6. Matera C, Warren WB, Moomjy M, et al: Prevalence of use of cocaine and other substances in an obstetric population. Am J Obstet Gynecol 1990; 163:797–801.
7. Slutsker L, Smith R, Higginson G, Fleming S: Recognizing illicit drug use by pregnant women: Reports from Oregon birth attendants. Am J Public Health 1993; 83:61–64.
8. Rizk B, Atterbury JL, Groome LJ: Reproductive risks of cocaine. Hum Reprod Update 1996; 2:43–55.
9. Sprauve ME: Substance abuse and HIV in pregnancy. Clin Obstet Gynecol 1996; 39:316–332.
10. Chazotte C, Youcah J, Freda MC: Cocaine using during pregnancy and low birth weight: The impact of prenatal care and drug treatment. Semin Perinatol 1995; 19:293–300.
11. Zuckerman B, Frank DA, Hingson R, et al: Effects of maternal marijuana and cocaine use on fetal growth. N Engl J Med 1989; 320:762–768.
12. King JC: Substance abuse in pregnancy. Symposium on Women's Healthcare. Substance Abuse in Pregnancy. 1997; 102:135–150.
13. Rodriguez EM, Mofenson LM, Chang BH, et al: Association of maternal drug use during pregnancy with maternal HIV culture positivity and perinatal HIV transmission. AIDS 1996; 10:273–282.
14. Frank DA, Zuckerman BS, Amaro H, et al: Cocaine use during pregnancy: Prevalence and correlates. Pediatrics 1988; 82:888–895.
15. Kline J, Ng SK, Schittini M, et al: Cocaine use during pregnancy: Sensitive detection by hair assay. Am J Public Health 1997; 87:352–358.
16. Fleming JA, Byck R, Barash PG: Pharmacology and therapeutic applications of cocaine. Anesthesiology 1990; 73:518–531.
17. Hatsukami DK, Fischman MW: Crack cocaine and cocaine hydrochloride. Are the differences myth or reality? JAMA 1996; 276:1580–1588.
18. Gold MS, Washton AM, Dackis CA: Cocaine abuse: Neurochemistry, phenomenology, and treatment. Nat Inst Drug Abuse Res Monogr Series 1985; 61:130–150.
19. National Institute of Drug Abuse: National Household Survey on Drug Abuse: Population Estimates 1991. Washington, DC: Government Printing Office, 1992.
20. Delaney DB, Larrabee KD, Monga M: Preterm premature rupture of membranes associated with recent cocaine use. Am J Perinatol 1997; 14:285–288.
21. Rozenak D, Diamant YZ, Yaffe H, et al: Cocaine: Maternal use during pregnancy and its effect on the mother, the fetus and the infant. Obstet Gynecol Survey 1990; 45:348–359.

22. Birnbach DJ, Stein DJ, Thomas K, et al: Cocaine abuse in the parturient: What are the anesthetic implications. Anesthesiology 1993; 79:A988.
23. Hans SL: Demographic and psychosocial characteristics of substance-abusing pregnant women. Clin Perinatol 1999; 26:55–74.
24. New York State Department of Health: Statewide planning and research cooperative. Neonatal drug-related discharges per 1,000 births. Albany NY: New York State, 1990.
25. Schutzman DL, Frankenfield-Chernicoff M, Clatterbaugh HE, et al: Incidence of intrauterine cocaine exposure in a suburban setting. Pediatrics 1991; 88:825–827.
26. Weisdorf T, Parran TV, Grahm A, Snyder C: Comparison of pregnancy specific interventions to a traditional treatment program for cocaine addicted pregnant women. J Subs Abuse Treat 1999; 16:39–45.
27. Furst CI, Beckman LI, Nakamura CY, Weiss M: Utilization of alcoholism treatment services. Los Angeles University of California at Los Angeles Alcohol Research Center, 1981.
28. Liang H: A profile of female clients admitted to publicly funded treatment in FY 1991. Boston: Report to the Massachusetts Department of Public Health by Health and Addictions Research Inc. January, 1992.
29. Bagasra O, Forman LJ, Howeedy A, Whittle P: A potential vaccine for cocaine abuse prophylaxis. Immunopharmacology 1992; 23:173–179.
30. Fox BS, Kantak KM, Edwards MA, et al: Efficacy of a therapeutic cocaine vaccine in rodent models. Nat Med 1996; 2:1129–1132.
31. Fox BS: Development of a therapeutic vaccine for the treatment of cocaine addiction. Drug Alcohol Depend 1997; 48:153–158.
32. Chavkin W: Drug addiction and pregnancy: Policy at a crossroad. Public Health Law 1990; 80:483–487.
33. Finkelstein N: Treatment programming for alcohol and drug dependent pregnant women. Int J Addictions 1993; 28:1275–1309.
34. MacGregor SN, Keith LG, Chasnoff IJ: Cocaine use during pregnancy: Adverse perinatal outcome. Am J Obstet Gynecol 1987; 157:686–690.
35. Dombrowski MP, Wolfe HM, Welch RA, et al: Cocaine abuse is associated with abruptio placentae and decreased birth weight, but not shorter labor. Obstet Gynecol 1991; 77:139–141.
36. Bernasko JW, Brown G, Mitchell JL, Matseoane SL: Spontaneous pneumothorax following cocaine use in pregnancy. Am J Emerg Med 1997; 15:107.
37. Mishra A, Landzberg BR, Parente JT: Uterine rupture in association with alkaloidal cocaine use. Am J Obstet Gynecol 1995; 173:243–244.
38. Iriye BK, Bristow RE, Hsu CD, et al: Uterine rupture associated with recent antepartum cocaine abuse. Obstet Gynecol 1994; 83:840–841.
39. Buehler BA: Cocaine: How dangerous is it during pregnancy. Nebraska Med J 1995; 80:116–117.
40. Lampley EC, Williams S, Myers SA: Cocaine-associated rhabdomyolysis causing renal failure in pregnancy. Obstet Gynecol 1996; 87:804–806.
41. Moen MD, Caliendo MJ, Marshall W, Uhler ML: Hepatic rupture in pregnancy associated with cocaine use. Obstet Gynecol 1993; 82:687–689.
42. Chao CR: Cardiovascular effects of cocaine during pregnancy. Semin Perinatol 1996; 20:107–114.
43. Burkett G, Yasin SY, Palow D, et al: Patterns of cocaine bingeing: Effect on pregnancy. Am J Obstet Gynecol 1994; 171:372–378.
44. Woods JR Jr, Plessinger MA: Pregnancy increases cardiovascular toxicity to cocaine. Am J Obstet Gynecol 1990; 162:529–534.
45. Handler A, Kistin N, Davis F, et al: Cocaine during pregnancy: Perinatal outcomes. Am J Epidemiol 1991; 133:818–824.
46. Tabor BL, Smith-Wallace T, Yonekura ML: Perinatal outcome associated with PCP versus cocaine abuse. Am J Drug Alcohol Abuse 1990; 16:337–348.
47. Center for Disease Control: Urogenital anomalies in the offspring of women using cocaine during early pregnancy. Morbid Mortal Wkly Rep 1989; 38:536–542.
48. Dixon SD, Bejar R: Echoencephalographic findings in neonates associated with maternal cocaine and metamphetamine use: Incidence and clinical correlates. J Pediatr 1989; 115:770–778.
49. Lester BM, LaGasse LL, Seifer R: Cocaine exposure and children: The meaning of subtle effects. Science 1998; 282:633–634.
50. Plessinger MA, Woods JR Jr: Maternal, placental and fetal pathophysiology of cocaine exposure during pregnancy. Clin Obstet Gynecol 1993; 36:267–278.
51. Dinsmoor MJ, Irons SJ, Christmas JT: Preterm rupture of membranes associated with recent cocaine use. Am J Obstet Gynecol 1994; 171:305–309.
52. Jasnosx KM, Hermansen MC, Snider C, Sang K: Congenital complete absence of the diaphragm: A rare variant of congenital diaphragmatic hernia. Am J Perinatol 1994; 11:340–343.
53. Mehta SK, Finkelhor RS, Anderson RL, et al: Transient myocardial ischemia in infants prenatally exposed to cocaine. J Pediatrics 1993; 122:945–949.
54. Bulbul ZR, Rosenthal DN, Kleinman CS: Myocardial infarction in the perinatal period secondary to maternal cocaine abuse. Arch Pediatr Adolesc Med 1994; 148:1092–1096.
55. Martinez A, Larabee K, Monga M: Cocaine is associated with intrauterine fetal death in women with suspected preterm labor. Am J Perinatology 1996; 13:163–166.
56. Little BB, Snell LM, Klein VR, et al: Cocaine abuse during pregnancy: Maternal and fetal implications. Obstet Gynecol 1989; 73:157–160.
57. Prasad PD, Leibach FH, Mahesh VB, et al: Human placenta as a target organ for cocaine action: Interaction of cocaine with the placental serotonin transporter. Placenta 1994; 15:267–278.
58. Krishna RB, Levitz M, Dancis J: Transfer of cocaine by the perfused human placenta: The effect of binding to serum proteins. Am J Obstet Gynecol 1993; 169:1418–1423.
59. ACOG Committee Opinion: Committee on Obstetrics: Maternal and Fetal Medicine Number 114. Int J Gynecol Obstet 1993; 41:102–105.
60. Campbell D, Parr MJ, Shutt LE: Unrecognized "crack" cocaine abuse in pregnancy. Br J Anaesth 1996; 77:553–555.
61. Towers CV, Pircon RA, Nageotte MP, et al: Cocaine intoxication presenting as preeclampsia and eclampsia. Obstet Gynecol 1993; 81:545–547.
62. Richardson GA, Day NL, McGauhey PJ: The impact of prenatal marijuana and cocaine use on the infant and child. Clin Obstet Gynecol 1993; 36:302–318.
63. Miller JM, Boudreaux MC, Regan FA: A case-control study of cocaine use in pregnancy. Am J Obstet Gynecol 1995; 172:180–185.
64. Hutchings DE: The puzzle of cocaine's effects following maternal use during pregnancy: Are there reconcilable differences? Neurotoxicol Teratol 1993; 15:281–286.
65. Kain ZN, Mayes LC, Ferris CA, et al: Cocaine-abusing parturients undergoing cesarean section. A cohort study. Anesthesiology 1996; 85:1028–1035.
66. Birnbach DJ, Stein DJ, Grunebaum A, et al: Cocaine screening of parturients without prenatal care: An evaluation of a rapid screening assay. Anesth Analg 1997; 84:76–79.
67. Grant T, Brown Z, Callahan C, et al: Cocaine exposure during pregnancy: Improving assessment with radioimmunoassay of maternal hair. Obstet Gynecol 1994; 83:524–531.
68. Oyler J, Darwin WD, Preston KL, et al: Cocaine disposition in meconium from newborns of cocaine-abusing mothers and urine of adult drug users. J Analyt Toxicol 1996; 20:453–462.
69. Kain ZN, Rimar S, Barash PG: Cocaine abuse in the parturient and effects on the fetus and neonate. Anesth Analg 1993; 77:835–845.
70. Kreek MJ: Cocaine, dopamine and the endogenous opioid system. J Addict Dis 1996; 15:73–96.
71. Unterwald EM, Horne-King K, Kreek MJ: Chronic cocaine alters brain mu opioid receptors. Brain Res 1992; 584:314–318.

72. Schindler CW, Tella SR, Erzouki HK, Goldberg SR: Pharmacological mechanisms in cocaine's cardiovascular effects. Drug Alcohol Depend 1995; 37:183–191.
73. Ramoska E, Sacchetti A: Propranolol induced hypertension in the treatment of cocaine intoxication. Ann Emerg Med 1985; 14:1112–1113.
74. Lange RA, Cigarroa RG, Flores ED, et al: Potentiation of cocaine-induced coronary vasoconstriction by beta-adrenergic blockade. Ann Intern Med 1990; 112:897–903.
75. Vertommen JD, Hughes SC, Rosen MA, et al: Hydralazine does not restore uterine blood flow during cocaine-induced hypertension in the pregnant ewe. Anesthesiology 1992; 76:580–587.
76. Hughes SC, Vertommen JD, Rosen MA, et al: Cocaine-induced hypertension in the ewe and response to treatment with labetalol. Anesthesiology 1991; 77:A1075.
77. Hollander JE: The management of cocaine-associated myocardial ischemia. N Engl J Med 1995; 333:1267–1271.
78. Derlet RW, Tseng CC, Albertson TE: Cocaine toxicity and the calcium channel blockers nifedipine and nimodipine in rats. J Emerg Med 1994; 12:1–4.
79. Williams RG, Kavanagh KM, Teo KK: Pathophysiology and treatment of cocaine toxicity: Implications for the heart and cardiovascular system. Can J Cardiology 1996; 12:95–301.
80. Birnbach DJ: Cardiovascular disease in the pregnant patient: A new risk factor. Cardiovasc Risk Factors 1994; 4:28–33.
81. Boylan JF, Cheng DC, Sandler AN, et al: Cocaine toxicity and isoflurane anesthesia: Hemodynamic, myocardial metabolic, and regional blood flow effects in swine. J Cardiothorac Vasc Anesth 1996; 10:772–777.
82. Murphy JL: Hypertension and pulmonary oedema associated with ketamine administration in a patient with a history of substance abuse. Can J Anaesthesia 1993; 40:160–164.
83. Jatlow P, Barash PG, Van Dyke C, et al: Cocaine and succinylcholine sensitivity: A new caution. Anesth Analg 1979; 58:235–238.
84. Samkoff LM, Daras M, Kleiman AR, Koppel BS: Spontaneous spinal epidural hematoma. Another neurologic complication of cocaine? Arch Neurol 1996; 53:819–821.
85. Nanji AA, Filipenko JD: Asystole and ventricular fibrillation associated with cocaine intoxication. Chest 1994; 85:132–133.
86. Stevens DC, Campbell JP, Carter JE, et al: Acid-base abnormalities associated with cocaine toxicity in emergency department patients. J Toxicol 1994; 32:31–39.
87. Hollander JE, Hoffman RS, Gennis P, et al: Nitroglycerin in the treatment of cocaine associated chest pain: Clinical safety and efficacy. J Toxicol Clin Toxicol 1994; 32:243–256.
88. Shih RD, Hollander JE, Burstein JL, et al: Clinical safety of lidocaine in patients with cocaine-associated myocardial infarction. Ann Emerg Med 1995; 26:702–706.
89. Spivey WH, Euerle B: Neurologic complications of cocaine abuse. Ann Emerg Med 1990; 19:1422–1428.
90. Wood M: Drugs and anesthesia: Pharmacology for anesthesiologists. In Wood M, Wood AJJ (eds). Drugs and the Sympathetic Nervous System, 2nd ed. Baltimore; Williams and Wilkins, 1990:375–405.
91. Ong BH: Hazards to health: Dextroamphetamine poisoning. N Eng J Med 1962; 266:1321–1322.
92. Delaney P, Estes M: Intracranial hemorrhage with amphetamine abuse. Neurology 1980; 30:1125–1128.
93. Harrington H, Heller HA, Dawson D, et al: Intracerebral hemorrhage and oral amphetamine. Arch Neurol 1983; 40:503–507.
94. Oro AS, Dixon SD: Perinatal cocaine and methamphetamine: Maternal and neonatal correlates. J Pediatr 1987; 111:571–578.
95. Eliot RH, Rees GB: Amphetamine ingestion presenting as eclampsia. Can J Anaesth 1990; 37:130–133.
96. Wagner CL, Katikaneni LD, Cox TH, et al: The impact of prenatal drug exposure on the neonate. Obstet Gynecol Clin North Am 1998; 25:169–194.
97. Eriksson M, Larsson G, Zetterstrom R: Amphetamine addiction and pregnancy. II: Pregnancy, delivery, and the neonatal period: Socio-economic aspects. Acta Obstet Gynecol Scand 1981; 60:253–259.
98. Eriksson M, Larsson G, Winbladh B, et al: The influence of amphetamine addiction on pregnancy and the newborn infant. Acta Paediatr Scand 1978; 67:95–99.
99. Levin JN: Amphetamine ingestion with biliary atresia. Pediatrics 1971; 79:130–131.
100. Little BB, Snell LM, Gilstrap LC: Methamphetamine abuse during pregnancy: Outcome and fetal effects. Obstet Gynecol 1988; 72:541–544.
101. Nelson MM, Forfar JO: Associations between drugs administered during pregnancy and congenital abnormalities of the fetus. Br Med J 1971; 1:523–527.
102. Oro AS, Dixon SD: Amphetamine addiction during pregnancy: 14-year follow up of growth and school performance. Acta Paediatrica 1996; 85:294–298.
103. Samuels SI, Maze A, Albright A: Cardiac arrest in a chronic amphetamine abuser. Anesth Analg 1979; 58:528–530.
104. Smith DS, Gutsche BB: Amphetamine abuse and obstetrical anesthesia. Anesth Analg 1980; 59:710–711.
105. Johnston RR, Way WL, Miller RD: Alteration of anesthetic requirement by amphetamine. Anesthesiology 1972; 36:357–363.
106. Henry JA: Ecstasy and the dance with death. BMJ 1992; 305:775.
107. Henry JA, Jeffreys KJ, Dawlings S: Toxicity and deaths from 3,4-methylenedioxymethamphetamine (ecstasy). Lancet 1992; 340:384–387.
108. Schwartz RH, Miller NS: MDMA (ecstasy) and the rave: A review. Pediatrics 1997; 100:705–708.
109. Campkin NJ, Davies UM: Treatment of ecstasy overdose with dantrolene. Anaesthesia 1993; 48:82–83.
110. Webb C, Williams V: Ecstasy intoxication: Appreciation of complications and the role of dantrolene. Anaesthesia 1992; 47:686–687.
111. Henry JA, Fallon JK, Kicman AT, et al: Low dose MDMA (ecstasy) induces vasopressin secretion. Lancet 1998; 351:1784.
112. Little BB, Snell LM, Klein VR, et al: Maternal and fetal effects of heroin addiction during pregnancy. J Reprod Med 1990; 35:159–165.
113. Ostrea EM, Brady M, Gause S, et al: Drug screening of newborns by meconium analysis: A large scale prospective epidemiological study. Pediatrics 1992; 89:107–113
114. National Institute on Drug Abuse: National Household Survey on Drug Abuse: Main Findings. Rockville, MD: Department of Health and Human Services, 1992. Publication No. 94-3012.
115. National Institute on Drug Abuse: National Household Survey of Drug Abuse: Population Estimates 1990. Rockville, MD: Department of Health and Human Services, 1991. Publication No. 91-1732.
116. Bell GL, Lau K: Perinatal and neonatal issues of substance abuse. Pediatric Clin North Am 1995; 42:261–275.
117. Kliman L: Drug dependence and pregnancy: Antenatal and intrapartum problems. Anaesth Intensive Care 1990; 18:358–360.
118. Rogriguez EM, Mofenson LM, Chang BH, et al: Association of maternal drug use during pregnancy with maternal HIV culture positivity and perinatal HIV transmission. AIDS 1996; 10:273–282.
119. Stoelting RK: Opioid agonists and antagonists. In Pharmacology and Physiology in Anesthetic Practice. Philadelphia: JB Lippincott 1987.
120. Weintraub SJ, Naulty JS: Acute abstinence syndrome after epidural injection of butorphanol. Anesth Analg 1985; 64:452–453.
121. Gold MS, Pottash AL, Extein I, Kleber HD: Clonidine in acute opiate withdrawal. N Eng J Med 1980; 302:1421–1422.
122. Wood PR, Soni N: Anaesthesia and substance abuse. Anaesthesia 1989; 44:672–680.
123. Brown HL, Britton KA, Mahaffey D, et al: Methadone maintenance in pregnancy: A reappraisal. Am J Obstet Gynecol 1998; 179:459–463.
124. Secker-Walker RH, Vacek PM, Flynn BS, Mead PB: Estimated gains in birth weight associated with reductions in smoking during pregnancy. J Reprod Med 1998; 43:967–974.
125. Prager K, Malin H, Spiegler D, et al: Smoking and drinking

behavior before and during pregnancy of married mothers of live-born infants and stillborn infants. Pub Health Rep 1984; 99:117–127.
126. Feng T: Substance abuse in pregnancy. Curr Opin Obstet Gynecol 1993; 5:16–23.
127. Kistin N, Handler A, Davis F, et al: Cocaine and cigarettes: A comparison of risks. Paediatr Perinatal Epidemiol 1996; 10:269–278.
128. Economides D, Braithwaite J: Smoking, pregnancy and the fetus. J R Soc Health 1994; 114:198–201.
129. Benowitz NL: Nicotine replacement therapy during pregnancy. JAMA 1991; 266:3174–3177.
130. Pearce AC, Jones RM: Smoking and anesthesia: Preoperative abstinence and perioperative morbidity. Anesthesiology 1984; 61:576–584.
131. Schneider NG, Ohmstead RE, Steinberg C, et al: Efficacy of buspirone in smoking cessation: A placebo controlled trial. Clin Pharmacol Ther 1996; 60:568–575.
132. Hughes JR, Goldstein MG, Hurt RD, et al: Recent advances in the pharmacotherapy of smoking. JAMA 1999; 28:72–76.
133. Jorenby DE, Leischow SJ, Nides MA, et al: A controlled trial of sustained release bupropion and nicotine patch or both for smoking cessation. N Engl J Med 1999; 340:685–691.
134. Hurt RD, Sachs DPL, Glover ED, et al: A comparison of sustained release bupropion and placebo for smoking cessation. N Engl J Med 1997; 337:1195–1202.
135. Ferry LH, Bruchette M: Efficacy of bupropion for smoking cessation in nondepressed smokers. J Addict Dis 1994; 13:249.
136. Heishman SJ, Henningfield JE, Kendler KS, et al: Conference summary: Society for Research on Nicotine and Tobacco Addiction 1998; 93:907–923.
137. Ascher JA, Cole JO, Colin J, et al: Bupropion: A review of its mechanism of antidepressant activity. J Clin Psychiatr 1995; 56:395–401.
138. Hebert S: Bupropion (Zyban, sustained-release tablets): Reported adverse reactions. CMAJ 1999; 160:1050–1105.
139. Humma LM, Swims MP: Bupropion mimics a transient ischemic attack. Ann Pharmacother 1999; 33:305–307.
140. Griffith JD, Carranza J, Griffith C, et al: Bupropion: Clinical assay for amphetamine-like abuse potential. J Clin Psychiatry 1983; 44:206–208.
141. Tucker WE Jr: Preclinical toxicology of buproprion: An overview. J Clin Psychiatry 1983; 44:60–62.
142. White AD, Andrews EB: The Pregnancy Registry Program Company at Glaxo Wellcome. J Allergy Clin Immunol 1999; 103:S362–S363.
143. DiFranza JR, Lew RA: Effect of maternal cigarette smoking on pregnancy complications and sudden infant death syndrome. J Fam Pract 1995; 40:385–394.
144. Wright LN, Thorp JM Jr, Kuller JA, et al: Transdermal nicotine replacement in pregnancy: Maternal pharmacokinetics and fetal effects. Am J Obstet Gynecol 1997; 176:1090–1094.
145. National Institute of Drug Abuse: National Household Survey on Drug Abuse. Population Estimates 1997. Washington, DC: Government Printing Office, 1998.
146. Press A, Done AK: Solvent sniffing: Physiological effects and community control measures. Pediatrics 1967; 39:451–461.
147. Jones HE, Balster RL: Inhalant abuse in pregnancy. Obstet Gynecol Clin North Am 1998; 25:153–167.
148. Wilkins-Haug L, Gabow PA: Toluene abuse during pregnancy: Obstetric complications and perinatal outcomes. Obstet Gynecol 1991; 77:504–509.
149. Grabski DG: Toluene sniffing produces cerebellar degeneration. Am J Psychiatry 1961; 118:461–462.
150. Keane JR: Toluene optic neuropathy. Ann Neurol 1978; 4:390.
151. Ehyai A, Freeman FR: Progressive optic neuropathy and sensorimotor hearing loss due to chronic glue sniffing. J Neurol Neurosurg Psychiatry 1983; 46:349–351.
152. Sasa M, Igarashi S, Miyazaki T, et al: Equilibrium disorders with diffuse brain atrophy in long-term toluene sniffing. Arch Otorhinolaryngol 1978; 221:163–169.
153. Reyes de la Rocha S, Brown MA, Fortenberry JD: Pulmonary function abnormalities in intentional spray paint inhalation. Chest 1987; 92:100–104.
154. Cunningham SR, Dalzell GWN, McGirr P, et al: Myocardial infarction and primary ventricular fibrillation after glue sniffing. Br Med J 1987; 294:739–740.
155. Murata K, Araki S, Yokoyama K, et al: Changes in autonomic function as determined by ECG R-R interval variability in sandal, shoe and leather workers exposed to *n*-hexane, xylene and toluene. Neurotoxicology 1994; 15:867–875.
156. Carlisle EJ, Donnelly SM, Vasuvattakul S, et al: Glue-sniffing and distal renal tubular acidosis: Sticking to the facts. J Am Soc Nephrol 1991; 1:1019–1027.
157. Pryor GT: A toluene-induced motor syndrome in rats resembling that seen in some solvent abusers. Neurotoxicol Teratol 1991; 13:387–400.
158. Hersh JH: Toluene embryopathy: Two new cases. J Med Genet 1989; 26:333–337.
159. Hersh JH, Podruch PE, Rogers G, et al: Toluene embryopathy. J Pediatr 1985; 106:922–927.
160. Ebrahim SH, Luman ET, Floyd RL, et al: Alcohol consumption by pregnant women in the United States during 1988–1995. Obstet Gynecol 1998; 92:187–192.
161. Beattie MC, Longabaugh R, Elliott G, et al: Effect of the social environment on alcohol involvement and subjective well-being prior to alcoholism treatment. J Stud Alcohol 1993; 54:283–296.
162. Pietrantoni M, Knuppel RA: Alcohol use in pregnancy. Clin Perinatol 1991; 18:93–111.
163. Guerri C, Renau-Piqueras J: Alcohol, astroglia, and brain development. Mol Neurobiol 1997; 15:65–81.
164. Pinazo-Duran MD, Renau-Piqueras J, Guerri C, et al: Optic nerve hypoplasia in fetal alcohol syndrome: An update. Eur J Ophthalmol 1997; 7:262–270.
165. Sampson PD, Streissguth AP, Bookstein FL, et al: Incidence of fetal alcohol syndrome and prevalence of alcohol-related neurodevelopmental disorder. Teratology 1997; 56:317–326.
166. Council on Scientific Affairs, American Medical Association: Fetal effects of maternal alcohol use. JAMA 1983; 249:2517–2521.
167. Edwards R: Anaesthesia and alcohol. Br Med J 1985; 291:423–424.
168. Swerdlow BN, Holley FO, Maitre PI, et al: Chronic alcohol intake does not change thiopental anesthetic requirement, pharmacokinetics, or pharmacodynamics. Anesthesiology 1990; 72:455–461.
169. Fried PA: Prenatal exposure to tobacco and marijuana: Effects during pregnancy, infancy, and early childhood. Clin Obstet Gynecol 1993; 36:319–337.
170. Mirochnick M, Meyer J, Frank DA, et al: Elevated plasma norepinephrine after in utero exposure to cocaine and marijuana. Pediatrics 1997; 99:555–559.
171. Fried PA, Watkinson B, Siegel LS: Reading and language in 9- to 12-year olds prenatally exposed to cigarettes and marijuana Neurotoxicol Teratol 1997; 19:171–183.
172. English DR, Hulse GK, Milne E, et al: Maternal cannabis use and birth weight: A meta-analysis. Addiction 1997; 92:1553–1560.
173. Zuckerman B, Frank DA, Hingson R, et al: Effects of maternal marijuana and cocaine on fetal growth. N Engl J Med 1989; 320:762–768.
174. Richardson GA, Day NL, McGauhey PJ: The impact of prenatal marijuana and cocaine use on the infant and child. Clin Obstet Gynecol 1993; 36:302–318.
175. Eyler FD, Behnke M: Early development of infants exposed to drugs perinatally. Clin Perinatol 1999; 26:107–150.

49

Acquired Immunodeficiency Syndrome and Obstetric Anesthesia

U. SINGH, FCA (SA)

D. A. ROCKE, MRCP, FRCP, FCA (SA), FRCA (HON)

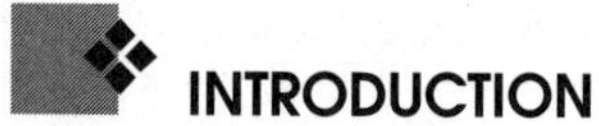

INTRODUCTION

The worldwide impact of human immunodeficiency virus (HIV) and acquired immunodeficiency syndrome (AIDS) is undisputed. Now well into the second decade, HIV and AIDS has become a global pandemic. As of June 30, 1997, a cumulative total of 1,644,183 AIDS cases had been reported to the World Health Organization (WHO), an 18% increase over the preceding year. Allowing for underdiagnosis, incomplete reporting, and reporting delays, approximately 8.4 million AIDS cases have occurred worldwide.[1] The WHO has provided a geographic breakdown of the worldwide distribution of adult HIV infection through mid-1997 (Fig. 49–1).[2] The majority of cases are from Sub-Saharan Africa, and by 2000 it was estimated that 90% of new AIDS cases would occur in the Third World. Worldwide, heterosexual intercourse is believed to account for more than 70% of all HIV transmission. The importance of various modes of transmission, however, varies greatly from one geographic area to another.[3] For example, an estimated 93% of HIV-infected people in Sub-Saharan Africa acquired the virus through heterosexual intercourse. In contrast, homosexual intercourse has been the dominant route of HIV transmission in areas such as Western Europe and North America. Conventional HIV education and prevention programs, which focus on homosexual men and injection drugs users, will be inadequate against heterosexually transmitted HIV.

The AIDS rate for black women in the United States is 17 times higher than for white women. Two major messages emerged from the third National Conference on Women and HIV in 1997.[4] First, women have become the most quickly increasing new group of AIDS patients in the United States. HIV infection was the third leading cause of death for all women in the United States in 1996[5] and the leading cause of death for black women. Secondly, the AIDS epidemic in the United States has reached a plateau for men but not for women. Although AIDS deaths had increased each year, in 1996 in the United States for the first time AIDS deaths decreased by 10%. AIDS prevalence substantially increased, however, reflecting this decline in AIDS deaths. About 80% of AIDS patients live in cities with a population of greater than half a million. In addition to their worldwide distribution, HIV infection and AIDS have become important causes of morbidity and mortality. In slightly more than a decade, HIV has emerged as the leading cause of death in the United States among persons between the ages of 25 and 44 years.[6, 7] HIV disease progression is also known to make virtually every organ system vulnerable to opportunistic disease.[8] The economic consequences are immense.

NATURAL HISTORY

Understanding the HIV replication cycle has allowed the development of various therapeutic options (Fig. 49–2). The first interaction of HIV and host cells is mediated by the viral gp120 envelope glycoprotein.[9] The critical linkage of gp120 with a specific cell surface

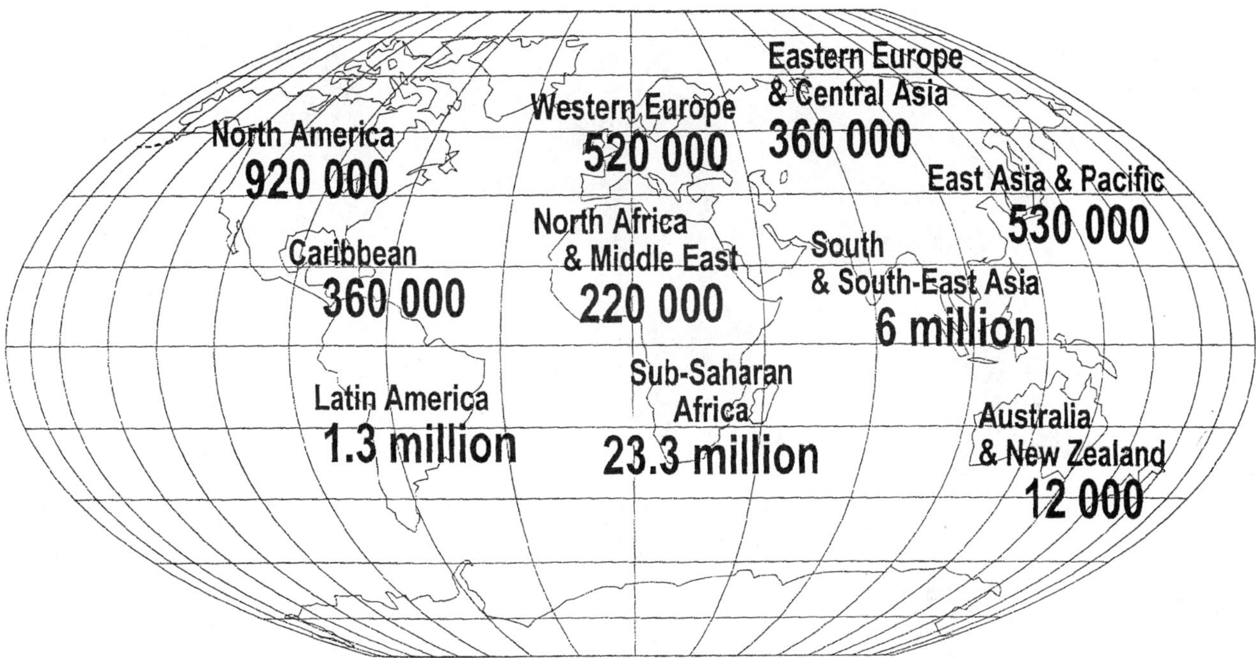

❖ **Figure 49–1** Adults and children estimated to be living with HIV/AIDS as of end of 1999. (From World Health Organization, December 1999.)

receptor, CD4, explains the affinity of HIV for CD4-bearing cells such as T lymphocytes, monocytes, and tissue macrophages.[8, 9] The CD4 T lymphocytes are the predominant target owing to the high number of CD4 molecules on the cell surface. Recent advances in the study of this fascinating virus include the identification of coreceptors such as the CXCR4 coreceptor on the helper T lymphocyte and the CCR5 coreceptor on the macrophage. These coreceptor molecules are essential for the process of fusion of the virus to the target cell. The HIV replication cycle begins after binding of the virus to cells.[9, 10] The viral RNA is then uncoated and reverse-transcribed into proviral DNA by the viral reverse-transcriptase enzyme.[8] The circularized proviral DNA translocates to the cell nucleus and is permanently integrated into the host's DNA by the viral integrase enzyme. Subsequently, the integrated viral genes may remain transcriptionally inactive or may be activated to be transcribed into genomic RNA and messenger RNA that are translated into viral proteins. Morphogenesis occurs at the cell membrane and the budding virion incorporates host cell proteins such as the major histocompatibility class antigens I and II into its lipid bilayer. As a final step, the viral proteins are cleaved by the HIV protease enzyme system.[10, 11]

The HIV protease is an important target for antiretroviral therapy. Protease inhibitors with a high affinity for the active site of the protease molecule interrupt cleavage of the gag and pol protein chains. These chains may subsequently assemble into incomplete noninfectious virus.

DISEASE PROGRESSION

Until recently, it was believed that HIV had a long latency period between infection and development of overt disease. Recent research has shown that the virus is active and replicating in certain tissues throughout the entire course of infection.[12] Hence, clinical latency does not necessarily imply virologic latency. Massive numbers of virus are produced each day, with a minimal production and clearance rate of 10 billion (10^{10}) virions per day.[13, 14] The half-life of virus particles is approximately 6 hours and the decay half-life of infected cells actively producing virus is approximately 1 to 6 days.[15] Over the course of infection, viral burden may rise from around 5000 virions/mL of plasma in early asymptomatic disease to between 100,000 and one million in patients with advanced disease.[16] Profound immunosuppression is accompanied by a decline in CD4+ T cell count and eventual disease progression. High levels of viral production appear to be balanced by viral clearance.[17]

Progression to AIDS may follow three variations: typical progressors, rapid progressors, or nonprogressors. The majority of patients (typical progressors) will develop AIDS within approximately 10 years of initial infection.[18] Rapid progressors (approximately

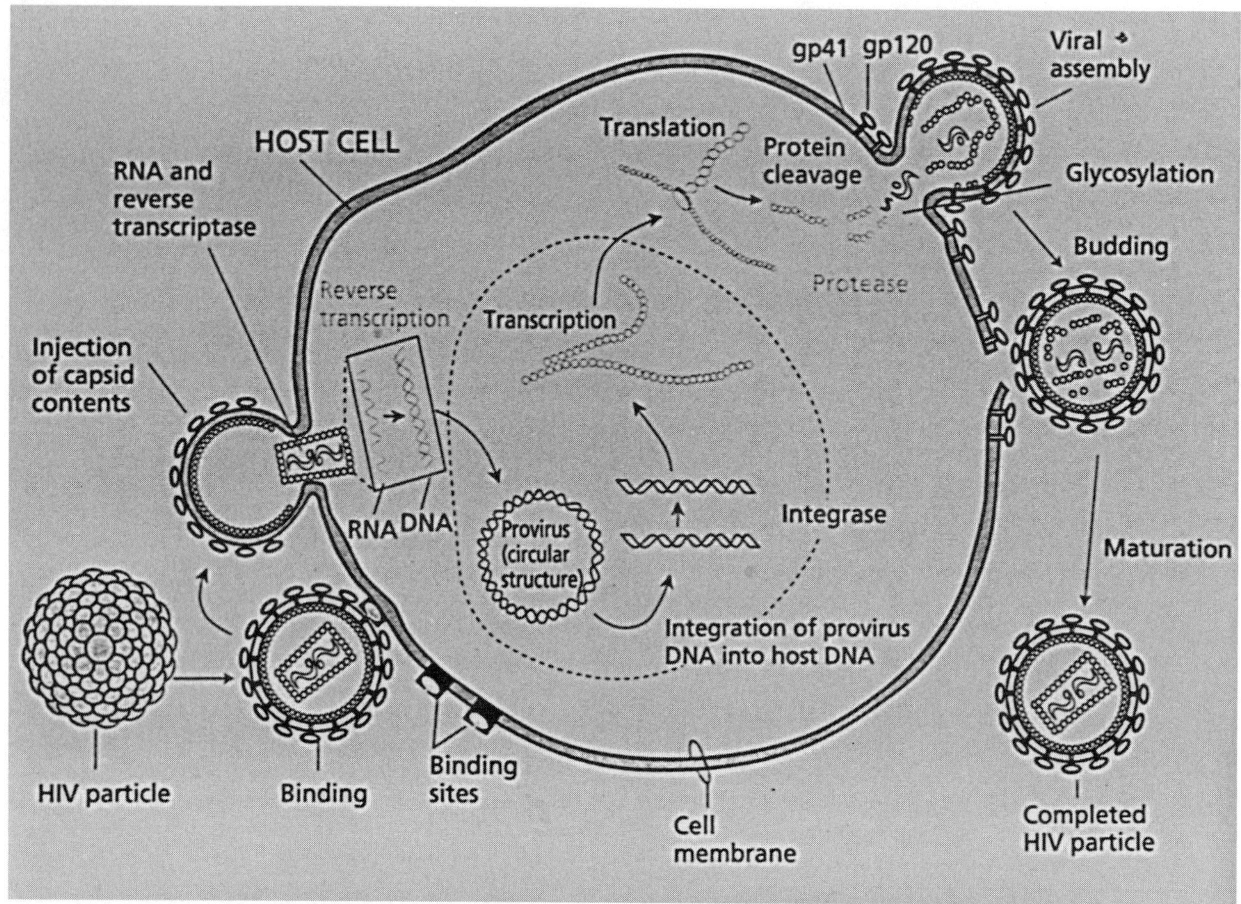

❖ **Figure 49–2** Understanding the replication cycle of the human immunodeficiency virus has allowed the development of various therapeutic options. (Adapted from Fauci AS, Lane HC: Human immunodeficiency virus (HIV) disease: AIDS and related disorders. *In* Isselbacher KJ, et al (eds): Harrison's Principles of Internal Medicine, 14th ed. New York, McGraw-Hill, 1994.)

10%) develop AIDS within 2 to 3 years.[18] A high and sustained viral load—the viral "set point"—following primary infection is a likely indicator of rapid disease progression. These patients may be infected with HIV strains that are more rapidly replicating and virulent. Nonprogressors constitute approximately 5% to 10% and may remain clinically asymptomatic with stable CD4+ T cell counts for 7 to 10 years after initial infection. Nonprogressors often present with lower viral load, which may indicate a more effective immune system or infection with less pathogenic strains.

DEFINITION AND CLASSIFICATION

The original definition of HIV/AIDS as prescribed by the Centers for Disease Control and Prevention (CDC), was intended for the purpose of surveillance and not for practical care. It has undergone several

Table 49–1 1993 Revised Classification System for Human Immunodeficiency Virus Infection and Expanded Acquired Immunodeficiency Syndrome Surveillance Case Definition for Adolescents and Adults

	Clinical Categories		
CD4+T Cell Categories	A Asymptomatic, Acute (Primary) HIV or PGL	B Symptomatic, Not A or C Conditions	C AIDS-Indicator Conditions
>500/μL	A1	B1	C1
200–499/μL	A2	B2	C2
<200/μL	A3	B3	C3

The shaded areas indicate the expanded AIDS surveillance case definition.
HIV, human immunodeficiency virus; PGL, progressive generalized lymphadenopathy.
Adapted from Morbidity Mortality Weekly Report 42(No. RR-17), December 18, 1992.

revisions since its inception and currently the 1993 Revised Classification System for HIV infection and Expanded AIDS Surveillance Case Definition for Adolescents and Adults is the version being used (Table 49–1). The classification system comprises a matrix of nine mutually exclusive categories, which stipulates that an HIV-infected individual with a CD4+ T cell count of $<200/\mu L$ has AIDS by definition, irrespective of his or her clinical condition. Furthermore, once an individual has demonstrated clinical features of category B or C, then upon resolution of the condition that individual may not return to his or her initial category.[8]

The attending clinician should, however, view HIV/AIDS as a clinical spectrum that begins with the primary infection, which may or may not be accompanied by the acute syndrome (Table 49–2). It is then followed by a period of asymptomatic infection, which is of variable duration (6 months to 10 years). Finally, the clinical picture culminates in the advanced form of the disease known as the clinical syndrome of AIDS.

DRUG THERAPY

In 1984, when the genetic structure of HIV was elucidated, it was immediately clear that there were three obvious targets for drug intervention. Three molecules, if blocked or inhibited, could disrupt the life cycle of the virus—the enzymes reverse transcriptase, protease, and integrase are the products of the HIV polygene. The third enzyme vital to the function of HIV, integrase, may also soon become a pharmacologic target. The availability of more numerous and more potent drugs to inhibit HIV replication has permitted the design of therapeutic strategies involving combinations of antiretroviral drugs that accomplish prolonged and near complete suppression of detectable HIV replication in many patients. In addition, more sensitive and reliable measurements of plasma viral load are better predictors of an individual's risk of progression to AIDS, time to death, and antiviral activity of potential therapeutic agents.

The HIV is a diploid virus; each virion carries two complete RNA genomic strands.[19] HIV RNA plasma assay may be determined by branched DNA or reverse transcriptase polymerase chain reaction (RT-PCR). The Food and Drug Administration has recently approved two newer assays of the RT-PCR that are accurate at low viral loads.[20] Baseline levels of HIV RNA have substantial predictive value for AIDS progression or death. The use of HIV RNA titer is helpful in decisions regarding the initiation of therapy and monitoring the effectiveness of treatment. Homologous recombination can occur when a cell is coinfected with two different but related strains. Recombination poses a problem with multidrug-resistant strains and the generation of a safe vaccine. Recombination may be an important HIV evolution strategy.

Table 49–2 CENTERS FOR DISEASE CONTROL CLASSIFICATION SYSTEM FOR HUMAN IMMUNODEFICIENCY VIRUS DISEASE

Group I	Acute HIV syndrome
Group II	Asymptomatic infection
Group III	Persistent generalized lymphadenopathy
Group IV	Other diseases
Subgroup A	Constitutional disease
Subgroup B	Neurologic disease
Subgroup C	Secondary infectious disease
Subgroup D	Secondary neoplasms
Subgroup E	Other conditions

Source: Fauci AS, Lane HC: Human immunodeficiency virus (HIV) disease: AIDS and related disorders. *In* Isselbacher KJ, et al (eds): Harrison's Principles of Internal Medicine, 14th ed. New York: McGraw-Hill, 1994.

Principles of Therapy

1. Regular periodic measurement of plasma HIV RNA levels and CD4+ T cell counts is necessary to determine the risk of disease progression and when to initiate or modify antiretroviral treatment regimens.
2. Using these tests, treatment should be individualized.
3. Maximum achievable suppression should be the goal of therapy. The single most important decision is the first drug regimen, as nothing else works as well.
4. Combination therapy is the best, used to optimal schedules and dosages.
5. Patients not meticulous about a drug schedule should not be prescribed indinavir.

Treatment should be commenced as soon as the diagnosis is established. Treatment is complicated by a long period between primary infection and appearance of clinical symptoms. The virus may become undetectable in the plasma but re-emerges on termination of therapy. The long-term safety of antiretroviral agents is unknown.

Nucleoside Reverse Transcriptase Inhibitors

Zidovudine (ZDV, formely called azidothymidine, or AZT) was the first antiretroviral drug approved by the Food and Drug Administration (FDA) for the treatment of HIV infection. It is the prototype drug in the nucleoside analogues. The efficacy of ZDV has been clearly established and its place in antiretroviral regimen is firmly rooted. In combination with other nucleoside analogues such as lamivudine and didanosine, ZDV is more effective as compared with monotherapy. The optimal dose has been extensively debated, which has resulted in the current recommendation of 200 mg three times a day in combination with other anti-retroviral agents. There are advantages to using ZDV, as it appears to improve neurologic symptoms and thrombocytopenia. The most frequently encountered side effects include fatigue, malaise, nausea, and headache, which eventually subside with ongoing usage. Bone marrow toxicity is perhaps the most alarming complication of ZDV, as macrocytic anemia and neutropenia may follow. Lamivudine is a cytidine analogue that is licensed only for use in conjunction with ZDV in situations in which ZDV is indicated, and to date they constitute the most potent combination of nucleosides. Although peripheral neuropathy and pancreatitis are the most important of the side effect profile of lamivudine, it is among the best tolerated of the nucleoside analogues.

Non-nucleoside Reverse Transcriptase Inhibitors

Nevirapine and delavirdine are the two main non-nucleoside analogues licensed for use that must be used in combination with other appropriate antiretroviral agents. Their use is associated with a maculopapular rash, which usually resolves over time. Non-nucleoside analogues have a possibly valuable role in future multidrug combinations.

Protease Inhibitors

The FDA has approved four protease inhibitors. Therapy is usually recommended on CD4+ T cell count, plasma HIV RNA level, or clinical status. Protease inhibitors are probably best reserved for those patients at higher progression risk. Viral resistance to protease inhibitors may develop after several months. Some protease inhibitors are insoluble and difficult to synthesize and have low oral availability. They have to be given in huge doses.

Protease inhibitors may precipitate hyperglycemia and diabetes mellitus.[21] Less than 1% may develop nonketotic hyperglycemia[22] 1 to 7 months after commencing treatment. Maximum serum glucose levels have been between 13.3 and 43.8 mmol/L. Patients respond to sulphonylurea or insulin. Most cases have been reported with indinavir, which has also been associated with nephrolithiasis. Another side effect of protease inhibitors is "Crix belly," characterized by elevated levels of triglycerides, cholesterol, and plasma glucose along with weight gain (18 kg or more). The condition tends to appear after 12 months of treatment.

Although protease inhibitors are expensive, when used in combination therapy with ZDV and lamivudine, they have been shown to reduce costs of inpatient and outpatient care as well as home health care. Nonadherence to long-term complex regimens can lead to emergence of resistant HIV strains. Before the practitioner offers protease inhibitors, the patient's living conditions should be stabilized and CD4 cell counts should indicate progression to AIDS. Those with a positive purified protein derivative skin test should be prescribed isoniazid. Those without a stable background should be offered two reverse transcriptase inhibitors. The emergence of resistant HIV strains should be closely monitored. Current research is into the efficacy of combinations of protease inhibitors.

The frequency of hypersensitivity reactions to protease inhibitors seems to be higher than that seen with nucleoside reverse transcriptase inhibitors.[23] The reactions are primarily cutaneous, including rash, erythema, fever, and urticaria. There may be a link to cytochrome P450-dependent drug interactions. The following drugs should not be given with indinavir: terfenadine, cisapride, astemizole, triazolam, midazolam, and rifampin.

Combination Anti-Retroviral Therapy

Only drug regimens that are expected to suppress HIV replication to undetectable levels should be studied in clinical trials or adopted in clinical practice.[24]

New guidelines for the treatment of HIV infection were published in early 2000.[25] Aggressive treatment, even in patients who are asymptomatic, with a three-drug regimen combining a protease inhibitor with two nucleoside reverse transcriptase inhibitors is recommended. An alternative to the three-drug regimen is the substitution of the protease inhibitors with nevirapine. Two-drug combinations are to be avoided and all monotherapy contraindicated except to prevent vertical transmission. Triple therapy should be started as soon as CD4+ T levels drop below 500/μL or HIV RNA levels exceed 20,000 copies/mL by polymerase chain reaction (PCR) assay. If viral load is not reduced 10-fold within 4 weeks and suppressed to undetectable levels within 4 months, a change in therapy is indicated. The triple-drug therapy requires 12 to 20 pills per day and has a cost of between US $10,000 and $12,000 annually.

Other therapeutic modalities under investigation include gene therapy,[26] monoclonal antibodies,[27] granulocyte colony stimulating factor,[28] interleukin-2, corticosteroids,[29] and cotrimaxazole.[30] Antisense compounds and oligonucleotides have also been designed to bind at various sites along the genome of HIV.

Treatment of Candidiasis and Other Aphthous Ulceration

Fungi, predominantly *Candida* species, are now among the most frequently isolated organisms in intensive care units and particularly so in AIDS patients. The most common cause of esophageal symptoms is candidiasis.[31] Odynophagia or dysphagia with oral candidiasis is an AIDS-defining diagnosis and can be treated empirically with a systemic azole. Weekly fluconazole (200 g) seems to be safe and effective in preventing oropharyngeal and vaginal candidiasis.[32] The second most frequent cause of oropharyngeal infection is cytomegalovirus, which produces either diffuse esophagitis or discrete ulcerations. Severe aphthous ulcers may respond to thalidomide, although rashes or excessive sedation may be problematic. Ganciclovir is a nucleoside analogue of guanisine, a homologue of acyclovir. It is used for treatment of cytomegalic retinitis.[33]

VERTICAL TRANSMISSION

Human immunodeficiency virus-1 may be transmitted from mother to infant during the antepartum, intrapartum, or postpartum period. In the United States, over 90% of reported cases of AIDS in children were acquired through vertical transmission.[34] During the 1990s the number of infants infected by transmission from their mother has greatly increased.[35] At the same time, research on vertical transmission has advanced to the stage where prevention of a large percentage of neonatal infection is a realistic possibility.[36] It is now accepted that pregnancy appreciably increases perinatal and maternal morbidity and mortality and significantly decreases survival time.

A particularly contentious issue is the screening for HIV infection in every pregnancy. The problem is getting consent to the HIV test. Antenatal HIV testing programs are also expensive. Limited resources should be channeled into places where prevention is most needed.[37] Education, appropriate management, and ongoing counseling and support are the cornerstones of treatment for HIV-positive pregnant women.[38] However, if a pregnant woman has access to antenatal treatment, knowledge of HIV status may be of great benefit.[37] Offering ZDV treatment to HIV-positive pregnant women decreases the number of pediatric HIV infections and reduces health care costs.[37] Caring for the HIV-infected child in the developed world is very expensive. Universal HIV counseling and voluntary HIV testing of pregnant women, coupled with ZDV treatment for HIV-positive pregnant women and their newborn infants to reduce vertical transmission would result in a net annual saving of US $426 million in the United States (1996). In the United States, the American Medical Association has approved a resolution calling for mandatory HIV testing for pregnant women and newborns. Without any treatment, the vertical transmission rate was 19% at 18 months in one French study.[39] The initial AIDS Controlled Trial Group (ACTG) 076 study showed that the likelihood of infant infection was reduced from 25% to 8% (a 70% reduction) when ZDV was administered to the mother prenatally and perinatally and to the infant during the first few weeks of life. The cost and difficulty of the ACTG 076 protocol has prompted efforts to make that intervention more accessible. ZDV prophylaxis for HIV-1-infected mothers, as defined by the ACTG 076 trial, is not possible in most parts of the world. Studies are underway to investigate whether briefer or less intense regimens are also effective. Globally feasible measures such as single-dose or short-course treatments, diet supplements, basic sanitation, and ways to minimize the time from membrane rupture to delivery are under study. In addition, in the developed world, combination therapy should be considered.

It is usually believed that fetal HIV transmission occurs either late in pregnancy or during labor and birth. Recent evidence suggests that it may occur much earlier and at a higher rate than previously thought. Based on limited data, ZDV use in the second and third trimesters of pregnancy was not associated with serious adverse effects in mothers or infants. Data are limited regarding the safety of ZDV during the first trimester. Whether lamivudine causes fetal toxicity is unknown. Transmission increases following amniocentesis and amnioscopy and in the presence of a sexually transmitted disease during pregnancy, preterm delivery, premature membrane rupture, hemorrhage during labor, and blood in the amniotic fluid. Immunologic, virologic, obstetric, and maternal factors influence vertical transmission; however, their relative contributions are not known. A higher frequency of HIV transmission during gestation may be associated with high maternal viral levels, decreased CD4+ cell counts, and stage of disease (primary infection and advanced maternal clinical HIV). Other factors increasing transmission include a lack of autologous neutralizing antibody. Viral load in cervicovaginal secretions may also be important. Thirty percent of HIV-positive women may have virus in cervicovaginal secretions. Other factors associated with intrapartum transmission include the mode of delivery, trauma (particularly for premature infants), the duration of ruptured membranes, and placental factors such as abruption or co-infections.[40] Transmission increases when the fetal membranes rupture more than 4 hours before delivery. In considering cesarean section, the known risks of the procedure must be balanced against its probable benefit in decreasing vertical transmission.[41] There is no current recommendation for cesarean section for the prevention of perinatal transmission.[40]

Maternal viral load is directly related to the risk of perinatal transmission and may be the most significant factor. Although maternal HIV-1 RNA levels are highly predictive of perinatal transmission, transmission also occurs with low levels of HIV RNA. Thus current data support the use of antenatal therapy at any level of plasma HIV RNA. While most research has been conducted with ZDV monotherapy, proposed trials include studies of a combination of ZDV/nevirapine during labor and delivery. Phase 1 trials with a combination of drugs including ZDV and lamivudine, alone and combined with several of the protease inhibitors, as well as other investigational nucleosides are under way.[40] The addition of nevirapine may lower vertical transmission to 2%.[41] ZDV therapy to interrupt vertical transmission of HIV is regrettably not widely used by HIV-infected pregnant women who are drug abusers.[42] Lack of adherence to chosen therapy was associated with continued cocaine use during pregnancy.

Women positive for HIV who have hepatitis C virus are more likely to transmit HIV infection to their infants.[43] Maternal hepatitis C virus may enhance transmission directly or is a marker for another cofactor such as maternal drug use. Co-infection may lead to increased HIV-1 expression or hepatitis C virus could modify the risk of vertical transmission through direct immunosuppression.

During antenatal care, monitoring for the earliest signs of opportunistic infection is important. HIV-positive women are prone to postnatal infectious complications. The recommendation that HIV-infected women should not breast-feed[44] is relevant to the first-world mother; however, in the context of the lack of proper water and sanitation facilities that is undeniable in some developing countries, this may not be a feasible option.

CLINICAL MANIFESTATIONS

Human immunodeficiency virus is indisputably a multisystem disease. In the earlier stages of the AIDS epidemic, the usual manifestations were opportunistic infections, unusual malignancies, and gastrointestinal symptoms. However, further research developments have led to a better understanding of the disease, which, together with improved drug therapy and increased longevity, have made HIV-mediated organ dysfunction a widely accepted entity. Index conditions for the diagnosis of AIDS in an HIV-positive patient are outlined in Table 49–3.

Neurologic Abnormalities

The neurologic system may be affected in a variety of ways (Table 49–4). Central nervous system (CNS) dysfunction is not unusual in the HIV-infected patient. Access to the nervous system is obtained early in the course of the infection,[45] as evidenced by the isolation of virions and antibodies in the cerebrospinal fluid. Hence HIV is described as a neurotropic virus. Most of the neurologic abnormalities seen during the initial infection are self-limited, although persistent dysfunction may occur. As the disease progresses to the advanced stage of clinical AIDS, significant neurologic deterioration becomes apparent. Up to 30% to 40% of patients newly diagnosed with AIDS have clinical evidence of neurologic dysfunction.[46] Neuropathology can present in various forms (see Table 49–4). The pathogenesis of these clinical conditions may be manifest as a primary effect of HIV or may be secondary to opportunistic infections or tumors.

Table 49–3 INDEX CONDITIONS FOR THE DIAGNOSIS OF ACQUIRED IMMUNODEFICIENCY SYNDROME IN A HUMAN IMMUNODEFICIENCY VIRUS (HIV)–POSITIVE PATIENT

Candidiasis of the bronchi, trachea, lungs
Candidiasis, esophageal
Cervical cancer, invasive
Coccidioidomycosis, disseminated or extrapulmonary
Cryptococcosis, extrapulmonary
Cryptosporidiosis, chronic intestinal (>1 month's duration)
Cytomegalovirus disease (other than liver, spleen, or lymph nodes)
Cytomegalovirus retinitis (with loss of vision)
HIV-related encephalopathy
Herpes simplex chronic ulcers (>1 month's duration), bronchitis, pneumonitis, esophagitis
Histoplasmosis, disseminated or extrapulmonary
Isophoriasis, chronic intestinal (>1 month's duration)
Kaposi's sarcoma
Burkitt's lymphoma (or equivalent term)
Immunoblastic lymphoma
Lymphoma of the brain, primary
Mycobacterium avium complex or *M. kansasii* infection, disseminated or extrapulmonary
Mycobacterium, any other species, infection pulmonary or extrapulmonary *Mycobacterium tuberculosis* infection, any site (pulmonary or extrapulmonary)
Pneumocystis carinii pneumonia
Pneumonia, recurrent
Progressive multifocal leukoencephalopathy
Recurrent *Salmonella* septicemia
Toxoplasmosis of the brain
Wasting syndrome due to HIV

Table 49–4 NEUROLOGIC MANIFESTATIONS OF HUMAN IMMUNODEFICIENCY VIRUS INFECTION

Early (Initial Infection)
Headache
Photophobia
Meningoencephalitis
Cognitive and affective changes
Cranial neuropathy
Peripheral neuropathy
Latent Phase
Demyelinating neuropathy
Cerebrospinal fluid abnormalities, even in asymptomatic patients
Late (Clinical Acquired Immunodeficiency Syndrome)
Meningitis
Diffuse encephalopathy
Focal brain lesions
Myelopathy (segmental or diffuse)
Peripheral neuropathy
Myopathy

Aseptic meningitis is generally an early manifestation of the disease and can range from headache and photophobia to frank encephalitis with cranial nerve involvement. Spontaneous resolution of this condition usually occurs within 2 to 4 weeks.

Encephalopathy of HIV, synonymous with terms such as *HIV-associated dementia* and *AIDS dementia complex*, is seen more frequently with disease progression. It may begin with increased forgetfulness and lack in concentration ability and can culminate in a vegetative state. Acute psychosis as a manifestation of AIDS dementia has been described in an obstetric patient.[47] In more severe forms of *AIDS dementia complex*, gait and sphincter disturbances may be present. Examination of cerebrospinal fluid will reveal nonspecific changes such as pleocytosis, which cannot be used as confirmation of the diagnosis. Markers such as β_2-microglobulin, quinolinic acid, and neopterin did initially show promise in this regard. These markers are elevated in the presence of encephalitis; however, convincing correlation with HIV neurologic involvement is still lacking. Structural neuroimaging techniques such as computed tomography and magnetic resonance imaging are most often normal in the early stages, as they require relatively large anatomic changes.[48] Dynamic or functional neuroimaging studies such as positron emission tomography or single photon emission computed tomography may display cortical and subcortical abnormalities in those with HIV-dementia, even in the asymptomatic patient.[49]

Spinal cord disease translates into a myelopathy. This is of special interest to the anesthesiologist, as neuraxial blockade plays a major role in the practice of obstetric anesthesia. Various mechanisms in the pathogenesis of spinal cord disease have been described, although the most frequent type is vacuolar myelopathy. The symptomatology relates to gait and sphincter disturbances. Affectation of the dorsal column of the spinal cord can result in sensory ataxia. Paresthesia and dysesthesia of the lower extremities may also manifest as an expression of spinal cord involvement. Hence, it is imperative that the anesthesiologist elicit the relevant symptoms and signs with subsequent documentation of preoperative neurologic deficits before proceeding with anesthesia.

Peripheral neuropathy is classically described as a distal sensory polyneuropathy that is perceived as a burning sensation of the lower extremities.[50] This clinical entity is an advanced feature of HIV and may be severe enough in some to limit ambulation. It is unresponsive to antiretroviral therapy and may in fact occur as a side effect of drugs such as didanosine, zalcitabine, and stavudine. Drug-induced peripheral neuropathy does, nonetheless, resolve following discontinuation of therapy.

Myopathy associated with HIV can range from an asymptomatic elevation in creatinine kinase and electromyographic changes[51] to a profound subacute wasting of muscle, especially proximal muscle groups.

Opportunistic infections include toxoplasmosis, cryptococcosis, JC virus (polymorphonuclear leukoencephalopathy), cytomegalovirus, mycobacterial tuberculosis, and HTLV-1 as a few examples. Toxoplasmosis infection of the CNS is well described in developed parts of the world. Diffuse encephalopathy with impairment of cognition and alertness are typical of this pathogen, and cerebral edema, if present, may improve dramatically with antibiotic therapy. *Cryptococcus neoformans* is an important cause of CNS morbidity and mortality in less developed countries. Neoplasms that are more frequently encountered in the CNS are Kaposi's sarcoma and primary CNS lymphoma.

Pulmonary Abnormalities

The respiratory system is the most common organ system affected. Hence, it is essential that an adequate evaluation of the chest is performed in the preoperative assessment of the HIV-infected parturient. Pulmonary involvement is usually due to opportunistic infections, the most prominent of which is *Pneumocystis carinii* pneumonia (PCP) in developed parts of the world. PCP is the initial AIDS-defining illness in 20% of patients. In the incipient stages of the HIV epidemic, this clinical entity had a uniformly fatal outcome,[52] whereas in recent years, comprehensive preventive and treatment measures have significantly reduced morbidity and mortality. This protozoal pathogen for the most part causes clinical disease when the CD4+ T cell count is less than 200/μL, thus indicating severe immunosuppression. The mild form of HIV-associated PCP follows an indolent course and must be entertained in the differential diagnosis in the context of vague symptoms like fever, pulmonary complaints, and loss of weight. The severe manifestation is similar to acute respiratory distress syndrome and the mortality is 60% if intubation and ventilatory support are required. Early initiation of steroids may decrease progression to respiratory failure and is indicated if the Pa_{O_2} is under 70 mm Hg. Glucocorticoids have shown clear benefit in severe cases by reducing the mortality and the number of patients who require ventilatory support by 50%.[53] Therapy must, however, have been initiated within 36 to 72 hours of the diagnosis.

Reactivation of latent pulmonary tuberculosis and bacterial pneumonia (e.g., pneumococcal pneumonia) are especially common in developing countries. In the recent past, however, the number of cases reported in developed societies has escalated. There has therefore been a resurgence of *Mycobacterium tuberculosis* infection in the United States, which is believed to be most likely directly related to the HIV epidemic. This clinical scenario has been further complicated by outbreaks of multidrug resistance, which has subsequently rendered its management significantly more difficult.

Mycobacterium avium complex, which comprises *M. avium* and M. *intracellulare,* is the third most common opportunistic infection seen in AIDS.[54] This disease complex is not unusual in the United States, and yet it is rarely seen on the African continent. *M. avium* complex typically occurs when the CD4+ T cell count is less than 100/μL. There is a disseminated form that may involve both the pulmonary system and extrapulmonary sites like the liver, lymph nodes, and bone marrow. The chest radiographic features in these individuals mainly include bilateral lower lobe infiltrates and, to a lesser extent, alveolar and nodular infiltrates. *M. kansasii* may also infect the lungs in a similar fashion to *M. tuberculosis,* so upper lobe cavitary lesions are not surprising.

Nonspecific interstitial pneumonitis is an entity peculiar to the patient with advanced HIV infection and must be considered in the differential diagnosis in a patient with faint bilateral interstitial infiltrates on the chest radiograph. Fortunately, this specific clinical condition follows a benign course that does not require therapeutic intervention.

Cardiovascular Abnormalities

Although cardiovascular involvement may be common in clinical AIDS (25–50% at autopsy),[55] only 6% of patients with AIDS develop symptoms. Dilated cardiomyopathy occurs in about 8% of patients with HIV infection, whereas the incidence of HIV cardiomyopathy in the obstetric seropositive population has not been determined. HIV cardiomyopathy marks the presence of progressive immunosuppression, as it correlates with helper-T cell counts of approximately 400/μL. The effect of pregnancy-induced reduction in systemic vascular resistance may in theory ameliorate this condition. However, the manner in which pregnancy and HIV cardiomyopathy coexist requires further investigation. Recent studies in the nonobstetric population suggest that early cardiologic evaluation is extremely useful, with the view to identification of those at risk so that therapy may then be instituted. Cardiac function may improve with conventional treatment regimens comprising digoxin, diuretics, and angiotensin converting enzyme inhibitors.[56] Myocarditis, which may be directly due to HIV or coxsackievirus group B, can present with nonspecific changes in the electrocardiogram. Pericardial disease may occur on the basis of Kaposi's sarcoma, tuberculosis, cryptococcosis, or lymphoma. The involvement of the pericardium has been associated with a reduction in survival time and necessitates preliminary echocardiography.[57] Nonbacterial thrombotic endocarditis has been reported and may account for unexplained embolic phenomena.

Renal Abnormalities

Although drug-induced nephropathy accounts for the majority of renal disease in patients with AIDS, HIV-associated nephropathy occurs in approximately 10% of patients with renal disease.[8] This condition has been described in both adults and children and may present early in the course of the infection. HIV nephropathy is characterized by focal segmental glomerulosclerosis, which can rapidly progress to end-stage renal failure. Heavy proteinuria is the typical finding on urinanalysis, whereas edema and hypertension are usually absent. This helps distinguish this entity from preeclampsia. To date, there has been no success in treatment, and end-stage renal failure appears inevitable within 12 months of the diagnosis. Sepsis, dehydration, and drug toxicity may also impair renal function. Antiretroviral agents and antimicrobial therapy mediating damage to the kidneys is well described. Some evidence has emerged that there may be an increased incidence of renal cell carcinoma in HIV-infected patients, but further studies are needed.

Gastrointestinal Abnormalities

The gastrointestinal system is commonly affected during HIV infection due to its susceptibility to opportunistic infections. Inspection of the oropharynx may reveal lesions such as candidiasis, oral hairy leukoplakia, aphthous ulcers, and Kaposi's sarcoma. Thalidomide has been found to improve aphthous lesions. This drug is largely avoided in the obstetric population, however. Esophageal involvement may translate into esophagitis or dysphagia, which may be of herpetic, cytomegaloviral, or candidal origin. This may present a problem of increased risk of regurgitation or aspiration, which is of particular interest to the anesthesiologist. HIV enteropathy is a syndrome characterized by chronic severe diarrhea for which no specific pathogen has been identified. Cachexia and electrolyte aberrations occur concomitantly with gastrointestinal tract involvement. Opportunistic infections of the liver may lead to abnormal liver function tests.

Hematologic Abnormalities

Abnormalities of the hematologic system have profound anesthetic implications and there are several mechanisms by which HIV affects the different cell lines. The effect of HIV on the blood film picture may be direct or secondary to opportunistic infections, tumor, or therapy.

Anemia is the most common finding. The normocytic normochromic variety of anemia will often reflect the impact of chronic infection on the red cells. Pregnancy, with its attendant physiologic dilutional anemia, may also play an additive role. Anemia is not an uncommon sequel following infection with mycobacteria, parvovirus B19, and fungi. Lymphoma and other forms of neoplastic disease may also give rise to anemia. AZT is known to inhibit erythroid maturation and hence significantly contributes to the macrocytic type of anemia in patients with AIDS. Antimicrobial agents with myelosuppressive properties such as trimethoprim and sulfamethoxazole may also compound the anemia. In some cases, the anemia may be severe enough to warrant chronic blood transfusions.[8]

Neutropenia is present in approximately 50% of seropositive patients. Although it may be mild in most asymptomatic seropositive patients, with disease progression it becomes sufficiently severe to render patients susceptible to infection and tumor. The impact of HIV on the white blood cell count of pregnant patients is largely determined by where in the spectrum of the disease the patient's condition lies. It therefore follows that the neutropenia is worsened with progression of the infection.

Thrombocytopenia, defined as a platelet count of less than 150,000/μL, is an early primary manifestation of HIV infection. The rate of incidental thrombocytopenia associated with normal pregnancy is widely quoted as 7%, and the condition is similar to HIV-induced thrombocytopenia with regard to its clinical significance. Reports of very low platelet counts in seropositive patients have been made in the context of abnormal bleeding, although such cases are not common. HIV thrombocytopenia resembles the clinical picture of idiopathic thrombocytopenic purpura.[8] The former does, however, improve following the commencement of antiretroviral therapy. Thrombocytopenia may also manifest as a side effect of medication.

Disseminated intravascular coagulopathy has been noted in severely immunocompromised HIV patients. It generally manifests in a low-grade form and explains the depressed levels of protein C.

Endocrine Abnormalities

Patients with AIDS may be unable to adequately respond to stress. Thyroid function may be abnormal, but clinical manifestations are unusual. Hyponatremia may occur in the setting of respiratory and CNS pathology, and may occur as an expression of the syndrome of inappropriate antidiuretic hormone secretion. At autopsy, many patients demonstrate adrenal gland involvement but only a minority manifest this clinically. Hence, the endocrine impairment may be evident only in those patients who present in late stages of the disease.

Immunologic Abnormalities

Traditionally, humoral and cell-mediated immunity are thought to be transiently suppressed during pregnancy.[58, 59] In the context of pregnancy and HIV infection, it was also believed that progression of symptomatology and the development of AIDS was hastened. This area of HIV research still remains unclear as a result of inconsistent findings and conflicting evidence in the literature. Some studies report a detrimental effect of pregnancy on immunity,[60, 61] while others contradict that the effect is significant.[62] The Women and Infants Transmission Study of 1997, a large, multicenter, longitudinal study, demonstrated stability in lymphocyte subsets during pregnancy and 1 year postpartum in HIV-infected women.[63]

The normal CD4-T cell count is quoted at 1000/μL and the helper-suppressor ratio at 2:1. Investigators have demonstrated lowered absolute helper cell counts and reversed helper-suppressor ratios in HIV-infected parturients.[45, 64] From these findings, it was concluded that synergism between pregnancy and HIV infection exists in affecting the depression in immune function. However, there is a growing body of evidence that this synergistic effect may not be clinically significant.[63] Vertical transmission is said to increase when CD4-T cell counts reach 400/μL and a further reduction to levels of approximately 300/μL results in the escalation of maternal complication rates.[65] The possibility of further immunosuppression and increased peripartum complications as a result of the administration of anesthesia in this clinical scenario has been addressed and refuted.[66]

Adverse drug reactions occur more frequently in the HIV-infected patient and appear to be more common with disease progression. These immunologically mediated drug allergies are an apparent paradox to the immunodeficient state that characterizes the disease. Although this entity manifests mainly as a cutaneous eruption, the incidence of true anaphylaxis is not increased, and one third of patients may therefore continue the use of the drug. This entity is a cause of huge concern regarding the emergence of multidrug resistance in the future.

Musculoskeletal Abnormalities

Wasting syndrome due to HIV is an AIDS-defining criterion. It is indicated by weight loss greater than 10%, together with intermittent or constant fever, chronic diarrhea, or fatigue of greater than 30 days' duration in the absence of another defined cause.[8] It is the current leading clinical indicator of AIDS in the United States. Histopathologic findings are in keeping with nonspecific myofiber degeneration and myositis, which are thought to be a direct effect of the virus. This has important pharmacokinetic implications to the anesthesiologist.

Pain Syndromes

A wide range of pain syndromes have been described in almost every organ system in seropositive patients, and the HIV-infected pregnant woman is not exempt from experiencing these pain-related syndromes. Chest pain, oral cavity pain, pain related to peripheral neuropathies, and musculoskeletal pain are encountered more frequently than other types. Pain is often due to specific organ pathology and must be actively excluded. Pain-related syndromes are described as chronic with acute intermittent exacerbations.[67] As the prescription of drugs is approached with much caution in pregnancy, it would not be surprising that pain is often undertreated in this patient population.

Ophthalmic Abnormalities

Generally, ophthalmic abnormalities present late in the disease and include conditions such as cytomegalovirus retinitis and retinal ischemia secondary to microvascular disease. Cytomegalovirus retinitis is the most common intraocular infection in AIDS patients and can progress to blindness following retinal destruction. Ganciclovir and foscarnet are effective in the treatment of this condition.

Opportunistic Infections

Pneumocystis carinii pneumonia is the most common opportunistic infection in developed countries, whereas in resource-poor countries, tuberculosis bears this title. The impact of opportunistic infections is the impairment of quality of life and reduction in lifespan in the HIV-infected patient, including the pregnant woman. Globally, tuberculosis is the leading cause of death among patients with AIDS and is therefore visualized as a poor prognosticator. The chest radiograph is abnormal in most patients and correlates with the degree of immunosuppression and stage of the disease.[68] CD4+ T cell counts in the region of 200/μL tend to be associated with hilar and mediastinal lymphadenopathy, whereas higher CD4+ T cell counts may present with cavitary lesions. Pleural involvement occurs more frequently in patients with HIV-related tuberculosis. Currently, the HIV/AIDS pandemic is largely responsible for the global resurgence of tuberculosis, which includes the United States. It should not be forgotten that tuberculosis is still a preventable disease and should therefore not account for the significant proportion of morbidity and mortality in patients with HIV infection.

Toxoplasmosis gondii is not an uncommon opportunistic pathogen, even in more affluent societies, and it primarily involves the central nervous system. Encouraging data have emerged regarding the use of didanosine in the treatment of toxoplasmosis. The use of dapsone, although reported, still requires further investigation. Thus, the anesthesiologist may be faced with patients who have either had prophylactic therapy instituted or required treatment of these pathogens in the context of pregnancy.

Cytomegalovirus encephalitis is a life-threatening infection and requires aggressive therapeutic intervention. Cidofovir, a nucleoside analogue of cytosine, is a recent development in the treatment of cytomegalovirus infection.

Neoplasms

Progressive HIV immunosuppression can lead to the development of malignant conditions. Lymphoproliferative tumors such as non-Hodgkin's lymphoma are usually of B-cell origin and may be intermediate or high grade in classification. The incidence of lymphoma related to Epstein-Barr virus is higher in the HIV population, and the condition may present as a primary central nervous system lymphoma. Kaposi's sarcoma, an affliction of mainly homosexual men, is uncommon in the obstetric population, and recent work has implicated human herpesvirus in its etiology.[69]

ANESTHETIC MANAGEMENT ISSUES

Assessment of Risk

There is a lack of information regarding the overall risk of anesthesia and surgery in the HIV-positive patient. At present, The American Society of Anesthesiologists (ASA) physical status assessment findings and the inherent surgical risk are considered together in the setting of pregnancy to provide a measure of the potential risk. Therefore, the presence of opportunistic infection, tumor, or organ dysfunction in conjunction with CDC staging and CD4+ T cell counts may be used as predictors of perioperative risk. A reliable clinical predictor of HIV-related immunosuppression is the presence of an opportunistic infection such as oral candidiasis, an easily identified opportunistic manifestation and useful indicator. Severe infections, advanced malignancies, and end-organ dysfunction complicate perioperative management and will require appropriate workup and therapeutic intervention prior to administration of anesthesia. Certainly the obstetric patient with AIDS should have a preoperative chest radiograph and electrocardiogram record available. Echocardiography is particularly useful in those patients who report cardiac symptoms and who demonstrate signs of cardiac involvement. Its role in the earlier stages of the infection, however, is yet to be fully validated.

Anesthetic Technique

Labor analgesia, mode of delivery, and post-delivery care of the HIV-infected parturient should be planned in collaboration with the obstetrics service. Caution has been expressed in the past regarding the administration of both regional anesthesia[70] and general anesthesia. In the seropositive parturient without clinical evidence of neurologic involvement, the potential for neurologic sequelae from regional techniques should not deter the anesthesiologist from employing neuraxial blockade for labor analgesia or cesarean section. It is widely accepted that the virus invades the CNS as early as the primary infection; therefore, regional techniques do not accelerate HIV progression to the nervous system. Neuraxial blockade is an invaluable technique in the armamentarium of the obstetric anesthesiologist, as it is useful in providing excellent labor analgesia with the potential to administer anesthesia for operative deliveries.[70]

Anesthesia for cesarean section must be tailored for the individual. Seropositivity per se does not dictate the preferred method of anesthesia. The most suitable method of anesthesia for cesarean section depends largely on the presence of comorbidity such as primary organ dysfunction, secondary infection, and neoplastic disease. Hence, it would be prudent to weigh the risks against the benefits when choosing the most suitable method of anesthesia.

Neurologic Considerations

Examination of the mental state of HIV-infected patients is essential in measuring baseline neurologic function and helps one in determining the validity of consent. Seropositive patients in the earlier stages of disease are generally in full control of their mental faculties and are capable of consenting to medical procedures.[71] The presence of AIDS dementia may preclude the patient's consenting to her own surgery. Full documentation of pre-existing neurologic deficits must be noted prior to anesthesia. The anesthesiologist may deem it more prudent to opt for a general anesthetic technique rather than regional anesthesia in the context of neurologic features from pre-existing spinal cord pathology. Spinal anesthesia is commonly performed in the obstetric population without adverse sequelae. Epidural blood patches may be safely used in the treatment of post–dural puncture headaches.

Neuroleptic drugs are not commonly prescribed in the obstetric population. However, in the context of acute psychosis, which may occur as a manifestation of AIDS dementia, the administration of butyrophenones may be necessary. The anesthesiologist must be wary of the increased incidence of extrapyramidal side effects in the HIV-infected patient who receives neuroleptic agents. Heightened sensitivity to benzodiazepines and opioids should also be anticipated, especially in patients with HIV-associated dementia. One may prescribe these agents if indicated, but caution needs to be exercised with regard to the dosage.

Pulmonary Considerations

The respiratory system is the most commonly affected in the HIV-infected patient and must be given adequate attention to avoid missing important pathology. The stress of the gravid uterus on the respiratory system with superimposed secondary infection renders the parturient more vulnerable to respiratory complications. Mild to moderate chest infections may benefit from the avoidance of general anesthesia. Regional anesthesia obviates the need to instrument the airway and its attendant complications, as the respiratory tract is often hyperreactive in this setting. Severe infections with concomitant respiratory failure generally are intolerant of even minor intercostal muscle blockade from regional anesthetic techniques. Postoperative ventilation may need to be considered in this instance.

The anesthesiologist must also be able to approach the chest radiograph that demonstrates bilateral diffuse interstitial infiltrates and offer a differential diagnosis.

Intraoperatively, a higher fraction of inspired oxygen may be needed by the parturient as a result of the combined effects of the pregnancy-induced reduction in functional residual capacity and secondary HIV-related pathology. Shunting within the alveolar-capillary unit is often increased, which may be reflected in decreased hemoglobin saturation. Thus, the proper evaluation of the impact of HIV on the respiratory system cannot be overemphasized.

Cardiovascular Considerations

The detection of a subclinical cardiomyopathy is critical in the assessment of the cardiac status of the HIV-infected patient, and preoperative echocardiography is indicated in those with cardiac symptoms. Carefully conducted epidural anesthesia is the preferred technique for both labor analgesia and cesarean section. The need for invasive monitoring will depend on the severity of cardiac disability. Electrocardiographic findings in patients with AIDS will often reveal abnormalities.

Renal Considerations

Meticulous attention must be paid to fluid balances, and urine output should be monitored. The use of central venous pressure monitoring may also be helpful in the management of fluids. Drugs with non–organ-dependent elimination are preferred, and nephrotoxic agents should be avoided.

Gastrointestinal Considerations

It is not uncommon to find oral lesions when examining the patient's mouth as part of the airway assessment. Mild to severe oral candidiasis and oral hairy leukoplakia may be noticed only when performing laryngoscopy for endotracheal intubation. Vomiting and diarrhea may be sufficiently severe to cause intravascular volume depletion and may require replacement of fluids prior to administration of anesthesia. Concomitant electrolyte abnormalities may occur and must also be searched for and corrected before anesthesia is begun.

Hematologic Considerations

The severity of anemia and the presence of coexisting conditions that may further impair oxygen-carrying capacity will dictate whether blood transfusions may be necessary. It is estimated that vaginal delivery is associated with blood loss of approximately 500 mL and cesarean section with the loss of 1000 mL of blood; therefore, the decision about blood transfusion, whether before or after delivery of the infant, will remain at the discretion of the anesthesiologist.

Neutropenia should alert the anesthesiologist to the inherent dangers of nosocomial infections. Strict aseptic technique must be adhered to with regard to the insertion of central venous monitor lines and arterial cannulation. There is a higher incidence of catheter sepsis in the seropositive population.

Thrombocytopenia is an early primary manifestation of HIV infection that improves with the use of zidovudine. It does not usually manifest with features of increased bleeding and its clinical relevance is yet to be fully elucidated. Platelet levels of 50,000 to 75,000/μL should be followed up by clinical examination to observe for petechiae, ecchymoses, or bleeding at intravenous or venipuncture sites. Investigations such as with thromboelastography may be useful prior to commencement of a regional anesthetic technique.

Pharmacologic Considerations

The appearance of cutaneous eruptions following drug administration under anesthesia is a cause for concern to the anesthesiologist. The dilemma lies in labeling the patient as being hypersensitive to the offending drug and the avoidance of its use in the future. Such situations must be clarified with further investigations that test for the presence of true hypersensitivity. As stated earlier, the incidence of true anaphylaxis is not increased.

The use of nondepolarizing muscle relaxants must be individually tailored in those patients who have generalized muscle wasting, as they require reduced dosages on the basis of reduced muscle mass.

Drug interactions have been recently described in the literature regarding the coadministration of certain antiretroviral agents, namely the protease inhibitors and anesthetic drugs such as fentanyl, alfentanil, and methadone. The nucleoside and non-nucleoside drugs are generally deemed safe.[72]

OCCUPATIONAL EXPOSURE

In 1996, the CDC's Hospital Infection Control Practices Advisory Committee revised the term "universal precautions" to "standard precautions." It is now widely accepted that the necessary safety measures must be taken when handling blood, blood products, tissue, and secretions of all patients, irrespective of their background history. Being careful only with known HIV-positive patients may lead to one being less than careful with those who are most infective, that is, those in the window period. Barrier protection must be sought with the use of gloves, gowns, facemasks, and eye-shields, as they reduce the risk considerably. The use of gloves prevents 98% of an anesthesiologist's contact with patient blood.[73]

Needlestick Injury

Percutaneous needle injury appears as the main area in which anesthesiologists must persevere to reduce exposure to potential pathogens. Contaminated needles should not be recapped by hand. The risk of transmission of HIV from a needlestick injury with HIV-infected blood is widely quoted as 0.32%.[74] This is a small but definite risk. All health institutions must have a protocol for managing a health care worker who has had a needlestick injury, and each health care worker must be aware of what to do (see Appendix A). Immediate access to antiretroviral drugs must be available. Drugs should be taken as soon as possible but at least within the first hour following the needlestick injury. The risk of seroconversion can, in this way, be reduced by 80%.[75] The choice of drug, combination of reverse transcriptase inhibitors, and addition of protease inhibitors will depend on availability, the type of injury, and whether there was any delay in the worker's taking the medication. The rationale underlying post-exposure prophylaxis is that chemoprophylaxis may prevent initial cellular infection and local propagation of HIV, and thus allow the host immune defenses to eliminate the introduction of the virus. The CDC, in collaboration with French and British public health authorities, has conducted a retrospective case control study using data reported to national surveillance systems in the United States, France, and the United Kingdom.[76] The conclusions reached were that three factors played a pivotal role in increasing the risk to the health care worker. The first factor is that the quantity of blood involved as indicated by visible contamination of the device by blood contributes to the risk, the second relates to the type of procedure for which the needle was used (arterial or venous cannulation), and the third factor involves the depth of the needlestick injury. Higher viral titers in patients with advanced HIV infection is also considered to appreciably increase the risk. It suffices to say that all health care workers must take the responsibility to minimize exposure to themselves and to their colleagues by handling potentially infective products safely and taking the necessary precautions with all patients.

Bi-directional infection, i.e., transmission of infection from a health care worker to a patient and vice versa, is a controversial issue. The risk to the patient is considerably lower than to the health care worker. In fact, it is believed to be extremely low[77] and thus virtually impossible to quantify. Therefore, there is a school of thought that suggests that retrospective notification of patients should not be done routinely. Mutual respect for human rights, however, is necessary in dealing with this controversy.

CONCLUSION

Anesthesiologists will be faced with an increasing number of HIV-infected parturients who may present with various aspects of this multisystem disease that have important implications to the administration of anesthesia. It cannot be overemphasized that all practicing anesthesiologists must be familiar with the disease. As drug therapy becomes more accessible to patients, its effect on the various organs and the potential interactions with anesthetic drugs will also be of increasing importance to the anesthesiologist. HIV is a foreboding disease. The impact it will have on world health and on world economy will depend on what can be achieved at the current stage of the pandemic. Countries that have the infrastructure to stem the tide of the disease through comprehensive prevention and awareness programs will avoid the disaster situation that awaits those countries that are unable to do the same. HIV/AIDS has been described as one of the greatest challenges in the history of modern medicine, "a disease that knows no borders and respects no moral code."[78]

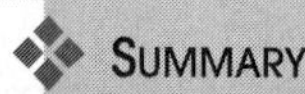

Summary

Key Points

- Women have become the fastest increasing new group of AIDS patients in the United States.
- Perinatal infant infection has been dramatically reduced, and monotherapy with ZDV is considered essential in the parturient.
- HIV-mediated organ dysfunction may be present and may have an impact on anesthetic management.
- Regional anesthesia is safe for use in the HIV-positive patient. CNS involvement occurs early, and there is no evidence that spinal anesthesia worsens the patient's neurologic status.

Key Reference

Hughes SC, Dailey PA, Landers D, et al: Parturients infected with human immunodeficiency virus and regional anesthesia: Clinical and immunologic response. Anesthesiology 1995; 82:32–37.

Case Stem

A 30-year-old pregnant woman with AIDS is scheduled for an elective cesarean section. Discuss the obstetric management of HIV and the possible anesthetic options. If regional anesthesia is selected and the patient develops a post–dural puncture headache, how will you treat it?

References

1. World Health Organization: Weekly Epidemiological Record. Geneva: WHO 1997;27:197–200.
2. World Health Organization: Global Programme on AIDS: The Current Global Situation of the HIV/AIDS Pandemic, 1st January, 1997. Geneva: WHO, 1997.
3. Mann JM, Taratola DJM, Netter TW: The HIV pandemic: Status and trends. *In* Mann JM, Tarantola DJM, Netter TW (eds): AIDS in the World. Cambridge, MA: Harvard University Press, 1992.
4. Phillips P: No Plateau for HIV/AIDS epidemic in US women. JAMA 1997; 277:1747–1749.
5. Centers for Disease Control and Prevention, U.S. Department of Health and Human Services/Public Health Service: Update: Mortality attributable to HIV infection among persons ages 25–44: United States, 1994. Morbid Mortal Wkly Rep 1996; 45:121–125.
6. Selik RM, Chu SY, Buehler JW: HIV infection as a leading cause of death among young adults in US cities and states. JAMA 1993; 269:2991–2994.
7. Singh GK, Yu SM: Trends and differentials in adolescent and young adult mortality in the United States, 1950 through 1993. Am J Public Health 1996; 86:560–564.

8. Fauci AS, Lane HC: Human immunodeficiency virus (HIV) disease: AIDS and related disorders. *In* Isselbacher KJ, et al (eds): Harrison's Principles of Internal Medicine, 14th ed. New York: McGraw-Hill, 1994.
9. Levy JA: HIV pathogenesis and long term survival. AIDS 1993; 7:1401–1410.
10. Crixivan product monograph: Current Antiretroviral Therapeutic Options. Merck & Co.
11. Fauci AS: The human immunodeficiency virus: Infectivity and mechanisms of pathogenesis. Science 1988; 239:617–622.
12. Heath SL, et al: Follicular dendritic cells and human immunodeficiency virus infectivity. Nature 1995; 377:740–744.
13. Ho DD, Neumann AU, Perelson AS: Rapid turnover of plasma virions and CD4 lymphocytes in HIV-1 infection. Nature 1995; 373:123–126.
14. Ho DD: Presentation Summary: HIV Pathogenesis. Improving the Management of HIV Disease 1996; 4:4–6.
15. Perelson AS, et al: HIV 1 dynamics in vivo: Virion clearance rate, infected cell life-span, and viral generation time. Science 1996; 271:1582–1586.
16. Merigan T: Individualization of therapy using viral markers. J AIDS Hum Retrovirol 1995; 10(suppl 1):S41–S46.
17. Vella S: HIV pathogenesis and treatment strategies. J AIDS Hum Retrovirol 1995; 10(suppl 1):S20–S23.
18. Haynes BF, Pantaleo G, Fauci AS: Toward an understanding of the correlates of protective immunity to HIV infection. Science 1996; 271:324–328.
19. Burke DS: Recombination in HIV: An important viral evolutionary strategy. Emerg Infect Dis 1997; 3:253–259.
20. Press D: Food and Drug Administration approval for two new molecular infectious disease assays. Mol Diagn 1999; 4:256.
21. Ault A: FDA warns of potential protease-inhibitor link to hyperglycaemia (news). Lancet 1997; 349:9068.
22. Dube MP, et al: Hyperglycaemia a possible late side effect of protease inhibitors. Lancet 1997; 350:713–714.
23. Bonfanti P, et al: Hypersensitivity reactions reported with HIV protease inhibitors. AIDS 1997; 11:1301–1302.
24. Feinberg M: Hidden dangers of incomplete suppression of antiretroviral therapy (commentary). Lancet 1997; 349:9063:1408.
25. Carpenter CC, Cooper DA, Fischl MA, et al: Antiretroviral therapy in adults: Updated recommendations of the International AIDS Society–USA Panel. JAMA 2000 19;283:381–390.
26. Martin R: Hybridon abandons GEM91, first generation anti-sense drug. PR Newswire downloaded July 25, 1997.
27. Reimann KA, Lin W, Bixler S, et al: A humanized form of a CD4-specific monoclonal antibody exhibits decreased antigen and prolonged half-life in Rhesus monkeys while retaining its unique biological and antiviral properties. AIDS Res Hum Retrovir 1997; 13:933–943.
28. Bohnlein E, et al: Granulocyte-colony stimulating factor (G-CSF) enriches stem cell population in HIV-infected patients. Blood 1997; 89:4299–4306.
29. Andrieu J-M, et al: Sustained increase in CD4 cell counts in asymptomatic human immunodeficiency virus type-1 seropositive patients treated with prednisolone for one year. J Infect Dis 1995; 171:523–530.
30. Caumes E, Guermonpitz G, Lecomte C, et al: Efficacy and desensitisation with sulfamethoxazole and trimethoprim in 48 previously hypersensitive patients infected with human immunodeficiency virus. Arch Dermatol 1997; 133:465–469.
31. Sharpstone D, Gazzard B: Gastrointestinal manifestations of HIV. Lancet 1996; 348:379–383.
32. Schuman P, Capps L, Peng G: Weekly fluconazole for prevention of mucosal candidiasis in women with HIV infection: A randomized, double-blind, placebo-controlled trial. Ann Intern Med 1997; 126:689–696.
33. Schwartz DH: Early treatment of HIV infection. N Engl J Med 1995; 333:1782.
34. Landers DV, Sweet LR: Reducing mother to infant transmission of HIV: The door remains open. N Engl J Med 1996; 334:1664–1665.
35. Luzuriaga K, Bryson Y, Krogstad P, et al: Combination treatment with zidovudine, didanosine and nevirapine in infants with human immunodeficiency virus type-1 infection. N Engl J Med 1997; 336:1343–1349.
36. Wilfert CM: Beginning to make progress against HIV [editorial]. N Engl J Med 1996; 335:1678–1680.
37. Noone A, Goldberg D: Antenatal HIV testing: What now? Despite guidelines, infections remain undetected [editorial]. Br Med J 1997; 314:1429–1430.
38. McIntyre JA: Management of HIV-positive pregnant women. CME 1996; 14:781–788.
39. McCarthy M: Can HIV-1 transmission be prevented during pregnancy and labour. Lancet 1996; 348:9033.
40. Bryson YJ: Improving the management of HIV disease. Int AIDS Soc USA 1996; 4:3.
41. Gelbe R: Nevirapine may reduce perinatal HIV transmission substantially. Reuters Health Information Services, Inc., July 29, 1997.
42. Andrew A, Wizma AA, et al: Zidovudine use reduces perinatal HIV type-1 transmission in an urban medical center. JAMA 1996:275:1504–1506.
43. Hershow RC, et al: HCV increase the rate of vertical HIV transmission. J Infect Dis 1997; 167:414–420.
44. Osborn JE: Prevention and Policy. Final comments after IXth International Conference on HIV/AIDS, Vancouver B.C. July 22, 1996, (via Internet).
45. Resnick L, Berger JR, Shapshak P, Tourtellotte WW: Neurology 1988; 38:9–14.
46. Kanzer MD: Neuropathology of AIDS. Crit Rev Neurobiol 1990; 5:313–362.
47. Birnbach DJ, Bourlier RA, Choi R, Thys DM: Anaesthetic management of caesarean section in a patient with active recurrent genital herpes and AIDS-related dementia. Br J Anaesthesiol 1995; 7:639–641.
48. Kramer EL, Sanger JJ: Brain imaging in acquired immunodeficiency syndrome dementia complex. Semin Nucl Med 1990; 20:353–363.
49. Ajmani A, Habte-Gabr E, Zarr M, et al: Cerebral blood flow SPECT with Tc-99m exametazine correlates in AIDS dementia complex stages: A preliminary report. Clin Nucl Med 1991; 16:656–659.
50. Leger JM, Bouche P, Bolgert F, et al: The spectrum of polyneuropathies in patients infected with HIV. J Neurol Neurosurg Psychiatry 1989; 52:1369–1374.
51. Report of Working Group: Nomenclature and research case definitions for neurologic manifestations of human immunodeficiency virus type-1 (HIV-1) infection. Neurology 1991; 41:778–785.
52. Minkoff H, Haynes deRegt R, Landesman S, Schwarz R: *Pneumocystis carinii* pneumonia with acquired immunodeficiency syndrome in pregnancy: A report of three maternal deaths. Obstet Gynecol 1986; 67:284–287.
53. Bozette A, Sattler FR, Chiu J, et al: A controlled trial of early adjunctive treatment with corticosteroids for *Pneumocystis carinii* pneumonia in the acquired immune deficiency syndrome. N Engl J Med 1990; 323:1351–1357.
54. Horsburgh CR: Advances in the prevention and treatment of *Mycobacterium avium* disease. N Engl J Med 1996; 313:377–383.
55. Cammarosano C, Lewis W: Cardiac lesions in acquired immune deficiency syndrome. J Am Coll Cardiol 1985; 5:703–706.
56. Barbaro G, Di Lorenzo G, Grisonorio B, et al: Incidence of dilated cardiomyopathy and detection of HIV in myocardial cells of HIV: Positive patients. N Engl J Med 1998; 339:1093–1099.
57. Heidenreich PA, et al: Pericardial effusion in AIDS: Incidence and survival. Circulation 1995; 92:3229–3234.
58. Barnett MA, Learmoth RP, Pihl E, Wood EC: T-helper lymphocyte depression in early human pregnancy. J Reprod Immunol 1983; 5:55–59.
59. Weinberg ED: Pregnancy-associated depression of cell-mediated immunity. Rev Infect Dis 1984; 6:814–820.
60. Burns DN, Nourjah P, Minkoff H, et al: Changes in CD4+ and CD8+ levels during pregnancy and post partum in women seropositive and seronegative for human immunodeficiency virus. Am J Obstet Gynecol 1996; 174:1461–1468.
61. Biggar RJ, Pahwa S, Minkoff H, et al: Immunosuppression in

pregnant women infected with human immunodeficieny virus. Am J Obstet Gynecol 1989; 161:1239–1244.
62. Brettle RP, Raab GM, Ross A, et al: HIV infection in women: Immunological markers and the influence of pregnancy. AIDS 1995; 9:1177–1184.
63. Tuomala RE, Kalish LA, Zorilla C, et al: The Women and Infants Transmission Study. Changes in Total, $CD4^+$, and $CD8^+$ lymphocytes during pregnancy and one year postpartum in HIV-infected women. Obstet Gynecol 1997; 6:967–973.
64. Landesman SH: Human immunodeficiency virus infection in women: An overview Semin Perinatol 1989; 13:2–6.
65. Minkoff HL, Henderson CE, Willoughby A: The influence of HIV serostatus on pregnancy outcome: Results of prospective case control study. Society of Perinatal Obstetricians, 10th meeting, Houston, 1990.
66. Gershon RY, Manning-Williams D: Anesthesia and the HIV infected parturient: A retrospective study. Int J Obstet Anesth 1997; 6:76–81.
67. Penfold J, Clark AJM: Pain syndromes in HIV infection. Can J Anesth 1992; 39:724–730.
68. Perlman DC, et al: Chest x-ray patterns vary with immunesuppression levels in HIV-related TB. Clin Infec Dis 1997; 25:242–246.
69. Greene ER: Spinal and epidural anesthesia in patients with AIDS. Anesth Analg 1986; 65:1090–1091.
70. Hughes SC, Dailey PA, Landers D, et al: Parturients infected with human immunodeficiency virus and regional anesthesia: Clinical and immunologic response. Anesthesiology 1995; 82:32.
71. Shapiro HM, Igor G, Weinger MB: AIDS and the central nervous system. Anesthesiology 1994; 80:187–200.
72. Hernandez Conte AT: Perioperative medicine and pain: Human immunodeficiency virus and potential anesthetic interaction. Semin Anesth 1998; 17:299–307.
73. Kristensen MS, Sloth E, Jensen TK: Relationship between anesthetic procedure and contact of anesthesia personnel with patient body fluids. Anesthesiology 1990; 73:619–624.
74. Gerberding JL: HIV transmission to providers and their patients. *In* Sande MA, Volberding PA (eds): The Medical Management of AIDS, 3rd ed. Philadelphia: WB Saunders, 1992:54–64.
75. Gerberding JL: Management of occupational exposure to blood borne viruses. N Engl J Med 1995; 332:444.
76. Centers for Disease Control and Prevention: Case control study of HIV seroconversion in health care workers after percutaneous exposure to HIV-infected blood: France, United Kingdom and United States, January 1988–August 1994. Morbid Mortal Wkly Rep.
77. Robert LM, Chamberland ME, Cleveland JL, et al: Investigations of patients of health care workers infected with HIV. Ann Intern Med 1995; 122:653–657.
78. Hughes SC: AIDS: The focus turns to women [editorial]. Int J Obstet Anesth 1993; 2:1–2.

APPENDIX A

MANAGEMENT OF NEEDLESTICK INJURY

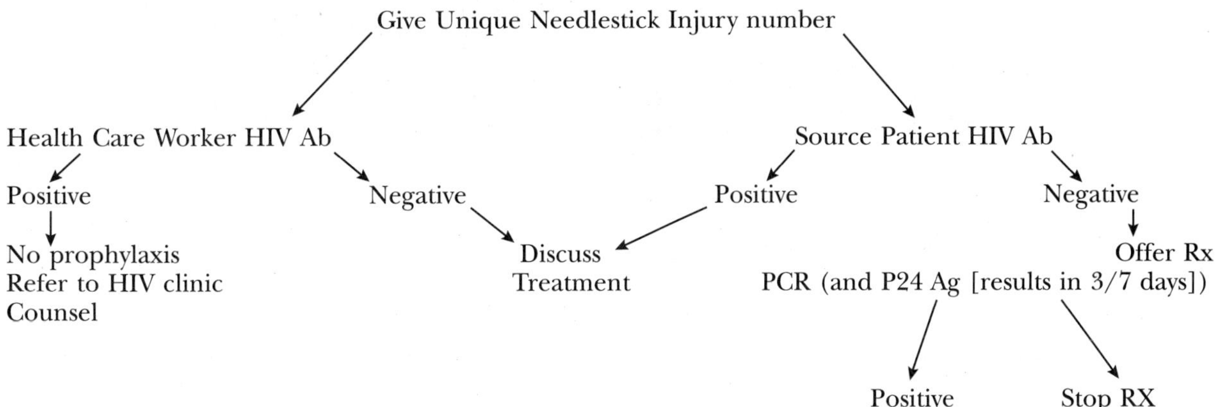

A. Institute STAT DOSE of antiretrovirals if patient is not pregnant.
B. Categorize risk:
   1. History of incident
      Hollow bore needle: ↑ risk
      Suture needle: ↓ risk
      Gloved: ↓ risk
      Visible blood: ↑ risk
   2. Viral load of source patient
      ↑ ↑ ↑ risk: ZDV + 3TC + indinavir
      ↑ ↑ risk: ZDV + 3TC
      AZT, 3TC, indinavir for:
      (1) All percutaneous injuries with hollow-bore instruments.
      (2) Very deep percutaneous injuries with non-hollow-bore needles that had visible blood in an ungloved health care worker.
      (3) Percutaneous and mucosal exposures with a high viral load > 10 000?
C. Explain health care worker must follow up results → seek treatments/sign statement/pregnancy test/resistance/side effects.
D. Do baseline biochemistry profile/Repeat twice weekly for 6/52 weeks.
   Full blood cell count
   Urea and creatinine
   Amylase
   Liver function test
E. Fill out appropriate compensation forms
F. Inform: Protease inhibitor as this medication is not on code.
G. Inform: breast-feeding/safe sex, avoid pregnancy for 4/52 weeks, counseling, no blood/organ donation.
H. HIV PCR + Ab 2 weeks, 1 month, 2 months, 3 months, 6 months, 12 months, 18 months.
   HCV PCR + Ab 2 weeks, 1 month, 3 months, 6 months, 12 months, 18 months.
I. Facilitate contact with hospital psychologists

Ab, antibody; HCV, hepatitis C virus; HIV, human immunodeficiency virus; PCR, polymerase chain reaction; Rx, treatment; 3TC; ZDV, zidovudine.

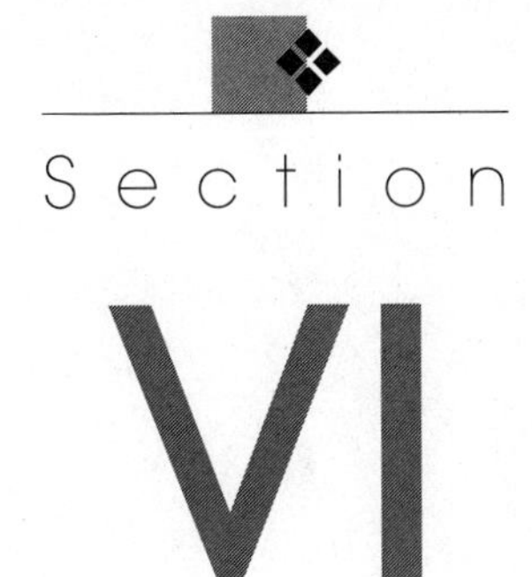

Related Considerations

50

Nausea and Vomiting

❖ TONY GIN, MD, MBCHB, Dipl HSM, FRCA, FANZCA

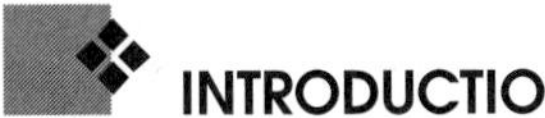

INTRODUCTION

Nausea and vomiting are common symptoms affecting nearly all women in early pregnancy. The majority of cases are managed by the women themselves and the symptoms mostly resolve by the 20th week of gestation.[1, 2] In up to 1% of pregnancies, persistent nausea and vomiting requires medical management to maintain adequate hydration and nutrition. The pathophysiology of this occurrence, known as hyperemesis gravidarum, is poorly understood and it is not related only to increased concentrations of human chorionic gonadotropin (hCG). In later pregnancy, heartburn and nausea are common symptoms that accompany the generalized relaxation of smooth muscle in the gastrointestinal system.[3]

The management of nausea and vomiting during early pregnancy has been influenced by concerns about teratogenicity ever since the thalidomide tragedy in the early 1960s. Further concerns about the antiemetic combination of doxylamine, dicyclomine, and pyridoxine (Debendox, Benedictin) led the manufacturer to voluntarily withdraw these products despite lack of evidence of teratogenicity in 33 million pregnancies. The U.S. Food and Drug Administration classifies drugs in pregnancy into five groups with regard to potential for birth defects. Antihistamines (e.g., cyclizine, diphenhydramine, doxylamine), and metoclopramide are class B (animal studies show no risk but human studies are inadequate *or* animal studies show some risk but are not supported by human studies), while the phenothiazines, droperidol, ondansetron and corticosteroids are class C (animal studies show risk but human studies are inadequate *or* no studies are available). Nevertheless, class B drugs are commonly used in early pregnancy and there are advocates for prompt pharmacologic treatment of nausea and vomiting to avoid the complications of hyperemesis. If a patient is hospitalized for hyperemesis, it is likely that many of the class B and C drugs previously listed will be used in any case.

Jewell and Young assessed the effectiveness of different methods of treating nausea and vomiting in early pregnancy.[4] They concluded that the antihistamines and the combination tablet Debendox were effective. Maternal side effects were minor and predictable, but there was little data on fetal outcome. Pyridoxine was effective in treating nausea, while P6 acupressure (over the Neiguan point just above the wrist on the forearm [between the palmaris longus and flexor carpi radialis]) was equivocal and the evidence for powdered ginger root taken orally was weak.

OVERVIEW

The incidence of postoperative nausea and vomiting (PONV) varies widely among different patient groups. Although medical complications are rare, PONV can be unpleasant, distressing, and embarrassing for the afflicted patient, causing dissatisfaction with otherwise successful surgery.[5] The management of PONV increases work in the recovery room and may lead to increased expense as a result of nursing workload and prolonged hospital stay.[6] There have been extensive reviews on PONV,[7, 8] and information relevant to obstetric anesthesia is summarized in the subsequent text.

Physiology. PONV has often been treated as a single entity because nausea was thought to be a symptom following low-intensity stimulation of the vomiting reflex. However, there may be different mechanisms for nausea and emesis, because emesis may occur without nausea and some drugs are more effective antinauseants than antiemetics.[9] There are also different higher centers involved in PONV and these may respond differently to different stimuli or antiemetic therapies. Many factors are thought to interact by increasing the threshold for other stimuli.[10] Vestibular stimulation may be one of the most important factors causing PONV. Transport of patients may cause PONV[11] by creating a mismatch of visual and vestibular input, similar to that in motion sickness. Patients with a history of motion sickness are more likely to suffer PONV, and patients often first notice nausea when they try to ambulate.[12] However, ondansetron, although not effective for motion sickness, is effective for PONV.

It is not clear why most general anesthetics apart from propofol, which has antiemetic properties,[13] should cause PONV.[10] Induction and maintenance of anesthesia with propofol, either with nitrous oxide or as part of total intravenous anesthesia, usually produces a lower incidence of PONV.[14, 15] In contrast to general anesthesia, regional anesthesia has a lower incidence of PONV. Nausea and vomiting usually only accompanies the use of neuraxial opioids, or hypotension secondary to sympathetic block.

Pain may be a cause of nausea, and adequate analgesia may relieve nausea.[16] However, opioids have a complex role in emesis.[10] Opioids can cause PONV, whatever the route of administration, and no opioid has been shown conclusively to cause more PONV than any other. Higher doses of opioids have antiemetic actions by depressing the vomiting center. A high incidence of PONV in patients receiving patient-controlled analgesia is an expected side effect that accompanies effective opioid analgesia.

Management. There is controversy regarding whether patients should be given antiemetic drugs prophylactically. If the incidence of PONV after a particular operation is low, it may not be necessary to give prophylaxis routinely. Logistic regression analysis has identified female gender, history of previous postoperative sickness, and history of motion sickness as the most important patient factors predicting PONV.[17, 18]

Although recent research has concentrated on evaluating antiemetic drugs, the avoidance of an emetic anesthetic technique is an obvious first step to reduce PONV. The use of regional anesthesia, propofol for induction of general anesthesia, and nonsteroidal anti-inflammatory drugs or local anesthetics for postoperative analgesia may reduce the incidence of PONV. Drug therapy has not been completely effective in preventing or treating PONV, and antiemetic drugs often have associated antihistaminic, anticholinergic, or antidopaminergic side effects.

Current Drug Therapy. A review of existing therapy concluded that the efficacy of existing antiemetics was generally poor.[19] Metoclopramide, despite its popularity, has not been superior to placebo in several well-controlled trials. It is best given intravenously near the end of anesthesia. Droperidol has also been studied extensively and is the most effective of the older antiemetics. Chlorpromazine, perphenazine, and cyclizine may be as efficacious but there are few confirmatory studies. Extrapyramidal side effects are uncommon but distressing. Transdermal hyoscine has minimal side effects, but more studies are required to prove its efficacy. For most of these drugs, doses used have been empiric and not based on pharmacokinetic knowledge. Not surprisingly, the duration of antiemetic effect has not been characterized. Some drugs may be more effective against nausea than emesis, but there is not a clear distinction during PONV to enable selective prescribing for nausea alone. Ephedrine, the active principle of the Chinese plant *Ma Huang*, is often used to treat hypotension associated with regional anesthesia, but it also has intrinsic antiemetic properties.[20]

The 5-hydroxytryptamine receptor-3 (5-HT_3) antagonists appear to be the most effective antiemetics available, with few side effects. Ondansetron was the first drug to be studied extensively, but there is now experience with granisetron, tropisetron, and dolasetron. Comparative studies have shown that generally ondansetron, 4 mg, is superior to metoclopramide, 10 mg,[21] but it has similar efficacy to droperidol, 0.625 mg or 1.25 mg.[22, 23] Comparisons between 5-HT_3 antagonists have been hampered by uncertainty over the appropriate equivalent doses. Ondansetron is more effective at preventing emesis than nausea and may fail to prevent PONV completely in 30% to 50% of patients. The specific 5-HT_3 antagonists should not be as effective when PONV is caused by other mechanisms. Ondansetron is considerably more expensive than other antiemetics, and it is important to assess the costs and benefits of new treatments. Most studies with ondansetron have concentrated on gynecologic patients and used barbiturates for induction of anesthesia rather than propofol. Other patient populations have a lower incidence of PONV and the cost-benefit considerations of ondansetron will be different.

The neurokinin (NK1) anatagonists are an exciting development in the treatment of PONV[24] because substance P appears to be an important transmitter in the vomiting center. The NK1 antagonists interrupt afferent inputs to the vomiting center and thus they have high efficacy whatever the stimulus for nausea and vomiting.

PONV and Postoperative Analgesia. During patient-controlled analgesia, antiemetics have been added to the opioid to decrease PONV. However, a recent review of this practice demonstrated that the results were not always convincing.[25] Although droperidol is effective, increased sedation is often reported and the benefits of adding droperidol to the opioid may be no different from giving a single dose of droperidol at the end of surgery.[26] No particular opioid was associated with a lower incidence of PONV.

Opioids administered into the intrathecal or extradural space may cause nausea and vomiting after systemic absorption of drug or via rostral spread in the cerebrospinal fluid. The incidence of emesis after epidural morphine can be as high as 40%.[27] Apart from conventional antiemetic drug treatment, careful titration of naloxone may reduce nausea.

Persistent PONV. After the initial dose of an antiemetic drug, the best treatment for patients continuing to have PONV is uncertain. It is logical to infer that combinations of antiemetic drugs with different modes of action may be more effective than single drug therapy. A look at recent comparative studies shows that one antiemetic usually still fails to prevent PONV in 20% to 40% of cases but that the combination of two antiemetics (usually ondansetron and droperidol) can reduce the incidence of PONV to between 4% and 15%.[28–30]

POSTOPERATIVE NAUSEA AND VOMITING IN OBSTETRIC ANESTHESIA

Early Pregnancy and Incidental Surgery During Pregnancy. As indicated earlier, there are no known fetal risks from using the standard antiemetic drugs in early pregnancy, but conclusive evidence is not available. The decision to give prophylaxis and treatment is usually an individual one influenced by the desire to minimize drug exposure versus the desire to avoid PONV.

Propofol is a popular induction agent for assisted reproduction procedures because of the associated rapid recovery and antiemetic effects. One report has suggested that patients for pronuclear stage embryo transfer anesthetized with a propofol regimen had lower pregnancy rates.[31] However, subsequent studies have questioned these findings.[32]

Patients for therapeutic abortion would be expected to have a very high incidence of PONV. However, it is difficult to find studies specifically indexed for this group of patients. The incidence of PONV was up to 50% in older studies,[33–35] and this has been greatly reduced by using propofol.[36, 37] There are no obvious differences in management of PONV compared with other gynecologic procedures.

Labor and Delivery. During labor, nausea and vomiting may occur for many reasons, including the use of nitrous oxide and meperidine for analgesia. Neuraxial opioids and hypotension caused by regional analgesia may also be contributing factors. The standard antiemetics have all been used to treat PONV. It is generally assumed that the placental transfer of these drugs is clinically insignificant and without known adverse effects, although only metoclopramide has been specifically studied using assessments of neonatal neurobehavior.[38, 39]

Cesarean Section. Nausea and vomiting is a special concern at cesarean section compared with other major surgical operations because acid aspiration is a particularly feared complication if regurgitation and emesis occur. Routine pharmacologic prophylaxis to reduce the volume and acidity of stomach contents is a standard practice. However, there is still the potential for aspiration whether this results from unexpected loss of consciousness during a regional anesthetic or excessive postoperative sedation after a general anesthetic. The Report on Confidential Enquiries into Maternal Deaths in the United Kingdom has recommended the use of a gastric tube to empty the stomach before extubation.[40]

Regional Anesthesia. There are many potential causes for nausea and vomiting during cesarean section under regional anesthesia. Some patients will already have reflux exacerbated by lying supine, and anxiety is known to be a predisposing factor for nausea and vomiting. Sodium citrate has a disagreeable taste to some women and may itself provoke vomiting. During the regional block, hypotension and neuraxial opioids can cause nausea and vomiting. During the operation, surgical manipulation may release gastrointestinal serotonin, stimulate vagal afferents, or directly compress the stomach. At delivery, hypotension caused by blood loss or rapid boluses of oxytocin, pain, and the use of supplemental opioids may all cause nausea and vomiting. Uterine exteriorization after delivery is commonly thought to increase the likelihood of pain and nausea, but a recent study in 194 women found no differences in these symptoms compared with leaving the uterus in situ.[41] To minimize nausea and vomiting, the main options for the anesthesiologist are to avoid hypotension, provide adequate analgesia, and use antiemetic drugs.

Hypotension is a common complication of epidural and intrathecal anesthesia and there are many regimens used in the prevention of it. Avoiding maternal hypotension significantly reduces the incidence of nausea and vomiting during spinal anesthesia.[42, 43] Hypotension is thought to trigger vomiting by causing hypoxemia of the vomiting center. Administration of oxygen decreases the incidence of emesis despite the presence of hypotension.[44] A higher segmental sympathetic block is associated with a higher incidence of hypotension, but a sufficiently high sensory block is also necessary for good intraoperative analgesia. Although neuraxial opioids can provide better analgesia and reduce pain and nausea caused by intra-abdominal manipulation,[45] they can themselves increase the incidence of nausea, particularly morphine and buprenorphine.[27, 46]

Antiemetic drugs are often used to minimize nausea and vomiting and there do not appear to be any differences in efficacy when they are used during epidural compared with spinal anesthesia. Some anesthesiologists wait until after delivery before giving antiemetic drugs, but there is no reason why the drugs cannot be given earlier for the greatest maternal benefit.

Metoclopramide is effective, and appears to have a better success rate during cesarean section, compared with its use for PONV in the general population. Metoclopramide, 0.15 mg/kg, reduced intraoperative nausea from 36% to 12%, and emesis from 15% to 0%,[47] while another study found that metoclopramide, 10 mg, reduced intraoperative nausea from 73% to 29%.[48] During spinal anesthesia, patients receiving metoclopramide had a lower incidence of nausea and vomiting both before and after delivery compared with the control group (14% vs. 81%).[39] In addition, all neonatal acid-base values were within normal limits and there were no significant differences in neurobehavioral examination results between the two groups. Droperidol, 2.5 mg, has been used successfully to reduce nausea from 40% to 12%,[49] but even droperidol, 0.5 mg, was effective in reducing nausea from 41% to 13%.[50] A comparative study showed that metoclopramide, 15 mg, and droperidol, 0.5 mg, were similarly effective during epidural anesthesia.[51]

In cesarean section patients under epidural anesthesia, ondansetron, 8 mg, and droperidol, 0.625 mg, had similar efficacy for lowering the incidence of nausea and vomiting.[52] In the ondansetron group, 15 of 16 patients were emesis-free and 11 of 16 nausea-free, while in the droperidol group, 14 of 16 were emesis-free and 12 of 16 were nausea-free.

A dose-ranging study showed that prophylactic use of granisetron in a minimum dose of 40 μg/kg was effective for preventing nausea and vomiting (14% incidence) during spinal anaesthesia.[53] The same group showed that granisetron (3 mg), droperidol (1.25 mg), and metoclopramide (10 mg) were equally effective for the prevention of intraoperative emesis (13–20%) but that granisetron was superior for 24-hour postoperative efficacy (7% vs. 20–23%).[54]

Acupressure was as effective as metoclopramide, 10 mg, to prevent nausea during spinal anesthesia.[55] However, propofol, 10 mg, given after delivery was ineffective for the treatment of intraoperative nausea and vomiting.[56, 57]

Postoperative Analgesia and PONV. The experience with PONV and different analgesic techniques is similar to that found after nonobstetric surgery. It is generally assumed that the transfer of antiemetic drugs into milk is clinically insignificant. Epidural morphine can provide better analgesia than patient-controlled analgesia, but the incidence of PONV can be high for both techniques.[58] Epidural fentanyl alone is associated with more nausea than when combined with bupivacaine, presumably because of the increased fentanyl dose required when it is used alone.[59] For the treatment of PONV associated with neuraxial opioids, success with droperidol,[60] transdermal hyoscine,[61] and acupressure[62] have all been recently reported. The use of intrathecal neostigmine has been associated with a high incidence of PONV that is dose related.[63–65] The addition of droperidol (10 mg) to morphine (60 mg) for patient-controlled analgesia following cesarean section under spinal anesthesia reduced the incidence of nausea and emesis, but could result in drowsiness, limiting the usefulness of the technique.[66]

Summary

Key Points

- Antihistamines, pyridoxine, and metoclopramide are thought to be the safest antiemetics to use in early pregnancy.
- During cesarean section under regional anesthesia, hypotension and discomfort from surgical manipulation are common causes of nausea and vomiting. Avoidance and early treatment of hypotension reduces the incidence of intraoperative nausea and vomiting. Prophylactic administration of metoclopramide or droperidol further reduces the incidence of nausea and vomiting.
- Management of persistent or severe nausea and vomiting should include combinations of antiemetics with different modes of actions. Alternative therapies such as acupressure should be considered in the patient with a history of PONV.

Key Reference

Lussos SA, Bader AM, Thornhill ML, Datta S: The antiemetic efficacy and safety of prophylactic metoclopramide for elective cesarean delivery during spinal anesthesia. Reg Anesth 1992; 17:126–130.

Case Stem

A parturient undergoing a cesarean section under spinal anesthesia begins to retch just after the start of the skin incision. Discuss the possible causes and management.

References

1. Broussard CN, Richter JE: Nausea and vomiting of pregnancy. Gastroenterol Clin North Am 1998; 27:123–151.
2. Nelson-Piercy C: Treatment of nausea and vomiting in pregnancy. Drug Saf 1998; 19:155–164.
3. Hytten F, Chamberlain G: The alimentary system. In Hytten F, Chamberlain G, eds. Clinical Physiology in Obstetrics, 2nd ed. Oxford, England: Blackwell; 1991:139–142.
4. Jewell D, Young G: Interventions for nausea and vomiting in early pregnancy (Cochrane Review). In: The Cochrane Library, Issue 1, 1999. Oxford: Update Software.
5. Van Wijk M, Smalhout B: A postoperative analysis of the patient's view of anaesthesia in a Netherlands teaching hospital. Anaesthesia 1990; 45:679–682.
6. Hirsch J: Impact of postoperative nausea and vomiting in the surgical setting. Anaesthesia 1994; 49(suppl):30–33.
7. Smith G, Rowbotham DJ: Supplement on postoperative nausea and vomiting. Br J Anaesth 1992; 69(suppl 1):1S–68S.
8. Watcha MF, White PF: Postoperative nausea and vomiting. Its etiology, treatment and prevention. Anesthesiology 1992; 77:162–184.
9. Hindle A: Ondansetron versus metoclopramide and droperidol: an unfair comparison. Anesth Analg 1993; 77:638–639.
10. Andrews PLR: Physiology of nausea and vomiting. Br J Anaesth 1992; 69(suppl 1):2S–19S.
11. Muir JJ, Warner MA, Offord KP, et al: Role of nitrous oxide and other factors in postoperative nausea and vomiting: a randomized and blinded prospective study. Anesthesiology 1987; 66:513–518.
12. Kamath B, Curran J, Hawkey C, et al: Anaesthesia, movement and emesis. Br J Anaesth 1990; 64:728–730.
13. Borgeat A, Wilder-Smith OHG, Saiah M, Rifat K: Subhypnotic doses of propofol possess direct antiemetic properties. Anesth Analg 1992; 74:539–541.
14. Sneyd JR, Carr A, Byrom WD, Bilski AJT: A meta-analysis of nausea and vomiting following maintenance of anaesthesia with propofol or inhalational agents. Eur J Anaesthesiol 1998; 15:433–445.
15. Tramér M, Moore A, McQuay H: Propofol anaesthesia and postoperative nausea and vomiting: quantitative systematic review of randomized controlled studies. Br J Anaesth 1997; 78:247–255.
16. Andersen R, Krogh K: Pain as a major cause for postoperative nausea. Can Anaesth Soc J 1976; 23:366–369.
17. Palazzo M, Evans R: Logistic regression analysis of fixed patient factors for postoperative sickness: a model for risk assessment. Br J Anaesth 1993; 70:135–140.
18. Haigh CG, Kaplan LA, Durham JM, et al: Nausea and vomiting after gynaecological surgery: a meta-analysis of factors affecting their incidence. Br J Anaesth 1993; 71:517–522.
19. Rowbotham DJ: Current management of postoperative nausea and vomiting. Br J Anaesth 1992; 69(suppl 1):46S–59S.

20. Rothenberg DM, Parnass SM, Litwack K, et al: Efficacy of ephedrine in the prevention of postoperative nausea and vomiting. Anesth Analg 1991; 72:58–61.
21. Diemunsch P, Conseiller C, Clyti N, Mamet JP, and the French Ondansetron Study Group: Ondansetron compared with metoclopramide in the treatment of established postoperative nausea and vomiting. Br J Anaesth 1997; 79:322–326.
22. Tang J, Watcha MF, White PF: A comparison of costs and efficacy of ondansetron and droperidol as prophylactic antiemetic therapy for elective outpatient gynecologic procedures. Anesth Analg 1996; 83:304–313.
23. Fortney JT, Gan TJ, Graczyk S, et al: A comparison of the efficacy, safety and patient satisfaction of ondansetron versus droperidol as antiemetics for elective outpatient surgical procedures. Anesth Analg 1998; 86:731–738.
24. Diemunsch P, Schoeffler P, Bryssine B, et al: Antiemetic activity of the NK1 receptor antagonist GR205171 in the treatment of established postoperative nausea and vomiting after major gynaecological surgery. Br J Anaesth 1999; 82:274–276.
25. Woodhouse A, Mather LE: Nausea and vomiting in the postoperative patient-controlled analgesia environment. Anaesthesia 1997; 52:770–775.
26. Gan TJ, Alexander R, Fennelly M, Rubin AP: Comparison of different methods of administering droperidol in patient-controlled analgesia in the prevention of postoperative nausea and vomiting. Anesth Analg 1995; 80:81–85.
27. Fuller JG, McMorland GH, Douglas MJ, Palmer L: Epidural morphine for analgesia after caesarean section: a report of 4880 patients. Can J Anaesth 1990; 37:636–640.
28. McKenzie R, Tantisira B, Karambelkar DJ, et al: Comparison of ondansetron with ondansetron plus dexamethasone in the prevention of postoperative nausea and vomiting. Anesth Analg 1994; 79:961–964.
29. McKenzie R, Uy NTL, Riley TJ, Hamilton DL: Droperidol/ondansetron combination controls nausea and vomiting after tubal banding. Anesth Analg 1996; 83:1218–1222.
30. Pueyo FJ, Carrascosa F, Lopez L, et al: Combination of ondansetron and droperidol in the prophylaxis of postoperative nausea and vomiting. Anesth Analg 1996; 83:117–122.
31. Vincent RD Jr, Syrop CH, Van Voorhis BJ, et al: An evaluation of the effect of anesthetic technique on reproductive success after laparoscopic pronuclear stage transfer: propofol/nitrous oxide versus isoflurane/nitrous oxide. Anesthesiology 1995; 82:352–358.
32. Beilin Y, Bodian CA, Mukherjee T, et al: The use of propofol, nitrous oxide or isoflurane does not affect the reproductive success rate following gamete intrafallopian transfer (GIFT): a multicenter pilot trial/survey. Anesthesiology 1999; 90:36–41.
33. Waldmann CS, Verghese C, Short SM, et al: The evaluation of domperidone and metoclopramide as antiemetics in day care abortion patients. Br J Clin Pharmacol 1985; 19:307–310.
34. Lim KS, Lim BL, Tee CS, Vengadasalam D: Nausea and vomiting after termination of pregnancy as day surgery cases: comparison of 3 different doses of droperidol and metoclopramide as anti-emetic prophylaxis. Singapore Med J 1991; 32:342–343.
35. Millar JM, Hall PJ: Nausea and vomiting after prostaglandins in day case termination of pregnancy: the efficacy of low dose droperidol. Anaesthesia 1987; 42:613–618.
36. Nathan N, Peyclit A, Lahrimi A, Feiss P: Comparison of sevoflurane and propofol for ambulatory anaesthesia in gynaecological surgery. Can J Anaesth 1998; 45:1148–1150.
37. Elhakim M, El-Sebiae S, Kaschef N, Essawi GH: Intravenous fluid and postoperative nausea and vomiting after day-case termination of pregnancy. Acta Anaesthesiol Scand 1998; 42:216–219.
38. Bylsma-Howell M, Riggs KW, McMorland GH, et al: Placental transport of metoclopramide: assessment of maternal and neonatal effects. Can Anaesth Soc J 1983; 30:487–492.
39. Lussos SA, Bader AM, Thornhill ML, Datta S: The antiemetic efficacy and safety of prophylactic metoclopramide for elective cesarean delivery during spinal anesthesia. Reg Anesth 1992; 17:126–130.
40. Department of Health: Report on Confidential Enquiries into Maternal Deaths in the United Kingdom, 1988–1990. London: Her Majesty's Stationery Office; 1994.
41. Edi-Osagie EC, Hopkins RE, Ogbo V, et al: Uterine exteriorisation at caesarean section: influence on maternal morbidity. Br J Obstet Gynaecol 1998; 105:1070–1078.
42. Datta S, Alper MH, Ostheimer GW, Weiss JB: Method of ephedrine administration and nausea and hypotension during spinal anesthesia for cesarean section. Anesthesiology 1982; 56:68–70.
43. Kang YG, Abouleish E, Caritis S: Prophylactic intravenous ephedrine infusion during spinal anesthesia for cesarean section. Anesth Analg 1982; 61:839–842.
44. Ratra CK, Badola RP, Bhargava KP: A study of factors concerned in emesis during spinal anaesthesia. Br J Anaesth 1972; 44:1208–1211.
45. Naulty JS, Datta S, Ostheimer GW, et al: Epidural fentanyl for post–cesarean delivery pain management. Anesthesiology 1985; 63:694–698.
46. Celleno D, Capogna G, Sebastini M, et al: Epidural analgesia during and after cesarean delivery: comparison of five opioids. Reg Anesth 1991; 16:79–83.
47. Chestnut DH, Vandewalker GE, Owen CL, et al: Administration of metoclopramide for prevention of nausea and vomiting during epidural anesthesia for elective cesarean section. Anesthesiology 1987; 66:563–566.
48. Danzer BI, Birnbach DJ, Stein DJ, et al: Does metoclopramide supplement postoperative analgesia using patient-controlled analgesia with morphine in patients undergoing elective cesarean delivery. Reg Anesth 1997; 22:424–427.
49. Santos A, Datta S: Prophylactic use of droperidol for control of nausea and vomiting during spinal anesthesia for cesarean section. Anesth Analg 1984; 63:85–87.
50. Mandell GL, Dewan DM, Howard G, Floyd HM: The effectiveness of low dose droperidol in controlling nausea and vomiting during epidural anesthesia for cesarean section. Int J Obstet Anesth 1992; 1:65–68.
51. Chestnut DH, Owen CL, Geiger M, et al: Metoclopramide versus droperidol for prevention of nausea and vomiting during epidural anesthesia for cesarean section. South Med J 1989; 82:1224–1227.
52. Pan PH, Moore CH: Intraoperative antiemetic efficacy of prophylactic ondansetron versus droperidol for cesarean section patients under epidural anesthesia. Anesth Analg 1996; 83:982–986.
53. Fujii Y, Tanaka H, Toyooka H: Granisetron prevents nausea and vomiting during spinal anaesthesia for caesarean section. Acta Anaesthesiol Scand 1998; 42:312–315.
54. Fujii Y, Tanaka H, Toyooka H: Prevention of nausea and vomiting with granisetron, droperidol and metoclopramide during and after spinal anaesthesia for caesarean section: a randomized, double-blind, placebo-controlled trial. Acta Anaesthesiol Scand 1998; 42:921–925.
55. Stein DJ, Birnbach DJ, Danzer BI, et al: Acupressure versus intravenous metoclopramide to prevent nausea and vomiting during spinal anesthesia for cesarean section. Anesth Analg 1997; 84:342–345.
56. Caba F, Echevarria M, Bernal-Davalos L, et al: Prophylaxis of intraoperative nausea and vomiting with sub-hypnotic dose of propofol during intradural anesthesia in cesarean section [in Spanish]. Rev Esp Anestesiol Reanim 1997; 44:262–266.
57. Shi JJ, Wang YP, Sun WZ, et al: The effect of low dose propofol for prevention of nausea and vomiting during spinal anesthesia for cesarean section. Acta Anaesthesiol Sin 1994; 32:95–98.
58. Eisenach JC, Grice SC, Dewan DM: Patient controlled analgesia following cesarean section: a comparison with epidural and intramuscular narcotics. Anesthesiology 1988; 68:444–448.
59. Cohen S, Lowenwirt I, Pantuck CB, et al: Bupivacaine 0.01% and/or epinephrine 0.5 μg/ml improve epidural fentanyl analgesia after cesarean section. Anesthesiology 1998; 89:1354–1361.
60. Sanansilp V, Areewatana S, Tonsukchai N: Droperidol and the side effects of epidural morphine after cesarean section. Anesth Analg 1998; 86:532–537.
61. Kotelko DM, Rottman RL, Wright WC, et al: Transdermal

scopolamine decreases nausea and vomiting following cesarean section in patients receiving epidural morphine. Anesthesiology 1989; 71:675–678.
62. Ho CM, Hseu SS, Tsai SK, Lee TY: Effect of P-6 acupressure on prevention of nausea and vomiting after epidural morphine for post–cesarean section pain relief. Acta Anaesthesiol Scand 1996; 40:372–375.
63. Pan PM, Huang CT, Wei TT, Mok MS: Enhancement of analgesic effect of intrathecal neostigmine and clonidine on bupivacaine spinal anesthesia. Reg Anesth Pain Med 1998; 23:49–56.
64. Krukowski JA, Hood DD, Eisenach JC, et al: Intrathecal neostigmine for post–cesarean section analgesia: dose response. Anesth Analg 1997; 84:1269–1275.
65. Chung CJ, Kim JS, Park HS, Chin YJ: The efficacy of intrathecal neostigmine, intrathecal morphine, and their combination for post–cesarean section analgesia. Anesth Analg 1998; 87:341–346.
66. Russell D, Duncan LA, Frame WT, et al: Patient-controlled analgesia with morphine and droperidol following caesarean section under spinal anaesthesia. Acta Anaesthesiol Scand 1996; 40:600–605.

51

Nerve Blocks in the Pregnant Patient

❖ JERRY D. VLOKA, MD, PHD
❖ ADMIR HADŽIĆ, MD, PHD
❖ LEON DROBNIK, MD, PHD

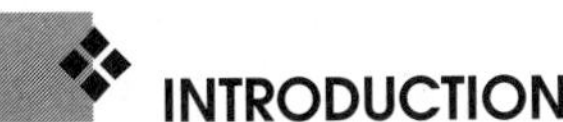

INTRODUCTION

The incidence of nonobstetric surgery during pregnancy has been estimated to range from 0.16%[1] to 2%[2]. However, since as many as one third to one half of conceived fetuses will not implant or otherwise will spontaneously miscarry, the true incidence of surgery during pregnancy has probably been underestimated. The most frequent surgical procedures related to pregnancy are the placement of a cervical suture (cerclage) for cervical incompetence, surgery for ovarian torsion, and orthopedic surgery for limb trauma. In the study by Mazze and Källén[3] most surgeries were done in the first trimester (42%), and less frequently in the second (35%), and third (23%) trimesters.

Because surgery during pregnancy is associated with an increased perinatal and maternal risk, it is important for the clinician to avoid techniques and drugs that could contribute to these risks. The apparent safety of the commonly used local anesthetics, (with the exception of cocaine hydrochloride,[4, 5]) and the ability to avoid general anesthesia, makes the use of local anesthesia and conduction blocks particularly appealing in this patient population. In addition to the relative safety of local anesthetics, performing surgery on awake patients confers an additional advantage with regard to airway protection and aspiration.

In this chapter we focus on the implications of local anesthetics in pregnancy and indications and techniques for various nerve blocks in the pregnant patient presenting for obstetric and nonobstetric surgery.

LOCAL ANESTHETICS IN PREGNANCY

Pregnancy is associated with profound physiologic changes that may influence disposition of drugs. For instance, cardiac output and blood volume increase early in the first trimester.[6, 7] Extravascular water content also increases.[8] In contrast, concentrations of plasma proteins (e.g., albumin, α_1-acid glycoprotein), which are important for drug binding, decrease during pregnancy.[9] Decreased protein binding associated with low albumin concentration during pregnancy may result in a greater fraction of unbound drug. These changes may affect the susceptibility of pregnant patients to the toxic effects of local anesthetics.

While early studies in mice suggested that the doses of lidocaine and bupivacaine required to produce convulsions is lower in pregnancy[10, 11] more recent evidence suggests that despite the aforementioned physiologic changes, pregnancy does not increase susceptibility of the central nervous system (CNS) to local anesthetic toxicity.[11–13] However, this may not be true for the more serious manifestations of local anesthetic toxicity. For instance, in 1979, Albright[14] reported several cases of cardiovascular collapse in pregnant women after unintentional intravascular injection of clinical doses of bupivacaine (5 patients) and etiodocaine (1 patient). It is especially disturbing that cardiac arrest occurred concurrently with, or shortly after, the onset of convulsions in otherwise healthy parturients, with most of these cases being fatal.[14, 15] With the removal of 0.75% bupivacaine from use as an epidural agent in the pregnant patient and with the routine use of incremental dosing of epidural local anesthetics in these patients, the incidence of local anesthetic–induced cardiac arrest has almost disappeared.

Additional factors that may place the parturient at a higher risk of severe complications of local anesthetic toxicity include reduced functional residual capacity and increased metabolic rate. This combination increases the risk of hypoxia during relatively brief periods of apnea or seizure activity.[16] Furthermore, aortocaval compression decreases the efficacy of closed-chest cardiac massage.[17] Finally, a large bolus of drug injected into an epidural vein may reach the heart rapidly through a dilated azygos system. Nevertheless, fatal cardiac arrest is rare in parturients who have received a toxic dose of lidocaine or mepivacaine.[14, 15]

Although the risk of local anesthetic toxicity is always present, toxic concentrations of local anesthetics resulting from absorption are rarely seen during properly conducted regional anesthesia.[18] The reported incidence of convulsions during obstetric regional anesthesia is low, varying from 0.03% to 0.5%.[19–21] Of note also is the lack of resultant maternal morbidity or mortality, suggesting that local anesthetic–induced toxic reactions, if properly treated, rarely result in permanent sequelae. Nevertheless, the reports of serious toxic reactions with bupivacaine and etidocaine suggest that when large doses of local anesthetics are required for a nerve block procedure, mepivacaine or lidocaine may be a better choice. Also, because 2-chloroprocaine is rapidly metabolized in the plasma, this agent might be most appropriate for short procedures in which profound muscle relaxation is not sought. Finally, epinephrine should be routinely used with local anesthetics to slow absorption and reduce peak drug levels because of its vasoconstrictive effect.[22] Its use, however, should be reconsidered in patients with preeclampsia, since vascular hypersensitivity in these patients may result in severe hypertension after injection of epinephrine-containing solutions of local anesthetics.[23]

Local Anesthetic Toxicity

Systemic toxicity owing to local anesthetics results from systemic absorption or intravascular injection of local anesthetic. While the toxicity most often involves the CNS, cardiovascular toxicity may also occur. Less common complications include tissue toxicity and hypersensitivity reactions. The tolerance to local anesthetics is affected by the rate of administration, the total dose of drug, and the physical status of the patient.[24]

The severity of CNS effects is directly proportional to the blood concentration of local anesthetic.[25] Initially, the patient may complain of numbness of the tongue, tinnitus, or lightheadedness. As plasma concentrations of lidocaine increase, more severe manifestations of CNS toxicity occur, including tremors, loss of consciousness, and convulsions. This is due to a selective blockade of central inhibitory neurons, which results in increased CNS excitation.[26] At still higher lidocaine concentrations, general CNS depression or coma may result from reversible blockade of inhibitory and excitatory neuronal pathways. Finally, depression of the brain stem cardiorespiratory centers may occur.

The relative toxicity of local anesthetics correlates with their potency. For instance, the mean toxic cumulative doses of lidocaine, etidocaine, and bupivacaine in awake dogs are 22 mg/kg, 8 mg/kg, and 5 mg/kg, respectively. This represents an approximate ratio of 4:2:1, which is similar to the relative anesthetic potency of these drugs.[27, 28] The commonly used local anesthetics, ranked from most to least toxic to the CNS, are bupivacaine, tetracaine, etidocaine, lidocaine, mepivacaine, and 2-chloroprocaine.[29]

The cardiovascular system is much more resistant to the toxic effects of local anesthetics than the CNS. Progressive depression of myocardial function and profound vasodilatation occur only at extremely high plasma concentrations of lidocaine or mepivacaine.[29] Prompt oxygenation, ventilation, and circulatory support usually prevents cardiac arrest after intravenous injection of clinical doses of these drugs.[30] In contrast, the more potent amide local anesthetics, bupivacaine and etidocaine, have a more narrow margin of safety.[30]

Prevention and Treatment of Local Anesthetic Toxicity

Early Recognition

- Careful observation of the patient, and monitoring of vital signs usually provides early warning of an impending reaction.

Prevention of the Progression of the Reaction

- Incremental injection of the local anesthetic helps detection of inadvertent intravenous injection.
- Discontinuation of drug, administration of supplemental oxygen, and maintenance of ventilation often limits the severity of the reaction.
- In patients exhibiting signs of CNS excitation, a small dose of thiopental (50 mg) may prevent convulsions. Although the depressant effect of the barbiturate may intensify the depressant effects of the local anesthetics, small doses of thiopental (50–100 mg), repeated as needed, are apparently safe.
- Prophylactic administration of a benzodiazepine in patients with advanced pregnancy may help reduce the incidence of convulsions with amide local anesthetics.[31]
- Oxygen should always be given by mask so that the patient is well oxygenated should a convulsion occur. This may prevent the anoxia and acidosis that ensue after a seizure, which may be deleterious for both the mother and the fetus.

If Convulsions Occur

- *The airway* should be cleared of foreign material and secretions. The patient should be hyperventilated with 100% oxygen.
- *When ventilation proves difficult* as a result of convulsions, muscle paralysis may be necessary by administering 60 to 80 mg of succinylcholine. Tracheal intubation with a cuffed endotracheal tube to facilitate ventilation and/or protect the airway from aspiration may also be necessary.
- *Support the circulation:* Elevation of the legs, displacement of the uterus to the left, and rapid administration of intravenous fluids and

vasopressors may be needed to support the depressed circulation. Because a high plasma concentration of local anesthetics may cause myocardial depression and vasodilatation, a mixed α- and β-agonist (e.g., ephedrine), may prevent or treat the arterial hypotension that may ensue.

Cardiac Arrest

- Cardiac arrest should be treated with external cardiac massage, defibrillation if necessary, sodium bicarbonate, and appropriate cardiotonic drugs. Left uterine displacement must be maintained. Failure to respond to these measures may require institution of full cardiovascular reanimation and/or prompt delivery of the fetus in order to make the resuscitative measures more efficient.[32]

Assessment of Fetal Well-Being

- As soon as possible after the initial resuscitation, the condition of the fetus should be assessed.
- Prompt maternal resuscitation usually restores uterine blood flow and fetal oxygenation and allows fetal excretion of local anesthetic to the mother via the placenta.[33]

Intraoperative Monitoring and Management

Placement of an intravenous catheter and initiation of an intravenous infusion is mandatory prior to placement of any regional block. The monitoring for block placement and for intraoperative monitoring should be similar to that used with general anesthesia. It should consist of a pulse oximeter, noninvasive blood pressure monitoring, and a three-lead electrocardiogram (ECG). In addition, most anesthesiologists and obstetricians prefer to monitor the fetal heart rate intraoperatively beginning at about 16 weeks' gestation.[34] Although the blocks can be placed in the holding area or in the operating room, the monitoring standards are the same in both areas. Immediate availability of equipment for resuscitation, such as equipment for airway management and suction catheters, is of paramount importance, regardless of location. Similarly, emergency medications, such as intravenous induction agents, short-acting muscle relaxants, and vasoactive agents (e.g., ephedrine, atropine) should be readily available at all times. Finally, positioning during block placement is important in order to avoid the hypotension that is frequently seen in pregnancy, with resultant impairment of venous return.[35, 36]

We prefer to premedicate these patients immediately prior to placement of the nerve block by using small, incremental doses of barbiturates and opioids, as necessary, for the patient's comfort.

Guidelines for Regional Anesthesia in Obstetrics

In an attempt to encourage quality patient care the House of Delegates of the American Society of Anesthesiologists approved the specific guidelines applying to the use of regional anesthesia during labor and delivery.[37–40] The same guidelines should apply to administration of any regional anesthetic in a pregnant patient.

Regional anesthesia should be initiated and maintained only in locations in which appropriate resuscitation equipment and drugs are immediately available to manage procedurally related problems. Resuscitation equipment (see Box) should include, but is not limited to, (1) sources of oxygen and suction equipment to maintain an airway, perform endotracheal intubation, and as a means to provide positive-pressure ventilation; (2) drugs; and (3) equipment for cardiopulmonary resuscitation. An intravenous infusion should be established before the initiation of regional anesthesia and maintained throughout the duration of the regional anesthetic. The patient's vital signs should be monitored by qualified personnel, and basic intraoperative monitoring should be routinely practiced.

RECOMMENDED RESUSCITATION EQUIPMENT IN THE RESUSCITATION CART FOR REGIONAL ANESTHESIA DURING LABOR AND DELIVERY

Oxygen and Suction Equipment

- Positive-pressure breathing apparatus
- Oxygen supply
- Suction equipment
- Laryngoscope and blades
- Endotracheal tubes
  - Adult: 6.5, 7, 7.5, 8
  - Infant: 2.5, 3, 3.5
- Stylets
- Oral and nasal airways
- Suction catheters
- Board for closed-chest massage

Drugs

- Ephedrine
- Atropine
- Calcium chloride
- Thiopental
- Midazolam
- Sodium bicarbonate
- Succinylcholine

Cardiopulmonary Resuscitation

- ECG monitor and defibrillator

Miscellaneous

- IV supplies, needles, plastic indwelling catheters

NERVE BLOCKS

Paracervical Block

Paracervical block is a relatively simple method for obtaining analgesia of the uterus and cervix. Common surgical indications for the use of a paracervical nerve block include termination of pregnancy, cervical cerclage, and pain relief during the first stage of labor. Paracervical block is an alternative anesthetic technique in many pregnant women who do not have access to, or reject the use of, epidural or spinal anesthesia. When used for labor analgesia, paracervical block does not adversely affect the progress of labor.

Sensory impulses from the upper vagina, cervix, and lower uterine segment are transmitted by visceral afferent nerve fibers that join the sympathetic chain at the L2 and L3 vertebrae, and enter the spinal cord at the T10 to L1 vertebrae. Local anesthetic is injected submucosally into the fornix of the vagina lateral to the cervix, with intention to block nerve transmission through the paracervical ganglion (Frankenhäuser's ganglion) which lies immediately lateral and posterior to the cervicouterine junction. Since pain from the first stage of labor results primarily from dilation of the cervix and distention of the lower uterine segment and upper vagina, paracervical block can be quite effective in achieving labor analgesia. The somatic sensory fibers from the perineum are, however, not blocked. Consequently, when used as a pain relieving method in labor, the analgesic potency derived from paracervical block is limited to the first stage of labor.

Technique

- The block is performed with the patient in the lithotomy position. The uterus is displaced leftward during the procedure, which may be accomplished by placing a folded pillow beneath the patient's right buttock.
- A needle is placed just below the vaginal mucosa (2–3 mm), lateral to the cervix at the 9 o'clock position (Fig. 51–1).[41]
- After aspiration for blood, 5 to 10 mL of low-concentration local anesthetic is injected.
- The fetal heart rate is monitored continuously during the next 5 to 10 minutes.[42]
- If there is no fetal bradycardia, the block is repeated on the other side just lateral to the cervix at the 9 o'clock position with the same volume of drug. The fetal heart rate and maternal blood pressure and pulse rate are monitored closely during the next 10 minutes.
- The duration of pain relief lasts from 40 minutes with 1.5% 2-chloroprocaine to 90 minutes with 1% mepivacaine. The block may be repeated at regular intervals.
- Because of its potential toxic effects, bupivacaine is not recommended for paracervical block anesthesia in obstetrics.
- Paracervical block is probably best avoided in cases of uteroplacental insufficiency or preexisting fetal heart rate tracing abnormalities.
- If the cervix has reached 8 cm of dilation, the block should be used with extreme caution, if at all, in order to prevent injection into the fetal scalp.

Choice of Local Anesthetic. Systemic local anesthetic toxicity, postpartum neuropathy,[43] and infection[44–46] have all been reported following paracervical block. Additional maternal complications include vasovagal syncope, laceration of the vaginal mucosa, and parametrial hematoma. However, the major disadvantage of paracervical block anesthesia is the relatively high frequency of fetal bradycardia following initiation of the block. This bradycardia is associated with decreased fetal oxygenation, fetal acidosis, and an increased likelihood of neonatal depression.[47] Bradycardia usually develops within 2 to 10 minutes and lasts from 3 to 30 minutes.[48] Fetal drug levels in infants with bradycardia are occasionally higher than those in simultaneously drawn maternal samples, suggesting that local anesthetics may reach the fetus by a more direct route than maternal systemic absorption.

While the exact etiology of bradycardia after paracervical block remains unclear, the evidence suggests that it is related to a combination of decreased uterine blood flow as a result of uterine vasoconstriction from the local anesthetic applied in close proximity to the artery,[49] and as a result of high fetal blood levels of local anesthetics, causing direct fetal CNS and myocardial depression.[22, 50] High fetal concentrations of local

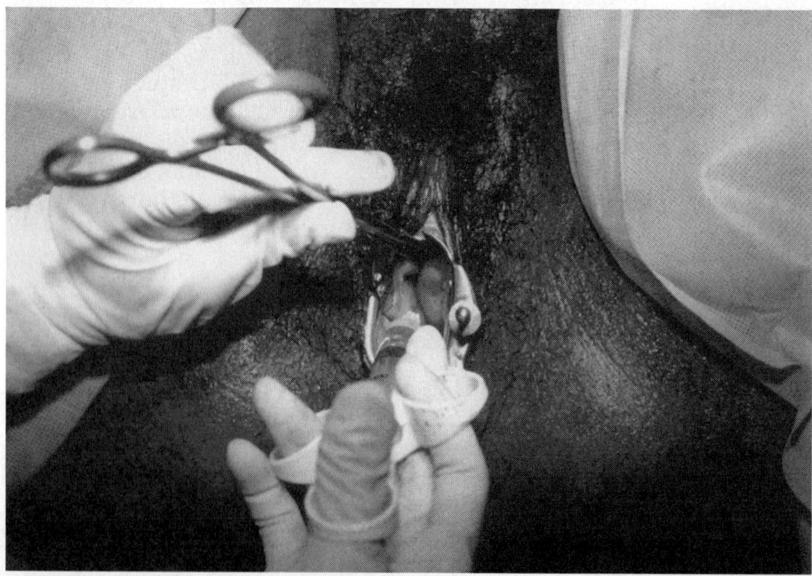

Figure 51–1 Paracervical block. A needle is placed just below the vaginal mucosa (2–3 mm), lateral to the cervix at the 9 o'clock position. After aspiration for blood, 5 to 10 mL of local anesthetic are injected.

anesthetics may also be the result of fetal acidosis and ion trapping.[51, 52] Other possible mechanisms include increased uterine activity following injection of local anesthetic (especially bupivacaine)[53] and reflex bradycardia resulting from manipulation of the fetal head, the uterus, or the uterine blood vessels during performance of the block.[50] Regardless of the etiology, fetal bradycardia associated with paracervical block does indicate fetal jeopardy and it is associated with increased neonatal morbidity and mortality.[54, 55] In the absence of fetal bradycardia, however, there are few adverse effects on the infant,[56] and doses of 100 mg of lidocaine have been reported to result in safe blood levels of lidocaine (below 5 μg/mL).[57, 58]

The choice of local anesthetic for paracervical block remains controversial. Published evidence suggests that fetal bradycardia occurs less frequently with 2-chloroprocaine than with amide local anesthetics.[59–61] 2-Chloroprocaine undergoes rapid enzymatic hydrolysis and thus has the shortest intravascular half-life among the local anesthetics used clinically. This rapid metabolism presents an advantage in the event of inadvertent intravascular or intrafetal injection. For instance, after paracervical block with 1% 2-chloroprocaine, only a trace of local anesthetic is detected in maternal or fetal samples. Nevertheless, while the North American manufacturers of bupivacaine have labeled bupivacaine as contraindicated for paracervical block, many European obstetricians prefer bupivacaine for its longer duration. Whatever the choice, however, the total volume of local anesthetic should be limited to 10 mL on each side, and the use of concentrated solutions of local anesthetics (e.g., 2% lidocaine or 3% 2-chloroprocaine) should be avoided.

Pudendal Block and Local Perineal Infiltration Anesthesia

The pudendal nerve includes somatic nerve fibers from the anterior division of the second, third, and fourth sacral nerves. These nerves provide sensory innervation for the lower vagina, vulva, and the perineum, as well as motor innervation to the perineal muscles and anal sphincters. Although the use of pudendal nerve block for vaginal delivery was first described in 1916,[62] the block was not frequently used until mid-1950s, when Klink[63] and Kohl[64] clarified the anatomy and improved the technique. Pudendal nerve block provides satisfactory analgesia for vaginal delivery and outlet forceps delivery. In contrast, the anesthesia for midforceps delivery, postpartum examination, repair of the upper vagina and cervix, and manual exploration of the uterine cavity is inadequate following pudendal block.[65] In addition, the transvaginal technique of pudendal nerve block results in frequent failure rate, approaching almost 50%.[66]

The timing of the block varies greatly between U.S. and European obstetricians. In the United States, the blocks are usually administered bilaterally just before delivery, reflecting the concern that pudendal block anesthesia prolongs the second stage of labor.[67] European obstetricians, however, tend to perform the block at the onset of the second stage of labor.[68]

Technique

- The transvaginal approach is most frequently used.
- A needle guide (Iowa trumpet or the Kobak needle guide) is routinely used to prevent vaginal and fetal injuries. The needle must protrude 1 to 1.5 cm beyond the needle guide.
- With the patient in the lithotomy position, the needle with the needle guide is typically introduced into the vagina by the left hand for a left pudendal block and by the right hand for a block on the right side.
- With the tip of the index finger palpating the ischial tuberosity, the needle is inserted through the vaginal mucosa and sacrospinous ligament immediately medial and posterior to the ischial spine. Then, 7 to 10 mL of local anesthetic (1% lidocaine, 1% mepivacaine, or 2% chloroprocaine) is injected in a blind manner, without routinely eliciting paresthesias. The technique is then repeated on the opposite side.
- Pudendal nerve block is associated with rapid maternal absorption of the local anesthetic.[67, 69] This rapid absorption of local anesthetics and the proximity of the pudendal artery warrants frequent aspiration before and during the procedure, and the avoidance of concentrated solutions of local anesthetics.
- The choice of local anesthetic, however, as well as the use of epinephrine to decrease the rate of absorption and/or prolong the duration of anesthesia remains a matter of personal preference.

Complications. Maternal complications are rare. Systemic local anesthetic toxicity, and infections, including vaginal and ischiorectal hematomas and subgluteal abscess, are among the most commonly reported complications.[45, 46]

Perineal Infiltration

Perineal infiltration with local anesthetic is probably the most commonly used local anesthetic technique for vaginal delivery. Since the perineal area is essentially devoid of major nerves, simple infiltration with a large volume of local anesthetic results in an almost immediate onset of anesthesia. Therefore, many obstetricians use perineal infiltration for repair of the episiotomy, perineal laceration, or as a supplement to ineffective pudendal or epidural block. Unfortunately, the anesthesia achieved with this technique is limited to the perineal area and does not provide any muscle relaxation.

Perineal infiltration results in significant absorption of local anesthetic, giving rise to blood levels even higher than those reported with pudendal and paracervical blocks.[70] Since 2-chloroprocaine is rapidly metabolized in plasma and thus reaches the fetus in minimal concentration, 2-chloroprocaine may be preferable to amide-type local anesthetics for antepartum perineal infiltration.[71]

Caudal Anesthesia

Since its introduction by Hingson and Edwards in 1942 for pain relief during the first stage of labor, caudal analgesia has been largely replaced by lumbar epidural analgesia, despite the reports of several large case series reporting high success rates with few complications.[21, 72, 73] The main problems with caudal analgesia is a high rate of failure to provide adequate analgesia owing to the numerous variations in the anatomy of the sacral hiatus. Additionally, the cephalad spread with the caudal epidural approach is frequently insufficient to provide adequate pain relief during the first stage of labor (i.e., to the T-10 sensory level), requiring a larger volume of local anesthetic solution. This, coupled with the relatively rich vasculature of the caudal epidural space, adds to a higher risk of local anesthetic toxicity. Furthermore, the inevitable blockade of the sacral nerve roots ensues rather early and may result in a higher forceps delivery rate and frequent failure of rotation of the fetal head from the occipitoposterior position.[74]

Caudal analgesia has been used as part of a two-catheter technique in some centers, despite the lack of clear evidence of its greater advantage. Although caudal anesthesia can be reliably used to provide perineal analgesia when delivery is imminent, or when an instrumental delivery is planned, even under these circumstances most anesthesiologists would probably use a low-dose local subarachnoid block or an intrathecal narcotic (e.g., sufentanil, 5–10 μg) for their ease of administration and more predictable results.

Local Infiltration Anesthesia for Cesarean Section

Infiltration of local anesthesia is a rarely used technique for cesarean section. While neuraxial anesthesia for cesarean section is undoubtedly superior with regard to patient comfort and efficacy, in an occasional patient local anesthesia may be the only viable option.[75] One example of this includes a patient with severe kyphoscoliosis and severe oropharyngeal edema presenting for emergency cesarean section. Another example is a case of profound fetal bradycardia without the presence of an anesthesiologist. Theoretic advantages of local anesthetic infiltration are that the patient is awake with protective airway reflexes, and the technique avoids hemodynamic changes, residual paralysis, and other disadvantages of central neuronal blockade. Most importantly, however, there is no delay with this technique and surgery can start almost immediately.

Most of the literature on this subject comes from lesser developed countries where there may be lack of anesthetic expertise, equipment, and/or supplies.[76–78] Local anesthetic infiltration is performed by the surgeon using large volumes (40–60 mL) of diluted solutions of local anesthetics. The injections are usually performed in various layers, depending on the stage of the operation. Ten milliliters of local anesthetic is injected immediately below the skin in the midline from the umbilicus to the pubis (Fig. 51–2*A*). Then 5 mL is injected into the rectus sheath at four points on either side. The needle should be felt passing through the anterior rectus sheath. Between 5 and 10 mL is infiltrated immediately below the linea alba after its exposure in order to anesthetize the parietal peritoneum. Alternatively, the peritoneum may be anesthetized by pouring in 10 mL of local anesthetic and employing gentle surgical manipulation of the peritoneum.[79] Once inside the peritoneal cavity, an additional 5 mL of local anesthetic is placed under the loose visceral peritoneum along the line of the proposed lower segment cut into the uterus (Fig. 51–2*B*).[76] Using a similar technique (0.5–1% prilocaine) and neuroleptanalgesia/sedation (e.g., droperidol, meperidine, and nalorphine), 80% of women in a study of 66 consecutive cesarean sections experienced only minimal discomfort during the procedure. Based on their experience with this method, Barker and Barker suggest that the surgical technique has to be somewhat modified when local infiltration is the sole anesthetic used.[76]

Other techniques have also been suggested by various authors, for example, a local field block of the lower abdominal wall,[80] or an "arrowhead" field block in which the T-10 to T-12 segments are blocked bilaterally in the midaxillary line with blocks of ilioinguinal and genitofemoral nerves.[81]

The use of various types and volumes of local anesthetic agents (prilocaine, 0.5%–1%; lidocaine, 0.25%–0.75% with epinephrine) have been reported to result in similar, satisfactory results. The total allowable dose of the agent used should be similar to those recommended for other regional anesthesia techniques.

Although clinical situations in which local infiltration anesthesia for cesarean section is indicated are rare in modern anesthesia practice, the published evidence suggests that this technique can be effective when general or neuraxial anesthesia may be contraindicated or undesirable.

Brachial Plexus Block

Brachial plexus anesthesia can be achieved in the pregnant patient by using either the interscalene, supraclavicular, or axillary approaches. Because the brachial plexus with each of these techniques is approached at a different level, the quality and distribution of anesthesia significantly vary. For instance, the brachial plexus block at the interscalene level provides better anesthesia for shoulder surgery (C4–C7) than the approach at the axilla (axillary block). Because surgery for trauma or elective surgery[82] of the hand and forearm are the most common indications for brachial plexus block in pregnancy, we limit the discussion of the brachial plexus blocks to the axillary block. Additionally, both the supraclavicular and interscalene approaches are associated with possible respiratory

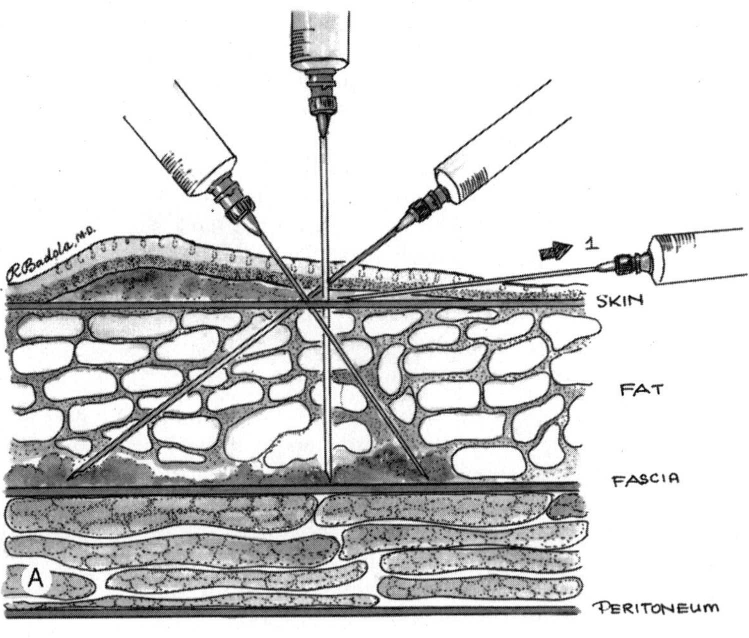

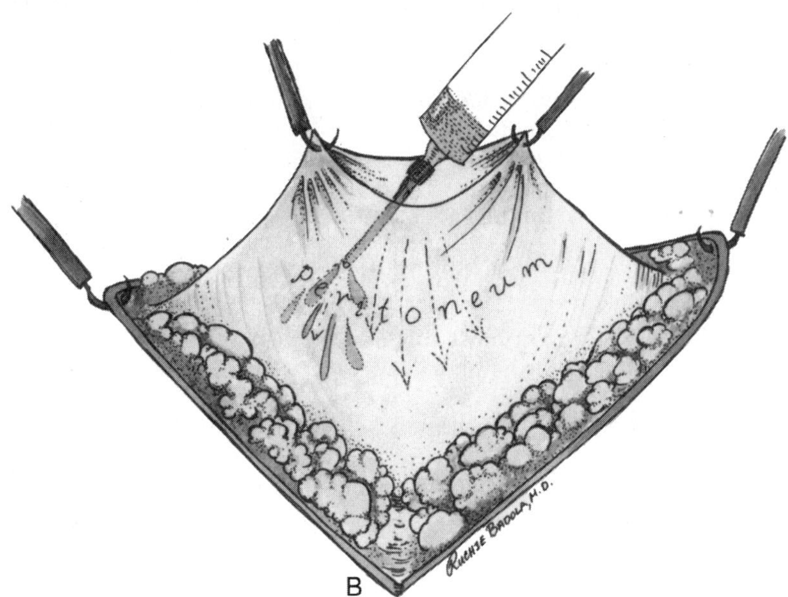

❖ **Figure 51–2** Local infiltration anesthesia for cesarean section. *A*, The skin and subcutanous tissue is infiltrated with local anesthetic in the midline from the umbilicus to the pubis. *B*, Once inside the peritoneal cavity, additional local anesthetic is placed under the loose visceral peritoneum along the line of the proposed lower segment cut into the uterus.

complications (pneumothorax and diaphragmatic paralysis) which makes them less suitable techniques in pregnant patients who have a need for substantially higher minute ventilation compared with nonpregnant patients.

Axillary Block

Indications for axillary block include surgery on the hand, wrist, forearm, and the elbow.

Technique

Several different approaches to axillary block have been described. Some authors, however, find that the transarterial axillary perivascular technique[83] is probably the easiest to perform and comparable in its success rate[84] and the incidence of complications to other approaches (paresthesia, nerve stimulator, midhumeral approach).

- The patient is placed in the supine position with arm abducted to 90 degrees and the forearm flexed and externally rotated so that the dorsum of the hand lies on the table next to the patient's head.
- The axillary pulse is palpated and followed proximally as far as possible. At this point, with the index and the third fingers pressing (fixing) the artery against the humerus, a needle (we prefer a 1.5 inch, 25-gauge needle) connected to two 20-mL syringes via a length of extension tubing and a stopcock is inserted just above the fingertips and toward the axilla.
- The needle is advanced until arterial blood appears in the hub of the needle during its

insertion, and then rapidly advanced until the inability to aspirate blood indicates that the needle penetrated the posterior arterial wall.
- While intermittently aspirating for blood to prevent inadvertent intravascular injection, two thirds of the planned dose is injected.
- The needle is then withdrawn first into the axillary artery and then carefully pulled back until blood return is no longer present. This indicates placement of the needle just outside the anterior wall of the axillary artery, where the remaining one third of the total local anesthetic dose is injected.

When the surgical procedure requires blockade of the musculocutaneous nerve, the needle must be placed as high in the axilla as possible and a larger volume of local anesthetic has to be used. Alternatively, local anesthetic can be injected into the substance of the coracobrachialis muscle by redirecting the needle above the axillary artery and advancing it until the humerus is contacted. The needle is then pulled back 1 cm and 10 mL of local anesthetic is injected.

Complications. Complications of axillary block are rare, but have included intravascular injection, local anesthetic toxicity, neurapraxia, and hematoma. As in all cases in which intravascular injection might occur, aspiration prophylaxis should be administered prior to initiation of the block.

Wrist Block

The indications for wrist block include surgery on the hand or fingers requiring short use of a tourniquet (<20 minutes). The block is, however, not recommended for surgery on the wrist. The technique centers around achieving anesthesia in the distribution of three separate nerves: median, radial, and ulnar nerves.

Technique

MEDIAN NERVE

- An assistant holds the wrist in gentle extension.
- The groove between the flexor carpi radialis and the palmaris longus tendons at the level of the middle crease of the wrist is palpated.
- A 25-gauge needle attached to a syringe with local anesthetic is inserted in the groove between the two tendons, with the needle pointing cephalad.
- At the depth of 5 to 10 mm the patient may report paresthesias.
- Regardless of presence or absence of paresthesias, 5 to 7 mL of local anesthetic of choice is injected.

RADIAL NERVE

- A 10-mL syringe with a 25-gauge, 1.5-inch-long needle is inserted just proximal to the styloid process of the radius, and local anesthetic is injected to raise a subcutaneous wheal halfway around the wrist, beginning at the palmaris longus and ending near the ulna on the dorsal aspect of the wrist.

ULNAR NERVE

- The wrist is held in slight extension. The block needle is inserted 5 to 10 mm immediately medial to the point of maximal pulsation of the ulnar artery and 5 to 7 mL of local anesthetic is injected.
- The latency of this block is about 10 minutes.

Wrist block provides sensory block of the hand and a motor block for the intrinsic muscles of the hand. The patient can still lift the arm, bend the elbow, and move the fingers.

Note: Epinephrine-containing solutions should not be used for wrist block.

Sciatic Nerve Block

Sciatic nerve block results in anesthesia of the posterior thigh and leg below the knee joint (with the exception of the medial aspect of the leg). Common techniques of sciatic nerve blockade include several different approaches: anterior,[85, 86] lateral,[87] and posterior.[88] Sciatic nerve block has been successfully used for surgical anesthesia and postoperative pain control for various operations above and below the knee.[89–91] However, in order to achieve satisfactory anesthesia in the anteromedial thigh, femoral or lumbar plexus blocks are also required.

Popliteal Block

Sciatic nerve block in the popliteal fossa (also called popliteal nerve block) is an anesthetic technique well-suited for operations below the knee.[89–91] While the prone position in which the classic posterior approach to popliteal block is performed is relatively contraindicated in advanced pregnancy,[92] two alternative approaches to popliteal block with a patient in the supine position have been reported to result in reliable anesthesia in the sciatic nerve distribution below the knee.[93, 94]

Popliteal Block: Lithotomy Approach

Technique

- With the patient in the supine position, the leg is flexed at both the hip and knee joints, and supported by an assistant (Fig. 51–3*A*).
- The anatomic landmarks of the popliteal fossa (popliteal crease inferiorly, the semimembranosus and semitendinosus muscles medially, and the long head of the biceps femoris muscle laterally) are readily identified in this position. The insulated needle, attached to a peripheral nerve stimulator, is inserted 7 cm above the popliteal crease, 1 cm lateral to the midline and directed 45 degrees cephalad (see Fig. 51–3*B*).

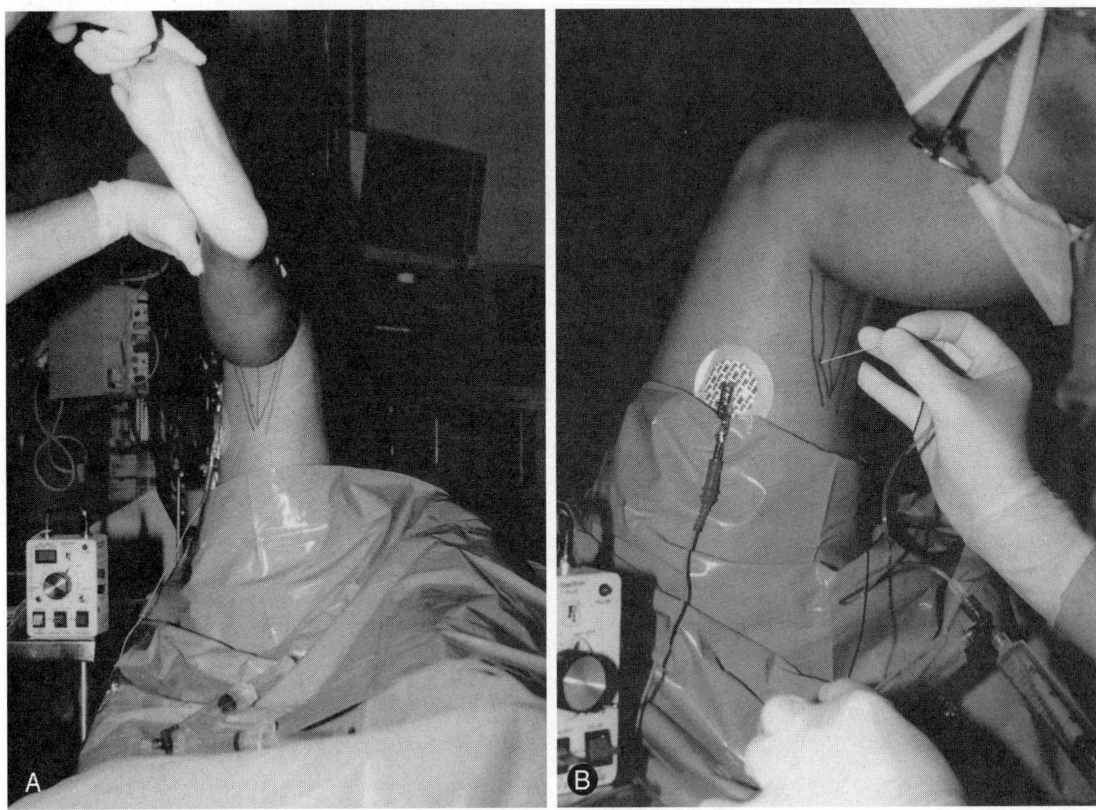

❖ **Figure 51–3** Popliteal block: lithotomy approach. *A*, With the patient in the supine position, the leg is flexed at both the hip and knee joints and supported by an assistant. *B*, An insulated needle, attached to a peripheral nerve stimulator, is inserted 7 cm above the popliteal crease, 1 cm lateral to the midline and directed 45 degrees cephalad in order to obtain stimulation of the popliteal nerve.

- On obtaining either dorsal or plantar flexion of the foot, using the output current of 0.4 mAmp or less, 30 to 40 mL of solution of local anesthetic is injected while intermittently aspirating for blood.
- When the nerve is not localized on the first needle insertion, the needle is slowly withdrawn to the skin and reinserted through the same skin puncture. The first reinsertion should be at an angle of 5 degrees, and the second at 10 degrees lateral to the initial insertion plane.
- Failure to obtain stimulation of the sciatic nerve should prompt removal of the needle. The needle is then reinserted through a new puncture site 5 mm lateral to the initial insertion site and same the maneuver is repeated. This technique is systematically repeated through new insertion sites in 5-mm incremental lateral insertions until the desired response is obtained.

Popliteal Block: Lateral Approach

Technique

- The lateral approach to popliteal block is also performed with the patient in the supine position and with the leg flexed at the knee joint.
- The leg is flexed at the knee joint, and the long axis of the foot is positioned at a 90-degree angle relative to the table.
- A 100-mm-long, insulated stimulating needle, attached to a low-output nerve stimulator, is inserted in a horizontal plane 7 cm cephalad to the most prominent point of the lateral femoral epicondyle, in the groove between the biceps femoris and the vastus lateralis muscles, until the shaft of the femoral bone is intentionally contacted (Fig. 51–4*A*). When the femur is not contacted within the depth of approximately 50 mm, the needle is reinserted 5 to 10 mm anterior (above) to the first insertion.
- After the femur is contacted, the needle is withdrawn to the skin, and redirected posteriorly at a 30-degree angle to the horizontal plane (see Fig. 51–4*B*).
- If stimulation of the sciatic nerve is not obtained, the needle is withdrawn to the skin and reinserted through the same skin puncture, first 5 to 10 degrees anterior and then 5 to 10 degrees posterior relative to the initial (30-degree) insertion plane.

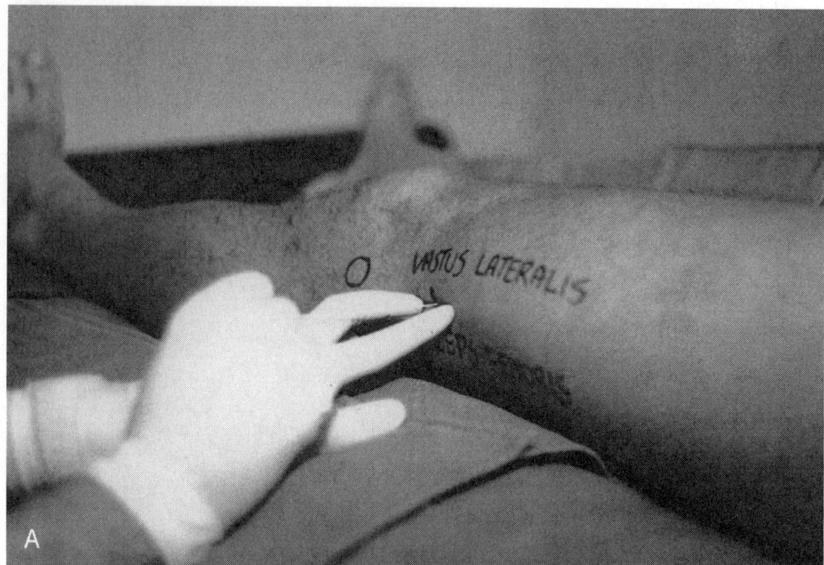

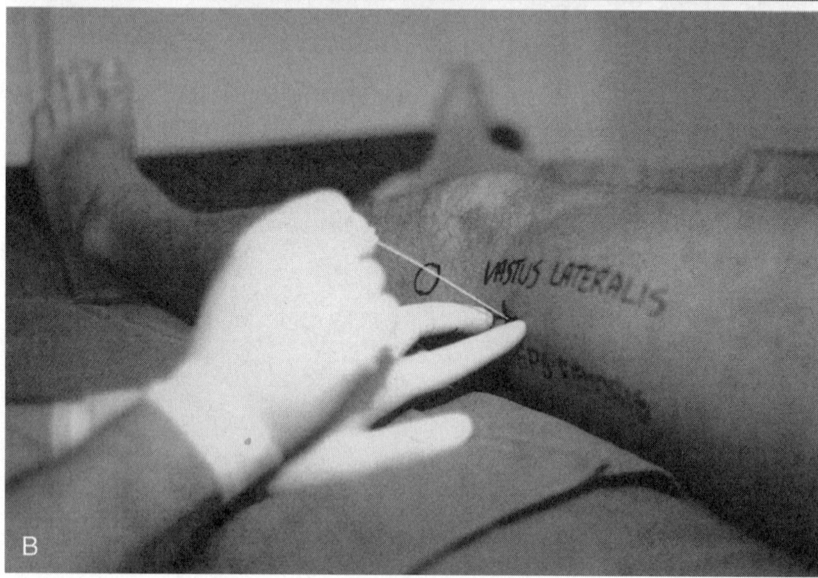

Figure 51–4 Popliteal block: lateral approach. *A*, A 100-mm-long needle, attached to a nerve stimulator, is inserted in a horizontal plane 7 cm cephalad to the most prominent point of the lateral femoral epicondyle, in the groove between the biceps femoris and the vastus lateralis muscles, until the shaft of the femoral bone is contacted. *B*, After the femur is contacted, the needle is withdrawn to the skin, and redirected posteriorly at a 30-degree angle to the horizontal plane and advanced until popliteal nerve stimulation is obtained.

- If the described redirections do not result in nerve localization, the same technique is simply repeated through new skin punctures in 5-mm increments posterior to the initial insertion plane.

In either technique, the reference electrode (positive +) should be connected to the lateral calf via an electrocadiographic (ECG) electrode. The initial current of 0.8 mA (2 Hz) is gradually decreased after obtaining an initial response to nerve stimulation. The localization of the nerve is considered successful when either tibial nerve stimulation (plantarflexion), or common peroneal stimulation (dorsal flexion) is obtained. The output current of the nerve stimulator is then gradually adjusted to the lowest current at which these responses are still observed. At this point, an inadvertent intravascular placement of the needle should be ruled out by gentle aspiration. Then, 30 mL of local anesthetic of choice is used. We routinely use 1.5% alkalinized mepivacaine (1 mEq of $NaHCO_3$ per 30 mL of mepivacaine) with 1:200,000 epinephrine when performing popliteal blocks for surgical anesthesia. Bupivacaine 0.25% with epinephrine using similar volumes is more appropriate for postoperative analgesia. When the surgery involves the medial aspect of the lower leg, supplementary block of the saphenous nerve is performed at the level of the tibial tuberosity or medial malleolus, using 8 to 10 mL 0.25% bupivacaine.

Femoral Nerve Block

Femoral nerve block confers anesthesia to the anteromedial thigh and medial aspect of the leg below the knee (saphenous nerve). Consequently, operations on the patella or anterior aspect of the knee joint, or a quadriceps muscle biopsy can all be performed under femoral block. The technique also provides superb analgesia after operations on the femur (e.g., femur fracture).

Technique

- A 22-gauge, 50-mm, short-bevel, insulated needle attached to a nerve stimulator (0.6 mA) is inserted adjacent to the lateral border of the femoral artery at the level of the inguinal crease (a skinfold 3 to 6 cm below and parallel to the inguinal ligament).[95]
- The needle is slowly advanced at an angle of 60 degrees cephalad to the horizontal plane while seeking a quadriceps muscle twitch. If a quadriceps muscle twitch is not obtained within a depth of 50 mm, the needle is withdrawn, redirected 10 degrees laterally and reinserted in the same fashion.
- If the above maneuver does not elicit a quadriceps muscle twitch, the subsequent needle insertions should be placed at increments of 5 mm lateral to the previous insertion sites. Once a quadriceps muscle twitch is obtained at less than 0.4 mA, the local anesthetic (20–30 mL of the desired local anesthetic) is injected.
- When the initial response is a sartorius muscle twitch, the quadriceps muscle twitch is sought by incrementally redirecting the needle laterally 10 degrees at a time, and advancing the needle 1 to 2 mm. The onset of blockade is typically within 3 to 5 minutes when the current is less than 0.4 mA, and it is documented by loss of sensation in the anterior thigh and saphenous nerve distribution, as well as the presence of quadriceps muscle relaxation.

Saphenous Nerve Block

The saphenous nerve is a branch of the femoral nerve and blocking it provides anesthesia to the medial aspect of the leg below the knee. It is routinely used in conjunction with popliteal nerve or sciatic nerve blocks for any operation below the knee. The technique consists of subcutaneous infiltration of 10 mL of local anesthetic of choice in a ring fashion between the anterior tibial tuberosity and the medial third of the popliteal crease.[96]

Ankle Block

Ankle block is indicated for any operation on the foot that does not require application of a tourniquet for a long period of time. Ankle block requires blocks of the four divisions of the sciatic nerve: deep peroneal, posterior tibial, superficial peroneal nerves, and the sural nerve. Additionally, the saphenous nerve (branch of the femoral nerve) has to be blocked at the ankle level.

Note: Epinephrine-containing solutions should not be used for ankle block.

Technique

Tibial Nerve

- The posterior tibial artery at the level of the medial malleolus is palpated and the skin at the midpoint between the Achilles tendon and the arterial pulse is anesthetized.
- A 1.5-inch long, 25-gauge needle is inserted behind the posterior tibial artery and advanced until the bone is contacted or paresthesias are induced.
- When paresthesias are induced, 7 mL of local anesthetic is deposited. However, if no paresthesias are induced after the bone is contacted, the needle is withdrawn 2 to 3 mm and 7 to 10 mL of local anesthetic is injected.

Deep Peroneal Nerve

- The deep peroneal nerve is anesthetized between the tendons of the extensor hallucis longus muscle medially and the anterior tibialis muscle laterally at the malleolar level. A 1.5-inch long, 25-gauge needle is inserted between the tendons and advanced until the bone is contacted or paresthesias are induced.
- When paresthesias are obtained, 7 mL of local anesthetic is injected.
- If no paresthesias are induced, the needle is withdrawn 2 to 3 mm and 7 to 10 mL of local anesthetic is injected.

Saphenous Nerve

- Five to 10 mL of local anesthetic is injected in a subcutaneous ring fashion around the great saphenous vein at the medial malleolus.

Superficial Peroneal Nerve

- Five to 10 mL of local anesthetic is injected between the lateral malleolus and extensor hallucis tendon.

Sural Nerve

- The sural nerve is blocked by injecting 5 to 10 mL of local anesthetic subcutaneously between the Achilles tendon and posterior border of the lateral malleolus.

Conclusion. A wide variety of nerve blocks and infiltration anesthesia present good alternatives to general and neuraxial anesthesia in many pregnant patients. These techniques allow one to use drugs with no laboratory or clinical evidence of teratogenesis, while possibly reducing maternal complications. Regardless of the technique used, however, avoidance of aortocaval compression, hypotension, acidosis, and hyperventilation constitute essential elements of sound anesthetic management in this setting. The patients should be adequately hydrated before administration of blocks that are likely to result in significant hypotension. Sedatives and analgesics with a history of safe use during pregnancy can be used for patient comfort. Beginning at 18 to 20 weeks' gestation, the pregnant patient should be transported on her side, and the uterus should be displaced leftward when she is positioned on the operating table. In addition to blood pressure, oxygen saturation, and ECG monitoring, fe-

❖ Summary

Key Points

- Surgery during pregnancy is associated with an increased perinatal and maternal risk. Anesthesiologists must be familiar with techniques and drugs that may decrease these risks. Maternal morbidity is associated with the underlying disease necessitating surgery as well as complications of anesthesia caused by the anatomic and physiologic changes of pregnancy.
- Local anesthesia and conduction blocks may be the optimal anesthetic option in the pregnant patient undergoing nonobstetric surgery.
- Regional anesthesia confers an additional advantage by providing surgical conditions while avoiding the use of general anesthesia.

Key Reference

Kort B, Katz VL, Watson WJ: The effect of nonobstetric operation during pregnancy. Surg Gynecol Obstet 1993; 177:371–376.

Case Stem

A pregnant patient at 24 weeks' gestation is scheduled for open reduction and internal fixation of a right ankle fracture. She has a history of asthma since childhood and has been intubated in the past. She also has a history of kyphoscoliosis, with Harrington rod placement at age 14. Discuss the obstetric and anesthetic implications.

tal heart rate and uterine activity should also be monitored both during and after surgery whenever technically feasible.[97, 98] Finally, equipment and drugs for resuscitation should be immediately available prior to placing any regional block.

References

1. Kort B, Katz VL, Watson WJ: The effect of nonobstetric operation during pregnancy. Surg Gynecol Obstet 1993; 177:371–376.
2. Brodsky JB, Cohen EN, Wu ML, et al: Surgery during pregnancy and fatal outcome. Am J Obstet Gynecol 1980; 138:1165–1167.
3. Mazze RI, Källén B: Reproductive outcome after anesthesia and operation during pregnancy: Am J Obstet Gynecol 1989; 161:1178–1185.
4. Fujinawa M, Mazze RI: Reproductive and teratogenic effects of lidocaine in Sprague-Dawley rats. Anesthesiology 1986; 65:626–632.
5. Abrams ME, Metters JS: Report on Confidential Enquiries into Maternal Deaths in the United Kingdom, 1985–87. London: Her Majesty's Stationary Office; 1991:73–87.
6. Lees MM, Taylor SH, Scott DB, Kerr MG: A study of cardiac output at rest throughout pregnancy. J Obstet Gynecol 1967; 74:319–328.
7. Lund CJ, Donovan JC: Blood volume during pregnancy. Am J Obstet Gynecol 1967; 98:393–403.
8. Hytten FE, Thomson AM, Taggart N: Total body water in normal pregnancy. J Obstet Gynaecol Br Commonw 1966; 73:553–561.
9. Song CS, Merkatz IR, Rifkind AB, et al: The influence of pregnancy and oral contraceptive steroids on the concentration of plasma proteins. Am J Obstet Gynecol 1970; 108:227–231.
10. Ravindran RS, Kim KC, Baldwin SJ: The effect of pregnancy on the threshold to local anesthetic induced convulsions in mice [abstract]. Anesthesiology 1982; 57:A700.
11. Santos AC, Pederson H, Harmon TW, et al: Does pregnancy alter the systemic toxicity of local anesthetics? Anesthesiology 1989; 70:991–995.
12. Morishima HO, Pedersen H, Finster M, et al: Bupivacaine toxicity in pregnant and nonpregnant ewes. Anesthesiology 1985; 63:134–139.
13. Morishima HO, Finster M, Arthur GR, Covino BG: Pregnancy does not alter lidocaine toxicity. Am J Obstet Gynecol 1990; 162:1320–1324.
14. Albright GA: Cardiac arrest following regional anesthesia with etidocaine and bupivacaine. Anesthesiology 1979; 51:285–287.
15. Marx GF: Cardiotoxicity of local anesthetics—the plot thickens [editorial]. Anesthesiology 1984; 60:3–5.
16. Archer GW, Marx GF: Arterial oxygenation during apnea in parturient woman. Br J Anaesth 1974; 46:358–360.
17. Kasten GW, Martin ST: Resuscitation from bupivacaine-induced cardiovascular toxicity during partial inferior vena cava occlusion. Anesth Analg 1986; 65:341–344.
18. Poppers J: Evaluation of local anesthetic agents for regional anesthesia in obstetrics. Br J Anaesth 1975; 47:322–327.
19. Adamson DH: Continuous epidural anesthesia in the community hospital. Can Anaesth Soc J 1973; 53:21–25.
20. Crawford JS: The second thousand epidural blocks in an obstetric hospital practice. Br J Anaesth 1972; 44:1277–1287.
21. Epstein HM, Sherline DM: Single injection caudal anesthesia in obstetrics. Obstet Gynecol 1969; 33:496–500.
22. Raiston DH, Schnider SM: The fetal and neonatal effects of regional anesthesia and obstetrics. Anesthesiology 1968; 48:34–64.
23. Hadžić A, Vloka JD, Patel N, Birnbach D: Hypertensive crisis after a successful placement of an epidural anesthetic in a hypertensive parturient. Reg Anesth 1995; 20:156–158.
24. Moore DC, Bridenbaugh LD, Thompson GE, et al: Factors determining dosages of amide-type local anesthetic drugs. Anesthesiology 1977; 47:263–268.
25. Carpenter RL, Mackey DC: Local anesthetics. In Barash PG, Cullen BF, Stoelting RK (eds): Clinical Anesthesia. Philadelphia: JB Lippincott; 1992:527.
26. de Jong RH, Robles R, Corbin RW: Central actions of lidocaine—synaptic transmission. Anesthesiology 1969; 30:19–23.
27. Liu PL, Feldman HS, Giasi R, et al: Comparative CNS toxicity of lidocaine, etidocaine, bupivacaine, and tetracaine in awake dogs following rapid intravenous administration. Anesth Analg 1983; 62:375–379.
28. Scott DB: Evaluation of the toxicity of local anesthetic agents in man. Br J Anaesth 1975; 47:56–60.
29. Covino BG, Vassalo HG: Local anesthetics: mechanisms of action and clinical use. New York: Grune & Stratton; 1976:126.
30. de Jong RH, Ronfeld RA, De Rosa RA: Cardiovascular effects of convulsant and supraconvulsant doses of amide local anesthetics. Anesth Analg 1982; 61:3–9.
31. de Jong RH, Bonin JD: Benzodiazepines protect mice from local anesthetic convulsions and deaths. Anesth Analg 1991; 60:385–389.
32. Marx GF: Cardiopulmonary resuscitation of late pregnant women. Anesthesiology 1982; 56:156.
33. Morishima HO, Adamsons K: Placental clearance of mepivacaine following administration to the guinea pig fetus. Anesthesiology 1967; 28:343–348.
34. Levinson G, Shnider SM: Anesthesia for surgery during pregnancy. In Schnider SM, Levinson G (eds): Anesthesia for Obstetrics. Baltimore: Williams & Wilkins; 1993: 259–280.
35. Marx GF, Bassell GM: Hazards of the supine position in pregnancy. Clin Obstet Gynecol 1982; 9:255–271.
36. Quiligan EJ, Tyler C: Postural effects on the cardiovascular

status in pregnancy: a comparison of the lateral and supine postures. Am J Obstet Gynecol 1978; 130:194–198.
37. American Society of Anesthesiology: Anesthesia Care Team (approved by the ASA House of Delegates, October 14, 1987).
38. American Academy of Pediatrics and American College of Obstetricians and Gynecologists: Guidelines for Perinatal Care. AAP; 1988.
39. American Society of Anesthesiology: Standards for Basic Intraoperative Monitoring (approved by the ASA House of Delegates, October 21, 1986; last amended, October 23, 1990.)
40. American Society of Anesthesiology: Standards for Postanesthesia Care (approved by the ASA House of Delegates, October 12, 1988; last amended, October 23 1990).
41. Jagerhorn M: Paracervical block in obstetrics: an improved injection method. Acta Obstet Gynecol Scand 1975; 54:9–27.
42. King JC, Sherline DM: Paracervical block with low doses of chloroprocaine: fetal and maternal effects. JAMA 1975; 231:56–57.
43. Gaylord TG, Pearson JW: Neuropathy following paracervical block in the obstetric patient. Obstet Gynecol 1982; 60:521–525.
44. Mercado AZ, Naz JF, Ataya KM: Postabortal paracervical abscess as a complication of paracervical block anesthesia. J Reprod Med 1989; 34:247–249.
45. Hibbard LT, Snyder EN, McVann RM: Subgluteal and retropsoal infection in obstetric practice. Obstet Gynecol 1972; 39:137–150.
46. Svancarek W, Chirino O, Schaefer G, Blythe JG: Retropsoas and subgluteal abscess following paracervical and pudendal anesthesia. JAMA 1977; 237:892–894.
47. Baxi LV, Petrie RH, James LS: Human fetal oxygenation following paracervical block. Am J Obstet Gynecol 1979; 135:1109–1112.
48. Parer JT: Handbook of Fetal Heart Monitoring. Philadelphia: WB Saunders; 1983:87.
49. Asling JH, Shnider SM, Margolis AJ, et al: Paracervical block in obstetrics. II. Etiology of fetal bradycardia following paracervical block anesthesia. Am J Obstet Gynecol 1970; 107:626–634.
50. Shnider SM, Asling JH, Holl JW, Margolis AS: Paracervical block anesthesia in obstetrics. I. Fetal complications and neonatal morbidity. 1970; 107:619–625.
51. Brown WU, Bell GC, Alper MH: Acidosis, local anesthetics, and the newborn. Obstet Gynecol 1976; 48:27–30.
52. Biehl D, Shnider SM, Levinson G, Calender K: Placental transfer of lidocaine: effects of fetal acidosis. Anesthesiology 1976; 48:27–30.
53. Fishburne JI, Greiss FC, Hopkinson R, Rhyne AL: Responses of the gravid uterine vasculature to arterial levels of local anesthetic agents. Am J Obstet Gynecol 1979; 133:753–756.
54. Grimes DA, Schulz KF, Cates W, et al: Local versus general anesthesia: which is safer for performing suction currettage abortions? Am J Obstet Gynecol 1979; 135:1030–1035.
55. Grimes DA, Cates W: Deaths from paracervical anesthesia used for first trimester abortion. N Engl J Med 1976; 295:1397–1399.
56. Jensen F, Qvist I, Brocks V, et al: Submucous paracervical blockade compared with intramuscular meperidine as analgesia during labor: a double-blind study. Obstet Gynecol 1984; 64:724–727.
57. Lucas JB, Reid PR, King TM: Plasma lidocaine levels following paracervical infiltration for aspiration abortion. Obstet Gynecol 1982; 60:506–508.
58. Kangas-Saarela T, Jouppila R, Poulakka J, et al: The effect of bupivacaine paracervical block on the neurobehavioural responses of newborn infants. Acta Anesthesiol Scand 1988; 32:566–570.
59. Weiss RR, Halevy S, Almonte RO, et al: Comparison of lidocaine and 2-chloroprocaine in paracervical block: clinical effects and drug concentrations in mother and child. Anesth Analg 1983; 62:168–173.
60. Phillipson EH, Kuhnert BR, Syracuse CB, et al: Intrapartum paracervical block anesthesia with 2-chloroprocaine. Am J Obstet Gynecol 1983; 146:16–22.
61. LeFevre ML: Fetal heart rate pattern and postparacervical fetal bradycardia. Obstet Gynecol 1984; 64:343–346.
62. King R: Perineal anesthesia in labor. Surg Gynecol Obstet 1916; 23:615–618.
63. Klink EW: Perineal nerve block: an anatomic and clinical study in the female. Obstet Gynecol 1953; 1:137–146.
64. Kohl GC: New method of pudendal nerve block. Northwest Med 1954; 53:1012–1013.
65. Hutchins CJ: Spinal anesthesia for instrumental delivery: a comparison with pudendal nerve block. Anaesthesia 1980; 35:376–377.
66. Scudamore JH, Yates MJ: Pudendal block—a misnomer? Lancet 1966; 1:23–24.
67. Zador G, Lindmark G, Nilson BA: Pudendal block in normal vaginal deliveries. Acta Obstet Gynecol Scand Suppl 1974; 34:51–64.
68. Langhoff-Roos J, Lindmark G: Analgesia and side-effects of pudendal block at delivery: a comparison of three local anesthetics. Acta Obstet Gynecol Scand 1985; 64:269–273.
69. Shnider SM, Way EL: Plasma levels of lidocaine (Xylocaine) in mother and newborn following obstetrical conduction anesthesia: clinical applications. Anesthesiology 1968; 29:951–958.
70. Philipson EH, Kuhnert BR, Syracuse CD: Maternal, fetal, and neonatal lidocaine levels following perineal infiltration. Am J Obstet Gynecol 1984; 149:403–407.
71. Philipson EH, Kuhnert BR, Syracuse CD: 2-Chloroprocaine for perineal infiltration. Am J Obstet Gynecol 1987; 157:1275–1278.
72. Dogu TS: Continous caudal analgesia and anesthesia for labor and vaginal delivery: a review of 4,071 confinements. Obstet Gynecol 1969; 33:92–97.
73. Moore DC, Bridenbaugh LD, Tucker GT: Caudal and epidural blocks with bupivacaine for childbirth: report of 657 parturients. Obstet Gynecol 1971; 37:667–676.
74. Moir DD: Local anesthetic techniques in obstetrics. Br J Anaesth 1986; 58:747–759.
75. Cooper MG, Feeney EM, Jospeh M, McGuiness JJ: Local anesthetic infiltration for Cesarean section. Anaesth Intensive Care 1989; 17:198–212.
76. Barker A, Barker M: Caesarean section under local anesthesia. Trop Doct 1976; 6:23–25.
77. Foster WH, Mjekevu T, Olsen G, et al: Low spinal anesthesia combined with local anesthesia for caesarean section—an evaluation. S Afr Med J 1983, 63:17–20.
78. Larsen JV, Barker A, Barker B, Brown RS: A technique combining neurolept-analgesia with local analgesia for caesarean section. S Afr Med J 1971; 45:750–751.
79. Macintosh RR, Bryce-Smith R: Local analgesia: abdominal surgery. Edinburgh: ES Livingstone; 1953:74–75.
80. Ranney B, Stanage WF: Advantages of local anaesthesia for ceasarean section. Obstet Gynecol 1975; 45:163–167.
81. Busby T: Local anesthesia for caesarean section. Am J Obstet Gynecol 1963; 87:399–404.
82. Stahl S, Blumenfeld Z, Yanritsky D: Carpal tunnel syndrome in pregnancy: indications for surgery. J Neurol Sci 1996; 136:182–184.
84. Cockings E, Moore PL, Lewis RC: Transarterial brachial plexus blockade using high doses of 1.5% mepivacaine. Reg Anesth 1987; 12:159–164.
85. Beck GP: Anterior approach to sciatic nerve block. Anesthesiology 1963; 24:222–224.
86. Raj PP, Parks RI, Watson TD, Jenkins MT: A new single position supine approach to sciatic-femoral nerve block. Anesth Analg 1975; 54:489–493.
87. Ichiyanagi K: Sciatic nerve block: lateral approach with the patient supine. Anesthesiology 1959; 20:601–604.
88. Moore DC: Block of sciatic and femoral nerves. In Moore DC (ed): Regional Block. Springfield, IL: CC Thomas; 1965:275–288.
89. Rorie DK, Byer DE, Nelson DO, et al: Assessment of block of the sciatic nerve in the popliteal fossa. Anesth Analg 1980; 59:371–376.
90. Gouverneur JM: Sciatic nerve block in the popliteal fossa with atraumatic needles and nerve stimulation. Acta Anaesth Belg 1985; 4:391–399.
91. Vloka JD, Hadžić A, Mulcare R, et al: Combined blocks of the sciatic nerve at the popliteal fossa and posterior cutaneous nerve of the thigh for short saphenous vein stripping in outpatients: an alternative to spinal anesthesia. J Clin Anesth 1997; 9:618–622.

92. Brown DL: Popliteal block. In Brown DL (ed): Atlas of Regional Anesthesia. Philadelphia: WB Saunders; 1992:109–113.
93. Vloka JD, Hadžić A, Koorn R, Thys DM: Supine approach to the sciatic nerve in the popliteal fossa. Can J Anaesth 1996; 43:964–967.
94. Hadžić A, Vloka JD: The lateral approach to popliteal nerve block: a comparison with the posterior approach. Anesthesiology 1998; 88:1480–1486.
95. Vloka JD, Hadžić A, Drobnik L, et al: Anatomical landmarks for femoral nerve block: a comparison of four needle insertion sites. Anesth Analg 1999; 89:1467–1470.
96. Kofoed H: Peripheral nerve blocks at the knee and ankle in operations for common foot disorders. Clin Orthop 1982; 168:97–101.
97. Biehl DR: Fetal monitoring during surgery unrelated to pregnancy. Can Anaesth Soc J 1985; 32:455–459.
98. Pederson H, Morishima HO, Finster M: Anesthesia for the pregnant woman undergoing surgery. Semin Anaesth 1982; 1:177–183.

52

Neonatal Resuscitation

❖ VALERIE A. ARKOOSH, MD

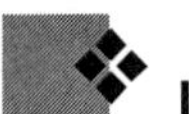

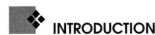

INTRODUCTION

At birth, numerous physiologic changes must occur for a fetus to successfully make the transition to a neonate. Despite the complexity of this process, only 6% of newborns born in the United States require life support in the delivery room.[1] This percentage rises quickly among newborns who weigh less than 1500 g. In Europe 2 to 6 per 1000 live births develop acute clinical sequelae of intrauterine asphyxia.[2] Of these, 25% of the moderate and 75% to 100% of the severe cases develop neurodevelopmental sequelae.[2] Delivery room personnel must understand the neonatal adaptations to extrauterine life, make provision for resuscitation, understand predictors of the need for resuscitation, and respond appropriately.

NEONATAL ADAPTATIONS TO EXTRAUTERINE LIFE[3, 4]

The fetus depends on placental blood flow for gas exchange. Pulmonary vascular resistance (PVR) is high, with 90% of right ventricular output shunting across the ductus arteriosus. Systemic vascular resistance (SVR) is low: 40% of cardiac output flows to the low-resistance placenta. During vaginal delivery, compression of the infant thorax expels fluid from the mouth and upper airways. With crying, the lungs fill with air, surfactant is released, and oxygenation is increased. These changes greatly decrease PVR. Simultaneously, clamping of the umbilical cord removes the low-resistance placental bed from the circulation, increasing SVR. Within minutes the right-to-left shunt across the foramen ovale and ductus arteriosus is substantially reduced.

Transient hypoxemia or acidosis is well tolerated by a normal newborn, and prompt intervention usually prevents any permanent sequelae. Prolonged neonatal hypoxemia or acidosis impedes the transition from fetal to neonatal physiology. The fetus/neonate initially responds to hypoxemia by redistributing blood flow to the heart, brain, and adrenal glands. Tissue oxygen extraction increases. Eventually, myocardial contractility and cardiac output decrease. Hypoxemia and acidosis promote patency of the ductus arteriosus, counteracting the normal neonatal increase in pulmonary artery blood flow. Ventilatory drive is reduced by indirect central nervous system depression and direct diaphragmatic depression. The net result of these physiologic responses is a neonate with persistent pulmonary hypertension and little or no ventilatory drive. Prompt intervention is necessary in these neonates.

PREPARATION FOR RESUSCITATION

Preparation for neonatal resuscitation encompasses a number of activities including acquisition and maintenance of the proper equipment; identification, education, and training of responding personnel; and development of contingency plans for additional personnel if needed. Equipment and medications should be organized together in one location in the delivery room, checked frequently for proper functioning and expiration date, and replenished immediately after use (Table 52–1).[1]

At least one person skilled in newborn resuscitation should attend every delivery. Additional personnel should be available if a high-risk delivery is anticipated. The importance of trained personnel who follow protocol-driven maneuvers is critical. In one hospital in China, neonatal mortality was reduced from 9.9% to 3.4% after the introduction of Neonatal Resuscitation Program Guidelines.[5] In the United States, an obstetric anesthesia workforce survey conducted by Hawkins and coworkers[6] in 1992 found that anesthesiologists performed neonatal resuscitation in less than 10% of cesarean deliveries. This percentage had decreased from 23% when a similar survey was administered in 1981. The remainder of resuscitations were performed by pediatricians, obstetricians, nurse specialists, family practitioners, respiratory therapists, or certified registered nurse anesthetists (CRNAs) not medically directed by an anesthesiologist. In a 1991 survey of mid-

Table 52–1 EQUIPMENT AND MEDICATIONS FOR NEONATAL RESUSCITATION

Suction Equipment	**Bag and Mask Equipment**
Bulb syringe	Neonatal resuscitation bag with pressure relief valve
Mechanical suction	Face masks: newborn and premature sizes
Suction catheters: 5F–10F	Oral airways
Meconium aspirator	Oxygen with flowmeter and tubing
Intubation Equipment	**Medications**
Laryngoscope	Epinephrine 1:10,000
Straight blades #0 and #1	Naloxone hydrochloride, 0.4 mg/mL or 1.0 mg/mL
Extra bulbs and batteries	Volume expander
Endotracheal tubes: 2.5–4.0 mm	Sodium bicarbonate 4.2% (5 mEq/10 mL)
Stylet	Dextrose 10%
Scissors and gloves	Sterile water and normal saline
Miscellaneous	
Radiant warmer	Umbilical artery catheterization tray
Stethoscope	Umbilical tape
Electrocardiograph	Umbilical catheters: 3.5F, 5F
Adhesive tape	Three-way stopcocks
Syringes and needles	Feeding tube: 5F
Alcohol sponges	

western community hospitals, routine involvement of anesthesia personnel in neonatal resuscitation was noted by 31% of respondents.[7] Looking forward, the need for anesthesia personnel to participate in neonatal resuscitation may increase as pediatric residents spend more time in primary care training and less in neonatology.

In determining need for personnel trained in neonatal resuscitation, practitioners in the United States can refer to Guideline VII of the American Society of Anesthesiology, Guidelines for Regional Anesthesia in Obstetrics (Appendix B). The guideline states: "Qualified personnel, other than the anesthesiologist attending the mother, should be immediately available to assume responsibility for resuscitation of the newborn. The primary responsibility of the anesthesiologist is to provide care to the mother. If the anesthesiologist is also requested to provide brief assistance in the care of the newborn, the benefit to the child must be compared to the risk to the mother."

ASSESSMENT OF RISK

With careful antepartum and intrapartum fetal assessment, the need for neonatal resuscitation can be predicted in about 80% of cases. Antepartum assessment includes evaluation for major fetal anomalies and identification of maternal factors that may influence fetal well-being (Table 52–2).[1, 3] Intrapartum events often predict the need for neonatal resuscitation (Table 52–3).[1, 3] Assessment must continue throughout labor since the clinical situation can change rapidly. Intrapartum evaluation includes fetal heart rate monitoring with, when indicated, fetal scalp or vibroacoustic stimulation, or fetal scalp blood sampling for pH determination.

Intrapartum fetal heart rate (FHR) monitoring is the first line of fetal assessment.[8] FHR monitoring is most reliable in confirming fetal well-being and is more than 90% accurate in predicting a 5-minute Apgar score greater than 7.[9, 10] In predicting fetal compromise, however, FHR monitoring has a false-positive rate of 35% to 50%.[10, 11] A recent study examined fetal heart rate strips of singleton infants with birthweights of at least 2500 grams and moderate to severe cerebral palsy and compared them with fetal heart rate strips from control children.[12] The 21 children with cerebral palsy who had multiple late decelerations or decreased heart rate variability represented 0.19% of the infants who had these fetal heart rate monitor findings. Thus, the false-positive rate in this patient population was 99.8%. Nonetheless, practitioners have little else with which to judge fetal well-being, and clinical decisions regarding delivery are often based on a careful evaluation of the FHR trace.

In the presence of a nonreassuring fetal heart rate trace, the practitioner may wish confirmatory studies of fetal well-being or the lack thereof. Digital stimulation of the fetal scalp or vibroacoustic stimulation through the maternal abdomen results in fetal heart

Table 52–2 MATERNAL AND FETAL FACTORS ASSOCIATED WITH NEED FOR RESUSCITATION

Maternal diabetes	Post-term gestation
Pregnancy-induced hypertension	Preterm gestation
Chronic hypertension	Multiple gestation
Previous Rh sensitization	Size-dates discrepancy
Previous stillbirth	Polyhydramnios
Bleeding in the second or third trimester	Oligohydramnios
Maternal infection	Maternal drug therapy, including reserpine, lithium carbonate, magnesium, adrenergic blocking drugs
Lack of prenatal care	
Maternal substance abuse	
Known fetal anomalies	

Table 52-3 INTRAPARTUM EVENTS ASSOCIATED WITH NEED FOR RESUSCITATION

Cesarean delivery	General anesthesia
Abnormal fetal presentation	Uterine tetany
Premature labor	Meconium-stained amniotic fluid
Rupture of membranes >24 h	Prolapsed cord
Chorioamnionitis	Abruptio placentae
Precipitous labor	Uterine rupture
Prolonged labor >24 h	Difficult instrumental delivery
Prolonged second stage >3–4 h	Maternal systemic narcotics within 4 h of delivery
Nonreassuring fetal heart rate patterns	

rate accelerations in a healthy, nonacidotic fetus. Fetal scalp pH determination can confirm or exclude fetal acidosis. A pH of less than 7.2 is considered abnormal, and if confirmed by a second measurement, may indicate the need for delivery.

Predictors of the need for endotracheal intubation include administration of general anesthesia to the mother and low infant weight.[13, 14] In growth-restricted infants, factors predicting low uterine artery pH and/or a 5-minute Apgar score less than 7 include preeclampsia, fetal distress, breech delivery, forceps use, older maternal age, amnioinfusion, general anesthesia, and nalbuphine use during labor.[14] In the presence of these risk factors, the available individual with the highest level of training in neonatal resuscitation should be called to perform the resuscitation.

RESPONSE

Intrapartum Resuscitation

Intrapartum resuscitation is attempted once fetal compromise is identified. Maternal factors that may impair oxygen delivery to the fetus must be identified and corrected if possible. These include maternal hypotension or decreased cardiac output secondary to aortocaval compression, sympathectomy, hemorrhage, or cardiac disease. Disease states that may interfere with maternal oxygenation, such as asthma, pneumonia, or pulmonary edema should be considered and if present, treated appropriately.

Attention must also be directed to the uterus because hyperstimulation, tetany, abruption, or rupture may interfere with blood flow to the fetus. Stopping oxytocin infusion or administering a tocolytic agent reduces uterine tone. Delivery is required if abruption or rupture are severe.

Umbilical cord prolapse should always be considered if fetal heart rate changes are sudden, severe, and prolonged. Oligohydramnios is a risk factor for umbilical cord compression and variable decelerations. Obstetricians are increasingly attempting saline amnioinfusion to alleviate cord compression.[15] Saline amnioinfusion is performed by infusing saline into the uterus via an intrauterine pressure catheter. Amnioinfusion is also being tried in cases of thick meconium in an attempt to dilute the meconium, in the hope of decreasing the severity of meconium aspiration syndrome.[16]

At Birth

The American Heart Association and the American Academy of Pediatrics together recommend the neonatal resuscitation protocol that follows. The first step in neonatal resuscitation is to minimize heat loss (Fig. 52–1).[17, 18] Depressed, asphyxiated infants often have an unstable thermal regulatory system. Additionally, cold stress leads to hypoxemia, hypercarbia, and metabolic acidosis, all of which promote persistence of the fetal circulation and hinder resuscitation. Within the first 20 seconds of life, the newborn should be dried, placed under a radiant warmer, and undergo suctioning of the mouth and nose (tracheal suctioning if meconium is present).

The second step (within 30 seconds of birth) is assessment of neonatal respiration. if the infant is gasping or apneic, begin positive-pressure ventilation (PPV) at a rate of 40 to 60 breaths/min with 100% oxygen.[18] Peak inspiratory pressures of 30 to 40 cm H_2O or higher are necessary for initial lung expansion.[17] The majority of infants requiring any resuscitation respond to these first two steps. Indications for endotracheal intubation include ineffective bag and mask ventilation, anticipated need for prolonged mechanical ventilation, or as a route for administration of medicine. With prolonged bag and mask ventilation, a nasal or orogastric tube should be inserted to decompress the stomach.

The third step is assessment of neonatal heart rate. Chest compressions are required in only 0.03% of deliveries.[17] Neonatal cardiac arrest is generally secondary to respiratory failure producing hypoxemia and tissue acidosis. The result of these metabolic changes is bradycardia, decreased cardiac contractility, and eventually cardiac arrest. Chest compressions should be instituted at a rate of 90 per minute when, after 15 to 30 seconds of PPV, the heart rate is below 60 or between 60 and 80 and not increasing.[18] Chest compressions should be stopped when heart rate is greater than 80. Chest compressions can be performed using either the thumb method or the two-finger method (Fig. 52–2). The depth of compressions should be approximately 1.5 to 2 cm. The ratio between chest compressions and ventilations should be 3:1, producing 90 compressions and 30 ventilations each minute. In practice, this equals thirty, 2-second cycles/min. A 2-second cycle consists of three chest compressions in 1.5 seconds, leaving 0.5 second for

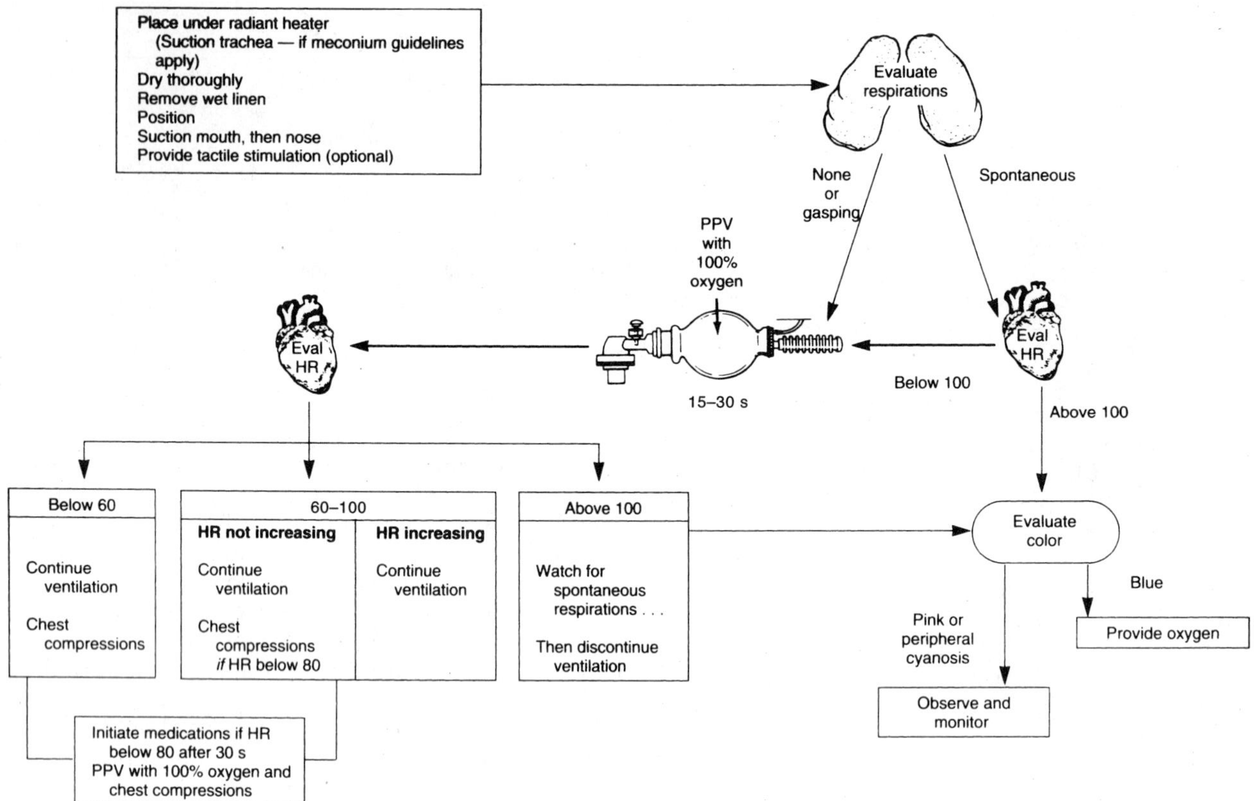

Figure 52–1 Overview of resuscitation in the delivery room. HR, heart rate; PPV, positive-pressure ventilation. (From Bloom RS, Cropley C [eds]: American Heart Association and American Academy of Pediatrics: *Textbook of Neonatal Resuscitation*. 1995: pp 0–5. Reprinted with permission from *Textbook of Neonatal Resuscitation* © 1995, 1987, 1990, 1994, American Heart Association.)

ventilation. In most neonates with adequate ventilation, cardiac function normalizes quickly.

The above three steps should all occur within the first minute of life. Although 1- and 5-minute Apgar scores (Table 52–4) are recorded as one way of assessing neonatal response to resuscitation, the practitioner *should not* wait for the 1-minute score to begin resuscitation. If the 5-minute score is less than 7, additional scores should be obtained every 5 minutes until 20 minutes have passed or until two successive scores are greater than or equal to 7.[19] In a study of stillborn infants, 66.6% were resuscitated and left the delivery room alive.[20] Of these, 39% survived beyond the neonatal period. Survival is unlikely if the Apgar score is 0 at greater than or equal to 10 minutes of age.[20]

Medications are indicated if, after adequate ventilation with 100% oxygen and chest compressions for 30 seconds, heart rate remains below 80 beats/min. Medications, doses, and routes of administration are given in Table 52–5. Naloxone hydrochloride is indicated specifically for neonatal respiratory depression caused by maternal opioid administration, but it should not be given to a neonate born of a narcotic-addicted mother as this can precipitate acute withdrawal in the neonate.[21] Sodium bicarbonate should only be used when ventilation is adequate (or respiratory acidosis will replace metabolic acidosis) *and* metabolic acidosis is documented or presumed, or all other measures have been unsuccessful.[17, 22] The use of blood volume expanders is rarely indicated and may be detrimental.[2, 23] Their use should be restricted to situations in which there is evidence of acute blood loss, such as fetomaternal hemorrhage, accompanied by clear signs of shock.[2, 23] Atropine is not indicated in

Table 52–4 **Apgar Scoring System**

Sign	0	1	2
Heart rate	Absent	<100	>100
Respiratory effort	Absent	Slow, irregular	Crying
Muscle tone	Flaccid	Some flexion of extremities	Active motion
Reflex irritability	No response	Grimace	Vigorous cry
Color	Blue, pale	Blue extremities	Completely pink

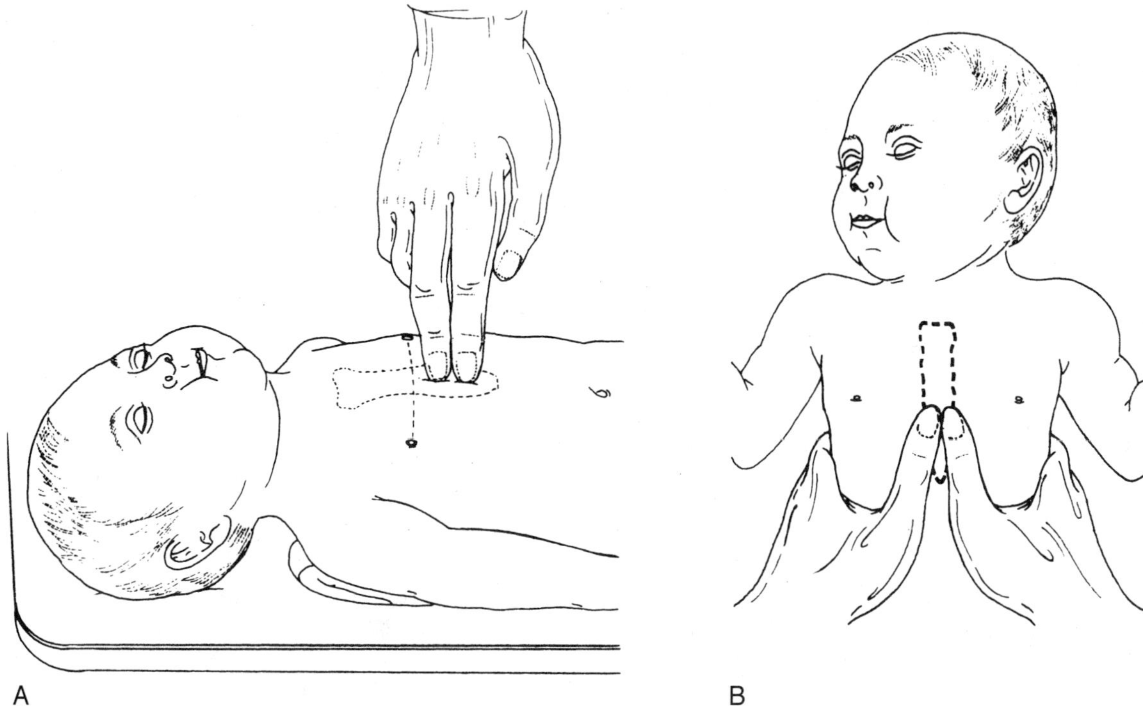

❖ **Figure 52–2** Positions for performing chest compressions. *A*, Two-finger method: the tips of the middle and index or ring fingers should be used for compression. *B*, Thumb method: the balls of the thumbs should be used for compression. (From Bloom RS, Cropley C (eds): American Heart Association and American Academy of Pediatrics: *Textbook of Neonatal Resuscitation*. 1995: pp 1–29. Reprinted with permission from *Textbook of Neonatal Resuscitation* © 1995, 1987, 1990, 1994, American Heart Association.)

neonatal resuscitation because vagal stimulation is rarely the cause of bradycardia in a newborn requiring resuscitation.[17] Direct laryngoscopy, however, may cause a transient decrease in heart rate.

Once the need for medications is established, there are three possible routes of administration: umbilical vein, peripheral veins, or endotracheal instillation. Endotracheal epinephrine effects are delayed up to 1 minute compared with intravenous administration.[24] Although increasing the dose of endotracheally administered epinephrine may be recommended in pediatric resuscitation, change in dose is not recommended in neonatal resuscitation.[21, 24] The larger dose of endotracheally administered epinephrine is associated with prolonged hypertension in an animal model.[24] Given the association between intraventricular hemorrhage and hypertension, the current recommendation is to administer the same dose of epinephrine (0.01 mg/kg) intravenously or endotracheally.[21, 24] If there is no response after endotracheal administration of epinephrine, intravenous access should be established as quickly as possible.

The umbilical vein is cannulated using a 3.5F or 5.0F radiopaque catheter with a single end-hole. The catheter should be inserted into the vein of the umbilical stump until the tip of the catheter is just below the skin level (Fig. 52–3). Free flow of blood should be present. If inserted too far, the catheter may enter the liver, which can be damaged by direct infusion of vasoactive drugs. Catheter location should be confirmed radiographically as soon as possible after insertion. Peripheral veins are adequate for resuscitation but may be difficult to cannulate in an emergency. While establishing intravenous access, both epinephrine and naloxone can be instilled into the trachea.

Neonatal Airway Management

Anatomic Considerations. There are five major differences between the neonatal and adult airway.[25] The neonate's tongue is relatively large in proportion to the mouth and can more easily obstruct the airway. The neonate's larynx is at the C3 to C4 level versus the C4 to C5 level in an adult. Because of this relatively acute angulation between the base of the tongue and the laryngeal opening, a straight laryngoscope blade facilitates visualization of the larynx. The neonate's epiglottis is narrower than the adult's and angled away from the axis of the trachea, rather than parallel to the tracheal axis. The axis of the vocal cords is perpendicular to the trachea in the adult. In the neonate the vocal cords have a lower attachment anteriorly than posteriorly. Because of this angulation, the endotracheal tube is more likely to be caught at the anterior commissure of the vocal cords. Finally, in the neonate, the narrowest portion of the larynx is below the vocal cords at the level of the cricoid cartilage. Thus, an endotracheal tube that passes easily through the vocal cords may meet resistance in the subglottic area.

Guidelines from the American Heart Association

Table 52-5 MEDICATIONS USED IN NEONATAL RESUSCITATION

MEDICATION	CONCENTRATION TO ADMINISTER	PREPARATION	DOSAGE/ ROUTE*	TOTAL DOSE/INFANT			RATE/PRECAUTIONS
				Weight		**Total mL**	
Epinephrine	1:10,000	1 mL	0.1–0.3 mL/kg IV or ET	1 kg		0.1–0.3 mL	Give rapidly
				2 kg		0.2–0.6 mL	May dilute with
				3 kg		0.3–0.9 mL	normal saline to 1–2
				4 kg		0.4–1.2 mL	mL if giving ET
				Weight		**Total mL**	
Volume expanders	Whole blood	40 mL	10 mL/kg IV	1 kg		10 mL	Give over 5–10 min
	5% Albumin-saline			2 kg		20 mL	
	Normal saline			3 kg		30 mL	
	Ringer's lactate			4 kg		40 mL	
				Weight	**Total Dose**	**Total mL**	
Sodium bicarbonate	0.5 mEq/mL (4.2% solution)	20 mL or two 10-mL prefilled syringes	2 mEq/kg IV	1 kg	2 mEq	4 mL	Give *slowly,* over at least 2 min
				2 kg	4 mEq	8 mL	Give only if infant is
				3 kg	6 mEq	12 mL	being effectively
				4 kg	8 mEq	16 mL	ventilated
				Weight	**Total Dose**	**Total mL**	
Naloxone hydrochloride	0.4 mg/mL	1 mL	0.1 mg/kg (0.25 mL/kg) IV, ET, IM, SQ	1 kg	0.1 mg	0.25 mL	
				2 kg	0.2 mg	0.50 mL	Give rapidly
				3 kg	0.3 mg	0.75 mL	IV, ET preferred
				4 kg	0.4 mg	1.00 mL	IM, SQ acceptable
	1.0 mg/mL	1 mL	0.1 mL/kg (0.1 mL/kg) IV, ET, IM, SQ	1 kg	0.1 mg	0.1 mL	
				2 kg	0.2 mg	0.2 mL	
				3 kg	0.3 mg	0.3 mL	
				4 kg	0.4 mg	0.4 mL	
				Weight		**Total μg/min**	
Dopamine	$\frac{6 \times \text{Weight (kg)} \times \text{Desired dose } (\mu g/kg/min)}{\text{Desired fluid (mL/h)}}$ = mg of dopamine per 100 mL of solution		Begin at 5 μg/kg/min (may increase to 20 μg/kg/min if necessary) IV	1 kg		5–10 μg/min	Give as a continuous infusion using an infusion pump
				2 kg		10–40 μg/min	Monitor heart rate and blood pressure closely
				3 kg		15–60 μg/min	Seek consultation
				4 kg		20–80 μg/min	

*IM, intramuscular; ET, endotracheal; IV, intravenous; SQ, subcutaneous.

From American Heart Association, American Academy of Pediatrics: Textbook of Neonatal Resuscitation. Dallas, TX: American Heart Association; 1994.

Correct

Catheter just below skin level

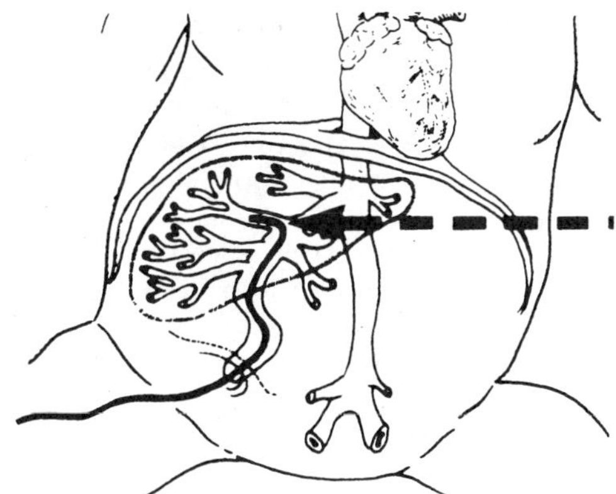

Figure 52–3 Umbilical vein catheter placement. (From Bloom RS, Cropley C (eds): American Heart Association and American Academy of Pediatrics: *Textbook of Neonatal Resuscitation*. 1995: pp 1–29. Reprinted with permission from *Textbook of Neonatal Resuscitation* © 1995, 1987, 1990, 1994, American Heart Association.)

and the American Academy of Pediatrics[18] caution against extreme extension or flexion of the neonate's head during resuscitation because, theoretically, stretching of the compliant trachea could produce airway obstruction. The ability to produce changes in tracheal diameter by changes in head position was studied in 18 healthy full-term infants using a flexible fiberoptic bronchoscope passed through an endotracheal tube positioned above the cricoid cartilage.[26] Video recordings were obtained with the anesthetized infant's head in neutral position, maximum possible extension, and maximum possible flexion. No patient had significant changes in tracheal dimension with changes in head position. This study does not eliminate another site, such as the hypopharynx, as susceptible to obstruction with extreme head positions.

Laryngeal Mask Airway (LMA). Recently, the size 1 LMA has been used successfully to resuscitate newborns requiring PPV at birth.[27–29] In a descriptive study by Paterson and associates,[27] eligible newborns weighed at least 2.5 kg and were of 35 weeks' gestation or greater. Twenty of 21 neonates were successfully resuscitated with the LMA. One neonate underwent tracheal intubation to facilitate administration of epinephrine. Time for LMA insertion averaged 8.6 seconds, circuit pressure at audible leak averaged 22 cm H_2O, and peak circuit pressure that was obtained averaged 37 cm H_2O. Gastric distention was not observed during the resuscitation procedure. The successful use of the LMA has also been described in neonates with Pierre-Robin syndrome in whom both bag and mask ventilation and endotracheal intubation had failed.[30, 31] Further studies are needed to assess the reliability of this technique of airway management in the neonate requiring resuscitation.

PRACTICAL ISSUES

Supplemental Oxygen. Although a high inspired oxygen concentration is recommended during resuscitation by most textbooks, there is evidence that this may not be absolutely necessary. In the Resair 2 Study asphyxiated newborn infants with birthweight greater than 999 grams were allocated to resuscitation with either room air or 100% oxygen.[2, 32] Eleven international sites participated in this study. Allocation to oxygen or room air was based on date of birth. Between the 288 infants in the room air group and the 321 infants in the oxygen group there were no differences in demographic data, mortality in the first 7 days of life, neonatal mortality, incidence of hypoxic-ischemic encephalopathy, or heart rate during resuscitation. Apgar scores were higher at 1 minute in the room air group; however, there were no significant differences at 5 minutes. Hopefully, future studies will specifically address the optimal use of oxygen during neonatal resuscitation.

Confirmation of Endotracheal Intubation. A disposable, colorimetric carbon dioxide detector can be used to accurately determine an endotracheal intubation during neonatal resuscitation.[33] Caution must be used though, because this detector does not identify a main stem bronchus intubation or an oropharyngeal intubation in spontaneously breathing patients. False-positive readings can be minimized by obtaining a reading only after 6 breaths have been given.

Airway Obstruction. Causes of airway obstruction in the newborn include choanal atresia, internal thyroglossal duct cysts, laryngeal and tracheal anomalies, and cardiovascular mediastinal anomalies. Congenital anomalies of the tracheobronchial tree include atresia, webs, tumors, and tracheomalacia. Aspiration of meconium and blood are documented causes of neonatal morbidity and mortality. Recently, a normal-appearing newborn infant who was unable to be resuscitated at birth was found at autopsy to have a fragment of decidual tissue in the larynx.[34] A diagnosis of tracheal obstruction caused by foreign body aspiration should be considered during resuscitations in which ventilation is inadequate or not possible.

Neonatal Hypoglycemia. Approximately 10% of healthy term neonates have transient hypoglycemia.[35] Other neonates at risk include those born of diabetic mothers or mothers who received a large amount of intravenous dextrose during labor. Macrosomic, premature, or postmature neonates also are prone to hypoglycemia. A dextrose strip is easily obtained for any infant at risk and should also be obtained from neonates who appear lethargic at birth without obvious cause. If the glucose level is less than 40 to 45 mg/dL, the neonate should be treated either with oral feedings (2–3 mL/kg 10% dextrose in water) or by intravenous infusion (8 mg/kg/min).

Pulse Oximeter Placement. The right-to-left shunt at the ductus arteriosus persists for some time after birth and may affect oxygen saturation readings obtained by pulse oximetry. Measurements of arterial oxygen saturation taken at birth simultaneously from the right hand and the right foot are consistently higher in the right hand.[36] An oxygen saturation measurement obtained from the right hand is a better index of neonatal cerebral oxygenation than that obtained from the lower extremities.

ETHICAL ASPECTS FOR THE OBSTETRIC ANESTHESIOLOGIST

When faced with the need to resuscitate a very low birthweight infant (<750 g), a stillborn infant, or an infant with severe congenital anomalies that may preclude long-term survival, the obstetric health care team may have conflicting feelings about how to proceed.[37] A survey of neonatologists in Alberta, Canada revealed that factors extremely important or important to the decision-making process include gestational age, birthweight, multiple anomalies, and parental requests.[38] Factors classified as not important include financial costs to parents, hospital, or society; medicolegal factors; the physician's own moral or religious beliefs; and potential adoption of the infant. There was disagreement concerning the importance of apnea and asystole at birth. Likelihood of neonatal death or severe handicap is also considered important, but only when these outcomes are greater than 75% certain to occur. Ideally, discussions are held between the parents, neonatology and obstetrics staff, and hospital ethics committee (when necessary) prior to delivery.[21] In the complete absence of such discussions, it is the author's personal opinion that it is best to attempt resuscitation.

❖ CONCLUSION Successful neonatal resuscitation requires an understanding of neonatal physiology and adequate preparation of personnel and supplies. Good antepartum and intrapartum assessment identifies the majority of infants who will require resuscitation. Those who frequent the delivery room, even when not designated as primary responders to neonatal resuscitations, should understand how to initiate neonatal resuscitation.

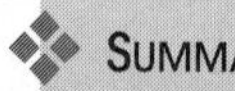

SUMMARY

Key Points

- In most cases, the need for neonatal resuscitation can be predicted by careful attention to antepartum history and intrapartum events.
- At least one person skilled in neonatal resuscitation and not directly involved in the care of the mother should be present at every delivery.
- The vast majority of neonates respond to warming, stimulation, gentle suctioning, and oxygen.
- Practitioners who frequent the delivery room should periodically review the algorithm for neonatal resuscitation.

Key Reference

Wimmer JE: Neonatal resuscitation. Pediatr Rev 1994; 15:255.

Case Stem

A female infant with estimated gestational age of 32 weeks is cyanotic and apneic and has a heart rate of 105 beats/min following an urgent cesarean delivery for a nonreassuring fetal heart rate strip. The mother had two prenatal visits and was hypertensive and tachycardic on arrival at the hospital. When she extracts the placenta, the obstetrician notes the presence of a moderate-sized placental abruption. Describe the risk factors for this infant and how you would proceed.

References

1. American Heart Association: Standards and guidelines for cardiopulmonary resuscitation and emergency care. JAMA 1992; 268:2276.
2. Saugstad OD: Practical aspects of resuscitating asphyxiated newborn infants. Eur J Pediatr 1998; 157(Suppl):S11.
3. Wimmer JE: Neonatal resuscitation. Pediatr Rev 1994; 15:255.
4. Ostheimer GW: Anaesthetists' role in neonatal resuscitation and care of the newborn. Can J Anaesth 1993; 40:R50.
5. Zhu XY, Fang HQ, Zeng SP, et al: The impact of the Neonatal Resuscitation Program Guidelines (NRPG) on the neonatal mortality in a hospital in Zhuhai, China. Singapore Med J 1997; 38:485.
6. Hawkins JL, Gibbs CP, Orleans M, et al: Obstetric anesthesia workforce survey—1981 versus 1992. Anesthesiology 1997; 87:135.
7. Heyman HJ, Joseph NJ, Salem MR, et al: Anesthesia personnel, neonatal resuscitation, and the courts [abstract]. Anesthesiology 1991; 75:A1074.
8. Guay J: Fetal monitoring and neonatal resuscitation: what the anaesthetist should know. Can J Anaesth 1991; 38:R83.
9. Krebs HB, Petres RE, Dunn LJ, et al: Intrapartum fetal heart rate monitoring. I. Classification and prognosis of fetal heart rate patterns. Am J Obstet Gynecol 1979; 133:762.
10. Schifrin BS, Dame L: Fetal heart rate patterns: prediction of Apgar score. JAMA 1972; 219:1322.

11. Tejani N, Mann LI, Bhakthavathsalan A: Correlation of fetal heart rate patterns and fetal pH with neonatal outcome. Obstet Gynecol 1976; 48:460.
12. Nelson KB, Dambrosia JM, Ting TY, et al: Uncertain value of electronic fetal monitoring in predicting cerebral palsy. N Engl J Med 1996; 334:613.
13. Parsons SJ, Sonneveld S, Nolan T: Is a paediatrician needed at all caesarean sections? J Paediatr Child Health 1998; 34:241.
14. Levy BT, Dawson JD, Toth PP, et al: Predictors of neonatal resuscitation, low Apgar scores, and umbilical artery pH among growth-restricted neonates. Obstet Gynecol 1998; 91:909.
15. Sivan E, Seidman DS, Barkai G, et al: The role of amnioinfusion in current obstetric care. Obstet Gynecol Surv 1992; 47:80.
16. Macri CJ, Schrimmer DB, Leung A, et al: Prophylactic amnioinfusion improves outcome of pregnancy complicated by thick meconium and oligohydramnios. Am J Obstet Gynecol 1992; 167:117.
17. Leuthner SR, Jansen RD, Hageman JR: Cardiopulmonary resuscitation of the newborn. Pediatr Clin North Am 1994; 41:893.
18. American Heart Association, American Academy of Pediatrics: Textbook of Neonatal Resuscitation. Dallas, TX: American Heart Association; 1994.
19. Jain L, Vidyasagar D: Controversies in neonatal resuscitation. Pediatr Ann 1995; 24:540.
20. Jain L, Ferre C, Vidyasagar D, et al: Cardiopulmonary resuscitation of apparently stillborn infants: survival and long-term outcome. J Pediatr 1991; 118:778.
21. Ginsberg HG, Goldsmith JP: Controversies in neonatal resuscitation. Clin Perinatol 1998; 25:1.
22. Hein HA: The use of sodium bicarbonate in neonatal resuscitation: help or harm? [Letter.] Pediatrics 1993; 91:496.
23. Roberton NRC: Use of albumin in neonatal resuscitation. Eur J Pediatr 1997; 156:428.
24. Frand MN, Honig KL, Hageman JR: Neonatal cardiopulmonary resuscitation: the good news and the bad. Pediatr Clin North Am 1998; 45:587.
25. Coté CJ, Todres ID: The pediatric airway. *In* Coté CJ, Ryan JF, Todres ID, Goudsouzian NG (eds): A Practice of Anesthesia for Infants and Children, 2nd ed. Philadelphia: WB Saunders; 1993:55.
26. Wheeler M, Roth AG, Dunham ME, et al: A bronchoscopic, computer-assisted examination of the changes in dimension of the infant tracheal lumen with changes in head position. Anesthesiology 1998; 88:1183.
27. Paterson SJ, Byrne PJ, Molesky MG, et al: Neonatal resuscitation using the laryngeal mask airway. Anesthesiology 1994; 80:1248.
28. Brimacombe J: The laryngeal mask airway for neonatal resuscitation [letter]. Pediatrics 1994; 93:874.
29. Lavies NG: Use of the laryngeal mask airway in neonatal resuscitation [letter]. Anaesthesia 1993; 48:352.
30. Denny NM, Desilva KD, Webber PA: Laryngeal mask airway for emergency tracheostomy in a neonate. Anaesthesia 1990; 45:895.
31. Baraka A: Laryngeal mask airway for resuscitation of a newborn with Pierre-Robin syndrome [letter]. Anesthesiology 1995; 83:645.
32. Saugstad OD, Rootwelt T, Aalen O: Resuscitation of asphyxiated newborn infants with room air or oxygen: an international controlled trial: The Resair 2 Study. Pediatrics 1998; 102:e1.
33. Roth B, Lundberg D: Disposable CO_2-detector, a reliable tool for determination of correct tracheal tube position during resuscitation of a neonate. Resuscitation 1997; 35:149.
34. van Wylick RC, Fletcher WA, MacRae BB, et al: Neonatal tracheal obstruction caused by aspiration of decidual tissue. Acta Paediatr 1998; 87:100.
35. Fanaroff AA, Martin RH (eds): Neonatal-Perinatal Medicine: Diseases of the Fetus and Infant, 5th ed. St. Louis: Mosby–Year Book; 1992.
36. Dimich I, Singh PP, Adell A, et al: Evaluation of oxygen saturation monitoring by pulse oximetry in neonates in the delivery system. Can J Anaesth 1991; 38:985.
37. Landwirth J: Ethical issues in pediatric and neonatal resuscitation. Ann Emerg Med 1993; 22:502.
38. Byrne PJ, Tyebkhan JM, Laing LM: Ethical decision-making and neonatal resuscitation. Semin Perinatol 1994; 18:36.

53

Critical Care Management of the Pregnant Patient

M. F. M. JAMES, MD, MBChB, FRCA

JOHN ANTHONY, MBChB, FCOG

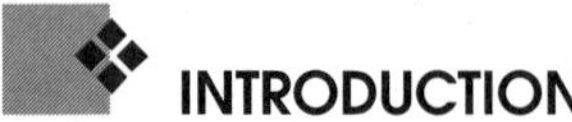

INTRODUCTION

Global maternal mortality rates indicate that half a million women die annually as a result of complications arising during pregnancy.[1] The incidence of mortality varies according to the socioeconomic development of different countries and may be partially preventable through development of infrastructure in poorer communities.[2] Developed nations report lower mortality rates but continue to focus on maternal deaths because many of them are associated with substandard care and some maternal deaths could be avoided by greater attention to critical care management.[3–8]

Obstetric critical care has been described as a discipline in its infancy.[9] The rate of occurrence of critical illness in pregnant patients is low, with published reports indicating an intensive care unit (ICU) admission rate of between 0.29% and 1.5% of deliveries in industrialized countries.[10–13] This low rate of ICU admission of obstetric patients frequently results in a relative inexperience in the management of the obstetric patient among critical care physicians and emphasizes the need for a team approach between obstetricians, anesthesiologists, and critical care physicians to meet the challenges posed by the critically ill pregnant patient. The majority of pregnant patients admitted to an ICU have complications related to the pregnancy, but in a significant proportion of patients the indication for ICU admission is unrelated to the pregnancy. A further group of patients have an underlying medical condition that has been aggravated by the pregnancy to the point at which ICU management is necessary. In developing countries, the greater incidence of obstetric complications may result in a higher admission rate to the ICU, but adequate data to assess the likely admission rate accurately are not available. Anesthetic complications may contribute significantly to ICU admissions. In one survey, anesthesia complications accounted for 13% of obstetric admissions to a general ICU, with general anesthesia having an incidence of a major complication resulting in ICU admission of 1 in 932, while regional anesthesia had an incidence of 1 in 4177.[14]

Interpreting data from the small number of reviews of ICU care of pregnant patients is fraught with difficulties, since criteria for admission to the ICU are frequently very different. Clearly, maternal mortality in any series depends to a very large degree on the criteria for ICU admission. In many units, complications simply requiring advanced monitoring are included in ICU admission data, whereas in others, notably the general ICUs, only life-threatening conditions qualify for admission. In reports from general ICUs, nonobstetric conditions feature prominently among the causes for ICU admission, whereas in obstetric units, obstetric causes for admission dominate. The spectrum of diseases requiring admission to two dedicated obstetric intensive care units (one in the United States and one in Africa) has been published.[12, 15] Hypertensive disease is the leading cause of morbidity and mortality followed by a variety of medical disorders complicating pregnancy (including sepsis), with obstetric hemorrhage accounting for about 10% of admissions.

It is difficult therefore to make any conclusive statements regarding overall prognosis in obstetric critical care, particularly since measures for comparison of disease severity have yet to be validated in this population (see later in chapter).

The alterations in maternal physiology and the

unique needs of the fetus place unusual demands on the critical care team. Furthermore, critical care of the obstetric patient is complicated by the fact that it frequently implies support of two patients with differing physiologic profiles and metabolic needs. Not only are the profiles of both patients different, but they are also continuously changing as pregnancy advances, independent of the disease process that has warranted ICU admission. Critical care of the obstetric patient requires an in-depth knowledge of both standard critical care practice and the special conditions pertaining to the pregnant patient. In particular, the changes in maternal cardiopulmonary physiology and the demands of the fetus need to be considered.

This chapter first briefly outlines important physiologic adaptations that occur during pregnancy in order to provide the framework against which the pathophysiologic events of pregnancy disorders can be measured. The diseases requiring critical care are divided into those that are incidental to pregnancy and those unique to pregnancy.

PREGNANCY PHYSIOLOGY

Physiologic Changes. Fetal growth and development is uniquely fostered by maternal physiologic adaptation. These include enhanced rates of peripheral oxygenation, the development of mild hypocarbia, increased renal clearance rates, metabolic changes characterized by accelerated starvation, and the development of a procoagulant clotting profile.

Physiologic hyperreninism increases aldosterone levels 10-fold.[16] This adaptation (among others) secures the retention of water and electrolytes by the kidneys and results in a 50% increase in plasma volume.[17, 18] Plasma volume expansion is matched by enhanced oxygen-carrying capacity brought about by a 14% to 28% increase in red cell mass.[19] Stroke volume and cardiac output rise by 40%, while blood pressure falls as a result of peripheral vasodilatation and because new vascular beds develop in the choriodecidual space.[20] The net effect of these changes is an accelerated rate of oxygen delivery to peripheral tissues. These changes exceed the requirements of pregnancy and the arteriovenous oxygen difference declines in normal pregnancy.[21] Fetal respiration is further facilitated by maternal physiologic hyperventilation leading to a partially compensated respiratory alkalosis. Typically the partial pressure of carbon dioxide in a pregnant woman falls by 15% with a reduction in plasma bicarbonate, although arterial pH remains unaltered.[22, 23] The arterial $PaCO_2$ reaches a nadir of 4 kPa (30 mm Hg) in the third trimester.

An 80% increase in effective renal plasma flow leads to a 50% rise in glomerular filtration.[24] These changes lead to increased excretion of glucose, vitamins, metabolites, and drugs. Serum levels of creatinine that exceed 80 μmol/L should be considered abnormal in pregnancy.

The changes that occur in coagulation are due to a number of mechanisms that include enhanced estrogen-dependent hepatic synthesis of fibrinogen and factors VII, VIII, X, and XIII.[25] The fibrinolytic system is impeded by increased levels of plasminogen activator inhibitor (PAI-1) and by altered binding of protein S, leading to physiologic resistance to activated protein C.[26] This expression of procoagulant activity in normal pregnancy is evident through increased circulating levels of thrombin–antithrombin III complexes.[25]

Effect of Gestational Age. The physiologic adaptation of pregnancy is progressive with increasing gestational age and reverts to normal at varying rates during and after the puerperium. The occurrence of labor contractions further augments these changes. Hence cardiac output rises progressively throughout pregnancy to a peak value of 7 L/min at approximately 32 weeks. Autotransfusion of blood from the choriodecidual circulation as well as catecholamine release during labor gives rise to peak values of 10 L/min.[27] Blood pressure (both systolic and diastolic) falls by 10% to 15% in the second trimester but rises again toward prepregnancy levels by the end of the third trimester with a further rise occurring in some patients during labor. After delivery, the contraction of the uterus leads to an increased preload, which can pose a risk to an impaired myocardium with the consequence that pulmonary edema frequently occurs at this time. The elevated cardiac output gradually declines over 2 to 3 weeks following delivery.

Anatomic Changes of Pregnancy and Their Effects on Pregnancy Physiology. The enlarging uterus may compress the inferior vena cava. It also displaces the diaphragm upward and has been implicated in partial ureteric obstruction.

Aortocaval compression is especially common in the third trimester and may lead to supine hypotension as a result of diminished venous return.[28] The adrenergic response to aortocaval compression may maintain (or increase) blood pressure, but diminished cardiac output can critically impair uterine perfusion, especially during labor. Regional anesthesia, which blocks the adrenergic response, may be associated with profound hypotension if the effects of aortocaval compression are ignored.

The diaphragm is displaced by the enlarging uterus, leading to a 10% to 20% reduction in residual volume and functional residual capacity (FRC). Tidal volume increases because of increased chest wall movement without any increase in respiratory rate. These latter changes are provoked by the action of progesterone on the respiratory center.[29] As pregnancy advances, the difference between closing capacity and FRC decreases owing to the increase in intra-abdominal pressure, and consequently airway closure and alveolar collapse become more likely, particularly in the supine position.[30, 31] Vasodilatation occurs throughout the respiratory tract resulting in upper airway hyperemia, edema, and fragility as well as increased vascular markings on the chest radiograph.

The renal tract shows evidence of ureteric dilatation, greater on the right than the left.[32] This may be due to the effects of progesterone on smooth muscle, although the ureteric contraction complex remains unaltered by pregnancy.[33] The enlarging uterus does not seem to obstruct the ureters, although they may be displaced laterally at the vesicoureteric junction.[34] Incompetence of the vesicoureteric sphincter may predispose to an increased risk of upper urinary tract infection.[33] Dilated ureters in pregnancy should not be misinterpreted as a sign of obstruction. The changes in the renal tract may persist to some extent for as long as 4 months postpartum.

Fetal Considerations. The fetus is totally dependent on uterine blood flow for its oxygen delivery and thus is especially at risk during maternal critical illness. Uterine blood flow may be varied by a number of factors. The uterine vasculature is normally maximally vasodilated, and uterine blood flow, and hence fetal oxygenation, is totally dependent on maternal cardiac output and blood pressure. Uterine vasoconstriction can occur in response to many events including maternal alkalosis, elevated catecholamine concentrations, and uterine contractions.

Gas exchange across the placenta is by simple diffusion, but transfer of oxygen is accelerated by the very low partial pressure of oxygen in the fetal circulation. However, despite the low partial pressure of oxygen in the fetus, the left shift of the oxyhemoglobin dissociation curve and the increased fetal hematocrit means that the oxygen content of fetal blood is relatively high. The fetus has no storage capacity for oxygen, and is therefore always at risk if placental oxygen delivery should fail, but there does appear to be a reasonable safety margin. It is worth noting that while high maternal inspired oxygen may result in only a small increase in oxygen partial pressure in the fetus, significant improvements in fetal saturation (and oxygen content) may be achieved because the fetal hemoglobin is operating on the steep part of the oxyhemoglobin dissociation curve.[35] The well-being of the fetus, therefore, demands that maternal cardiac output, uterine blood flow, and maternal Pa_{O_2} are all maintained at close to, or above, normal values for pregnancy during critical care management.

CRITICAL CARE CONSIDERATIONS

Scoring Systems in Critically Ill Pregnant Women. Evaluating the likely outcome of critical illness in an obstetric population is difficult, largely because the scoring systems used to evaluate patient status during critical illness—such as the Acute Physiological and Chronic Health Evaluation (APACHE II)—have not been properly validated in an obstetric population. Mortality in obstetric patients needing critical care has been described as being higher than in nonobstetric patients,[36] appropriate,[37] and lower[10, 38] than predicted using clinical experience and various scoring systems. Differences in the normal physiology of pregnancy may bias the scoring systems, resulting in higher scores than the actual severity of the disease warrants.[39] The relative rarity of obstetric critical care patients may result in higher than normal ratings on the Therapeutic Intervention Scoring System (TISS), which may simply reflect greater than normal physician involvement in the pregnant critically ill patient than that which would occur in a nonobstetric admission.[40] In the obstetric ICU at our institution (Groote Schuur Hospital), a study of the Simplified Acute Physiology Score (SAPS) showed good prediction of maternal morbidity, but not of mortality. The failure to predict mortality was related to the very low death rate (1.96%) in the study group of 661 women admitted to the obstetric ICU over a 3-year period (JA Penny, M Bloch, J Anthony, personal communication, 1999). In trauma, the Revised Trauma Score has been shown to be a poor predictor of adverse pregnancy outcome.[41] No definitive statements regarding the predictability of outcome in pregnant patients in the ICU can therefore be made until the scoring systems in use have been properly evaluated in an obstetric population. This makes comparison of therapeutic techniques and their outcome difficult.

Pharmacology and Radiologic Exposure. In addition to normal critical care considerations, management of the critically ill obstetric patient requires consideration of pharmacology peculiar to the pregnant patient, the appropriate use of monitoring, and awareness of the altered metabolic needs of both mother and fetus. Specific consideration needs to be given to potential hazards of standard ICU procedures, particularly radiologic ones, which may exert a detrimental effect on mother or fetus. Radiologic procedures are often an essential part of the management of critically ill patients, but in the pregnant patient the risk of radiation exposure to the fetus must be considered. Radiologic hazards to the fetus include fetal death, malformations, and an increase in the incidence of childhood cancers, notably leukemia. However, although the increase in risk is statistically significant, in real terms the magnitude of the hazard is quite small, with an expected increase in incidence of childhood malignancy of the order of 0.1%.[10] Exposure of the fetus to radiation doses of less than 5 rad is not associated with an increase in the incidence of congenital abnormalities, but above 15 rad the risk of malformations is markedly increased. It has been estimated that a single chest radiograph exposes the fetus to a dose of around 0.001 rad, whereas pelvic computed tomography scans deliver a large radiation dose of around 5 rad. The dose of radiation received by the fetus can be reduced by the use of abdominal shielding and well-collimated beams. Plain chest films necessary for diagnosis and safe management of the pregnant patient should not be withheld on the basis of undue concern over fetal exposure.[42]

Monitoring. Hemodynamic monitoring may be particularly valuable in the obstetric patient, and a low threshold should be used for the placement of intra-arterial lines. The ease of access to blood gas analysis and continuous blood pressure measurement, coupled with the low morbidity, make arterial lines potentially invaluable. Pulmonary artery catheterization is more controversial. Indications for the placement of a pulmonary artery catheter (PAC) are similar to those in nonpregnant patients with the exception of severe preeclampsia, for which there is no analogous condition in the nonpregnant state. The current controversy regarding the use of PACs is far from resolved, and current evidence is insufficient to conclude that PAC use alters ICU mortality and morbidity,[43] although there has been recent support for PAC use in patients with unclear hemodynamic and metabolic profiles.[44] Apart from problems relating to complications of catheter placement, serious concerns have been expressed regarding the satisfactory interpretation of data, and user knowledge of how to apply PAC-derived measurements in the clinical situation is frequently suboptimal.[45] However, if PAC monitoring is to be used, consideration must be given to the variations from normal caused by the pregnant state, and interpretation of data must be made with these physiologic changes in mind. Corrections for body surface area may not be valid in pregnancy, as nomograms for body surface area in pregnancy are not available.[10] Specific consideration can be given to the use of PACs in obstetrics in severe preeclampsia and maternal cardiac disease in which measurement of left ventricular filling pressures and cardiac output may assist during the marked hemodynamic changes that can occur during labor and delivery. A review of the pulmonary artery catheters used in the management of preeclamptic patients admitted to our obstetric ICU revealed that most catheters were inserted for the management of patients in renal failure (56%), followed by pulmonary edema (32%), and eclampsia (6%) (WM Gilbert, J Anthony, personal communication, 1999). There is some evidence that the incidence of complications of pulmonary artery catheterization may be lower in pregnant patients than in other ICU populations because of their young age and absence of comorbid conditions.[10] In the Groote Schuur obstetric ICU, 95 catheters inserted over a 3-year period gave rise to 3 complications (2 cases of venous thrombosis and 1 case of cellulitis).[45a] A recent consensus meeting reached the conclusion that PAC monitoring does not reduce complications and mortality in patients with preeclampsia but conceded that it may be useful in oliguria unresponsive to fluids, pulmonary edema, and resistant hypertension.[46] As with many of the conclusions of this meeting, the evidence on which this statement was based has been considered to be weak and we subscribe to the view that hemodynamic monitoring has a role to play in the management of selected critically ill pregnant women, predominantly among those admitted with severe preeclampsia.

Fetal monitoring may include monitoring of fetal heart rate (FHR), fetal biophysical profile, and ultrasound examination combined with Doppler velocimetry of the fetoplacental circulation and fetal middle cerebral artery blood flow. Continuous FHR monitoring is particularly useful in situations in which changes in fetal well-being may affect clinical decisions in the critically patient. However, interpretation of the data obtained can be difficult, and the expert input of an experienced obstetrician is required for their proper evaluation. This is particularly important when the pregnant patient is sent to an ICU outside of the labor and delivery suite. A detailed description of FHR monitoring and its implications is discussed in Chapter 5.

GENERAL PRINCIPLES OF CRITICAL CARE IN PREGNANCY

The general principles of managing the critically ill obstetric patient are determined primarily by the nature of the underlying illness rather than specifically by the fact that the patient is pregnant. Details of the specific management of all of the possible conditions that can arise concurrently with pregnancy is beyond the scope of this chapter, but there are certain basic principles that can be considered together with their possible application in pregnancy.

Respiratory Management

Respiratory failure is one of the more common causes of admission of pregnant patients to an intensive care unit. The cause of the ventilatory failure may be related to pregnancy, particularly the complications of preeclampsia leading to pulmonary edema, amniotic fluid embolism, and pulmonary edema following the use of tocolytics. In addition, pregnant patients are particularly susceptible to pulmonary thromboembolic disease and may also suffer from aspiration of gastric contents, especially in association with general anesthesia. The increased metabolic demands of pregnancy may also lead to an exacerbation of preexisting conditions such as myasthenia gravis and asthma. In both of these preexisting conditions, reports exist of pregnancy almost equally having no influence on, improving, or worsening the underlying condition. Other neurologic complications that may lead to respiratory failure in pregnancy include coincidental Guillain-Barré syndrome, subarachnoid hemorrhage, and the rare but catastrophic condition, pituitary apoplexy.[47] Adult respiratory distress syndrome (ARDS) in pregnancy may arise from many causes, including lung infection, trauma, hemorrhagic complications of pregnancy, amniotic fluid embolism, and smoke inhalation, although the most common causes are hemorrhage, infection, and toxemia.[48]

In managing the respiratory function of a pregnant patient, consideration must be given to the underlying physiology. By far the most important consideration for the fetus is the maintenance of oxygen delivery. The use of therapeutic maneuvers and medications to treat the underlying disease process should always take priority over considerations of injury to the unborn child, since hypoxia represents a far greater risk for the unborn child than any of the complications of pharmacology.

Positive-Pressure Ventilation. In judging the adequacy of ventilatory therapy in the pregnant patient, the physiologic changes in blood gases need to be considered, notably the decrease in arterial carbon dioxide tension. Hyperventilation with a resultant further decrease in carbon dioxide tension should probably be avoided, as hypocarbia adversely affects uterine blood flow and consequently the supply of oxygen to the fetus in experimental animals. However, in humans the danger is less conclusively established. Improvements in fetal pH have been noted with moderate hyperventilation, and reductions in fetal pH have been observed only in association with extreme hyperventilation with a reduction in maternal Pa_{CO_2} to levels of 2 kPa (17 mm Hg). Where pressure considerations permit, tidal volumes of 10 to 15 mL/kg should be used, and the ventilator rate adjusted to achieve an appropriate Pa_{CO_2}. The diminution in uterine blood flow associated with hyperventilation is probably multifactorial arising from both the hemodynamic consequences of positive-pressure ventilation and the acid-base changes. Complications of ventilation therapy in pregnant patients have been reported to be very common (81%), of which half are due to direct lung injury resulting in pneumothorax and pneumomediastinum.[48] Management of the adult respiratory distress syndrome (ARDS) in the pregnant patient is complicated by the preexisting reduction of FRC and by the increased oxygen demand of the patient. The anemia of pregnancy may further compromise oxygen delivery to both mother and fetus during intensive care management, in which positive-pressure ventilation may decrease cardiac output. The general trend in modern intensive care management is to minimize ventilatory pressures during positive-pressure ventilation, aiming at permissive hypercapnia rather than using excessively high inflation pressures to achieve normal carbon dioxide tensions. However, given the decreased chest wall compliance in the pregnant patient, it may be acceptable to allow a higher maximum plateau pressure in these patients and a figure of 35 cm H_2O has been regarded as acceptable in the ventilated, pregnant patient.[49]

Respiratory Infections. Drugs used to treat respiratory infections, including most antibiotics, appear to have little implication for fetal injury, with the exception of the tetracyclines, which should be used only if exceptional circumstances demand their administration. Question marks exist regarding some antibiotics including aminoglycosides and vancomycin, but these drugs should not be withheld when the clinical benefit to the mother, with possible improvement in fetal oxygen delivery, outweighs any potential risk. Acyclovir has been used in the treatment of varicella pneumonia in pregnancy without apparent harm to the fetus.

Asthma. The use of catecholamines in severe asthma is well established, and improvement in maternal ventilatory status in severe asthma probably outweighs the potential disadvantages to uterine blood flow, which are considered in more detail later under the management of hemodynamic problems. Corticosteroids have been widely used in the pregnant patient with asthma and are generally regarded as safe, whereas theophyllines should be regarded as secondary therapy only,[50] and may not have any benefit in terms of decreasing response times to therapy and shortening hospital stay.[51] In severe asthma, consideration may be given to the use of magnesium sulfate, which has been shown to enhance bronchodilatation and to improve weaning in asthmatic patients.[52] Interestingly, there is one report of severe asthma in a pregnant patient in the first trimester, in whom intractable bronchospasm improved markedly on termination of the pregnancy.[53]

Hemodynamic and Vascular Management

Uterine blood flow is, as noted previously, almost entirely passively dependent on maternal blood pressure and cardiac output; therefore, maintaining reasonable hemodynamic stability in the critically ill patient is clearly a major consideration for both mother and fetus. It is of particular concern in disease states in which hemodynamic disturbances are characteristic of the condition, notably Guillain-Barré syndrome, tetanus, and pheochromocytoma. In all of these diseases, the instability of the autonomic nervous system may produce dramatic swings in blood pressure together with arrhythmias. There have, however, been no detailed reports of the management of these conditions, as their occurrence in pregnancy is relatively rare. The use of magnesium sulfate for the control of the hemodynamic disturbances of both tetanus[54] and pheochromocytoma[55] has been well established, and this agent would be a logical choice in these conditions. It is possible that magnesium sulfate infusions may also be of value in managing the autonomic instability of Guillain-Barré syndrome, but there are no reports of its use in this condition.

Inotropic and Vasoactive Agents. Hemodynamic support of the pregnant patient raises the question of the safety of vasoactive and inotropic agents in this patient population. The first consideration must always depend on adequate volume replacement and patient position to avoid aortocaval compression before pharmacologic means of supporting the blood pressure are considered. A notable exception to this general rule is hypotension associated with amniotic fluid embolus, in which positive inotropic support is necessary from the outset. All of the commonly used catecholamines—epinephrine, norepinephrine, and dopamine—have been shown to decrease uterine blood flow in experimental animals, but dobutamine is more controversial with some studies suggesting that uterine blood flow may be increased during dobutamine infusion. Ephedrine is by far the most widely recommended of the catecholamines for the treatment of maternal hypotension and there is extensive experience with the use of this agent in the treatment of maternal hypotension associated with regional anesthesia. The use of the phosphodiesterase inhibitors is less clear. Amrinone has no beneficial effect on uterine blood flow in pregnant primates,[55a] and its use may be associated with cardiac arrhythmias and worsening hypoxia in a patient treated with this drug during pregnancy.[55b] There are no reports of the use of milrinone in obstetric patients.

Arrhythmias. The changes in autonomic, hemodynamic, and hormonal function in pregnancy may all predispose to the increased incidence of cardiac arrhythmias during pregnancy, but treatment of arrhythmias should be reserved for those with hemodynamic consequences.[56] Digoxin and quinidine have been extensively used in pregnancy without adverse effects on the fetus. Calcium channel blockers have been used recently in the management of preeclampsia with favorable results, although concerns have been expressed regarding their cardiovascular safety in combination with magnesium.[57, 58] However, other studies have failed to show significant interactions,[59] and the problem has been described as being more of a theoretic one.[60] The combination may, however, result in neuromuscular weakness.[61] Adenosine is effective in treating arrhythmias involving the atrioventricular node and has been successfully used in pregnancy to treat supraventricular tachycardia and Wolff-Parkinson-White syndrome. However, it can cause bronchospasm and should be avoided in patients with asthma. Disopyramide, lidocaine, and flecainide have all been used in pregnancy, but experience with these agents in the treatment of arrhythmias in pregnancy is limited. Disopyramide has been associated with induction of premature labor, and lidocaine may cause neonatal behavioral abnormalities. A number of concerns have been expressed regarding the safety of β-adrenergic blocking agents, including fetal hypotension and bradycardia, hypoglycemia, hyperbilirubinemia, and intrauterine growth retardation. The real risk of these complications has not been established, but it seems advisable to avoid long-term use of β-adrenergic blocking agents in cases of known intrauterine growth retardation.[56] Amiodarone has an extremely long half-life (>50 days) and carries risks of neonatal hypothyroidism. Its use should be reserved for the treatment of life-threatening arrhythmias unresponsive to other therapies.

Hypertension. The treatment of hypertension in pregnancy is extensively covered later in this chapter as well as in Chapter 38. Alphamethyl dopa has a long and established place in the management of hypertension in the pregnant patient, but the angiotensin-converting enzyme inhibitors should be avoided in pregnancy because they may lead to the development of renal dysfunction in the fetus. There are no reports of the use of angiotensin-II receptor blockers in pregnancy. In acute hypertensive crises, particularly those of endocrine origin, magnesium sulfate may be a very valuable agent. Its use in pheochromocytoma in pregnancy has been described,[55] and the management of pheochromocytoma in pregnancy has been recently reviewed.[62] Sodium nitroprusside is highly effective in controlling severe hypertension, but it does not improve uterine perfusion and carries risks of fetal toxicity and iatrogenic hypotension. It should be used for short-term control of hypertensive crises only when other options have been exhausted; if it is used, invasive monitoring is mandatory. Diazoxide is a powerful vasodilator, but it is no longer as popular as it once was, largely because of the uncontrollable nature of the hypotension that it occasionally causes, and the occasional maternal and neonatal hypoglycemia that may result.[63]

Cardiopulmonary Arrest. External cardiac massage is not as efficient in the pregnant patient, particularly in the third trimester, owing to caval compression impeding venous return and obstruction to massage caused by the engorged breasts. Lateral tilt improves the venous return, but it may cause difficulties with positioning of the patient and decreases the efficiency of chest compressions; left lateral manual displacement of the uterus may be preferable. The difficulties of ensuring venous return from the lower half of the body means that the femoral route should not be used for resuscitative drugs. If the fetus is viable, early delivery may produce good fetal outcome, as well as improving maternal survival. The decision must be made early, as the operation should be started within 4 to 5 minutes of arrest.

Coagulation. Pregnancy induces a hypercoagulable state, and this, coupled with venous stasis in the pelvic veins and legs, leads to an increased risk of venous thromboembolic disease in pregnancy. Pulmonary thromboembolism now accounts for 15% to 20% of maternal mortality. Patients with cardiac disease—notably those with atrial fibrillation and prosthetic cardiac valves—may require continuous anticoagulant therapy. Warfarin must be avoided during the first trimester, as severe fetal abnormalities are associated with exposure to the coumarin derivatives early in pregnancy; even in later pregnancy, the safety of warfarin is not fully established. Heparin has a long history of safety in pregnancy and should always be the first choice in the ICU, not only because of its lack of fetal effects, but also because it can be readily reversed should operative delivery become imperative. Prophylactic anticoagulation should always be considered in the critically ill pregnant patient, and low-dose heparin should be given to all pregnant patients in the ICU unless contraindicated. The dangers of a combination of low molecular weight heparins and regional anesthesia must be borne in mind when analgesia and operative delivery are considered. Other measures to limit the risk of deep venous thrombosis, including mobilization exercises and intermittent leg compression, should also be considered.

TRAUMA IN PREGNANCY

Trauma is one of the leading causes of nonobstetric death in women of reproductive age and occurs in 6% to 7% of all pregnancies,[64] although less than 1% of all pregnant women require hospitalization for trauma-related injuries.[42] Motor vehicle injuries account for the majority of major injuries, with assault and falls being the next most common, possibly because of the anatomic and physiologic changes in pregnancy interfering with coordination and balance. The mortality secondary to trauma among pregnant women is not greater than that seen in the nonpregnant population, but there is significant risk to the fetus, with fetal death exceeding maternal mortality by between three- and ninefold.[65] Hemorrhage and head injury account for the majority of maternal fatalities, while fetal death is associated with maternal hemodynamic shock, maternal head injury, pelvic fractures, and hypoxemia. Maternal tolerance of blood loss is probably increased by the physiologic changes in pregnancy, particularly the expanded blood volume. However, the compensatory mechanisms invoked by hemorrhage may delay the overt manifestations of shock until severe hemodynamic decompensation occurs, with catastrophic results for the fetus. Since uterine blood flow is markedly affected by catecholamines, physiologic responses to stress and trauma may result in excessive reductions in uterine blood flow, despite adequately maintained maternal arterial pressures. As in other causes of ICU admission, scoring systems devised for the nonpregnant state do not accurately predict either maternal or fetal outcome.[66]

General Principles. Resuscitation should follow normal trauma guidelines, with particular emphasis on airway protection and adequate ventilation, given the poor tolerance for even brief periods of inadequate ventilation in the pregnant state. Airway management consideration must include an awareness of the increased aspiration risk in the pregnant patient. Nasal intubation, if absolutely necessary, must be performed with great care because of the increased vascularity of airway mucous membranes. Aggressive fluid resuscitation of the injured mother should be undertaken, bearing in mind the increased blood volume and elevated cardiac output in the pregnant state. Every effort should be made to ensure support of the fetal circulation without resort to inotropic or vasoconstrictor agents. Maternal position is crucial, and the supine position should be avoided if at all possible to minimize the risks of aortocaval compression.

Uterine Injury. The gravid uterus renders the pregnant woman uniquely susceptible to intra-abdominal injuries with blunt abdominal trauma. As gestation advances, the uterus becomes progressively more susceptible to trauma, and the uterus itself may pose a risk to other intra-abdominal organs, particularly the urinary bladder. Uterine rupture is fortunately rare, occurring in less than 1% of all cases of maternal trauma. Where uterine rupture does occur, the consequences are grave, with maternal mortality of the order of 10% and fetal mortality approaching 100%. Even without uterine rupture, uterine distortion associated with severe trauma may result in placental separation, owing to the relatively inelastic nature of the placenta compared with the uterus. This can lead to fetomaternal hemorrhage caused by transplacental transfer of blood from the fetus to the mother. This results in fetal anemia, and FHR abnormalities. Fetal death may result from hypoxia aggravated by the development of fetal anemia. Transplacental hemorrhage can be detected by the Kleihauer-Betke test, which identifies the presence of fetal hemoglobin in the maternal circulation. Fetomaternal hemorrhage in the presence of Rhesus incompatibility may lead to maternal sensitization, and Rh immune globulin should be considered for all Rh D–negative women suffering this complication. Abruptio placentae is usually diagnosed clinically when massive placental separation has taken place. Small, concealed episodes of retroplacental bleeding are more likely to present with pain and uterine irritability, detectable by means of cardiotocography. Ultrasound is useful in the diagnosis of premature rupture of the membranes leading to the loss of amniotic fluid, although clinical examination is usually sufficient to establish the diagnosis. Close monitoring of fetal well-being is essential, as early delivery of a viable fetus may offer the best outcome for both mother and child.

As pregnancy advances, the uterus becomes particularly vulnerable to penetrating abdominal injury, which has been associated with perinatal mortality rates of up to 50%.[67] However, upper abdominal injuries may be associated with severe visceral injuries to bowel, liver, and spleen. Conservative management of abdominal penetration may be considered if the following criteria are satisfied: (1) stable maternal vital signs and (2) no evidence of fetal distress in the case of a viable fetus.[67] If exploratory laparotomy is undertaken, simple uterine closure is usually sufficient for simple penetrating wounds of the uterus. Each individual case must be judged on its merits, and generalizations are difficult to make.

Burns. Burn injury in pregnancy represents a major hazard to both mother and fetus. Major burns in which more than 10% of the body surface area (BSA) is burned are further classified into moderate (10–19% BSA), severe (20–39% BSA), and critical (>40% BSA). The severity of the burn injury is also determined by the depth of the burn, the site of the injury (face, hands, or perineum increasing the severity rating) and associated injuries, particularly pulmonary damage. The pregnancy is at risk because of an increased chance of spontaneous abortion and because of intrauterine death. The former is thought to be partly due to increased uterine activity as a consequence of the high levels of prostaglandins found in burned patients. The source of these prostaglandins is the increased release of phospholipase A from burned tissue, leading to increased breakdown of arachidonic acid and prostaglandin production.[68] Fetal death may be due to decreased uterine perfusion secondary to shock, or it may be due to hypoxia secondary to maternal hypoxemia as a result of pulmonary injury, ARDS, or increased oxygen demand caused by the burn. The outcome of critically burned obstetric patients is poor for both mother and fetus, with maternal mortality in the range of 60% being reported and fetal loss of up to 100%.

Severe burns in pregnancy require immediate, aggressive fluid resuscitation as needed, and the Parkland Hospital formula is often used. In this regimen, Ringer's lactate is administered at a rate of 4 mL/kg/BSA burn over the first 24 hours, with half given in the first 8 hours and the remainder over the next 16 hours. It is imperative that normal maternal hemodynamics be maintained together with objective signs of adequate tissue perfusion, such as urine output, which should be sustained around 0.5 to 1.0 mL/kg/h. Oxygen administration during the resuscitation phase is advisable. FHR monitoring should be undertaken to detect early evidence of fetal compromise. Carbon monoxide poisoning may affect the fetus to a greater extent than the mother, as fetal hemoglobin has an even higher affinity for carbon monoxide. Suspected carbon monoxide inhalation should be treated with 100% oxygen with positive-pressure ventilation if necessary, and hyperbaric oxygen may be considered if the intoxication is severe (carboxyhemoglobin levels >20%, neurologic changes in the mother, or overt fetal distress).[64] Early tangential wound excision and grafting within the first 3 to 7 days after the injury has been associated with improved maternal and fetal survival.[69] In the early stages of gestation, tocolysis may be considered to control preterm labor, but it should not be embarked on in the presence of maternal sepsis or placental abruption.[68] In cases in which the fetus is viable, early delivery is advocated and has been associated with excellent maternal and fetal survival, even in critical burns.[70] As in other forms of injury, consideration must be given to maternal positioning in the ICU, and the supine position should be avoided whenever possible. Wound dressings should not contain povidone-iodine, as the iodine can be extensively absorbed and adversely affect fetal thyroid function.

PREECLAMPSIA

Definition. Preeclampsia is recognized as a reversible clinical syndrome characterized by sustained hypertension (diastolic pressure >90 mm Hg) and proteinuria (>300 mg/24 h) during the latter half of pregnancy. Delivery of the fetus always secures remission of the disease.[71]

The features that define preeclampsia may be the only clinical manifestations of the syndrome. The disease may, however, present as a syndrome of multiorgan failure (including neurologic, renal, liver, hematologic, cardiorespiratory, and fetoplacental abnormalities). Other clinical features such as seizures and renal failure may overshadow hypertension and proteinuria in these patients, although the latter markers of the disease are invariably present.

Incidence and Contribution to Mortality Statistics. Preeclampsia affects 2% to 6% of pregnant women. The peak incidence is among women in their first pregnancy, while chronic hypertension, diabetes, antiphospholipid syndrome, multiple pregnancy, and gestational trophoblastic disease are all independent risk factors for the development of preeclampsia.[72, 73]

Preeclampsia is among the leading causes of maternal mortality in both the developing and the developed world.[72–77] In South Africa the initial reports arising from a statutory confidential enquiry into maternal deaths identified hypertensive disease as the single most common obstetric cause of death among South African women.[8] The last published British *Report on Confidential Enquiries into Maternal Deaths* ranked hypertensive deaths as the second most common problem in the United Kingdom.[7] Disturbingly, both the South African and the British reports noted that 80% of these deaths were associated with substandard care and were potentially avoidable.

Eclampsia with or without evidence of intracranial hemorrhage is the single most lethal complication of preeclampsia/eclampsia. Deaths have also been associated with pulmonary edema, hemolysis, elevated liver enzymes, and low platelets (HELLP) syndrome, renal failure, and the development of hypovolemia (commonly caused by concurrent abruptio placentae; rarely it occurs as a result of a ruptured liver hematoma).[8]

Pathophysiology. The pathogenesis of preeclampsia is incompletely understood. Genetic predisposition is implicated, and women whose mothers or siblings have developed eclampsia are at increased risk themselves.[78–82] Those who develop the disease follow a hierarchical pathophysiologic pattern, with the earliest anatomic changes being evident in the blood vessels of the placental bed. These vessels normally dilate after the 16th week of pregnancy as a result of trophoblastic invasion. In preeclamptic women the vessels fail to dilate and develop additional forms of pathology, the most characteristic of which is acute atherosis.[83–86] This lesion is analogous to atherosclerosis and gives rise to partial luminal obstruction of the artery by lipid-laden myointimal cells. Simultaneously there may be evidence of endothelial perturbation and altered vascular reactivity; these events precede the clinical disease. The second phase consists of clinical disease in which hypertension, proteinuria, and intrauterine fetal growth restriction become evident. Biochemically, these patients have persistent evidence of deranged endothelial and platelet function manifesting in numerous ways.[87–93] Impaired prostacyclin production with augmented release of a host of vasoconstrictors (including platelet-derived thromboxane, endothelin, serotonin, and possibly catecholamines) leads to a rising peripheral vascular resistance.[88–92] Endothelial perturbation triggers the expression of cell adhesion molecules that interact with activated leukocytes and platelets.[94–96] Platelet turnover increases and may develop into overt thrombocytopenia in some patients. The activated platelets release a range of cytokines that mediate intravascular coagulation, manifesting as increasing levels of circulating thrombin–antithrombin III complexes, falling antithrombin III levels, and increased levels of fibrin degradation products.[25, 97] Although the clinical disease may follow a largely indolent course, the third phase of the disease is recognized by the development of fulminant multiorgan failure.

Multiorgan failure in severe preeclampsia can be attributed to widespread ischemia. Postmortem studies reveal evidence of vascular injury (commonly fibrinoid necrosis), hemorrhage, and ischemic necrosis in the liver, brain, kidney, and placenta.[98–103] Widespread vascular injury is associated with the development of interstitial edema. This leads to intravascular dehydration, intensified peripheral vasospasm, and diminished cardiac output. The rate of oxygen delivery to the peripheral tissues is critically low in acute severe preeclampsia and aggravates diminished perfusion through the damaged vasculature.[104–106]

Clinical Presentation. Most women suffering from preeclampsia have non–life-threatening disease that resolves on delivery. Severe disease needs to be carefully characterized, and those patients deserve close attention. The need for intensive care is evident from the maternal mortality reports that highlight eclampsia, pulmonary complications, HELLP syndrome, and renal failure as the leading causes of death.[7, 8]

Eclampsia. Eclampsia is defined as the occurrence of generalized tonic-clonic epileptiform seizures in a pregnant patient with proteinuric hypertension. Most seizures occur before delivery, although 40% of those who have a seizure do so within the first 24 hours postpartum. Late postpartum eclampsia, an unusual entity, has also been described and is the occurrence of seizure activity between 48 hours and 4 weeks after delivery.[107–109] Eclampsia may be preceded by prodromal symptoms: typically headaches and visual disturbances (blurred vision, photopsia, scotomata, and diplopia).[110, 111] The blood pressure at the time of seizure activity varies. Patients may initially have a seizure with blood pressure that is mildly elevated or even normal.[112] More commonly they have moderate to severe hypertension. The seizure itself is associated with a surge in blood pressure and a fall in peripheral oxygen saturation during the tonic-clonic phase. The occurrence of severe hypertension has been clearly linked to the risk of cerebrovascular hemorrhage.[113]

The differential diagnosis of seizure activity in pregnancy is extensive and ranges from the obvious (epilepsy) to rare but important conditions that include systemic lupus erythematosus, thrombotic thrombocytopenic purpura, amniotic fluid embolus, cerebral venous thrombosis, malaria, and cocaine intoxication.[114–117]

Pulmonary Complications. Pulmonary complications frequently lead to critical care admission. They include the development of upper airway edema, pulmonary edema, and aspiration pneumonia. Patients with severe preeclampsia are predisposed to the development of pulmonary edema because of low oncotic pressure, leaky capillaries, and left ventricular dysfunction. Rapid plasma volume expansion has been shown repeatedly to cause a sharp rise in left-sided filling pressures, often without any changes in central venous pressure. This rise occurs despite evidence of normal systolic ventricular function and is a reflection of reduced ventricular compliance during diastole. Diastolic dysfunction cannot be detected in the absence of invasive monitoring and is therefore often ignored by attending physicians. Consequently, iatrogenic fluid overload (even with small amounts of fluid) is a frequent cause of pulmonary edema among these patients.

Occasionally patients present with evidence of cardiomyopathy, although this is not typical of the disease and may be indistinguishable from other forms of pulmonary edema without echocardiography or invasive monitoring. Occult valvular disease may also precipitate pulmonary edema in pregnancies complicated by hypertension.

Atelectasis may occur in the critically ill preeclamptic patient, either postoperatively or among patients with HELLP syndrome, who often splint the right hemidiaphragm because of pain associated with subdiaphragmatic pathology. Aspiration pneumonia must also be considered in the differential diagnosis of any woman with eclampsia who develops respiratory distress.

Adult respiratory distress syndrome (ARDS) is often cited as a complication of preeclampsia. This is unlikely to be a primary complication of the disease but may follow aspiration pneumonia or prolonged ventilation. Mabie and coworkers[48] reported the occurrence of ARDS in an obstetric intensive care unit. Over a 6-year period, 16 cases of respiratory distress attributable to ARDS were diagnosed (having excluded fluid overload and left ventricular dysfunction). Four of these 16 cases were linked to preeclampsia/eclampsia. Three of these 4 cases had additional complications that may have contributed to the development of ARDS (including aspiration pneumonia, lupus nephritis, sepsis, and a ruptured liver hematoma with massive blood transfusion). The fourth case had pulmonary edema that developed into ARDS after the patient experienced a respiratory arrest.

Laryngeal edema may be present in severe preeclampsia at the time of first presentation or may develop during the course of the disease. It is of particular importance in relation to the decisions that need to be made concerning anesthesia for delivery, as well as the need for postoperative ventilation in patients having general anesthesia.

HELLP Syndrome. First described by Weinstein[101] in 1982, this syndrome consists of a subset of patients with preeclampsia who develop hepatic ischemia giving rise to periportal hemorrhage and necrosis. They also have evidence of microangiopathic hemolytic anemia and thrombocytopenia. Hence the mnemonic, HELLP standing for: *h*emolysis, *e*levated *l*iver enzymes, and *l*ow *p*latelets. These patients often complain of epigastric pain which, in the setting of mild hypertension, may be mistaken for dyspepsia. Patients with severe HELLP syndrome are usually very obviously ill: they may have associated renal failure (characterized by rising urea, creatinine, and the passage of small quantities of blood-stained or cola-colored urine) and are at increased risk for seizures.

The differential diagnosis of hepatic derangement in pregnancy extends to include conditions that may mimic preeclampsia, such as thrombotic thrombocytopenic purpura and acute fatty liver of pregnancy.[118, 119] Obstetric cholestasis and viral hepatitis may enter the differential in milder cases of HELLP syndrome. Distinguishing between these conditions may be difficult, but the hallmark of preeclamptic disease is that it resolves after delivery.[120]

A rare but serious complication of the HELLP syndrome is the development of a subcapsular liver hematoma. The surface of the liver in HELLP syndrome generally shows evidence of multiple petechial hemorrhages. These lesions may enlarge and become confluent. A ruptured hematoma may be associated with right upper quadrant pain and sudden hypovolemia.

Renal Complications. The renal pathology that gives rise to renal failure includes intrinsic renal abnormalities, typically characterized by the lesion of glomerular capillary endotheliosis.[102] This condition is one in which the glomeruli are partially obstructed by lipid-laden mesangial cells. Prerenal ischemia caused by a combination of vasospasm and low cardiac output creates a cycle of ischemia that may end in acute tubular necrosis. Those patients most susceptible to acute tubular necrosis are those who have underlying preeclamptic changes with superimposed hypovolemia caused by abruptio placentae or ruptured subcapsular liver hematoma. Hemoglobinuria from patients with the HELLP syndrome may also give rise to renal impairment.

The presentation of renal impairment in acute severe preeclampsia is commonly that of oliguria with or without hematuria. However, while perinatal mortality associated with maternal renal failure is high, the prognosis of the mother with renal failure associated with preeclampsia is remarkably good. In a local study of renal failure in gestational proteinuric hypertension, perinatal mortality was 45% (33 of 73 patients). However, although 7 women (10%) required dialysis in the short term, none required long-term dialysis or kidney transplant and there were no maternal deaths (AJ Drakeley, P Le Roux, J Penny, J Anthony, personal communication, 1999). In another study, perinatal mortality was 40%, but maternal mortality from pregnancy-related renal failure was less than 2% (1 of 57 patients).[121]

Principles of Management. A few general critical care principles of management apply to the management of all preeclamptic women. Severe preeclampsia is an ischemic condition, partially correctable by hemodynamic manipulation.[122] Plasma volume expansion and vasodilatation are generic to all other specific interventions. The other sine qua non of management is that all forms of severe preeclampsia are reversible on delivery of the fetus.

Plasma Volume Expansion. Restoration of the circulating plasma volume increases ventricular filling pressures, stroke volume, and cardiac output.[105, 122] It also accelerates the rate of oxygen delivery to the peripheral tissues. Plasma volume expansion by itself decreases systemic vascular resistance, although blood pressure is unlikely to fall because the cardiac output rises simultaneously. Small amounts of fluid (300 mL) may be used as a fluid challenge in patients with evidence of oliguria or as a prelude to vasodilatation. Left ventricular diastolic dysfunction complicates fluid management in severe preeclampsia, and central venous pressure monitoring is misleading. Blind fluid challenges should be limited, and any patient with severe disease needing more than two fluid challenges should be considered a candidate for invasive hemodynamic monitoring.

Vasodilatation. Vasodilatation may be imperative among patients with severe hypertension who are at risk for cerebrovascular hemorrhage (mean arterial pressures >140 mm Hg). Vasodilatation at less severe levels of hypertension may increase perfusion, providing plasma volume expansion takes place either before or during vasodilatation. Without plasma volume expansion, vasodilatation alone may increase the risk of oliguric renal failure and fetal distress because intravascular dehydration precludes an adequate increase in cardiac output as the vessels dilate.

Many drugs have been used as vasodilators. They include

1. Hydralazine. Hydralazine is an effective direct-acting vasodilator infused in normal saline at a rate of 2.5 to 7.5 mg/h after an initial loading dose of 5 to 10 mg. The tachycardia that commonly follows the administration of hydralazine is usually a result of an inadequate preload, although there are reports of increased levels of norepinephrine associated with the administration of the drug. Although hydralazine is an old drug, it is effective and free from adverse drug interactions.
2. Calcium channel blockers. Dihydropyridine calcium channel blockers, such as nifedipine, are effective vasodilators and have a rapid onset of action. Hypotensive episodes can result from an inadequate preload, although drug interactions, especially between nifedipine and magnesium sulfate, are described in several anecdotal reports.[57, 61] These episodes may reflect the negative inotropic properties of both drugs, although individual susceptibility based on impaired left ventricular function probably also plays a role.

   Nimodipine, a second-generation dihydropyridine calcium channel blocker used to prevent ischemic neurologic deficit in patients with subarachnoid hemorrhage, has been used in the management of a small number of women with eclampsia.[123–126] Because it acts as a vasodilator and inhibitor of calcium transport in neuronal tissue, it may have anticonvulsant properties. Insufficient data exist to justify the use of nimodipine for this indication, although a randomized study is in progress.

3. Labetalol. Intravenous labetalol has combined α- and β-blocking properties. The mechanism of action (in the doses commonly required to reduce blood pressure) is that of negative chronotropism. The use of labetalol should be confined to the treatment of patients who have hypertension on the basis of a high cardiac output.[127] One group has reported a reduction in the incidence of ventricular arrhythmias in patients treated with labetalol; ventricular arrhythmias are, however, rarely observed clinically.[128]
4. Other drugs. Nitroglycerin, an arteriolar dilator and venodilator, diminishes venous return leading to a fall in left ventricular preload and may be specifically indicated in the management of pulmonary edema. Potent antihypertensive drugs such as sodium nitroprusside are virtually never required in the management of severe preeclampsia.[129]

Specific Aspects of Management

Eclampsia. Prevention of recurrent seizures, control of the airway to prevent aspiration pneumonia, control of severe hypertension, and termination of the pregnancy constitute the main therapeutic goals in the treatment of eclampsia.

Seizure Prophylaxis. The drug of choice for seizure prophylaxis is magnesium sulfate. Randomized evidence clearly demonstrates a significantly lower risk of recurrent seizures when magnesium sulfate is compared with phenytoin and benzodiazepines used for the same indication.[130–132] Magnesium sulfate is a weak calcium channel blocker that also regulates intracellular calcium flux through the *N*-methyl-D-aspartate receptor in neuronal tissue and may inhibit ischemic neuronal damage brought about by anion flux through this receptor.[133–135] Parenterally administered magnesium may result in systemic vasodilatation and improved cardiac output as well as cerebral vasodilatation distal to the middle cerebral artery. Retinal artery vasospasm has been reversed by magnesium sulfate infusion.[136–138] The myocardial effects of parenteral magnesium include slowing of the cardiac conduction times; in high doses magnesium is significantly negatively inotropic.[139, 140] Intravenous magnesium sulfate reduces serum calcium levels, possibly as a result of increased renal magnesium and calcium excretion.[141, 142] Falling serum calcium levels inhibit acetylcholine release at the motor end plate, the extent of which is directly related to the level of the serum magnesium and inversely proportional to the calcium concentration.[143, 144] This inhibition of acetylcholine release is the origin of magnesium sulfate toxicity that can lead to neuromuscular blockade and respiratory arrest.[145, 146] The therapeutic level of serum magnesium remains controversial; higher serum levels of magnesium may be associated with greater anticonvulsant efficacy but also greater toxicity.

The Collaborative Eclampsia Trial regimen of a 4-g loading dose followed by a constant infusion of 1 g/h was shown to be effective and safe. The kidney excretes magnesium sulfate, and impaired renal function should alert the clinician to the possibility of toxicity, even with low-dosage regimens. Magnesium sulfate (even at therapeutic levels) may give rise to weakness in patients with myasthenia gravis and other neuromuscular disorders, whose diseases are unmasked by the drug.[147]

Patients who experience recurrent seizures despite magnesium sulfate are best managed by intubation and ventilation while sedated by a continuous high-dose benzodiazepine or thiopental infusion. These patients may have cerebral edema, and care should be taken to maintain a mean arterial pressure in excess of 100 mm Hg in order to preserve cerebral blood flow in the face of raised intracranial pressure.[148]

Control of the Airway. Postural control together with suctioning the airway is an important first aid measure. Recognition of the need for ventilatory care is the next priority. Patients who have recurrent seizures or persistent postictal coma are better managed by endotracheal intubation and elective ventilation in order to protect the airway. Ventilatory care should be maintained for a minimum of 24 hours postpartum, until the patient is fully conscious and upper airway edema has resolved. Patients with upper airway edema who require endotracheal intubation for any reason should not be extubated until there is clear evidence that the laryngeal edema has resolved. The latter should be established by testing the patient's ability to breathe past the deflated cuff of the obstructed tube.

Control of Blood Pressure. Severe hypertension increases the risk of hypertensive encephalopathy. Cerebral edema and raised intracranial pressure increase the risk of cerebral ischemia when the perfusion pressure falls below 100 mm Hg. Control of blood pressure is imperative, but iatrogenic hypotension must be avoided.[148]

Obstetric Management. The mode of delivery is an empiric obstetric decision. Vaginal delivery may be contemplated providing the patient has no complicating features other than a single seizure. Induction of labor should not be protracted, and an arbitrary time limit should be set to attain a vaginal delivery.[149]

Renal Failure. Prerenal ischemia commonly gives rise to oliguria (a urine output of <30 mL/h). Providing that the patient is not already in positive fluid balance, plasma volume expansion should be attempted. If two fluid challenges fail to improve the urinary output, low-dose dopamine should be commenced at an infusion rate of 1 to 5 μg/kg/min. Low-dose dopamine (1–5 μg/kg/min) is thought to act as a selective renal artery vasodilator. Although of questionable benefit in general critical care, several randomized studies have demonstrated efficacy of low-dose dopamine without adverse effects in the oliguric preeclamptic patient.[150, 151]

Patients who fail to respond to either of these measures require more intensive monitoring. Pulmonary artery catheters are a useful adjunct in securing optimum ventricular preload and afterload.[152] The volume-replete vasodilated patient who remains oliguric has intrinsic renal pathology, usually acute tubular necrosis. A single large dose of furosemide (0.5–1.0 g intravenously) may convert these patients to high-output renal failure. Should this measure also fail, care must be taken to avoid fluid overload and the patient should be prepared for dialysis.[129]

ACUTE LUNG INJURY. Patients who present with respiratory distress are frequently a diagnostic challenge. In cases in which the diagnosis remains in doubt after clinical examination and special investigation, echocardiography or pulmonary artery catheterization is indicated.

Pulmonary edema must be managed according to the hemodynamic findings.[153, 154] In the absence of iatrogenic fluid overload, afterload reduction may be the most important aspect of management.

The development of localized lung signs and purulent sputum should alert the clinician to the possibility of aspiration pneumonia. Radiologic findings may vary from normal lung fields to unilateral shadowing, atelectasis, and collapse. Bronchoscopy may be necessary if aspiration of particulate matter is suspected. Treatment with broad-spectrum (including anaerobic) antibiotic coverage is the keystone to management.

HELLP SYNDROME. The management of HELLP syndrome is primarily obstetric. The complications associated with HELLP syndrome (renal failure, eclampsia, and respiratory distress) may independently necessitate critical care. Clinically significant metabolic and hematologic aberrations are unusual in uncomplicated HELLP syndrome. Hypoglycemia may occur in some cases but is more characteristic of acute fatty liver of pregnancy (which may be confused with HELLP syndrome). Coagulopathy is equally uncommon. Thrombocytopenia and impaired platelet function can both give rise to surgically impaired coagulation. Prolonged partial thromboplastin times and International Normalized Ratios (INRs) are more likely to occur in association with acute fatty liver than with HELLP syndrome.

Delivery always cures HELLP syndrome. The thrombocytopenia should attain a nadir within 72 hours of delivery.[120] Persistent thrombocytopenia should lead to a search for sepsis or folate deficiency. If no such cause can be found for persistent thrombocytopenia, the original diagnosis must be reconsidered. Thrombotic thrombocytopenic purpura and systemic lupus erythematosus are two of the main differential diagnoses.[119]

THE HYPOVOLEMIC PATIENT. Hypovolemia complicates preeclampsia commonly as a result of abruptio placentae, occasionally as a result of obstetric hemorrhage, and rarely following rupture of a subcapsular liver hematoma. It is a particular challenge because the preeclamptic patient may already have impaired peripheral oxygenation, now further diminished by decreasing cardiac output. Resuscitation is rendered difficult by the preeclamptic patient's predisposition to develop pulmonary edema. Yet the coincident occurrence of hypovolemia and preeclampsia as a cause of maternal mortality cannot be ignored. These patients therefore should be identified as critically ill mothers who will benefit from adequate resuscitation under the appropriate guidance of invasive hemodynamic monitoring.

ANESTHETIC CONSIDERATIONS. Many critically ill patients who have preeclampsia require operative delivery. The choice of anesthesia is influenced by the specific circumstance.[155] With regard to general anesthesia the hypertensive surge associated with endotracheal intubation is undesirable in women already severely hypertensive, and the possibility of failed intubation also exists, especially in relation to patients with upper airway edema following eclamptic seizures. Regional anesthesia presents theoretic difficulty with the measurement of preload in patients who already have impaired peripheral oxygenation. Other concerns may arise from coagulopathy and thrombocytopenia.

Failed intubation remains a dominant concern and regional anesthesia (despite the potential problems and in the absence of randomized trials) remains the first-choice method of anesthesia. General anesthesia is nevertheless indicated in patients with eclampsia and in those who have a demonstrable coagulopathy. Patients with platelet counts of less than 100,000/L should be investigated further for their coagulation status before regional anesthesia is attempted. The pressor response to intubation has been controlled by the use of a bolus dose of magnesium sulfate either alone or in combination with alfentanil given immediately after induction.[156, 157] Remifentanil may also be valuable in this situation, but no studies currently exist.

MISCELLANEOUS CONDITIONS

There are a number of conditions requiring intensive care in which little difference occurs in the management between pregnant and nonpregnant patients. These conditions are outlined briefly with an emphasis on those aspects relevant to pregnancy management.

Thrombotic Thrombocytopenic Purpura. Thrombotic thrombocytopenic purpura (TTP) is a condition of relevance to obstetric intensivists because it constitutes one of the principal differential diagnoses of HELLP syndrome.[158]

TTP is part of a spectrum of microangiopathic conditions that includes hemolytic uremic syndrome (HUS). There is no clear distinction between these entities, although TTP may occur during pregnancy whereas HUS is more likely to occur 6 weeks to 6 months postpartum. TTP presents with a clinical pentad of features: microangiopathic hemolytic anemia, fever, neurologic disturbance, renal impairment, and thrombocytopenia are all prerequisite to the diagnosis. The neurologic features of the syndrome may be transitory and may present only during the clinical course of the disease. Mild hypertension and proteinuria may make the condition clinically indistinguishable from HELLP syndrome. The response of the two conditions to delivery differs. Whereas HELLP syndrome invariably resolves, delivery has no effect on the clinical course of TTP. Other diagnostic features that may help to distinguish between the two conditions include evidence of marked hemolysis on examination of the peripheral blood smear (this is more characteristic of TTP than HELLP).

Without appropriate management TTP has a high mortality rate. Treatment consists of plasmapheresis, infusion of fresh-frozen plasma, and high-dose steroids.

Acute Fatty Liver of Pregnancy. Acute fatty liver of pregnancy (AFLP) is a condition of the third trimester characterized by microvesicular fatty infiltration of the liver.[158] The incidence of the disease is increasing, probably as a result of increased surveillance and the identification of milder cases. The quoted incidence is approximately 1 in 12,000 deliveries. Mortality rates are also falling because of improvements in critical care and because of the inclusion of milder cases in statistical records. Mortality rates are currently below 20%.[118, 159]

The severity of AFLP varies, with some patients presenting with mild right upper quadrant discomfort associated with prodromal nausea and vomiting. Others rapidly develop fulminant liver failure leading to coma. The development of a depressed level of consciousness may be attributed to either hypoglycemia or the onset of hepatic encephalopathy. The former complication is a particularly common feature of AFLP and should alert the clinician to the possible diagnosis. More than 50% of affected patients have symptoms and signs attributable to preeclampsia (hypertension and proteinuria), which may make the distinction from HELLP syndrome difficult. Jaundice is often present at the time of diagnosis.

Liver enzymes are elevated with transaminases elevated severalfold, although values above 1000 IU/L may occur in severe cases. Hematologically, patients with AFLP have deranged coagulation. Prolonged partial thromboplastin time and INR along with microangiopathic hemolytic anemia are all consistent with the diagnosis. Neutrophil leukocytosis and elevated levels of fibrin degradation products as a result of disseminated intravascular coagulation may all be present.

Management principles revolve around delivery and supportive therapy. Delivery should be effected as rapidly as possible, once the diagnosis has been established. Underlying coagulopathy may complicate operative delivery, and regional anesthesia is contraindicated. Standard supportive therapy includes maintenance of the blood glucose level, correction of the coagulopathy, the use of lactulose to limit the effects of intestinal bacteria, and the administration of vitamin K to mother and baby. Intubation and ventilation may become necessary in the comatose mother who cannot protect her airway.

Associated complications that may develop include renal failure and pancreatitis; these conditions need to be treated accordingly.

Amniotic Fluid Embolus. This is a rare but lethal condition in which the mother develops an anaphylactoid response to the presence of amniotic fluid in the circulation. It has been suggested that the name is a misnomer and that the syndrome is more appropriately named the "anaphylactoid syndrome of pregnancy."[117]

The clinical syndrome is diagnosed every 1 in 8000 to 1 in 80,000 pregnancies. Owing to the rarity of the condition, a national registry of cases was opened in the United States; this remains the most authoritative single source of information about this condition.[117]

The condition usually presents during labor but may occur during cesarean delivery. Rarely, it can manifest immediately after birth. There are no known demographic predisposing factors and the onset of the syndrome bears no relationship to the route of delivery or other obstetric determinants, such as prior amniotomy and oxytocin administration. The onset of the syndrome is usually abrupt. Hypotension is universally present and almost all patients develop pulmonary edema with cyanosis. The other cardinal clinical feature is the development of profound coagulopathy, which should immediately alert the attending obstetrician to the diagnosis. Approximately 50% of patients develop seizures, although seizures are the single most common presenting symptom in patients who develop amniotic fluid embolus before delivery of the fetus. There is a high risk of cardiopulmonary arrest.

The pathophysiology of amniotic fluid embolus is poorly understood but appears to be immunologically mediated and bears a striking resemblance to anaphylactic or septic shock. Hemodynamically, affected patients all have markedly impaired left ventricular function.[160]

These patients have a very poor prognosis. In the American national registry, 61% of the patients died and only 15% survived neurologically intact. Diagnosis therefore must be prompt; resuscitation invariably needs to be commenced in situ (usually the labor ward or operating room suite). Inotropic support must be introduced early (by implication, the attending physicians need to recognize that hypotension is related to both hypovolemia and left ventricular failure). Massive, continuous transfusion may be necessary to control bleeding related to coagulopathy. Obstetric intervention in the form of hysterectomy may be necessary to control bleeding in patients undergoing cesarean section. Intubation and ventilation along with pulmonary artery catheterization are essential adjuncts to intensive care management.

Obstetric Hemorrhage. This occurs as a result of bleeding from the placental site or as a consequence of trauma to the genital tract. The latter includes uterine rupture and lower genital tract injuries associated with childbirth. Severe antepartum hemorrhage is managed by delivery, while postpartum bleeding is likely to require a range of pharmacologic and surgical interventions.

The obstetric patient in shock is resuscitated, using blood component therapy, as for any other hypovolemic intensive care patient. Abruptio placentae presents a special challenge because the coagulopathy is the result of blood loss as well as of the release of thromboplastin from the placental bed. This gives rise to disseminated intravascular coagulation. Patients may develop hypertension, proteinuria, and renal failure indistinguishable from preeclampsia. Preeclamptic patients are also at increased risk for developing abruptio placentae and are especially susceptible to the effects of hypovolemia. If there is doubt about the diagnosis, the patient should be managed as if she had preeclampsia, with fluid management, monitoring, and seizure prophylaxis for preeclampsia instituted.

The pharmacologic control of postpartum hemorrhage from the placental bed after delivery depends on the use of a range of oxytocic drugs. Oxytocin can be administered as an infusion of 20 U in a liter of saline; parenteral ergonovine may also be used (0.5 mg), although caution should be exercised in hypertensive patients because ergonovine may induce contraction of vascular smooth muscle. Prostaglandin $F_{2\alpha}$ may be administered directly into the uterus by transabdominal injection. This drug may cause both vasospasm and bronchospasm if administered intravenously, and care should be taken to restrict the dose to a total of 3 to 4 mg without any intravenous extravasation. Misoprostol has been suggested as an oxytocic agent for the control of postpartum hemorrhage (600 μg orally). Insufficient evidence currently exists to allow any recommendation that this drug should be routinely used, although it may constitute a final option, prior to surgery, in cases in which other treatments have failed.

The timing and the mode of surgical intervention are a question of individual obstetric judgment. The need to conserve reproductive function may dictate a progressive surgical approach that begins with stepwise devascularization of the uterus, proceeding to internal iliac artery ligation and ultimately hysterectomy. Interventional radiologic techniques such as internal iliac artery embolization may also play a role in management.

❖ **CONCLUSION** Pregnant women sometimes become critically ill and require intensive care. This chapter has focused on care of the mother and has largely ignored the issue of obstetric judgment and surgical intervention that more often than not attends the management of these patients. The responsibility for care of these women must be multidisciplinary and the argument in favor of dedicated obstetric intensive care units is founded on these considerations. It is likely that these ICUs are viable only in centers that serve a very large obstetric population or that have a large referral network. Because obstetric ICUs are likely to remain uncommon, physicians practicing general intensive care medicine have to remain cognizant of pregnancy and its influence on the principles of critical care management.

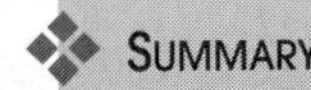

SUMMARY

Key Points

- Critical care of the obstetric patient requires good teamwork between obstetricians, critical care specialists, and anesthesiologists.
- The management of critical illness in obstetrics requires a knowledge of the physiology of pregnancy, an understanding of the pathology of the disease process, and awareness of the consequences of therapeutic maneuvers for mother and fetus.
- The use of therapeutic maneuvers and medications to treat the disease process should always take priority over considerations of possible fetal injury, since maternal damage represents a far greater risk to the fetus than any pharmacologic considerations.

Key Reference

Lapinsky SE, Kruczynski K, Seaward GR, et al: Critical care management of the obstetric patient. Can J Anaesth 1997; 44:325–329.

Case Stem

A previously healthy 24-year-old is admitted at 32 weeks' gestation complaining of severe right upper quadrant pain. The pain responds well to meperidine, but an hour later she suffers a grand mal seizure. Her blood pressure is 180/105 mm Hg. Emergency C-section is performed under general anesthesia, during which she develops a severe coagulopathy and hypovolemic shock. The patient requires massive transfusion and does not regain consciousness at the end of surgery. Discuss the differential diagnosis and management.

References

1. Royston E, Armstrong S: Causes of maternal death. *In* Royston E, Armstrong S (eds): Preventing Maternal Deaths. Geneva: World Health Organization; 1989:75–106.
2. Huque AA, Koblinsky MA: Maternal mortality: levels, trends and determinants. *In* Mother Care Project, 10th ed. Arlington, VA: John Snow, Inc; 1991.
3. Department of Health and Social Security: Report on Confidential Enquiries into Maternal Deaths, 1979–1981. London: Her Majesty's Stationery Office; 1986.
4. Department of Health and Social Security: Report on Confidential Enquiries into Maternal Deaths, 1982–1984. London: Her Majesty's Stationery Office; 1989.
5. Department of Health and Social Security: Report on Confidential Enquiries into Maternal Deaths, 1985–1987. London: Her Majesty's Stationery Office; 1991.
6. Department of Health and Social Security: Report on Confidential Enquiries into Maternal Deaths, 1988–1990. London: Her Majesty's Stationery Office; 1994.
7. Department of Health and Social Security: Report on Confidential Enquiries into Maternal Deaths, 1991–1993. London: Her Majesty's Stationery Office; 1996.
8. Department of Health: First Interim Report on Confidential Enquiries into Maternal Deaths in South Africa. Pretoria Department of Health; 1998.
9. Scarpinato L: Obstetric critical care [editorial; comment]. Crit Care Med 1998; 26:433.
10. Lapinsky SE, Kruczynski K, Seaward GR, et al: Critical care management of the obstetric patient. Can J Anaesth 1997; 44:325–329.
11. de Mello WF, Restall J: The requirement of intensive care

support for the pregnant population [letter; comment]. Anaesthesia 1990; 45:888.
12. Mabie WC, Sibai BM: Treatment in an obstetric intensive care unit. Am J Obstet Gynecol 1990; 162:1–4.
13. Graham SG, Luston MC: The requirement for intensive care support for the pregnant population. Anaesthesia 1989; 44:581–584.
14. Stephens ID: ICU admissions from an obstetrical hospital. Can J Anaesth 1991; 38:677–681.
15. Johanson RB, Anthony J, Dommisse J: Obstetric intensive care at Groote Schuur Hospital. Obstet Gynecol 1995; 15:174–177.
16. Geelhoed GW, Vander AJ: Plasma renin activities during pregnancy and parturition. J Clin Endocrinol Metab 1968; 28:412–415.
17. Pirani BBK, Campbell DM, MacGillivray I: Plasma volume in normal first pregnancy. J Obstet Gynaecol Br Commonw 1973; 80:884–887.
18. Nolten WE, Erlich EM: Sodium and mineralocorticoids in normal pregnancy. Kidney Int 1980; 18:162–172.
19. Taylor DJ, Lind T: Red cell mass during and after normal pregnancy. Br J Obstet Gynaecol 1979; 86:364–370.
20. Huckabee WE: Uterine blood flow. Am J Obstet Gynecol 1962; 84:1623–1633.
21. Bader RA, Bader ME, Rose DJ, Braunwald E: Hemodynamics at rest and during exercise in normal pregnancy as studied by cardiac catheterization. J Clin Invest 1995; 34:1524–1536.
22. Eng M, Butler J, Bonica JJ: Respiratory function in pregnant obese women. Am J Obstet Gynecol 1975; 123:241–245.
23. Lucius H, Gahlenbeck H, Kleine HO, et al: Respiratory functions, buffer system, and electrolyte concentrations of blood during human pregnancy. Respir Physiol 1970; 9:311–317.
24. Dunlop W, Davison JM: Renal haemodynamics and tubular function in human pregnancy. Baillieres Clin Obstet Gynaecol 1987; 1:769–787.
25. Halligan A, Bonnar J, Sheppard B, et al: Haemostatic fibrinolytic and endothelial variables in normal pregnancies and pre-eclampsia. Br J Obstet Gynaecol 1994; 101:488–492.
26. Lefkowitz JB, Clarke SH, Barbour LA: Comparison of protein S functional and antigenic assay in normal pregnancy. Am J Obstet Gynecol 1996; 175:657–660.
27. Robson SC, Dunlop W, Boys RJ, Hunter S: Cardiac output during labour. BMJ 1994; 295:1169–1172.
28. Howard BK, Goodson JH, Mengert WR: Supine hypotensive syndrome in late pregnancy. Obstet Gynecol 1953; 1:371–377.
29. de Swiet M: The respiratory system. In Hytten FE, Leitch I (eds): Clinical Physiology in Obstetrics. Oxford: Blackwell Scientific Publications, 1980: 79–100.
30. Craig DB, Toole MA: Airway closure in pregnancy. Can Anaesth Soc J 1975; 22:665–672.
31. Awe RJ, Nicotra MB, Newsom TD, Viles R: Arterial oxygenation and alveolar-arterial gradients in term pregnancy. Obstet Gynecol 1979; 53:182–186.
32. Cietak KA, Newton JR: Serial qualitative maternal nephrosonography in pregnancy. Br J Radiol 1985; 58:399–400.
33. Mattingly RF, Barkowf HI: Clinical implications of ureteral reflux in pregnancy. Clin Obstet Gynecol 1978; 21:263–273.
34. Lindheimer MD, Katz AL: The kidney in pregnancy. *In* Brenner BM, Rector FCJ (eds): The Kidney. Philadelphia: WB Saunders; 1970:1253–1259.
35. Meschia G: Supply of oxygen to the fetus. J Reprod Med 1979; 23:160–165.
36. Collop NA, Sahn SA: Critical illness in pregnancy: an analysis of 20 patients admitted to a medical intensive care unit [see comments]. Chest 1993; 103:1548–1552.
37. el-Solh AA, Grant BJ: A comparison of severity of illness scoring systems for critically ill obstetric patients. Chest 1996; 110:1299–1304.
38. Lewinsohn G, Herman A, Leonov Y, Klinowski E: Critically ill obstetric patients: outcome and predictability. Crit Care Med 1994; 22:1412–1414.
39. Scarpinato L, Gerber D: Critically ill obstetrical patients: outcome and predictability [letter; comment]. Crit Care Med 1995; 23:1449–1451.
40. Lewinsohn G, Leonov Y, Klinowski E: Critically ill obstetric patients: outcome and predictability [letter]. Crit Care Med 1995; 23:1450–1451.
41. Biester EM, Tomich PG, Esposito TJ, Weber L: Trauma in pregnancy: normal Revised Trauma Score in relation to other markers of maternofetal status—a preliminary study. Am J Obstet Gynecol 1997; 176:1206–1210.
42. Critchlow JF: Obstetric problems in the intensive care unit. in: Rippe JM, Irwin RS, Fink MP, Cerra FB (eds): Intensive Care Medicine, 3rd ed. Boston: Little, Brown, 1996:1846–1853.
43. Becker KJ: Resolved: A pulmonary artery catheter should be used in the management of the critically ill patient. Con [comment; review]. J Cardiothorac Vasc Anesth 1998; 12:1–6.
44. Staudinger T, Locker GJ, Laczika K, et al: Diagnostic validity of pulmonary artery catheterization for residents at an intensive care unit. J Trauma 1998; 44:902–906.
45. Vender JS: Resolved: A pulmonary artery catheter should be used in the management of the critically ill patient. Pro [see comments; review]. J Cardiothorac Vasc Anesth 1998; 12 (Suppl):12.
45a. Gilbert WM, Towner DR, Field NT, Anthony J: The safety and utility of pulmonary artery catheterization in severe pre-eclampsia/eclampsia. Am J Obstet Gynecol 2000; 175 (in press).
46. Anonymous: Pulmonary artery catheter consensus conference: consensus statement [see comments; review]. Crit Care Med 1997; 25:910–925.
47. Raps EC, Galetta SL, Flamm ES: Neuro-intensive care of the pregnant woman [review]. Neurol Clin 1994; 12:601–611.
48. Mabie WC, Barton JR, Sibai BM: Adult respiratory distress syndrome in pregnancy. Am J Obstet Gynecol 1992; 167:955–957.
49. Lapinsky SE, Kruczynski K, Slutsky AS: Critical care in the pregnant patient [review]. Am J Resp Crit Care Med 1995; 152:427–455.
50. Dombrowski MP: Pharmacologic therapy of asthma during pregnancy [review]. Obstet Gynecol Clin North Am 1997; 24:559–574.
51. Wendel PJ, Ramin SM, Barnett-Hamm C, et al: Asthma treatment in pregnancy: a randomized controlled study. Am J Obstet Gynecol 1996; 175:150–154.
52. Frakes MA, Richardson LE: Magnesium sulfate therapy in certain emergency conditions [review]. Am J Emerg Med 1997; 15:182–187.
53. Shanies HM, Venkataraman MT, Peter T: Reversal of intractable acute severe asthma by first-trimester termination of pregnancy. J Asthma 1997; 34:169–172.
54. James MF, Manson ED: The use of magnesium sulphate infusions in the management of very severe tetanus. Intensive Care Med 1985; 11:5–12.
55. James MF, Huddle KR, Owen AD, Van der Veen BW: Use of magnesium sulphate in the anaesthetic management of phaeochromocytoma in pregnancy. Can J Anaesth 1988; 35:178–182.
55a. Fishburne JIJ, Dormer KJ, Payne GG, et al: Effects of amrinone and dopamine on uterine blood flow and vascular responses in the gravid baboon. Am J Obstet Gynecol 1988; 158:829–837.
55b. Jelsema RD, Bhatia RK, Ganguly S: Use of intravenous amrinone in the short-term management of refractory heart failure in pregnancy. Obstet Gynecol 1991; 78:935–936.
56. Yau G, Oh TE: Severe cardiac disease in pregnancy. 1997:499–506.
57. Waisman GD, Mayorga LM, Camera MI, et al: Magnesium plus nifedipine: potentiation of hypotensive effect in preeclampsia? [See comments.] Am J Obstet Gynecol 1988; 159:308–309.
58. Davis WB, Wells SR, Kuller JA, Thorp JMJ: Analysis of the risks associated with calcium channel blockade: implications for the obstetrician-gynecologist [review] Obstet Gynecol Surv 1997; 52:198–201.
59. Fenakel K, Fenakel G, Appelman Z, et al: Nifedipine in the treatment of severe preeclampsia. Obstet Gynecol 1991; 77:331–337.
60. Idama TO, Lindow SW: Magnesium sulphate: a review of clinical pharmacology applied to obstetrics [review]. Br J Obstet Gynaecol 1998; 105:260–268.

61. Ben-Ami M, Giladi Y, Shalev E: The combination of magnesium sulphate and nifedipine: a cause of neuromuscular blockade. Br J Obstet Gynaecol 1994; 101:262–263.
62. O'Riordan JA: Pheochromocytomas and anesthesia. Int Anesthesiol Clin 1997; 35:99–127.
63. Gin T, Ngan Kee WD: Obstetric Emergencies. 1997;494–498.
64. Mighty H: Trauma in pregnancy [review]. Crit Care Clin 1994; 10:623–634.
65. Drost TF, Rosemurgy AS, Sherman HF, et al: Major trauma in pregnant women: maternal/fetal outcome. J Trauma 1990; 30:574–578.
66. Kissinger DP, Rozycki GS, Morris JAJ, et al: Trauma in pregnancy: predicting pregnancy outcome [published erratum appears in Arch Surg 1991; 126:1524]. Arch Surg 1991; 126:1079–1086.
67. Moise KJJ, Belfort MA: Damage control for the obstetric patient [review]. Surg Clin North Am 1997; 77:835–852.
68. Polko LE, McMahon MJ: Burns in pregnancy [review]. Obstet Gynecol Surv 1998; 53:50–56.
69. Prasanna M, Singh K: Early burn wound excision in "major" burns with "pregnancy": a preliminary report. Burns 1996; 22:234–237.
70. Ullmann Y, Blumenfeld Z, Hakim M, et al: Urgent delivery, the treatment of choice in term pregnant women with extended burn injury. Burns 1997; 23:157–159.
71. Davey DA, MacGillivray I: The classification and definition of the hypertensive disorders of pregnancy [see comments]. Am J Obstet Gynecol 1988; 158:892–898.
72. MacGillivray I: Some observations on the incidence of pre-eclampsia. J Obstet Gynaecol Br Commonw 1958; 65:536–539.
73. MacGillivray I: The Hypertensive Disease of Pregnancy. Place: Publisher; 1983: xx–xx.
74. Duley L: Maternal mortality associated with hypertensive disorders of pregnancy in Africa, Asia, Latin America and the Caribbean [see comments; review]. Br J Obstet Gynaecol 1992; 99:547–553.
75. World Health Organization: Geographic variation in the incidence of hypertension in pregnancy. Am J Obstet Gynecol 1988; 158:80–83.
76. Hogberg U, Innala E, Sandstrom A: Maternal mortality in Sweden, 1980–1988. Obstet Gynecol 1994; 84:240–244.
77. Bashir A, Aleem M, Mustansar M: A 5-year study of maternal mortality in Faisalabad City, Pakistan. Int J Gynaecol Obstet 1995; 50(suppl 2):S93–S96.
78. Chesley LC, Annitto JE, Cosgrove RA: The familial factor in toxemia of pregnancy. Obstet Gynecol 1968; 32:303–311.
79. Chesley LC, Cooper DW: Genetics of hypertension in pregnancy: possible single gene control of pre-eclampsia and eclampsia in the descendants of eclamptic women. Br J Obstet Gynaecol 1986; 93:898–908.
80. Cooper DW, Liston WA: Genetic control of severe pre-eclampsia. J Med Genet 1979; 16:409–416.
81. Humphrey KE, Harrison GA, Cooper DW, et al: HLA-G deletion polymorphism and pre-eclampsia/eclampsia. Br J Obstet Gynaecol 1995; 102:707–710.
82. Harrison GA, Humphrey KE, Jones N, et al: A genomewide linkage study of preeclampsia/eclampsia reveals evidence for a candidate region on 4q. Am J Hum Genet 1997; 60:1158–1167.
83. Robertson WB, Brosens I, Dixon HG: The pathological response of the vessels of the placental bed to hypertensive pregnancy. J Pathol Bacteriol 1967; 93:581–592.
84. Pijnenborg R, Anthony J, Davey DA, et al: Placental bed spiral arteries in the hypertensive disorders of pregnancy. Br J Obstet Gynaecol 1991; 98:648–655.
85. Pijnenborg R: The placental bed. Hypertension in Pregnancy 1996; 15:7–23.
86. Robertson WB, Brosens I, Dixon G: Uteroplacental vascular pathology. Eur J Obstet Gynecol Reprod Biol 1975; 5:47–65.
87. Roberts JM, Taylor RN, Musci TJ, et al. Preeclampsia: an endothelial cell disorder. Am J Obstet Gynecol 1989; 161:1200–1204.
88. McCarthy AL, Woolfson RG, Raju SK, Poston L: Abnormal endothelial cell function of resistance arteries from women with preeclampsia. Am J Obstet Gynecol 1993; 168:1323–1330.
89. Nova A, Sibai BM, Barton JR, et al: Maternal plasma level of endothelin is increased in preeclampsia. Am J Obstet Gynecol 1991; 165:724–727.
90. Clark BA, Halvorson L, Sachs B, Epstein FH: Plasma endothelin levels in preeclampsia: elevation and correlation with uric acid levels and renal impairment. Am J Obstet Gynecol 1992; 166:962–968.
91. Walsh SW: Preeclampsia: an imbalance in placental prostacyclin and thromboxane production. Am J Obstet Gynecol 1985; 152:335–340.
92. Gujrati VR, Shanker K, Vrat S, et al: Novel appearance of placental nuclear monoamine oxidase: biochemical and histochemical evidence for hyperserotonomic state in preeclampsia-eclampsia. Am J Obstet Gynecol 1996; 175:1543–1550.
93. Redman CW: Platelets and the beginnings of preeclampsia [editorial; comment]. N Engl J Med 1990; 323:478–480.
94. Lyall F, Greer IA, Boswell F, et al: The cell adhesion molecule, VCAM-1, is selectively elevated in serum in pre-eclampsia: does this indicate the mechanism of leucocyte activation? [See comments.] Br J Obstet Gynaecol 1994; 101:485–487.
95. Halim A, Kanayama N, El Maradny E, et al: Plasma P selectin (GMP-140) and glycocalicin are elevated in preeclampsia and eclampsia: their significances. Am J Obstet Gynecol 1996; 174:272–277.
96. Halim A, Kanayama N, El Maradny E, et al: Correlated plasma elastase and sera cytotoxicity in eclampsia: a possible role of endothelin-1–induced neutrophil activation in preeclampsia-eclampsia. Am J Hypertens 1996; 9:33–38.
97. Taylor RN, Casal DC, Jones LA, et al: Selective effects of preeclamptic sera on human endothelial cell procoagulant protein expression. Am J Hypertens 1991; 165:t–10.
98. Sheehan H, Lynch J: Cerebral lesions. *In* Sheehan H, Lynch J (eds): Pathology of Toxemia of Pregnancy. Baltimore: Williams & Wilkins; 1973:524–553.
99. Donaldson JO: The brain in eclampsia. Hypertension Pregnancy 1994; 13:115–133.
100. Richards AM, Graham DI, Bullock MRR: Clinicopathological study of neurological complications due to hypertensive disorders in pregnancy. J Neurol Neurosurg Psychiatry 1999; 51:416.
101. Weinstein L: Syndrome of hemolysis, elevated liver enzymes and low platelet count: a severe consequence of hypertension in pregnancy. Am J Obstet Gynecol 1982; 142:159–167.
102. Spargo BH, McCartney C, Winemiller R: Glomerular capillary endotheliosis in toxemia of pregnancy. Arch Pathol 1959; 13:593–599.
103. Barton JR, Sibai BM: Cerebral pathology in eclampsia [review]. Clin Perinatol 1991; 18:891–910.
104. Visser W, Wallenburg HC: Central hemodynamic observations in untreated preeclamptic patients. Hypertension 1991; 17:1072–1077.
105. Belfort MA, Anthony J, Kirshon B: Respiratory function in severe gestational proteinuric hypertension: the effects of rapid volume expansion and subsequent vasodilatation with verapamil. Br J Obstet Gynaecol 1991; 98:964–972.
106. Belfort MA, Saade GR, Wasserstrum N, et al: Acute volume expansion with colloid increases oxygen delivery and consumption but does not improve the oxygen extraction in severe pre-eclampsia. J Matern Fetal Med 1995; 4:57–64.
107. Douglas KA, Redman CW: Eclampsia in the United Kingdom [see comments]. BMJ 1994; 309:1395–1400.
108. Lubarsky SL, Barton JR, Friedman SA, et al: Late postpartum eclampsia revisited [review]. Obstet Gynecol 1994; 83:502–505.
109. Tetzschner T, Felding C: Postpartum eclampsia: impossible to eradicate? Clin Exp Obstet Gynecol 1994; 21:74–76.
110. Duncan R, Hadley D, Bone I, et al: Blindness in eclampsia: CT and MR imaging. J Neurol Neurosurg Psychiatry 1989; 52:899–902.
111. Chang WN, Lui CC, Chang JM: CT and MRI findings of eclampsia and their correlation with neurologic symptoms. Chin Med J (Engl) 1996; 57:191–197.
112. Lindheimer MD: Pre-eclampsia-eclampsia 1996: preventable? Have disputes on its treatment been resolved? [Review.] Curr Opin Nephrol Hypertens 1996; 5:452–458.
113. Unal M, Senakayli OC, Serce K: Brain MRI findings in two

cases with eclampsia [review]. Australas Radiol 1996; 40:348–350.
114. Hauser WA, Kurland LT: The epidemiology of epilepsy in Rochester, Minnesota 1935 through 1967. Epilepsia 1975; 16:1–66.
115. Towers CV, Pircon RA, Nageotte MP, et al: Cocaine intoxication presenting as preeclampsia and eclampsia. Obstet Gynecol 1993; 81:545–547.
116. Gamba G: Acute thrombocytopaenias and thrombotic thrombocytopaenic purpura: differential diagnosis. Transfus Sci 1992; 13:13–16.
117. Clark SL, Hankins GD, Dudley DA, et al: Amniotic fluid embolism: analysis of the national registry [see comments]. Am J Obstet Gynecol 1995; 172:t–67.
118. Kaplan MM: Acute fatty liver of pregnancy [review]. N Engl J Med 1985; 313:367–370.
119. Atlas M, Barkai G, Menczer J, et al: Thrombotic thrombocytopaenic purpura in pregnancy. Br J Obstet Gynaecol 1982; 89:476–479.
120. Chandran R, Serra-Serra V, Redman CW: Spontaneous resolution of pre-eclampsia-related thrombocytopaenia. Br J Obstet Gynaecol 1992; 99:887–890.
121. Ventura JE, Villa M, Mizraji R, Ferreiros R: Acute renal failure in pregnancy. Renal Failure 1997; 19:217–220.
122. Wallenburg HC: Hemodynamics in hypertensive pregnancy. *In* Rubin PC (ed): Hypertension in Pregnancy. New York: Elsevier Science; 1988.
123. Belfort MA, Carpenter RJJ, Kirshon B, et al: The use of nimodipine in a patient with eclampsia: color flow Doppler demonstration of retinal artery relaxation. Am J Obstet Gynecol 1993; 169:204–206.
124. Anthony J, Mantel G, Johanson R, Dommisse J: The haemodynamic and respiratory effects of intravenous nimodipine used in the treatment of eclampsia. Br J Obstet Gynaecol 1996; 103:518–522.
125. Hongo K, Kobayashi S: Calcium antagonists for the treatment of vasospasm following subarachnoid haemorrhage [review]. Neurol Res 1993; 15:218–224.
126. Horn EH, Filshie M, Kerslake RW, et al: Widespread cerebral ischaemia treated with nimodipine in a patient with eclampsia. BMJ 1990; 301:794–794.
127. Wasserstrum N, Cotton DB: Hemodynamic monitoring in severe pregnancy-induced hypertension. Clin Perinatol 1986; 13:781–799.
128. Bhorat IE, Naidoo DP, Rout CC, Moodley J: Malignant ventricular arrhythmias in eclampsia: a comparison of labetalol with dihydralazine. Am J Obstet Gynecol 1993; 168:1292–1296.
129. Linton DM, Anthony J: Critical care management of severe pre-eclampsia. Intensive Care Med 1997; 23:248–255.
130. Coetzee EJ, Dommisse J, Anthony J: A randomised controlled trial of intravenous magnesium sulphate versus placebo in the management of women with severe pre-eclampsia. Br J Obstet Gynaecol 1998; 105:300–303.
131. Anonymous: Which anticonvulsant for women with eclampsia? Evidence from the Collaborative Eclampsia Trial. Lancet 1995; 345:1455–1463.
132. Anthony J, Johanson RB, Duley L: Role of magnesium sulfate in seizure prevention in patients with eclampsia and pre-eclampsia [review]. Drug Saf 1996; 15:188–199.
133. Altura BT, Altura BM: Interactions of Mg and K on cerebral vessels—aspects in view of stroke: review of present status and new findings. Magnesium 1984; 3:195–211.
134. de Jonge MC, Traber J: Nimodipine: cognition, aging, and degeneration [review]. Clin Neuropharmacol 1993; 16(suppl 1):S25–S30.
135. Lipton SA, Rosenberg PA: Excitatory amino acids as a final common pathway for neurologic disorders [see comments; review]. N Engl J Med 1994; 330:613–622.
136. Naidu S, Payne AJ, Moodley J, et al: Randomised study assessing the effect of phenytoin and magnesium sulphate on maternal cerebral circulation in eclampsia using transcranial Doppler ultrasound. Br J Obstet Gynaecol 1996; 103:111–116.
137. Belfort MA, Moise KJJ: Effect of magnesium sulfate on maternal brain blood flow in preeclampsia: a randomized, placebo-controlled study. Am J Obstet Gynecol 1992; 167:661–666.
138. Belfort MA, Saade GR, Moise KJJ: The effect of magnesium sulfate on maternal retinal blood flow in preeclampsia: a randomized placebo-controlled study. Am J Obstet Gynecol 1992; 167:1548–1553.
139. Kulick DL, Hong R, Ryzen E, et al: Electrophysiologic effects of intravenous magnesium in patients with normal conduction systems and no clinical evidence of significant cardiac disease. Am Heart J 1988; 115:367–373.
140. Arsenian MA: Magnesium and cardiovascular disease. Prog Cardiovasc Dis 1993; 35:271–310.
141. Smith LGJ, Burns PA, Schanler RJ: Calcium homeostasis in pregnant women receiving long-term magnesium sulfate therapy for preterm labor. Am J Obstet Gynecol 1992; 167:45–51.
142. Cruikshank DP, Chan GM, Doerrfeld D: Alterations in vitamin D and calcium metabolism with magnesium sulfate treatment of preeclampsia. Am J Obstet Gynecol 1993; 168:1170–1176.
143. Mordes JP, Wacker WC: Excess magnesium. Pharmacol Rev 1978; 29:273–300.
144. Ramanathan J, Sibai BM, Pillai R, Angel JJ: Neuromuscular transmission studies in preeclamptic women receiving magnesium sulfate. Am J Obstet Gynecol 1988; 158:40–46.
145. Richards A, Stather-Dunn L, Moodley J: Cardiopulmonary arrest after the administration of magnesium sulphate: a case report. S Afr Med J 1985; 67:145.
146. Swartjes JM, Schutte MF, Bleker OP: Management of eclampsia: cardiopulmonary arrest resulting from magnesium sulfate overdose. Eur J Obstet Gynecol Reprod Biol 1992; 47:73–75.
147. Bashuk RG, Krendel DA: Myasthenia gravis presenting as weakness after magnesium administration. Muscle Nerve 1990; 13:708–712.
148. Richards AM, Moodley J, Graham DI, Bullock MR: Active management of the unconscious eclamptic patient. Br J Obstet Gynaecol 1986; 93:554–562.
149. Anthony J, Johanson R, Dommisse J: Critical care management of severe preeclampsia. Fetal Maternal Med Rev 1994; 6:219–229.
150. Kirshon B, Lee W, Mauer MB, Cotton DB: Effects of low-dose dopamine therapy in the oliguric patient with preeclampsia. Am J Obstet Gynecol 1988; 159:604–607.
151. Mantel GD, Makin JD: Low dose dopamine in postpartum pre-eclamptic women with oliguria: a double-blind, placebo-controlled, randomised trial. Br J Obstet Gynaecol 1997; 104:1180–1183.
152. Clark SL, Greenspoon JS, Aldahl D, Phelan JP: Severe preeclampsia with persistent oliguria: management of hemodynamic subsets. Am J Obstet Gynecol 1986; 154:490–494.
153. Clark SL, Cotton DB: Clinical indications for pulmonary artery catheterization in the patient with severe preeclampsia [see comments]. Am J Obstet Gynecol 1988; 158:453–458.
154. Lee W, Rokey R, Cotton DB: Noninvasive maternal stroke volume and cardiac output determinations by pulsed Doppler echocardiography. Am J Obstet Gynecol 1988; 158:505–510.
155. Neumark J: Anaesthesia for caesarean section. Curr Opin Anaesthesiol 1996; 9:202–206.
156. Allen RW, James MF, Uys PC: Attenuation of the pressor response to tracheal intubation in hypertensive proteinuric pregnant patients by lignocaine, alfentanil and magnesium sulphate. Br J Anaesth 1991; 66:216–223.
157. Ashton WB, James MF, Janicki P, Uys PC: Attenuation of the pressor response to tracheal intubation by magnesium sulphate with and without alfentanil in hypertensive proteinuric patients undergoing caesarean section. Br J Anaesth 1991; 67:741–747.
158. Fagan EA: Disorders of the liver, biliary system and pancreas. *In* de Swiet M (ed): Medical Disorders in Obstetric Practice. Oxford, England: Blackwell Scientific Publications; 1989:426–520.
159. Pereira SP, O'Donohue J, Wendon J, Williams R: Maternal and perinatal outcome in severe pregnancy-related liver disease. Hepatology 1997; 26:1258–1262.
160. Clark SL, Cotton DB, Gonik B, et al: Central hemodynamic alterations in amniotic fluid embolism. Am J Obstet Gynecol 1988; 158:1124–1126.

54

Maternal Mortality

❖ TREVOR THOMAS, MD, FRCA

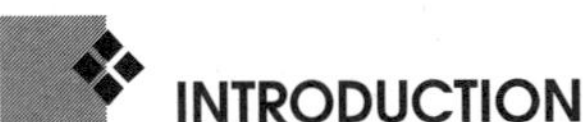

INTRODUCTION

Maternal mortality is an important factor in maternal health worldwide. At present, the World Health Organization (WHO)[1] estimates that "in every minute of every day a woman dies of pregnancy-related complications somewhere in the world—nearly 600,000 deaths each year." These women often die because of poor public health measures and inadequate care during their pregnancy. The majority of these deaths occur among the developing nations of the world. Those parturients delivering in Western Europe and North America are in fact a very privileged population by international standards. The risk of death is greatest in Sub-Saharan Africa, the Horn of Africa, and the adjacent regions of the Arabian Peninsula, India, and Afghanistan. The comparative risks of the inhabitants of these countries compared with the best of the United States, Canada, and Western Europe is so great that it is difficult to imagine.[1] To collect such figures accurately, a commonly accepted definition of maternal death must exist. The most widely accepted definitions come from the *International Classification of Diseases* (ICD). The *International Classification of Diseases* in its ninth *Revision* (ICD9) defines a *maternal death* as "the death of a woman while pregnant or within 42 days of termination of a pregnancy, from any cause related to or aggravated by the pregnancy or its management, but not from accidental or incidental causes." *Direct obstetric deaths* are defined as "those resulting from obstetric complications of the pregnant state (pregnancy, labour and puerperium), from interventions, omissions, incorrect treatment, or from a chain of events resulting from any of the above." *Indirect obstetric deaths* are defined as "those resulting from previous existing disease, or disease that developed during pregnancy and which was not due to direct obstetric causes, but which was aggravated by the physiological effects of pregnancy." The tenth *Revision of the Classification of Diseases* (ICD10) has introduced a new category of pregnancy-related death that is defined as "the death of a woman while pregnant or within 42 days of termination of pregnancy, irrespective of the cause of death." This new definition has been introduced for use in cases in which the cause of death cannot be identified precisely. It is hoped that the introduction of this new definition will improve the collection of data on maternal deaths.

Retrieval of the information on which the figures are based is difficult, and the results are known to be inaccurate. Under-reporting is common, even in the developed world. Bouvier-Colle et al.[2] report that the discrepancy in France between the number of maternal deaths registered by ICD9 coding and those retrieved by examination of other classifications of death in the National Statistics shows a potential error of greater than 50%. Similarly, in the United Kingdom it has been shown that the National Record of maternal deaths kept by the Registrar General underestimates maternal mortality by approximately 30%.[3] Between 1985 and 1993, the Registrar General was aware of 485 maternal deaths, whereas the system of confidential inquiries into maternal deaths identified 689 deaths. It is interesting to note the variability of retrieval. The Registrar General identified 78% of maternal deaths between 1985 and 1987, whereas between 1991 and 1993 only 60% were identified by the National Registration System. The figures from both France and the United Kingdom, where reporting maternal deaths is encouraged, illustrate the difficulty of identifying the true size of the problem of maternal mortality worldwide. If under-reporting of this scale occurs in such well organized and regulated systems, we must suspect that the true maternal mortality throughout the world probably exceeds 1 million women each year.

NATIONAL VARIABILITY

The geographic variability in maternal mortality rates seen on an international scale also exists within national boundaries. There are few countries within which the methods of gathering information are sufficiently accurate to allow such comparisons; the United Kingdom is one. It is densely populated and has such a well-established and accurate method of collecting information on maternal deaths that this comparison is possible (Fig. 54–1). Even in the narrow confines of such a small country, it is worth noting that regional mortality rates varied from 5.3 to 13 per 100,000 maternities. The fact that maternal risk is some two times greater in one region of the United Kingdom than in

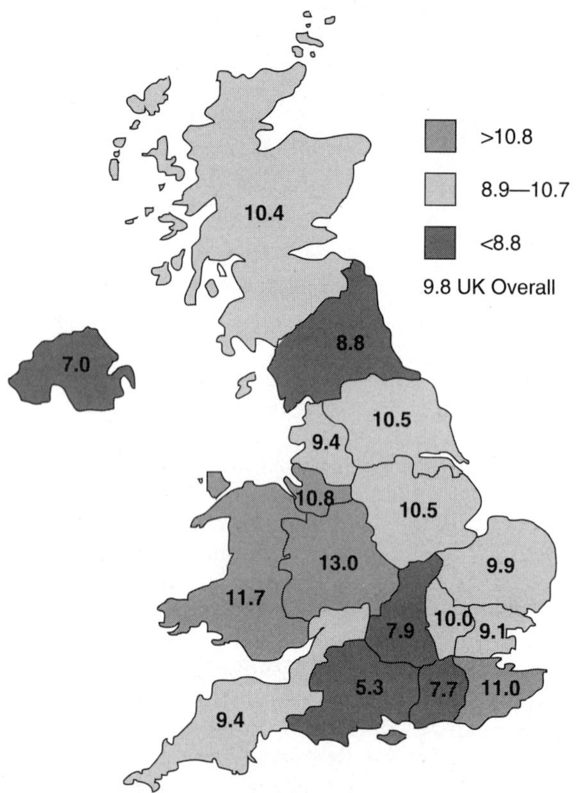

❖ **Figure 54–1** Variability in maternal mortality rates within the various regions of the United Kingdom. (Data from the *Report on Confidential Enquiries into Maternal Deaths for the Triennium 1991–1993*. Her Majesty's Stationery Office.)

another must indicate variations in the standard of care as well as in the population being cared for. Closer scrutiny of the changing international and national death rates can give us some insight into the risks that result in maternal death. While making this scrutiny, we must always remember the factors that lead to under-reporting and to inaccurate or incorrect attribution of the cause of death. These factors include the following:

1. Differences in definitions
2. Differences in death certification procedures
3. Social factors
    a. The consequences of blame
    b. The social status of women
    c. Religious factors
4. Legal considerations
5. Professional considerations

The discrepancy introduced by changing definitions and methods of inquiry is also a significant factor. Mortality data from Sweden[4] show clearly the effect of using different ICD classifications (Table 54–1).

The use of birth and death certificate comparisons had no effect on Swedish totals, but in the United States it added 27% to the registration totals.[5]

CAUSE OF DEATH

Collection of total numbers of maternal deaths is difficult, and accurate identification of the cause of death more so. Perhaps the simplest illustration of this difficulty is to consider a hypothetical case of a woman of 40 in her fourth pregnancy who is admitted to an obstetric unit suffering from gestational hypertension. On admission, signs of fetal distress are noted and an emergency cesarean section is undertaken under general anesthesia. The patient suffers a major obstetric hemorrhage during the operation and is subsequently admitted to an intensive care unit, where she dies with adult respiratory distress syndrome (ARDS). The immediate registerable cause of death may be ARDS, but the problems leading up to the pulmonary problem are as much to blame. The cause of death in such a case could as easily be attributed in maternal mortality inquiries or reviews to hypertension, to hemorrhage, or to ARDS. The fact that treatment of her various problems was poorly carried out by any one, or more, of the many departments involved may easily escape attention and the proper attribution of risk may never be achieved.

To overcome these problems, a reliable, confidential system of collecting data must exist. Any such system must be able to demonstrate and guarantee the following features:

1. A regionally based network of informants and assessors
2. A method of confidentiality that will convert the regionally generated information into anonymous nationally collated data
3. A two-tier system of assessment:
    a. At a regional level
    b. At a national level
4. A system of reporting that is immune from legal subpoena

The declared aims of such a system should be

1. To assess and inform
2. To identify solutions
3. To improve outcome
4. To improve assessment
5. To produce a regular public report on the information collected

Table 54–1 Effect of Changing International Classification of Disease (ICD) Definitions on Recovered Maternal Death Numbers*

Version	Recovered Deaths (%)
ICD8	100
ICD9	161
ICD10	177

*ICD8 total = 100% and late deaths are excluded.

Data from Högberg U, Innala E, Sandström A: Maternal mortality in Sweden, 1980–1988. Obstet Gynecol 1994; 84:240–245.

RISK MANAGEMENT

European and American Confidential Inquiries into Maternal Deaths

A national system of confidential medical inquiry into maternal deaths originated in the United Kingdom in 1928. This short-lived arrangement relied on information collected by Medical Officers of Health throughout England and Wales. It produced two reports, the first in 1930 and the second in 1932. This method of inquiry continued until the end of 1951 and summaries of the inquiries made appeared in Annual Reports from the Ministry of Health "on the state of the public health." One important feature of this predecessor of the triennial *Reports on Confidential Enquiries into Maternal Deaths* that we now have was the assessment of a primary *avoidable* factor in each of the maternal deaths reported. In 1928, the inquiries identified a maternal mortality rate in England and Wales of 4.4 per 1000 total births. By 1951, that rate had fallen to 0.8 per 1000 births. The marked improvement, together with the consequences of the Second World War, may have resulted in part from a decrease in the proportion of maternal deaths assessed, a problem encountered in reverse in the United States (see later discussion) in 1987. By 1951, reports were actually received on only about 60% of the total maternal deaths registered in the United Kingdom. By this time, a major defect of the system had been identified. There was no consultant or specially qualified practitioner nominated to assist medical officers in their assessment of cases of unusual difficulty. In 1949, the subject was discussed at the Twelfth British Congress on Obstetrics and Gynaecology. Reports were received of a method of inquiry used in the United States of America in which investigations were carried out by a local committee of experts who subsequently published case reports and comments in medical journals. Consultations between the Royal College of Obstetricians and Gynaecologists, the Society of Medical Officers of Health, and the Minister of Health resulted in the creation of the system of inquiry that we are familiar with today. It was designed to include all who might contribute information on a maternal death. The family doctor, Medical Officer of Health, midwife, obstetrician, and, subsequently, anesthesiologists and pathologists were included in the team that was to collect, assess, and report on all maternal deaths that occurred in England and Wales. The model was adopted by Scotland and Northern Ireland in subsequent years, and eventually, from 1985, all three reports were amalgamated to give an overall picture of events in the United Kingdom. In the *Report on Confidential Enquiries for 1988 through 1990*,[6] the results of a European initiative were published. Several European and international sources had been approached, to collect as much information as possible on crude maternal death rates, definitions, registration and verification procedures, and, perhaps most importantly, the denominator data on which all such mortality figures are based. National administrators of those countries with membership in the European College of Obstetrics and Gynaecology were approached, as were secretaries of national societies of obstetrics and gynecology. This European survey found that all countries had a national mortality data collection agency and some had regional agencies. The latter tended to produce more complete and reliable data. Statutory notification of maternal deaths, together with hospital reports, personal local knowledge, and various methods of verification of death certificates were all used to collect crude maternal death figures. A specific question on pregnancy was included in the death certification procedures of four countries, Denmark, Germany, the Irish Republic, and Scotland. Five countries carried out specific inquiries into individual deaths, Hungary, the Irish Republic, the Netherlands, Romania, and the United Kingdom. In a further four countries, Belgium, France, Germany, and Norway, inquiries were carried out only in some regions. The inquiries themselves varied from the confidential and anonymized analysis carried out in the United Kingdom to a system used in Romania in which, it would seem, a risk of criminal proceedings was integral to the inquiry. The results of the inquiries in the various countries were not necessarily published. The reliability of data collected under the threat of criminal proceedings must be viewed with considerable reservation. Indeed, the Romanian figures are made up mainly of abortion-related deaths; of the 148 deaths per 100,000 live births, 128 were attributed to abortion. In spite of reservations over the results, the picture that emerges is that in Western Europe mortality rates are roughly 7 or 8 per 100,000 live births, whereas in Eastern Europe the mortality rate is generally higher, varying from about 11 to 44 per 100,000 (excluding Romania). In many of the surveys, it was not possible to identify the cause of death, and even a relatively simple event, such as hemorrhage, is not accurately represented in the tables of this publication.

In the United States, similar attempts to quantify maternal mortality rates have been made over many years. A National Pregnancy-Related Mortality Surveillance System was set up in 1987. It has collected information both retrospectively and prospectively in collaboration with the American College of Obstetrics and Gynecology and state health departments. National death files, state health department files, maternal mortality review committee files, and individual and media reports have all been used. The results of this initiative showed a decreasing maternal mortality rate between 1979 and 1987. However, when prospective collection of information began, the mortality rate apparently increased from 7.2 per 100,000 live births in 1987 to 10 per 100,000 live births in 1990. The American surveillance system makes wide-ranging inquiries using death certification, state registration, and information from professionals in the field of obstetrics to maximize collection of mortality figures. The results have been reviewed.[5] The increase is probably due to more complete collection of information rather than a genuine worsening of maternal health. However, it may be significant that increases in the number of maternal deaths have also been recorded in the

U.K. *Confidential Enquiries* for 1988 through 1990.[6] These latter increases in the number of deaths accompany changing birth rates, however, and the overall mortality rate is essentially unchanged.

Berg et al.[5] point out that, in spite of the apparent increase, the prospective American figures, like the retrospective ones, are likely to underestimate the total maternal mortality by some 50%. This underestimate is similar in proportion to that attaching to the official registration mechanisms in Western Europe. The figures that are available from the U.S. Surveillance System show considerable similarity between these causes of death and those found in European maternal mortality reports. It is impossible to say whether the unreported deaths would materially affect the balance of importance of individual causes of death. Given similarities to the European experience, it is likely that they would not. In 1997, Hawkins et al.[7] reported the results of the first study of anesthesia-related maternal mortality in the United States. Again, similarities between U.K. and U.S. data were noted. Differences were also present and deserve comment.

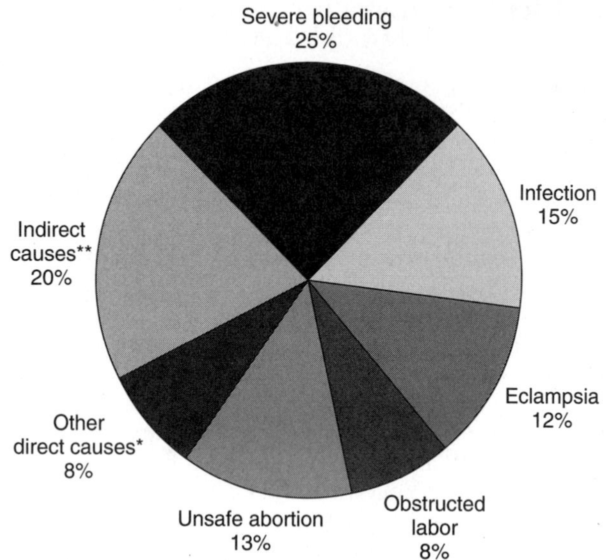

❖ **Figure 54–2** Causes of maternal death in the developing world. (From World Health Organization and World Bank.)

The Anesthesiologist's Role

Documenting the details of maternal death can provide information to show which risk factors are most frequently responsible for maternal fatalities. When these factors are accurately quantified, resources can be directed to reduce the risk or treat its consequences. This ideal can, of course, be achieved only when sufficient resources are made available by those responsible, whether government, insurers, or the profession itself. Examination of the detail contained in other available mortality inquiries and reports shows major differences in the nature of risk between the developing and the developed world, but some similarities also exist. Extraction of information from WHO statistics[1, 8] shows that, as far as can be ascertained in the developing world, infection, abortion, and obstructed labor cause approximately one third of maternal deaths. A further 20% are due to indirect causes, which include anemia, malaria, and heart disease. However, maternal hemorrhage accounts for 25% of maternal mortality in the developing world, just as it does in the developed world (Fig. 54–2).

The principles of good risk management are as follows:

1. Identify risks
2. Assess the frequency and gravity of risk
3. Respond to eliminate or combat the risk

Application of risk management strategies will allow us to improve our care and the clinical outcomes for our patients.

Reports from the United Kingdom, Western Europe, the United States, and Australia reveal a common set of factors that increase maternal risk. They are as follows:

1. Increasing maternal age
2. Increasing parity
3. Maternal hemorrhage
4. Maternal hypertension
5. Maternal thromboembolism (excluding amniotic fluid embolism)
6. Administration of anesthesia
7. Sociogeographic factors, such as racial origin

The most complete and detailed analyses of mortality in a sufficiently large population over a sufficiently long period of time are the reports of *Confidential Enquiries into Maternal Deaths* from the British Isles. This series of triennial reports has run from 1952. It has varied a little in style, content, and definitions over the 40-plus years covered. The original report covered England and Wales only. The first Northern Irish report appeared in 1956 and the first Scottish report in 1965. From the 1985–1987 report onward, the United Kingdom as a whole was covered in a single report. This mine of information will be the main source for subsequent comments on individual causative factors of importance to obstetric anesthesiologists in this chapter. Additional comments will be derived from Berg et al.,[5] Högberg et al.,[4] and Shearman,[9] all of whom have reported recently on trends of maternal mortality in the developed world.

Extrapolations can easily be made from the assessment of risk using these sources, and individual or local variations of practice and risk can be noted. For instance, the *Confidential Enquiry* series identifies increasing maternal age as a risk factor. Attention is drawn to it particularly in the confidential inquiries for 1990 through 1993.[3] In Sweden, a similar effect is noted,[4] but in this Swedish report the effect of age is magnified, especially when combined with parity. In Sweden, age greater than 35 years increased the risk of maternal death fivefold, and, with the interaction of parity, it was shown that primiparae older than 35 had a 20-fold greater risk of dying than women younger than 35 with a parity of two to three. The major risk factors listed differ in their relative importance, not only from nation to nation but also with time. Consideration of the time element is important for any risk analysis because medical care of the parturient also changes with time. Comparisons can therefore be made between variation in practice and changing mortality. Such comparisons are not easily amenable to statistical analysis, partly because it is difficult to collect denominator data and partly because changes in practice are haphazard in their rate of introduction and rarely occur singularly. Nevertheless, some correlations of changing practice with improving mortality are very convincing, such as the change from magnesium trisilicate antacid prophylaxis to a combination of sodium citrate 0.3 molar plus histamine-2 receptor blocking drugs prior to anesthesia. This has been associated with an almost complete abolition of anesthesia-related aspiration of gastric contents as a cause of maternal death (see later).

Comparisons between national statistics are more difficult and probably less reliable because the populations and social environments differ as well as do medical methods.

Given the similarity of reported problems in the developed world, it is reasonable to use the detailed U.K. figures as the basis for risk management strategies. They clearly show that the main causes of death are as follows:

1. Hemorrhage
2. ARDS
3. Hypertension
4. Thromboembolism
5. Anesthesia
6. Cardiac disease (recorded as indirect deaths)

To gauge the importance of these factors for obstetric anesthesia services, it is necessary first to define the anesthesiologist's role and second to apply good risk management principles. Originally, obstetric anesthesiologists simply provided anesthesia for operative obstetrics. In the United Kingdom in the years following World War II, general anesthesia was almost invariably used, whereas in the United States and on the European mainland, regional anesthetic techniques were used quite freely. Practice in the United Kingdom has changed substantially, and epidural and subarachnoid anesthesia are now freely used as well. Such changes influence maternal mortality substantially (see later).

The original, almost singular, role of obstetric anesthesiologists has now broadened, and most obstetric anesthesia services provide the following:

1. Anesthesia for operative obstetrics
2. Regional analgesia for pain relief in labor
3. Cardiopulmonary resuscitation of the parturient
4. High dependency and intensive care of the sick parturient
5. Treatment during maternal hemorrhage
6. Assessment and control of the cardiovascular system in parturients suffering hypertensive disease of pregnancy or with cardiac problems

In these circumstances, the anesthesiologist's particular skills are now seen as invaluable. However, the expanded role confers an increased responsibility and an increasing likelihood that the obstetric anesthesiologist will be held responsible for maternal fatalities. The scale of obstetric anesthesiologist involvement has recently been assessed by the United Kingdom Audit Commission.[10] Even their economic analysis revealed that obstetric anesthesiologists were involved in the treatment of approximately 38% of all mothers in the United Kingdom. The interunit range shown by their inquiry varied from 10% to 60% of mothers, and these figures largely ignored the care given to the sick parturients by obstetric anesthesiologists. Figures can also be extracted from the triennial *Reports on Confidential Enquiries into Maternal Deaths (CEMD)* for the United Kingdom. In the triennium 1988 through 1990,[6] the report identified extensive anesthetic input into the care of the sick mother. Approximately 18% of all deceased parturients had been cared for in an intensive care unit for some time before their deaths. Approximately 25% had suffered major obstetric hemorrhage, and a further 38% had received anesthesia for cesarean section. There is obvious overlap between these categories, but these bald statistics probably indicate that obstetric anesthesia services are involved in the care of at least 50% of mothers who died.

Anesthesia-Related Mortality

Overall, maternal mortality rates have improved almost constantly in the developed world for the last 50 years. Anesthesia has not kept pace with the best of these improvements, nor even the average for most of that time. In the United Kingdom, in the decade between 1970 and 1981, there was a rapid decrease in deaths from ruptured uterus, infection, and, following the 1967 Act, abortion. These improvements threw the importance of anesthesia as a cause of maternal death into stark relief. When anesthetic deaths were expressed as a percentage of all direct maternal deaths, the figures rose from 10.9% in 1970 to 12.6% in 1981. However, between 1970 and 1981 the actual number of deaths per triennium, directly attributable to anesthesia, fell, from 37 (in 1970–1972)[11] to 22 (in 1979–1981).[12] Put another way, the quality of anesthesia care was not improving as quickly as were other elements of obstetric care. When this disturbing factor became known, closer attention was paid to the anesthesia-related mortality data.

The application of basic risk management principles showed that the main areas of risk were as follows:

1. Aspiration of gastric contents
2. Failure to intubate the trachea
3. Poor postoperative care
4. Misuse of drugs and equipment

In addition, the great majority of deaths occurred in mothers receiving general anesthesia for emergency procedures (Fig. 54–3). Other contributing factors, clearly identified in the 1979 through 1981 CEMD,[13] included a failure of communication between obstetric and anesthetic services such that demand for emergency anesthesia became extremely urgent, leaving no time for prophylaxis, preparation, or any opportunity for anesthesia options to be explored. In addition, the anesthesiologists involved were often junior, called from other theater activities, with little experience to guide them in such circumstances, and easily bullied into hurried decisions. Discussion of this problem formed part of the deliberations of the U.K. Government's Social Services Committee in 1979. In their subsequent report, the Committee recommended that "Anaesthetists below the grade of registrar—i.e., those with less than 12 months' experience—are not allowed to give a general or an epidural anaesthetic to any pregnant woman unless properly supervised."[14] The Social Services Committee made a number of other valuable and influential recommendations as a result of risk identification, and changes in obstetric anesthesia services were accelerated. More anesthesiologists of more senior, experienced standing were deployed in obstetric units, and operating theater equipment and staffing were also improved to match standards in other surgical areas.

Equally significant changes of practice occurred and were guided by information contained in the *CEMD* reports. There was a swing away from general anesthesia, which had been shown to be higher risk than regional anesthesia for operative obstetrics. The improvement of anesthesia-related mortality that followed in the 12 years between 1981 and 1993 was impressive (see Fig. 54–3).

Those general anesthesia procedures that were performed benefited from the changing attitudes toward prophylaxis against pulmonary acid aspiration. In the *CEMD* report for 1979 through 1981,[12] eight parturients died from Mendelson's (acid aspiration) syndrome. Of these mothers, five had received the then widely used magnesium trisilicate antacid prophylaxis. The use of sodium citrate as a nonparticulate antacid for parturients had first been reported in 1973.[13] The virtues of sodium citrate were confirmed by Holdsworth et al.[15] and the dangers of magnesium trisilicate were shown by Gibbs et al.[16] The use and advantages of histamine-2 receptor blockers appeared in reports shortly thereafter.[17, 18] Largely as a result of these various reports, the use of sodium citrate, together with H_2 receptor blockers, became commonplace. Since the mid-1980s, the total number of anesthesia-related deaths due to aspiration of gastric content has declined, and the *CEMD* has not reported any maternal deaths in parturients who have received a correctly timed regimen of H_2 blockers with sodium citrate. These changes were not simply fortuitous, but were in fact an example of good risk management, comprising the identification of cause and the reduction of risk.

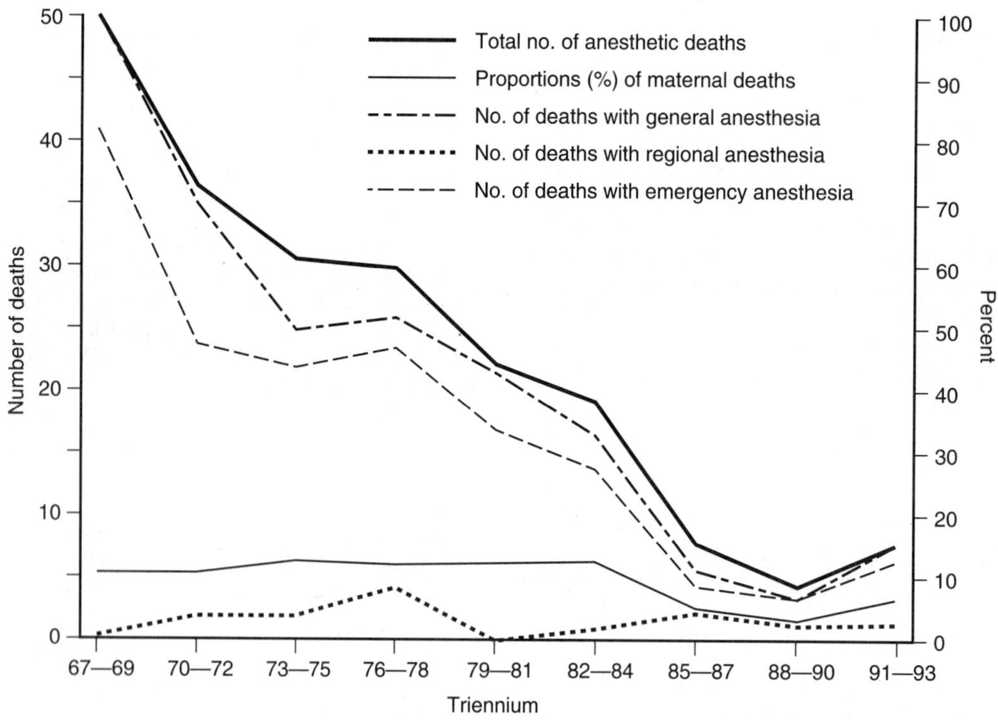

Figure 54–3 Maternal mortality due to anesthesia between 1967 and 1993. Comparison of total mortality with that due to general anesthesia, that occurring in emergency cases, and that due to regional anesthesia. (From Holdcroft AH, Thomas TA: Principles and Practice of Obstetric Anaesthesia. London: Blackwell, 1999.)

The first analysis of anesthesia-related maternal mortality in the U.S. appeared in 1997.[7] The study was based on information collected by the Centers for Disease Control and Prevention (CDC) through their National Pregnancy Mortality Surveillance System. The period studied ran from 1979 to 1990, and information was further subdivided into periods between 1979 to 1984 and 1985 to 1990. The U.S. figures are therefore derived in a very different way from the U.K. figures. A number of assumptions and extrapolations are made in the former, which also suffers from the under-reporting commented on by Berg et al.[5] Nevertheless, comparison of the causes of death and changes occurring over time in anesthesia-related maternal mortality bear an uncanny resemblance to the U.K. experience in many particulars. There are, however, two interesting, and perplexing, differences between the trends in the U.K. and U.S.. The overall decrease in anesthesia-related mortality is seen in both sets of figures (Table 54–2). The rate of change over the decade seems different, with the U.K. statistics decreasing by some 80% and the U.S. ones by 60%. However, the mortality rate of 4.3 per million births from which the U.S. figures start is probably underestimated by anything from 35% to 50%, so the changes are probably very similar. The causes of death in the two countries are also similar. Problems with the maintenance of airways and aspiration of gastric contents predominate in general anesthesia–related deaths. One marked difference is noticeable in regional anaesthesia–related deaths, however. The U.S. data show that 50% of regional anesthesia deaths before 1984 were due to local anesthetic toxicity. After withdrawal of bupivacaine 0.75%, in 1984, fewer such cases have occurred, although significant numbers were reported. In the U.K. on the other hand, where bupivacaine 0.75% was used relatively infrequently and fractionated epidural dosing was common, very few local anesthetic toxicity fatalities have been recorded. In the decade in question, there were only two deaths, which might have been due to local anesthetic toxicity but, even in these two cases, a degree of uncertainty exists in the diagnosis.

The really surprising aspect of the U.S. figures is the lack of improvement in general anesthesia-related deaths. In the U.K., an improvement of some 70% can be seen (see Table 54–2), whereas the U.S. figures appear largely unchanged. This difference could be due to the fact that the number of general anesthetic procedures is declining in the United Kingdom, whereas it is remaining constant in the U.S. Unfortunately, obtaining reliable information about the numbers of anesthetics and their nature is extremely difficult in both countries. In the United Kingdom, we have an indication that the percentage of general anesthetics given for cesarean delivery has declined but, because of the increase in cesarean section rate, the reduction in the number of general anesthetics is much smaller.[19] Russell is in the process of repeating his survey, and, so far, the indications are that general anesthesia usage is continuing to decline (personal communication, 1999). Hawkins et al.,[20] on the other hand, used national work force surveys conducted in 1981[21] and 1992 to estimate the proportion of general and regional anesthetics administered for cesarean section during their study period. Detailed criticisms were made of this methodology[22] in an editorial of 1997. Chestnut[22] points out that the number of general anesthetics given is likely to have been underestimated in both these surveys, so, as in the U.K. experience, the number of general anesthetics given in the United States will have declined by a much smaller proportion than expected. Given the similarity of the denominator figures that are intrinsic in these comments, it is baffling to see the apparent difference in rate of change of mortality due to general anesthesia between the two countries. Hawkins highlights the fact that the risk of deaths from general anesthesia actually increased in the United States from 20 per million in 1979 to 32.3 per million in 1990. The reasons for the difference are difficult to understand. The methods of general anesthesia, drugs for general anesthesia, monitoring standards, and techniques in general seem to be very similar. Possibilities are that a difference in population treated causes the discrepancy or that the proportion of cases treated as emergencies is markedly different between the two countries. We know that patients with darker skin color account for some 50% of maternal deaths in both the United Kingdom and the United States. In the latter it may be that the darker-skinned population make up a greater proportion of those patients receiving general anesthetics. Equally, it may be that interspecialty communication is not as good in the United States, leading to a greater urgency in a higher proportion of poorly prepared or sick parturients. Both the U.K. *CEMD* reports and an earlier U.S.

Table 54–2

ANESTHESIA-RELATED MATERNAL MORTALITY (ARMM)	UK			USA		
	1979–1981	1988–1990	% Change	1979–1984	1985–1990	% Change
Rate/million pregnancies/ births	8.7	1.7	−80	4.3	1.7	−60
Number of deaths						
General anesthesia	2.2	4	−70	33	32	−3
Regional anesthesia	1	1	0	19	9	−50

report[23] emphasize the significant increase in risk that occurs when a patient presents as an emergency case. Emergency anesthesia is more likely to be general rather than regional in nature because of urgency of demand. Thus we have a compounding of risk with both urgent demand and the use of general anesthesia.

Close, timely collaboration between obstetricians and obstetric anesthesiologists is essential to ensure early recognition of potential risk. Such good teamwork will allow appropriate prophylactic measures to be instituted and a sensible choice of anesthetic made. In addition, participation in obstetric anesthesia services by experienced anesthesiologists and use of the fullest range of patient monitoring available is essential if we are to further reduce the toll of deaths from general anesthesia.

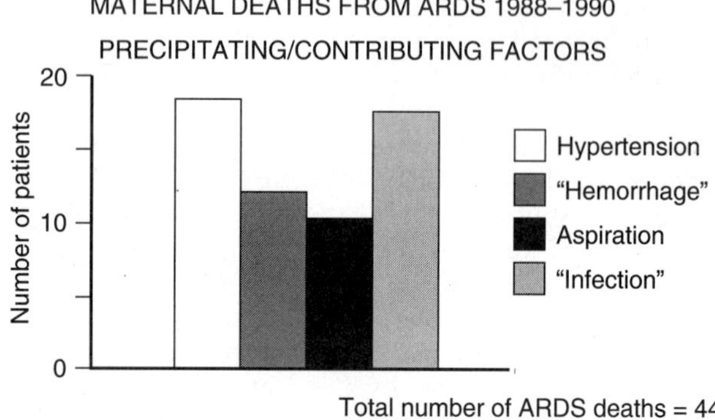

❖ **Figure 54–5** Precipitating or contributing factors leading to adult respiratory distress syndrome fatalities in the United Kingdom from 1988 to 1990.

Adult Respiratory Distress Syndrome

Aspiration followed by ARDS still occurs, however. In the *CEMD* of 1988 through 1990, at least 44 parturients died from ARDS; all were treated in an intensive care unit for varying lengths of time before their deaths. However, aspiration is not the only event that can trigger ARDS. Eighteen of the patients suffered from gestational hypertension, and in 12 the precipitating factor was obstetric hemorrhage. Ten mothers were known to have aspirated prior to their admission to the intensive care unit, and combinations of trigger factors must be particularly lethal. This was the first clear identification of ARDS as a cause of maternal mortality. Breakdown of the statistics is shown in Figures 54–4 and 54–5. It is now recognized that aspiration and ARDS are risk factors for parturients other than those receiving anesthesia. All parturients should be given H_2 blockers prophylactically as soon as they enter one of the risk groups, unless a contraindication to the drug exists. The risk groups are those suffering from the following conditions:

1. Hypertensive disease of pregnancy
2. Obstetric hemorrhage
3. Chest infections

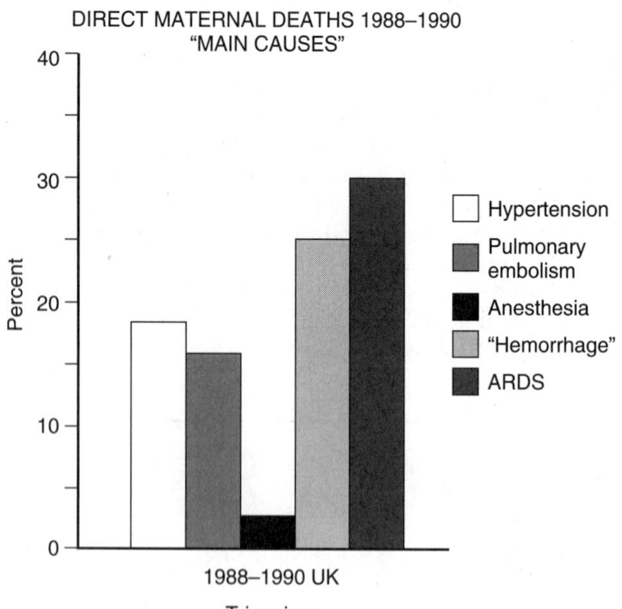

❖ **Figure 54–4** The relative importance of five major contributing causes of maternal mortality in the United Kingdom between 1988 and 1990. Each of the bars shows the percentage contribution made by these five causes of death. It demonstrates the overwhelming importance of adult respiratory distress syndrome as a cause of death.

The high dependency or intensive care of these mothers differs from that of nonpregnant women. Many parturients are especially susceptible to pulmonary edema before the development of ARDS. Once pulmonary edema is established, continuing high pulmonary capillary pressures, the use of high FIO_2, and high airway pressures during ventilation treatment to maintain high oxygen saturation rates lead inexorably to a downward spiral into ARDS, multiorgan failure, and death. Meticulous control of pulmonary capillary pressures, avoidance of overtransfusion, careful assessment of renal function, and acceptance of lower than usual SaO_2 will lessen the risks to these mothers and give sufficient time for the normal postpartum physiologic diuretic response to become established and the cardiovascular system to resume normal functions in most parturients.

Control of intravenous infusion fluids and their type and volume is of particular importance to those parturients suffering from the effects of hemorrhage. Treatment of maternal hemorrhage is now clearly a responsibility for obstetric anesthesiologists.

Hemorrhage

In both the developing and the developed world, hemorrhage is the underlying causative factor in at least 25% of maternal deaths. A few of these fatalities occur in the home, particularly in the early pregnancy deaths associated with ectopic pregnancy, and these cannot be addressed by improvements in hospital services and protocols. Most hemorrhage deaths, however, occur in the hospital. The contribution made by hemorrhage to the U.K. maternal mortality rates over a 20-year period are shown in Figure 54–6. The figures for each

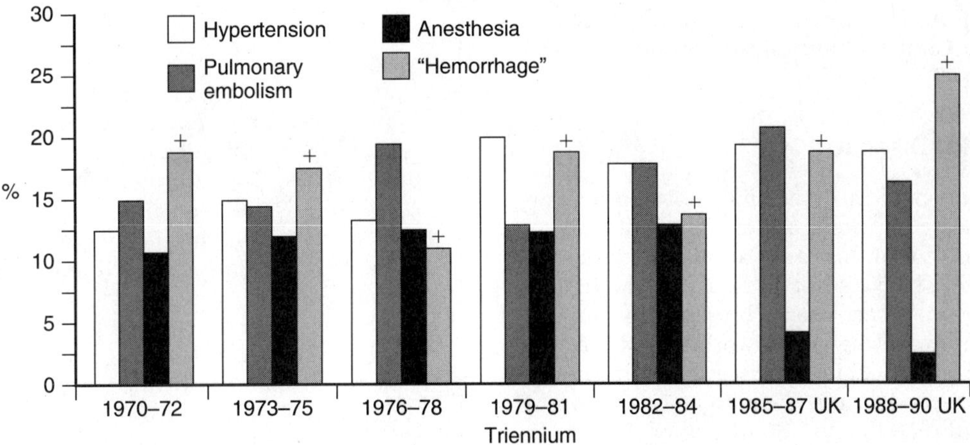

❖ **Figure 54-6** The true contribution made by hemorrhage to maternal mortality between 1970 and 1990 in the United Kingdom. The proportion of deaths due to hemorrhage is compared with the proportion of deaths due to hypertension, pulmonary embolism, and anesthesia. The total number of deaths due to hemorrhage has been produced by the addition of individual cases from various chapters of the Reports on Confidential Enquiries into Maternal Deaths (from Her Majesty's Stationery Office) for the same period.

triennium in this illustration have been culled from the various chapters of *CEMD* reports and show that, in some 3-year periods, hemorrhage caused more deaths than either the hypertensive disease of pregnancy or a thromboembolism.

When the sequelae of obstetric hemorrhage and its treatment, such as ARDS, are included in the statistics, the true importance of bleeding in parturients becomes apparent. Once the risk is properly understood, measures can be put in place to address the problem. These often take the form of protocols.

The protocols are often derived from, or loosely based on, published advice such as that in *CEMD* reports from 1979 through 1993. But however good the protocols, improvements in outcome will only be achieved if the advice is thoroughly known to all the staff of the unit and is acted upon. Too often protocols are ignored because individuals think they know better. A number of basic observations apart from the protocol itself are perhaps pertinent here.

1. Maternal hemorrhage is often, and should always be considered to be, partially or completely covert and therefore not directly measurable.
2. Maternal systemic blood pressure will only decrease when blood loss is already 25% of total blood volume or more. Once started, the decrease can be very rapidly progressive.
3. Other clinical signs and symptoms of hemorrhage should therefore be used as an indicator that blood loss is occurring. The signs and symptoms to be sought are
   a. Pallor
   b. Tachycardia
   c. Sweating
   d. Fearfulness
   e. Oliguria
4. Measurement of central venous pressure will usually confirm the diagnosis and will provide a useful method for controlling intravenous fluid replacement therapy. It will only be successful in the latter context if a maximum of 6 cm H_2O is used as the upper limit of central venous pressure that is to be tolerated. Central venous pressure must not be used (elevated) as a means of "driving" the kidneys. Diuresis postpartum is a physiologic event that awaits hormonal changes. It may not occur for 48 hours. Diuretics may help the unwary anesthesiologist who has ignored this physiologic fact and overloaded the patient to the point of pulmonary edema.

Excessive fluid replacement, especially with crystalloid and colloid solutions, contributes to maternal deaths from ARDS and also to considerable maternal morbidity, often involving intensive care. Early involvement of senior experienced obstetric anesthesiologists will often prevent such excesses. Good protocols should demand that senior staff are informed and involved in the management of cases of obstetric hemorrhage (see earlier discussion).

The monitoring and management of the cardiovascular system during pregnancy and labor demands knowledge and experience of the pregnant patient's physiology in other situations than hemorrhage. Cardiac disease is an important risk factor causing indirect maternal deaths in substantial numbers of women in both the developing and the developed world. A considerable proportion of cardiac deaths occur in parturients who have received an anesthetic for cesarean delivery. Approximately 10% of all cesarean-related maternal deaths in the United Kingdom are caused by cardiac disease. Choice of anesthesia can be critical in such cases.

Cardiovascular Disease

The contribution made to maternal mortality by cardiovascular disease is often underestimated because maternal deaths due to this cause are usually classified as indirect deaths. They do not form part of the figures derived solely from direct deaths but are the cause of substantial mortality around the world. In the developing world, congenital heart disease and acquired valvular heart disease form a very large proportion of the 20% of indirect deaths identified by WHO. In the developed world, cardiovascular disease is probably becoming increasingly important as a cause of maternal death (Fig. 54–7). In the United Kingdom in the 3-year period of 1991 through 1993, all forms of cardiovascular disease contributed to increasing mortality. The majority of the deaths involved rupture of aneurysms of the thoracic aorta. When these cases are added to the deaths due to rupture of the splenic artery and subarachnoid blood vessels, and to "intracerebral bleeds," the total number of indirect deaths due to spontaneous rupture of a major blood vessel rises to 30. Specific cardiac disease contributed a further 31 deaths, so the cardiovascular system actually accounted for 61 indirect deaths in that 3-year period.

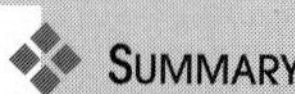

Summary

Key Points

- During every minute of each day, somewhere in the world a woman dies of pregnancy-related complications.
- In the last 20 years, anesthesiologists have achieved significant improvements in the quality of care and, in the Western world, have significantly reduced anesthesia-related mortality.
- The improvements are due to the rational application of risk management principles, better understanding of the parturient, and improved communication with and monitoring of the patient, but most of all, the deployment of more anesthesiologists with better training and experience.

Key Reference

Hawkins JL, Koonin LM, Palmer SK, Gibbs CP: Anesthesia-related deaths during obstetric delivery in the U.S., 1979–1990. Anesthesiology 1997; 86:277–284.

Case Stem

Discuss the advances in obstetric anesthesia that have occurred during the past 20 years and outline the steps that can be taken to further decrease maternal mortality in your country.

CONCLUSION

Anesthesiologists have, in the last 20 years, achieved significant improvements in the quality of their care of parturients. They have done so by the application of the principles of risk management. The first step in this approach has used maternal mortality data as a measure of the standard of care. To be a truly effective risk management tool, the data must be complete, accurate, and detailed. The history of the U.K. experience in their reports on *Confidential Enquiries into Maternal Deaths* shows how such a data set can be used to

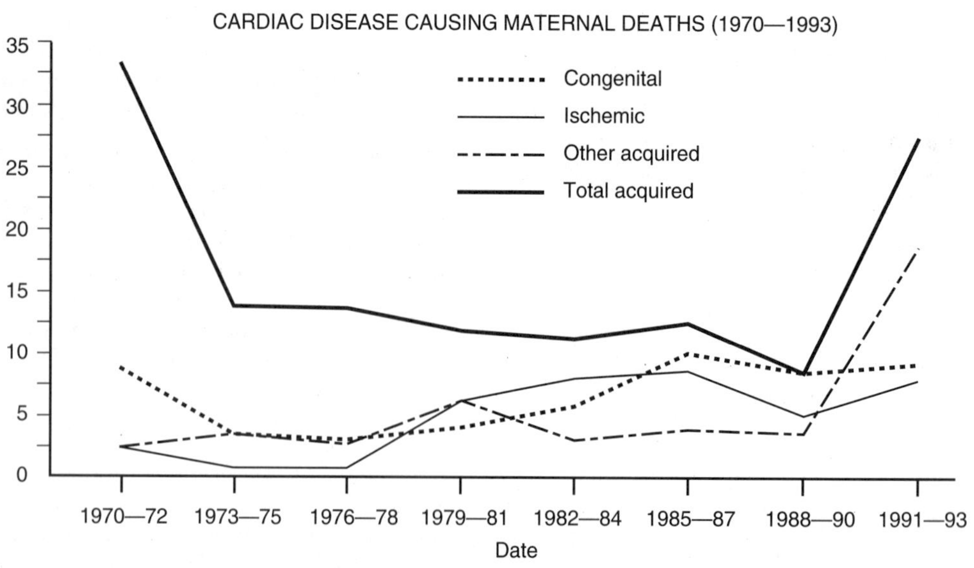

Figure 54–7 The contribution made by various forms of cardiac disease to indirect maternal mortality in the United Kingdom between 1970 and 1993.

good effect. It is encouraging that other countries are following suit.

It is of some relevance to see how important it is to continue the monitoring system even when the number of fatalities becomes very small. In the U.K. 1991 through 1993 triennium, anesthesia-related maternal mortality increased, from 1.7, in 1988 to 1990, to 3.5 deaths per million pregnancies. The numbers of deaths are, of course, very small, so it would be foolish to read too much into the change. Nevertheless, the causes of the increased numbers of deaths remain unchanged. Dark-skinned parturients are at greater risk than white. Most of the fatalities involve inadequate monitoring, inexperienced anesthesiologists, or use of general anesthesia in emergency cases.

The most recent figures are awaited. It is hoped that they will not show further worsening. Whatever the mortality rate, the information will be valuable, especially if it still contains evidence of avoidable factors in many deaths. The collection of national mortality statistics around the world will help our understanding of the risks our patients run even though they may throw up apparent anomalies from time to time. We, as obstetric anesthesiologists, can do better by heeding the invaluable information that can be made available to us through reliable maternal mortality data.

References

1. The World Health Organisation with the World Bank: Maternal Health Around the World. 1997.
2. Bouvier-Colle MH, Varnoux N, Costes P, Hatton F: Reasons for the under-reporting of maternal mortality in France, as indicated by a survey of all deaths among women of childbearing age. Int J Epidemiol 1991; 20:717–721.
3. UK Health Departments: Report on Confidential Enquiries into Maternal Deaths in the U.K., 1991–1993. London: Her Majesty's Stationery Office, 1996.
4. Högberg U, Innala E, Sandström A: Maternal mortality in Sweden, 1980–1988. Obstet Gynecol 1994; 84:240–245.
5. Berg CJ, Atrash HK, Koonin LM, Tucker M: Pregnancy-related mortality in the United States, 1987–1990. Obstet Gynecol 1996; 88:162–167.
6. UK Health Departments: Report on Confidential Enquiries into Maternal Deaths in the United Kingdom, 1988–1990. London: HMSO, 1994.
7. Hawkins JL, Koonin LM, Palmer SK, Gibbs CP: Anesthesia-related deaths during obstetric delivery in the United States, 1979–1990. Anesthesiology 1997; 86:277–284.
8. Abou Zahr C, Royston E: Maternal Mortality: A Global Factor Book. Geneva: World Health Organisation; 1991.
9. Shearman RP: Trends in maternal mortality in Australia: relevance in current practice. Aust N Z J Obstet Gynaecol 1990; 30:15–17.
10. The Audit Commission: Anaesthesia under Examination, the Efficiency and Effectiveness of Anaesthesia and Pain Relief Services in England and Wales. A National Report. Oxford, England. 1997.
11. Department of Health and Social Security: Report on Health and Social Subjects 11: Report on Confidential Enquiries into Maternal Deaths in England and Wales, 1970–1972. London. HMSO, 1975.
12. Department of Health and Social Security: Report on Health and Social Subjects 29: Report on Confidential Enquiries into Maternal Deaths in England and Wales, 1979–1981. London: HMSO, 1986.
13. Lahiri SK, Thomas TA, Hodgson RMH: Single dose antacid therapy for the prevention of Mendelson's syndrome. Br J Anaesth 1973; 45:1143–1146.
14. Second Report from the Social Services Committee, Session 1979–80. Perinatal and Neonatal Mortality, Vol. 1. London: HMSO, 1980.
15. Holdsworth JD, Johnson K, Maskall G, et al: Mixing of antacids with stomach contents: another approach to the prevention of acid aspiration (Mendelson's) syndrome. Anaesthesia 1980; 35:641–650.
16. Gibbs CP, Schwarz DJ, Wynne JW, et al: Antacid pulmonary aspiration in the dog. Anesthesiology 1979; 51:380–385.
17. Dundee JW, Moore J, Johnston JR, McCaughey W: Cimetidine and obstetric anaesthesia. Lancet 1981; 2:252.
18. McAuley DM, Moore J, McCaughey W, et al: Ranitidine as an antacid before elective caesarean section. Anaesthesia 1983; 38:108–114.
19. Brown GW, Russell IF: A survey of anaesthesia for caesarean section. Int J Obstet Anesth 1995; 4:214–218.
20. Hawkins JL, Gibbs CP, Orleans M, et al: Obstetric anesthesia workforce survey, 1981 versus 1992. Anesthesiology 1997; 87:135–143.
21. Gibbs CP, Krischer J, Peckham BM, et al: Obstetric anesthesia: a national survey. Anesthesiology 1986; 65:298–306.
22. Chestnut DH: Anesthesia and maternal mortality. Anesthesiology 1997; 86:273–276.
23. Endler GC, Mariona FG, Sokol J, Stevenson LB: Anesthesia-related maternal mortality in Michigan, 1972–1984. Am J Obstet Gynecol 1988; 159:187–193.

55

Ethical Issues and Consent in Obstetric Anesthesia

❖ DAVID CROOKE, MBBS, BA, MBIOMED E, FANZCA

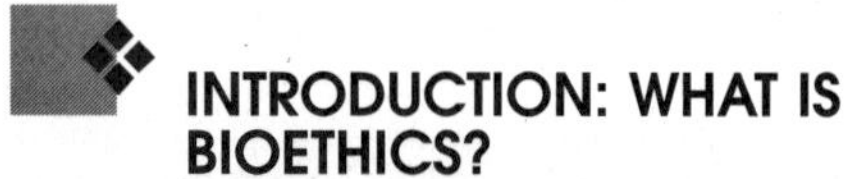

INTRODUCTION: WHAT IS BIOETHICS?

Bioethics, medical ethics, nursing ethics, moral philosophy, and ethics are interrelated entities, which in turn are related to ethical, legal, and cultural aspects of the society in which we live. Bioethics purports to be a "rational and systematic reflection on the various moral, legal and social problems brought on by the extraordinary development of medicine and the other sciences of life."[1] At one level, bioethics may be seen as yet another subspecialty in medicine; however, in reality ethical issues permeate all of medicine. Anesthesiologists need a working knowledge of bioethics along with certain related skills in addressing clinical ethical problems as they arise.

There are a diversity of views regarding the nature of bioethics; its methods; and importantly, how bioethics is to be taught to young doctors and nurses. Health administrators in Australia see the most prominent bioethical issues as making not for resuscitation (NFR) orders; the treatment of human immunodeficiency virus (HIV) antibody–positive and acquired immunodeficiency syndrome (AIDS) patients; differences between caregivers belonging to different professional groups; and the allocation of health care resources.[2]

Although the theory of bioethical analysis may be complex and multifarious, clinical bioethical reflection has two practical hallmarks. First, it is very particular in orientation, tied ineluctably to the individual case, its context, and particular detail. Ethical generalizations or universals are frequently tautologic (e.g., "murder is wrongful killing"), they may serve only as vignettes, and finally the relevance of the ethical universal to a particular ethical case needs to be established. Beware that the language employed in ethical discussion may carry implicit moral judgment and covertly bias debate. Consider, for example, the abortion debate. Abortion will always seem wrong when described as "murder" in an antiabortionist argument. Alternatively, abortion may seem acceptable when a pro-choice argument contrasts maternal rights and responsibilities with first trimester fetal rights and responsibilities. Alternatively, abortion may seem justified and medically indicated when described as abortion for fetal trisomy 18 or for maternal primary pulmonary hypertension in a medical argument. There will always be a range of views on the issue of abortion.[3] Bioethical analysis often involves consideration of the context and detail of particular ethical clinical problems.

The second hallmark of ethical inquiry is the strong requirement for human judgment:

> Moral judgments are judgments, not deductions; they are not themselves deduced; they can be supported, defended, argued for or against, justified or established, but not deduced.[4]

This contrasts with a scientistic model of applied ethics which uses a relevant ethical theory or "covering law" along with relevant empiric facts to move deductively to an apparently deterministic ethical conclusion. This form of ethical reasoning resembles certain forms of scientific reasoning and is frequently invalid in ethics. Universal theories and covering laws in science have a very different status to theories in ethics. Universal theories in ethics do not necessarily have priority over particular cases in ethics. Judgment, interpretation, and compromise are always required in deciding which universal ethical assertions are relevant to or bear on a particular clinical scenario. This judgment and interpretation involve consideration of the particular details of a given ethical scenario in the light of any relevant universal imperatives and similar cases. This process of reflection involves interplay between the particular details of a case and universal ethical tenets.

The subjective versus objective distinction has limited use in bioethics. Traditional ideals in ethics such as impartiality and the objective viewpoint in ethical decision making have more recently been criticized as being covertly biased, or simply irrelevant to the complex context of a particular case.[5] However, it is important that decisions concerning ethical questions not be made along self-interested lines. Appropriate impartiality, along with declarations of conflicts of interest, is very important.

In bioethics, then, there is no algorithm or consistent method to be used in ethical inquiry. The products of ethical inquiry are not deterministic, but, rather, they need to be argued for and asserted. Although bioethics does not offer universal solutions to bioethical problems, when provided with an adequately described particular clinical ethical problem, bioethical inquiry offers the following: sense can be made of the range of positions and responses to the problem; rival positions in responding to a problem can usually be sorted into stronger and weaker positions; and points of tension and difficulty in a debate are better appreciated, so that relations between the various peoples in the debate are sustained.

THEORY AND PRACTICE IN BIOETHICS

An ethical theory is a general ethical statement, which is abstract and removed from individual cases but which can bear on particular cases and clinical practice. There is much interplay between so-called theory and practice, that is, general ethical universals and particular ethical scenarios. Among the many ethical theories, there is no theory that necessarily has privilege in bioethics. The following ethical theories may have relevance in ethical debate[6, 7]: naturalism, absolutism, deontologism, principlism, consequentialism, utilitarianism, proportionalism, contextualism, feminist ethics, virtue ethics, and intuitivism, and are briefly outlined in passing.

Bioethical practice is implicit in much of medical practice. This implicit everyday ethics may be thought of as clinical practical wisdom acquired in apprenticeship, or tacitly acquired clinical practice from mentors who manifest good ethical practice. This relates to so-called *intuitivism,* everyday ethical decision making that we all have to employ in performing clinical work. Underpinning this everyday working ethics, more critical thinking or a body of ethical/legal "theory" is required, for use by the practitioner in analyzing more difficult cases. Hare[8] proposed these two levels of ethical functioning for medical practitioners within psychiatry.

One such ethical theory is that of *principlism.* For many reasons, awareness of bioethical issues is increasing. Beauchamp and Childress championed principlism, or the "theory of principles," in their book *Principles of Biomedical Ethics*[9] and this had a significant impact on bioethics and the teaching of bioethics. You will recognize beneficence and non-maleficence as, respectively, doing good for and avoiding harm to the patient. Respect for patient autonomy entails facilitating, as much as is possible, the patient's right to self-determination. Respect for justice involves treating patients justly with respect to the law and broader societal issues and touches issues of resource allocation. Veracity involves truth-telling, especially when directly asked by the patient. Confidentiality involves appropriately respecting patient information. The principlism that Beauchamp and Childress publicized is a useful, easily articulated ethical starting point; furthermore, it is consonant with the analytical nature of medicine. This theory equips people with an explicit language and awareness through which to begin to analyze an ethical problem. Concerns for beneficence and non-maleficence are of course not independent, and the greater the degree of medical intervention, the heavier is a doctor's concern to avoid harming the patient. As we see in a later example concerning consent, when these principles are in tension different people can resolve the tensions in different ways, leading to a sense of relativism. It is important that ethical theory be conjoined with clinical common sense and a process of talking with others, ethical reflection, and careful consideration of tensions between these principles.

Another such critical ethical theory is *utilitarianism.* The utilitarian family of ethical systems[10, 11] has evolved since the time of Bentham. It is well known that the utilitarian's aim is to provide the "greatest good for the greatest number of people"; however, the nature of goodness still needs to be defined for any utilitarian analysis. Each form of utilitarianism has a definition of the "value criteria," or what is to count as good, along with a method of how to measure this good across a population. Older forms of utilitarianism, such as hedonistic utilitarianism, had hedonism and immediate pleasure as the value criteria. More contemporary forms of utilitarianism have "preference satisfaction" or "social welfare" as the value criteria. Alterations in these value criteria lead to somewhat different utilitarian theories.

Utilitarianism certainly attracts strong criticism. For example, Williams argues that in a serious way utilitarianism misrepresents the nature of human beings.[12] The notion of humans acting out of a universal concern as utilitarian agents, stripped of other human feelings, aspirations, and motives, is a misrepresentation of what it is to be human. Glover[13] describes a related problem, whereby "the utilitarian view makes people replaceable." It is not that utilitarian concerns will not bear on an ethical analysis of the situation, but rather that they do not tell the whole story.

Rule utilitarianism contrasts with *act utilitarianism,* and is a major variant within the family of utilitarian theories. Particular action is guided by "rules," which are not simply rules of thumb such as an act utilitarian would readily acknowledge. The rules themselves are what is grounded in the utilitarian analysis, in what is a clear two-stage procedure, as in Austin's dictum[14]: "Our rules would be fashioned on utility; our conduct, on our rules." The entire grounding and status of moral "rules" in utilitarian ethical systems can be problematic.

The nature of "good" and how to recognize it can vary considerably between the different utilitarian theories. Entities such as theologic concerns, absolutes, duty, conscience, principles, intentions, feelings, and obligations within particular relationships lose their primary significance and become relevant only because of their consequences and strictly utilitarian outcome. Utilitarianism belongs to bureaucracy and the hospital and state level. For many practitioners, utilitarianism is an inappropriate form of critical ethical thinking at the individual doctor-patient level.

Utilitarian arguments are part of a larger group of ethical theories referred to as *consequentialism*, which focuses on the consequences of actions, rather than anything intrinsic to the action, in assessing the ethical propriety of a given action. Nonutilitarian consequentialism has no strict value criteria and no strict method of measuring the good across a population. Doctors frequently consider the ethical consequences of their actions for individual patients, sometimes referred to as the "micro" ethical level. Hospital administrations and government health departments have ethical concerns that relate to small and large populations, referred to as "meso" and "macro" ethical levels. Clearly there can be tensions within and between these levels. For example, a micro level concern for patient confidentiality is in tension with a macro level concern for reporting of AIDS-related disease to the government public health unit. Consequentialist arguments are relevant in bioethical debate concerning extremely premature newborns. Some of these bioethical scenarios are most upsetting for all those concerned, so whatever the outcome of critical ethical reflection and theorization, all staff actions must be carried out with great sensitivity and respect for patients, family, and staff.[15] Consequentialist arguments are also relevant to the very controversial issue of euthanasia.[16]

Absolutism and *deontologism* contrast sharply with consequentialism. In these theories the moral value of actions is more implicit to the action and less dependent on the consequences of an action. Consider an extreme example of a pregnant woman who is brain dead after a fatal subarachnoid hemorrhage at 28 weeks' gestation. Does this fetus have a right to life? In attempting to answer this question, a clear notion of the nature of a "right" is required. A "right" is innate; it generates a corresponding duty in other agents and is frequently embodied in a law. Rights may be strong or weak, absolute or relative. Some argue that a fetus has either no rights or weak rights, while many others argue that a fetus has a very strong right to life. Others ask questions such as "rights to what?" A range of answers is possible, such as rights to actual life, to quality of life, or to autonomy. In this example then of a brain dead mother, the gestation is most important in the ethical analysis. At the extremes of gestation it is easier to decide on the ethically proper action in this sad ethical scenario. Other examples concerning limits to resuscitation effort in newborns of extreme prematurity are again familiar to most anesthesiologists. A very challenging example involves the ethical propriety of using tissues and organs from anencephalic newborns for organ transplantation. Sound ethical arguments in favor of using anencephalic newborns as organ donors are sustainable,[17] but in practice this may be very upsetting for staff involved in such procedures and could be difficult to implement because of polarization of views on this topic.

Contextualism and *feminist theories*[18] highlight the importance of the situation and context surrounding a particular situation or ethical scenario. Thus the details of an individual case become very important in deciding on ethically proper medical actions. Contextualism[19] is related to *proportionalism*. Such theories are not systematic, but relate to a practical wisdom concerned with gaining a judicious mix of all the relevant theories, interested parties, circumstances, and details. Human *virtues*[20] are important in the professional setting. The psychiatrist Dr. A. Meares has used poetry as a medium for ethical reflection.[21]

In conclusion, medical practitioners should have two levels of ethical functioning, a robust everyday intuitive ethical sense coupled with a deeper awareness and ability to critically reflect on more difficult ethical problems. Practitioners should try to have awareness of a number of ethical theories,[22] and be sensitive to the differing levels[23] and styles[24] of ethical theory. Ethical argument often involves balancing multiple tensions and fuzzy issues rather than "black and white" issues. Human judgment has a vital role. Bioethical reflection and analysis is complex, unmeasurable in the scientific sense, and necessarily pragmatic.

PROFESSIONALISM AND PROFESSIONAL REGULATION

Medical practitioners are professional people. Professionalism entails a public undertaking to act in a particular manner and respect certain standards; sometimes this is tacit, while other medical graduations involve the graduands taking a public oath. These standards usually relate to the legal requirements of the state and also to standards set by the medical profession itself. A doctor's conscience and the requirements of the state can sometimes be in tension. An extreme example concerns the conduct of doctors in Nazi Germany during World War II. A more contemporary example of conflict of interest or tension involves medical practitioners adopting a small business person role in the community, or being directly employed by a health insurance company. The point here is that doctors, as individuals and as a group, have unique responsibilities and duties to contribute to their society in a number of ways and these duties carry associated special authorities and limited rights such as professional autonomy.

The colleges and associations representing anesthetists have collective responsibilities to maintain standards within the profession, to facilitate the functioning of the particular professional group within a society, and generally to maintain the integrity of the medical profession[25]:

> A "responsible profession" should regularly debate the dimensions of its professional responsibility and [associated] ethical implications. The final product is not a document, but [an ongoing] dialogue. Within a profession, ethics [entails] . . . a collective undertaking by which practical wisdom is developed . . . [and there exists ongoing] shared critical reflection . . . not entirely from a process of imposed teaching . . .

So these colleges representing anesthesiologists may have examinations and criteria for fellowship along with maintenance of standards programs for members. Colleges may have an explicit code of ethics embodied in a particular document[26] or a set of more general documents such as guidelines, policies, and procedures.

Directors of anesthetic departments in hospitals have collective responsibilities that are similar to the previously noted responsibilities of the anesthesia associations, but have additional ethical responsibilities to trainee anesthesiologists in the department. There are also ethical aspects to continuous quality improvement or quality assurance activity within the department. Consider, for example, the director of a small hospital with an obstetric epidural service. What annual number of epidurals is required to maintain staff proficiency in the management of epidural analgesia?

INFORMED CONSENT IN OBSTETRIC ANESTHESIA

Understanding consent in clinical medicine requires an awareness of some foundation concepts such as the "doctor-patient relationship" and "duty of care." Understanding the modern multidisciplinary team is also important.

Valid patient consent is best seen as a clinical process. This process entails a triad of patient competence to give consent, appropriate information disclosure with comprehension and understanding, and finally appropriate patient voluntariness. Events associated with the process include documentation, and a clear patient signal indicating consent. This signal can be in three forms: implied consent, verbal consent, and written consent. These discrete events are evidence of an underlying valid consent process. If the underlying process is seriously flawed, a signed consent form has little worth. Also, having signed a consent form and started treatment, any patient who later feels the risk disclosure was inadequate may freely withdraw or vary the consent.

The principles of bioethics are relevant to consent. Specifically, beneficence and respect for autonomy are in opposition sometimes. Consider a patient with strong predictors of difficult intubation, who wants general anesthesia for a nonelective cesarean section. An anesthesiologist who strongly but respectfully guides the patient into accepting a spinal anesthetic is allowing beneficence to trump patient autonomy. In doing so the anesthesiologist may be seen as acting paternalistically. Paternalism involves violation of a bioethical principle with intention to benefit the patient and avoid a great harm. Absent or borderline patient consent is involved, and there must be reasonable belief that the patient's desires are "irrational" or that later, when the patient is better able to consent, the treatment will be understood or endorsed.[27]

Paternalism can be very overt in psychiatry and public health. Subtle forms of paternalism are more widespread, for example, in the way we present information or outline treatment options to patients. It is inevitable that there are limited paternalist aspects to anesthesia and medicine. When we identify paternalism in our actions we should ask—Is it appropriate? Consider the limited paternalism regarding airway management for anesthesia in a cesarean section patient. The anesthesiologist, having the airway expertise and the responsibility of safely managing the airway, appropriately has major input into what happens. Consider the limited paternalism during a bad "cord-prolapse" scenario: In transit to the operating room the patient is hurriedly told what will happen, along with remarks such as "We have to do a cesarean section now to save your baby." Frequently doctors may not ask such patients if they have questions and will take consent as implied by their compliance with treatment. Consider, in contrast, a patient with severe nonreassuring cardiotocographic (CTG) patterns who, despite obstetric advice, maintains an explicit refusal to consent to cesarean section.[28] Assuming solid patient comprehension and understanding of the consequences of refusal, a forced cesarean section will probably be seen legally as trespass, and ethically perhaps as inappropriate paternalism. However, if it was thought the patient was "irrational," psychotic, or not fully comprehending the situation, the doctors—for better or worse—would have to make some difficult decisions. The obstetrician would lead the way here and try to establish the nature of the patient's objection to surgery, unless the primary objection was actually to anesthesia.

The Doctor-Patient Relationship. Valid consent processes occur within a special relationship—the *doctor-patient relationship* (DPR). If you have any experience with epidural childbirth complicated by obstetric palsy, you will understand the importance of the doctor-patient relationship. The association of the epidural with the nerve palsy is usually not causal. Despite this, the situation is very difficult: Through the patient's eyes the needle in the back appears to be the cause of the nerve injury, especially if benign catheter paresthesia was present. Satisfactory resolution of this difficult situation requires three things: (1) An effective DPR; (2) a prior disclosure to both the patient and her partner that covered the remote risk of nerve injury in childbirth, with or without an epidural; and (3) early involvement by an experienced neurologist is essential.

Conceptions of the doctor-patient relationship are embedded in our culture and idealized by some, such that anger and bereavement can occur when a complex reality fails to measure up. The media is involved in the DPR, and this can sometimes contribute to unrealistic patient expectation.

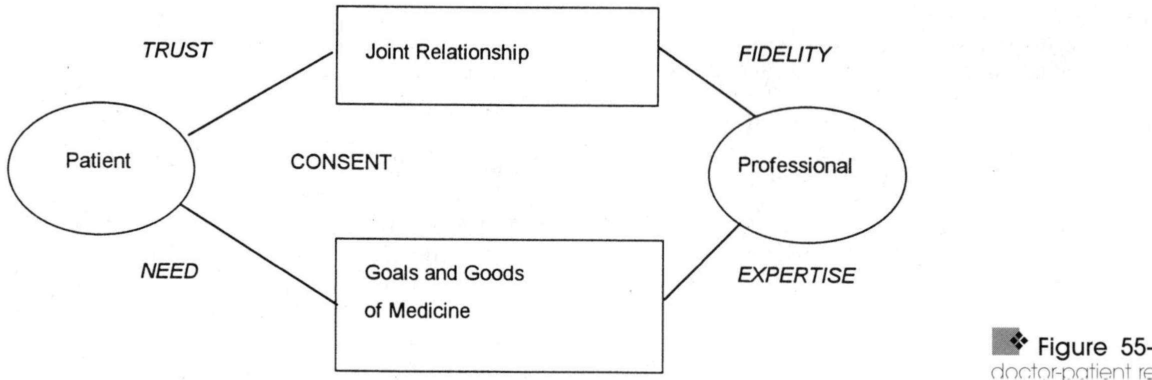

❖ **Figure 55–1** The doctor-patient relationship.

Figure 55–1 is a model[29] of the doctor-patient relationship. In this adequate model, the goals and goods of medicine are bridled to meet the consenting patient's need, under the guide of professional expertise. Despite the potential power imbalance, the DPR has a joint nature. Fidelity may be thought of as any reasonable balancing of the bioethical principles. Trust and joint relationship are not jargon terms here; the analogy of getting into a boat is apt, talking with the pilot and perhaps encountering unexpected weather.

In considering a private obstetric DPR developing over some months, this model seems authentic. What of the anesthetic DPR? Often, the anesthesiologist first encounters a patient when called to the labor room, and there is little time to build the anesthetic DPR. Many factors contribute to patient expectation before meeting the anesthetic doctor—antenatal classes, obstetricians, midwives, the media, and past patient experience. Midwives talk with patients about their analgesia options and usually help set realistic patient expectation. Through anesthetic department liaison with the antenatal clinic, antenatal educators, and midwives, information disclosure can commence well before this particular anesthesiologist meets the patient in the labor room. What can this anesthesiologist do in that short time to build an effective DPR and to gain valid patient consent for treatment?

The Multidisciplinary Team—Balancing Different Perspectives. It is important to recognize that we work within a multidisciplinary team (MDT). There is more than one doctor-patient relationship and more than one discipline involved in obstetric patients. The triad of patient, midwife, and obstetrician is familiar. When the anesthesiologist becomes involved, there is the potential for a range of different perspectives. Sometimes there is tension within the multidisciplinary team that needs careful consideration. Not all tension is negative. The anesthesiologist's aim is to function effectively within the multidisciplinary team. To understand the MDT we need a concept of the single discipline, such as midwifery or anesthesia. Disciplines are perhaps similar to a Kuhnian paradigm which involves[30]:

> . . . cônceptual frameworks . . . with substantive working rules . . . laws and "looser" elements: general theories . . . a common fund of . . . concepts . . ., rules of "evidence," standards for confirmation and dis-confirmation, a coherent tradition, and a shared sense concerning the significant questions along with accepted techniques for solving them.

The multidisciplinary team is not a cozy homogeneous group of multidisciplined individuals. An effective MDT is a heterogeneous group of individuals from different disciplines who have some joint commitment to work together—hopefully there is a healthy diversity of views and some constructive tensions within. Tensions between individuals in the MDT often originate from differences between the disciplines themselves. The process of fairly addressing these tensions within the team and not suppressing them can improve the quality of patient care, avert simple mistakes, and reduce medicolegal risk. Balancing the different perspectives within the team is sometimes tricky, and patients are sometimes perplexed by the different views. Examining the range of responses to an issue within the MDT is often helpful. In legal action against an anesthesiologist, the midwife's and obstetrician's view of events can be very important.

Where possible, view tensions in the MDT constructively. Working effectively with other members of the MDT is important. In many hospitals after an epidural block is placed the midwife or obstetric nurse checks on maternal and fetal responses to the block. Prior to leaving, the anesthesiologist should check that the midwife is happy with the observations and that the correct expectations of the block are in place. It also helps to check that top-up or infusion orders are clear—after all, it is the midwife who will be responsible for the patient's epidural after the anesthesiologist leaves.

In the event of a bad outcome, or later complaint and legal action, an understanding of the MDT helps to preserve cohesion and buffer staff stresses, to avoid traditional doctor-nurse polarization, and to make sense of the different perspectives that exist within the team. The day a midwife says to the anesthesiologist, prior to an epidural, "I am not happy with the consent here doctor," you know that the multidisciplinary team is functioning effectively.

Duties of Care in Anesthesia. In anesthesia there are "duties of care" concerning the way we perform standard medical procedures. These duties include the need to:

1. Gather patient history.
2. Examine the patient.
3. Use medical tests.
4. Reach diagnosis and differential diagnoses.
5. Present options and information, disclose risk, and seek consent.
6. Perform treatment(s).
7. Maintain documentation.
8. Follow up patient problems and manage complications.

Prior to placing an epidural in the obstetric unit, the history taking is routine but important because the anesthesiologist's manner at that stage builds the doctor-patient relationship. Discussion of the obstetric context with the obstetrician and midwife and also checking the CTG is usual. Anesthetists are not CTG experts, but if there is concern get an obstetric review prior to the epidural, especially if the CTG straps are removed during placement of the epidural. On examination the anesthesiologist may check the airway and lumbar spine. Pathology such as the platelet count may be checked. In my view, the fact that patients are in pain does not justify overlooking these duties of care, nor falling below the expected standards of care. Patients and their partners usually witness the anesthesiologist taking reasonable care while performing these standard medical procedures, even if briefly. So when the anesthesiologist presents information, discloses risks, and seeks consent, it is manifestly based on standard medical procedure.

How much information and risk disclosure should we provide? The quality and quantity, along with the manner and styles of risk disclosure, vary greatly between anesthesiologists. Patient's questions and involvement alter the nature of the consent process and discussions of risk disclosure. Using a postal questionnaire, Bush[31] compared the self-reported practice of 150 U.S. and UK anesthesiologists in obtaining informed consent. The U.S. group were keener on a separate written consent and discussed more of the risks and benefits relating to general anesthesia than the UK group. The approach to regional anesthesia was more uniform between the U.S. and the UK anesthesiologists.

Lanigan and Reynolds[32] used a postal questionnaire to study risk disclosure in the practice of 523 UK and Irish anesthesiologists. The questionnaire comprised a fictitious cesarean section case history and a list of sample statements to determine the level of consensus among anesthesiologists concerning treatment options and appropriate risk information. For type of anesthesia, 63% advised a regional, 32% after discussion would allow the mother a choice of anesthesia, and 5% would advise general anesthesia. The levels of consensus concerning risk disclosure were conveyed using an analytic method with graphical output. This method determined the points of focal agreement and consensus among anesthesiologists (Fig. 55–2).

For regional anesthesia there was general agreement on disclosing perioperative discomfort, hypotension, conversion to general anesthesia, partial blockade, weak legs, and accidental dural tap, while anesthesiologists were generally against discussion of paraplegia. Discussion of backache and micturition difficulties with regional blockade was optional. For general anesthesia there was general agreement in favor of disclosing postoperative pain. While there was diversity of opinion on whether to disclose deep vein thrombosis, awareness, aspiration, and hypoxia, most anesthesiologists would indicate to the patient that regional anesthesia was safer than general anesthesia.

Commencing a discussion on risk information with the patient, using a standard risk disclosure is helpful. If patients say they do not want to be told of risks, basic risk information should be imparted implicitly—within a description of what will happen and how the patient can help. General risk disclosure needs to be supplemented by particular disclosures and information unique to the particular situation. A good discussion with the patient and her partner is the guide. Anxious patients do not need less information, but rather a sensitive presentation. Appropriately imparting real anesthetic options, setting risk information in context, and allaying anxiety are all central to the art of medicine.

It is important to ask patients and their partners for their questions. Patients who ask questions tend to receive more information. When patients have no questions or say they know all about epidurals, the anesthesiologist can ask patients some questions to check their understanding and contrive some discussion. If patients seem ambivalent in obstetric unit epidural situations, they may need some time to consider their options or to discuss things with the midwife. Generally verbal consent to proceed should be explicitly asked for, with the midwife in attendance. In my view, for routine cases, working on the quality of a public verbal consent seems quite adequate. Other institutions may use a separate written consent form for epidurals in labor; however, if the underlying consent process is flawed, a signed form can mean little.

In contrast, consent processes for clinical trials and research are different. The bioethical principles can have multiple aspects, so beneficence with respect to that subject, the population, and future patients may need more delicate balancing. Despite ethics committees,[33] different time pressures, and written consent forms, striking a working balance in clinical trials is also demanding.

In clinical practice, striking a working balance between information-giving, respect for patient self-determination, and "getting on with the necessary" can be a challenge. Despite this we should not see consent in obstetric anesthesia as unduly difficult.[34] Generally, we use the same principles in seeking consent as we do throughout clinical medicine.[35] Practically, in obstetric anesthesia, with exhausted patients in significant pain, a doctor who acts in accordance with accepted medical practice and in the patient's best interests is unlikely to be found to have acted unlawfully, even despite borderline consent.

Achieving an effective doctor-patient relationship is the key in obstetric anesthesia. Such patients are "in partnership" with their doctors, are easier to work with in difficult situations, and are likely to have better

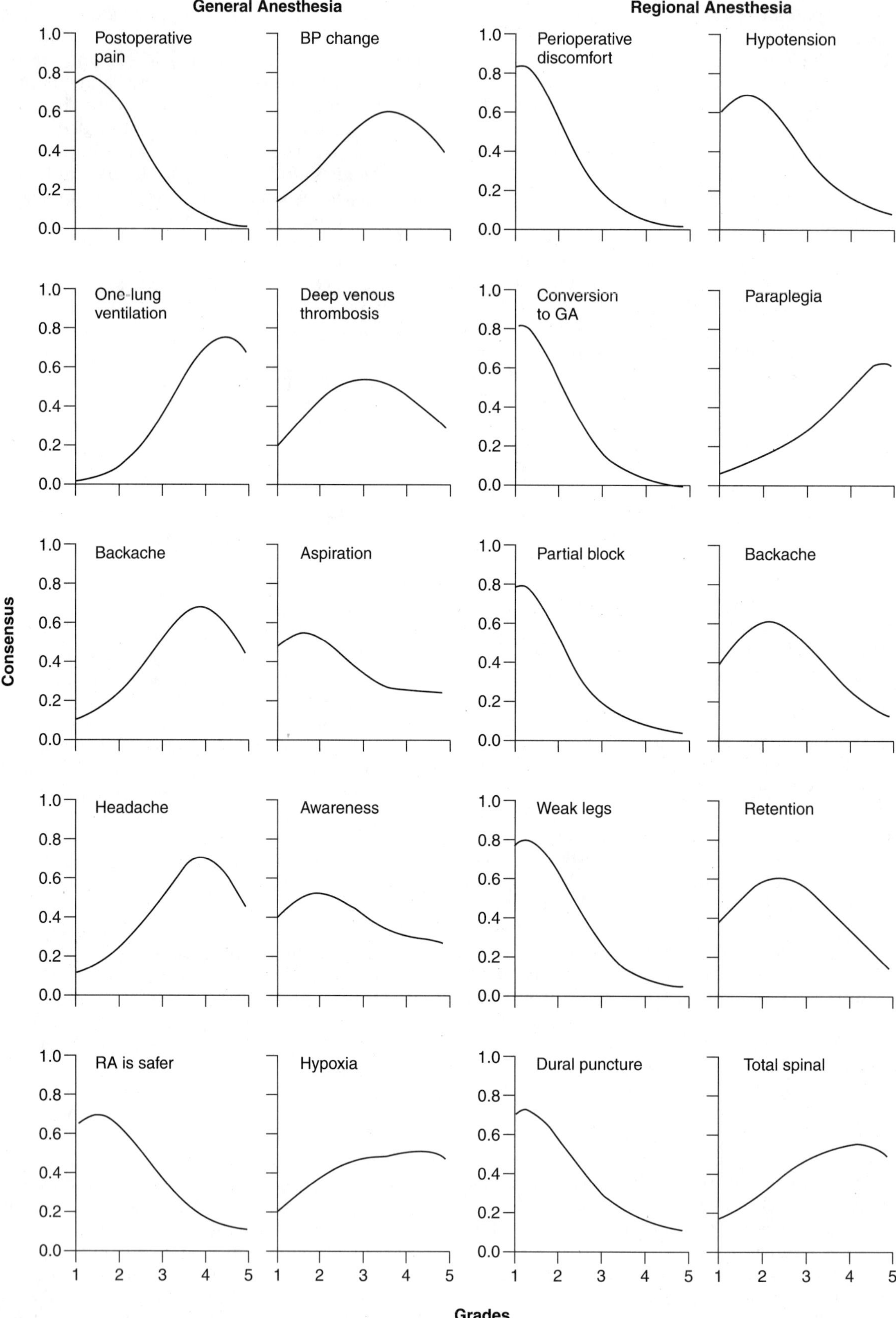

Figure 55–2 Consensus agreement on the delivery of risk information on anesthesia to a mother awaiting elective cesarean section. Grades: 1 = must be mentioned; 2 = worth mentioning; 3 = optional; 4 = not worth mentioning; 5 = must not be mentioned unless specifically asked. Consensus = 1.0 = full agreement.

patient satisfaction. Later, if problems occur, both patient and doctor benefit.

Medicolegal Background to Consent. Medicolegally speaking, patients and their partners need information in making informed choices concerning their well-being. In providing this information, doctors are empowering patients and respecting the legal principle of patient self-determination. In elective cases, patients should be informed of all information that is likely to influence their particular decision. *Material risks* need disclosure. A risk is material if[36]:

> . . . in the circumstances of the particular case, a reasonable [or ordinary] person in the patient's position, if warned of the risk would be likely to attach significance to it *or* if the medical practitioner is, or should reasonably be, aware that the particular patient, if warned of the risk, would be likely to attach significance to it.

Clearly patient self-determination is sometimes not possible. Within Australia, if treatment is of an urgent lifesaving nature and consent cannot be obtained, consent is not required—although prior patient directives do need attention. Within Australia, if treatment is of an urgent lifesaving nature and consent can be obtained, consent should be "good enough" to proceed, especially when patient compliance for a regional block is required. Always doctors should act reasonably in light of the situation.

Legal action against a doctor may involve three potential considerations: professional negligence; trespass or assault in the absence of valid consent; and uncommonly, breach of contract.[37] Serious failures of informed consent usually involve allegations of professional negligence. In action for negligence, where a duty of care exists, there is implicit an expected standard of care. The law determines that a doctor's actions have reached the expected standard of care in several ways. An older *Bolam principle* stated that "if a doctor had acted in accordance with a reasonable and competent body of professional opinion," then she or he had met the standard of care. In asserting that the medical profession determines standards of care, the Bolam test is appropriate in judging how we may use medical tests, examine patients, and so on. Specialist examinations and continuing medical education can be seen as keeping us up-to-date with a reasonable and competent body of professional opinion.

However, when considering how a doctor presents information, discloses risk, and seeks patient consent, the 1992 Australian High Court case of *Rogers* v *Whitaker* is exemplary. This legal case indicated the Bolam test was outmoded within Australia. The High Court of Australia signaled that in assessing the standard of care concerning provision of information to a given patient, the doctor's medical perspective alone is inadequate. In presenting such information and in seeking patient consent we are always treating on a case by case basis. The plaintiff Whitaker was blind in the right eye following a 1946 accident. In 1984, the proposed surgery carried possible functional and cosmetic benefit for the blind eye. In extraordinary preoperative questioning concerning the remote possibility of damage to her good eye, the complication of sympathetic ophthalmia was not mentioned. Rogers operated, and postoperatively Whitaker suffered this rare complication and became bilaterally blind. It is clear that Rogers had indeed failed in his duty to warn the patient of a material risk.

Negligence is not failure to achieve a good outcome, nor failure to disclose all remote risks. Whitaker's negligence action was successful despite several challenges, because it fulfilled all four necessary legal conditions. First, a duty of care existed to inform Whitaker of the risk of sympathetic ophthalmia. There was failure to inform Whitaker, so a breach of duty or deficient standard of care was present. Actual injury was suffered by the patient in that Whitaker became bilaterally blind. The final requirement, that legal causation be satisfied, is the most complex of the criteria for professional negligence. This involves establishing that breech of duty led to patient injury and in *Rogers* v *Whitaker* it was clear that, if informed of the risk, Whitaker would have refused surgery.[38]

The evidence was that Whitaker questioned Rogers extensively concerning complications, so much so that he became annoyed. Even the most remote, known risk of postoperative blindness was likely to influence Whitaker's decision to have surgery. Experts later debated the probability of the complication, but the number was irrelevant, since sympathetic ophthalmia was a material risk and needed disclosure. In this case the courts determined the appropriate standard of care concerning risk disclosure.

The concept of patient self-determination entails a notion of freedom including both freedom to choose and freedom to refuse. Consider an adult Jehovah's Witness with a major postpartum hemorrhage who needs surgery. If the patient was to hear "We will not operate unless you have a blood transfusion," her freedom to refuse transfusion would be unreasonably compromised.

Clear advanced directives such as that of the adult Jehovah's Witness are usually very binding. To knowingly transfuse an adult Jehovah's Witness patient can result in allegations of trespass and assault. Legally this is very different from negligence. The patient does not have to prove injury or causation—only that consent to treatment received was absent. Usually action for trespass is not appropriate in seeking compensation for medical injury. Advanced directives are perhaps the exception and there certainly are successful findings of trespass against doctors who have transfused Jehovah's Witness patients.

What of a woman with a written advanced directive not to have an epidural in labor who then requests an epidural when in extreme labor pain? Perhaps the patient's refusal did not cover the later circumstance. Another written consent overriding the previous written directive is of little use.

In obstetrics there is clear potential for patient misunderstanding, and sometimes patients are left with grievances. Inevitably legal action occurs. British courts place a strong emphasis on evidence of approved medical action, while North American courts champion informed choice and the patient's right to be given information, regardless of usual practices. Australian courts are between these two poles.

In my view systematic, multidisciplinary, postanesthesia rounds are the best single response to concerns about quality of informed consent in obstetric anesthesia. Patient consent and comprehension that was "good enough" for a rushed procedure last night can today be strengthened and improved in the postanesthesia round. In this setting good medicine and good law usually converge.

❖ **Conclusion** Clinician awareness of the ethical dimensions to medical practice is vital to the art of medicine. It is important that clinicians have mature professional approaches to tensions and ethical problems within medicine. A certain knowledge base is required, but thereafter sustaining a reflective dialogue with colleagues and even patients is required. Guardianship tribunals, medical boards, and medical defense organizations usually provide support and help for clinicians tackling ethical problems. The clinician must first, however, recognize and identify the ethical problem. Awareness of the character of bioethical problems helps clinicians to better recognize ethical problems in our everyday work.[39]

There is no single ethical theory or deterministic approach to bioethics that will return the correct answer to ethical problems. There are instead a number of correct approaches and methods of tackling ethical problems in clinical practice. Awareness of context and important cultural and legal aspects to ethical problems help us to gain a complete appreciation of a particular ethical problem. After discussion, debate, and reflection concerning ethical issues and a clinical problem, human judgment and practical wisdom are always required for bioethics to deliver an outcome.

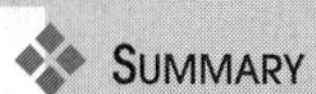

Summary

Key Points

- Despite a diversity of views regarding the nature of bioethics, value judgments and bioethical concerns permeate all levels of medicine and health care.
- Ethical argument often involves balancing multiple tensions and unclear issues, with human judgment playing a vital role.
- Bioethical and legal issues underpin the notion of (informed) consent in medicine within the context of the doctor-patient relationship.
- Balancing the different perspectives within the multidisciplinary team is essential in sustaining good-quality health care.

Key Reference

Fulford KWM, Gillett G, Soskice JM (eds): Medicine and Moral Reasoning. New York: Cambridge University Press; 1994.

Case Stem

An educated and articulate term parturient has a severe "nonreassuring" fetal heart rate tracing and, despite strong obstetric advice, continues to communicate an explicit refusal to consent to cesarean section. How should the medical team approach this situation?

References

1. Reichlin M: Observations on the epistemological status of bioethics. J Med Philos 1994; 19:79–102.
2. McNeill P, Walters JD, Webster I: Ethical issues in Australian hospitals. Med J Aust 1994; 160:63–65.
3. Siedlecky S, Wyndham D: Populate and Perish—Australian Women's Fight for Birth Control. Allen and Unwin; 1990.
4. Benjamin M: Judgement and the art of compromise. Thinking, the Journal of Philosophy for Children 1992; 9(4):2–7.
5. Nagel T: The View from Nowhere. New York: Oxford University Press; 1986.
6. Reich WT(ed): Encyclopaedia of Bioethics. New York: The Free Press; 1978.
7. Singer P(ed): A Companion to Ethics. Cambridge, MA: Blackwell; 1991.
8. Hare RM: The philosophical basis of psychiatric ethics. *In* Bloch S, Chodoff P (eds): Psychiatric Ethics, 2nd ed. New York: Oxford University Press; 1991.
9. Beauchamp T, Childress J: Principles of Biomedical Ethics. New York: Oxford University Press; 1983.
10. Lyons D: Forms and Limits of Utilitarianism. New York: Oxford University Press; 1965.
11. Singer P: Practical Ethics. New York: Cambridge University Press; 1979.
12. Smart JJC, Williams B: Utilitarianism—For and Against. Cambridge University Press; 1973:99.
13. Glover J: Causing Death and Saving Lives. New York: Penguin Books; 1977:71–73.
14. Mackie JL: Ethics: Inventing Right and Wrong. Santa Barbara, CA: Pelican; 1977:136.
15. Clark SE, Marley J: Good grief. Med J Aust 1993; 158:834–841.
16. Burgess MM: The medicalization of dying. J Med Philos 1993; 18:269–279.
17. Singer P: Rethinking Life and Death. The Text Publishing Company; 1994.
18. Cole EB, Coultrap-McQin S (eds): Explorations in Feminist Ethics: Theory and Practice. Indiana University Press; 1992.
19. Ladd J: Positive and negative euthanasia. *In* White JE (ed): Contemporary Moral Problems. West Publishing; 1985:58–69.
20. May WF: The virtues in a professional setting. *In* Fulford KWM (eds): Medicine and Moral Reasoning. New York: Cambridge University Press; 1994:75–90.
21. Meares A: A Way of Doctoring. Melbourne: Hill of Content; 1985.
22. Lovat TJ: Main streams of bioethical thought. Baillieres Clin Obstet Gynaecol 1991; 5:511–528.
23. Seanor D, Fotion N: Levels of moral thinking. *In* Hare and Critics: Essays on Moral Thinking. Arlington, VA: Clarendon Paperbacks; 1990.
24. Williams B: Ethics and the limits of philosophy. *In* Styles of Ethical Theory. 1985: 71–92.
25. Walsh ML: Ethics—a professional responsibility. *In* Australian Anaesthesia, 1992. Continuing Education for Anaesthetists from the Australian and New Zealand College of Anaesthetists. ANZCA; 1992:138.
26. Pargiter R, Bloch S: Developing a code of ethics for psychiatry: the Australasian experience. Aust N Z J Psychiatry 1994; 28:188–196.

27. Committee on Medical Education: A Casebook in Psychiatric Ethics. Brunner/Mazel; 1990.
28. Phelan JP: The maternal abdominal wall: a fortress against fetal health care? South California Law Review 1991; 65:461–490.
29. Verbal communication, G. Gleeson, PhD, 1997, John Plunkett Centre for Ethics, St. Vincent's Hospital, Sydney, Australia.
30. Kuhn TS: Structure of Scientific Revolutions. Chicago: University of Chicago Press; 1962:10–11, 43–44.
31. Bush DJ: A comparison of informed consent for obstetric anaesthesia in the USA and the UK. Int J Obstet Anaesth 1995; 4:1–6.
32. Lanigan C, Reynolds F: Risk information supplied by obstetric anaesthetists in Britain and Ireland to mothers awaiting elective caesarean section. Int J Obstet Anaesth 1995; 4:7–13.
33. Blake D: The hospital ethics committee—health care's moral conscience or white elephant? Hastings Cent Rep 1992; January–February:6–11.
34. Gild WM: Informed consent: a review. Anesth Analg 1989; 68:649–653.
35. Grice SC, Eisenach JC, Dewan MD, Robinson ML: Evaluation of informed consent for anaesthesia for labor and delivery. ASA Abstract no. A664. Anesthesiology 1988; 69:3A.
36. Skene L: Law and Medical Practice: Rights, Duties, Claims and Defences, paragraph 6.14. Stoneham, MA: Butterworths; 1998: 142.
37. Staunton P, Whyburn B: Nursing and the Law, 4th ed. Philadelphia: WB Saunders/Balliere Tindall; 1997:99.
38. Staunton P, Whyburn B: Nursing and the Law, 4th ed. Philadelphia: WB Saunders/Balliere Tindall; 1997.
39. Thomas G: An Introduction to Ethics: Five Central Problems of Moral Judgement. Indianapolis: Hackett Pub Co; 1993.

56

Patient Satisfaction: Capturing Patients' Perspective in the Evaluation of Obstetric Care

❖ PETER SALMON, MSc, DPhil

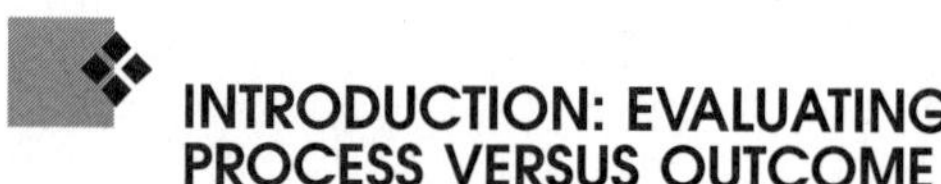

INTRODUCTION: EVALUATING PROCESS VERSUS OUTCOME

Systematic evaluation is intrinsic to good quality care because it allows clinicians and managers to monitor their performance and to maintain or improve their skills or service. Evaluation also meets the pressure for cost-effectiveness from public and private funders of care. Traditionally, evaluation has focused on outcomes, in particular mortality and morbidity, which have the advantage of being unambiguous and important. These criteria are, however, insufficient in areas where outcomes are less clear-cut, such as in palliative care or management of chronic disease. In these areas, evaluation of outcome is still possible, but it is necessary to turn to the patient for the answers in the form of subjective quality of life. Other areas of health care present an even greater challenge to evaluation because patients are normally healthy both before and after intervention. These include screening procedures and, of course, obstetric care. In these areas, evaluation according to the *outcome* for the patient is normally uninformative. Therefore evaluation necessarily focuses on the *process* of care.

THE CONCEPT OF SATISFACTION

In practice, the usual way of evaluating the process of obstetric care has been by asking the patient how satisfied she is. At first sight, the answers are very encouraging. The modal position of patients' ticks on a 100-mm visual analogue line is typically within a few millimeters of the "satisfied" end.[1–4] Given a scale of 10, the modal response is typically 10 and hardly any patient scores less than 8.[5] When patients are asked if they are satisfied, 95% report that they are.[6] In many published studies, these uniform responses have been carefully documented and dutifully subjected to statistical comparisons, even in situations in which groups that have received different care differed by only a whisker. One response is that the present chapter should stop here. The process of care is as good as it can be; well done.

Another response is that something is wrong with these findings. High satisfaction is not, of course, confined to obstetrics but recurs across medical care. At the very least, such uniform responses provide no information, just as an examination that everyone passes is uninformative. Surely, it is odd that patients do not differ in their precise *level* of satisfaction, even if they are all satisfied. Therefore, the consistency of findings of high satisfaction sounds a warning. It is wise to examine carefully the background to the use of satisfaction ratings so as to be clear on exactly what they tell us.

Consumerism in Health Care

In broad terms, three distinct sets of assumptions influence the way that clinical care is thought of and evaluated.[7] The concept of satisfaction belongs to only one of these sets. Traditionally, clinical care is regarded as an activity that brings together an inexpert (patient) with an expert (doctor). The role of each is well-defined: the doctor should gather information and make a decision and should then ensure that the patient does what she is told. As a reaction to this view, an alternative has developed in which doctor and patient are each seen as experts, albeit with different areas of expertise. According to this view, the doctor should use good communication skills to help the patient disclose her concerns and should address psychosocial concerns as readily as biomedical ones. The third view is consumerism: that health care brings a consumer (patient) together with a service-provider (doctor). It is from this view that the concept of satisfaction has emanated. Clinicians and theorists alike have seen in customer satisfaction an appealing way of simplifying the complexities of evaluating care. They have even gone so far as to claim that "customer satisfaction" should be regarded as an element of health status.[8]

Problems with the Concept of Satisfaction

Clearly, consumerism is the framework within which health care is delivered in countries where patients freely choose their doctors and payment is by fee-for-service. However, it is doubtful that consumerism is valid as a model of what health care is about at the level of the consulting room, labor ward, or delivery suite. For consumerism and satisfaction to be validly applied to health care, satisfaction must be a function of health care. Consider an analogy. Satisfaction is the main function of visiting a restaurant. There are simpler and cheaper ways of finding nutrition, but we visit the restaurant to be pampered and satisfied. Because of this, we normally weigh up the service we have received and decide whether or not we are satisfied with it. Therefore, without blinking, we complete the satisfaction questionnaire that is left with the bill. By contrast, we visit a supermarket to keep ourselves alive and nourished and not for satisfaction. A satisfaction questionnaire given with the till receipt would take us aback. Because we did not *go* to be satisfied we had not thought about whether or not we *were* satisfied. Cosmetic surgery aside, medical care is arguably closer to the supermarket than the restaurant. Obstetricians are consulted to deliver healthy babies to healthy mothers, not to provide satisfaction. Therefore, most patients probably do not have a consumerist concept of satisfaction in relation to obstetric care, any more than to health care in general. Satisfaction or dissatisfaction is simply not an issue for them because they do not approach medical care with the kinds of consumerist expectations with which they approach the consumption of luxury goods and services.[8]

There are further problems with the concept of satisfaction as applied to medical care. In particular, few patients are competent to evaluate its technical quality. They do not have the knowledge and most have insufficient experience of childbirth. An additional problem is that hospital patients' notorious tendency to passivity and acquiescence in the face of doctors' authority is incompatible with feeling dissatisfied.[8] Without the potential for dissatisfaction, there can be no satisfaction. Feelings of satisfaction and dissatisfaction with medical care do, of course, sometimes arise, just as they occasionally do in a supermarket. However, this usually only occurs when there have been gross departures from what patients, or shoppers, regard as normal,[9] such as a particularly rude doctor or checkout operator.

Understanding Patients' Responses to Satisfaction Questionnaires

Probably the main occasion when patients think about whether they are satisfied is when they are asked how satisfied they are. That is, being asked about satisfaction creates the concept in the patient's mind. However, patients' answers indicate that their concept of satisfaction is not necessarily the same as the concept of satisfaction that exists in the clinician's mind. As observed earlier, patients' responses to simple satisfaction questions typically indicate extremely high levels of satisfaction. Very few patients identify themselves as dissatisfied.[8, 10] The main thing this tells us is that in formal surveys, just as in individual consultations, patients are reluctant to criticize their clinicians. When principles of good questionnaire design are adhered to so that, in particular, questions are less transparent,[11] more variable responses are obtained. The resulting scores do seem to measure a property of the patient-clinician relationship that is clinically important. Patients who say they are satisfied are the most likely to comply with treatment advice.[7] There is also some evidence that they have a better clinical outcome.[12] However, the satisfaction scores depend more on interpersonal than technical aspects of care.[10] It seems that, whereas patients are not competent to evaluate technical aspects of care, they do evaluate the psychosocial aspects. It follows that it would be possible for a scurrilous or technically poor clinician to satisfy a patient by careful attention to communication and relationship skills. Additional influences on how satisfied patients say they are further weaken the value of these ratings as indicators of quality of care.[10] The satisfied patients tend to be older or less well educated.[13] They are healthier, at least in terms of mental health,[14, 15] and happier with the world in general.[12] In summary, therefore, when patients respond positively to a simple question about satisfaction, they can mean a multitude of different things (Fig. 56–1).

APPROACHES TO CAPTURING PATIENTS' PERSPECTIVE: SATISFACTION IN CONTEXT

Clearly, satisfaction does not provide a simple way of capturing patients' perspective to evaluate quality of care. This does not mean that it should have no place in evaluation. However, it should be adopted more cautiously and with the knowledge that it is one imper-

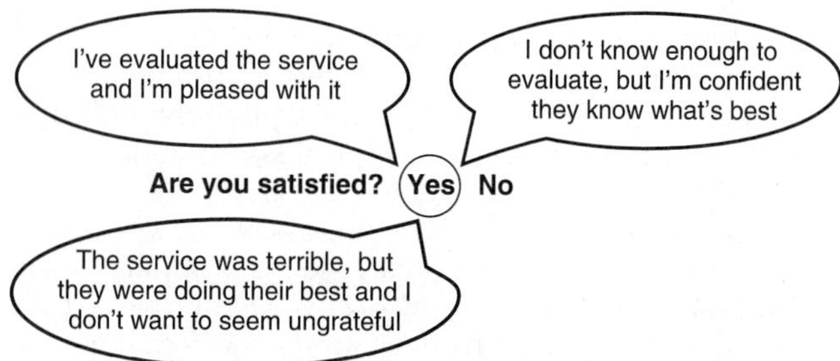
I've evaluated the service and I'm pleased with it
I don't know enough to evaluate, but I'm confident they know what's best
Are you satisfied? Yes No
The service was terrible, but they were doing their best and I don't want to seem ungrateful

❖ **Figure 56–1** The diverse meanings of "being satisfied." When patients are asked simple questions about satisfaction, positive responses are typical, but they arise for many reasons, 8.

fect approach out of a wide range of approaches that can be taken (Fig. 56–2).

Using Objective Criteria

The simplest approach is just to identify some objective criteria that indicate quality care. For example, criteria might include brevity of waiting times, cleanliness of the clinic, or readability of written information that is provided. In practice, many items find their way onto such lists because they have the stamp of a consumer orientation or because the experts that derived the lists thought they mattered to patients. Unfortunately, clinicians and experts do not reliably detect their patients' concerns.[16, 17] Therefore the criteria that clinicians choose often differ from what patients think are most important. As well as being inaccurate in assessing individual patients' concerns, different professions evidently have different biases (Table 56–1).[17] Therefore, rather than relying on experts, another way of choosing objective criteria is to find the "average" patient's view of what is important by surveying a representative sample of patients. For example, the items that patients surveyed by Drew et al.[17] rated as most important could be used to compare different settings, or to check on maintenance of quality of care over time in a single setting.

In principle, objective quality criteria like these could be observed by clinicians, managers, or outside personnel. However, there are obvious advantages to recruiting patients as the observers, given their close-up view. Patients' views of care do not depend only on its objective characteristics. Those views are influenced, in particular, by the patients' expectations and their history of related treatment. Therefore, patients' subjective evaluation of discrete elements of their care can be more informative than purely objective observations. For example, in one recording scheme of this kind, hospital inpatients are asked how adequate or inadequate they find the cleaning of the ward, visiting arrangements, level of noise, food, pain control, and the nurses' and doctors' behavior.[18]

Patients' Experience of Care

The focus on discrete elements of care is useful for some purposes. In particular, it can help identify specific problematic—or positive—aspects of the way that care is delivered. However, it is never possible to ensure that all important elements have been enquired about, and there is no completely acceptable way of weighing the relative importance of different elements of care in contributing to patients' overall experience of care. Therefore, an alternative approach is to ask directly about patients' experience of their care.

Identifying the Components of Experience

Patients' experience is complex to measure because it is multifaceted and resists being captured in a single question. Indeed, the words or expressions that patients use to describe any experience of health care are vast in number. Nevertheless, this diversity of terms normally reflects a limited number of underlying components of experience. To understand this, a helpful analogy is the experience of color. Most of us think that we see a limitless number of hues around us. In reality, we see only three colors. Every hue that can be seen results from a different combination of the primary colors: red, yellow, and blue. In the same way,

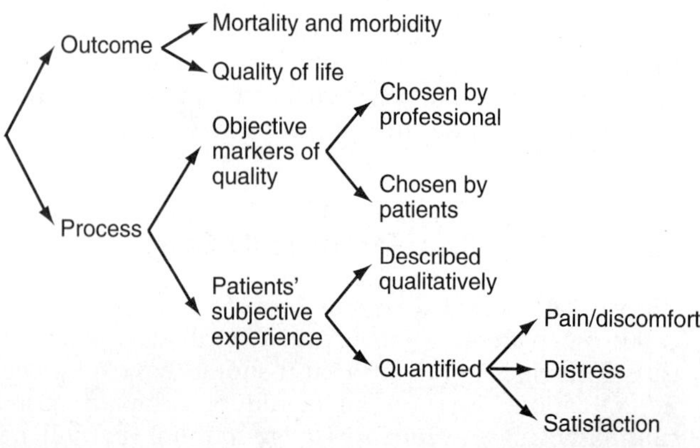

❖ **Figure 56–2** Choices in using patients' perspective to evaluate care. Satisfaction ratings provide only one of several ways in which patients' perspective can be sought.

Table 56-1 IMPORTANCE OF EACH OF 40 ITEMS TO WOMEN'S EXPERIENCE OF CHILDBIRTH IN HOSPITAL, AS RATED BY MOTHERS, MIDWIVES, AND OBSTETRICIANS*

MOTHERS	MIDWIVES	OBSTETRICIANS	ITEM
1	7	1	Baby being healthy
4	3	10	Being shown how to control gas and air
6	20	17	Being told major risks of procedures
8	1	6	Every procedure explained beforehand
11	17	13	Friend or relative present
14	6	11	Being able to hold baby right away
15	9	9	Being told how treatments will feel
20	39	34	Being delivered by qualified staff
24	13	25	Ward rest hour
31	34	31	Being delivered without forceps
37	35	32	Not having an episiotomy

*Items ranked according to their mean ratings by each group. Data from Drew NC, Salmon P, Webb L: Mothers', midwives' and obstetricians' views on the features of obstetric care which influence satisfaction with childbirth. Br J Obstet Gynaecol 1989: 96:1084–1088.

apparently different subjective experiences of care can reflect variations in a small number of underlying components. The components of patients' experience of clinical care can be identified and scored by a combination of careful interviewing and statistical analysis. Examining the sequence of steps taken in two reports shows how this can be applied to childbirth.[19, 20]

The first step was to find out how patients normally describe their experience. Therefore, a small sample of patients was interviewed about their experience of childbirth so that the words and phrases they used to describe it could be noted. Removing synonyms and esoteric terms left 20 different words or phrases. Each was written in opposite forms and given a scale, resulting in a questionnaire that was completed by 110 patients postnatally. A statistical technique (principal components analysis) was used to identify clusters of items that patients tended to answer in the same way. These clusters indicated three separate components of the patients' experience: "worry," "physical discomfort," and "fulfillment/satisfaction." Patients were given scores for their experiences on each component (by summing the scores on the items belonging to the relevant cluster). These scores were used to explore how patients' experience of childbirth was related to factors in patients' history and in the care that they received. For instance, delivery was less distressing in those who had attended antenatal classes, but more distressing in women whose pregnancy was unplanned or in whom a previous pregnancy had been terminated.

These components of experience probably apply quite generally to medical and surgical procedures, since similar ones have emerged in endoscopy and surgery.[20, 21] Nevertheless, different groups of patients use very different language for different procedures. Therefore, it is important to carry out the complete sequence of steps for any procedure that is to be evaluated and in each population in which it is to be evaluated. The results in one procedure cannot simply be generalized to another.

The Independence of the Components of Experience

Components that result from this kind of statistical procedure are independent. This means that, for example, whether or not a patient is in pain does not correlate with whether she is satisfied and emotionally calm; conversely, a patient could be dissatisfied but in no pain at all. Because the components are independent, procedures that are intended to improve one component can have unpredicted effects on others. For example, childbirth by cesarean section is less painful for the mother than is vaginal delivery, but it is also more distressing and less satisfying.[19] Because different components of experience can be affected differently, it will often be impossible to classify an intervention as improving or worsening patients' experience overall. Similarly, it will often be impossible to classify a particular patient as having a good or bad experience. Different components would point to different answers. To produce a single score, the scores on each component could simply be added together. However, this would mean assuming that each component matters equally to patients. In practice, one or another component has normally been regarded as most important. Traditionally, care surrounding medical and surgical procedures has been geared to minimizing pain and discomfort, and sometimes emotional distress. Increasingly, however, the strengthening influence of consumerism means that patient satisfaction is seen as the key dimension.

Qualitative versus Quantitative Evaluation of Experience

Questionnaire surveys of patients' views tend to perpetuate assumptions about how patients view their care. This happens because any questionnaire only finds out what the questions ask, so users of a questionnaire can only find out about things that the designers of the questionnaire had thought of. Another way of expressing this is that questionnaires can "censor" what pa-

Table 56–2 Patients' Evaluation of Patient-Controlled Analgesia

Question	Rating	Responses (N)
How did you feel about PCA?	Extremely positive	83
	Fairly positive	79
	Neutral	28
	Fairly negative	6
	Extremely negative	4
How much control did you have?	Complete	51
	Quite a lot	86
	Some	47
	A little	11
	None	3
	Missing response	2

tients reveal[8] because patients often have things to communicate that are not included in any questionnaire. Qualitative methods therefore have an important place in evaluation because they can identify aspects of patients' experience that had not previously been appreciated. Recent evaluation of patient-controlled analgesia (PCA) in postoperative patients illustrates how this approach can give rise to answers that are quite different from those that questionnaires provide. A questionnaire survey of 200 patients found the results in Table 56–2, which supported the usual assumption that patients are extremely satisfied with PCA because it gives them control over their pain relief.[22] However, a qualitative study in which 26 similar patients at the same hospital were prompted to talk about their experience of PCA in their own way suggested different conclusions.[23] Although most patients described PCA enthusiastically, about a third described it negatively (e.g., "about as effective as pissing into the wind"). Only one patient spontaneously said anything about feeling in control. Instead, most volunteered that they liked PCA because it saved them from bothering the nurses. When prompted to talk about control, no patient was very positive about it (e.g., "when you're in pain you don't care whether you're in control"). Indeed, other comments showed problems with PCA that *restricted* patients' control over pain relief: one third of patients described side-effects or fears about addiction that stopped them from using PCA as much as they wished and others feared addiction or overdose if they used it "too much."

CONCLUSION

This chapter is too brief to teach a reader how to use patients' perspective to evaluate obstetric care. However, it provides a framework for the decisions that researchers and clinicians face when deciding how care should be evaluated, and when evaluating evaluations that are reported by others. At the very least, it should be clear that simple questions that ask whether patients are satisfied are rarely informative. Beyond this, it should be apparent that different approaches are available that can expose clinicians and researchers to the patients' perspective. Psychologic and statistical techniques can help identify and quantify what *can* be measured, but they do not avoid the necessity for decisions about what *will* be measured in practice. These decisions require value judgments, and these judgments expose assumptions about the purpose of health care. Because evaluation depends on value judgments as well as science, it should be expected that ideas about how care should be evaluated will change over time. For example, it might be that the continuing emphasis on assessing satisfaction with obstetric anesthesia care will gradually change patients' priorities so that, in the future, satisfaction becomes as important for patients as it already is for researchers and managers.

References

1. Collis RE, Davies DWL, Aveling W: Randomised comparison of combined spinal-epidural and standard epidural analgesia in labour. Lancet 1995; 345:1413–1416.
2. Davies SJ, Paech MJ, Welch H, et al: Maternal experience during epidural or combined spinal-epidural anesthesia for cesarian section: A prospective, randomized trial. Anesth Analg 1997; 85:607–613.
3. Price C, Lafreniere L, Brosnan C, Findley I: Regional analgesia in early active labour: Combined spinal epidural vs. epidural. Anaesthesia 1998; 53:951–955.
4. Swart M, Sewell J, Thomas D: Intrathecal morphine for Caesarian section: An assessment of pain relief, satisfaction and side-effects. Anaesthesia 1997; 52:364–381.
5. Mould TAJ, Chong S, Spencer JAD, Gallivan S: Women's involvement with the decision preceding their caesarian section and their degree of satisfaction. Br J Obstet Gynaecol 1996; 103:1074–1077.
6. Ranta P, Spalding M, Kangas-Saarela T, et al: Maternal expectations and experiences of labour pain: Options of 1091 Finnish parturients. Acta Anaesthesiol Scand 1995; 39:60–66.
7. Roter DL, Hall JA: Doctors Talking with Patients/Patients Talking with Doctors: Improving Outcomes in Medical Visits. Westport, CT: Auburn House, 1992.
8. Williams B: Patient satisfaction: A valid concept? Soc Sci Med 1994; 38:509–516.
9. Nelson EC, Larson C: Patients' good and bad surprises: How do they relate to overall patient satisfaction. Q Rev Bull 1993; 19:89–94.
10. Fitzpatrick R: Scope and measurement of patient satisfaction. In Fitzpatrick R, Hopkins A (eds): Measurement of Patients' Satisfaction with Their Care. London: Royal College of Physicians, 1993: 1–17.
11. Oppenheim AN: Questionnaire Design, Interviewing and Attitude Measurement. London: Pinter, 1992.
12. Fitzpatrick R, Hopkins A: Patient satisfaction in relation to clinical care: A neglected contribution. In Fitzpatrick R, Hopkins A (eds): Measurement of Patients' Satisfaction with Their Care. London: Royal College of Physicians, 1993: 77–86.
13. Hall J, Dornan M: Patient sociodemographic characteristics as predictors of satisfaction with medical care: A meta-analysis. Soc Sci Med 1990; 30:811–818.
14. Cleary P, Edgman-Levitan S, Roberts M, et al: Patients evaluate their hospital care: A national survey. Health Affairs 1991; 10:254–267.
15. Marshall GN, Hays RD, Mazel R: Health status and satisfaction with health care: Results from the medical outcomes study. J Consult Clin Psychol 1996; 64:380–390.
16. Bradley C, Brewin CR, Duncan SL: Perceptions of labour: discrepancies between midwives' and patients' ratings. Br J Obstet Gynaecol 1983; 90:1176–1179.
17. Drew NC, Salmon P, Webb L: Mothers', midwives' and obstetricians' views on the features of obstetric care which influence satisfaction with childbirth. Br J Obstet Gynaecol 1989; 96:1084–1088.

18. Gritzner C: The CASPE patient satisfaction system. *In* Fitzpatrick R, Hopkins A (eds): Measurement of Patients' Satisfaction with Their Care. London: Royal College of Physicians, 1993: 33–41.
19. Salmon P, Drew NC: Multi-dimensional assessment of women's experience of childbirth: Relationship to obstetric procedure, antenatal preparation and obstetric history. J Psychosom Res 1992; 36:317–327.
20. Salmon P, Shah R, Berg S, Williams C: Evaluating customer satisfaction with colonoscopy. Endoscopy 1994; 26:342–346.
21. Johnston M: Dimensions of recovery from surgery. Int Rev Appl Psychol 1984; 33:505–520.
22. Chumbley GM, Hall GM, Salmon P: Patient-controlled analgesia: An assessment by 200 patients. Anaesthesia 1998; 53:216–221.
23. Taylor NM, Hall GM, Salmon P: Patients' experiences of patient-controlled analgesia. Anaesthesia 1996; 51:525–528.

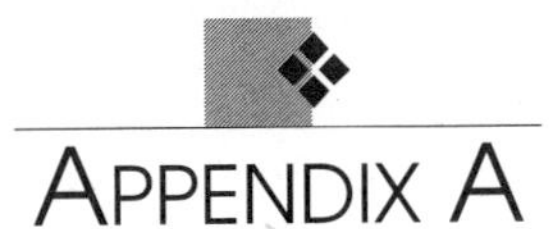

Appendix A

Regional Anesthesia in the Third World: Is It an Option?

❖ Saywan Lim, MBBS (Singapore), FFARCS (Ireland), FRCA (England), FANZCA, FRCPS (Glasgow), FRACP (Hon), FACP (Hon), FAMM (Malaysia)

This is an international textbook, with chapters being written by obstetric anesthesiologists from every corner of the world. But is regional anesthesia and analgesia an option for parturients in Third World countries, where resources are sometimes quite suboptimal? In considering this question, it would appear necessary to first have an idea of the healthcare and the political and socioeconomic scenario generally prevailing in Third World countries. These countries differ from one another in many ways, and each has different priorities, but there are certain themes running through the healthcare delivery systems of nearly all Third World countries that permit some generalizations.

Good health is a most precious possession. In recent times, however, it is no longer considered a luxury for only the wealthy. In fact, good health has been recognized as a basic right and therefore should be beyond the need for economic justification. Unfortunately, the stark truth remains that good health is generally foreign to Third World countries, where socioeconomic conditions are often characterized by widespread poverty, malnutrition, crime, drug and alcohol dependence, and prostitution. In these countries, far too often healthcare is given a very low priority. Poverty is inescapably linked with illiteracy, lack of education, poor nutrition, overcrowded housing, unsafe water, and improper disposal of sewage. Poor sanitary conditions are a way of life and are reflected in the recurrent epidemics of gastrointestinal diseases. The combination of all of these factors, coupled with often substandard medical care for women and infants, is undoubtedly responsible for the elevated perinatal and infant death rates.

Unfortunately, when it comes to providing healthcare for Third World countries, there are often insufficient resources to meet everyone's needs. If the wealthiest nations in the world cannot fulfil all their expectations for healthcare, how can the poorest nations be expected to? All health decisions involve a choice: a compromise between alternatives that are usually conflicted within the bounds of restricted funds. Thus, the provision of good healthcare is often determined by the financial resources of the government and its determination to implement measures to eliminate poverty, provide education, increase employment, raise the standard of living, erect housing for the indigent, ensure nutrition for children, and provide a safe water supply and proper disposal of sewage. When children cannot eat and people are living on the street, where does epidural analgesia for labor fit in?

Beyond improvements in the standard of living and public health provisions, Third World countries in search of good health for their citizens must, within budgetary constraints, establish a practical healthcare delivery system of primary care centers and secondary institutions for patients who require hospitalization. When one considers the inevitable lack of human and material resources, the definition of "adequate" healthcare must change. Notwithstanding the inherent difficulties, medical treatment for pregnant women must be part of the medical system in a country that is to have a future. Despite the rather depressing scenario of lack of trained personnel, facilities, and supplies in most Third World countries, the overriding concern in the delivery of anesthesia to obstetric patients remains the same everywhere in the world: Some form of anesthesia should be provided to those who request or need it; and if anesthesia is to be provided, it must be performed safely.

CHOICE OF ANESTHESIA IN THE THIRD WORLD

The choice of anesthetic technique is often dictated by the facilities available and dependent on the preference and training of the anesthesia provider. The old aphorism that the anesthetic is only as safe as the anesthetist holds very true, as education and experience with a particular technique will significantly contribute to a safe outcome. Even without any constraints of facilities and resources, the use of regional anesthesia has tremendously grown throughout the world. While one may argue endlessly about the advantages of spending limited healthcare dollars on regional versus general anesthesia, in Third World countries where technologic resources are often unavailable, the fully awake appearance of those patients who have received regional anesthesia for their operations conveys an added element of safety and suggests an advantage. Physicians in Third World countries cannot always provide regional anesthesia, either because patients refuse or because resources are lacking. But when the patient does not object to the administration of a regional anesthetic and when the needles and local anesthetics are available, anesthesiologists throughout the world agree that it is safer to have a parturient awake.

ANESTHETIC PRACTICE IN THIRD WORLD COUNTRIES

Reports from Africa[1] and Asia,[2] where the majority of Third World countries exist, indicate that owing to manpower shortages, limited training opportunities, and lack of equipment and drugs, the majority of anesthetics are administered by nonphysicians, quite often without the supervision of physicians. As Third World countries invariably report that as many as 80% of the population live in rural areas, the anesthetics are for procedures undertaken predominantly in rural-based centers. Poorly staffed and equipped recovery rooms and less than satisfactory blood banks add to the problems encountered by obstetric patients in these countries.

The delivery of a safe and effective anesthetic for obstetric patients in the face of inadequate funding, poor training, and poor facilities and with the majority of anesthetics being administered by nonphysicians is characterized by the following:

1. Ambient air is used as carrier gas. Oxygen enrichment is provided by oxygen concentrators or cylinder oxygen, when available. Draw-over machines are commonly used, as opposed to constant flow machines, and equipment is generally low-tech in order to reduce problems of maintenance.
2. Patients are spontaneously breathing. Controlled ventilation is used only when absolutely essential and hand-bagging is common.
3. Single-drug anesthesia is usually utilized. Balanced anesthesia and polypharmacy are deemed inappropriate. Diethyl ether and ketamine remain popular agents.
4. Regional anesthesia is employed predominantly. Most are spinals, but there are also peripheral blocks. Only rarely are epidurals with a catheter technique used.

The regular reports emanating from Third World countries of insufficient and irregular oxygen supply and inadequate maintenance of anesthetic equipment have resulted in a reliance on anesthetic techniques that require a minimum of equipment, without forsaking the basic principles of safe practice in managing patients. Spinal anesthesia for cesarean section meets all of these demands while reducing the costs involved in the purchase and maintenance of current equipment and drugs for the administration of general anesthesia. Thus, it should come as no surprise that the use of local and regional anesthesia techniques is widely used in Third World countries and is growing in popularity.

In the face of uncertain and insufficient supplies of oxygen, prudence directs that the limited resources of oxygen be hoarded for major surgery and resuscitation purposes, and local and regional anesthetic techniques should be more widely utilized to provide analgesia and anesthesia for the obstetric patient in Third World countries. It cannot be overemphasized, however, that even in economically poorer countries, safety is the expected outcome following the administration of any anesthetic, and the usual precautions of monitoring of patients and the availability of resuscitation equipment must be satisfied in every case.

Statistically, with the population rising at the rate of 2% to 3% (despite the human immunodeficiency virus [HIV] epidemic), it is evident that birth rates in Third World countries continue to outnumber those

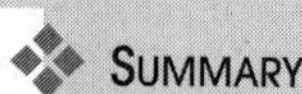

SUMMARY

Key Points

- During every minute of every day, somewhere in the world a woman dies of pregnancy-related complications.
- In the last 20 years, anesthesiologists have achieved significant improvements in the quality of care and in the Western World, resulting in significantly reduced anesthesia-related mortality.
- The improvements are due, in part, to the sensible application of risk management principles, better understanding of the parturient, and improved communication and monitoring, but most of all, they are due to the deployment of more anesthesiologists with better training and experience.

Key Reference

Hawkins JL, Koonin LM, Palmer SK, Gibbs CP: Anesthesia-related deaths during obstetric delivery in the United States, 1979–1990. Anesthesiology 1997; 86:277–284.

Case Stem

Discuss the advances in obstetric anesthesia that have occurred during the past 20 years and outline the steps that can be taken to further decrease maternal mortality in your country.

in more developed countries. Therefore, one can assume that there is a greater need for obstetric analgesia and anesthesia services in Third World countries than elsewhere. Thus, the requirement of a safe yet reliable anesthetic in conditions where oxygen supplies are limited favors the choice of regional anesthesia techniques. Reports from practitioners in Third World countries consistently support the popularity of regional anesthesia and should come as no surprise. Education and greater availability of the necessary equipment and local anesthetics are necessary if this popularity is to continue.

One is tempted to feel that the main factor holding back the increased use of regional anesthesia in Third World countries is the lack of training to enable practitioners to effect regional blockade. Reports from Africa have pointed to the lack of trained medical practitioners and consequently the heavy reliance on "clinical officers" to administer clinical care, including anesthetics. This lack of trained personnel has resulted in fewer operative procedures being effected in Africa and probably other Third World countries. It is to the credit of the World Federation of Societies of Anesthesiologists that since 1980, refresher courses have been conducted under its auspices to provide better training to Third World practitioners and nonphysicians who continue to provide the majority of anesthetics to obstetric patients in these parts of the world. Hopefully, further inroads will occur to allow greater education and availability of textbooks such as this to find their way into these countries and aid in the education of a new generation of anesthesia providers.

References

1. Egan E: The provision of anaesthesia in east Africa—a conundrum. Middle East J Anaesthesiol 1993; 12:165–170.
2. Rahardjo E: The anaesthesia service in Indonesia. World Anaesth 1998; 2:12.

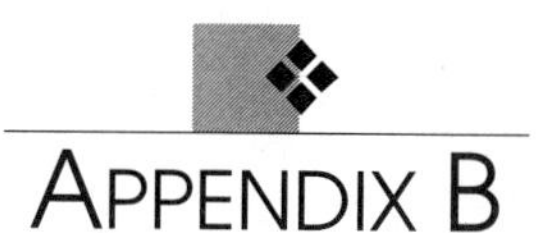

APPENDIX B

Practice Guidelines for Obstetrical Anesthesia

A Report by the American Society of Anesthesiologists Task Force on Obstetrical Anesthesia

PRACTICE guidelines are systematically developed recommendations that assist the practitioner and patient in making decisions about health care. These recommendations may be adopted, modified, or rejected according to clinical needs and constraints.

Practice guidelines are not intended as standards or absolute requirements. The use of practice guidelines cannot guarantee any specific outcome. Practice guidelines are subject to periodic revision as warranted by the evolution of medical knowledge, technology, and practice. The guidelines provide basic recommendations that are supported by analysis of the current literature and by a synthesis of expert opinion, open forum commentary, and clinical feasibility data.

Developed by the Task Force on Obstetrical Anesthesia: Joy L. Hawkins, M.D. (Chair), Denver, Colorado; James F. Arens, M.D., Galveston, Texas; Brenda A. Bucklin, M.D., Omaha, Nebraska; Robert A. Caplan, M.D., Seattle, Washington; David H. Chestnut, M.D., Birmingham, Alabama; Richard T. Connis, Ph.D., Woodinville, Washington; Patricia A. Dailey, M.D., Hillsborough, California; Larry C. Gilstrap, M.D., Houston, Texas; Stephen C. Grice, M.D., Alpharetta, Georgia; Nancy E. Oriol, M.D., Boston, Massachusetts; Kathryn J. Zuspan, M.D., Edina, Minnesota.

Submitted for publication October 29, 1998. Accepted for publication October 29, 1998. Supported by the American Society of Anesthesiologists, under the direction of James F. Arens, M.D., Chairman of the Ad Hoc Committee on Practice Parameters. Approved by the House of Delegates, October 21, 1998. Effective date January 1, 1999. A list of the articles used to develop these guidelines is available by writing to the American Society of Anesthesiologists.

Address reprint requests to American Society of Anesthesiologists: 520 North Northwest Highway, Park Ridge, IL 60068-2573.

Key words: Anesthesia cesarean section; analgesia labor and delivery.

Anesthesiology 1999; 90-600-11

A. Purposes of the Guidelines for Obstetrical Anesthesia

The purposes of these Guidelines are to enhance the quality of anesthesia care for obstetric patients, reduce the incidence and severity of anesthesia-related complications, and increase patient satisfaction.

B. Focus

The Guidelines focus on the anesthetic management of pregnant patients during labor, non-operative delivery, operative delivery, and selected aspects of postpartum care. The intended patient population includes, but is not limited to intrapartum and postpartum patients with uncomplicated pregnancies or with common obstetric problems. The Guidelines do not apply to patients undergoing surgery during pregnancy, gynecological patients or parturients with chronic medical disease (e.g., severe heart, renal or neurological disease).

C. Application

The Guidelines are intended for use by anesthesiologists. They also may serve as a resource for other anesthesia providers and health care professionals who advise or care for patients who will receive anesthesia care during labor, delivery and the immediate postpartum period.

D. Task Force Members and Consultants

The ASA appointed a Task Force of 11 members to review the published evidence and obtain consultant opinion from a representative body of anesthesiologists and obstetricians. The Task Force members consisted of anesthesiologists in both private and academic practices from various geographic areas of the United States.

The Task Force met its objective in a five-step process. First, original published research studies relevant to these issues were reviewed and analyzed. Second, Consultants from various geographic areas of the United States who practice or work in various settings (e.g., academic and private practice) were asked to participate in opinion surveys and review and comment on drafts of the Guidelines. Third, the Task Force held two open forums at major national meetings to solicit input from attendees on its draft recommendations. Fourth, all available information was used by the Task Force in developing the Guideline recommendations. Finally, the Consultants were surveyed to assess their opinions on the feasibility of implementing the Guidelines.

E. Availability and Strength of Evidence

Evidence-based guidelines are developed by a rigorous analytic process. To assist the reader, the Guidelines make use of several descriptive terms that are easier to understand than the technical terms and data that are used in the actual analyses. These descriptive terms are defined below:

The following terms describe the availability of scientific evidence in the literature.

Insufficient: There are too few published studies to investigate a relationship between a clinical intervention and clinical outcome.

Inconclusive: Published studies are available, but they cannot be used to assess the relationship between a clinical intervention and a clinical outcome because the studies either do not meet predefined criteria for content as defined in the "Focus of the Guidelines," or do not meet research design or analytic standards.

Silent: There are no available studies in the literature that address a relationship of interest.

The following terms describe the strength of scientific data.

Supportive: There is sufficient quantitative information from adequately designed studies to describe a statistically significant relationship ($p < 0.01$) between a clinical intervention and a clinical outcome, using the technique of meta-analysis.

Suggestive: There is enough information from case reports and descriptive studies to provide a directional assessment of the relationship between a clinical intervention and a clinical outcome. This type of qualitative information does not permit a statistical assessment of significance.

Equivocal: Qualitative data have not provided a clear direction for clinical outcomes related to a clinical intervention and (1) there is insufficient quantitative information or (2) aggregated comparative studies have found no quantitatively significant differences among groups or conditions.

The following terms describe survey responses from Consultants for any specified issue. Responses are weighted as agree = +1, undecided = 0 or disagree = −1.

Agree: The average weighted responses must be equal to or greater than +0.30 (on a scale of −1 to 1) to indicate agreement.

Equivocal: The average weighted responses must be between −0.30 and +0.30 (on a scale of −1 to 1) to indicate an equivocal response.

Disagree: The average weighted responses must be equal to or less than −0.30 (on a scale of −1 to 1) to indicate disagreement.

Guidelines

I. Perianesthetic Evaluation.

1. History and Physical Examination. The literature is silent regarding the relationship between anesthesia-related obstetric outcomes and the performance of a focused history and physical examination. However, there is suggestive data that a patient's medical history and/or findings from a physical exam may be related to anesthetic outcomes. The Consultants and Task Force agree that a focused history and physical examination may be associated with reduced maternal, fetal and neonatal complications. The Task Force agrees that the obstetric patient benefits from communication between the anesthesiologist and the obstetrician.

Recommendations: The anesthesiologist should do a focused history and physical examination when consulted to deliver anesthesia care. This should include a maternal health history, an anesthesia-related obstetric history, an airway examination, and a baseline blood pressure measurement. When a regional anesthetic is planned, the back should be examined. Recognition of significant anesthetic risk factors should encourage consultation with the obstetrician.

2. Intrapartum Platelet Count. A platelet count may indicate the severity of a patient's pregnancy-induced hypertension. However, the literature is insufficient to assess the predictive value of a platelet count for anesthesia-related complications in either uncomplicated parturients or those with pregnancy-induced hypertension. The Consultants and Task Force both agree that a routine platelet count in the healthy parturient is not necessary. However, in the patient with pregnancy-induced hypertension, the Consultants and Task Force both agree that the use of a platelet count may reduce the risk of anesthesia-related complications.

Recommendations: A specific platelet count predictive of regional anesthetic complications has not been determined. The anesthesiologist's decision to order or require a platelet count should be individualized and based upon a patient's history, physical examination and clinical signs of a coagulopathy.

3. Blood Type and Screen. The literature is silent regarding whether obtaining a blood type and screen is associated with fewer maternal anesthetic complications. The Consultants and Task Force are equivocal regarding the routine use of a blood type and screen to reduce the risk of anesthesia-related complications.

Recommendations: The anesthesiologist's decision to order or require a blood type and screen or cross-match should be individualized and based on anticipated hemorrhagic complications (e.g., placenta previa in a patient with previous uterine surgery).

4. Perianesthetic Recording of the Fetal Heart Rate. The literature suggests that analgesic/anesthetic agents may influence the fetal heart rate pattern. There is insufficient literature to demonstrate that perianesthetic recording of the fetal heart rate prevents fetal complications. However, both the Task Force and Consultants agree that perianesthetic recording of the fetal heart rate reduces fetal and neonatal complications.

Recommendations: The fetal heart rate should be monitored by a qualified individual before and after administration of regional analgesia for labor. The Task Force recognizes that *continuous* electronic recording of the fetal heart rate may not be necessary in every clinical setting[1] and may not be possible during placement of a regional anesthetic.

II. Fasting in the Obstetric Patient.

1. Clear Liquids. Published evidence is insufficient regarding the relationship between fasting times for clear liquids and the risk of emesis/reflux or pulmonary aspiration during labor. The Task Force and Consultants agree that oral intake of clear liquids during labor improves maternal comfort and satisfaction. The Task Force and Consultants are equivocal whether oral intake of clear liquids increases maternal risk of pulmonary aspiration.

Recommendations: The oral intake of modest amounts of clear liquids may be allowed for uncomplicated laboring patients. Examples of clear liquids include, but are not limited to, water, fruit juices without pulp, carbonated beverages, clear tea, and black coffee. The volume of liquid ingested is less important than the type of liquid ingested. However, patients with additional risk factors of aspiration (e.g., morbid obesity, diabetes, difficult airway), or patients at increased risk for operative delivery (e.g., nonreassuring fetal heart rate pattern) may have further restrictions of oral intake, determined on a case-by-case basis.

2. Solids. A specific fasting time for solids that is predictive of maternal anesthetic complications has not been determined. There is insufficient published evidence to address the safety of *any* particular fasting period for solids for obstetric patients. The Consultants agree that a fasting period for solids of 8 hours or more is preferable for uncomplicated parturients undergoing *elective* cesarean delivery. The Task Force recognizes that in laboring patients the timing of delivery is uncertain; therefore compliance with a predetermined fasting period is not always possible. The Task Force supports a fasting period of at least 6 hours before elective cesarean delivery.

Recommendations: Solid foods should be avoided in laboring patients. The patient undergoing elective cesarean delivery should undergo a fasting period for solids consistent with the hospital's policy for nonobstetric patients undergoing elective surgery. Both the amount and type of food ingested must be considered when determining the timing of surgery.

III. Anesthesia Care for Labor and Vaginal Delivery.

A. Overview of Recommendations. Anesthesia care is not necessary for all women for labor and/or delivery. For women who request pain relief for labor and/or delivery, there are many effective analgesic techniques available. Maternal request represents sufficient justification for pain relief, but the selected analgesia technique depends on the medical status of the patient, the progress of the labor, and the resources of the facility. When sufficient resources (e.g., anesthesia and nursing staff) are available, epidural catheter techniques should be one of the analgesic options offered. The primary goal is to provide adequate maternal analgesia with as little motor block as possible when regional analgesia is used for uncomplicated labor and/or vaginal delivery. This can be achieved by the administration of local anesthetic at low concentrations. The concentration of the local anesthetic may be further reduced by the addition of narcotics and still provide adequate analgesia.

B. Specific Recommendations

1. Epidural anesthetics:

a. Epidural local anesthetics. The literature supports the use of single-bolus epidural local anesthetics for providing greater quality of analgesia compared to *parenteral opioids*. However, the literature indicates a reduced incidence of spontaneous vaginal delivery associated with single-bolus epidural local anesthetics. The literature is insufficient to indicate causation. Compared to *single-injection spinal opioids* the literature is equivocal regarding the analgesic efficacy of single-bolus epidural local anesthetics. The literature suggests that epidural local anesthetics compared to spinal opioids are associated with a lower incidence of pruritus.

The literature is insufficient to compare the incidence of other side-effects.

b. Addition of opioids to epidural local anesthetics. The literature supports the use of epidural local anesthetics with opioids, when compared with *equal* concentrations of epidural local anesthetics without opioids for providing greater quality and duration of analgesia. The former is associated with reduced motor block and an increased likelihood of spontaneous delivery, possibly as a result of a reduced total dose of local anesthetic administered over time.##

The literature is equivocal regarding the analgesic efficacy of *low* concentrations of epidural local anesthetics with opioids compared to *higher* concentrations of epidural local anesthetics without opioids. The literature indicates that low concentrations of epidural local anesthetics with opioids compared to higher concentrations of epidural local anesthetics are associated with reduced motor block.

No differences in the incidence of nausea, hypotension, duration of labor, or neonatal outcomes are found when epidural local anesthetics with opioids were compared to epidural local anesthetics without opioids. However, the literature indicates that the addition of opioids to epidural local anesthetics results in a higher incidence of pruritus. The literature is insufficient to determine the effects of epidural local anesthetics with opioids on other maternal outcomes (e.g., respiratory depression, urinary retention).

The Task Force and majority of Consultants are supportive of the case-by-case selection of an analgesic technique for labor. The subgroup of Consultants reporting a preferred technique, when all choices are available, selected an epidural local anesthetic technique. When a low concentration of epidural local anesthetic is used, the Consultants and Task Force agree that the addition of an opioid(s) improves analgesia and maternal satisfaction without increasing maternal, fetal or neonatal complications.

Recommendations: The selected analgesic/anesthetic technique should reflect patient needs and preferences, practitioner preferences or skills, and available resources. When an epidural local anesthetic is selected for labor and delivery, the addition of an opioid may allow the use of a lower concentration of local anesthetic and prolong the duration of analgesia. Appropriate resources for the treatment of complications related to epidural local anesthetics (e.g., hypotension, systemic toxicity, high spinal anesthesia) should be available. If opioids are added, treatments for related complications (e.g., pruritus, nausea, respiratory depression) should be available.

c. Continuous Infusion Epidural Techniques (CIE). The literature indicates that effective analgesia can be maintained with a low concentration of local anesthetic with an epidural infusion technique. In addition, when an opioid is added to a local anesthetic infusion, an even lower concentration of local anesthetic provides effective analgesia. For example, comparable analgesia is found, with a reduced incidence of motor block, using bupivacaine infusion concentrations of *less than* 0.125% with an opioid compared to bupivacaine concentrations *equal to* 0.125% without an opioid.*** No comparative differences are noted for incidence of instrumental delivery.

The literature is equivocal regarding the relationship between different local anesthetic infusion regimens and the incidence of nausea or neonatal outcome. However, the literature suggests that local anesthetic infusions with opioids are associated with a higher incidence of pruritus.

The Task Force and Consultants agree that infusions using low concentrations of local anesthetics with or without opioids provide equivalent analgesia, reduced motor block, and improved maternal satisfaction when compared to higher concentrations of local anesthetic.

Recommendations: Adequate analgesia for uncomplicated labor and delivery should be provided with the secondary goal of producing as little motor block as possible. The lowest concentration of local anesthetic infusion that provides adequate maternal analgesia and satisfaction should be used. For example, an infusion concentration of bupivacaine equal to or greater than 0.25% is unnecessary for labor analgesia for most patients. The addition of an opioid(s) to a low concentration of local anesthetic may improve analgesia and minimize motor block. Resources for the treatment of potential complications should be available.

2. Spinal Opioids With or Without Local Anesthetics. The literature suggests that spinal opioids with or without local anesthetics provide effective labor analgesia without significantly altering the incidence of neonatal complications. There is insufficient literature to compare spinal opioids with parenteral opioids. However, the Consultants and Task Force agree that spinal opioids provide improved maternal analgesia compared to parenteral opioids.

The literature is equivocal regarding analgesic efficacy of spinal opioids compared to epidural local anesthetics. The Consultants and Task Force agree that spinal opioids provide equivalent analgesia compared to epidural local anesthetics. The Task Force agrees that the rapid onset of analgesia provided by single-injection spinal techniques may be advantageous for selected patients (e.g., those in advanced labor).

Recommendations: Spinal opioids with or without local anesthetics may be used to provide effective, although time-limited, analgesia for labor. Resources for

---

##No meta-analytic differences in the likelihood of spontaneous delivery were found when studies using morphine or meperidine were added to studies using only fentanyl or sufentanil.

***References to bupivacaine are included for illustrative purposes only, and because bupivacaine is the most extensively studied local anesthetic for CIE. The Task Force recognizes that other local anesthetic agents are equally appropriate for CIE.

the treatment of potential complications (e.g., pruritus, nausea, hypotension, respiratory depression) should be available.

3. Combined Spinal-Epidural Techniques. Although the literature suggests that combined spinal-epidural techniques (CSE) provide effective analgesia, the literature is insufficient to evaluate the analgesic efficacy of CSE compared to epidural local anesthetics. The literature indicates that use of CSE techniques with opioids when compared to epidural local anesthetics with or without opioids results in a higher incidence of pruritus and nausea. The Task Force and Consultants are equivocal regarding improved analgesia or maternal benefit of CSE versus epidural techniques. Although the literature is insufficient to evaluate fetal and neonatal outcomes of CSE techniques, the Task Force and Consultants agree that CSE does not increase the risk of fetal or neonatal complications.

Recommendations: Combined spinal-epidural techniques may be used to provide rapid and effective analgesia for labor. Resources for the treatment of potential complications (e.g., pruritus, nausea, hypotension, respiratory depression) should be available.

4. Regional Analgesia and Progress of Labor. There is insufficient literature to indicate whether timing of analgesia related to cervical dilation affects labor and delivery outcomes. Both the Task Force and Consultants agree that cervical dilation at the time of epidural analgesia administration does not impact the outcome of labor.

The literature indicates that epidural analgesia may be used in a trial of labor for previous cesarean section patients without adversely affecting the incidence of vaginal delivery. However, randomized comparisons of epidural versus other specific anesthetic techniques were not found, and comparison groups were often confounded.

Recommendations: Cervical dilation is not a reliable means of determining when regional analgesia should be initiated. Regional analgesia should be administered on an individualized basis.

5. Monitored or Stand-by Anesthesia Care for Complicated Vaginal Delivery. Monitored anesthesia care refers to instances in which an anesthesiologist has been called upon to provide specific anesthesia services to a particular patient undergoing a planned procedure.[2] For these Guidelines, stand-by anesthesia care refers to the availability of the anesthesiologist in the facility, in the event of obstetric complications. The literature is silent regarding the subject of monitored or stand-by anesthesia care in obstetrics. However, the Task Force and Consultants agree that monitored or stand-by anesthesia care for complicated vaginal delivery reduces maternal, fetal, and neonatal complications.

Recommendations: Either monitored or stand-by anesthesia care, determined on a case-by-case basis for complicated vaginal delivery (e.g., breech presentation, twins, and trial of instrumental delivery), should be made available when requested by the obstetrician.

IV. Removal of Retained Placenta.

1. Anesthetic Choices. The literature is insufficient to indicate whether a particular type of anesthetic is more effective than another for removal of retained placenta. The literature is also insufficient to assess the relationship between a particular type of anesthetic and maternal complications. The Task Force and Consultants agree that spinal or epidural anesthesia (i.e., regional anesthesia) is associated with reduced maternal complications and improved satisfaction when compared to general anesthesia or sedation/analgesia. The Task Force recognizes that circumstances may occur when general anesthesia or sedation/analgesia may be the more appropriate anesthetic choice (e.g., significant hemorrhage).

Recommendations: Regional anesthesia, general endotracheal anesthesia, or sedation/analgesia may be used for removal of retained placenta. Hemodynamic status should be assessed before giving regional anesthesia to a parturient who has experienced significant bleeding. In cases involving significant maternal hemorrhage, a general anesthetic may be preferable to initiating regional anesthesia. Sedation/analgesia should be titrated carefully due to the potential risk of pulmonary aspiration in the recently delivered parturient with an unprotected airway.

2. Nitroglycerin for Uterine Relaxation. The literature suggests and the Task Force and Consultants agree that the administration of nitroglycerin is effective for uterine relaxation during removal of retained placental tissue.

Recommendations: Nitroglycerin is an alternative to terbutaline sulfate or general endotracheal anesthesia with halogenated agents for uterine relaxation during removal of retained placental tissue. Initiating treatment with a low dose of nitroglycerin may relax the uterus sufficiently while minimizing potential complications (e.g., hypotension).

V. Anesthetic Choices for Cesarean Delivery.

The literature suggests that spinal, epidural or CSE anesthetic techniques can be used effectively for cesarean delivery. When compared to regional techniques, the literature indicates that general anesthetics can be administered with shorter induction-to-delivery times. The literature is insufficient to determine the relative risk of maternal death associated with general anesthesia compared to other anesthetic techniques. However, the literature suggests that a greater number of maternal deaths occur when general anesthesia is administered. The literature indicates that a larger proportion of neonates in the general anesthesia groups, compared to those in the regional anesthesia groups, are assigned Apgar scores of less than 7 at one and five minutes. However, few studies have utilized randomized comparisons of general versus regional anesthesia, resulting in potential selection bias in the reporting of outcomes.

The literature suggests that maternal side effects associated with regional techniques may include hypotension, nausea, vomiting, pruritus and postdural puncture headache. The literature is insufficient to examine the comparative merits of various regional anesthetic techniques.

The Consultants agree that regional anesthesia can be administered with fewer maternal and neonatal complications and improved maternal satisfaction when compared to general anesthesia. The consultants are equivocal about the possibility of increased maternal complications when comparing spinal or epidural anesthesia with CSE techniques. They agree that neonatal complications are not increased with CSE techniques.

Recommendations: The decision to use a particular anesthetic technique should be individualized based on several factors. These include anesthetic, obstetric and/or fetal risk factors (e.g., elective versus emergency) and the preferences of the patient and anesthesiologist. Resources for the treatment of potential complications (e.g., airway management, inadequate analgesia, hypotension, pruritus, nausea) should be available.

VI. Postpartum Tubal Ligation.

There is insufficient literature to evaluate the comparative benefits of local, spinal, epidural or general anesthesia for postpartum tubal ligation. Both the Task Force and Consultants agree that epidural, spinal and general anesthesia can be effectively provided without affecting maternal complications. Neither the Task Force nor the Consultants agree that local anesthetic techniques provide effective anesthesia, and they are equivocal regarding the impact of local anesthesia on maternal complications. Although the literature is insufficient, the Task Force and Consultants agree that a postpartum tubal ligation can be performed safely within eight hours of delivery in many patients.

Recommendations: Evaluation of the patient for postpartum tubal ligation should include assessment of hemodynamic status (e.g., blood loss) and consideration of anesthetic risks. The patient planning to have an elective postpartum tubal ligation within 8 hours of delivery should have no oral intake of solid foods during labor, and postpartum until the time of surgery. Both the timing of the procedure and the decision to use a particular anesthetic technique (i.e., regional versus general) should be individualized, based on anesthetic and/or obstetric risk factors and patient preferences. The anesthesiologist should be aware that an epidural catheter placed for labor may be more likely to fail with longer postdelivery time intervals. If a postpartum tubal ligation is to be done before the patient is discharged from the hospital, the procedure should not be attempted at a time when it might compromise other aspects of patient care in the labor and delivery area.

VII. Management of Complications.

1. Resources for Management of Hemorrhagic Emergencies. The literature suggests that the availability of resources for hemorrhagic emergencies is associated with reduced maternal complications. The Task Force and Consultants agree that the availability of resources for managing hemorrhagic emergencies is associated with reduced maternal, fetal and neonatal complications.

Recommendations: Institutions providing obstetric care should have resources available to manage hemorrhagic emergencies *(Table 1)*. In an emergency, the use of type-specific or O negative blood is acceptable in the parturient.

2. Equipment for Management of Airway Emergencies. The literature suggests, and the Task Force and Consultants agree that the availability of equipment for the management of airway emergencies is associated with reduced maternal complications.

Recommendations: Labor and delivery units should have equipment and personnel readily available to manage airway emergencies. Basic airway management equipment should be immediately available during the initial provision of regional analgesia *(Table 2)*. In addition, portable equipment for difficult airway management should be readily available in the operative area of labor and delivery units *(Table 3)*.

3. Central Invasive Hemodynamic Monitoring. There is insufficient literature to indicate whether pulmonary artery catheterization is associated with improved maternal, fetal or neonatal outcomes in patients with pregnancy-related hypertensive disorders. The literature is silent regarding the management of obstetric patients with central venous catheterization alone. The literature suggests that pulmonary artery

Table 1. SUGGESTED RESOURCES FOR OBSTETRIC HEMORRHAGIC EMERGENCIES*

1. Large bore iv catheters
2. Fluid warmer
3. Forced air body warmer
4. Availability of blood bank resources
5. Equipment for infusing iv fluids and/or blood products rapidly. Examples include (but are not limited to) hand squeezed fluid chambers, hand inflated pressure bags, and automatic infusion devices.

*The items listed represent suggestions. The items should be customized to meet the specific needs, preferences, and skills of the practitioner and healthcare facility.

Table 2. SUGGESTED RESOURCES FOR AIRWAY MANAGEMENT DURING INITIAL PROVISION OF REGIONAL ANESTHESIA*

1. Laryngoscope and assorted blades
2. Endotracheal tubes, with stylets
3. Oxygen source
4. Suction source with tubing and catheters
5. Self-inflating bag and mask for positive pressure ventilation
6. Medications for blood pressure support, muscle relaxation, and hypnosis

*The items listed represent suggestions. The items should be customized to meet the specific needs, preferences, and skills of the practitioner and healthcare facility.

catheterization has been used safely in obstetric patients; however, the literature is insufficient to examine specific obstetric outcomes. The Task Force and Consultants agree that it is not necessary to use central invasive hemodynamic monitoring routinely for parturients with severe preeclampsia.

Recommendations: The decision to perform invasive hemodynamic monitoring should be individualized and based on clinical indications that include the patient's medical history and cardiovascular risk factors. The Task Force recognizes that not all practitioners have access to resources for utilization of central venous or pulmonary artery catheters in obstetric units.

4. Cardiopulmonary Resuscitation. The literature is insufficient to evaluate the efficacy of CPR in the obstetric patient during labor and delivery. The Task Force is supportive of the immediate availability of basic and advanced life-support equipment in the operative area of labor and delivery units.

Recommendations: Basic and advanced life-support equipment should be immediately available in the operative area of labor and delivery units. If cardiac arrest occurs during labor and delivery, standard resuscitative measures and procedures, including left uterine displacement, should be taken. In cases of cardiac arrest, the American Heart Association has stated the following: "Several authors now recommend that the decision to perform a perimortem cesarean section should be made rapidly, with delivery effected within 4 to 5 minutes of the arrest."[3]

Table 3. SUGGESTED CONTENTS OF A PORTABLE UNIT FOR DIFFICULT AIRWAY MANAGEMENT FOR CESAREAN SECTION ROOMS*

1. Rigid laryngoscope blades and handles of alternate design and size from those routinely used†
2. Endotracheal tubes of assorted size
3. Laryngeal mask airways of assorted sizes
4. At least one device suitable for emergency nonsurgical airway ventilation. Examples include (but are not limited to), retrograde intubation equipment, a hollow jet ventilation stylet or cricothyrotomy kit with or without a transtracheal jet ventilator, and the esophageal-tracheal combitube.
5. Endotracheal tube guides. Examples include (but are not limited to) semirigid stylets with or without a hollow core for jet ventilation, light wands, and forceps designed to manipulate the distal portion of the endotracheal tube.
6. Equipment suitable for emergency surgical airway access
7. Topical anesthetics and vasoconstrictors

*The items listed represent suggestions. The items should be customized to meet the specific needs, preferences, and skills of the practitioner and healthcare facility.

†The Task Force believes fiberoptic intubation equipment should be readily available.

Adapted from Practice guidelines for management of the difficult airway: A report by the American Society of Anesthesiologists Task Force on Management of the Difficult Airway. Anesthesiology 1993; 78:599–602.

References

1. Guidelines for Perinatal Care, 4th ed. American Academy of Pediatrics and American College of Obstetricians and Gynecologists, 1997, p 100–102
2. American Society of Anesthesiologists: Position on monitored anesthesia care, ASA Standards, Guidelines and Statements. Park Ridge, IL, American Society of Anesthesiologists, October 1997, pp 20–21
3. Guidelines for cardiopulmonary resuscitation and emergency cardiac care: recommendations of the 1992 national conference. JAMA 1992; 268:2249

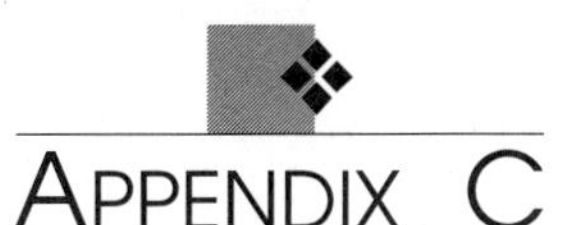

APPENDIX C

Society for Obstetric Anesthesia and Perinatology: Outline of Curriculum Goals for Anesthesia Residents Completing Clinical Anesthesia Year 3

GENERAL ISSUES

1. Ability to function as part of a team with obstetricians, nursing staff, nurse midwives, neonatologists, and pediatricians to provide optimal medical, obstetric, and anesthetic care for parturients and their fetuses or neonates
2. Familiarity with the ASA guidelines pertaining to obstetric anesthesia

I. Maternal Physiology

A. Knowledge

1. Maternal physiology: time course and changes during gestation
   a. Cardiovascular adaptations to pregnancy
   b. Pulmonary, respiratory, and airway changes

c. Gastrointestinal, hematologic, and renal changes
2. Maximum allowable concentration (MAC) and local anesthetic adjustments during pregnancy
3. Approach to CPR in a parturient, awareness of need for delivery of baby

II. Fetal and Placental Physiology

A. Knowledge

1. Placental development, structure and inability to autoregulate placental flow
2. Placental gas exchange, nutrient transport, drug transfer
3. Antenatal fetal evaluation (growth, fluid, positions, biophysical profile)
4. Fetal circulation
5. Fetal and neonatal effects of maternally administered anesthetic drugs
6. Fetal adaptations to hypoxia
7. Fetal heart rate patterns during labor and their response to hypoxia or asphyxia

B. Skills

1. Ability to describe impact on fetus of drop in maternal cardiac output
2. Ability to interpret obstetric information about fetus
3. Ability to interpret fetal heart rate patterns during labor

III. Neonatal Physiology

A. Knowledge

1. Intrapartum fetal resuscitation
2. Neonatal physiologic adaptations to extrauterine life
3. Resuscitation of the newborn—NALS protocol

B. Skills

1. Can predict the likelihood of need for resuscitation
2. Recognizes neonate needing resuscitation
3. Can initiate resuscitation of a neonate

IV. Patterns and Obstetric Management of Labor

A. Knowledge

1. Physiology of labor and the smooth muscle of the uterus
2. Definition of the stages of labor and their typical duration
3. Effect of uterine contractions on placental exchange and fetal oxygenation
4. Indications for analgesia during labor
5. Effect of analgesia on labor and delivery
6. Effect on labor of maternal hydration, position, hyperventilation, hypotension

B. Skills

1. Recognize and treat uterine hypertonus or hyperstimulation

V. Obstetric Indications for and Management of Urgent Abdominal Deliveries

A. Knowledge

1. Obstetric indications for abdominal delivery and classification according to urgency
2. Inherent maternal anesthetic risk of urgent or emergent delivery
3. Surgical and anesthetic management of bleeding during delivery, including drug therapy, surgical maneuvers, transfusion therapy

B. Skills

1. Facility in the institution of rapid-sequence general anesthesia
2. Ability to manage a difficult airway (e.g., may include facility with fiberoptic, awake, retrograde wire intubation or cricothyrotomy)
3. Facility and safe practice in instituting urgent regional anesthesia

VI. Local Anesthetics for Obstetrics

A. Knowledge

1. General principles of local anesthetic pharmacology
2. Treatment of systemic local anesthetic toxicity, including maternal seizure or cardiotoxicity
3. Response to total or near-total spinal
4. Effect of local anesthetics on the uterus and fetus
5. Effect of vasoconstrictors and other local anesthetic additives on the uterus and fetus
6. Placental transfer and fetal uptake (potential for fetal ion trapping)
7. Fetal and newborn local anesthetic toxicity
8. Potential for maternal local anesthetic neurotoxicity

B. Skills

1. Ability to make logical choice of local anesthetic and dosage for labor analgesia or cesarean delivery
2. Ability to describe and perform steps in resuscitation from toxicity

VII. Neuraxial Opioids for Obstetrics

A. Knowledge

1. General principles of neuraxial opioid pharmacology
2. Treatment of opioid side effects and toxicity, including maternal respiratory arrest
3. Effect of opioids on the uterus and fetus
4. Interaction between neuraxial opioids and local anesthetics

B. Skills

1. Ability to make logical choice of opioid and dosage for labor analgesia, cesarean delivery, or postcesarean pain management
2. Ability to describe and perform steps in resuscitation from respiratory arrest

VIII. Regional Anesthesia for Obstetrics

A. Knowledge

1. Pain pathways involved in labor and delivery
2. Options available for maternal comfort
3. Contraindications to regional anesthesia
4. Management of alterations in the cardiovascular and respiratory systems caused by neuraxial analgesia or anesthesia

5. Approach to inadequate regional anesthesia during labor or operative delivery
6. Convert labor analgesia to anesthesia for operative delivery
7. Complications of regional anesthesia and their treatment: post–dural puncture headache, maternal backache, maternal nerve palsy, epidural abscess or hematoma

B. Skills

1. Demonstrates aseptic technique for major regional blocks
2. Performs safe and effective subarachnoid and epidural blockade for labor analgesia, operative delivery, and postpartum tubal ligation
3. Demonstrates adequate documentation of regional techniques and subsequent maternal and fetal monitoring
4. Facility performing epidural blood patch

IX. General Anesthetics for Obstetrics

A. Knowledge

1. Indications for general endotracheal anesthesia (GETA)
2. Ventilatory requirements of parturients
3. Medication choices for induction and maintenance and the appropriate doses for cesarean delivery
4. Impact on the fetus of the induction-to-delivery and uterine incision–to–delivery intervals

B. Skills

1. Ability to develop a plan for GETA based on the physiologic and physical changes of pregnancy
2. Ability to recognize and outline management of a difficult airway based on physical examination of neck, oropharynx, and body habitus
3. Ability to outline a failed intubation plan following the ASA algorithm
4. Ability to recognize pulmonary aspiration of gastric contents and outline a plan for the postanesthetic care unit (PACU) and postoperative care of a patient who has aspirated

X. Obstetric Complications and Their Management

A. Knowledge

1. Understand management of maternal ante- or postpartum hemorrhage (uterine rupture, abruption or atony, placenta previa or accreta, retained placenta)
2. Understand treatment for maternal embolic events—amniotic fluid, air, or thrombus

XI. Medical Diseases During Pregnancy and Their Perioperative Management

A. For Each of the Following Disease Categories:

1. General understanding of how the disease impacts on pregnancy
2. General understanding of how pregnancy impacts on the disease
3. General understanding of the obstetric implications and management of the disease
4. Ability to communicate the anesthetic implications of the disease to nonanesthesiologist colleagues attending the patient
5. Assess the severity of disease and evaluate the need for patient transfer to a high-risk facility
6. Describe the anesthetic management of the patient for vaginal or cesarean delivery

B. Hypertensive Disorders of Pregnancy

1. Knowledge

a. Classification of hypertensive disorders during pregnancy
b. Epidemiology of preeclampsia—risk factors
c. Pathophysiology of preeclampsia as a multisystem disease
d. Medical/obstetric management of preeclampsia
   (1) term vs. preterm fetus
   (2) mild vs. severe disease
   (3) assessment of fetal well-being
   (4) seizure prophylaxis; magnesium sulfate effects
   (5) antihypertensive therapy
   (6) management of oliguria
   (7) indications for invasive monitoring
e. Anesthetic selection for and management of the preeclamptic parturient
   (1) labor and vaginal delivery
   (2) abdominal delivery—nonurgent
   (3) abdominal delivery—urgent

2. Skills

a. Ability to diagnose the parturient with preeclampsia
b. Ability to identify the patient requiring invasive monitoring
c. Ability to effectively treat the patient with an eclamptic seizure

C. Morbid Obesity

1. Skills

a. Ability to perform successful regional anesthesia techniques in morbidly obese parturients

D. Respiratory Disease

1. Knowledge

a. Asthma
b. Adult respiratory distress syndrome (ARDS)

E. Cardiac Disease

1. Knowledge

a. Understand when invasive monitors are needed for delivery and postpartum care
   (1) congenital heart disease

(a) left-to-right shunts
(b) right-to-left shunts (tetralogy of Fallot)
(c) pulmonary hypertension (Eisenmenger's syndrome)
(d) coarctation of aorta
(2) idiopathic hypertrophic subaortic stenosis (IHSS)
(3) ischemic heart disease
(4) valvular heart disease
(a) aortic stenosis
(b) aortic insufficiency
(c) mitral stenosis
(d) mitral regurgitation
(5) peripartum cardiomyopathy

F. Endocrine Disease
1. Knowledge
a. Diabetes mellitus
b. Thyroid disease
(1) hyperthyroidism
(2) hypothyroidism
2. Skills
a. Ability to manage glucose control in the parturient during cesarean or vaginal delivery

G. Hematologic and Coagulation Disorders
1. Knowledge
a. Anemias
b. Coagulation disorders

H. Neurologic Disease
1. Knowledge
a. Multiple sclerosis
b. Spinal cord injury
c. Myasthenia gravis
d. Seizure disorders
e. Subarachnoid hemorrhage or vascular malformations

I. Substance Abuse and Infection with Human Immunodeficiency Virus (HIV)
1. Knowledge
a. Substance abuse
(1) ethanol abuse
(2) opioid abuse and barbiturate use
(3) cocaine abuse
b. HIV infection

J. Miscellaneous Disorders
1. Renal disease
2. Liver disease
3. Musculoskeletal disorders
4. Scoliosis
5. Rheumatoid arthritis
6. Spina bifida cystica
7. Autoimmune disorders
8. Prior back surgery, including Harrington rod placement

XII. Anesthetic Management of Nonobstetric Surgery During Pregnancy
A. Knowledge
1. Considerations for elective surgery during pregnancy
2. Understand when and which medicines may be teratogens
3. Considerations for trauma or emergency surgery during pregnancy
4. Understand when fetal monitoring is needed during maternal surgery
5. Physiology of pregnancy as it might impact cardiovascular, respiratory, and transfusion decisions during surgery
B. Skills
1. Ability to discuss risks of elective surgery with patients and colleagues

XIII. Ethical Issues
A. Knowledge
1. Awareness of potential for maternal-fetal conflicts of interest (e.g., general anesthesia for emergency cesarean delivery in the setting of perceived fetal jeopardy)
2. Respect for all moral and religious points of view (e.g., Jehovah's Witness patient)
3. Awareness of fetal development and current limits of viability
B. Skills
1. Recognizes own ethical attitudes versus patient's moral concerns and is willing to arrange for nonprejudicial transfer of care, if necessary
2. Recognizes need for timely consultation regarding difficult moral or legal issues

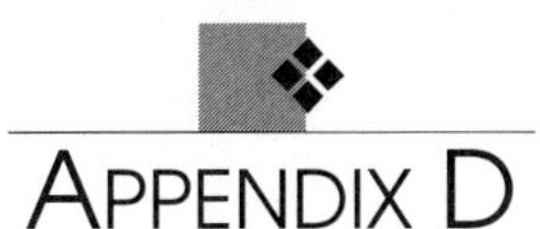

APPENDIX D

Australian and New Zealand College of Anaesthetists

Review E3 (1994)

THE SUPERVISION OF TRAINEES IN ANAESTHESIA

Supervision is defined as being performed by an anaesthetist who possesses the Diploma of FANZCA or a qualification acceptable to the Council.

1. CATEGORIES OF SUPERVISION

There are four such categories, viz.:

1. Supervisor rostered for one trainee and available solely to that trainee.
2. Supervisor rostered to supervise two trainees who are in operating theatres in close proximity. The supervisor must be fully conversant with the nature of the patients on both lists and able to provide one-to-one supervision of each as appropriate.
3. The supervisor is available either in the operating suite or the Hospital but is not exclusively available for a specific trainee.
4. The supervisor is not in the Hospital but is on call within reasonable travelling time and is exclusively rostered for the period in question. This category of supervision applies mainly to out of hours cases. Consultation must be available at all times.

Note: In the above, the term "theatre" includes any anaesthetising location in the Hospital.

2. MINIMUM SUPERVISION LEVELS

2.1 ***General***

2.1.1 In order to ensure adequate supervision of trainees, Departments must employ at least one full-time equivalent (FTE) specialist anaesthetist for each trainee. There should be no more than two non-specialist anaesthetists (including trainees) for each FTE specialist anaesthetist employed.

2.1.2 Supervision at category 1 or 2 level may be appropriate at any stage of training and should be encouraged since it gives the best opportunities for teaching and training techniques.

2.1.3 Supervision at category 1 or 2 levels should average at least 25% of all work done by trainees.

2.1.4 Supervision at category 4 level should not average more than 30% of all work done by trainees.

2.1.5 Out of hours work should comprise between 25% and 50% of any trainee's workload during the first four years of training.

2.1.6 At all stages of training, a supervisor must attend an anaesthetic whenever a trainee requests assistance. Conversely, a supervisor should attend an anaesthetic whenever this is deemed desirable.

2.1.7 All trainees must be supervised at category 1 level during a familiarisation period in any working area with which they are unfamiliar.

2.2 ***First Year Trainee***

2.2.1 Supervision at category 1 level should be provided for all cases during an initial period varying in length according to the trainee's previous experience and their development of skills and judgement. For trainees without previous anaesthetic experience, this will need to be for at least four months.

2.2.2 Supervision at category 1 and 2 levels should be provided for most of the in-hours cases for the rest of the year.

2.2.3 After the initial period, the supervisor should be notified of all out of hours cases. At least 25% of out of hours cases should be supervised at category 1 or 2 level. The supervisor should attend for all patients with conditions such as the following:

2.2.3.1 Patients requiring major resuscitation.

2.2.3.2 Patients with serious medical illness.

2.2.3.3 Debilitated patients.

2.2.3.4 Children under the age of ten years.

2.2.3.5 Surgery which poses special anaesthetic problems.

2.2.3.6 Any other high risk patients.

2.2.3.7 Any patients who the trainee does not feel competent to anaesthetise.

2.3 ***Second Year Trainee***

2.3.1 Supervision at category 1 and 2 levels should be provided for about half the in-hours case load.

2.3.2 Supervision at category 1 and 2 levels should be provided for at least 20% of the out of hours case load.

2.3.3 The supervisor should be advised of all young children, all seriously ill patients and any patients posing special problems for the anaesthetist.

2.4 ***Third Year Trainee***

2.4.1 Supervision at category 3 level may be appropriate for many of the in hours cases except where new areas of practice are encountered. In areas such as cardiothoracic, obstetric and major paediatric anaesthesia, category 1 supervision is normally appropriate.

2.4.2 For out of hours work, the supervisor should be advised of all young children, all seriously ill patients or those providing special problems for the anaesthetist.

2.4.3 It should be the supervisor's decision whether to attend the anaesthetic or not. Attendance on trainee request remains obligatory.

2.5 ***Fourth Year Trainee***

2.5.1 Supervision at category 3 level is appropriate for all work previously encountered but it may still be necessary for supervision to be at category 1 level for new work experiences.

2.5.2 For out of hours work, consultation can be at the discretion of the trainee although consultation (and where necessary supervision) remains essential for unfamiliar clinical situations.

2.6 ***Provisional Fellow***

2.6.1 Consultation and appropriate supervision must be available at all times.

This policy document has been prepared having regard to general circumstances, and it is the responsibility of the practitioner to have express regard to the particular circumstances of each case, and the application of this policy document in each case.

Policy documents are reviewed from time to time, and it is the responsibility of the practitioner to ensure that the practitioner has obtained the current version. Policy documents have been prepared having regard to the information available at the time of their preparation, and the practitioner should therefore have regard to any information, research or material which may have been published or become available subsequently.

Whilst the College endeavours to ensure that policy documents are as current as possible at the time of their preparation, it takes no responsibility for matters arising from changed circumstances or information or material which may have become available subsequently.

Promulgated: 1989
Reviewed: 1994
Date of current document: Oct 1994

THE DUTIES OF AN ANAESTHETIST

1. PREAMBLE

These guidelines represent the views of the Australian and New Zealand College of Anaesthetists as to the duties of an anaesthetist. In hospitals with College approved training posts, specialist staff have additional educational duties. It is accepted that not all of these duties will be carried out by every anaesthetist.

2. CLINICAL DUTIES

2.1 Providing anaesthesia and other appropriate consultative services.

2.2 Carrying out pre-operative assessment and continuing management of patients (see College Policy Documents *'The Pre-Anaesthetic Consultation'* (P7) and *'Responsibilities of Anaesthetists in the Post-Operative Period'* (P20)).

2.3 Supervising anaesthesia trainees and other staff as appropriate.

2.4 Supervising the Recovery Area.

2.5 Supervising the anaesthesia component of the work of the Day Care Surgery Unit (see College Policy Document *'Guidelines for the Care of Patients Recovering from Anaesthesia Related to Day Surgery'* (P15)).

2.6 Organising and managing an acute pain service.

2.7 Associating with a Pain Management Unit where appropriate (see College Policy Document *'Minimum Standards for Pain Management Units'* (P25)).

2.8 Providing an acute resuscitation service for medical, surgical and trauma emergencies.

2.9 Supervising and/or assisting with managing patients in the Intensive Care Unit.

2.10 Providing a consultative service in respect of pre-operative assessment and management.

2.11 Supervising or managing cardiopulmonary bypass as appropriate.

2.12 Such other clinical services as may be necessary and appropriate to the specialty.

3. OTHER PROFESSIONAL DUTIES

3.1 Assisting with administrative duties relating to the proper functioning of the Department and the Hospital.

3.2 Providing and participating in appropriate educational activities for

3.2.1 anaesthetic trainees
3.2.2 intern and resident medical staff
3.2.3 medical students
3.2.4 trainee and postgraduate nurses
3.2.5 anaesthetic nurses and/or technicians
3.2.6 recovery area nurses
3.2.7 operating room nurses
3.2.8 other health professionals
3.2.9 interested community groups in subjects such as "basic life support".

3.3 Supervising the preparation of teaching material.

3.4 Participating in peer review and quality improvement activities to ensure and review the quality of patient care (see College Policy Document *'Quality Assurance'* (E9)).

3.5 Participating in continuing medical education to maintain personal knowledge and skills as established in the College's Maintenance of Standards Programme. Amongst objectives of this education, it is necessary to ensure that practice of anaesthesia is consistent with personal safety.

3.6 Contributing to activities of professional associations.

3.7 Participating in research and reviews on drugs, equipment, clinical management and techniques, physiological, pharmacological and other matters relevant to anaesthesia, pain relief, resuscitation and intensive care. These activities may include assistance to trainees with their formal project.

3.9 Contributing to advisory services as a member of Hospital Committees, Health Commissions and other organisations.

3.10 Contributing to professional anaesthesia related organisations.

3.11 Participating in activities to safeguard the well-being of colleagues.

4. THE APPORTIONMENT OF TIME BETWEEN CLINICAL AND OTHER PROFESSIONAL DUTIES

All anaesthetists should have a commitment to the continuing medical education of themselves and their colleagues. On average 10% of the normal working week should be allowed for this activity to ensure that personal professional standards are maintained. All anaesthetists also have commitments to administration, quality assurance and other educational duties. Time must be set aside for these duties which may be distributed throughout the staff of a department or practice group to allow for expertise to be effectively utilised.

4.1 ***The Director of Anesthesia***

4.1.1 The Director has a prime responsibility to ensure that the Department of Anaesthesia functions safely and effectively. Consequently administration comprises a significant part of the workload. In order to maintain a high personal standard of patient care, a minimum of 40% of the normal working week should be devoted to the activities outlined in sections 2.1–2.12 inclusive. This allows up to 60% of the normal working week to be scheduled for duties outlined in sections 3.1–3.11.

4.1.2 If the Director is not a full time appointee, appropriate time must be provided for clinical and administrative duties and personal continuing education needs.

4.2 *The Deputy Director of Anaesthesia*

4.2.1 In large Departments, a Deputy Director should be appointed to assist the Director with the administration of the Department.

4.2.2 Under these circumstances the Director and Deputy Director will between them ensure that a minimum of 40% of their joint working week is devoted to activities outlined in sections 2.1–2.12, and up to 60% to activities outlined in sections 3.1–3.11.

4.3 *The Whole Time or Staff Anaesthetist*

As well as responsibilities for clinical duties, the whole time or staff anesthetist must have a commitment to teaching, to personal continuing medical education, to administration, quality assurance and other activities. In order to ensure a high quality of patient care, a minimum of 30% of a normal working week should be devoted to other professional activities as outlined in sections 3.1–3.11 inclusive.

4.4 *The Visiting Anaesthetist*

Provision should be made for the administrative and educational duties and responsibilities of visiting anaesthetists.

4.5 *The Trainee Anaesthetist*

The trainee is not a specialist—the trainee is a specialist-in-training. The supervision of the trainee is an essential component of the training experience (see College Policy Document *'The Supervision of Trainees in Anaesthesia'* (E3)). They should be assigned educational and administrative responsibilities appropriate to their level of training.

5. CONCLUSION

All staff must have sufficient exposure to clinical duties to maintain their skills. They must also have sufficient time set aside for other professional duties as defined in this document to ensure a high standard of practice both at a departmental or group level as well as on an individual basis.

RELATED DOCUMENTS

P7 The Pre-Anaesthetic Consultation

P15 Guidelines for the Care of Patients Recovering from Anaesthesia

P20 Responsibilities of Anaesthetists in the Post-Operative Period

P25 Minimum Standards for Pain Management Units

E3 The Supervision of Trainees in Anaesthesia

E9 Quality Assurance

This policy document has been prepared having regard to general circumstances, and it is the responsibility of the practitioner to have express regard to the particular circumstances of each case, and the application of this policy document in each case.

Policy documents are reviewed from time to time, and it is the responsibility of the practitioner to ensure that the practitioner has obtained the current version. Policy documents have been prepared having regard to the information available at the time of their preparation, and the practitioner should therefore have regard to any information, research or material which may have been published or become available subsequently.

Whilst the College endeavours to ensure that policy documents are as current as possible at the time of their preparation, it takes no responsibility for matters arising from changed circumstances or information or material which may have become available subsequently.

Promulgated: 1990
Reviewed: 1995
Date of current document: Oct 1995

RECOMMENDED MINIMUM FACILITIES FOR SAFE ANAESTHETIC PRACTICE IN OPERATING SUITES

The safe provision of anaesthesia requires appropriate staff, facilities and equipment for proper patient safety. These are specified in this Document.

1. PRINCIPLES OF ANAESTHETIC CARE

1.1 Anaesthesia should be administered only by medical practitioners with appropriate training in anaesthesia or by trainees supervised according to College Policy Documents. *'The Supervision of Trainees in Anaesthesia'* (E3) and *'Privileges in Anaesthesia'* (P2).

1.2 Every patient presenting for anaesthesia should have a pre-anaesthetic consultation by a medical practitioner who has appropriate training in anaesthesia. See College Policy Document *'Pre-anaesthetic Consultation'* (P7).

1.3 Appropriate monitoring of physiological variables must occur during anaesthesia. See College Policy Document *'Monitoring During Anaesthesia'* (P18).

2. STAFFING

2.1 In addition to the nursing staff required by those carrying out the operative procedure, there must be:

2.1.1 An assistant to the anaesthetist. See College Policy Document *'Minimum Assistance for the Safe Conduct of Anaesthesia'* (P8).

2.1.2 Adequate assistance in positioning the patient.

2.1.3 Adequate technical assistance to ensure proper servicing of all equipment used.

3. OPERATING SUITES

3.1 ***Anaesthetic Equipment***

3.1.1 Essential requirements are listed below. Where a range of equipment is recommended, the hospital is expected to provide the type most suitable to its needs.

3.1.2 Each hospital must designate:

3.1.2.1 One (or more) specialists to advise on the choice and maintenance of anesthetic equipment.

3.1.2.2 One (or more) of its nursing or technical staff to be responsible for the organisation of cleaning, maintenance and servicing of anaesthetic equipment.

3.1.3 There must be an anaesthetic machine for each anaesthetising location which is capable of delivering oxygen and nitrous oxide as well as other anaesthetic agents which are in common use. Essential equipment includes:

3.1.3.1 Suitable calibrated vaporisers for the delivery of inhalational anaesthetic agents.

3.1.3.2 A range of suitable breathing systems.

3.1.3.3 Breathing systems suitable for paediatric use if children are to be anaesthetised.

3.1.3.4 Medical air where this is clinically necessary.

3.1.4 Safety devices which must be present on every machine include:

3.1.4.1 An indexed gas connection system.

3.1.4.2 A reserve supply of oxygen.

3.1.4.3 An oxygen supply failure warning device. See College Policy Document *'Monitoring During Anaesthesia'* (P18).

3.1.4.4 A breathing system high pressure relief valve.

3.1.4.5 An oxygen concentration analyser with appropriate alarm limits. See College Policy Document *'Monitoring During Anaesthesia'* (P18).

3.1.4.6 Every anaesthetic machine purchased after 1 January 1996 shall have a device to prevent the supply of a hypoxic gas mixture whenever nitrous oxide is administered.

3.1.4.7 Every anaesthetic machine purchased after 1 January 1996 shall have an approved non-slip connection for the common gas outlet whenever a circle system is in use.

3.1.5 A separate means of inflating the lungs with oxygen must be provided in each anaesthetising location. This apparatus should comply with the current requirements of the relevant national Standards. Its oxygen supply should be independent of the anaesthetic machine.

3.1.6 Suction apparatus must be available for the exclusive use of the anaesthetist at all times together with appropriate hand pieces and endotracheal suction catheters. This apparatus should comply with the current requirements of the relevant national Standards. Provision must be made for an alternative suction system in the event of primary suction failure.

3.1.7 In every anaesthetising location there must be:

3.1.7.1 Appropriate protection for the anaesthesia team against biological contaminants. This shall include disposable gloves and eye shields.

3.1.7.2 A stethoscope

3.1.7.3 A sphygmomanometer

3.1.7.4 Monitoring equipment complying with College Policy Document *'Monitoring During Anaesthesia'* (P18). Special problems are encountered in magnetic resonance imaging facilities. See College Policy Document *'Recommended Minimum Facilities for Safe Anaesthetic Practice in Organ Imaging Units'* (T3).

3.1.7.5 An appropriate range of face masks.

3.1.7.6 An appropriate range of oropharyngeal, nasopharyngeal and laryngeal mask airways.

3.1.7.7 Two laryngoscopes with a range of suitable blades.

3.1.7.8 An appropriate range of endotracheal tubes and connectors.

3.1.7.9 A range of endotracheal tube introducers.

3.1.7.10 Inflating syringe and clamps.

3.1.7.11 Magill's forceps.

3.1.7.12 A suitable range of adhesive and other tapes.

3.1.7.13 Scissors.

3.1.7.14 Sterile endotracheal lubricant.

3.1.7.15 Vascular tourniquets.

3.1.7.16 Intravenous infusion equipment with an appropriate range of cannulae and solutions.

3.1.7.17 Means for the safe disposal of items contaminated with biological fluids as well as of "sharps" and waste glass.

3.1.7.18 Equipment suitable for the establishment of subarachnoid, epidural or regional nerve blocks.

3.1.8 In each anaesthetising location there should be available:

3.1.8.1 Equipment for managing difficult intubations.

3.1.8.2 Equipment for automatic ventilation of the lungs incorporating alarms as specified in College Policy Document *'Monitoring During Anaesthesia'* (P18).

3.1.8.3 Equipment for the direct measurement of arterial and venous pressures.

3.1.8.4 Equipment for the rapid infusion of fluids.

3.1.8.5 Equipment to minimise patient heat loss by warming of infused fluids and the body surface.

3.1.8.6 Equipment to warm and humidify gases administered during anaesthesia.

3.1.8.7 Provision for scavenging of anaesthetic gases and vapours with interface equipment which precludes over-pressurisation of the anaesthesia breathing circuit.

3.1.8.8 Interpleural drainage sets.

3.1.8.9 A cardiac defibrillator with capacity for synchronised cardioversion.

3.1.9 Other requirements for safe anaesthesia include:

3.1.9.1 Appropriate lighting for the clinical observation of patients which complies with the current requirements of the relevant national Standards.

3.1.9.2 Emergency lighting.

3.1.9.3 Telephone/Intercom to communicate with persons outside the anaesthetising location.

3.1.9.4 Refrigeration facilities for the storage of drugs and biological products.

3.1.9.5 The means to maintain room temperature in the anaesthetising location within the range of 18–28°C.

3.1.9.6 Patient transfer trolleys/beds as specified in College Policy Document *'Guidelines for the Care of Patients Recovering from Anaesthesia'* (P4).

3.2 ***Drugs***

3.2.1 In addition to the drugs and agents commonly used in anaesthesia, drugs necessary for the management of conditions which may complicate or co-exist with anaesthesia must also be available:

Anaphylaxis
Cardiac arrhythmias
Cardiac arrest
Pulmonary oedema
Hypotension
Hypertension
Bronchospasm
Respiratory depression
Hypoglycaemia
Hyperglycaemia
Adrenal dysfunction
Raised intracranial pressure
Uterine atony
Blood coagulopathy
Malignant hyperpyrexia

3.2.2 In making an appropriate selection of

drugs for the management of these conditions, advice should be sought as in 3.1.2.1.

3.2.3 Appropriate mechanisms must exist for the regular replacement of these drugs after use and/or their expiry date has been reached.

3.2.4 A basic supply of dantrolene should be rapidly available to all anaesthetising locations with further doses being available on request.

3.3 ***Routines for Checking, Cleaning and Servicing Equipment***

3.3.1 Regular sterilising, cleaning and housckccping routines for the care of equipment should be established.

3.3.2 Documented servicing of the anaesthetic machine and medical gas equipment by an appropriate organisation must be carried out at least twice a year. After any modification to the gas distribution system, gas analysis and flow measurement must be carried out and documented before use.

3.3.3 A copy of the College Policy Document *'Protocol for Checking an Anaesthetic Machine Before Use'* (T2) or a similar document should be available on each anaesthetic machine.

3.4 ***Recovery Area***

3.4.1 Recovery from anaesthesia should take place under appropriate supervision in a designated area which conforms with College Policy Document *'Guidelines for the Care of Patients Recovering from Anaesthesia'* (P4).

3.4.2 Contingency plans should exist which would allow rapid patient transfer in an emergency from the operating suite or recovery areas under adequate medical supervision.

This policy document has been prepared having regard to general circumstances, and it is the responsibility of the practitioner to have express regard to the particular circumstances of each case, and the application of this policy document in each case.

Policy documents are reviewed from time to time, and it is the responsibility of the practitioner to ensure that the practitioner has obtained the current version. Policy documents have been prepared having regard to the information available at the time of their preparation, and the practitioner should therefore have regard to any information, research or material which may have been published or become available subsequently.

Whilst the College endeavours to ensure that policy documents are as current as possible at the time of their preparation, it takes no responsibility for matters arising from changed circumstances or information or material which may have become available subsequently.

Promulgated: 1989
Reviewed: 1994
Date of current document: Oct 1995

PROTOCOL FOR CHECKING THE ANAESTHETIC MACHINE

1. INTRODUCTION

1.1 The regulated supply of gases and vapours for anaesthesia and the provision of controlled ventilation for the patient are the main functions of the anaesthetic machine or workstation. Because oxygenation and ventilation are essential for every patient and because even a brief failure to maintain them may cause irreparable harm, every machine must be regularly and thoroughly checked to ensure that all functions are correctly maintained.

1.2 There must be a reserve facility to maintain oxygenation and ventilation of a patient should failure of the primary systems occur.

1.3 To ensure early detection of any failure in the anaesthetic machine, it is essential that appropriate alarms are present in the machine and that there is monitoring of the state of the patient as specificed in College Policy Document P18 *Monitoring during Anaesthesia.*

1.4 This protocol incorporates three components:

1.4.1 **Level One check.** This is very detailed and is required on any new machine and on all machines after the required regular servicing.

1.4.2 **Level Two check.** This should be performed at the start of each anaesthetic session.

1.4.3 **Level Three check.** This should be performed immediately before commencing each subsequent anaesthetic.

Each check must be derived specifically for the machine under test and the Anaesthesia Department (on behalf of the hospital administration) is responsible for the training and accreditation of the personnel involved with each test.

1.5 Accreditation for checking the anaesthetic machine requires:

1.5.1 **Level One.** Attendance at a manufacturer's course or by attendance at a programme developed jointly by the hospital's Bioengineering and Anaesthesia Departments.

1.5.2 **Levels Two and Three.** Checks must follow protocols specifically developed for the machine under test. All personnel must be trained in correct procedures and accredited to perform them by the Anaesthesia Department. The specific protocols should be attached to the machine.

2. PROTOCOLS

Level One check. This must be performed on new anaesthetic machines before they enter service and following all service inspections, which must be performed at regular and specified intervals.

2.1.1 The Hospital, Anaesthesia Department or body responsible for the equipment shall keep a detailed record of the equipment and the checking procedures. This process requires that a checklist be maintained. The checklist will be based on manufacturer's guidelines, and on Biomedical Engineers and Anaesthesia Department recommendations. The protocols shall describe checking and calibration protocols and the intervals at which these must be performed.

2.1.2 The anaesthetic machine must have a prominent label to advise of past service(s) and to indicate when the next check is due. This label must be visible to the anaesthetist.

2.1.3 **Gas Delivery System.** The check shall include:

2.1.3.1 Quantifying and minimising leaks

2.1.3.2 Excluding crossed pipelines within the machine

2.1.3.3 Ascertaining the correct functioning of non-return valves thoughout the system

2.1.3.4 Ascertaining the integrity of oxygen failure prevention and warning devices

2.1.4 **Anaesthetic Vapour Delivery System.** The check shall include:

2.1.4.1 The method and accuracy of vapour output and delivery devices

2.1.4.2 The calibration of vapour output devices and monitors

2.1.5 A formal check of compliance of all components of the machine or part of the machine (after servicing of that part in accordance with AS3551) with the relevant Australian or New Zealand standard is essential.

2.1.6 The check specified above must be undertaken by a suitably qualified person. The check must be recorded with inclusion of information as to what was checked, and by whom.

Level Two check. This check must be undertaken by a suitably qualified person (such as an anaesthetist, technician or nurse) in accordance with a protocol specific for the particular machine. Thus several different protocols may be required in a single hospital. These will serve to verify the correct functioning of the anaesthesia machine before it is used for patient care. Equipment required for the tests must be available on each machine.

2.2.1 **High Pressure System.**

2.2.1.1 Check oxygen cylinder supply. Ensure that cylinder content is sufficient for its intended purpose.

2.2.1.2 Check that piped gas supplies (where present) are at the specified pressures and that following high pressure system checks, the cylinders are turned off.

2.2.1.3 Check gas pipeline connections. Confirm correct pipeline supply using an oxygen analyser or multigas analyser.

2.2.2 **Low Pressure System.**

2.2.2.1 Check control valves and flow meters. Turn on each gas and observe the appropriate operation of the corresponding flow meter. Check the functioning of any interactive anti-hypoxic device.

2.2.2.2 Check that any required vaporiser is present:

2.2.2.2.1 Check that adequate anaesthetic liquid is present

2.2.2.2.2 Ensure that the vaporiser filling ports are closed.

2.2.2.2.3 Check correct seating and locking of a detachable vaporiser.

2.2.2.2.4 Test for circuit leaks for each vaporiser in both on and off positions

2.2.2.2.5 Ensure power is available for electrically operated vaporisers

2.2.2.3 Check for pre-circuit leaks using a method sensitive to 100 ml/minute and appropriate for the specific machine.

2.2.2.4 **Breathing systems.** Check the general status to ensure correct assembly and absence of leaks. The precise protocol will depend on the anaesthesia circuit to be used.

2.2.2.4.1 In the circle system check its integrity and the functioning of unidirectional valves.

This can be accomplished with a breathing bag on the patient limb of the Y-piece. Ventilate the system manually using an appropriate fresh gas flow. Observe inflation and deflation of the attached breathing bag and check for normal system resistance and compliance. Observe movement of unidirectional valves. Check function of adjustable pressure limiting (APL) valve by ensuring easy gas spill through APL when the two breathing bags are squeezed.

2.2.2.4.2 Perform leak test on circle with breathing bag attached to Y-piece and fresh gas flow of 300 ml/min. Pressure of more than 30 cm. of water is necessary to exclude significant leaks but requires the presence of a machine pressure relief valve set to 50–60 cm. of water and an incircuit pressure gauge.

2.2.3 **Automatic Ventilation Sytem.** This should be checked according to the manufacturer's recommendations. This test protocol must be present on the machine. A test lung (such as a suitably compliant bag) may be used to check the function of the ventilator. Where practicable, gas flow should be reduced to check for leaks. The functioning of disconnection and high pressure alarms should be checked at this time.

2.2.4 **Scavenging System.** This should be checked after connection to APL valve and ensuring a free gas flow. If there is negative pressure in any part of the system, ensure that this does not lead to emptying of the breathing system. With the patient outlet occluded, a full breathing system should not empty with the APL valve open.

2.2.5 **Emergency Ventilation System.** Verify the presence and functioning of an alternative method of providing oxygen and of controlled ventilation (such as a self-inflating bag).

2.2.6 **Other Apparatus to Be Used.** This should be checked according to specified protocols. Attention should be given to:

2.2.6.1 Equipment used for airway maintenance and intubation of the trachea.

2.2.6.2 Suction apparatus
2.2.6.3 Gas analysis devices
2.2.6.4 Monitoring equipment. Special attention should be paid to alarm limits and any necessary calibration
2.2.6.5 Intravenous infusion devices
2.2.6.6 Devices to reduce hypothermia during anaesthesia
2.2.6.7 Breathing circuit humidifiers
2.2.6.8 Breathing circuit filters

2.2.7 **Final check.** Ensure vaporisers are turned off and that the breathing system is purged with air or oxygen as appropriate.

2.3 **Level Three check.** Immediately before commencement of each anaesthetic, the anaesthetist should:

2.3.1 Check a changed vaporiser using the protocol outlined in 2.2.2.2.
2.3.2 Check a changed breathing circuit using the protocol outlined in 2.2.2.4.
2.3.3 Check that equipment as specified in 2.2.6 is ready for the next case.

This policy document has been prepared having regard to general circumstances, and it is the responsibility of the practitioner to have express regard to the particular circumstances of each case, and the application of this policy document in each case.

Policy documents are reviewed from time to time, and it is the responsibility of the practitioner to ensure that the practitioner has obtained the current version. Policy documents have been prepared having regard to the information available at the time of their preparation, and the practitioner should therefore have regard to any information, research or material which may have been published or become available subsequently.

Whilst the College endeavours to ensure that policy documents are as current as possible at the time of their preparation, it takes no responsibility for matters arising from changed circumstances or information or material which may have become available subsequently.

Promulgated: 1984
Reviewed: 1990
Date of current document: Oct 1996

RECOMMENDED MINIMUM FACILITIES FOR SAFE ANAESTHETIC PRACTICE IN DELIVERY SUITES

The safe provision of anaesthesia requires appropriate staff, facilities and equipment for proper patient safety. These are specified in this Document.

1. PRINCIPLES OF ANAESTHETIC CARE

1.1 Anaesthesia should be administered only by medical practitioners with appropriate training in anaesthesia or by trainees supervised according to College Policy Documents *'The Supervision of Trainees in Anaesthesia'* (E3) and *'Privileges in Anaesthesia'* (P2).

1.2 Every patient presenting for anaesthesia should have a pre-anaesthetic consultation by a medical practitioner who has appropriate training in anaesthesia. See College Policy Document *'Pre-anaesthetic Consultation'* (P7).

1.3 Appropriate monitoring of physiological variables must occur during anaesthesia. See College Policy Document *'Monitoring During Anaesthesia'* (P18).

2. STAFFING

2.1 In addition to the nursing staff required by those carrying out the obstetric or the operative procedure, there must be:

2.1.1 An assistant to the anaesthetist. See College Policy Document *'Minimum Assistance for the Safe Conduct of Anaesthesia'* (P8). For the establishment and management of epidural blockade for analgesia in labour, the presence of a midwife trained and competent in obstetric epidural management is required.

2.1.2 Adequate assistance in positioning the patient.

2.1.3 Adequate technical assistance to ensure proper servicing of all equipment used.

2.1.4 At the time of delivery, there must be a medical practitioner with appropriate training in the resuscitation and care of the neonate with sole responsibility for that task.

3. DELIVERY SUITES

3.1 ***Anaesthetic Equipment***

3.1.1 Where general anaesthesia, sedation or major regional blockade are utilised, equipment must comply with the requirements set out below as well as with College Policy Document *'Sedation for Diagnostic and Minor Surgical Procedures'* (P9). Where a range of equipment is recommended, the hospital is expected to provide the type most suitable to its needs. Where patients are transferred to another facility for operative delivery, anaesthetic and resuscitative equipment is still essential for the management of complications of epidural and other major regional blockade.

3.1.2 Each hospital must designate:

3.1.2.1 One (or more) specialists to advise on the choice and maintenance of anaesthetic equipment.

3.1.2.2 One (or more) of its nursing or technical staff to be responsible for the organisation of cleaning, maintenance and servicing of anaesthetic equipment.

3.1.3 There must be an anaesthetic machine for each anaesthetising location which is capable of delivering air, oxygen, nitrous oxide as well as other anaesthetic agents which are in common use. Essential equipment includes:

3.1.3.1 Suitable calibrated vaporisers for the delivery of inhalational anaesthetic agents.

3.1.3.2 A range of suitable breathing systems.

3.1.3.3 Medical air where this is clinically necessary.

3.1.4 Safety devices which must be present on every machine include:

3.1.4.1 An indexed gas connection system.

3.1.4.2 A reserve supply of oxygen.

3.1.4.3 An oxygen supply failure warning device. See College Policy Document *'Monitoring During Anaesthesia'* (P18).

3.1.4.4 A breathing system high pressure relief valve.

3.1.4.5 An oxygen concentration analyser with appropriate alarm limits. See College Policy Document *'Monitoring During Anaesthesia'* (P18).

3.1.4.6 Every anaesthetic machine purchased after 1 January 1996 shall have a device to prevent the supply of a hypoxic gas mixture whenever nitrous oxide is administered.

3.1.4.7 Every anaesthetic machine purchased after 1 January 1996 shall have an approved non-slip connection for the common gas outlet whenever a circle system is in use.

3.1.5 A separate means of inflating the lungs with oxygen must be provided in each anaesthetising location. This apparatus should comply with the current requirements of the relevant national Standards. Its oxygen supply should be independent of the anaesthetic machine.

3.1.6 Suction apparatus must be available for the exclusive use of the anaesthetist at all times together with appropriate hand pieces and endotracheal suction catheters. This apparatus should comply with the current requirements of the relevant national Standards. Provision must be made for an alternative suction system in the event of primary suction failure.

3.1.7 In every anaesthetising location there should be:

- 3.1.7.1 Appropriate protection for the anaesthesia team against biological contaminants. This shall include disposable gloves and eye shields.
- 3.1.7.2 A stethoscope
- 3.1.7.3 A sphygmomanometer
- 3.1.7.4 Monitoring equipment complying with College Policy Document *'Monitoring During Anaesthesia'* (P18).
- 3.1.7.5 An appropriate range of face masks.
- 3.1.7.6 An appropriate range of oropharyngeal, nasopharyngeal and laryngeal mask airways.
- 3.1.7.7 Two laryngoscopes with a range of suitable blades.
- 3.1.7.8 An appropriate range of endotracheal tubes and connectors.
- 3.1.7.9 A range of endotracheal tube introducers.
- 3.1.7.10 Inflating syringe and clamps.
- 3.1.7.11 Magill's forceps.
- 3.1.7.12 A suitable range of adhesive and other tapes.
- 3.1.7.13 Scissors.
- 3.1.7.14 Sterile endotracheal lubricant.
- 3.1.7.15 Vascular tourniquets.
- 3.1.7.16 Intravenous infusion equipment with an appropriate range of cannulae and solutions.
- 3.1.7.17 Means for the safe disposal of items contaminated with biological fluids as well as of 'sharps' and waste glass.
- 3.1.7.18 Equipment suitable for the establishment of subarachnoid, epidural or regional nerve blocks.
- 3.1.7.19 Provision for scavenging of anaesthetic gases and vapours with interface equipment which precludes over-pressurisation of the anaesthesia breathing circuit.
- 3.1.7.20 A cardiac defibrillator with capacity for synchronised cardioversion.

3.1.8 In every anaesthetising location there should be available:

- 3.1.8.1 Equipment for managing difficult intubations.
- 3.1.8.2 Equipment for automatic ventilation of the lungs incorporating alarms as specified in College Policy Document *'Monitoring During Anaesthesia'* (P18).
- 3.1.8.3 Equipment for the direct measurement of arterial and venous pressures.
- 3.1.8.4 Equipment for the rapid infusion of fluids.
- 3.1.8.5 Equipment to minimise patient heat loss by warming of infused fluids and the body surface.
- 3.1.8.6 Equipment to warm and humidify gases administered during anaesthesia.
- 3.1.8.7 Interpleural drainage sets.

3.1.9 Other requirements for safe anaesthesia include:

- 3.1.9.1 Appropriate lighting for the clinical observation of patients which complies with the current requirements of the relevant national Standards.
- 3.1.9.2 Emergency lighting.
- 3.1.9.3 Telephone/Intercom to communicate with persons outside the anaesthetising location.
- 3.1.9.4 Refrigeration facilities for the storage of drugs and biological products.
- 3.1.9.5 The means to maintain room temperature in the anaesthetising location within the range of 18–28°C.
- 3.1.9.6 Patient transfer trolleys/beds as specified in College Policy Document *'Guidelines for the Care of Patients Recovering from Anaesthesia'* (P4).

3.1.10 In each delivery room there must be:

- 3.1.10.1 Apparatus for the administration of inhalational analgesia with a minimum of 30% oxygen.
- 3.1.10.2 Suction apparatus for the exclusive use of the anaesthetist which is separate from that required for the resuscitation of the neonate.
- 3.1.10.3 Separate oxygen outlets and suitable attachments for administering oxygen to the mother and to the neonate.

3.2 ***Drugs***

3.2.1 In addition to the drugs and agents commonly used in anaesthesia, drugs necessary for management of conditions which may complicate or co-exist with anaesthesia must also be available:

Anaphylaxis
Cardiac arrhythmias
Cardiac arrest
Pulmonary oedema
Hypotension
Hypertension
Bronchospasm
Respiratory depression
Hypoglycaemia
Hyperglycaemia
Adrenal dysfunction
Raised intracranial pressure
Uterine atony
Blood coagulopathy
Malignant hyperpyrexia

3.2.2 In making an appropriate selection of drugs for the management of these conditions, advice should be sought as in 3.1.2.1.

3.2.3 Appropriate mechanisms must exist for the regular replacement of these drugs after use and/or their expiry date has been reached.

3.2.4 A basic supply of dantrolene should be rapidly available to all anaesthetising locations with further doses being available on request.

3.3 ***Routines for Checking, Cleaning and Servicing Equipment***

3.3.1 Regular sterilising, cleaning and housekeeping routines for the care of equipment should be established.

3.3.2 Documented servicing of the anaesthetic machine and medical gas equipment by an appropriate organisation must be carried out at least twice a year. After any modification in the gas distribution system, gas analysis and flow measurement must be carried out and documented before use.

3.3.3 A copy of the College Policy Document *'Protocol for Checking an Anaesthetic Machine Before Use'* (T2) or a similar document should be available on each anaesthetic machine.

3.4 ***Recovery Area***

3.4.1 Recovery from anaesthesia should take place under appropriate supervision in a designated area which conforms with College Policy Document *'Guidelines for the Care of Patients Recovering from Anaesthesia'* (P4).

3.4.2 Contingency plans should exist which would allow rapid patient transfer in an emergency from the delivery suite or recovery areas to another appropriate area under adequate medical supervision.

3.5 ***Neonatal Resuscitation Equipment***

3.5.1 A suitable range of equipment must be available for:

3.5.1.1 Administration of oxygen to the neonate.

3.5.1.2 Intubation and ventilation of the neonate.

3.5.1.3 Clearing of the airway of the neonate.

3.5.1.4 Administration of intravenous fluids and drugs.

3.5.1.5 Maintenance of the neonate's temperature.

3.5.2 An appropriate range of drugs must be available.

3.5.3 It is recommended that each hospital designate:

3.5.3.1 One (or more) medical practitioners with appropriate training and qualifications to advise on the choice and maintenance of equipment and drugs required for the resuscitation and care of the neonate.

3.5.3.2 One or more of its nursing or technical staff to be responsible for the organisation of cleaning, servicing and maintenance of this equipment.

This policy document has been prepared having regard to general circumstances, and it is the responsibility of the practitioner to have express regard to the particular circumstances of each case, and the application of this policy document in each case.

Policy documents are reviewed from time to time, and it is the responsibility of the practitioner to ensure that the practitioner has obtained the current version. Policy documents have been prepared having regard to the information available at the time of their preparation, and the practitioner should therefore have regard to any information, research or material which may have been published or become available subsequently.

Whilst the College endeavours to ensure that policy documents are as current as possible at the time of their preparation, it takes no responsibility for matters arising from changed circumstances or information or material which may have become available subsequently.

Promulgated: 1989
Reviewed: 1994
Date of current document: Oct 1995

MAJOR REGIONAL ANAESTHESIA

1. GENERAL PRINCIPLES

1.1 Major Regional Anaesthesia is an anaesthetic technique which can produce significant physiological changes or local anaesthetic toxicity and which may cause patient morbidity or mortality (e.g. epidural or spinal blockage, plexus blockade, intravenous regional blockade).

1.2 Major regional anaesthesia should be undertaken only by medical practitioners with adequate experience in the technique or by those in a supervised training programme. Such persons must understand the relevant anatomy, physiology, pharmacology and complications of the particular block. They must be able to recognise and promptly treat any complications of the block.

1.3 The Australian and New Zealand College of Anaesthetists does not approve of one person assuming the dual responsibility of both the operator and the anaesthetist for any forms of major regional anaesthesia.

1.4 Management of major regional anaethesia should include secure intravenous access, patient monitoring in accordance with Policy Document P18 "Monitoring During Anaesthesia" and appropriate sedation.

1.5 The anaesthetist should be in attendance throughout the procedure, or until the block is successful, the condition of the patient is stable and the potential for acute toxicity of the local anaesthetic has passed.

1.6 To ensure that standards of patient care are satisfactory, equipment and staffing of the area in which the patient is being managed should satisfy the requirements of the following Australian and New Zealand College of Anaesthetists Policy Documents:

- T1 "Recommended Minimum Facilities for Safe Anaesthetic Practice in Operating Suites"
- T6 "Recommended Minimum Facilities for Safe Anaesthetic Practice in Delivery Suites"
- P2 "Privileges in Anaesthesia"
- P4 "Guidelines for the Care of Patients Recovering from Anaesthesia"
- P9 "The Use of Sedation for Diagnostic and Minor Surgical Procedures".

2. SPECIFIC PRINCIPLES FOR POSTOPERATIVE EPIDURAL ANALGESIA MANAGEMENT

The placement of an epidural catheter and the administration of the initial dose of local anaesthetic or opioid is the responsibility of the anaesthetist performing the procedure.

2.1 Should the anaesthetist delegate the further administration of epidural analgesia to another person it is the responsibility of the anaesthetist to hand over properly the patient's management to that person and to satisfy himself or herself of the competence of that person to manage the epidural analgesia and carry out the administration procedures. Adequate medical records documenting the time, dose and subsequent effects must be kept.

2.2 Competency should be established by:

2.2.1 A form of accreditation which certifies that the person who will be performing the epidural administration has carried out a sufficient number of similar administrations satisfactorily under supervision, and

2.2.2 Enquiry of the person to establish familiarity with and knowledge of the procedure and subsequent management, including the management of complications.

2.3 No person should be required to carry out any such procedure if uncertain of their competence to do so.

2.4 All patients must have secure intravenous access throughout the duration of the epidural analgesia.

February 1993

GUIDELINES FOR THE CARE OF PATIENTS RECOVERING FROM ANAESTHESIA

1. GENERAL PRINCIPLES

1.1 Recovery from anaesthesia should take place under supervision in an area designated for the purpose.

1.2 This area should be close to where the anaesthetic was administered.

1.3 The staff working in this area must be trained for their role and able to contact supervising medical staff promptly when the need arises.

1.4 In some situations (for example, paediatric hospitals) minor variations in these Guidelines may be appropriate.

2. THE RECOVERY AREA

2.1 ***Design Features***

2.1.1 The area should be part of the operating or procedural suite. Access should be available to medical staff who are not in operating suite clothing, so that they may continue to supervise the patient's care. Provision should be made for rapid evacuation of patients from the area in an emergency.

2.1.2 It should have ventilation to operating theatre standards.

2.1.3 The space allocated per bed/trolley should be at least 9 square metres. There must be easy access to the patient's head.

2.1.4 The number of bed/trolley spaces must be sufficient for expected peak loads and there should be at least 1.5 spaces per operating room.

2.1.5 Each bed space must be provided with:

2.1.5.1 an oxygen outlet

2.1.5.2 a vacuum outlet complying with the current requirements of the relevant national Standards.

2.1.5.3 two General Power Outlets

2.1.5.4 lighting to allow accurate detection of cyanosis

2.1.5.5 emergency lighting

2.1.5.6 appropriate facilities for mounting and operating any necessary equipment and for the patient's chart.

2.1.6 Space must be provided for a nursing station, storage of drugs, of clean linen as well as a utility room.

2.1.7 There must be appropriate facilities for scrubbing up for procedures.

2.1.8 There should be a wall clock with a sweep second hand or analogue display clearly visible from each bed space.

2.1.9 Communication facilities should include:

2.1.9.1 an emergency call system to areas such as the Department of Anaesthesia.

2.1.9.2 a telephone and access to the Hospital paging system.

2.1.10 There should be easy access for portable X-Ray equipment with appropriate power outlets provided in the area. There should also be an X-Ray viewing box.

2.1.11 An emergency power supply should be available in the area.

3. EQUIPMENT AND DRUGS

3.1 Each bed space should be provided with:

3.1.1 oxygen flowmeter and patient oxygen delivery systems

3.1.2 suction equipment including a receiver, appropriate hand pieces and a range of suction catheters

3.1.3 a pulse oximeter

3.1.4 a sphygmomanometer which may be automated and include cuffs suitable for all patients

3.1.5 a stethoscope

3.1.6 a means of measuring body temperature

3.2 Within the recovery area there must be:

3.2.1 a means of inflating the lungs with oxygen in a ratio of one per two bed spaces, but with a minimum of two such devices

3.2.2 airway management and intubation drugs and equipment

3.2.3 emergency and resuscitative drugs

3.2.4 a range of I.V. equipment and fluids and a means of warming those fluids

3.2.5 drugs for pain control

3.2.6 a range of syringes and needles

3.2.7 electrocardiographs with a minimum of 1 to 3 bed spaces.

3.3 There should be easy access to:

3.3.1 a 12 lead electrocardiograph

3.3.2 a monitor for measurement of direct arterial and venous pressures

3.3.3 a capnometer

3.3.4 a defibrillator

3.3.5 a neuromuscular function monitor

3.3.6 a bronchoscope with sucker and grasping forceps

3.3.7 a warming cupboard
3.3.8 a refrigerator for drugs and blood
3.3.9 a patient warming device
3.3.10 a procedure light
3.3.11 a simple surgical tray
3.3.12 blood gas and electrolyte measuring
3.3.13 diagnostic imaging services

3.4 The recovery trolley/bed must:
3.4.1 have a firm base and mattress
3.4.2 tilt from one or both ends both head up and head down at least 15 degrees
3.4.3 be easy to manoeuvre
3.4.4 have efficient and accessible brakes
3.4.5 provide for sitting the patient up
3.4.6 have secure side rails which must be able to be dropped below the base or be easily removed
3.4.7 have an I.V. pole
3.4.8 have provision for mounting monitoring equipment, patient ventilation equipment, oxygen cylinders, underwater seal drains and suction apparatus during transport of patients.

4. STAFFING

4.1 Staff trained in the care of patients recovering from anaesthesia must be present at all times.

4.2 A registered nurse trained in recovery area care should be in charge.

4.3 Trainee nurses and registered nurses who are not experienced in the care of patients recovering from anaesthesia must be supervised.

4.4 The ratio of registered nurses to patients needs to be flexible so as to provide no less than one nurse to three patients, and one nurse to each patient who has not recovered protective reflexes or consciousness.

5. MANAGEMENT AND SUPERVISION

5.1 Written protocols for management should be established. The Director of Anaesthesia, or the Anaesthetist-in-Charge, should be responsible for the medical aspects of these policies.

5.2 A written routine for checking the equipment and drugs must be established.

5.3 Observations should be recorded at appropriate intervals and should include state of consciousness, oxygen saturation, respiratory rate, pulse rate, blood pressure and temperature.

5.4 All patients should remain until they are considered safe to be discharged from the recovery area according to established criteria.

5.5 The anaesthetist responsible for the patient should:
5.5.1 accompany the patient until transfer to recovery area staff is completed
5.5.2 provide written and verbal instructions to the recovery area staff
5.5.3 specify the type of apparatus and the flow rate to be used for oxygen therapy
5.5.4 remain in the vicinity until the patient is safe to be left in the care of recovery area staff
5.5.5 supervise the recovery period and authorise the patient's discharge from the recovery area. It is recognised that in some circumstances it may be necessary for the anaesthetist previously responsible for the patient to delegate these duties to a trained recovery area nurse or to another anaesthetist who should be fully informed of the clinical state of the patient.

5.6 The practitioner responsible for the patient's overall care should be available to consult with the anaesthetist should the need arise in the recovery period and, where appropriate, to authorise the discharge of the patient.

This policy document has been prepared having regard to general circumstances, and it is the responsibility of the practitioner to have express regard to the particular circumstances of each case, and the application of this policy document in each case.

Policy documents are reviewed from time to time, and it is the responsibility of the practitioner to ensure that the practitioner has obtained the current version. Policy documents have been prepared having regard to the information available at the time of their preparation, and the practitioner should therefore have regard to any information, research or material which may have been published or become available subsequently.

Whilst the College endeavours to ensure that policy documents are as current as possible at the time of their preparation, it takes no responsibility for matters arising from changed circumstances or information or material which may have become available subsequently.

Promulgated: 1989
Reviewed: 1994
Date of current document: June 1995

MINIMUM ASSISTANCE REQUIRED FOR THE SAFE CONDUCT OF ANAESTHESIA

The presence of a trained assistant during the conduct of anaesthesia is a major contributory factor to safe patient management. The assistant must have undertaken appropriate training to enable them to provide effective support to the anaesthetist. The duties of anaesthetists and thus of their assistants will range from the straightforward in the management of a minor case to the complex during some anaesthesia procedures. The guidelines that follow are therefore stated in general terms to establish both the practical and educational responsibilities of a competent assistant to the anaesthetist.

1. PRINCIPLES

1.1 Trained assistance for the anaesthetist is essential for the safe and efficient conduct of anaesthesia.

1.2 This assistance requires:

1.2.1 The presence of an assistant during preparation for and induction of anaesthesia. The assistant must remain under the immediate direction of the anaesthetist until instructed that their services are no longer required.

1.2.2 The presence of an assistant at short notice if required during the maintenance of anaesthesia.

1.2.3 The presence of an assistant at the conclusion of anaesthesia.

1.3 These principles apply wherever the anaesthetic is given.

1.4 Institutions in which anaesthetics are given must provide a service which ensures the availability and maintenance of anaesthesia equipment in accordance with College Policy Documents on recommended minimum facilities for safe anaesthetic practice. The relevant College Policy Documents are:

T1 "Recommended Minimum Facilities for Safe Anaesthetic Practice in Operating Suites"

T2 "Protocol for Checking an Anaesthetic Machine Before Use"

T3 "Recommended Minimum Facilities for Safe Anaesthetic Practice in Organ Imaging Units"

T4 "Recommended Minimum Facilities for Safe Anaesthetic Practice for Electro Convulsive Therapy (ECT)"

T5 "Recommended Minimum Facilities for Safe Anaesthetic Practice in Dental Surgeries"

T6 "Recommended Minimum Facilities for Safe Anaesthetic Practice in Delivery Suites"

1.5 Staff employed for the above purposes must be trained as defined below for this role.

2. DEPLOYMENT OF ASSISTANTS

2.1 The deployment of assistants in accordance with 1.2, should be specified by management protocols.

2.2 The nature and workload of the anaesthetic service will determine the number and status of assistants.

2.3 The duties of an assistant should be specified in an appropriate job description.

2.4 Whilst assisting the anaesthetist, the assistant is wholly and exclusively responsible to that anaesthetist.

2.5 The assistant is an essential member of the staff establishment in every area in which anaesthetics are given.

2.6 There must be appropriate staffing establishment and rosters for assistants. Assistance must be available for both elective and emergency anaesthesia in all locations where it is performed.

2.7 Where a number of assistants are employed, an appropriately trained member of their group should be designated as being in charge.

3. EDUCATIONAL REQUIREMENTS FOR ASSISTANTS

An adequately trained assistant to the anaesthestist must have attended and completed a training course which has as a minimum the following criteria:

3.1 Eligibility

3.1.1 Those without previous health sector experience must have the Higher School Certificate or its equivalent.

3.1.2 Those with nursing experience must hold a certificate as an Enrolled Nurse or a Registered Nurse.

3.1.3 Registered Nurses and Enrolled Nurses must be in current clinical employment or have been so employed within one year of acceptance into a training course.

3.2 Course of Instruction

At a minimum this will include:

3.2.1 A course of lectures of at least 150 hours, established by an appropriate and recognised Institution of Learning. A significant amount of the lecture material must be prepared and delivered by anaesthetists. A distance learning course is appropriate when conditions demand this.

3.2.2 Practical instruction supervised by trained anaesthetists which should be documented in a log book as a record describing the type of instruction received and experience gained.

3.2.3 Completion of assignments appropriate to the curriculum which are suitable for presentation to trainees and supervisors.

3.2.4 Successful completion of internal assessments and designated examinations.

3.3 Duration of the Course

3.3.1 For those without previous hospital experience, two years of full time study.

3.3.2 For those with Registered Nurse or Enrolled Nurse qualifications, one year full time or two years part time study.

3.3.3 For those employed as trainee assistants, two years part time study.

3.3.4 The course should not exceed three years.

An addendum sets out a potential course outline.

THE HANDOVER OF RESPONSIBILITY DURING AN ANAESTHETIC

During an anaesthetic, the major responsibility of the anaesthetist is to provide care for the patient. This requires the continuous presence of the anaesthetist. In certain circumstances, it is necessary for the anaesthetist to hand over that responsibility to a colleague. Specific procedures must be followed. Handovers will not compromise patient safety provided that these procedures are followed. In prolonged anaesthetics, handover may be advantageous to the patient by preventing undue fatigue of the anaesthetist.

1. Temporary relief of the anaesthetist

This is necessary when the primary anaesthetist must leave the patient but will return to resume management of the anaesthetic.

1.1 The primary anaesthetist will leave only while the patient is in a stable state and no potentially adverse events are likely to occur.

1.2 The primary anaesthetist must be satisfied as to the competence of the relieving anaesthetist to provide care and must have explained all facts relevant to safe management.

1.3 The primary anaesthetist must be available to return at short notice.

2. Permanent handover of responsibility for care

This is necessary when the primary anaesthetist must leave the patient under the care of another anaesthetist for the remainder of the anaesthetic.

2.1 The primary anaesthetist will only hand over responsibility at a time when the clinical status of the patient is appropriate.

2.2 The primary anaesthetist must be satisfied as to the competency of the relieving anaesthetist to assume management of the case. The handover procedure must include a briefing as to the patient's pre-operative status, events during the anaesthetic and discussion of any foreseeable problems.

2.3 The relieving anaesthetist has responsibility to be fully conversant with the patient's present and ongoing anaesthetic management and must indicate a willingness to accept that responsibility.

3. Protocol for transfer of responsibility

The following items must also be considered by the primary and the relieving anaesthetists:

3.1 The patient's health status having regard to past history and the present condition.

3.2 Observations of the patient according to College Policy Document P18—*Monitoring During Anaesthesia* as shown by the anaesthetic record.

3.3 A check to ensure correct functioning of the anaesthesia machine and any other equipment which is interfaced to the patient as well as of all monitoring devices in use.

3.4 The provision of information about the handover to the surgeon and (in the case of a trainee) the consultant anaesthetist.

This policy document has been prepared having regard to general circumstances, and it is the responsibility of the practitioner to have express regard to the particular circumstances of each case, and the application of this policy document in each case.

Policy documents are reviewed from time to time, and it is the responsibility of the practitioner to ensure that the practitioner has obtained the current version. Policy documents have been prepared having regard to the information available at the time of their preparation, and the practitioner should therefore have regard to any information, research or material which may have been published or become available subsequently.

Whilst the College endeavours to ensure that policy documents are as current as possible at the time of their preparation, it takes no responsibility for matters arising from changed circumstances or information or material which may have become available subsequently.

Promulgated: 1994
Date of current document: Oct 1994

GUIDELINES FOR THE CONDUCT OF EPIDURAL ANALGESIA IN OBSTETRICS

PREAMBLE

Epidural analgesia is a safe and effective method of pain relief in labour, provided appropriate precautions are taken as follows:

1. Epidural puncture and/or cannulation of the epidural space should be carried out only by persons with adequate training and experience in the technique.
2. Such persons must be:
   2.1 Readily available to supervise the management of the epidural.
   2.2 Competent to deal with the occasional life-threatening and other complications which may arise from the injection of agents into the epidural or sub-arachnoid space.
3. An appropriately trained person must be present to assist the anaesthetist whilst performing the epidural block.
4. Once epidural analgesia has been established, and the response of the patient to the agent or agents has been assessed by the anaesthetist, further doses to maintain analgesia may be administered by other suitably trained medical or nursing staff, provided that:
   4.1 The dose has been prescribed by the anaesthetist;
   4.2 The anaesthetist delegating the "top-up" procedure is satisfied that the person who will carry out the task is competent to do so and competent to appropriately monitor the patient and her fetus;
   4.3 The person carrying out these tasks is satisfied that he or she is competent to do so;
   4.4 Appropriate equipment and skilled staff are readily available to treat complications and any adverse reactions; and
   4.5 Written instructions and management guidelines are provided.
5. All patients undergoing epidural analgesia must be nursed in an area appropriately equipped with staff able to:
   5.1 Monitor both the patient and fetus;
   5.2 Detect the extent of the block and any adverse effects; and
   5.3 Judge the necessity for top-up doses.
6. A record must be made of the procedure, the clinical and other observations and the instructions delegated to other staff.
7. All patients receiving epidural analgesia must have an intravenous infusion inserted before the institution of the block and the infusion must be left in situ for the duration of the block.
8. Satisfactory and safe epidural analgesia can be produced by continuous or patient-controlled epidural infusion of local anaesthetic alone, opioid alone or local anaesthetic-opioid mixtures. The same principles of management should apply when epidural analgesia is administered by these methods.
9. At all times the ultimate responsibility for the management of epidural analgesia remains that of the anaesthetist who performs the procedure or a delegated specialist anaesthetist.
10. All patients having epidural analgesia in labour must be admitted under the direct care and supervision of a registered medical practitioner.

February 1993

MONITORING DURING ANAESTHESIA

INTRODUCTION

Monitoring of certain fundamental physiological variables during anaesthesia is essential. Clinical judgement will determine how long this monitoring should be continued following completion of anaesthesia.

The Health Care Facility in which the procedure is being performed is responsible for provision of equipment for anaesthesia and monitoring on the advice of one or more designated specialist anaesthetists, and for effective maintenance of this equipment (see College Policy Document *'Recommended Minimum Facilities for Safe Anaesthetic Practice in Operating Suites'* (T1)).

Some or all of the recommendations in this document may need to be exceeded depending on the physical status of the patient, the type and complexity of the surgery to be performed as well as the requirements of anaesthesia.

The described monitoring must always be used in conjunction with careful clinical observation by the anaesthetist as there are circumstances in which equipment may not detect unfavourable clinical developments.

The following recommendations refer to patients undergoing general anaesthesia or major regional anaesthesia for diagnostic or therapeutic procedures and should be interpreted in conjunction with other Policy Documents published by the Australian and New Zealand College of Anaesthetists.

1. PERSONNEL

Clinical monitoring by a vigilant anaesthetist is the basis of safe patient care during anaesthesia. This should be supplemented by appropriate devices to assist the anaesthetist.

A medical practitioner whose sole responsibility is the provision of anaesthetic care for that patient must be constantly present from induction of anaesthesia until safe transfer to Recovery Room staff or Intensive Care Unit has been accomplished. This medical practitioner must be appropriately trained in Anaesthesia, or be a Trainee Anaesthetist supervised in accordance with College Policy Document *'The Supervision of Trainees in Anaesthesia'* (E3).

In exceptional circumstances brief absences of the person primarily responsible for the anaesthetic may be unavoidable. In such circumstances that person may temporarily delegate observation of the patient to an appropriately qualified person who is judged to be competent for the task. Permanent handover of responsibility must be to an anaesthetist who is able to accept continued responsibility for the care of the patient (see College Policy Document *'Handover of Responsibility during an Anaesthetic'* (P10)).

The individual anaesthetist is responsible for monitoring the patient and should ensure that appropriate monitoring equipment is available. Some procedures necessitate special monitoring (e.g. MRI scanning) or remote monitoring to reduce hazard to staff (e.g. radiological procedures) (see College Policy Document *'Recommended Minimum Facilities for Safe Anaesthetic Practice in Organ Imaging Facilities'* (T3)).

2. PATIENT MONITORING

2.1 ***Circulation***

The circulation must be monitored at frequent and clinically appropriate intervals by detection of the arterial pulse and measurement of arterial blood pressure by indirect or direct means.

2.2 ***Ventilation***

Ventilation must be monitored continuously by both direct and indirect means.

2.3 ***Oxygenation***

Oximetric values must be interpreted in conjunction with clinical observation of the patient. Adequate lighting must be available to aid with assessment of patient colour.

3. EQUIPMENT

3.1 ***Oxygen Supply Failure Alarm***

An automatically activated device to monitor oxygen supply pressure and to warn of low pressure must be fitted to the anaesthetic machine. This device should shut off the nitrous oxide supply and be capable of maintaining oxygen flow for a limited period (see College Policy Document *'Recommended Minimum Facilities for Safe Anaesthetic Practice in Operating Suites'* (T1)).

3.2 ***Oxygen Analyser***

A device incorporating an audible signal to warn of low oxygen concentrations, correctly fitted in the breathing system, must be in continuous operation for every patient when an anaesthetic machine is in use.

3.3 ***Pulse Oximeter***

Pulse oximetry provides evidence of the level of oxygen saturation of the haemoglobin of arterial blood and identifies arterial pulsation at the site of application. A pulse oximeter must be in use for every anaesthetised patient.

3.4 ***Breathing System Disconnection or Ventilator Failure Alarm***

When an automatic ventilator is in use, a device capable of warning promptly of a breathing system disconnection or ventilator failure must be in continuous operation. This device must be automatically activated.

3.5 ***Electrocardiograph***
Equipment to monitor and continually display the electrocardiograph must be available for every anaesthetised patient.

3.6 ***Temperature Monitor***
Equipment to monitor temperature continuously must be available for every anaesthetised patient.

3.7 ***Carbon Dioxide Monitor***
A monitor of carbon dioxide level in inhaled and exhaled gases must be exclusively available for every patient.

3.8 ***Neuromuscular Function Monitor***
Equipment to monitor neuromuscular function must be available for every patient in whom neuromuscular blockade has been induced.

3.9 ***Volatile Anaesthetic Agent Monitor***
Equipment to monitor the concentration of inhaled anaesthetics must be exclusively available for every patient undergoing general anaesthesia. This recommendation should be implemented as soon as possible but in any case no later than 1 January 1998.

3.10 ***Other Equipment***
When clinically indicated, equipment to monitor other physiological variables such as cardiac output should be available.

RELATED DOCUMENTS

T1 Recommended Minimum Facilities for Safe Anaesthetic Practice in Operating Suites
T3 Recommended Minimum Facilities for Safe Anaesthetic Practice in Organ Imaging Facilities
E3 The Supervision of Trainees in Anaesthesia
P10 Handover of Responsibility During an Anaesthetic

This policy document has been prepared having regard to general circumstances, and it is the responsibility of the practitioner to have express regard to the particular circumstances of each case, and the application of this policy document in each case.

Policy documents are reviewed from time to time, and it is the responsibility of the practitioner to ensure that the practitioner has obtained the current version. Policy documents have been prepared having regard to the information available at the time of their preparation, and the practitioner should therefore have regard to any information, research or material which may have been published or become available subsequently.

Whilst the College endeavours to ensure that policy documents are as current as possible at the time of their preparation, it takes no responsibility for matters arising from changed circumstances or information or material which may have become available subsequently.

Promulgated: 1990
Reviewed: 1990
Date of current document: Oct 1995

RESPONSIBILITIES OF THE ANAESTHETIST IN THE POST-OPERATIVE PERIOD

1. The anaesthetist has major responsibility for the management of the patient recovering from anaesthesia. During this time, responsibility is shared with the surgeon or other consultant for consultative advice with respect to:

1.1 monitoring (including clinical observations)
1.2 pain relief
1.3 fluid therapy
1.4 respiratory therapy

2. The anaesthetist has responsibility for ensuring that the patient recovers safely from anaesthesia in an area appropriately equipped and staffed for that purpose (see College Policy Document P4 'Guidelines for the Care of Patients Recovering from Anaesthesia').

This responsiblity includes:

2.1 A formal handover of responsibility to recovery area staff with appropriate briefing as to management protocols. Such a handover of care should only occur when the anaesthetist considers that the patient is safe to leave, particularly with regard to cardio-respiratory stability.

2.2 Availability to deal with any unexpected problems or ensuring that another nominated anaesthetist or other consultant is available and has necessary information about the patient.

2.3 Ensuring that the patient remains in the recovery facility until safe for discharge to a ward. Where transfer to an intensive care unit or high dependency unit is necessary, responsibility for care remains with the anaesthetist until this transfer is complete.

2.4 Ensuring that there will be adequate post-operative care of the patient after discharge from the recovery area.

3. When a patient is to be discharged from medical care on the same day that an anaesthetic has been administered, the anaesthetist must ensure that the patient and his/her caregivers understand the principles of post-anaesthesia care (see College Policy Document P15 'Guidelines for the Perioperative Care of Patients Selected for Day Care Surgery').

4. The anaesthetist has a responsibility to:

4.1 Ensure that any adverse effects which may be related to anaesthesia are recognised, managed and documented appropriately.

4.2 Audit outcomes of his/her anaesthesia care and include these in quality assurance or peer review processes.

4.3 Ensure that patients and/or caregivers are aware of any matters relevant to the conduct of anaesthesia particularly when these may impact on future health care.

This policy document has been prepared having regard to general circumstances, and it is the responsibility of the practitioner to have express regard to the particular circumstances of each case, and the application of this policy document in each case.

Policy documents are reviewed from time to time, and it is the responsibility of the practitioner to ensure that the practitioner has obtained the current version. Policy documents have been prepared having regard to the information available at the time of their preparation, and the practitioner should therefore have regard to any information, research or material which may have been published or become available subsequently.

Whilst the College endeavours to ensure that policy documents are as current as possible at the time of their preparation, it takes no responsibility for matters arising from changed circumstances or information or material which may have become available subsequently.

Promulgated: 1990
Reviewed: 1996
Date of current document: Feb 1996

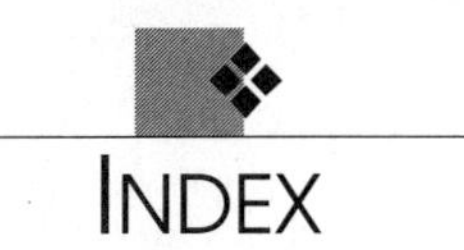

INDEX

Note: Page numbers in *italics* refer to illustrations; page numbers followed by t refer to tables.

D

Q

R

ISBN 0-443-06560-8